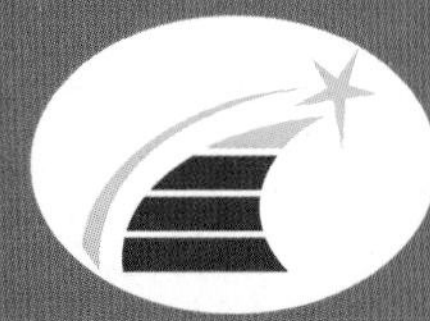

2024 ICD-10-PCS

BUCK'S

Jackie L. Koesterman, CPC
Coding and Reimbursement Specialist
JDK Medical Coding EDU
Grand Forks, North Dakota

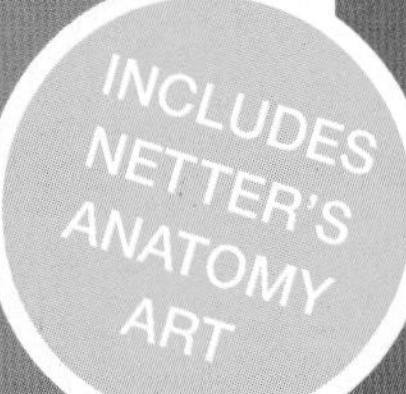

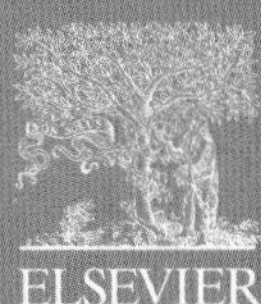

ELSEVIER

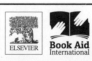

Elsevier
3251 Riverport Lane
St. Louis, Missouri 63043

BUCK'S 2024 ICD-10-PCS ISBN: 978-0-443-11183-9

International Standard Book Number: 978-0-443-11183-9

Content Strategist: Laura Klein
Content Development Manager: Danielle Frazier
Senior Content Development Specialist: Joshua S. Rapplean
Publishing Services Manager: Deepthi Unni
Project Manager: Nayagi Anandan
Senior Book Designer: Maggie Reid

Printed in Canada

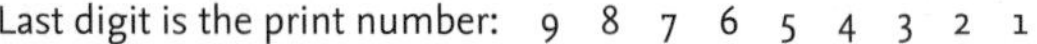
Last digit is the print number: 9 8 7 6 5 4 3 2 1

DEDICATION

To all who require of themselves the highest level of accuracy, integrity, and professionalism. You enhance our profession and are a tremendous asset to health care. May this manual be of assistance to you.

With Greatest Admiration.

Carol J. Buck, MS

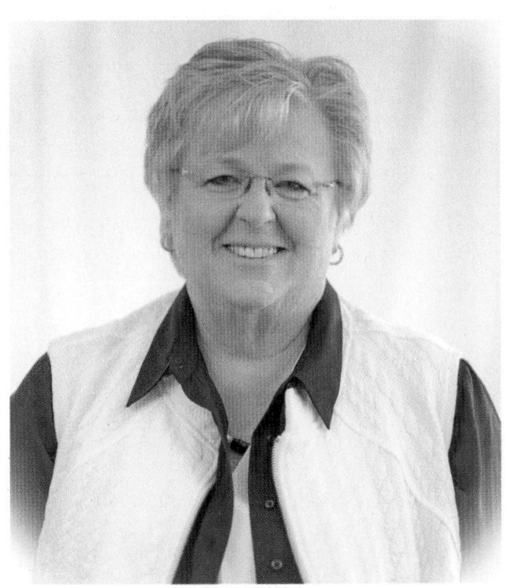

DEVELOPMENT OF THIS EDITION

Lead Technical Collaborator

Jackie L. Koesterman, CPC
Coding and Reimbursement Specialist
JDK Medical Coding EDU
Grand Forks, North Dakota

Query Team

Patricia Cordy Henricksen, MS, CHCA, CPC-I, CPC, CCP-P, ASC-PM
AAPC-Approved Instructor
Auditing, Coding, and Education Specialist
Soterion Medical Services
Lexington, Kentucky

CONTENTS

SYMBOLS AND CONVENTIONS

Annotated

Throughout the manual, revisions, additions, and deleted codes or words are indicated by the following symbols:

New and revised content from the previous edition are indicated by green font.

~~deleted~~ Deletions from the previous edition are struck through.

ICD-10-PCS Table Symbols

Throughout the manual information is indicated by the following symbols:

♀ ♂ **Sex conflict:** *Definitions of Medicare Code Edits* (MCE) detects inconsistencies between a patient's sex and any diagnosis or procedure on the patient's record. For example, a male patient with cervical cancer (diagnosis) or a female patient with a prostatectomy (procedure). In both instances, the indicated diagnosis or the procedure conflicts with the stated sex of the patient. Therefore, the patient's diagnosis, procedure, or sex is presumed to be incorrect.

Non-covered: There are some procedures for which Medicare does not provide reimbursement. There are also procedures that would normally not be reimbursed by Medicare but due to the presence of certain diagnoses are reimbursed.

Limited Coverage: For certain procedures whose medical complexity and serious nature incur extraordinary associated costs, Medicare limits coverage to a portion of the cost.

DRG Non-OR A **non-operating room procedure that does affect MS-DRG assignment** is indicated by a purple highlight.

Non-OR A **non-operating room procedure that does not affect MS-DRG assignment** is indicated by a yellow highlight.

Combination: Certain combinations of procedures are treated differently than their constituent codes.

Hospital-Acquired Condition: Some procedures are always associated with Hospital Acquired Conditions (HAC) according to the MS-DRG.

Coding Clinic: American Hospital Association's *Coding Clinic*® citations provide reference information to official ICD-10-PCS coding advice.

OGCR The ***Official Guidelines for Coding and Reporting*** symbol includes the placement of a portion of a guideline as that guideline pertains to the code by which it is located. The complete OGCR are located in the Introduction.

[ ] Brackets below the tables enclose the alphanumeric options for Non-covered, Limited Coverage, DRG Non-OR, Non-OR, and HAC.

Note: The final FY2024 MS-DRG and Medicare Code Edits were unavailable at the time of printing. Proposed new DRG Non-OR procedures were available and have been included below the appropriate tables with "(proposed)" appearing behind the codes. Please check codingupdates.com for final FY2024 MS-DRG and MCE information.

GUIDE TO THE 2024 UPDATES

The ICD-1Ø-PCS codes that have changed are shown in the lists below.
If you would like to see this information in table format, please visit codingupdates.com for a complete listing.

2024 ICD-10-PCS New, Revised, and Deleted Codes

NEW CODES

- Ø2HW3RZ
- Ø2PW3RZ
- Ø2WW3RZ
- ØCSSØZZ
- ØCSS7ZZ
- ØCSS8ZZ
- ØDH17JZ
- ØDH27JZ
- ØDH37JZ
- ØWHCØGZ
- ØWHC3GZ
- ØWHC4GZ
- ØWPCØGZ
- ØWPC3GZ
- ØWPC4GZ
- ØWPCXGZ
- ØWWCØGZ
- ØWWC3GZ
- ØWWC4GZ
- ØWWCXGZ
- 5AØ9B5K
- 5AØ9C5K
- 5AØ9D5K
- 8EØUØEN
- 8EØU3EN
- 8EØU4EN
- 8EØU7EN
- 8EØU8EN
- 8EØWØEN
- 8EØW3EN
- 8EØW4EN
- 8EØW7EN
- 8EØW8EN
- XØ5
- XØ51329
- X2H
- X2HØ3R9
- X2H13R9
- X2H2ØR9
- X2H3ØR9
- X2H63V9
- X2HK3V9
- X2HLØF9
- X2HMØF9
- X2HXØF9
- X2KH3D9
- X2KH3E9
- X2KJ3D9
- X2KJ3E9
- X2U
- X2U4Ø79
- X2UQØP9
- X2URØP9
- XNHGØF9
- XNHHØF9
- XNR
- XNR8ØD9
- XNRLØ99
- XNRMØ99
- XRGJØB9
- XRGKØB9
- XRGLØB9
- XRGMØB9
- XWØ13L9
- XWØ13S9
- XWØ33K9
- XWØ33P9
- XWØ33Q9
- XWØ33R9
- XWØ43K9
- XWØ43P9
- XWØ43Q9
- XWØ43R9
- XWØ53T9
- XWØDXJ9
- XWØDXN9
- XW133H9
- XW143H9
- XX2
- XX2ØX89
- XX2F3W9
- XXE2X19
- XXE5XY9

REVISED CODES

- XRGAØR7
- XRGA3R7
- XRGA4R7
- XRGBØR7
- XRGB3R7
- XRGB4R7
- XRGCØR7
- XRGC3R7
- XRGC4R7
- XRGDØR7
- XRGD3R7
- XRGD4R7
- XWØØX27
- XWØ1X27

DELETED CODES

- XV5
- XV5Ø8A4
- XWØ33G4
- XWØ33H4
- XWØ43G4
- XWØ43H4

Introduction

ICD-10-PCS Official Guidelines for Coding and Reporting

2024

The Centers for Medicare and Medicaid Services (CMS) and the National Center for Health Statistics (NCHS), two departments within the U.S. Federal Government's Department of Health and Human Services (DHHS) provide the following guidelines for coding and reporting using the International Classification of Diseases, 10th Revision, Procedure Coding System (ICD-10-PCS). These guidelines should be used as a companion document to the official version of the ICD-10-PCS as published on the CMS website. The ICD-10-PCS is a procedure classification published by the United States for classifying procedures performed in hospital inpatient health care settings.

These guidelines have been approved by the four organizations that make up the Cooperating Parties for the ICD-10-PCS: the American Hospital Association (AHA), the American Health Information Management Association (AHIMA), CMS, and NCHS.

These guidelines are a set of rules that have been developed to accompany and complement the official conventions and instructions provided within the ICD-10-PCS itself. They are intended to provide direction that is applicable in most circumstances. However, there may be unique circumstances where exceptions are applied. The instructions and conventions of the classification take precedence over guidelines. These guidelines are based on the coding and sequencing instructions in the Tables, Index and Definitions of ICD-10-PCS, but provide additional instruction. Adherence to these guidelines when assigning ICD-10-PCS procedure codes is required under the Health Insurance Portability and Accountability Act (HIPAA). The procedure codes have been adopted under HIPAA for hospital inpatient healthcare settings. A joint effort between the healthcare provider and the coder is essential to achieve complete and accurate documentation, code assignment, and reporting of diagnoses and procedures. These guidelines have been developed to assist both the healthcare provider and the coder in identifying those procedures that are to be reported. The importance of consistent, complete documentation in the medical record cannot be overemphasized. Without such documentation accurate coding cannot be achieved.

Table of Contents

Conventions

A1

ICD-10-PCS codes are composed of seven characters. Each character is an axis of classification that specifies information about the procedure performed. Within a defined code range, a character specifies the same type of information in that axis of classification.

Example: The fifth axis of classification specifies the approach in sections 0 through 4 and 7 through 9 of the system.

A2

One of 34 possible values can be assigned to each axis of classification in the seven-character code: they are the numbers 0 through 9 and the alphabet (except I and O because they are easily confused with the numbers 1 and 0). The number of unique values used in an axis of classification differs as needed.

Example: Where the fifth axis of classification specifies the approach, seven different approach values are currently used to specify the approach.

A3

The valid values for an axis of classification can be added to as needed.

Example: If a significantly distinct type of device is used in a new procedure, a new device value can be added to the system.

A4
As with words in their context, the meaning of any single value is a combination of its axis of classification and any preceding values on which it may be dependent.
Example: The meaning of a body part value in the Medical and Surgical section is always dependent on the body system value. The body part value Ø in the Central Nervous body system specifies Brain and the body part value Ø in the Peripheral Nervous body system specifies Cervical Plexus.
A5
As the system is expanded to become increasingly detailed, over time more values will depend on preceding values for their meaning.
Example: In the Lower Joints body system, the device value 3 in the root operation Insertion specifies Infusion Device and the device value 3 in the root operation Replacement specifies Ceramic Synthetic Substitute.
A6
The purpose of the alphabetic index is to locate the appropriate table that contains all information necessary to construct a procedure code. The PCS Tables should always be consulted to find the most appropriate valid code.
A7
It is not required to consult the index first before proceeding to the tables to complete the code. A valid code may be chosen directly from the tables.
A8
All seven characters must be specified to be a valid code. If the documentation is incomplete for coding purposes, the physician should be queried for the necessary information.
A9
Within a PCS table, valid codes include all combinations of choices in characters 4 through 7 contained in the same row of the table. In the example below, ØJHT3VZ is a valid code, and ØJHW3VZ is *not* a valid code.
A1Ø
"And," when used in a code description, means "and/or," except when used to describe a combination of multiple body parts for which separate values exist for each body part (e.g., Skin and Subcutaneous Tissue used as a qualifier, where there are separate body part values for "Skin" and "Subcutaneous Tissue").
Example: Lower Arm and Wrist Muscle means lower arm and/or wrist muscle.
A11
Many of the terms used to construct PCS codes are defined within the system. It is the coder's responsibility to determine what the documentation in the medical record equates to in the PCS definitions. The physician is not expected to use the terms used in PCS code descriptions, nor is the coder required to query the physician when the correlation between the documentation and the defined PCS terms is clear.
Example: When the physician documents "partial resection" the coder can independently correlate "partial resection" to the root operation Excision without querying the physician for clarification.

Medical and Surgical Section Guidelines (section Ø)

B2. Body System
General guidelines
B2.1a
The procedure codes in the general anatomical regions body systems expressed concern with the coding options based on 1) the Index entry and Device Key for Brachytherapy seeds that instructs to use Radioactive Element and 2) published coding advice for the GammaTile™ collagen implant for which a new code was created effective XXXX that describes Insertion with radioactive element and for which a corresponding Index entry exists. Anatomical Regions, General, Anatomical Regions, Upper Extremities and Anatomical Regions, Lower Extremities can be used when the procedure is performed on an anatomical region rather than a specific body part or on the rare occasion when no information is available to support assignment of a code to a specific body part.
Examples: Chest tube drainage of the pleural cavity is coded to the root operation Drainage found in the body system Anatomical Regions, General. Suture repair of the abdominal wall is coded to the root operation Repair in the body system Anatomical Regions, General.
Amputation of the foot is coded to the root operation Detachment in the body system Anatomical Regions, Lower Extremities.
B2.1b
Where the general body part values "upper" and "lower" are provided as an option in the Upper Arteries, Lower Arteries, Upper Veins, Lower Veins, Muscles and Tendons body systems, "upper" or "lower" specifies body parts located above or below the diaphragm respectively.
Example: Vein body parts above the diaphragm are found in the Upper Veins body system; vein body parts below the diaphragm are found in the Lower Veins body system.

B3. Root Operation
General guidelines
B3.1a
In order to determine the appropriate root operation, the full definition of the root operation as contained in the PCS Tables must be applied.
B3.1b
Components of a procedure specified in the root operation definition or explanation as integral to that root operation are not coded separately. Procedural steps necessary to reach the operative site and close the operative site, including anastomosis of a tubular body part, are also not coded separately.

SECTION: Ø **MEDICAL AND SURGICAL**
BODY SYSTEM: J **SUBCUTANEOUS TISSUE AND FASCIA**
OPERATION: H **INSERTION:** Putting in a nonbiological appliance that monitors, assists, performs, or prevents a physiological function but does not physically take the place of a body part

Body Part	Approach	Device	Qualifier
S Subcutaneous Tissue and Fascia, Head and Neck V Subcutaneous Tissue and Fascia, Upper Extremity W Subcutaneous Tissue and Fascia, Lower Extremity	Ø Open 3 Percutaneous	1 Radioactive Element 3 Infusion Device Y Other Device	Z No Qualifier
T Subcutaneous Tissue and Fascia, Trunk	Ø Open 3 Percutaneous	1 Radioactive Element 3 Infusion Device V Infusion Pump Y Other Device	Z No Qualifier

Examples: Resection of a joint as part of a joint replacement procedure is included in the root operation definition of Replacement and is not coded separately. Laparotomy performed to reach the site of an open liver biopsy is not coded separately. In a resection of sigmoid colon with anastomosis of descending colon to rectum, the anastomosis is not coded separately.

Multiple procedures

B3.2

During the same operative episode, multiple procedures are coded if:

a. The same root operation is performed on different body parts as defined by distinct values of the body part character. *Examples:* Diagnostic excision of liver and pancreas are coded separately.
b. The same root operation is repeated in multiple body parts, and those body parts are separate and distinct body parts classified to a single ICD-10-PCS body part value. *Examples:* Excision of the sartorius muscle and excision of the gracilis muscle are both included in the upper leg muscle body part value, and multiple procedures are coded. Extraction of multiple toenails are coded separately.
c. Multiple root operations with distinct objectives are performed on the same body part. *Example:* Destruction of sigmoid lesion and bypass of sigmoid colon are coded separately.
d. The intended root operation is attempted using one approach, but is converted to a different approach. *Example:* Laparoscopic cholecystectomy converted to an open cholecystectomy is coded as percutaneous endoscopic Inspection and open Resection.

Discontinued or incomplete procedures

B3.3

If the intended procedure is discontinued or otherwise not completed, code the procedure to the root operation performed. If a procedure is discontinued before any other root operation is performed, code the root operation Inspection of the body part or anatomical region inspected. *Example:* A planned aortic valve replacement procedure is discontinued after the initial thoracotomy and before any incision is made in the heart muscle, when the patient becomes hemodynamically unstable. This procedure is coded as an open Inspection of the mediastinum.

Biopsy procedures

B3.4a

Biopsy procedures are coded using the root operations Excision, Extraction, or Drainage and the qualifier Diagnostic. *Examples:* Fine needle aspiration biopsy of fluid in the lung is coded to the root operation Drainage with the qualifier Diagnostic. Biopsy of bone marrow is coded to the root operation Extraction with the qualifier Diagnostic. Lymph node sampling for biopsy is coded to the root operation Excision with the qualifier Diagnostic.

Biopsy followed by more definitive treatment

B3.4b

If a diagnostic Excision, Extraction, or Drainage procedure (biopsy) is followed by a more definitive procedure, such as Destruction, Excision or Resection at the same procedure site, both the biopsy and the more definitive treatment are coded. *Example:* Biopsy of breast followed by partial mastectomy at the same procedure site, both the biopsy and the partial mastectomy procedure are coded.

Overlapping body layers

B3.5

If root operations such as, Excision, Extraction, Repair or Inspection are performed on overlapping layers of the musculoskeletal system, the body part specifying the deepest layer is coded.
Example: Excisional debridement that includes skin and subcutaneous tissue and muscle is coded to the muscle body part.

Bypass procedures

B3.6a

Bypass procedures are coded by identifying the body part bypassed "from" and the body part bypassed "to." The fourth character body part specifies the body part bypassed from, and the qualifier specifies the body part bypassed to.
Example: Bypass from stomach to jejunum, stomach is the body part and jejunum is the qualifier.

B3.6b

Coronary artery bypass procedures are coded differently than other bypass procedures as described in the previous guideline. Rather than identifying the body part bypassed from, the body part identifies the number of coronary arteries bypassed to, and the qualifier specifies the vessel bypassed from.
Example: Aortocoronary artery bypass of the left anterior descending coronary artery and the obtuse marginal coronary artery is classified in the body part axis of classification as two coronary arteries, and the qualifier specifies the aorta as the body part bypassed from.

B3.6c

If multiple coronary arteries are bypassed, a separate procedure is coded for each coronary artery that uses a different device and/or qualifier.
Example: Aortocoronary artery bypass and internal mammary coronary artery bypass are coded separately.

Control vs. more specific root operations

B3.7

The root operation Control is defined as, "Stopping, or attempting to stop, postprocedural or other acute bleeding." Control is the root operation coded when the procedure performed to achieve hemostasis, beyond what would be considered integral to a procedure, utilizes techniques (e.g. cautery, application of substances or pressure, suturing or ligation or clipping of bleeding points at the site) that are not described by a more specific root operation, such as Bypass, Detachment, Excision, Extraction, Reposition, Replacement, or Resection. If a more specific root operation definition applies to the procedure performed, then the more specific root operation is coded instead of Control.
Example: Silver nitrate cautery to treat acute nasal bleeding is coded to the root operation Control.
Example: Liquid embolization of the right internal iliac artery to treat acute hematoma by stopping blood flow is coded to the root operation Occlusion.
Example: Suctioning of residual blood to achieve hemostasis during a transbronchial cryobiopsy is considered integral to the cryobiopsy procedure and is not coded separately.

Excision vs. Resection

B3.8

PCS contains specific body parts for anatomical subdivisions of a body part, such as lobes of the lungs or liver and regions of the intestine. Resection of the specific body part is coded whenever all of the body part is cut out or off, rather than coding Excision of a less specific body part.
Example: Left upper lung lobectomy is coded to Resection of Upper Lung Lobe, Left rather than Excision of Lung, Left.

Excision for graft

B3.9

If an autograft is obtained from a different procedure site in order to complete the objective of the procedure, a separate procedure is coded, except when the seventh character qualifier value in the ICD-10-PCS table fully specifies the site from which the autograft was obtained.

Examples: Coronary bypass with excision of saphenous vein graft, excision of saphenous vein is coded separately.

Replacement of breast with autologous deep inferior epigastric artery perforator (DIEP) flap, excision of the DIEP flap is not coded separately. The seventh character qualifier value Deep Inferior Epigastric Artery Perforator Flap in the Replacement table fully specifies the site of the autograft harvest.

Fusion procedures of the spine

B3.10a

The body part coded for a spinal vertebral joint(s) rendered immobile by a spinal fusion procedure is classified by the level of the spine (e.g., thoracic). There are distinct body part values for a single vertebral joint and for multiple vertebral joints at each spinal level.

Example: Body part values specify Lumbar Vertebral Joint, Lumbar Vertebral Joints, 2 or More and Lumbosacral Vertebral Joint.

B3.10b

If multiple vertebral joints are fused, a separate procedure is coded for each vertebral joint that uses a different device and/or qualifier.

Example: Fusion of lumbar vertebral joint, posterior approach, anterior column and fusion of lumbar vertebral joint, posterior approach, posterior column are coded separately.

B3.10c

Combinations of devices and materials are often used on a vertebral joint to render the joint immobile. When combinations of devices are used on the same vertebral joint, the device value coded for the procedure is as follows:

- If an interbody fusion device is used to render the joint immobile (containing bone graft or bone graft sustitute), the procedure is coded with the device value Interbody Fusion Device
- If bone graft is the *only* device used to render the joint immobile, the procedure is coded with the device value Nonautologous Tissue Substitute or Autologous Tissue Substitute
- If a mixture of autologous and nonautologous bone graft (with or without biological or synthetic extenders or binders) is used to render the joint immobile, code the procedure with the device value Autologous Tissue Substitute

Examples: Fusion of a vertebral joint using a cage style interbody fusion device containing morsellized bone graft is coded to the device Interbody Fusion Device. Fusion of a vertebral joint using a bone dowel interbody fusion device made of cadaver bone and packed with a mixture of local morsellized bone and demineralized bone matrix is coded to the device Interbody Fusion Device.

Fusion of a vertebral joint using both autologous bone graft and bone bank bone graft is coded to the device Autologous Tissue Substitute.

Inspection procedures

B3.11a

Inspection of a body part(s) performed in order to achieve the objective of a procedure is not coded separately.

Example: Fiberoptic bronchoscopy performed for irrigation of bronchus, only the irrigation procedure is coded.

B3.11b

If multiple tubular body parts are inspected, the most distal body part (the body part furthest from the starting point of the inspection) is coded. If multiple non-tubular body parts in a region are inspected, the body part that specifies the entire area inspected is coded.

Examples: Cystoureteroscopy with inspection of bladder and ureters is coded to the ureter body part value. Exploratory laparotomy with general inspection of abdominal contents is coded to the peritoneal cavity body part value.

B3.11c

When both an Inspection procedure and another procedure are performed on the same body part during the same episode, if the Inspection procedure is performed using a different approach than the other procedure, the Inspection procedure is coded separately.

Example: Endoscopic Inspection of the duodenum is coded separately when open.

Excision of the duodenum is performed during the same procedural episode.

Occlusion vs. Restriction for vessel embolization procedures

B3.12

If the objective of an embolization procedure is to completely close a vessel, the root operation Occlusion is coded. If the objective of an embolization procedure is to narrow the lumen of a vessel, the root operation Restriction is coded.

Examples: Tumor embolization is coded to the root operation Occlusion, because the objective of the procedure is to cut off the blood supply to the vessel.

Embolization of a cerebral aneurysm is coded to the root operation Restriction, because the objective of the procedure is not to close off the vessel entirely, but to narrow the lumen of the vessel at the site of the aneurysm where it is abnormally wide.

Release procedures

B3.13

In the root operation Release, the body part value coded is the body part being freed and not the tissue being manipulated or cut to free the body part.

Example: Lysis of intestinal adhesions is coded to the specific intestine body part value.

Release vs. Division

B3.14

If the sole objective of the procedure is freeing a body part without cutting the body part, the root operation is Release. If the sole objective of the procedure is separating or transecting a body part, the root operation is Division.

Examples: Freeing a nerve root from surrounding scar tissue to relieve pain is coded to the root operation Release. Severing a nerve root to relieve pain is coded to the root operation Division.

Reposition for fracture treatment

B3.15

Reduction of a displaced fracture is coded to the root operation Reposition and the application of a cast or splint in conjunction with the Reposition procedure is not coded separately. Treatment of a nondisplaced fracture is coded to the procedure performed.

Examples: Casting of a nondisplaced fracture is coded to the root operation Immobilization in the Placement section.

Putting a pin in a nondisplaced fracture is coded to the root operation Insertion.

Transplantation vs. Administration
B3.16
Putting in a mature and functioning living body part taken from another individual or animal is coded to the root operation Transplantation. Putting in autologous or nonautologous cells is coded to the Administration section.
Example: Putting in autologous or nonautologous bone marrow, pancreatic islet cells or stem cells is coded to the Administration section.

Transfer procedures using multiple tissue layers
B3.17
The root operation Transfer contains qualifiers that can be used to specify when a transfer flap is composed of more than one tissue layer, such as a musculocutaneous flap. For procedures involving transfer of multiple tissue layers including skin, subcutaneous tissue, fascia or muscle, the procedure is coded to the body part value that describes the deepest tissue layer in the flap, and the qualifier can be used to describe the other tissue layer(s) in the transfer flap.
Example: A musculocutaneous flap transfer is coded to the appropriate body part value in the body system Muscles, and the qualifier is used to describe the additional tissue layer(s) in the transfer flap.

Excision/Resection followed by replacement
B3.18
If an excision or resection of a body part is followed by a replacement procedure, code both procedures to identify each distinct objective, except when the excision or resection is considered integral and preparatory for the replacement procedure.
Examples: Mastectomy followed by reconstruction, both resection and replacement of the breast are coded to fully capture the distinct objectives of the procedures performed. Maxillectomy with obturator reconstruction, both excision and replacement of the maxilla are coded to fully capture the distinct objectives of the procedures performed. Excisional debridement of tendon with skin graft, both the excision of the tendon and the replacement of the skin with a graft are coded to fully capture the distinct objectives of the procedures performed. Esophagectomy followed by reconstruction with colonic interposition, both the resection and the transfer of the large intestine to function as the esophagus are coded to fully capture the distinct objectives of the procedures performed.
Examples: Resection of a joint as part of a joint replacement procedure is considered integral and preparatory for the replacement of the joint and the resection is not coded separately. Resection of a valve as part of a valve replacement procedure is considered integral and preparatory for the valve replacement and the resection is not coded separately.

Detachment procedures of extremities
B3.19
The root operation Detachment contains qualifiers that can be used to specify the level where the extremity was amputated. These qualifiers are dependent on the body part value in the "upper extremities" and "lower extremities" body systems. For procedures involving the detachment of all or part of the upper or lower extremities, the procedure is coded to the body part value that describes the site of the detachment.
Example: An amputation at the proximal portion of the shaft of the tibia and fibula is coded to the Lower leg body part value in the body system Anatomical Regions, Lower Extremities, and the qualifier High is used to specify the level where the extremity was detached.

The following definitions were developed for the Detachment qualifiers

Body Part	Qualifier	Definition
Upper arm and upper leg	1	High: Amputation at the proximal portion of the shaft of the humerus or femur
	2	Mid: Amputation at the middle portion of the shaft of the humerus or femur
	3	Low: Amputation at the distal portion of the shaft of the humerus or femur
Lower arm and lower leg	1	High: Amputation at the proximal portion of the shaft of the radius/ulna or tibia/fibula
	2	Mid: Amputation at the middle portion of the shaft of the radius/ulna or tibia/fibula
	3	Low: Amputation at the distal portion of the shaft of the radius/ulna or tibia/fibula
Hand and Foot	Ø	Complete*
	4	Complete 1st Ray
	5	Complete 2nd Ray
	6	Complete 3rd Ray
	7	Complete 4th Ray
	8	Complete 5th Ray
	9	Partial 1st Ray
	B	Partial 2nd Ray
	C	Partial 3rd Ray
	D	Partial 4th Ray
	F	Partial 5th Ray
Thumb, finger, or toe	Ø	Complete: Amputation at the metacarpophalangeal/metatarsal-phalangeal joint
	1	High: Amputation anywhere along the proximal phalanx
	2	Mid: Amputation through the proximal interphalangeal joint or anywhere along the middle phalanx
	3	Low: Amputation through the distal interphalangeal joint or anywhere along the distal phalanx

*When coding amputation of Hand and Foot, the following definitions are followed:
Complete: Amputation through the carpometacarpal joint of the hand, or through the tarsal-metatarsal joint of the foot.
Partial: Amputation anywhere along the shaft or head of the metacarpal bone of the hand, or of the metatarsal bone of the foot.

GUIDELINES (ICD-10-PCS)

B4. Body Part

General guidelines

B4.1a

If a procedure is performed on a portion of a body part that does not have a separate body part value, code the body part value corresponding to the whole body part.

Example: A procedure performed on the alveolar process of the mandible is coded to the mandible body part.

B4.1b

If the prefix "peri" is combined with a body part to identify the site of the procedure, and the site of the procedure is not further specified, then the procedure is coded to the body part named. This guideline applies only when a more specific body part value is not available.

Examples: A procedure site identified as perirenal is coded to the kidney body part when the site of the procedure is not further specified. A procedure site described in the documentation as peri-urethral, and the documentation also indicates that it is the vulvar tissue and not the urethral tissue that is the site of the procedure, then the procedure is coded to the vulva body part.

A procedure site documented as involving the periosteum is coded to the corresponding bone body part.

B4.1c

If a procedure is performed on a continuous section of an arterial or venous single vascular body part, code the body part value corresponding to the anatomically most proximal (closest to the heart) portion of the arterial or venous body part.

Example: A procedure performed on a continuous section of artery from the femoral artery to the external iliac artery with the point of entry at the femoral artery is coded to the external iliac body part. A procedure performed on a continuous section of artery from the femoral artery to the external iliac artery with the point of entry at the external iliac artery is also coded to the external iliac artery body part.

Branches of body parts

B4.2

Where a specific branch of a body part does not have its own body part value in PCS, the body part is typically coded to the closest proximal branch that has a specific body part value.

In the cardiovascular body systems, if a general body part is available in the correct root operation table, and coding to a proximal branch would require assigning a code in a different body system, the procedure is coded using the general body part value.

Example: A procedure performed on the mandibular branch of the trigeminal nerve is coded to the trigeminal nerve body part value.

Bilateral body part values

B4.3

Bilateral body part values are available for a limited number of body parts. If the identical procedure is performed on contralateral body parts, and a bilateral body part value exists for that body part, a single procedure is coded using the bilateral body part value. If no bilateral body part value exists, each procedure is coded separately using the appropriate body part value.

Examples: The identical procedure performed on both fallopian tubes is coded once using the body part value Fallopian Tube, Bilateral. The identical procedure performed on both knee joints is coded twice using the body part values Knee Joint, Right and Knee Joint, Left.

Coronary arteries

B4.4

The coronary arteries are classified as a single body part that is further specified by number of arteries treated. One procedure code specifying multiple arteries is used when the same procedure is performed, including the same device and qualifier values.

Examples: Angioplasty of two distinct coronary arteries with placement of two stents is coded as Dilation of Coronary Artery, Two Arteries with Two Intraluminal Devices.

Angioplasty of two distinct coronary arteries, one with stent placed and one without, is coded separately as Dilation of Coronary Artery, One Artery with Intraluminal Device, and Dilation of Coronary Artery, One Artery with no device.

Tendons, ligaments, bursae and fascia near a joint

B4.5

Procedures performed on tendons, ligaments, bursae and fascia supporting a joint are coded to the body part in the respective body system that is the focus of the procedure. Procedures performed on joint structures themselves are coded to the body part in the joint body systems.

Examples: Repair of the anterior cruciate ligament of the knee is coded to the knee bursae and ligament body part in the bursae and ligaments body system. Knee arthroscopy with shaving of articular cartilage is coded to the knee joint body part in the Lower Joints body system.

Skin, subcutaneous tissue and fascia overlying a joint

B4.6

If a procedure is performed on the skin, subcutaneous tissue or fascia overlying a joint, the procedure is coded to the following body part:

- Shoulder is coded to Upper Arm
- Elbow is coded to Lower Arm
- Wrist is coded to Lower Arm
- Hip is coded to Upper Leg
- Knee is coded to Lower Leg
- Ankle is coded to Foot

Fingers and toes

B4.7

If a body system does not contain a separate body part value for fingers, procedures performed on the fingers are coded to the body part value for the hand. If a body system does not contain a separate body part value for toes, procedures performed on the toes are coded to the body part value for the foot.

Example: Excision of finger muscle is coded to one of the hand muscle body part values in the Muscles body system.

Upper and lower intestinal tract

B4.8

In the Gastrointestinal body system, the general body part values Upper Intestinal Tract and Lower Intestinal Tract are provided as an option for the root operations such as Change, Inspection, Removal and Revision. Upper Intestinal Tract includes the portion of the gastrointestinal tract from the esophagus down to and including the duodenum, and Lower Intestinal Tract includes the portion of the gastrointestinal tract from the jejunum down to and including the rectum and anus.

Example: In the root operation Change table, change of a device in the jejunum is coded using the body part Lower Intestinal Tract.

B5. Approach

Open approach with percutaneous endoscopic assistance

B5.2a

Procedures performed using the open approach with percutaneous endoscopic assistance are coded to the approach Open.

Example: Laparoscopic-assisted sigmoidectomy is coded to the approach Open.

Percutaneous endoscopic approach with hand-assistance or extension of incision
B5.2b
Procedures performed using the percutaneous endoscopic approach with hand-assistance, or with an incision or extension of an incision to assist in the removal of all or a portion of a body part, or to anastomose a tubular body part with or without the temporary exteriorization of a body structure, are coded to the approach value Percutaneous Endoscopic.
Examples: Hand-assisted laparoscopic sigmoid colon resection with exteriorization of a segment of the colon for removal of specimen with return of colon back into abdominal cavity is coded to the approach value percutaneous endoscopic.
Laparoscopic sigmoid colectomy with extension of stapling port for removal of specimen and direct anastomosis is coded to the approach value percutaneous endoscopic.
Laparoscopic nephrectomy with midline incision for removing the resected kidney is coded to the approach value percutaneous endoscopic.
Robotic-assisted laparoscopic prostatectomy with extension of incision for removal of the resected prostate is coded to the approach value percutaneous endoscopic.

External approach
B5.3a
Procedures performed within an orifice on structures that are visible without the aid of any instrumentation are coded to the approach External.
Example: Resection of tonsils is coded to the approach External.
B5.3b
Procedures performed indirectly by the application of external force through the intervening body layers are coded to the approach External.
Example: Closed reduction of fracture is coded to the approach External.

Percutaneous procedure via device
B5.4
Procedures performed percutaneously via a device placed for the procedure are coded to the approach Percutaneous.
Example: Fragmentation of kidney stone performed via percutaneous nephrostomy is coded to the approach Percutaneous.

B6. Device
General guidelines
B6.1a
A device is coded only if a device remains after the procedure is completed. If no device remains, the device value No Device is coded. In limited root operations, the classification provides the qualifier values Temporary and Intraoperative, for specific procedures involving clinically significant devices, where the purpose of the device is to be utilized for a brief duration during the procedure or current inpatient stay. If a device that is intended to remain after the procedure is completed requires removal before the end of the operative episode in which it was inserted, both the insertion and removal of the device should be coded.
B6.1b
Materials such as sutures, ligatures, radiological markers and temporary post-operative wound drains are considered integral to the performance of a procedure and are not coded as devices.
B6.1c
Procedures performed on a device only and not on a body part are specified in the root operations Change, Irrigation, Removal and Revision, and are coded to the procedure performed.
Example: Irrigation of percutaneous nephrostomy tube is coded to the root operation Irrigation of indwelling device in the Administration section.

Drainage device
B6.2
A separate procedure to put in a drainage device is coded to the root operation Drainage with the device value Drainage Device.

Obstetric Section Guidelines (section 1)

C. Obstetrics Section
Products of conception
C1
Procedures performed on the products of conception are coded to the Obstetrics section. Procedures performed on the pregnant female other than the products of conception are coded to the appropriate root operation in the Medical and Surgical section.
Example: Amniocentesis is coded to the products of conception body part in the Obstetrics section. Repair of obstetric urethral laceration is coded to the urethra body part in the Medical and Surgical section.

Procedures following delivery or abortion
C2
Procedures performed following a delivery or abortion for curettage of the endometrium or evacuation of retained products of conception are all coded in the Obstetrics section, to the root operation Extraction and the body part Products of Conception, Retained. Diagnostic or therapeutic dilation and curettage performed during times other than the postpartum or post-abortion period are all coded in the Medical and Surgical section, to the root operation Extraction and the body part Endometrium.

Radiation Therapy Section Guidelines (section D)

D. Radiation Therapy Section
Brachytherapy
D1.a
Brachytherapy is coded to the modality Brachytherapy in the Radiation Therapy section. When a radioactive brachytherapy source is left in the body at the end of the procedure, it is coded separately to the root operation Insertion with the device value Radioactive Element.
Example: Brachytherapy with implantation of a low dose rate brachytherapy source left in the body at the end of the procedure is coded to the applicable treatment site in section D, Radiation Therapy, with the modality Brachytherapy, the modality qualifier value Low Dose Rate, and the applicable isotope value and qualifier value. The implantation of the brachytherapy source is coded separately to the device value Radioactive Element in the appropriate Insertion table of the Medical and Surgical section. The Radiation Therapy section code identifies the specific modality and isotope of the brachytherapy, and the root operation Insertion code identifies the implantation of the brachytherapy source that remains in the body at the end of the procedure.
Exception: Implantation of Cesium-131 brachytherapy seeds embedded in a collagen matrix to the treatment site after resection of brain tumor is coded to the root operation Insertion with the device value Radioactive Element, Cesium-131 Collagen Implant. The procedure is coded to the root operation Insertion only, because the device value identifies both the implantation of the radioactive element and a specific brachytherapy isotope that is not included in the Radiation Therapy section tables.
D1.b
A separate procedure to place a temporary applicator for delivering the brachytherapy is coded to the root operation Insertion and the device value Other Device.
Examples: Intrauterine brachytherapy applicator placed as a separate procedure from the brachytherapy procedure is coded to Insertion of Other Device, and the brachytherapy is coded separately using the modality Brachytherapy in the Radiation Therapy section.
Intrauterine brachytherapy applicator placed concomitantly with delivery of the brachytherapy dose is coded with a single code using the modality Brachytherapy in the Radiation Therapy section.

New Technology Section Guidelines (section X)

E. New Technology Section

General guidelines

E1.a

Section X codes fully represent the specific procedure described in the code title, and do not require additional codes from other sections of ICD-10-PCS. When section X contains a code title which fully describes a specific new technology procedure, and is the only procedure performed, only the section X code is reported for the procedure. There is no need to report an additional code in another section of ICD-10-PCS.

Example: XW043A6 Introduction of Cefiderocol Anti-infective into Central Vein, Percutaneous Approach, New Technology Group 6, can be coded to indicate that Cefiderocol Anti-infective was administered via a central vein. A separate code from table 3E0 in the Administration section of ICD-10-PCS is not coded in addition to this code.

E1.b

When multiple procedures are performed, New Technology section X codes are coded following the multiple procedures guideline.

Examples: Dual filter cerebral embolic filtration used during transcatheter aortic valve replacement (TAVR), X2A5312 Cerebral Embolic Filtration, Dual Filter in Innominate Artery and Left Common Carotid Artery, Percutaneous Approach, New Technology Group 2, is coded for the cerebral embolic filtration, along with an ICD-10-PCS code for the TAVR procedure.

An extracorporeal flow reversal circuit for embolic neuroprotection placed during a transcarotid arterial revascularization procedure, a code from table X2A, Assistance of the Cardiovascular System is coded for the use of the extracoporeal flow reversal circuit, along with an ICD-10-PCS code for the transcarotid arterial revascularization procedure.

F. Selection of Principal Procedure

The following instructions should be applied in the selection of principal procedure and clarification on the importance of the relation to the principal diagnosis when more than one procedure is performed:

1. Procedure performed for definitive treatment of both principal diagnosis and secondary diagnosis
   a. Sequence procedure performed for definitive treatment most related to principal diagnosis as principal procedure.
2. Procedure performed for definitive treatment and diagnostic procedures performed for both principal diagnosis and secondary diagnosis
   a. Sequence procedure performed for definitive treatment most related to principal diagnosis as principal procedure
3. A diagnostic procedure was performed for the principal diagnosis and a procedure is performed for definitive treatment of a secondary diagnosis.
   a. Sequence diagnostic procedure as principal procedure, since the procedure most related to the principal diagnosis takes precedence.
4. No procedures performed that are related to principal diagnosis; procedures performed for definitive treatment and diagnostic procedures were performed for secondary diagnosis
   a. Sequence procedure performed for definitive treatment of secondary diagnosis as principal procedure, since there are no procedures (definitive or nondefinitive treatment) related to principal diagnosis.

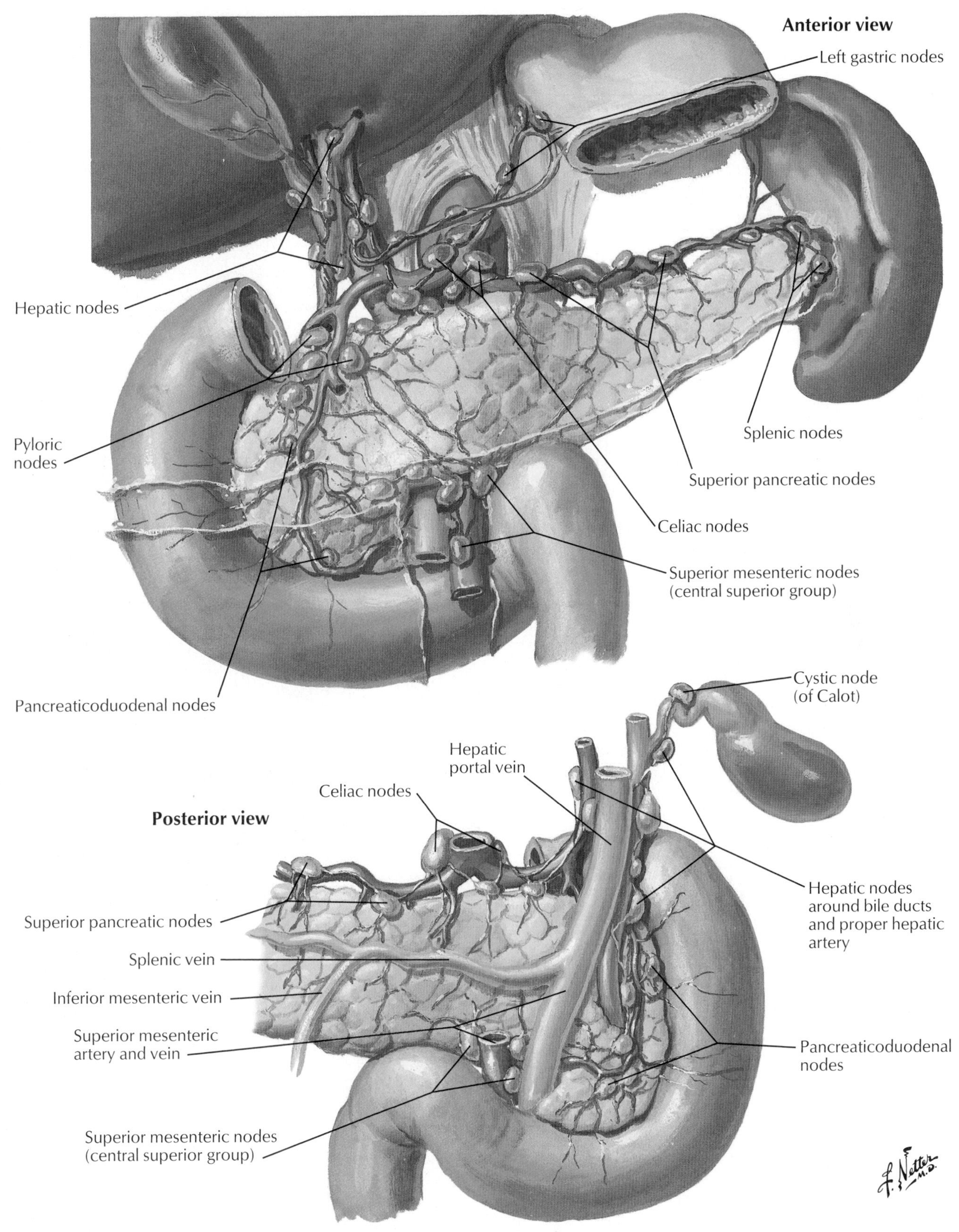
Anterior view
Left gastric nodes
Hepatic nodes
Pyloric nodes
Splenic nodes
Superior pancreatic nodes
Celiac nodes
Superior mesenteric nodes (central superior group)
Pancreaticoduodenal nodes
Cystic node (of Calot)
Hepatic portal vein
Celiac nodes
Posterior view
Superior pancreatic nodes
Splenic vein
Inferior mesenteric vein
Superior mesenteric artery and vein
Superior mesenteric nodes (central superior group)
Hepatic nodes around bile ducts and proper hepatic artery
Pancreaticoduodenal nodes
F. Netter M.D.

ANATOMY ILLUSTRATIONS

Plate 1 Lymph Vessels and Nodes of Pancreas.

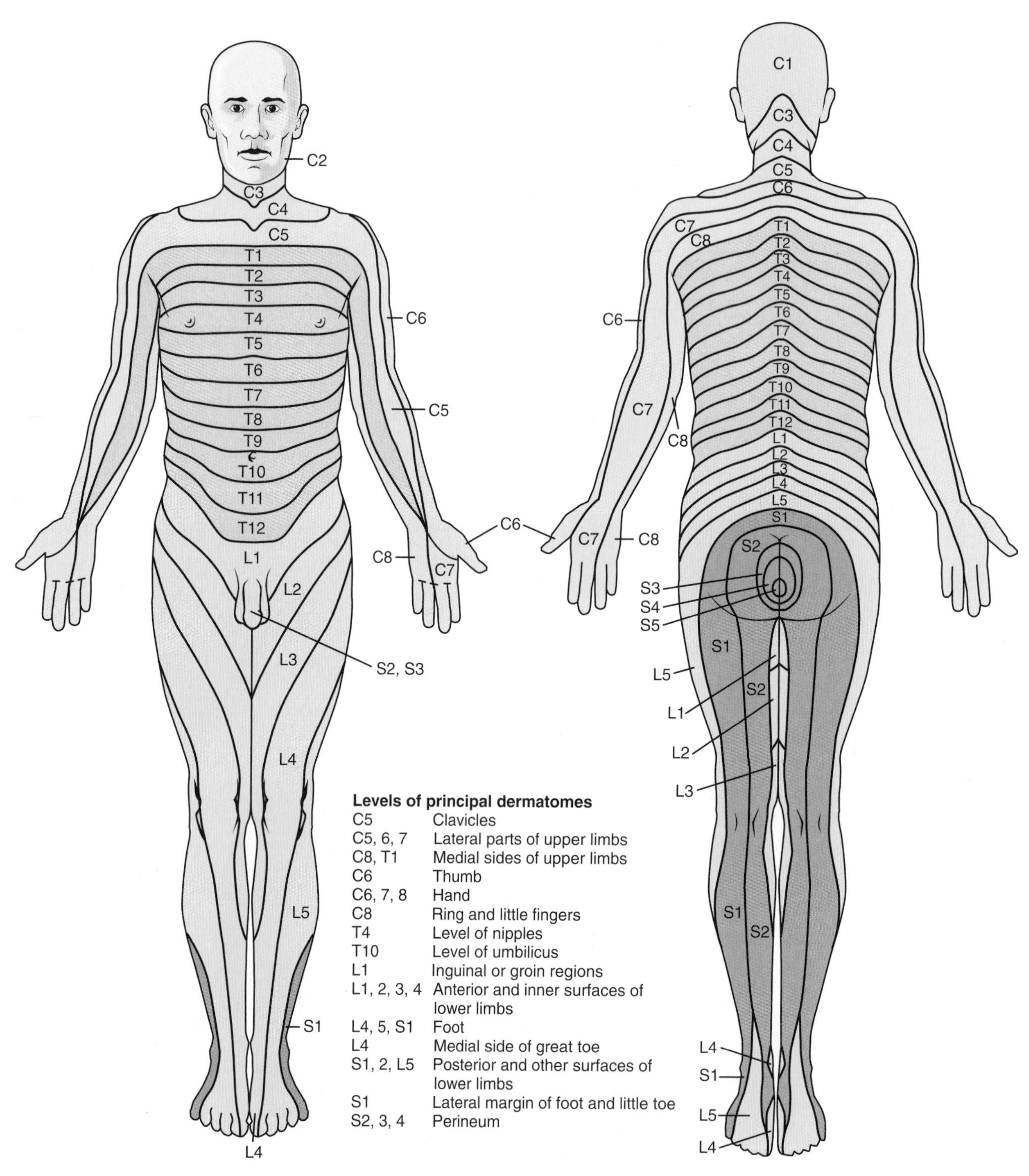
C2
C3
C4
C5
T1
T2
T3
T4
C6
T5
T6
T7
C5
T8
T9
T10
T11
T12
C6
L1
C8
C7
L2
S2, S3
L3
L4
L5
S1
L4
C1
C3
C4
C5
C6
C7
C8
T1
T2
T3
T4
T5
T6
T7
T8
T9
T10
T11
T12
L1
L2
L3
L4
L5
S1
C6
C7
C8
C6
C7
C8
S2
S3
S4
S5
S1
L5
S2
L1
L2
L3
S1
S2
L4
S1
L5
L4
Levels of principal dermatomes
C5 Clavicles
C5, 6, 7 Lateral parts of upper limbs
C8, T1 Medial sides of upper limbs
C6 Thumb
C6, 7, 8 Hand
C8 Ring and little fingers
T4 Level of nipples
T10 Level of umbilicus
L1 Inguinal or groin regions
L1, 2, 3, 4 Anterior and inner surfaces of lower limbs
L4, 5, S1 Foot
L4 Medial side of great toe
S1, 2, L5 Posterior and other surfaces of lower limbs
S1 Lateral margin of foot and little toe
S2, 3, 4 Perineum

Plate 2 Schematic demarcation of Dermatomes. (Miller MD, Hart JA, MacKnight JM: Essential Orthopaedics, ed 2, Philadelphia, 2020, Elsevier.)

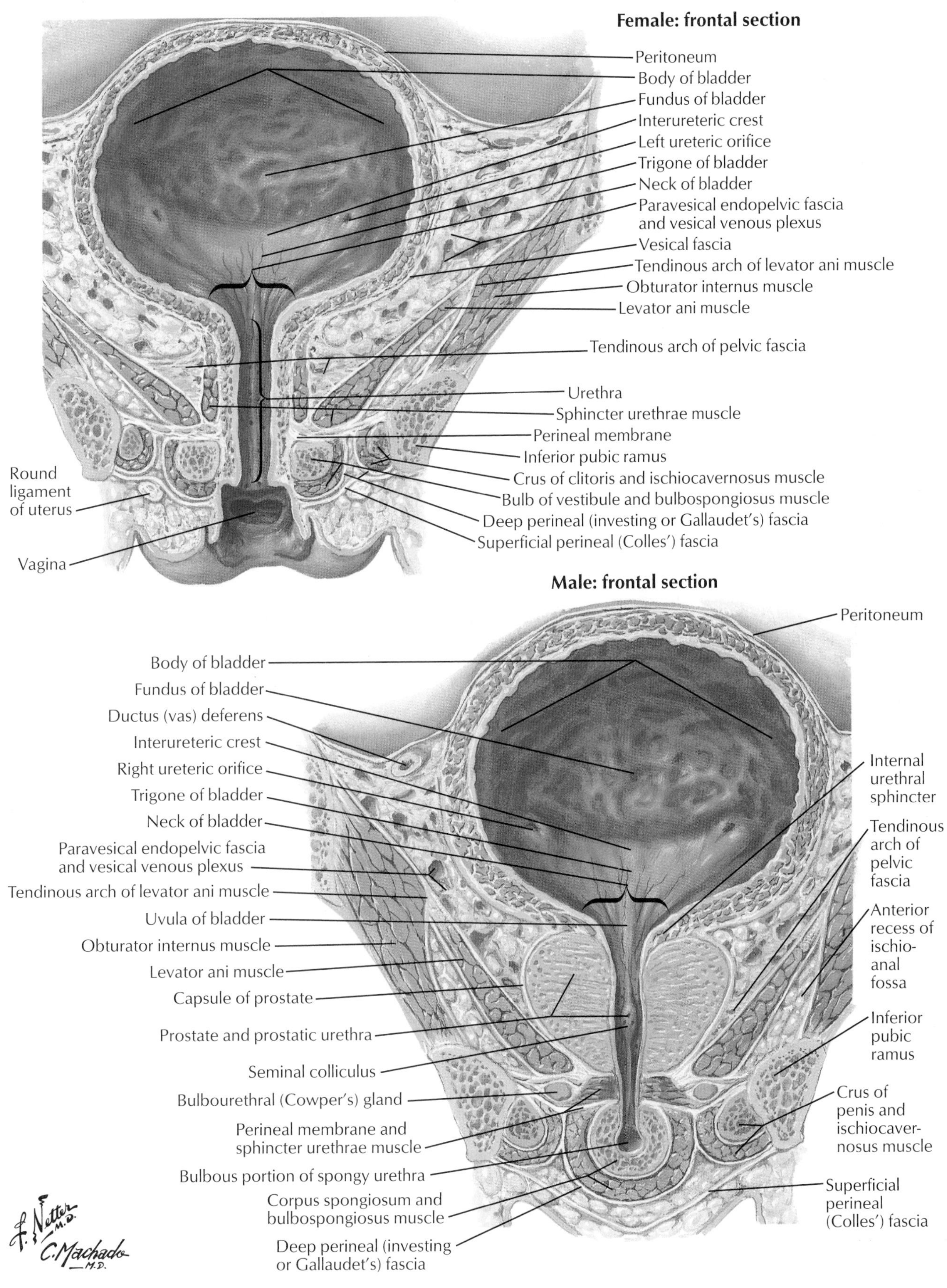
Female: frontal section
Peritoneum
Body of bladder
Fundus of bladder
Interureteric crest
Left ureteric orifice
Trigone of bladder
Neck of bladder
Paravesical endopelvic fascia and vesical venous plexus
Vesical fascia
Tendinous arch of levator ani muscle
Obturator internus muscle
Levator ani muscle
Tendinous arch of pelvic fascia
Urethra
Sphincter urethrae muscle
Perineal membrane
Inferior pubic ramus
Crus of clitoris and ischiocavernosus muscle
Bulb of vestibule and bulbospongiosus muscle
Deep perineal (investing or Gallaudet's) fascia
Superficial perineal (Colles') fascia
Round ligament of uterus
Vagina
Male: frontal section
Peritoneum
Body of bladder
Fundus of bladder
Ductus (vas) deferens
Interureteric crest
Right ureteric orifice
Trigone of bladder
Neck of bladder
Paravesical endopelvic fascia and vesical venous plexus
Tendinous arch of levator ani muscle
Uvula of bladder
Obturator internus muscle
Levator ani muscle
Capsule of prostate
Prostate and prostatic urethra
Seminal colliculus
Bulbourethral (Cowper's) gland
Perineal membrane and sphincter urethrae muscle
Bulbous portion of spongy urethra
Corpus spongiosum and bulbospongiosus muscle
Deep perineal (investing or Gallaudet's) fascia
Internal urethral sphincter
Tendinous arch of pelvic fascia
Anterior recess of ischio-anal fossa
Inferior pubic ramus
Crus of penis and ischiocaver-nosus muscle
Superficial perineal (Colles') fascia
F. Netter M.D.
C. Machado M.D.

Plate 3 Urinary Bladder: Female and Male. (Copyright 2023 Elsevier Inc. All rights reserved. www.netterimages.com. Image ID: 4714)

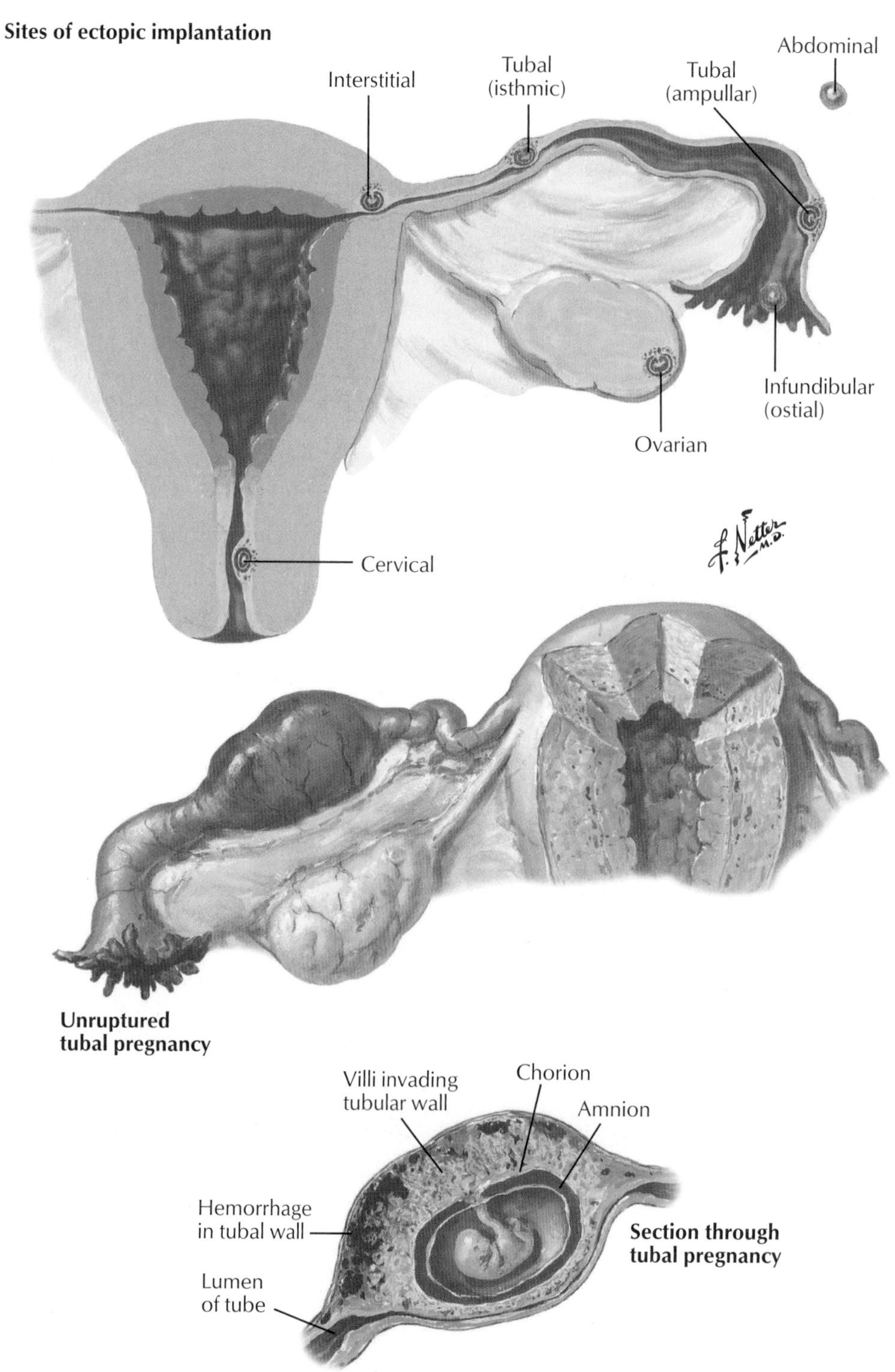
Sites of ectopic implantation
Interstitial
Tubal (isthmic)
Tubal (ampullar)
Abdominal
Infundibular (ostial)
Ovarian
Cervical
Unruptured tubal pregnancy
Villi invading tubular wall
Chorion
Amnion
Hemorrhage in tubal wall
Section through tubal pregnancy
Lumen of tube

Plate 4 Ectopic Pregnancy.

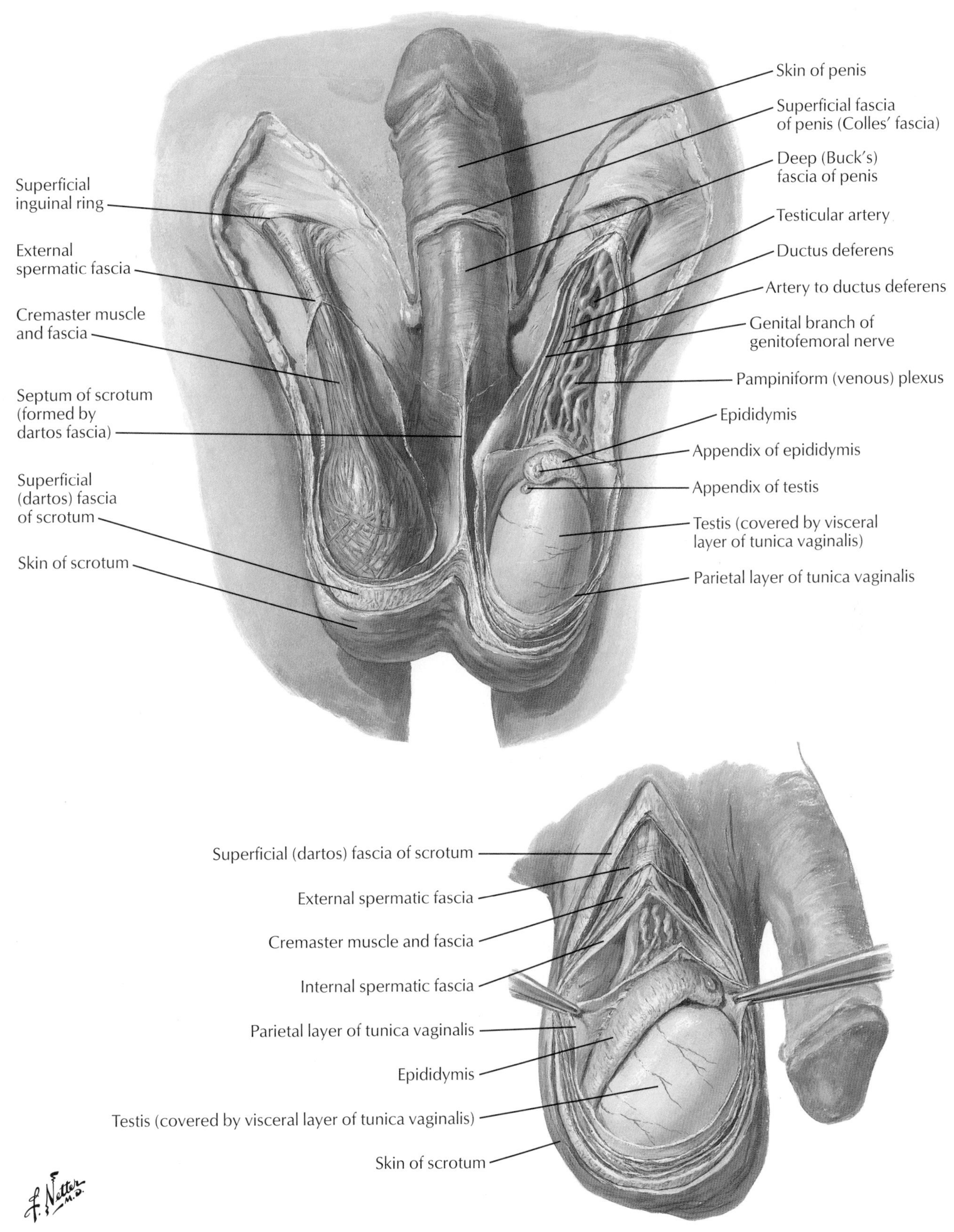
Skin of penis
Superficial fascia of penis (Colles' fascia)
Deep (Buck's) fascia of penis
Testicular artery
Ductus deferens
Artery to ductus deferens
Genital branch of genitofemoral nerve
Pampiniform (venous) plexus
Epididymis
Appendix of epididymis
Appendix of testis
Testis (covered by visceral layer of tunica vaginalis)
Parietal layer of tunica vaginalis
Superficial inguinal ring
External spermatic fascia
Cremaster muscle and fascia
Septum of scrotum (formed by dartos fascia)
Superficial (dartos) fascia of scrotum
Skin of scrotum
Superficial (dartos) fascia of scrotum
External spermatic fascia
Cremaster muscle and fascia
Internal spermatic fascia
Parietal layer of tunica vaginalis
Epididymis
Testis (covered by visceral layer of tunica vaginalis)
Skin of scrotum

Plate 5 Scrotum and Contents.

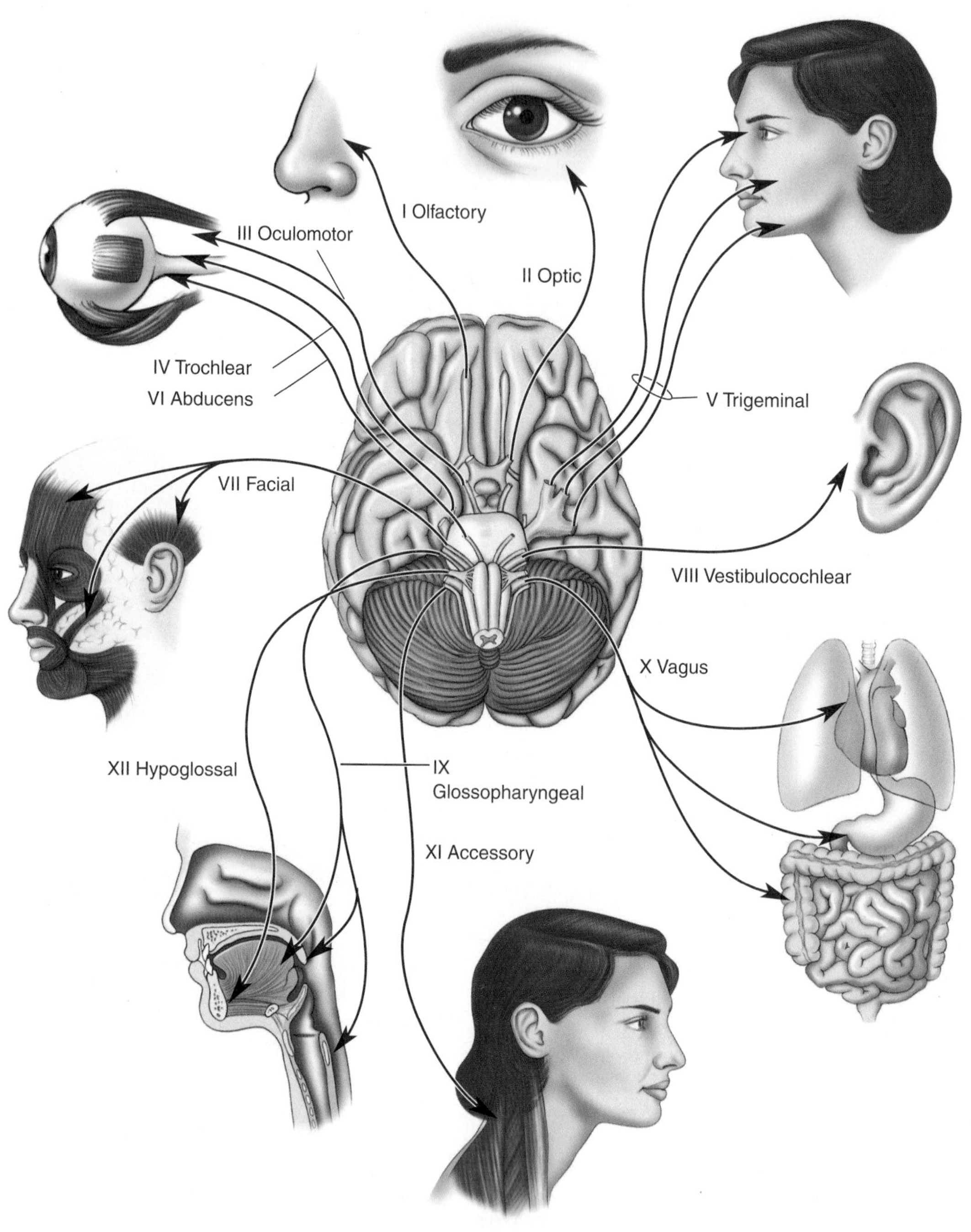

Plate 6 Cranial Nerves (12 pairs) are known by their numbers (Roman numerals) and names. (Herlihy BL: The Human Body in Health and Illness, ed 6, St. Louis, 2018, Elsevier.)

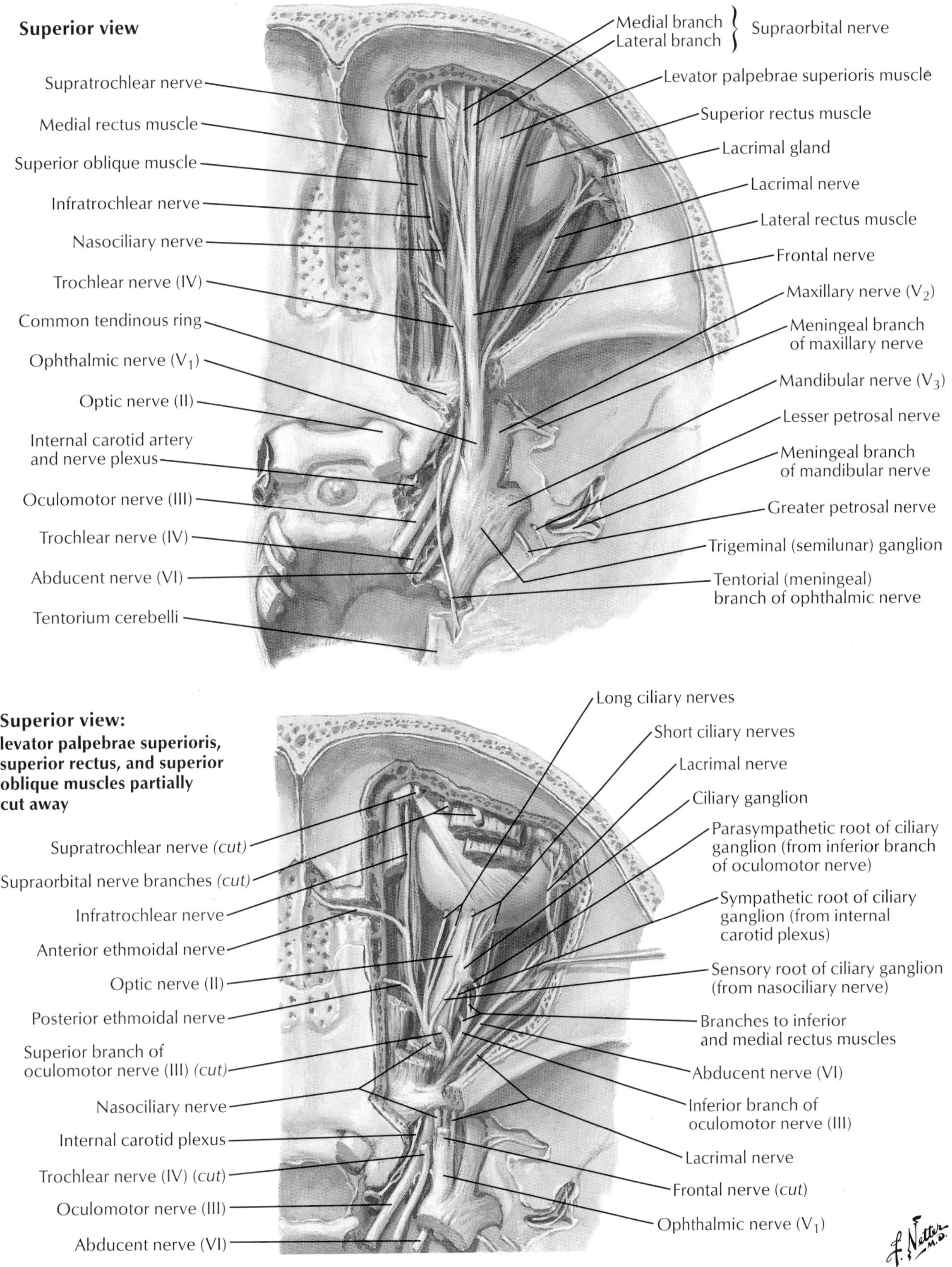
Superior view
Medial branch
Lateral branch
Supraorbital nerve
Supratrochlear nerve
Levator palpebrae superioris muscle
Medial rectus muscle
Superior rectus muscle
Superior oblique muscle
Lacrimal gland
Infratrochlear nerve
Lacrimal nerve
Lateral rectus muscle
Nasociliary nerve
Frontal nerve
Trochlear nerve (IV)
Maxillary nerve (V_2)
Common tendinous ring
Meningeal branch of maxillary nerve
Ophthalmic nerve (V_1)
Mandibular nerve (V_3)
Optic nerve (II)
Lesser petrosal nerve
Internal carotid artery and nerve plexus
Meningeal branch of mandibular nerve
Oculomotor nerve (III)
Greater petrosal nerve
Trochlear nerve (IV)
Trigeminal (semilunar) ganglion
Abducent nerve (VI)
Tentorial (meningeal) branch of ophthalmic nerve
Tentorium cerebelli
Superior view: levator palpebrae superioris, superior rectus, and superior oblique muscles partially cut away
Long ciliary nerves
Short ciliary nerves
Lacrimal nerve
Ciliary ganglion
Supratrochlear nerve (cut)
Parasympathetic root of ciliary ganglion (from inferior branch of oculomotor nerve)
Supraorbital nerve branches (cut)
Infratrochlear nerve
Sympathetic root of ciliary ganglion (from internal carotid plexus)
Anterior ethmoidal nerve
Sensory root of ciliary ganglion (from nasociliary nerve)
Optic nerve (II)
Posterior ethmoidal nerve
Branches to inferior and medial rectus muscles
Superior branch of oculomotor nerve (III) (cut)
Abducent nerve (VI)
Nasociliary nerve
Inferior branch of oculomotor nerve (III)
Internal carotid plexus
Lacrimal nerve
Trochlear nerve (IV) (cut)
Frontal nerve (cut)
Oculomotor nerve (III)
Ophthalmic nerve (V_1)
Abducent nerve (VI)
F. Netter M.D.

Plate 7 Nerves of Orbit.

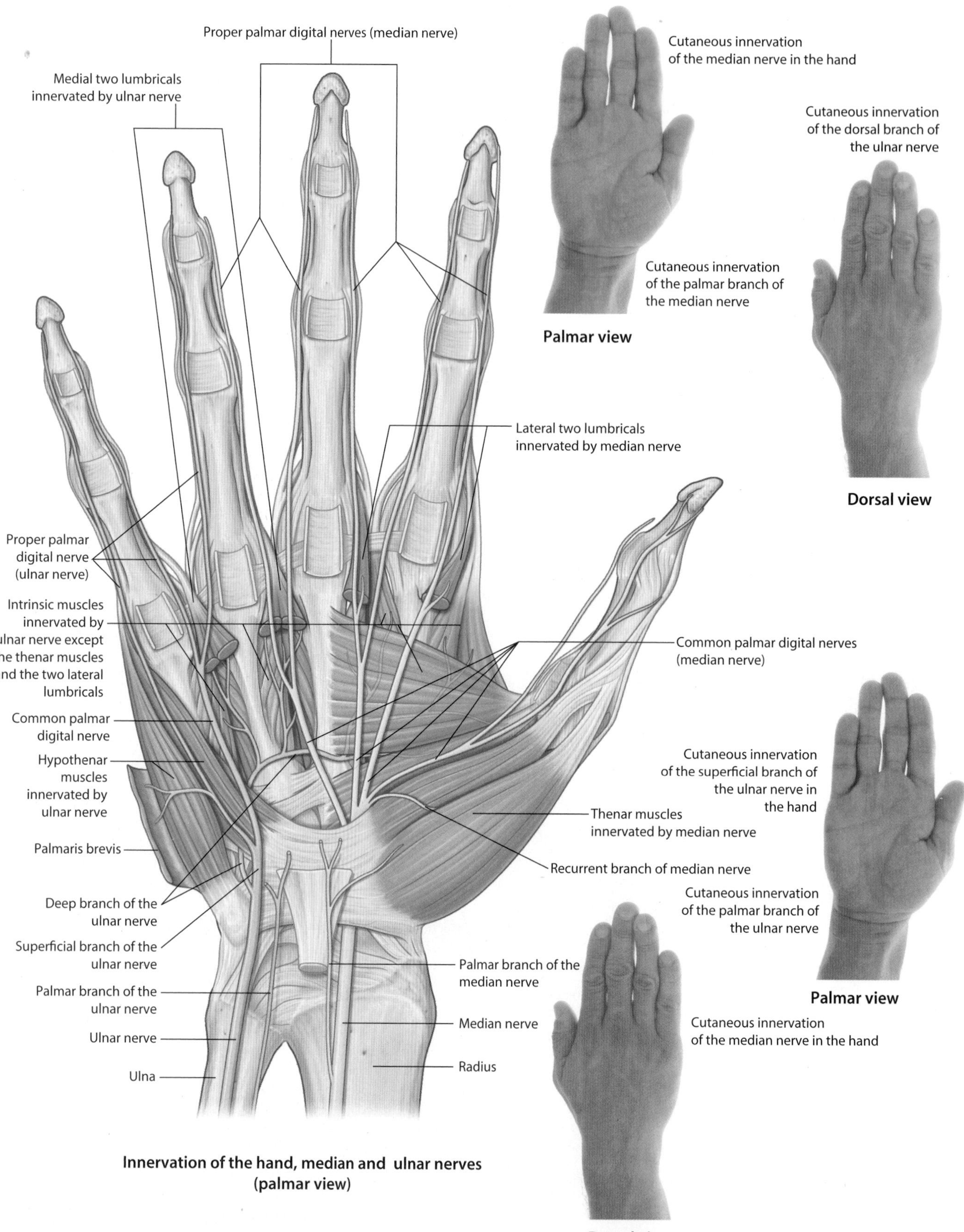
Proper palmar digital nerves (median nerve)
Medial two lumbricals innervated by ulnar nerve
Lateral two lumbricals innervated by median nerve
Proper palmar digital nerve (ulnar nerve)
Intrinsic muscles innervated by ulnar nerve except the thenar muscles and the two lateral lumbricals
Common palmar digital nerve
Hypothenar muscles innervated by ulnar nerve
Palmaris brevis
Deep branch of the ulnar nerve
Superficial branch of the ulnar nerve
Palmar branch of the ulnar nerve
Ulnar nerve
Ulna
Common palmar digital nerves (median nerve)
Thenar muscles innervated by median nerve
Recurrent branch of median nerve
Palmar branch of the median nerve
Median nerve
Radius
Innervation of the hand, median and ulnar nerves (palmar view)
Cutaneous innervation of the median nerve in the hand
Cutaneous innervation of the palmar branch of the median nerve
Palmar view
Cutaneous innervation of the dorsal branch of the ulnar nerve
Dorsal view
Cutaneous innervation of the superficial branch of the ulnar nerve in the hand
Cutaneous innervation of the palmar branch of the ulnar nerve
Palmar view
Cutaneous innervation of the median nerve in the hand
Dorsal view

Plate 8 Innervation of the Hand: Median and Ulnar Nerves. (From Drake RL, Vogl AW, Mitchell AWM, Tibbitts RM, Richardson PE: Gray's Atlas of Anatomy, ed 2, Philadelphia, 2015, Churchill Livingstone.)

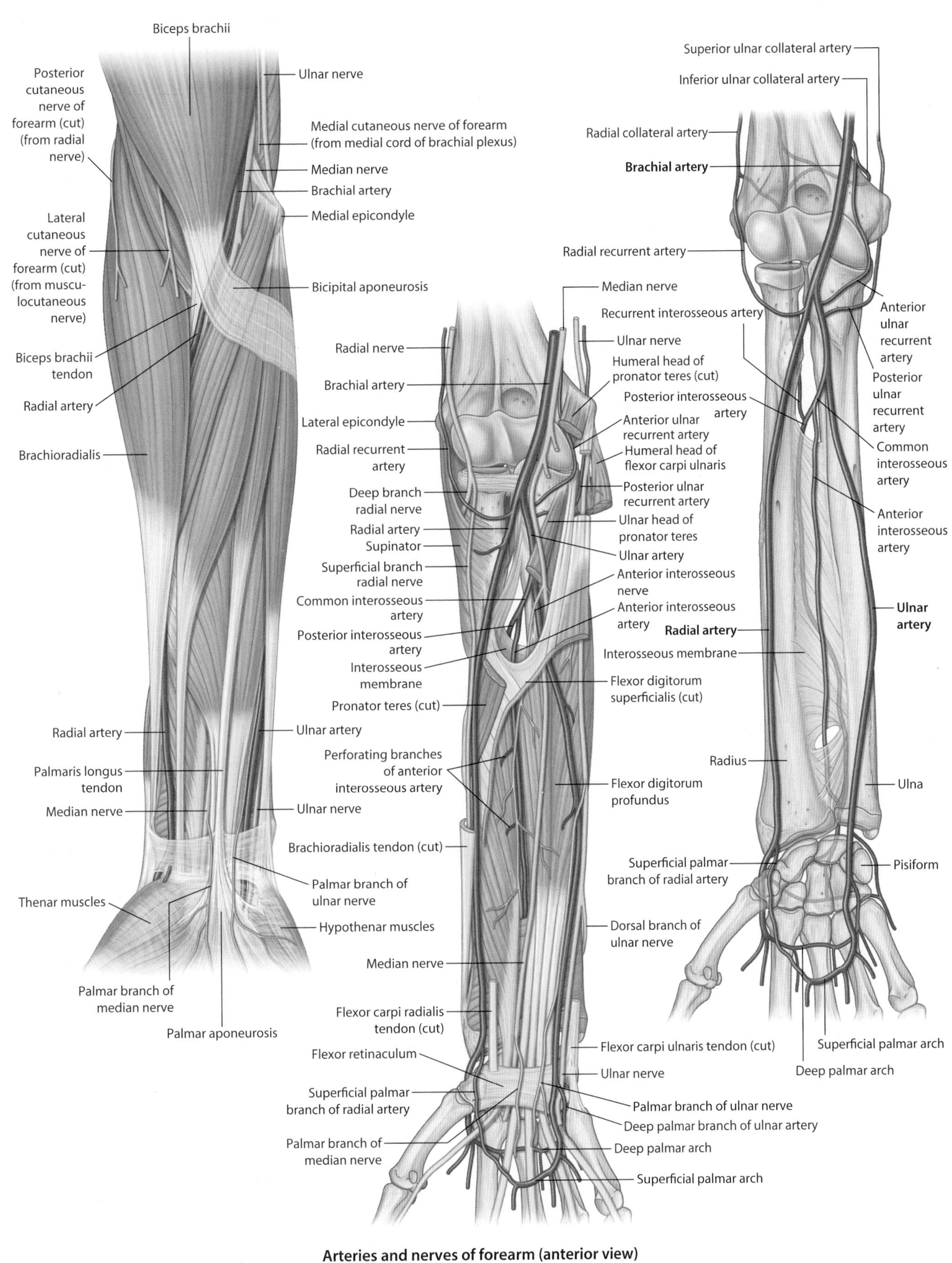

Biceps brachii
Posterior cutaneous nerve of forearm (cut) (from radial nerve)
Ulnar nerve
Medial cutaneous nerve of forearm (from medial cord of brachial plexus)
Median nerve
Brachial artery
Medial epicondyle
Lateral cutaneous nerve of forearm (cut) (from musculocutaneous nerve)
Bicipital aponeurosis
Biceps brachii tendon
Radial artery
Brachioradialis
Radial artery
Ulnar artery
Palmaris longus tendon
Median nerve
Ulnar nerve
Thenar muscles
Palmar branch of ulnar nerve
Hypothenar muscles
Palmar branch of median nerve
Palmar aponeurosis
Radial nerve
Brachial artery
Lateral epicondyle
Radial recurrent artery
Deep branch radial nerve
Radial artery
Supinator
Superficial branch radial nerve
Common interosseous artery
Posterior interosseous artery
Interosseous membrane
Pronator teres (cut)
Perforating branches of anterior interosseous artery
Brachioradialis tendon (cut)
Median nerve
Flexor carpi radialis tendon (cut)
Flexor retinaculum
Superficial palmar branch of radial artery
Palmar branch of median nerve
Median nerve
Recurrent interosseous artery
Ulnar nerve
Humeral head of pronator teres (cut)
Posterior interosseous artery
Anterior ulnar recurrent artery
Humeral head of flexor carpi ulnaris
Posterior ulnar recurrent artery
Ulnar head of pronator teres
Ulnar artery
Anterior interosseous nerve
Anterior interosseous artery
Interosseous membrane
Flexor digitorum superficialis (cut)
Flexor digitorum profundus
Dorsal branch of ulnar nerve
Flexor carpi ulnaris tendon (cut)
Ulnar nerve
Palmar branch of ulnar nerve
Deep palmar branch of ulnar artery
Deep palmar arch
Superficial palmar arch
Superior ulnar collateral artery
Inferior ulnar collateral artery
Radial collateral artery
Brachial artery
Radial recurrent artery
Anterior ulnar recurrent artery
Posterior ulnar recurrent artery
Common interosseous artery
Anterior interosseous artery
Radial artery
Ulnar artery
Radius
Ulna
Superficial palmar branch of radial artery
Pisiform
Superficial palmar arch
Deep palmar arch

Arteries and nerves of forearm (anterior view)

Plate 9 Arteries and Nerves of the Forearm (Anterior View). (From Drake RL, Vogl AW, Mitchell AWM, Tibbitts RM, Richardson PE: Gray's Atlas of Anatomy, ed 2, Philadelphia, 2015, Churchill Livingstone.)

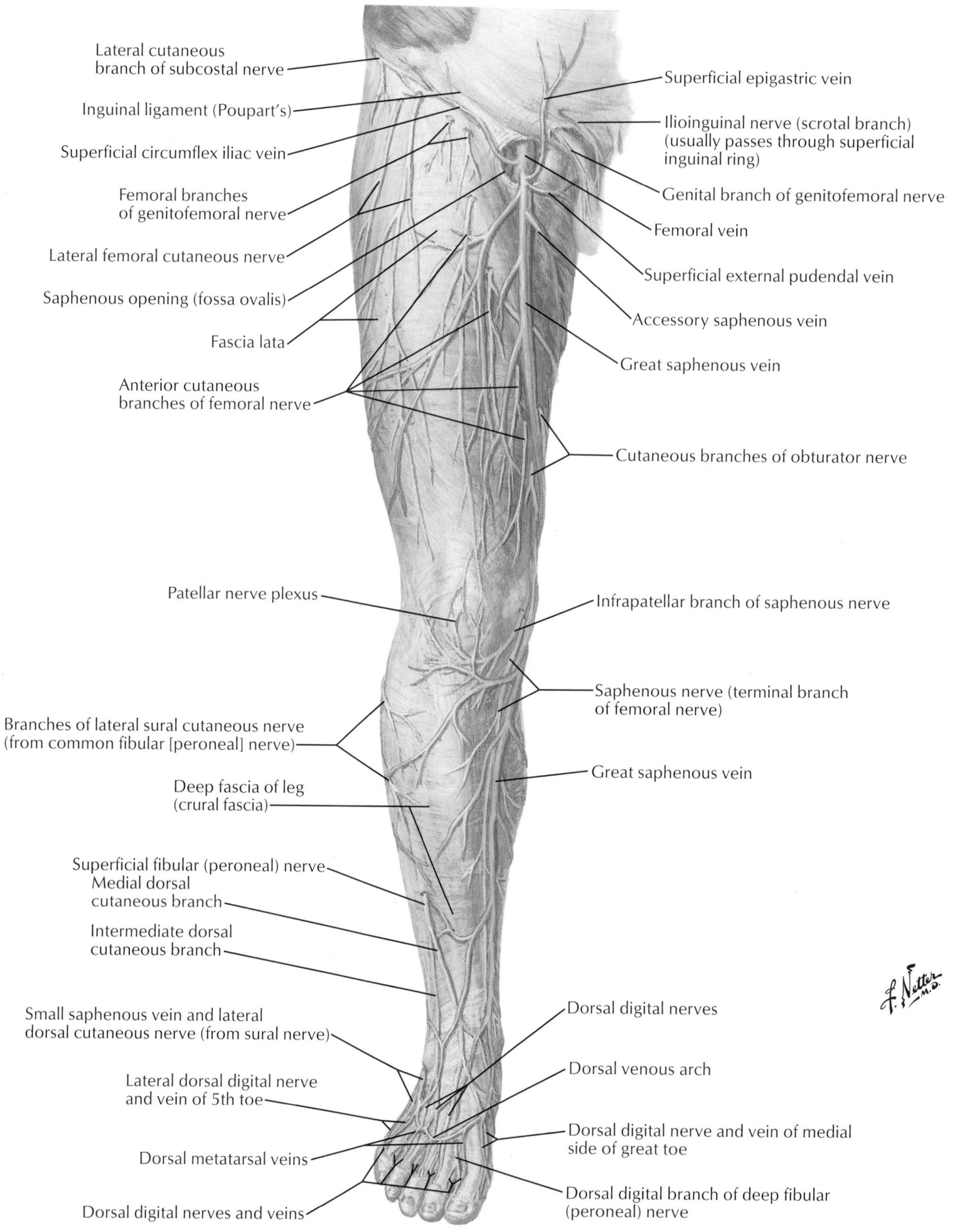
Lateral cutaneous branch of subcostal nerve
Inguinal ligament (Poupart's)
Superficial circumflex iliac vein
Femoral branches of genitofemoral nerve
Lateral femoral cutaneous nerve
Saphenous opening (fossa ovalis)
Fascia lata
Anterior cutaneous branches of femoral nerve
Superficial epigastric vein
Ilioinguinal nerve (scrotal branch) (usually passes through superficial inguinal ring)
Genital branch of genitofemoral nerve
Femoral vein
Superficial external pudendal vein
Accessory saphenous vein
Great saphenous vein
Cutaneous branches of obturator nerve
Patellar nerve plexus
Infrapatellar branch of saphenous nerve
Saphenous nerve (terminal branch of femoral nerve)
Branches of lateral sural cutaneous nerve (from common fibular [peroneal] nerve)
Great saphenous vein
Deep fascia of leg (crural fascia)
Superficial fibular (peroneal) nerve
Medial dorsal cutaneous branch
Intermediate dorsal cutaneous branch
Small saphenous vein and lateral dorsal cutaneous nerve (from sural nerve)
Lateral dorsal digital nerve and vein of 5th toe
Dorsal metatarsal veins
Dorsal digital nerves and veins
Dorsal digital nerves
Dorsal venous arch
Dorsal digital nerve and vein of medial side of great toe
Dorsal digital branch of deep fibular (peroneal) nerve
F. Netter M.D.

Plate 10 Superficial Nerves and Veins of Lower Limb: Anterior View. (Copyright 2023 Elsevier Inc. All rights reserved. www.netterimages.com. Image ID: 4846.)

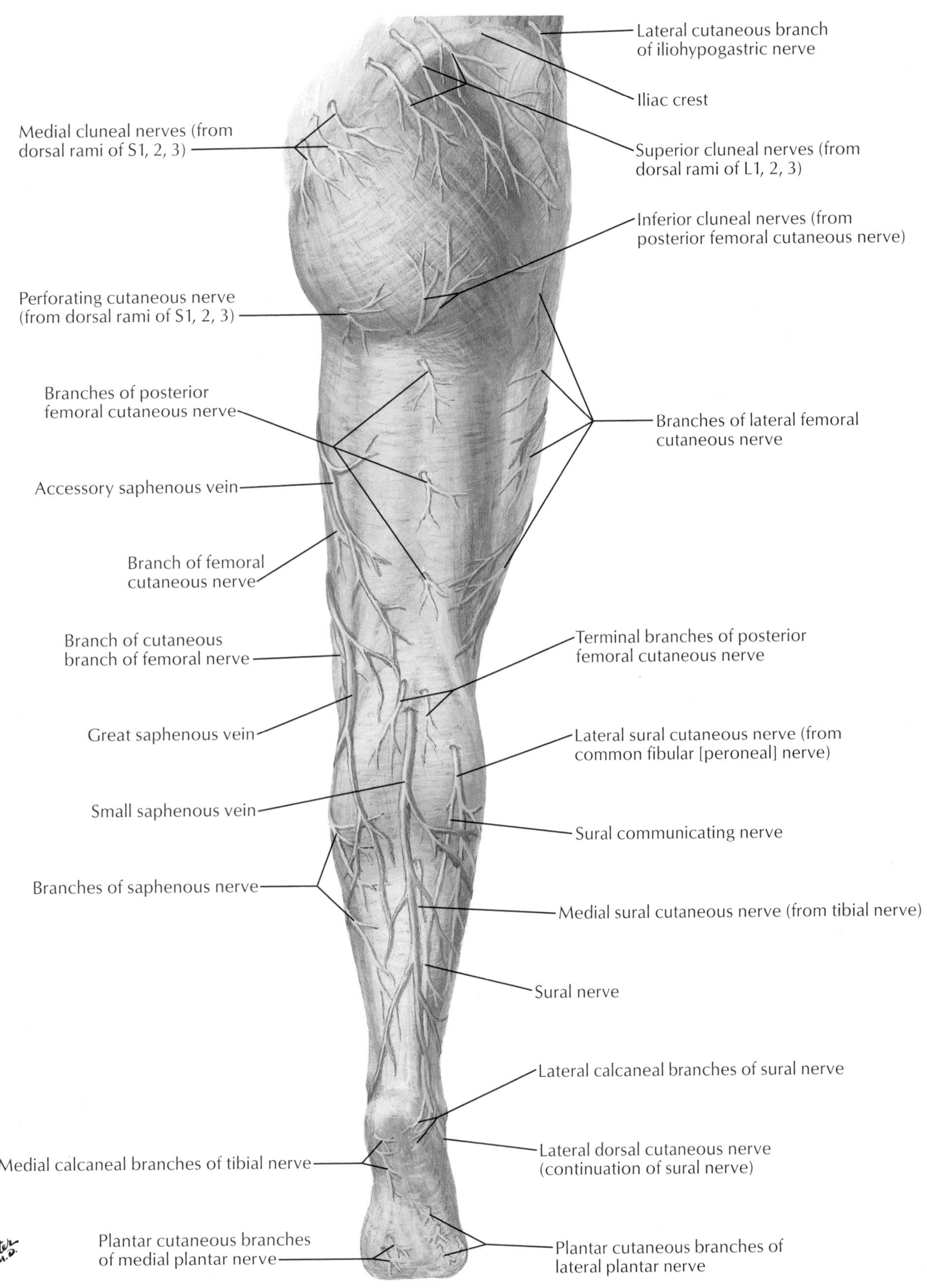
Lateral cutaneous branch of iliohypogastric nerve
Iliac crest
Medial cluneal nerves (from dorsal rami of S1, 2, 3)
Superior cluneal nerves (from dorsal rami of L1, 2, 3)
Inferior cluneal nerves (from posterior femoral cutaneous nerve)
Perforating cutaneous nerve (from dorsal rami of S1, 2, 3)
Branches of posterior femoral cutaneous nerve
Branches of lateral femoral cutaneous nerve
Accessory saphenous vein
Branch of femoral cutaneous nerve
Branch of cutaneous branch of femoral nerve
Terminal branches of posterior femoral cutaneous nerve
Great saphenous vein
Lateral sural cutaneous nerve (from common fibular [peroneal] nerve)
Small saphenous vein
Sural communicating nerve
Branches of saphenous nerve
Medial sural cutaneous nerve (from tibial nerve)
Sural nerve
Lateral calcaneal branches of sural nerve
Medial calcaneal branches of tibial nerve
Lateral dorsal cutaneous nerve (continuation of sural nerve)
Plantar cutaneous branches of medial plantar nerve
Plantar cutaneous branches of lateral plantar nerve
F. Netter M.D.

Plate 11 Superficial Nerves and Veins of Lower Limb: Posterior View. (www.netterimages.com. Image ID: 4669.)

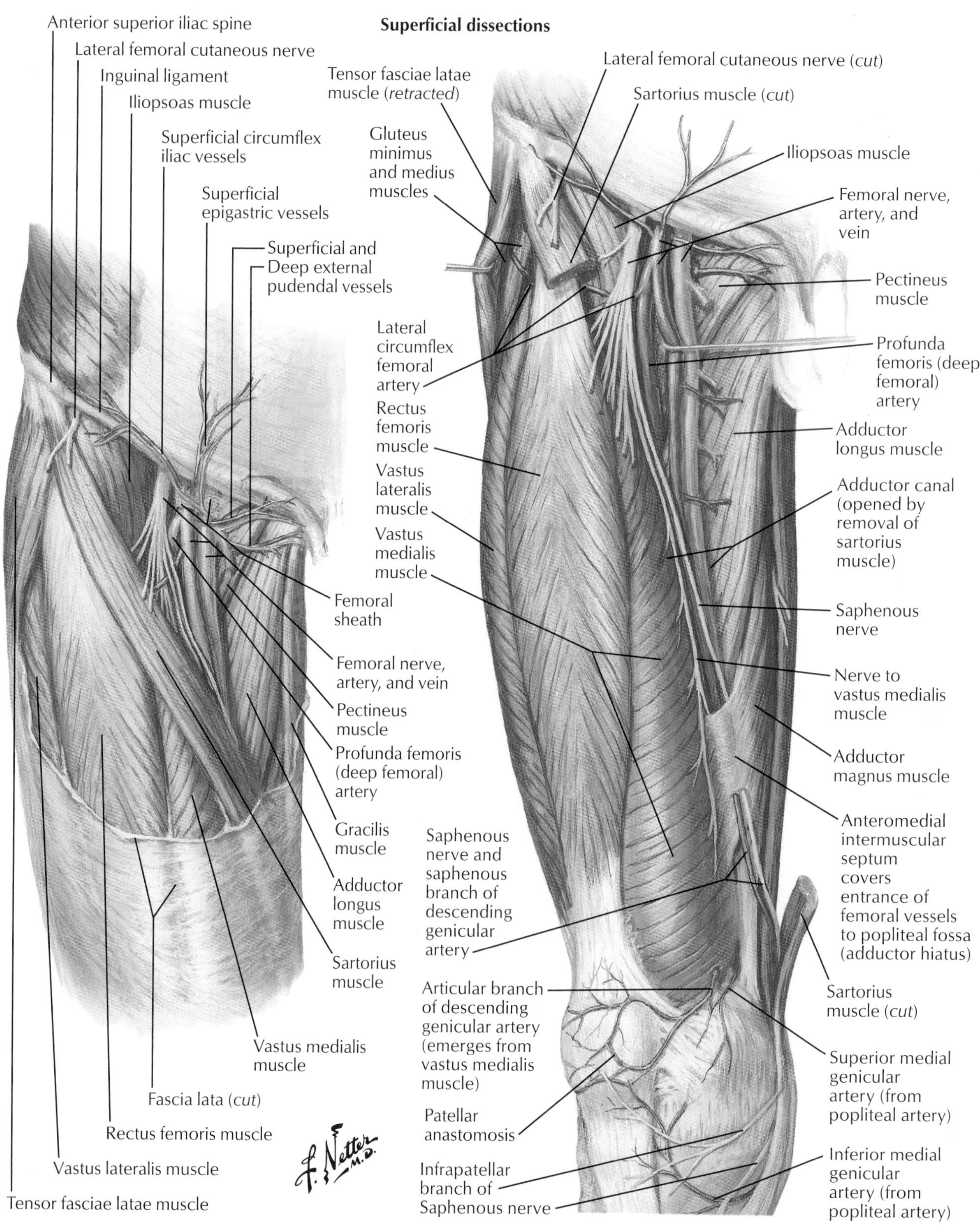
Superficial dissections
Anterior superior iliac spine
Lateral femoral cutaneous nerve
Inguinal ligament
Iliopsoas muscle
Superficial circumflex iliac vessels
Superficial epigastric vessels
Superficial and Deep external pudendal vessels
Femoral sheath
Femoral nerve, artery, and vein
Pectineus muscle
Profunda femoris (deep femoral) artery
Gracilis muscle
Adductor longus muscle
Sartorius muscle
Vastus medialis muscle
Fascia lata (cut)
Rectus femoris muscle
Vastus lateralis muscle
Tensor fasciae latae muscle
Tensor fasciae latae muscle (retracted)
Gluteus minimus and medius muscles
Lateral circumflex femoral artery
Rectus femoris muscle
Vastus lateralis muscle
Vastus medialis muscle
Saphenous nerve and saphenous branch of descending genicular artery
Articular branch of descending genicular artery (emerges from vastus medialis muscle)
Patellar anastomosis
Infrapatellar branch of Saphenous nerve
Lateral femoral cutaneous nerve (cut)
Sartorius muscle (cut)
Iliopsoas muscle
Femoral nerve, artery, and vein
Pectineus muscle
Profunda femoris (deep femoral) artery
Adductor longus muscle
Adductor canal (opened by removal of sartorius muscle)
Saphenous nerve
Nerve to vastus medialis muscle
Adductor magnus muscle
Anteromedial intermuscular septum covers entrance of femoral vessels to popliteal fossa (adductor hiatus)
Sartorius muscle (cut)
Superior medial genicular artery (from popliteal artery)
Inferior medial genicular artery (from popliteal artery)
F. Netter M.D.

Plate 12 Arteries and Nerves of Thigh: Anterior Views.

Deep dissection

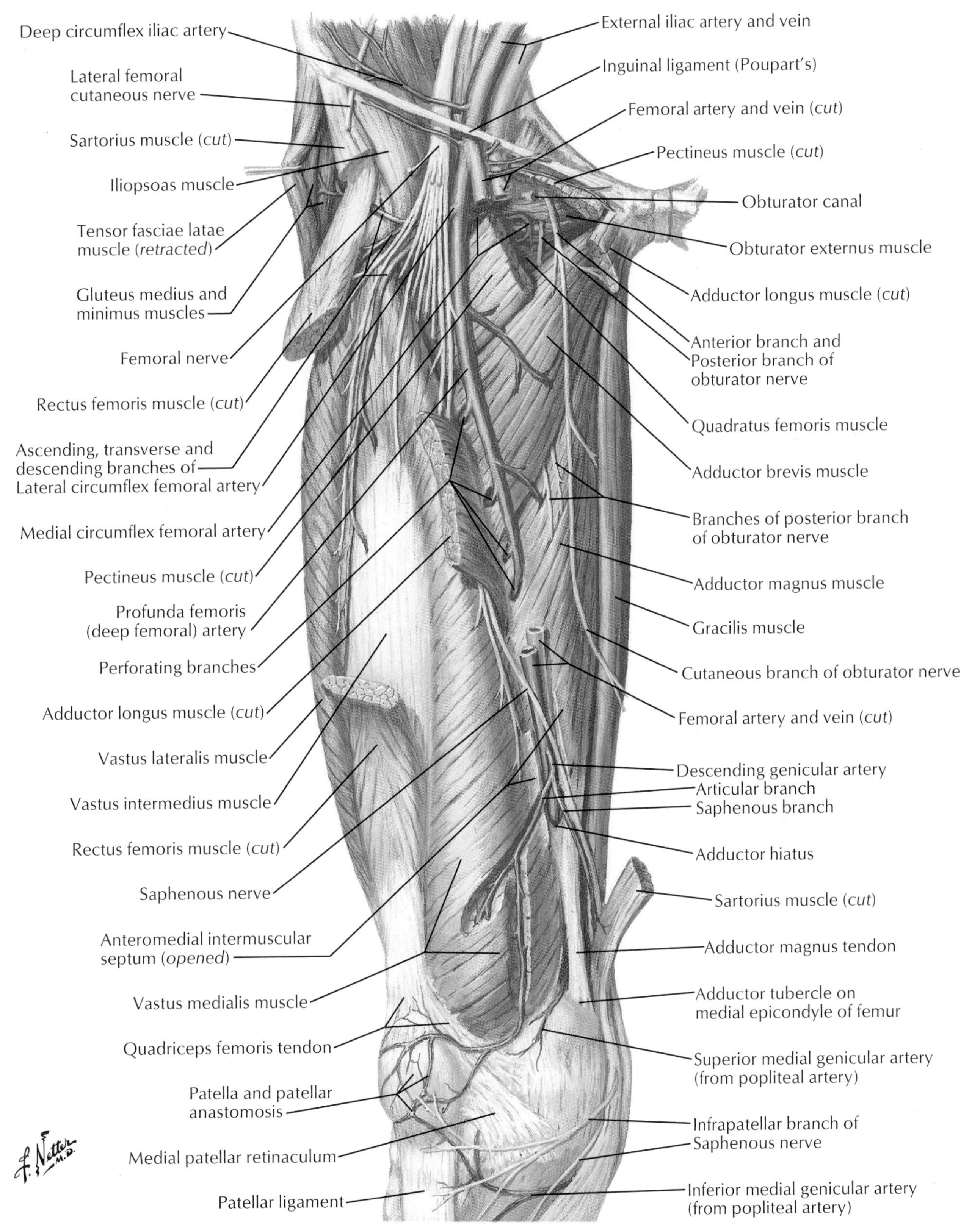

Deep circumflex iliac artery
Lateral femoral cutaneous nerve
Sartorius muscle (cut)
Iliopsoas muscle
Tensor fasciae latae muscle (retracted)
Gluteus medius and minimus muscles
Femoral nerve
Rectus femoris muscle (cut)
Ascending, transverse and descending branches of Lateral circumflex femoral artery
Medial circumflex femoral artery
Pectineus muscle (cut)
Profunda femoris (deep femoral) artery
Perforating branches
Adductor longus muscle (cut)
Vastus lateralis muscle
Vastus intermedius muscle
Rectus femoris muscle (cut)
Saphenous nerve
Anteromedial intermuscular septum (opened)
Vastus medialis muscle
Quadriceps femoris tendon
Patella and patellar anastomosis
Medial patellar retinaculum
Patellar ligament
External iliac artery and vein
Inguinal ligament (Poupart's)
Femoral artery and vein (cut)
Pectineus muscle (cut)
Obturator canal
Obturator externus muscle
Adductor longus muscle (cut)
Anterior branch and
Posterior branch of obturator nerve
Quadratus femoris muscle
Adductor brevis muscle
Branches of posterior branch of obturator nerve
Adductor magnus muscle
Gracilis muscle
Cutaneous branch of obturator nerve
Femoral artery and vein (cut)
Descending genicular artery
Articular branch
Saphenous branch
Adductor hiatus
Sartorius muscle (cut)
Adductor magnus tendon
Adductor tubercle on medial epicondyle of femur
Superior medial genicular artery (from popliteal artery)
Infrapatellar branch of Saphenous nerve
Inferior medial genicular artery (from popliteal artery)
F. Netter M.D.

Plate 13 Arteries and Nerves of Thigh: Posterior View. (Copyright 2023 Elsevier Inc. All rights reserved. www.netterimages.com. Image ID: 49316.)

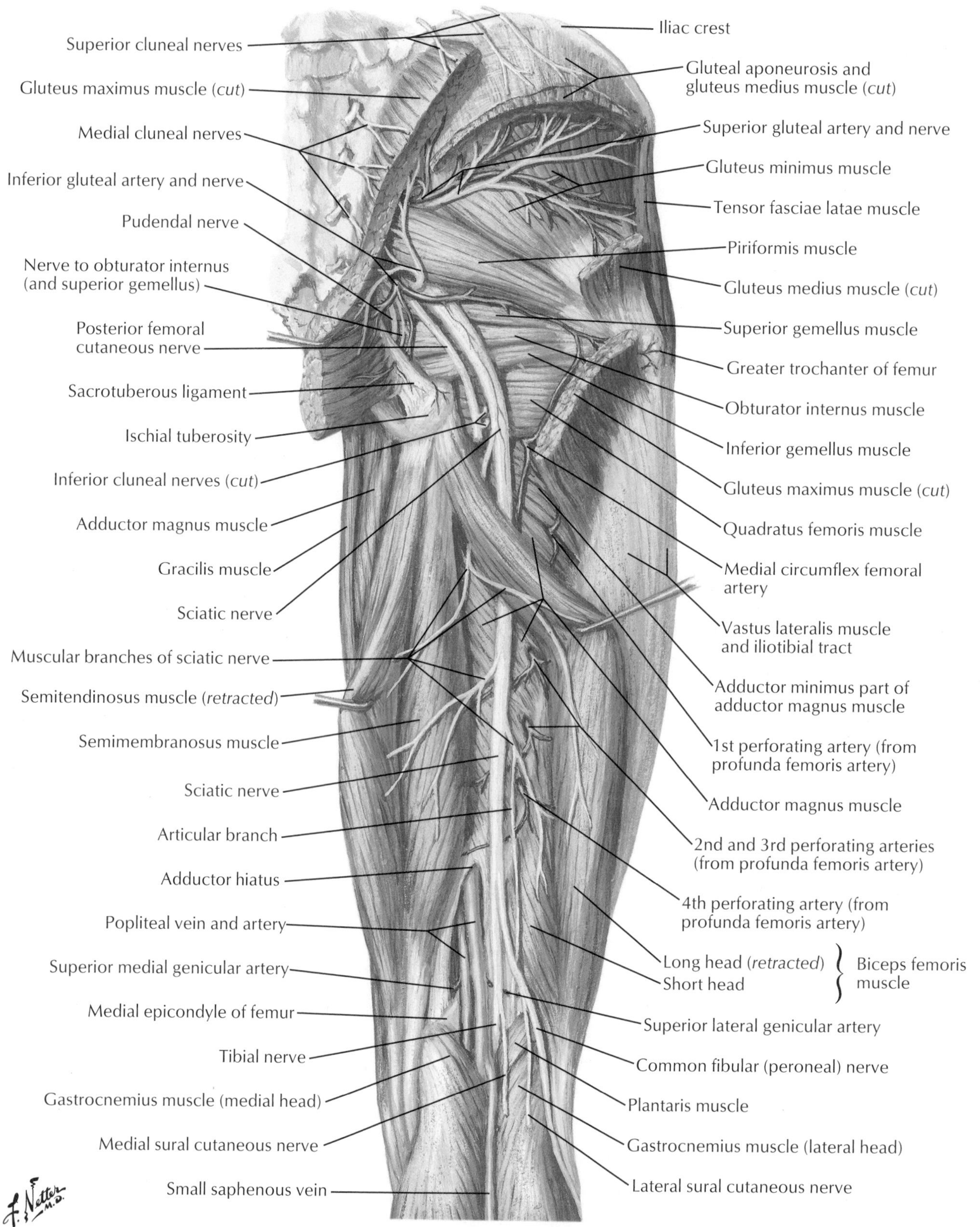
Deep dissection
Superior cluneal nerves
Gluteus maximus muscle (*cut*)
Medial cluneal nerves
Inferior gluteal artery and nerve
Pudendal nerve
Nerve to obturator internus (and superior gemellus)
Posterior femoral cutaneous nerve
Sacrotuberous ligament
Ischial tuberosity
Inferior cluneal nerves (*cut*)
Adductor magnus muscle
Gracilis muscle
Sciatic nerve
Muscular branches of sciatic nerve
Semitendinosus muscle (*retracted*)
Semimembranosus muscle
Sciatic nerve
Articular branch
Adductor hiatus
Popliteal vein and artery
Superior medial genicular artery
Medial epicondyle of femur
Tibial nerve
Gastrocnemius muscle (medial head)
Medial sural cutaneous nerve
Small saphenous vein
Iliac crest
Gluteal aponeurosis and gluteus medius muscle (*cut*)
Superior gluteal artery and nerve
Gluteus minimus muscle
Tensor fasciae latae muscle
Piriformis muscle
Gluteus medius muscle (*cut*)
Superior gemellus muscle
Greater trochanter of femur
Obturator internus muscle
Inferior gemellus muscle
Gluteus maximus muscle (*cut*)
Quadratus femoris muscle
Medial circumflex femoral artery
Vastus lateralis muscle and iliotibial tract
Adductor minimus part of adductor magnus muscle
1st perforating artery (from profunda femoris artery)
Adductor magnus muscle
2nd and 3rd perforating arteries (from profunda femoris artery)
4th perforating artery (from profunda femoris artery)
Long head (*retracted*)
Short head
Biceps femoris muscle
Superior lateral genicular artery
Common fibular (peroneal) nerve
Plantaris muscle
Gastrocnemius muscle (lateral head)
Lateral sural cutaneous nerve
F. Netter M.D.

Plate 14 Arteries and Nerves of Thigh: Posterior View.

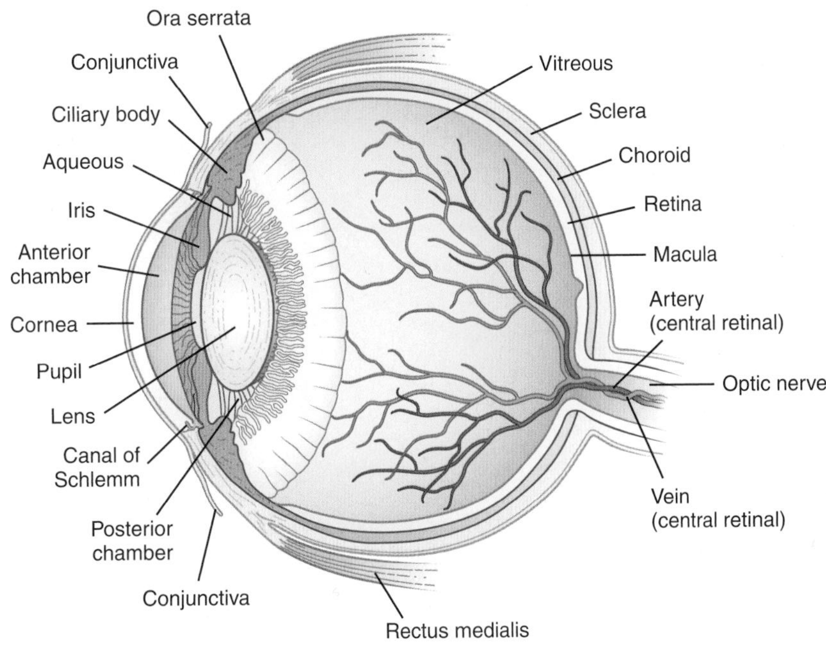
Ora serrata
Conjunctiva
Ciliary body
Aqueous
Iris
Anterior
chamber
Cornea
Pupil
Lens
Canal of
Schlemm
Posterior
chamber
Conjunctiva
Rectus medialis
Vitreous
Sclera
Choroid
Retina
Macula
Artery
(central retinal)
Optic nerve
Vein
(central retinal)

Plate 15 Anatomy of the eye. (Dehn RW, Asprey DP: Essential Clinical Procedures, ed 3, Philadelphia, 2013, Saunders.)

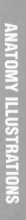

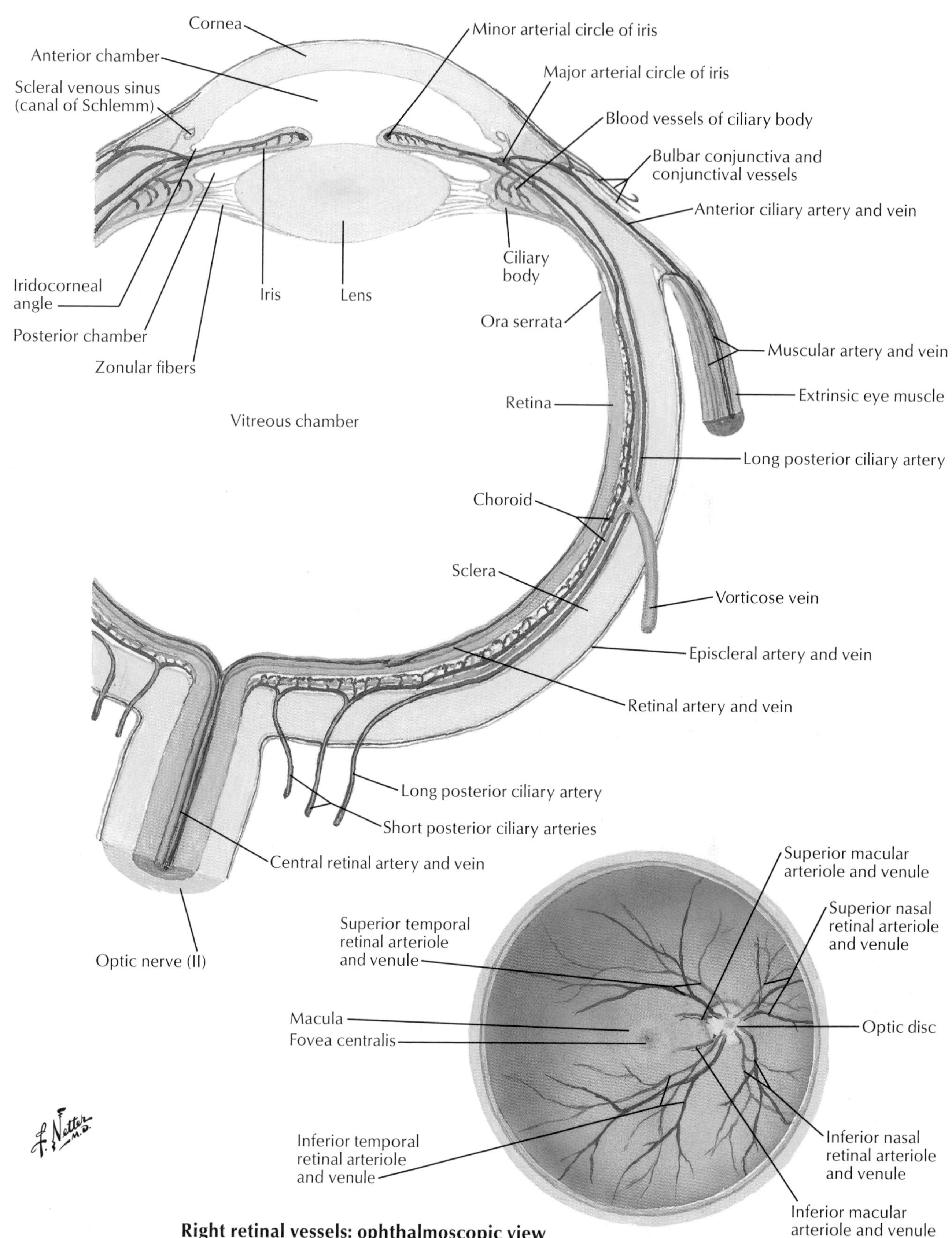

Right retinal vessels: ophthalmoscopic view

Plate 16 Intrinsic Arteries and Veins of Eye.

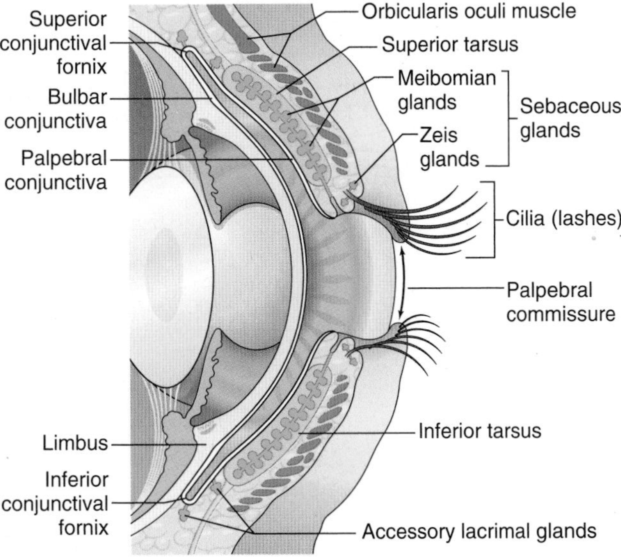
Superior conjunctival fornix
Bulbar conjunctiva
Palpebral conjunctiva
Limbus
Inferior conjunctival fornix
Orbicularis oculi muscle
Superior tarsus
Meibomian glands
Zeis glands
Sebaceous glands
Cilia (lashes)
Palpebral commissure
Inferior tarsus
Accessory lacrimal glands

Plate 17 Anatomy of the conjunctiva and eyelids. (Kumar V, Abbas AK, Aster JC: Robbins and Cotran Pathologic Basis of Disease, ed 9, Philadelphia, 2015, Saunders.)

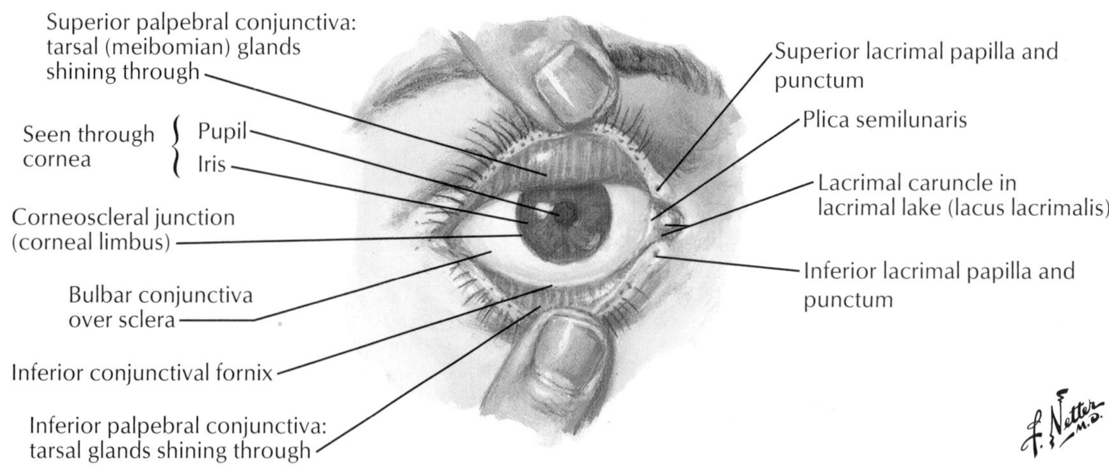
Superior palpebral conjunctiva: tarsal (meibomian) glands shining through
Seen through cornea
Pupil
Iris
Corneoscleral junction (corneal limbus)
Bulbar conjunctiva over sclera
Inferior conjunctival fornix
Inferior palpebral conjunctiva: tarsal glands shining through
Superior lacrimal papilla and punctum
Plica semilunaris
Lacrimal caruncle in lacrimal lake (lacus lacrimalis)
Inferior lacrimal papilla and punctum
F. Netter M.D.

Plate 18 Eyelid.

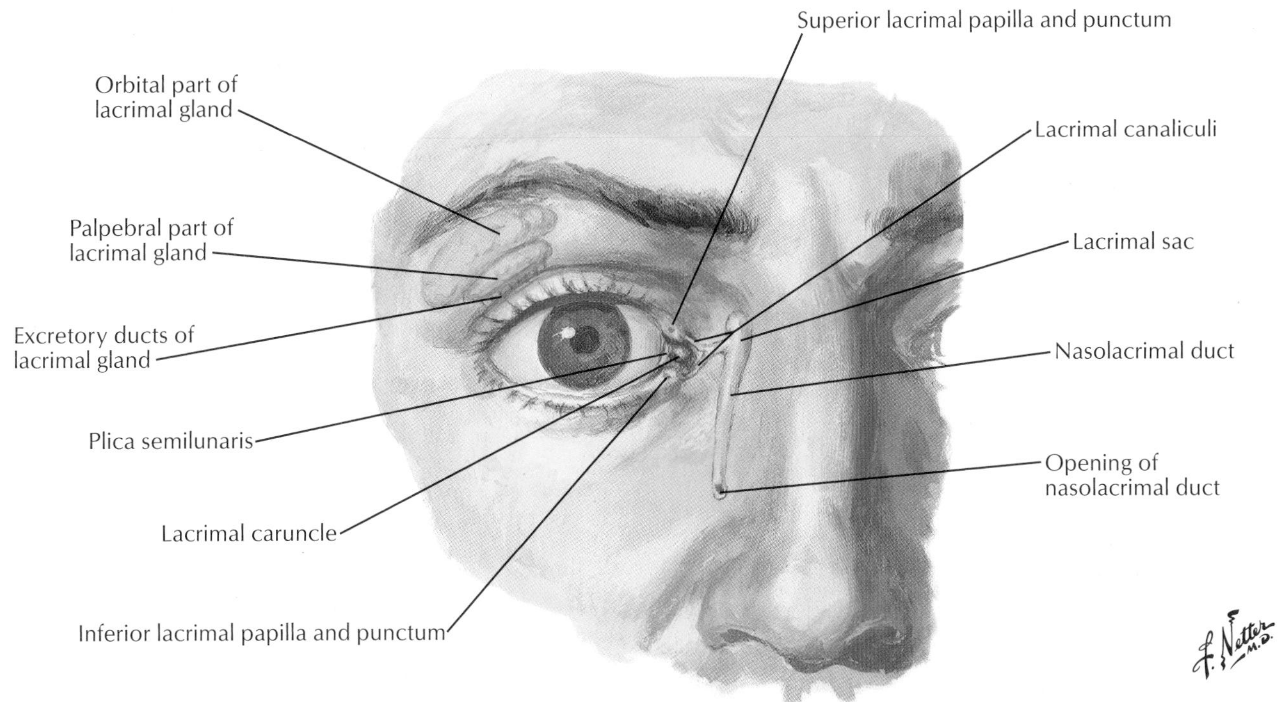
Superior lacrimal papilla and punctum
Orbital part of lacrimal gland
Lacrimal canaliculi
Palpebral part of lacrimal gland
Lacrimal sac
Excretory ducts of lacrimal gland
Nasolacrimal duct
Plica semilunaris
Opening of nasolacrimal duct
Lacrimal caruncle
Inferior lacrimal papilla and punctum
F. Netter M.D.

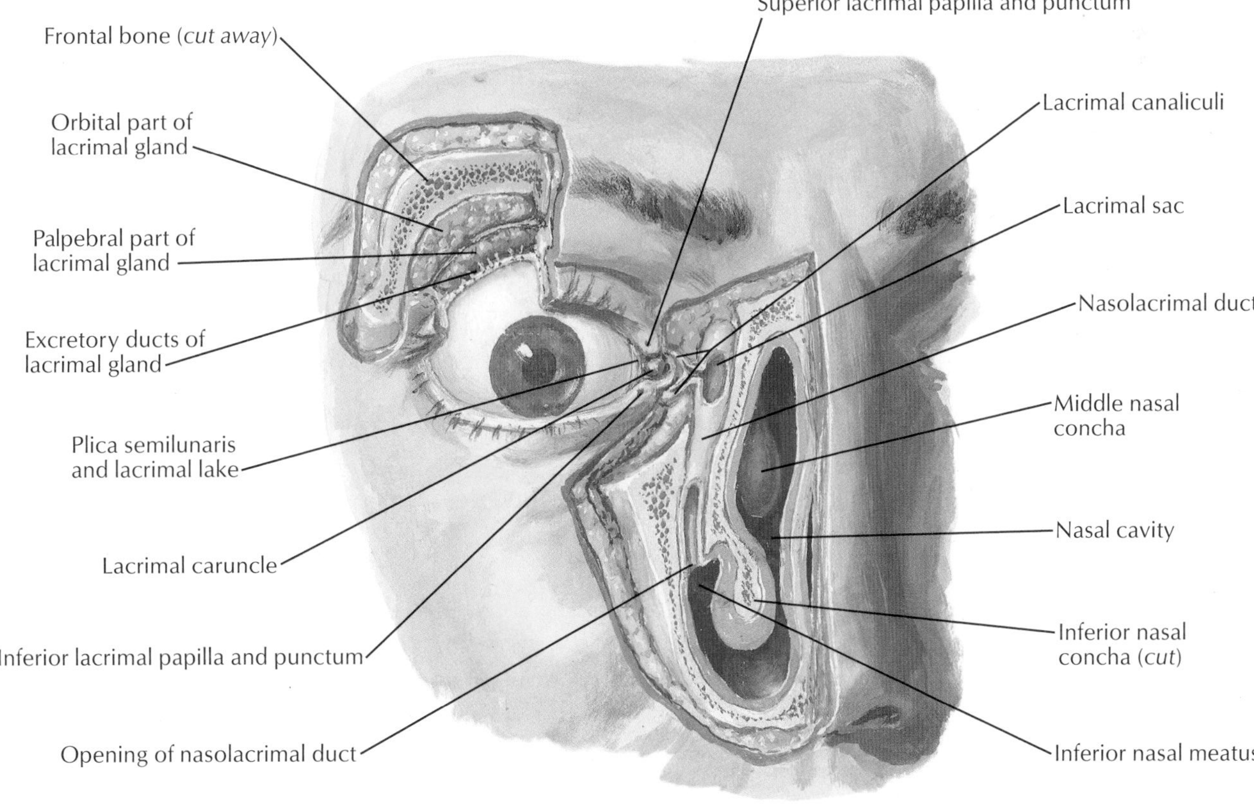
Superior lacrimal papilla and punctum
Frontal bone (*cut away*)
Lacrimal canaliculi
Orbital part of lacrimal gland
Lacrimal sac
Palpebral part of lacrimal gland
Nasolacrimal duct
Excretory ducts of lacrimal gland
Middle nasal concha
Plica semilunaris and lacrimal lake
Nasal cavity
Lacrimal caruncle
Inferior nasal concha (*cut*)
Inferior lacrimal papilla and punctum
Opening of nasolacrimal duct
Inferior nasal meatus

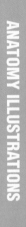

ANATOMY ILLUSTRATIONS

Plate 19 Lacrimal Apparatus.

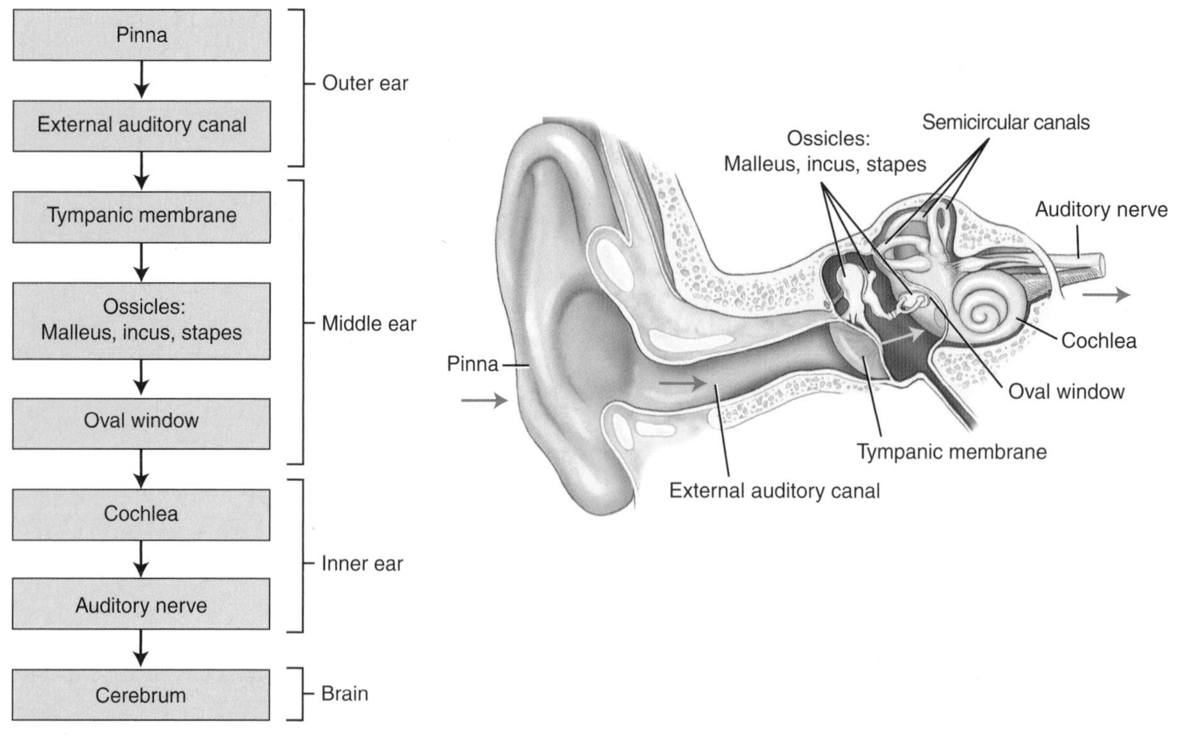

Plate 20 Pathway of Sound. (LaFleur Brooks D, LaFleur Brooks M: Basic Medical Language, ed 4, St. Louis, 2013, Mosby.)

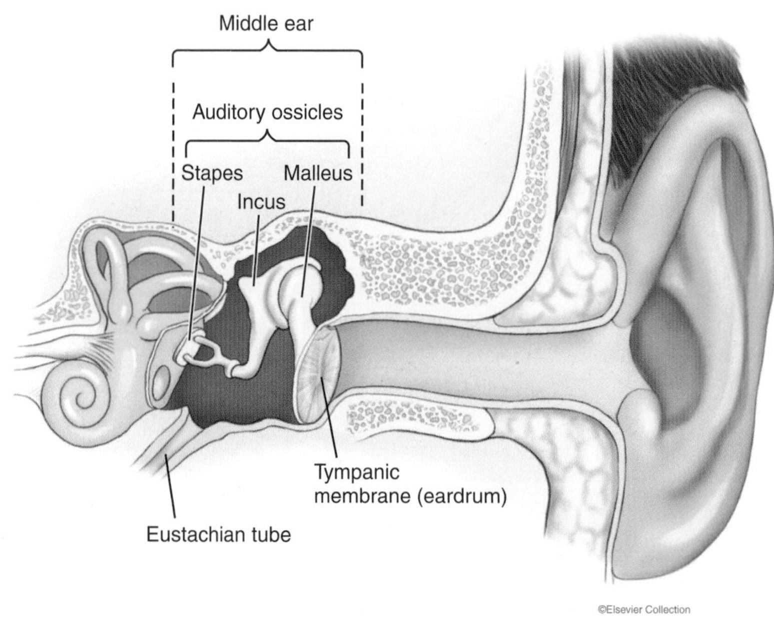

Plate 21 Middle ear structures. (©Elsevier Collection.)

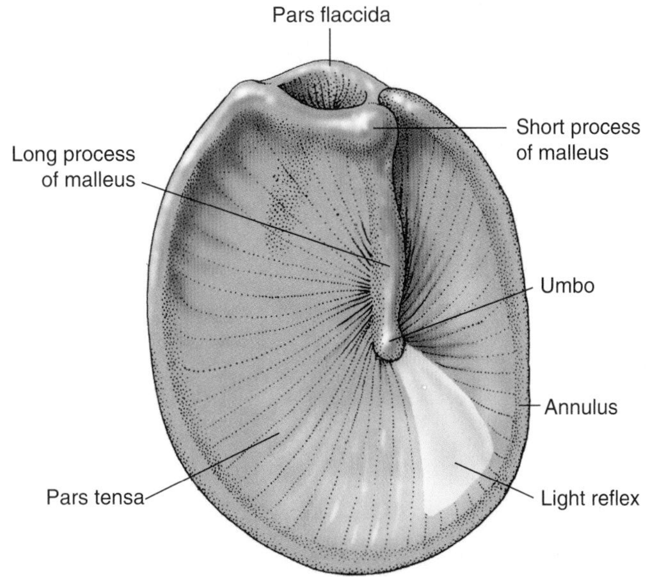
RIGHT TYMPANIC MEMBRANE
Pars flaccida
Short process of malleus
Long process of malleus
Umbo
Annulus
Pars tensa
Light reflex

Plate 22 Structural landmarks of tympanic membrane. (Ignatavicius DD, Workman ML: Medical-Surgical Nursing: Patient-Centered Collaborative Care, ed 7, St. Louis, 2013, Saunders.)

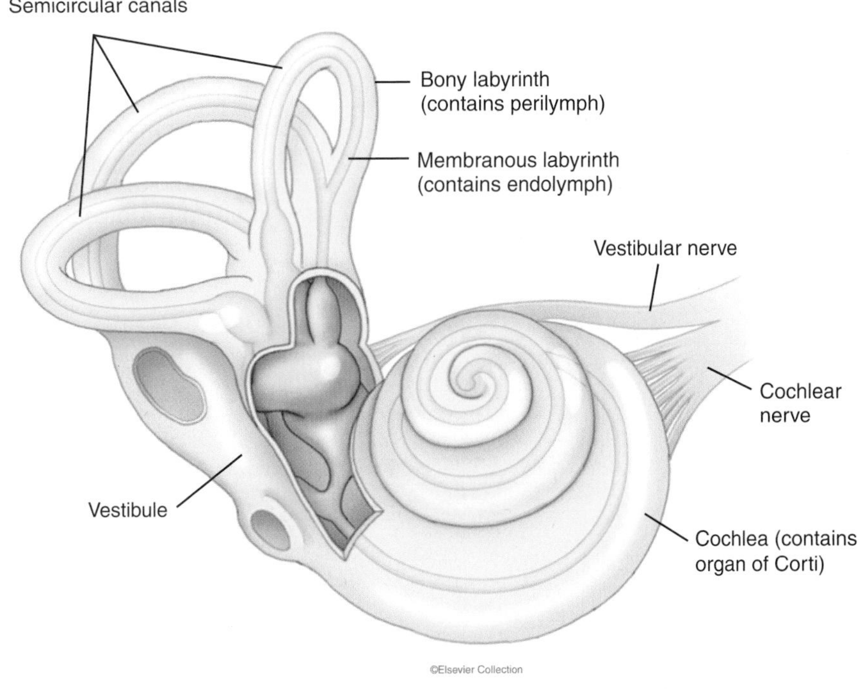
Semicircular canals
Bony labyrinth (contains perilymph)
Membranous labyrinth (contains endolymph)
Vestibular nerve
Cochlear nerve
Vestibule
Cochlea (contains organ of Corti)
©Elsevier Collection

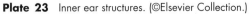

Plate 23 Inner ear structures. (©Elsevier Collection.)

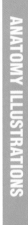

ANATOMY ILLUSTRATIONS

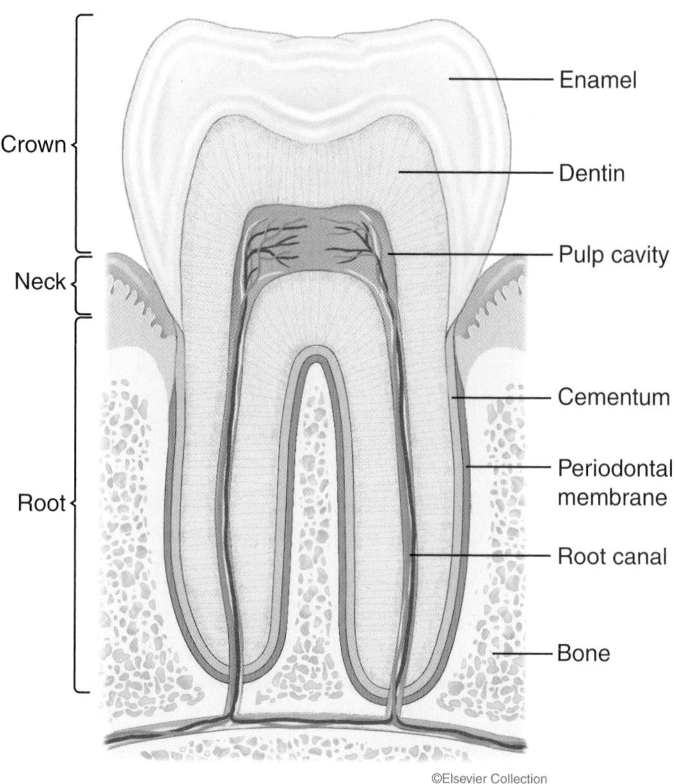
Crown
Neck
Root
Enamel
Dentin
Pulp cavity
Cementum
Periodontal membrane
Root canal
Bone
©Elsevier Collection

Plate 24 The Tooth. (©Elsevier Collection).

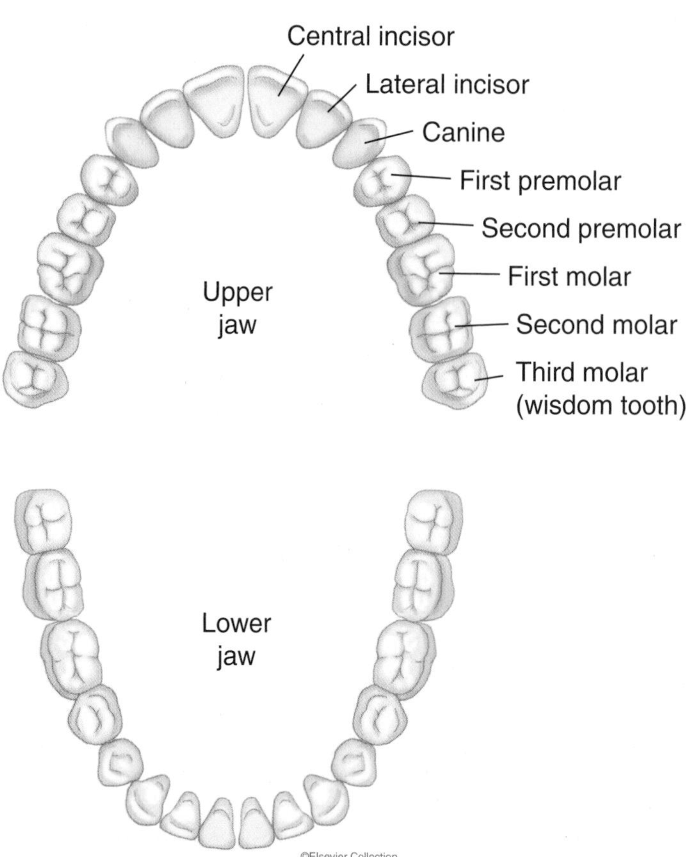
Central incisor
Lateral incisor
Canine
First premolar
Second premolar
First molar
Second molar
Third molar (wisdom tooth)
Upper jaw
Lower jaw
©Elsevier Collection

Plate 25 Adult Teeth. (©Elsevier Collection).

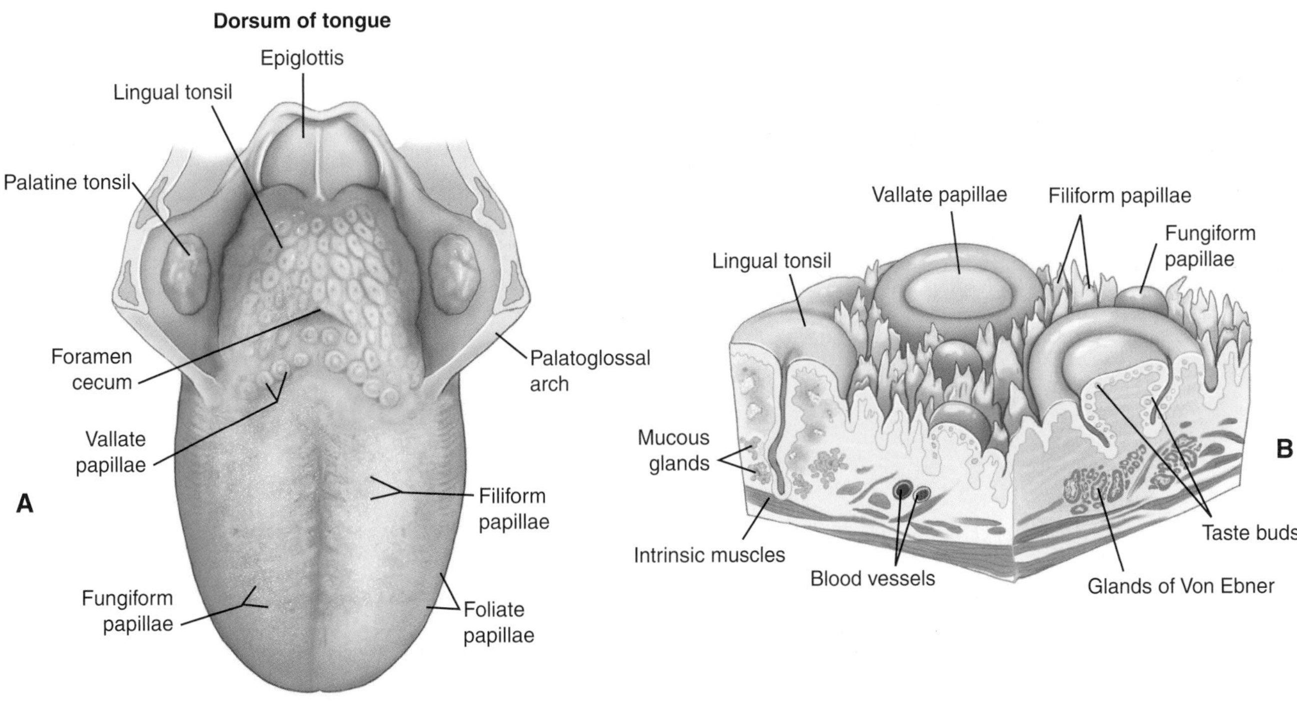
Dorsum of tongue
Epiglottis
Lingual tonsil
Palatine tonsil
Foramen cecum
Palatoglossal arch
Vallate papillae
A
Filiform papillae
Fungiform papillae
Foliate papillae
Vallate papillae
Filiform papillae
Fungiform papillae
Lingual tonsil
Mucous glands
B
Intrinsic muscles
Blood vessels
Taste buds
Glands of Von Ebner
© Elsevier Collection

Plate 26 A, Dorsal view of tongue showing the roughened large lingual tonsils on the posterior of the tongue and the foliate papillae on the side. B, Section of dorsal of the tongue showing a cutaway through lingual papillae and showing von Ebner's glands at the base of the vallate papilla. (Brand RW, Isselhard DE: Anatomy of Orofacial Structures: A Comprehensive Approach, ed 8, St. Louis, 2019, Elsevier.)

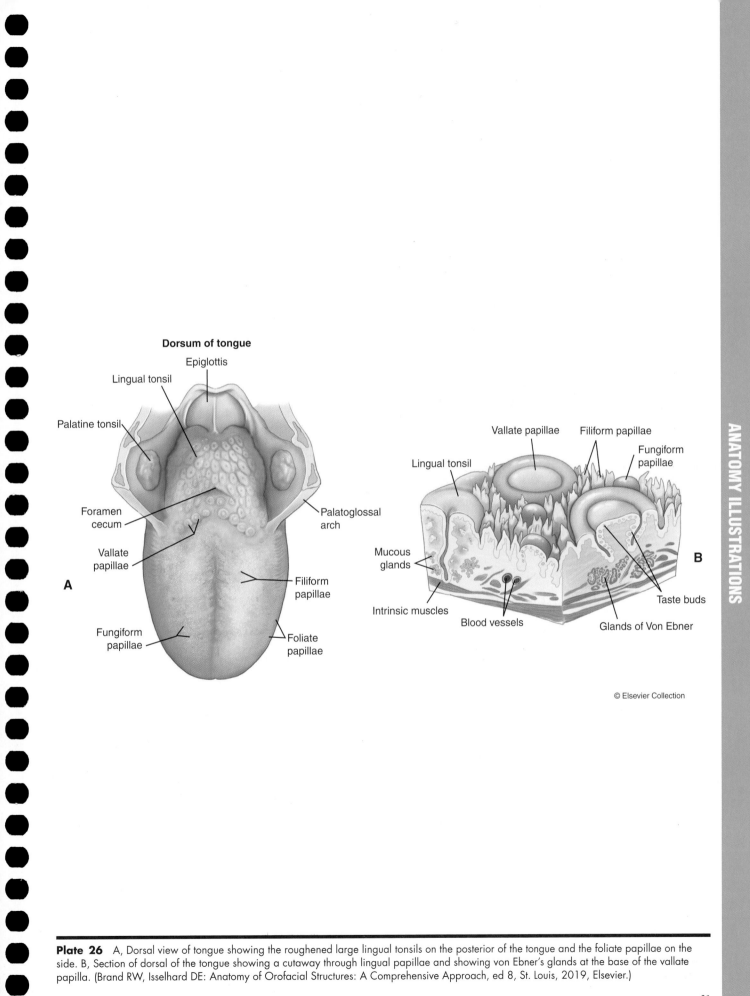

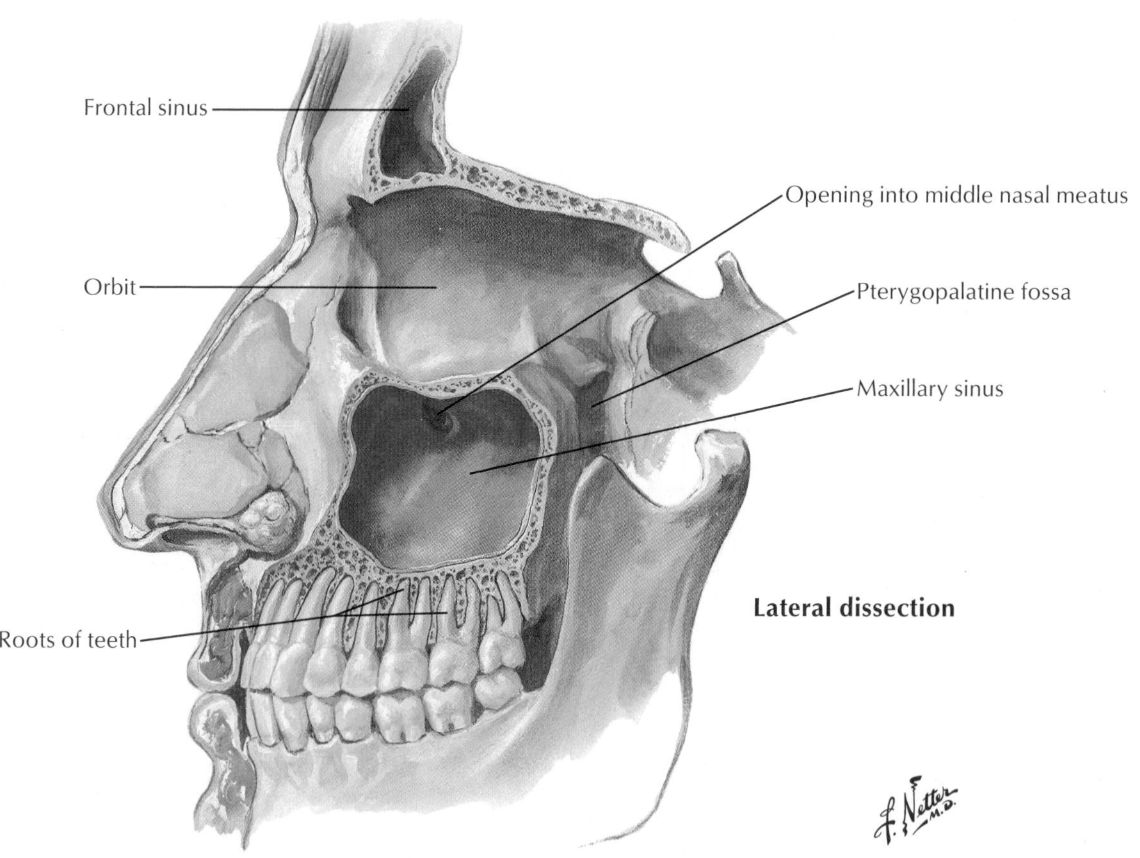
Frontal sinus
Opening into middle nasal meatus
Orbit
Pterygopalatine fossa
Maxillary sinus
Lateral dissection
Roots of teeth

Plate 27 Paranasal Sinuses.

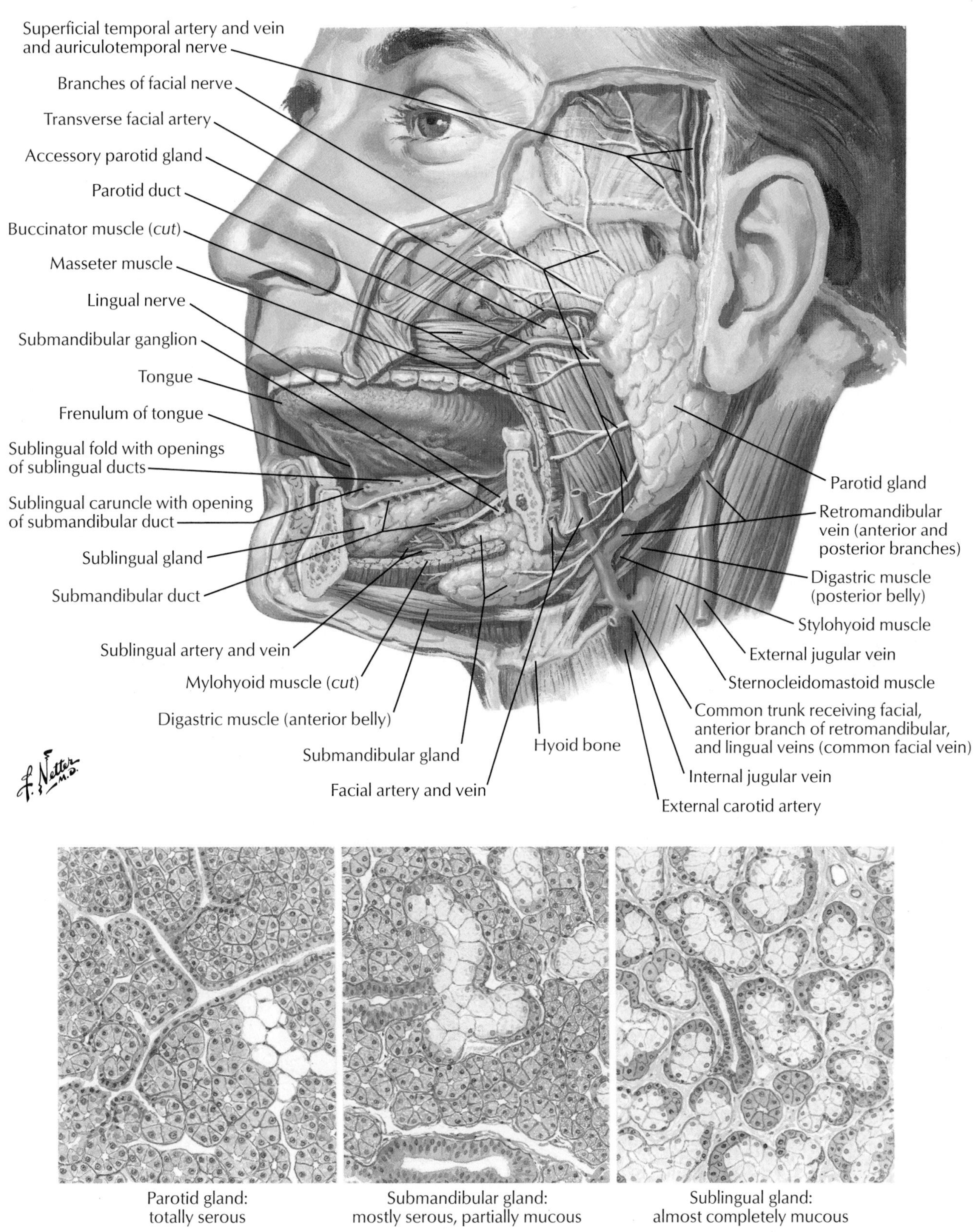
Superficial temporal artery and vein and auriculotemporal nerve
Branches of facial nerve
Transverse facial artery
Accessory parotid gland
Parotid duct
Buccinator muscle (cut)
Masseter muscle
Lingual nerve
Submandibular ganglion
Tongue
Frenulum of tongue
Sublingual fold with openings of sublingual ducts
Sublingual caruncle with opening of submandibular duct
Sublingual gland
Submandibular duct
Sublingual artery and vein
Mylohyoid muscle (cut)
Digastric muscle (anterior belly)
Submandibular gland
Facial artery and vein
Hyoid bone
Parotid gland
Retromandibular vein (anterior and posterior branches)
Digastric muscle (posterior belly)
Stylohyoid muscle
External jugular vein
Sternocleidomastoid muscle
Common trunk receiving facial, anterior branch of retromandibular, and lingual veins (common facial vein)
Internal jugular vein
External carotid artery
F. Netter M.D.
Parotid gland: totally serous
Submandibular gland: mostly serous, partially mucous
Sublingual gland: almost completely mucous

Plate 28 Salivary Glands. (Copyright 2023 Elsevier Inc. All rights reserved. www.netterimages.com. Image ID: 4396.)

Coronary Arteries: Arteriographic Views

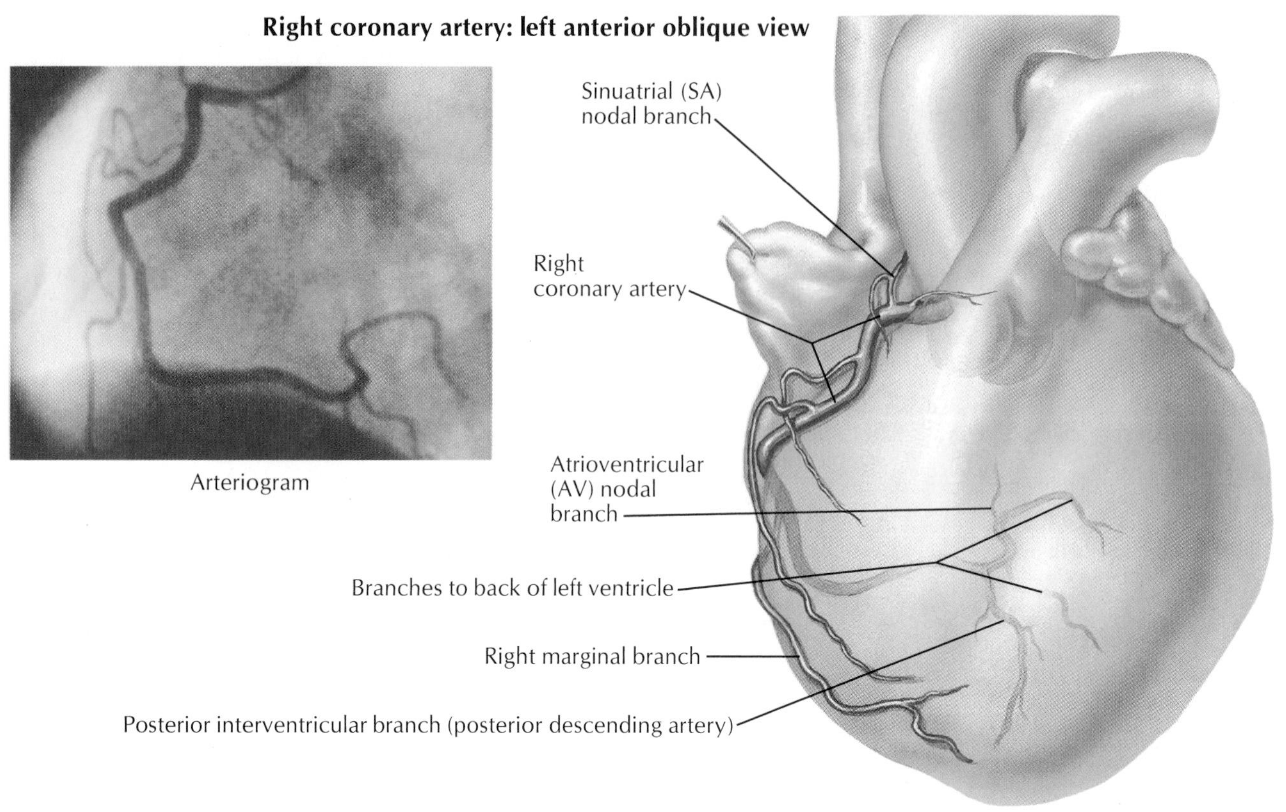
Right coronary artery: left anterior oblique view
Sinuatrial (SA) nodal branch
Right coronary artery
Atrioventricular (AV) nodal branch
Branches to back of left ventricle
Right marginal branch
Posterior interventricular branch (posterior descending artery)
Arteriogram

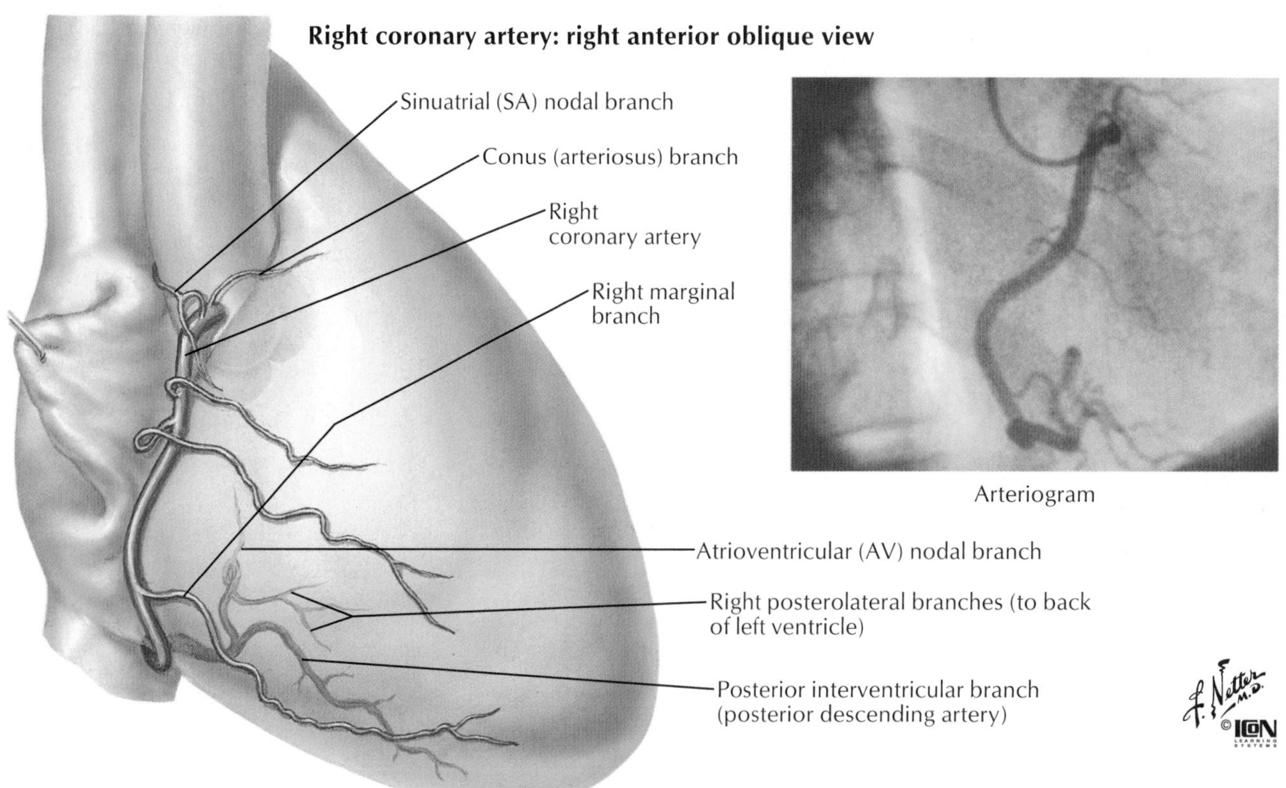
Right coronary artery: right anterior oblique view
Sinuatrial (SA) nodal branch
Conus (arteriosus) branch
Right coronary artery
Right marginal branch
Atrioventricular (AV) nodal branch
Right posterolateral branches (to back of left ventricle)
Posterior interventricular branch (posterior descending artery)
Arteriogram
F. Netter M.D.
©ICON LEARNING SYSTEMS

Plate 29 Coronary Arteries: Arteriographic Views. (www.netterimages.com. Image ID: 4725.)

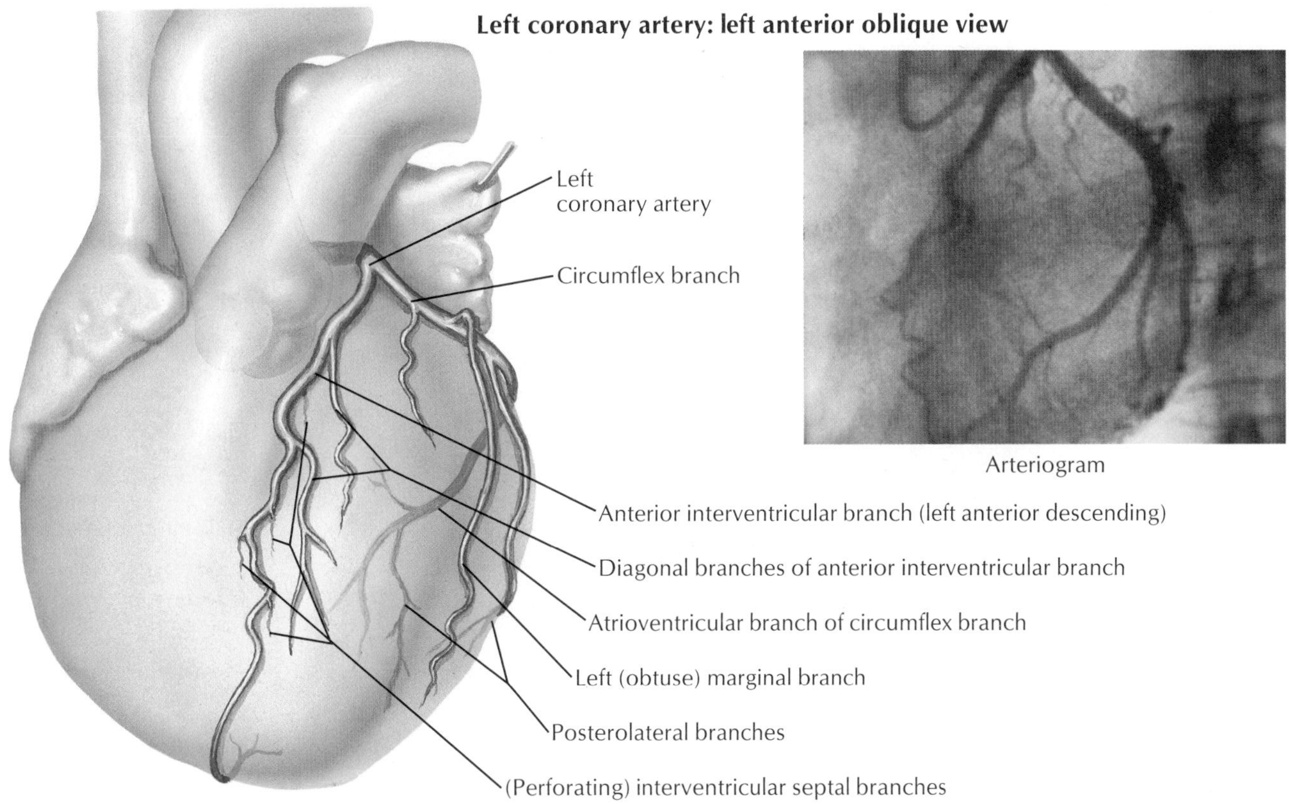
Left coronary artery: left anterior oblique view
Left
coronary artery
Circumflex branch
Arteriogram
Anterior interventricular branch (left anterior descending)
Diagonal branches of anterior interventricular branch
Atrioventricular branch of circumflex branch
Left (obtuse) marginal branch
Posterolateral branches
(Perforating) interventricular septal branches

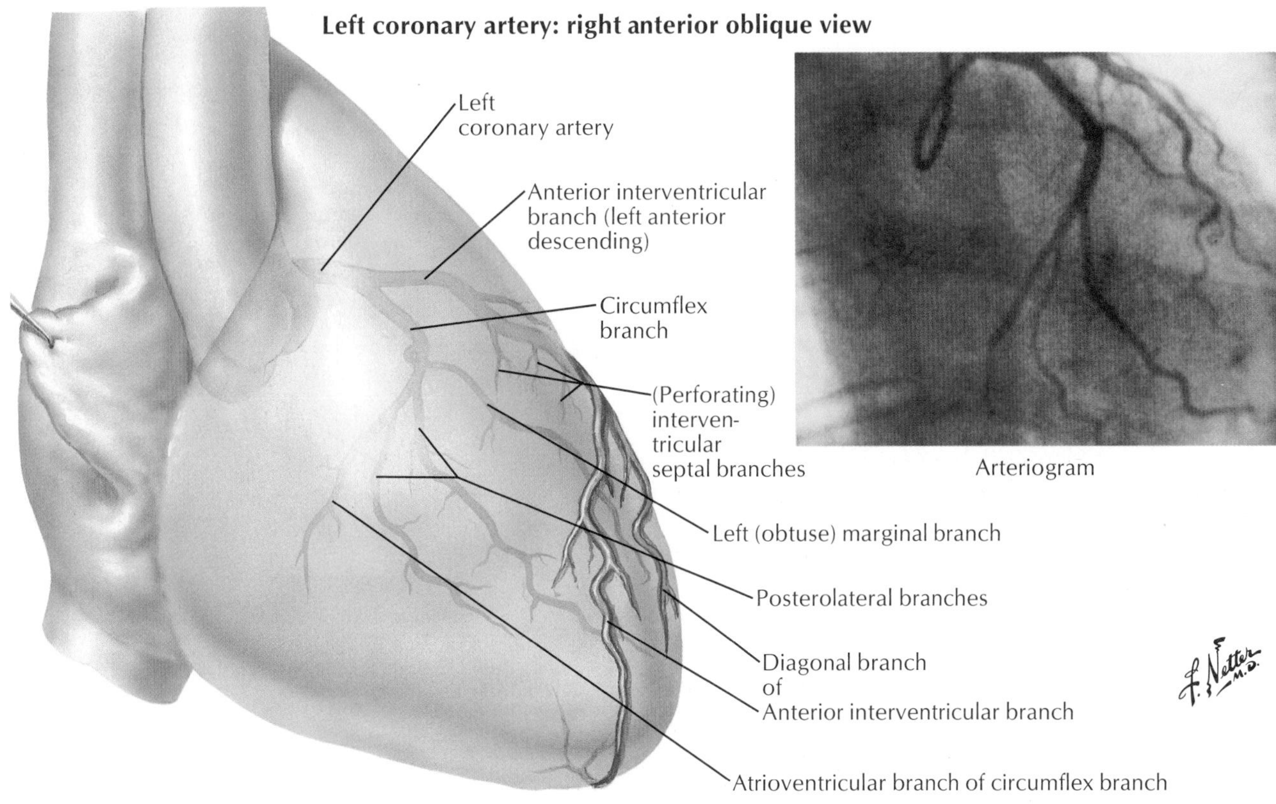
Left coronary artery: right anterior oblique view
Left
coronary artery
Anterior interventricular
branch (left anterior
descending)
Circumflex
branch
(Perforating)
interven-
tricular
septal branches
Arteriogram
Left (obtuse) marginal branch
Posterolateral branches
Diagonal branch
of
Anterior interventricular branch
Atrioventricular branch of circumflex branch

ANATOMY ILLUSTRATIONS

Plate 30 Coronary Arteries: Arteriographic Views.

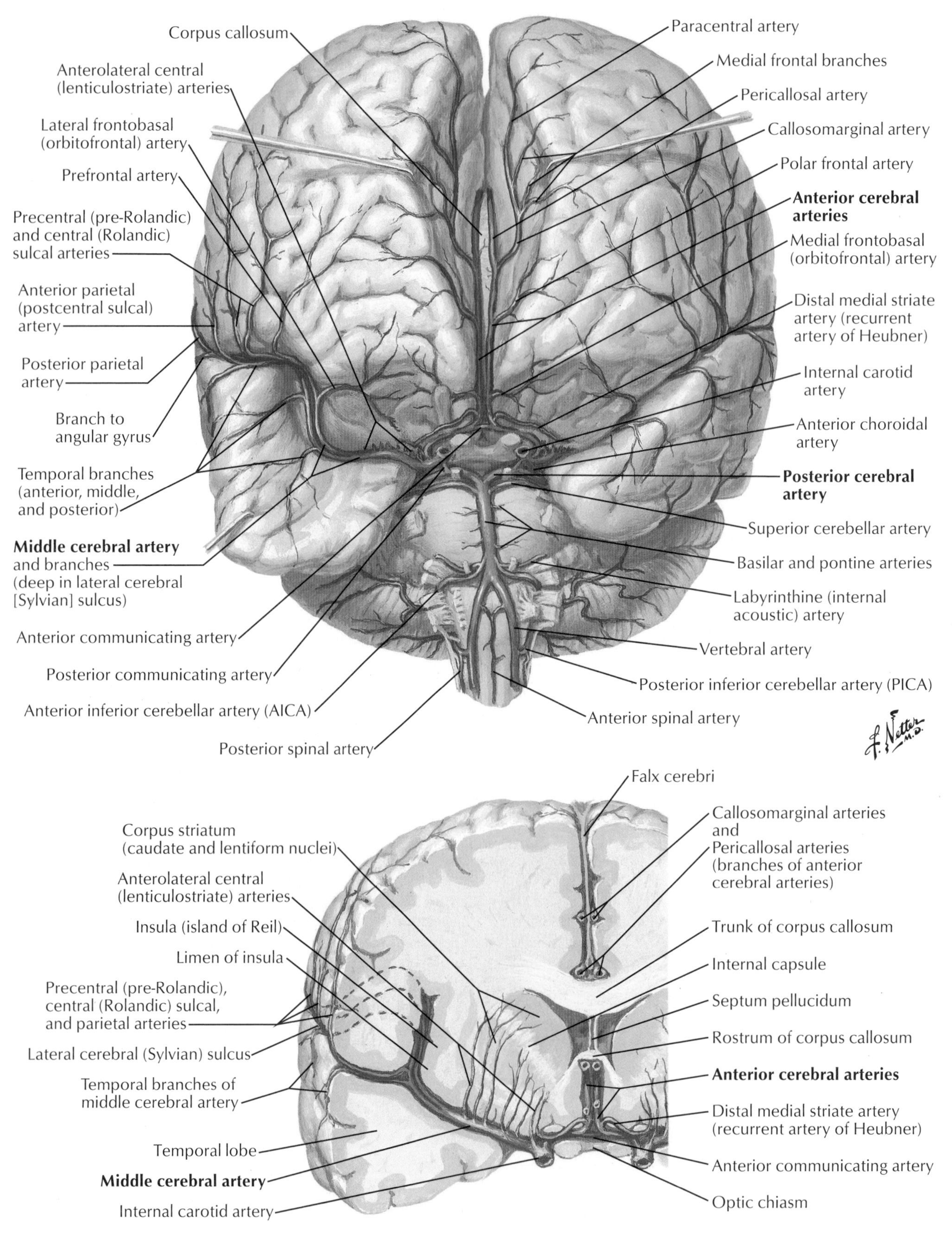
Corpus callosum
Anterolateral central (lenticulostriate) arteries
Lateral frontobasal (orbitofrontal) artery
Prefrontal artery
Precentral (pre-Rolandic) and central (Rolandic) sulcal arteries
Anterior parietal (postcentral sulcal) artery
Posterior parietal artery
Branch to angular gyrus
Temporal branches (anterior, middle, and posterior)
Middle cerebral artery and branches (deep in lateral cerebral [Sylvian] sulcus)
Anterior communicating artery
Posterior communicating artery
Anterior inferior cerebellar artery (AICA)
Posterior spinal artery
Paracentral artery
Medial frontal branches
Pericallosal artery
Callosomarginal artery
Polar frontal artery
Anterior cerebral arteries
Medial frontobasal (orbitofrontal) artery
Distal medial striate artery (recurrent artery of Heubner)
Internal carotid artery
Anterior choroidal artery
Posterior cerebral artery
Superior cerebellar artery
Basilar and pontine arteries
Labyrinthine (internal acoustic) artery
Vertebral artery
Posterior inferior cerebellar artery (PICA)
Anterior spinal artery
F. Netter M.D.
Falx cerebri
Corpus striatum (caudate and lentiform nuclei)
Anterolateral central (lenticulostriate) arteries
Insula (island of Reil)
Limen of insula
Precentral (pre-Rolandic), central (Rolandic) sulcal, and parietal arteries
Lateral cerebral (Sylvian) sulcus
Temporal branches of middle cerebral artery
Temporal lobe
Middle cerebral artery
Internal carotid artery
Callosomarginal arteries and Pericallosal arteries (branches of anterior cerebral arteries)
Trunk of corpus callosum
Internal capsule
Septum pellucidum
Rostrum of corpus callosum
Anterior cerebral arteries
Distal medial striate artery (recurrent artery of Heubner)
Anterior communicating artery
Optic chiasm

Plate 31 Arteries of Brain: Frontal View and Section.

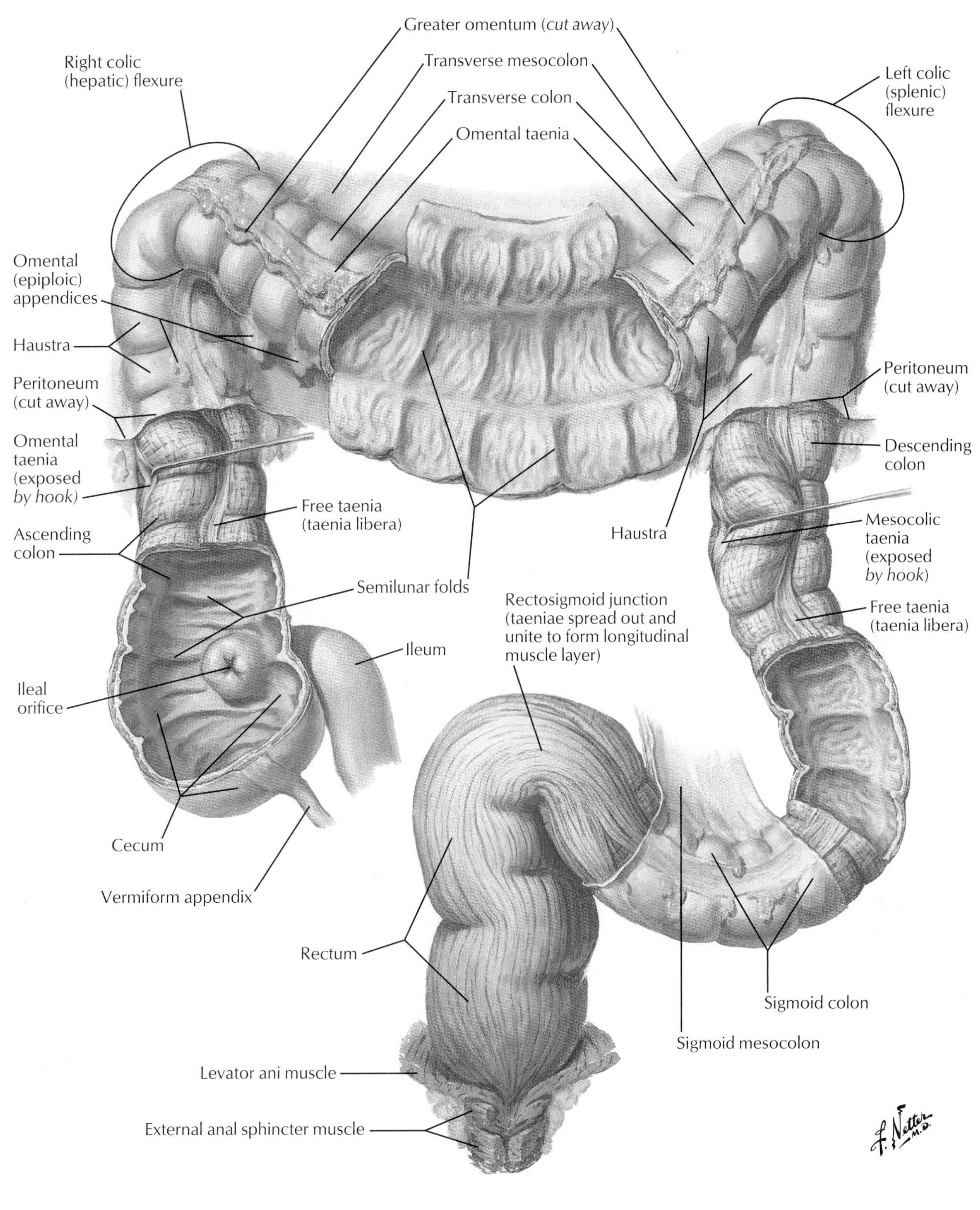
Greater omentum (cut away)
Transverse mesocolon
Transverse colon
Omental taenia
Right colic
(hepatic) flexure
Left colic
(splenic)
flexure
Omental
(epiploic)
appendices
Haustra
Peritoneum
(cut away)
Omental
taenia
(exposed
by hook)
Ascending
colon
Free taenia
(taenia libera)
Semilunar folds
Ileum
Ileal
orifice
Cecum
Vermiform appendix
Rectum
Levator ani muscle
External anal sphincter muscle
Haustra
Peritoneum
(cut away)
Descending
colon
Mesocolic
taenia
(exposed
by hook)
Free taenia
(taenia libera)
Rectosigmoid junction
(taeniae spread out and
unite to form longitudinal
muscle layer)
Sigmoid colon
Sigmoid mesocolon
F. Netter M.D.

Plate 32 Mucosa and Musculature of Large Intestine. (Copyright 2023 Elsevier Inc. All rights reserved. www.netterimages.com. Image ID: 4778.)

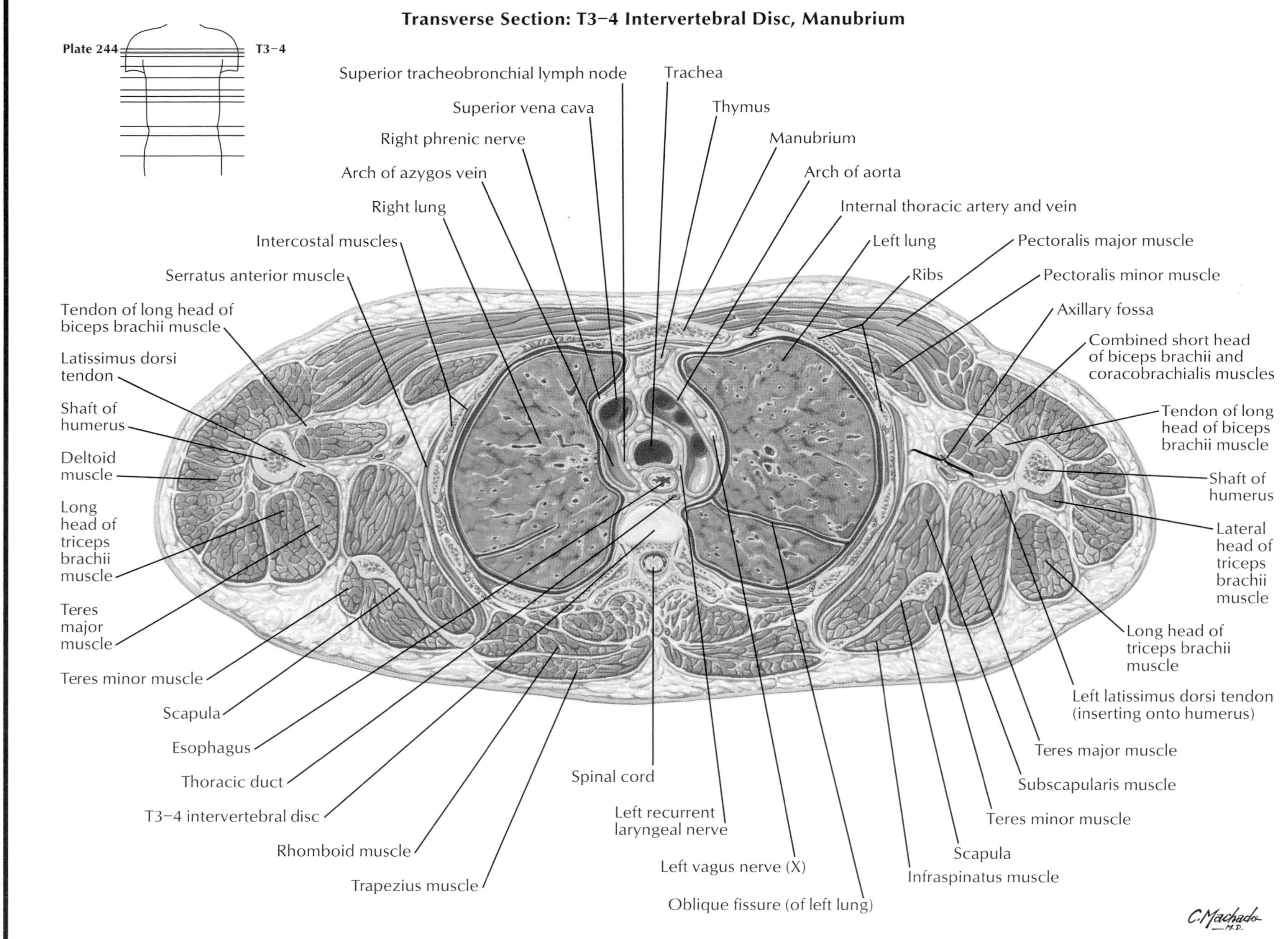
Transverse Section: T3–4 Intervertebral Disc, Manubrium
Plate 244
T3–4
Superior tracheobronchial lymph node
Superior vena cava
Right phrenic nerve
Arch of azygos vein
Right lung
Intercostal muscles
Serratus anterior muscle
Tendon of long head of biceps brachii muscle
Latissimus dorsi tendon
Shaft of humerus
Deltoid muscle
Long head of triceps brachii muscle
Teres major muscle
Teres minor muscle
Scapula
Esophagus
Thoracic duct
T3–4 intervertebral disc
Rhomboid muscle
Trapezius muscle
Trachea
Thymus
Manubrium
Arch of aorta
Internal thoracic artery and vein
Left lung
Ribs
Pectoralis major muscle
Pectoralis minor muscle
Axillary fossa
Combined short head of biceps brachii and coracobrachialis muscles
Tendon of long head of biceps brachii muscle
Shaft of humerus
Lateral head of triceps brachii muscle
Long head of triceps brachii muscle
Left latissimus dorsi tendon (inserting onto humerus)
Teres major muscle
Subscapularis muscle
Teres minor muscle
Scapula
Infraspinatus muscle
Spinal cord
Left recurrent laryngeal nerve
Left vagus nerve (X)
Oblique fissure (of left lung)
C. Machado M.D.

Plate 33 Cross Section of Thorax at T3-4 Disc Level. (www.netterimages.com. Image ID: 4880.)

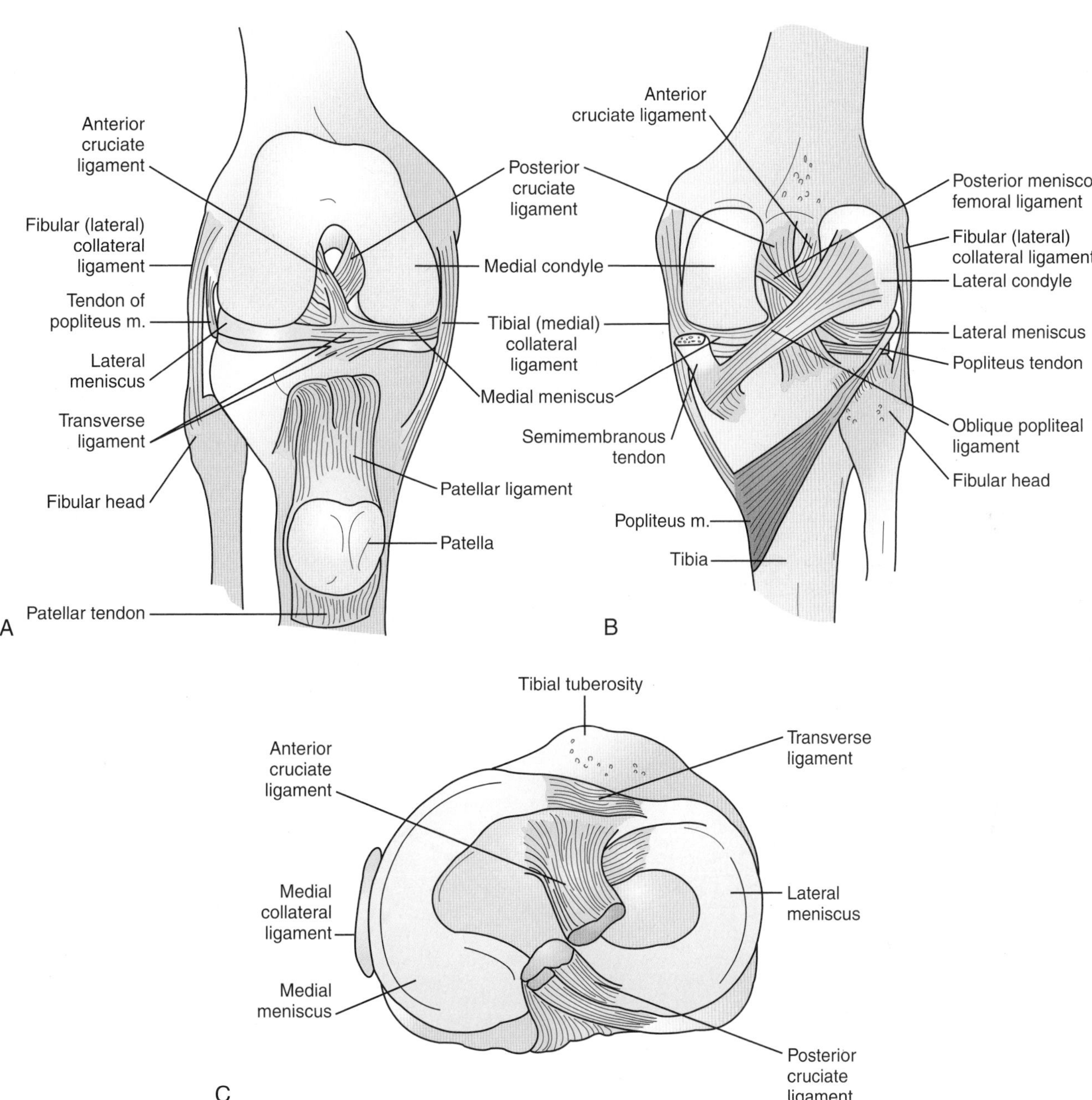

Anterior cruciate ligament
Fibular (lateral) collateral ligament
Tendon of popliteus m.
Lateral meniscus
Transverse ligament
Fibular head
Patellar tendon
A
Posterior cruciate ligament
Medial condyle
Tibial (medial) collateral ligament
Medial meniscus
Patellar ligament
Patella
Anterior cruciate ligament
Semimembranous tendon
Popliteus m.
Tibia
B
Posterior menisco-femoral ligament
Fibular (lateral) collateral ligament
Lateral condyle
Lateral meniscus
Popliteus tendon
Oblique popliteal ligament
Fibular head
Tibial tuberosity
Anterior cruciate ligament
Transverse ligament
Medial collateral ligament
Lateral meniscus
Medial meniscus
Posterior cruciate ligament
C

Plate 34 Knee joint opened; anterior, posterior, and proximal views. A, Anterior view of the knee joint, opened by folding the patella and patellar ligament inferiorly. On the lateral side is the fibular collateral ligament, separated by the popliteal tendon from the lateral meniscus. On the medial side, the tibial collateral ligament is attached to the medial meniscus. The anterior and posterior cruciate ligaments are seen between the femoral condyles. B, Posterior view of the opened knee joint with a more complete view of the posterior cruciate ligament. C, The femur is removed, showing the proximal (articular) end of the right tibia. On the medial side is the gently curved medial meniscus; on the lateral side is the more tightly curved lateral meniscus. The anterior end of the medial meniscus is anchored to the surface of the tibia by the transverse ligament. The cut ends of the anterior and posterior cruciate ligaments are shown, as well as the meniscofemoral ligament. (Fritz S: Mosby's Essential Sciences for Therapeutic Massage: Anatomy, Physiology, Biomechanics, and Pathology, ed 5, St. Louis, 2017, Elsevier.)

Paramedian (sagittal) dissection

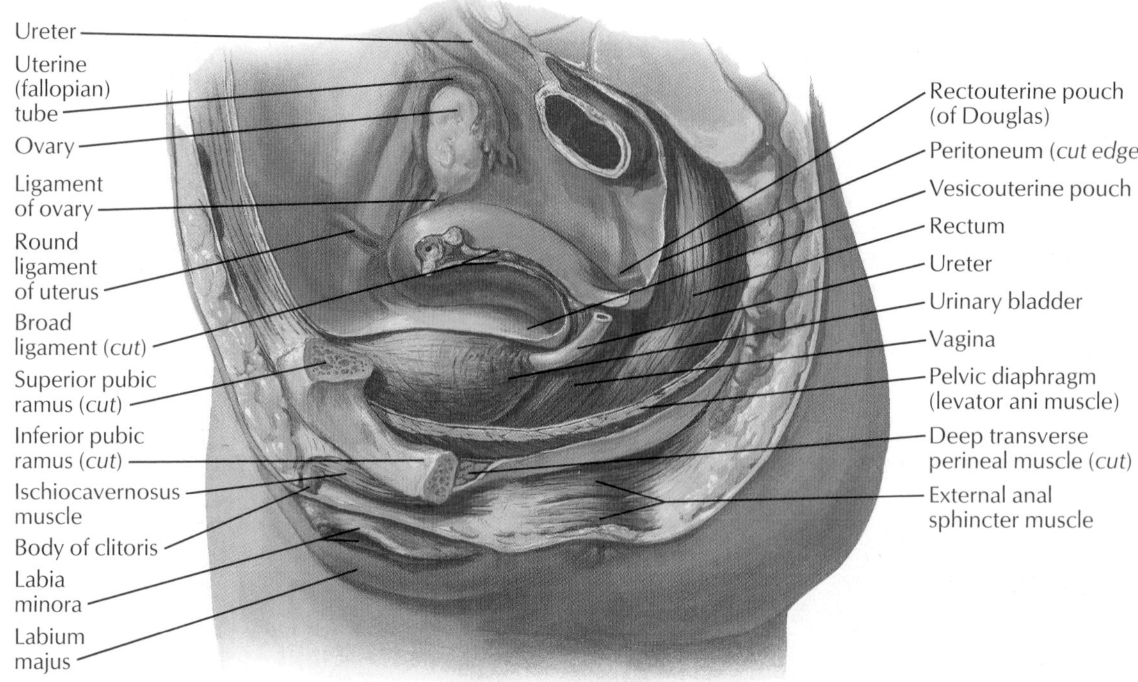
Ureter
Uterine (fallopian) tube
Ovary
Ligament of ovary
Round ligament of uterus
Broad ligament (cut)
Superior pubic ramus (cut)
Inferior pubic ramus (cut)
Ischiocavernosus muscle
Body of clitoris
Labia minora
Labium majus
Rectouterine pouch (of Douglas)
Peritoneum (cut edge)
Vesicouterine pouch
Rectum
Ureter
Urinary bladder
Vagina
Pelvic diaphragm (levator ani muscle)
Deep transverse perineal muscle (cut)
External anal sphincter muscle

Median (sagittal) section

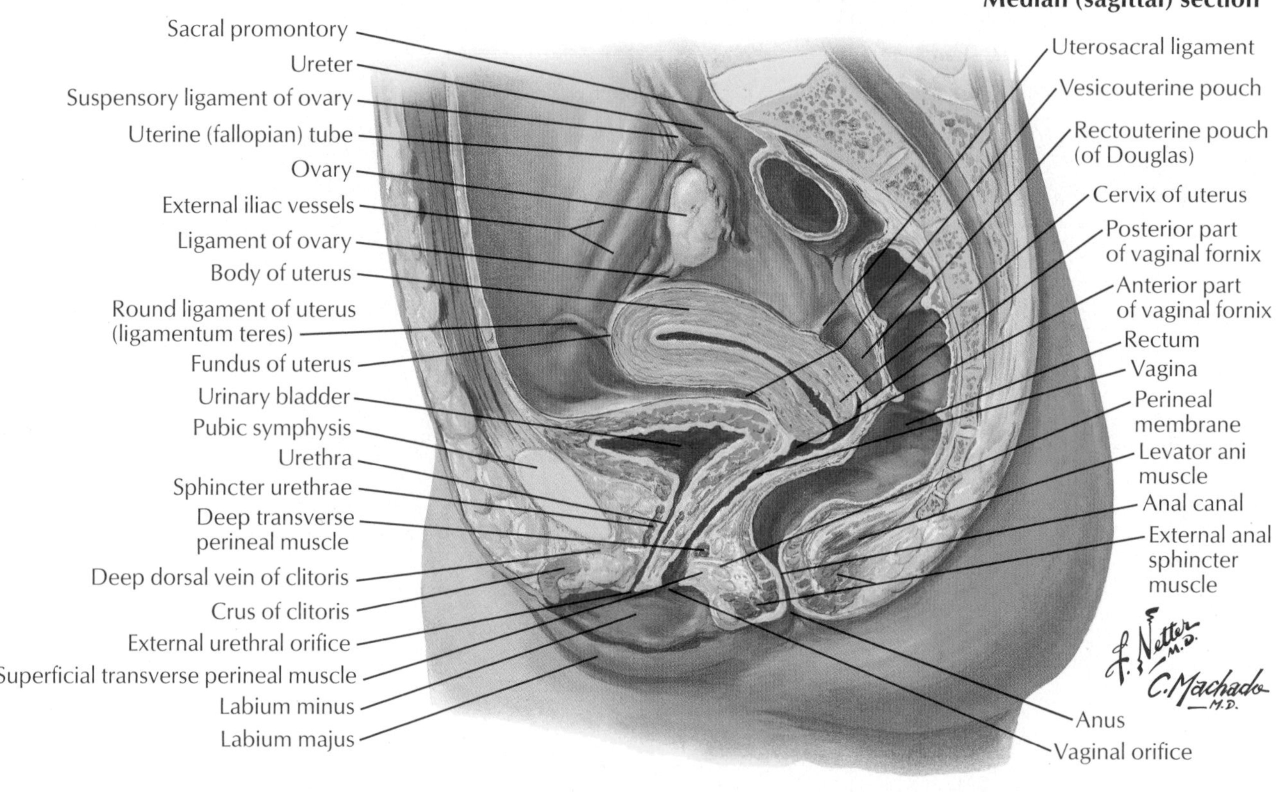
Sacral promontory
Ureter
Suspensory ligament of ovary
Uterine (fallopian) tube
Ovary
External iliac vessels
Ligament of ovary
Body of uterus
Round ligament of uterus (ligamentum teres)
Fundus of uterus
Urinary bladder
Pubic symphysis
Urethra
Sphincter urethrae
Deep transverse perineal muscle
Deep dorsal vein of clitoris
Crus of clitoris
External urethral orifice
Superficial transverse perineal muscle
Labium minus
Labium majus
Uterosacral ligament
Vesicouterine pouch
Rectouterine pouch (of Douglas)
Cervix of uterus
Posterior part of vaginal fornix
Anterior part of vaginal fornix
Rectum
Vagina
Perineal membrane
Levator ani muscle
Anal canal
External anal sphincter muscle
F. Netter M.D.
C. Machado M.D.
Anus
Vaginal orifice

Plate 35 Pelvic Viscera and Perineum: Female. (www.netterimages.com. Image ID: 4463.)

TABLES

Medical and Surgical

SECTION: Ø MEDICAL AND SURGICAL
BODY SYSTEM: Ø CENTRAL NERVOUS SYSTEM AND CRANIAL NERVES
OPERATION: 1 BYPASS: Altering the route of passage of the contents of a tubular body part

Body Part	Approach	Device	Qualifier
6 Cerebral Ventricle	Ø Open 3 Percutaneous 4 Percutaneous Endoscopic	7 Autologous Tissue Substitute J Synthetic Substitute K Nonautologous Tissue Substitute	Ø Nasopharynx 1 Mastoid Sinus 2 Atrium 3 Blood Vessel 4 Pleural Cavity 5 Intestine 6 Peritoneal Cavity 7 Urinary Tract 8 Bone Marrow A Subgaleal Space B Cerebral Cisterns
6 Cerebral Ventricle	Ø Open 3 Percutaneous 4 Percutaneous Endoscopic	Z No Device	B Cerebral Cisterns
U Spinal Canal	Ø Open 3 Percutaneous 4 Percutaneous Endoscopic	7 Autologous Tissue Substitute J Synthetic Substitute K Nonautologous Tissue Substitute	2 Atrium 4 Pleural Cavity 6 Peritoneal Cavity 7 Urinary Tract 9 Fallopian Tube

Coding Clinic: 2Ø21, Q2, P19; 2Ø13, Q2, P37 – ØØ163J6
Coding Clinic: 2Ø18, Q4, P86 – ØØ1UØJ2
Coding Clinic: 2Ø19, Q4, P22 – ØØ163JA

SECTION: Ø MEDICAL AND SURGICAL
BODY SYSTEM: Ø CENTRAL NERVOUS SYSTEM AND CRANIAL NERVES
OPERATION: 2 CHANGE: Taking out or off a device from a body part and putting back an identical or similar device in or on the same body part without cutting or puncturing the skin or a mucous membrane

Body Part	Approach	Device	Qualifier
Ø Brain E Cranial Nerve U Spinal Canal	X External	Ø Drainage Device Y Other Device	Z No Qualifier

Non-OR All Values

SECTION: Ø MEDICAL AND SURGICAL
BODY SYSTEM: Ø CENTRAL NERVOUS SYSTEM AND CRANIAL NERVES
OPERATION: 5 DESTRUCTION: Physical eradication of all or a portion of a body part by the direct use of energy, force, or a destructive agent

Body Part	Approach	Device	Qualifier
Ø Brain W Cervical Spinal Cord X Thoracic Spinal Cord Y Lumbar Spinal Cord	Ø Open 3 Percutaneous 4 Percutaneous Endoscopic	Z No Device	3 Laser Interstitial Thermal Z No Qualifier
1 Cerebral Meninges 2 Dura Mater 6 Cerebral Ventricle 7 Cerebral Hemisphere 8 Basal Ganglia 9 Thalamus A Hypothalamus B Pons C Cerebellum D Medulla Oblongata F Olfactory Nerve G Optic Nerve H Oculomotor Nerve J Trochlear Nerve K Trigeminal Nerve L Abducens Nerve M Facial Nerve N Acoustic Nerve P Glossopharyngeal Nerve Q Vagus Nerve R Accessory Nerve S Hypoglossal Nerve T Spinal Meninges	Ø Open 3 Percutaneous 4 Percutaneous Endoscopic	Z No Device	Z No Qualifier

Non-OR ØØ5[ØFGHJKLMNPQRSWXY][Ø34]ZZ

Coding Clinic: 2021, Q2, P18 – ØØ5[WX]ØZZ
Coding Clinic: 2021, Q3, P17 – ØØ5CØZZ
Coding Clinic: 2022, Q1, P5Ø – ØØ5K3ZZ

SECTION: Ø MEDICAL AND SURGICAL
BODY SYSTEM: Ø CENTRAL NERVOUS SYSTEM AND CRANIAL NERVES
OPERATION: 7 DILATION: Expanding an orifice or the lumen of a tubular body part

Body Part	Approach	Device	Qualifier
6 Cerebral Ventricle	Ø Open 3 Percutaneous 4 Percutaneous Endoscopic	Z No Device	Z No Qualifier

Coding Clinic: 2017, Q4, P4Ø – ØØ764ZZ

SECTION: Ø MEDICAL AND SURGICAL
BODY SYSTEM: Ø CENTRAL NERVOUS SYSTEM AND CRANIAL NERVES
OPERATION: 8 DIVISION: Cutting into a body part, without draining fluids and/or gases from the body part, in order to separate or transect a body part

Body Part	Approach	Device	Qualifier
Ø Brain 7 Cerebral Hemisphere 8 Basal Ganglia F Olfactory Nerve G Optic Nerve H Oculomotor Nerve J Trochlear Nerve K Trigeminal Nerve L Abducens Nerve M Facial Nerve N Acoustic Nerve P Glossopharyngeal Nerve Q Vagus Nerve R Accessory Nerve S Hypoglossal Nerve W Cervical Spinal Cord X Thoracic Spinal Cord Y Lumbar Spinal Cord	Ø Open 3 Percutaneous 4 Percutaneous Endoscopic	Z No Device	Z No Qualifier

SECTION: Ø MEDICAL AND SURGICAL
BODY SYSTEM: Ø CENTRAL NERVOUS SYSTEM AND CRANIAL NERVES
OPERATION: 9 DRAINAGE: *(on multiple pages)*
Taking or letting out fluids and/or gases from a body part

Body Part	Approach	Device	Qualifier
Ø Brain 1 Cerebral Meninges 2 Dura Mater 3 Epidural Space, Intracranial 4 Subdural Space, Intracranial 5 Subarachnoid Space, Intracranial 6 Cerebral Ventricle 7 Cerebral Hemisphere 8 Basal Ganglia 9 Thalamus A Hypothalamus B Pons C Cerebellum D Medulla Oblongata F Olfactory Nerve G Optic Nerve H Oculomotor Nerve J Trochlear Nerve K Trigeminal Nerve L Abducens Nerve M Facial Nerve N Acoustic Nerve P Glossopharyngeal Nerve Q Vagus Nerve R Accessory Nerve S Hypoglossal Nerve T Spinal Meninges U Spinal Canal W Cervical Spinal Cord X Thoracic Spinal Cord Y Lumbar Spinal Cord	Ø Open 3 Percutaneous 4 Percutaneous Endoscopic	Ø Drainage Device	Z No Qualifier

DRG Non-OR ØØ9[3TWXY]3ØZ
Non-OR ØØ9U[34]ØZ

Coding Clinic: 2Ø15, Q2, P3Ø – ØØ9WØØZ
Coding Clinic: 2Ø18, Q4, P85 – ØØ9UØØZ

SECTION: Ø MEDICAL AND SURGICAL
BODY SYSTEM: Ø CENTRAL NERVOUS SYSTEM AND CRANIAL NERVES
OPERATION: 9 DRAINAGE: *(continued)*
Taking or letting out fluids and/or gases from a body part

Body Part	Approach	Device	Qualifier
Ø Brain 1 Cerebral Meninges 2 Dura Mater 3 Epidural Space, Intracranial 4 Subdural Space, Intracranial 5 Subarachnoid Space, Intracranial 6 Cerebral Ventricle 7 Cerebral Hemisphere 8 Basal Ganglia 9 Thalamus A Hypothalamus B Pons C Cerebellum D Medulla Oblongata F Olfactory Nerve G Optic Nerve H Oculomotor Nerve J Trochlear Nerve K Trigeminal Nerve L Abducens Nerve M Facial Nerve N Acoustic Nerve P Glossopharyngeal Nerve Q Vagus Nerve R Accessory Nerve S Hypoglossal Nerve T Spinal Meninges U Spinal Canal W Cervical Spinal Cord X Thoracic Spinal Cord Y Lumbar Spinal Cord	Ø Open 3 Percutaneous 4 Percutaneous Endoscopic	Z No Device	X Diagnostic Z No Qualifier

DRG Non-OR ØØ933ZZ
Non-OR ØØ9[Ø123456789ABCDFGHJKLMNPQRSU][34]ZX
Non-OR ØØ9U[34]ZZ
Non-OR ØØ9[TWXY]3[XZ]

Coding Clinic: 2Ø15, Q3, P12-13 – ØØ9[46]3ØZ

SECTION: Ø MEDICAL AND SURGICAL
BODY SYSTEM: Ø CENTRAL NERVOUS SYSTEM AND CRANIAL NERVES
OPERATION: B EXCISION: Cutting out or off, without replacement, a portion of a body part

Body Part	Approach	Device	Qualifier
Ø Brain 1 Cerebral Meninges 2 Dura Mater 6 Cerebral Ventricle 7 Cerebral Hemisphere 8 Basal Ganglia 9 Thalamus A Hypothalamus B Pons C Cerebellum D Medulla Oblongata F Olfactory Nerve G Optic Nerve H Oculomotor Nerve J Trochlear Nerve K Trigeminal Nerve L Abducens Nerve M Facial Nerve N Acoustic Nerve P Glossopharyngeal Nerve Q Vagus Nerve R Accessory Nerve S Hypoglossal Nerve T Spinal Meninges W Cervical Spinal Cord X Thoracic Spinal Cord Y Lumbar Spinal Cord	Ø Open 3 Percutaneous 4 Percutaneous Endoscopic	Z No Device	X Diagnostic Z No Qualifier

Non-OR ØØB[Ø126789ABCDFGHJKLMNPQRS][34]ZX

Coding Clinic: 2015, Q1, P13 – ØØBØØZZ
Coding Clinic: 2016, Q2, P13 – ØØB[MRS]ØZZ
Coding Clinic: 2016, Q2, P18 – ØØB7ØZZ
Coding Clinic: 2021, Q3, P17 – ØØBCØZZ

SECTION: Ø MEDICAL AND SURGICAL
BODY SYSTEM: Ø CENTRAL NERVOUS SYSTEM AND CRANIAL NERVES
OPERATION: C EXTIRPATION: Taking or cutting out solid matter from a body part

Body Part	Approach	Device	Qualifier
Ø Brain 1 Cerebral Meninges 2 Dura Mater 3 Epidural Space, Intracranial 4 Subdural Space, Intracranial 5 Subarachnoid Space, Intracranial 6 Cerebral Ventricle 7 Cerebral Hemisphere 8 Basal Ganglia 9 Thalamus A Hypothalamus B Pons C Cerebellum D Medulla Oblongata F Olfactory Nerve G Optic Nerve H Oculomotor Nerve J Trochlear Nerve K Trigeminal Nerve L Abducens Nerve M Facial Nerve N Acoustic Nerve P Glossopharyngeal Nerve Q Vagus Nerve R Accessory Nerve S Hypoglossal Nerve T Spinal Meninges U Spinal Canal W Cervical Spinal Cord X Thoracic Spinal Cord Y Lumbar Spinal Cord	Ø Open 3 Percutaneous 4 Percutaneous Endoscopic	Z No Device	Z No Qualifier

Coding Clinic: 2Ø15, Q1, P12 – ØØCØØZZ
Coding Clinic: 2Ø19, Q3, P4; 2Ø16, Q2, P29; 2Ø15, Q3, P11 – ØØC4ØZZ
Coding Clinic: 2Ø15, Q3, P13 – ØØC74ZZ
Coding Clinic: 2Ø16, Q4, P28 – ØØCØØZZ
Coding Clinic: 2Ø17, Q4, P48 – ØØCUØZZ
Coding Clinic: 2Ø19, Q2, P37 – ØØCØ4ZZ

SECTION: Ø MEDICAL AND SURGICAL
BODY SYSTEM: Ø CENTRAL NERVOUS SYSTEM AND CRANIAL NERVES
OPERATION: D EXTRACTION: Pulling or stripping out or off all or a portion of a body part by the use of force

Body Part	Approach	Device	Qualifier
Ø Brain 1 Cerebral Meninges 2 Dura Mater 7 Cerebral Hemisphere C Cerebellum F Olfactory Nerve G Optic Nerve H Oculomotor Nerve J Trochlear Nerve K Trigeminal Nerve L Abducens Nerve M Facial Nerve N Acoustic Nerve P Glossopharyngeal Nerve Q Vagus Nerve R Accessory Nerve S Hypoglossal Nerve T Spinal Meninges	Ø Open 3 Percutaneous 4 Percutaneous Endoscopic	Z No Device	Z No Qualifier

Non-OR ØØDC[Ø34]ZZ

Coding Clinic: 2Ø15, Q3, P14 – ØØD2ØZZ
Coding Clinic: 2Ø21, Q4, P4Ø – ØØD[Ø7]ØZZ

SECTION: Ø MEDICAL AND SURGICAL
BODY SYSTEM: Ø CENTRAL NERVOUS SYSTEM AND CRANIAL NERVES
OPERATION: F FRAGMENTATION: Breaking solid matter in a body part into pieces

Body Part	Approach	Device	Qualifier
3 Epidural Space, Intracranial 4 Subdural Space, Intracranial 5 Subarachnoid Space, Intracranial 6 Cerebral Ventricle U Spinal Canal	Ø Open 3 Percutaneous 4 Percutaneous Endoscopic X External	Z No Device	Z No Qualifier

ØØF[3456]XZZ
Non-OR ØØF[3456]XZZ

SECTION: Ø MEDICAL AND SURGICAL
BODY SYSTEM: Ø CENTRAL NERVOUS SYSTEM AND CRANIAL NERVES
OPERATION: H INSERTION: Putting in a nonbiological appliance that monitors, assists, performs, or prevents a physiological function but does not physically take the place of a body part

Body Part	Approach	Device	Qualifier
Ø Brain ⊞	Ø Open	1 Radioactive Element 2 Monitoring Device 3 Infusion Device 4 Radioactive Element, Cesium-131 Collagen Implant M Neurostimulator Lead Y Other Device	Z No Qualifier
Ø Brain ⊞	3 Percutaneous 4 Percutaneous Endoscopic	1 Radioactive Element 2 Monitoring Device 3 Infusion Device M Neurostimulator Lead Y Other Device	Z No Qualifier
6 Cerebral Ventricle ⊞ E Cranial Nerve ⊞ U Spinal Canal ⊞ V Spinal Cord ⊞	Ø Open 3 Percutaneous 4 Percutaneous Endoscopic	1 Radioactive Element 2 Monitoring Device 3 Infusion Device M Neurostimulator Lead Y Other Device	Z No Qualifier

⊞ ØØHØ[Ø34]MZ
⊞ ØØH[6EUV][Ø34]MZ
DRG Non-OR ØØH[O3][Ø3][24]Z
DRG Non-OR ØØH[6UV]32Z
Non-OR ØØH[UV][Ø34]3Z

Coding Clinic: 2020, Q2, P15 – ØØH633Z
Coding Clinic: 2020, Q2, P17 – ØØHUØ3Z

SECTION: Ø MEDICAL AND SURGICAL
BODY SYSTEM: Ø CENTRAL NERVOUS SYSTEM AND CRANIAL NERVES
OPERATION: J INSPECTION: Visually and/or manually exploring a body part

Body Part	Approach	Device	Qualifier
Ø Brain E Cranial Nerve U Spinal Canal V Spinal Cord	Ø Open 3 Percutaneous 4 Percutaneous Endoscopic	Z No Device	Z No Qualifier

Non-OR ØØJE3ZZ
Non-OR ØØJ[EUV][Ø3][2Y]Z

Coding Clinic: 2017, Q1, P5Ø – ØØJU3ZZ
Coding Clinic: 2019, Q2, P37 – ØØJØØZZ
Coding Clinic: 2021, Q2, P18 – ØØJØ4ZZ

SECTION: Ø MEDICAL AND SURGICAL
BODY SYSTEM: Ø CENTRAL NERVOUS SYSTEM AND CRANIAL NERVES
OPERATION: K MAP: Locating the route of passage of electrical impulses and/or locating functional areas in a body part

Body Part	Approach	Device	Qualifier
Ø Brain 7 Cerebral Hemisphere 8 Basal Ganglia 9 Thalamus A Hypothalamus B Pons C Cerebellum D Medulla Oblongata	Ø Open 3 Percutaneous 4 Percutaneous Endoscopic	Z No Device	Z No Qualifier

SECTION: Ø MEDICAL AND SURGICAL
BODY SYSTEM: Ø CENTRAL NERVOUS SYSTEM AND CRANIAL NERVES
OPERATION: N RELEASE: Freeing a body part from an abnormal physical constraint by cutting or by the use of force

Body Part	Approach	Device	Qualifier
Ø Brain 1 Cerebral Meninges 2 Dura Mater 6 Cerebral Ventricle 7 Cerebral Hemisphere 8 Basal Ganglia 9 Thalamus A Hypothalamus B Pons C Cerebellum D Medulla Oblongata F Olfactory Nerve G Optic Nerve H Oculomotor Nerve J Trochlear Nerve K Trigeminal Nerve L Abducens Nerve M Facial Nerve N Acoustic Nerve P Glossopharyngeal Nerve Q Vagus Nerve R Accessory Nerve S Hypoglossal Nerve T Spinal Meninges W Cervical Spinal Cord X Thoracic Spinal Cord Y Lumbar Spinal Cord	Ø Open 3 Percutaneous 4 Percutaneous Endoscopic	Z No Device	Z No Qualifier

Coding Clinic: 2017, Q2, P24; 2015, Q2, P22 – ØØNWØZZ
Coding Clinic: 2016, Q2, P29 – ØØNØØZZ
Coding Clinic: 2017, Q3, P1Ø – ØØNCØZZ
Coding Clinic: 2018, Q4, P1Ø – ØØNM4ZZ
Coding Clinic: 2019, Q1, P29 – ØØNYØZZ
Coding Clinic: 2019, Q2, P2Ø – ØØNW3ZZ

Ø: M/S Ø: CENTRAL NERVOUS SYSTEM AND CRANIAL NERVES K: MAP N: RELEASE

SECTION: Ø MEDICAL AND SURGICAL
BODY SYSTEM: Ø CENTRAL NERVOUS SYSTEM AND CRANIAL NERVES
OPERATION: P REMOVAL: Taking out or off a device from a body part

Body Part	Approach	Device	Qualifier
Ø Brain V Spinal Cord	Ø Open 3 Percutaneous 4 Percutaneous Endoscopic	Ø Drainage Device 2 Monitoring Device 3 Infusion Device 7 Autologous Tissue Substitute J Synthetic Substitute K Nonautologous Tissue Substitute M Neurostimulator Lead Y Other Device	Z No Qualifier
Ø Brain V Spinal Cord	X External	Ø Drainage Device 2 Monitoring Device 3 Infusion Device M Neurostimulator Lead	Z No Qualifier
6 Cerebral Ventricle U Spinal Canal	Ø Open 3 Percutaneous 4 Percutaneous Endoscopic	Ø Drainage Device 2 Monitoring Device 3 Infusion Device J Synthetic Substitute M Neurostimulator Lead Y Other Device	Z No Qualifier
6 Cerebral Ventricle U Spinal Canal	X External	Ø Drainage Device 2 Monitoring Device 3 Infusion Device M Neurostimulator Lead	Z No Qualifier
E Cranial Nerve	Ø Open 3 Percutaneous 4 Percutaneous Endoscopic	Ø Drainage Device 2 Monitoring Device 3 Infusion Device 7 Autologous Tissue Substitute M Neurostimulator Lead Y Other Device	Z No Qualifier
E Cranial Nerve	X External	Ø Drainage Device 2 Monitoring Device 3 Infusion Device M Neurostimulator Lead	Z No Qualifier

Non-OR ØØP[ØV]X[Ø23M]Z
Non-OR ØØP6X[Ø3]Z
Non-OR ØØPEX[Ø23]Z
Non-OR ØØPUX[Ø23M]Z
Non-OR ØØP[Ø6EUV][3X][Ø23M]Z

SECTION: Ø MEDICAL AND SURGICAL
BODY SYSTEM: Ø CENTRAL NERVOUS SYSTEM AND CRANIAL NERVES
OPERATION: Q REPAIR: Restoring, to the extent possible, a body part to its normal anatomic structure and function

Body Part	Approach	Device	Qualifier
Ø Brain 1 Cerebral Meninges 2 Dura Mater 6 Cerebral Ventricle 7 Cerebral Hemisphere 8 Basal Ganglia 9 Thalamus A Hypothalamus B Pons C Cerebellum D Medulla Oblongata F Olfactory Nerve G Optic Nerve H Oculomotor Nerve J Trochlear Nerve K Trigeminal Nerve L Abducens Nerve M Facial Nerve N Acoustic Nerve P Glossopharyngeal Nerve Q Vagus Nerve R Accessory Nerve S Hypoglossal Nerve T Spinal Meninges W Cervical Spinal Cord X Thoracic Spinal Cord Y Lumbar Spinal Cord	Ø Open 3 Percutaneous 4 Percutaneous Endoscopic	Z No Device	Z No Qualifier

Coding Clinic: 2Ø13, Q3, P25 – ØØQ2ØZZ

SECTION: Ø MEDICAL AND SURGICAL
BODY SYSTEM: Ø CENTRAL NERVOUS SYSTEM AND CRANIAL NERVES
OPERATION: R REPLACEMENT: Putting in or on biological or synthetic material that physically takes the place and/or function of all or a portion of a body part

Body Part	Approach	Device	Qualifier
1 Cerebral Meninges 2 Dura Mater 6 Cerebral Ventricle F Olfactory Nerve G Optic Nerve H Oculomotor Nerve J Trochlear Nerve K Trigeminal Nerve L Abducens Nerve M Facial Nerve N Acoustic Nerve P Glossopharyngeal Nerve Q Vagus Nerve R Accessory Nerve S Hypoglossal Nerve T Spinal Meninges	Ø Open 4 Percutaneous Endoscopic	7 Autologous Tissue Substitute J Synthetic Substitute K Nonautologous Tissue Substitute	Z No Qualifier

SECTION: Ø MEDICAL AND SURGICAL
BODY SYSTEM: Ø CENTRAL NERVOUS SYSTEM AND CRANIAL NERVES
OPERATION: S REPOSITION: Moving to its normal location, or other suitable location, all or a portion of a body part

Body Part	Approach	Device	Qualifier
F Olfactory Nerve G Optic Nerve H Oculomotor Nerve J Trochlear Nerve K Trigeminal Nerve L Abducens Nerve M Facial Nerve N Acoustic Nerve P Glossopharyngeal Nerve Q Vagus Nerve R Accessory Nerve S Hypoglossal Nerve W Cervical Spinal Cord X Thoracic Spinal Cord Y Lumbar Spinal Cord	Ø Open 3 Percutaneous 4 Percutaneous Endoscopic	Z No Device	Z No Qualifier

SECTION: 0 MEDICAL AND SURGICAL
BODY SYSTEM: 0 CENTRAL NERVOUS SYSTEM AND CRANIAL NERVES
OPERATION: T RESECTION: Cutting out or off, without replacement, all of a body part

Body Part	Approach	Device	Qualifier
7 Cerebral Hemisphere	0 Open 3 Percutaneous 4 Percutaneous Endoscopic	Z No Device	Z No Qualifier

SECTION: 0 MEDICAL AND SURGICAL
BODY SYSTEM: 0 CENTRAL NERVOUS SYSTEM AND CRANIAL NERVES
OPERATION: U SUPPLEMENT: Putting in or on biological or synthetic material that physically reinforces and/or augments the function of a portion of a body part

Body Part	Approach	Device	Qualifier
1 Cerebral Meninges 2 Dura Mater 6 Cerebral Ventricle F Olfactory Nerve G Optic Nerve H Oculomotor Nerve J Trochlear Nerve K Trigeminal Nerve L Abducens Nerve M Facial Nerve N Acoustic Nerve P Glossopharyngeal Nerve Q Vagus Nerve R Accessory Nerve S Hypoglossal Nerve T Spinal Meninges	0 Open 3 Percutaneous 4 Percutaneous Endoscopic	7 Autologous Tissue Substitute J Synthetic Substitute K Nonautologous Tissue Substitute	Z No Qualifier

Coding Clinic: 2018, Q1, P9; 2017, Q3, P11 – 00U20KZ
Coding Clinic: 2021, Q3, P17 – 00U20KZ

SECTION: Ø MEDICAL AND SURGICAL
BODY SYSTEM: Ø CENTRAL NERVOUS SYSTEM AND CRANIAL NERVES
OPERATION: W REVISION: Correcting, to the extent possible, a portion of a malfunctioning device or the position of a displaced device

Body Part	Approach	Device	Qualifier
Ø Brain V Spinal Cord	Ø Open 3 Percutaneous 4 Percutaneous Endoscopic	Ø Drainage Device 2 Monitoring Device 3 Infusion Device 7 Autologous Tissue Substitute J Synthetic Substitute K Nonautologous Tissue Substitute M Neurostimulator Lead Y Other Device	Z No Qualifier
Ø Brain V Spinal Cord	X External	Ø Drainage Device 2 Monitoring Device 3 Infusion Device 7 Autologous Tissue Substitute J Synthetic Substitute K Nonautologous Tissue Substitute M Neurostimulator Lead	Z No Qualifier
6 Cerebral Ventricle U Spinal Canal	Ø Open 3 Percutaneous 4 Percutaneous Endoscopic	Ø Drainage Device 2 Monitoring Device 3 Infusion Device J Synthetic Substitute M Neurostimulator Lead Y Other Device	Z No Qualifier
6 Cerebral Ventricle U Spinal Canal	X External	Ø Drainage Device 2 Monitoring Device 3 Infusion Device J Synthetic Substitute M Neurostimulator Lead	Z No Qualifier
E Cranial Nerve	Ø Open 3 Percutaneous 4 Percutaneous Endoscopic	Ø Drainage Device 2 Monitoring Device 3 Infusion Device 7 Autologous Tissue Substitute M Neurostimulator Lead Y Other Device	Z No Qualifier
E Cranial Nerve	X External	Ø Drainage Device 2 Monitoring Device 3 Infusion Device 7 Autologous Tissue Substitute M Neurostimulator Lead	Z No Qualifier

Non-OR ØØW[ØV]X[Ø237JKM]Z
Non-OR ØØW[6U]X[Ø23JM]Z
Non-OR ØØWEX[Ø237M]Z

SECTION: Ø MEDICAL AND SURGICAL
BODY SYSTEM: Ø CENTRAL NERVOUS SYSTEM AND CRANIAL NERVES
OPERATION: X TRANSFER: Moving, without taking out, all or a portion of a body part to another location to take over the function of all or a portion of a body part

Body Part	Approach	Device	Qualifier
F Olfactory Nerve G Optic Nerve H Oculomotor Nerve J Trochlear Nerve K Trigeminal Nerve L Abducens Nerve M Facial Nerve N Acoustic Nerve P Glossopharyngeal Nerve Q Vagus Nerve R Accessory Nerve S Hypoglossal Nerve	Ø Open 4 Percutaneous Endoscopic	Z No Device	F Olfactory Nerve G Optic Nerve H Oculomotor Nerve J Trochlear Nerve K Trigeminal Nerve L Abducens Nerve M Facial Nerve N Acoustic Nerve P Glossopharyngeal Nerve Q Vagus Nerve R Accessory Nerve S Hypoglossal Nerve

SECTION: Ø MEDICAL AND SURGICAL
BODY SYSTEM: 1 PERIPHERAL NERVOUS SYSTEM
OPERATION: 2 CHANGE: Taking out or off a device from a body part and putting back an identical or similar device in or on the same body part without cutting or puncturing the skin or a mucous membrane

Body Part	Approach	Device	Qualifier
Y Peripheral Nerve	X External	Ø Drainage Device Y Other Device	Z No Qualifier

Non-OR Ø12YX[ØY]Z

SECTION: Ø MEDICAL AND SURGICAL
BODY SYSTEM: 1 PERIPHERAL NERVOUS SYSTEM
OPERATION: 5 DESTRUCTION: Physical eradication of all or a portion of a body part by the direct use of energy, force, or a destructive agent

Body Part	Approach	Device	Qualifier
Ø Cervical Plexus 1 Cervical Nerve 2 Phrenic Nerve 3 Brachial Plexus 4 Ulnar Nerve 5 Median Nerve 6 Radial Nerve 8 Thoracic Nerve 9 Lumbar Plexus A Lumbosacral Plexus B Lumbar Nerve C Pudendal Nerve D Femoral Nerve F Sciatic Nerve G Tibial Nerve H Peroneal Nerve K Head and Neck Sympathetic Nerve L Thoracic Sympathetic Nerve M Abdominal Sympathetic Nerve N Lumbar Sympathetic Nerve P Sacral Sympathetic Nerve Q Sacral Plexus R Sacral Nerve	Ø Open 3 Percutaneous 4 Percutaneous Endoscopic	Z No Device	Z No Qualifier

Non-OR Ø15[Ø234569ACDFGHQ][Ø34]ZZ
Non-OR Ø15[18BR]3ZZ

SECTION: Ø MEDICAL AND SURGICAL
BODY SYSTEM: 1 PERIPHERAL NERVOUS SYSTEM
OPERATION: 8 DIVISION: Cutting into a body part, without draining fluids and/or gases from the body part, in order to separate or transect a body part

Body Part	Approach	Device	Qualifier
Ø Cervical Plexus 1 Cervical Nerve 2 Phrenic Nerve 3 Brachial Plexus 4 Ulnar Nerve 5 Median Nerve 6 Radial Nerve 8 Thoracic Nerve 9 Lumbar Plexus A Lumbosacral Plexus B Lumbar Nerve C Pudendal Nerve D Femoral Nerve F Sciatic Nerve G Tibial Nerve H Peroneal Nerve K Head and Neck Sympathetic Nerve L Thoracic Sympathetic Nerve M Abdominal Sympathetic Nerve N Lumbar Sympathetic Nerve P Sacral Sympathetic Nerve Q Sacral Plexus R Sacral Nerve	Ø Open 3 Percutaneous 4 Percutaneous Endoscopic	Z No Device	Z No Qualifier

SECTION: Ø MEDICAL AND SURGICAL
BODY SYSTEM: 1 PERIPHERAL NERVOUS SYSTEM
OPERATION: 9 DRAINAGE: Taking or letting out fluids and/or gases from a body part

Body Part	Approach	Device	Qualifier
Ø Cervical Plexus 1 Cervical Nerve 2 Phrenic Nerve 3 Brachial Plexus 4 Ulnar Nerve 5 Median Nerve 6 Radial Nerve 8 Thoracic Nerve 9 Lumbar Plexus A Lumbosacral Plexus B Lumbar Nerve C Pudendal Nerve D Femoral Nerve F Sciatic Nerve G Tibial Nerve H Peroneal Nerve K Head and Neck Sympathetic Nerve L Thoracic Sympathetic Nerve M Abdominal Sympathetic Nerve N Lumbar Sympathetic Nerve P Sacral Sympathetic Nerve Q Sacral Plexus R Sacral Nerve	Ø Open 3 Percutaneous 4 Percutaneous Endoscopic	Ø Drainage Device	Z No Qualifier
Ø Cervical Plexus 1 Cervical Nerve 2 Phrenic Nerve 3 Brachial Plexus 4 Ulnar Nerve 5 Median Nerve 6 Radial Nerve 8 Thoracic Nerve 9 Lumbar Plexus A Lumbosacral Plexus B Lumbar Nerve C Pudendal Nerve D Femoral Nerve F Sciatic Nerve G Tibial Nerve H Peroneal Nerve K Head and Neck Sympathetic Nerve L Thoracic Sympathetic Nerve M Abdominal Sympathetic Nerve N Lumbar Sympathetic Nerve P Sacral Sympathetic Nerve Q Sacral Plexus R Sacral Nerve	Ø Open 3 Percutaneous 4 Percutaneous Endoscopic	Z No Device	X Diagnostic Z No Qualifier

Non-OR Ø19[Ø12345689ABCDFGHKLMNPQR]3ØZ
Non-OR Ø19[Ø12345689ABCDFGHKLMNPQR]3ZZ
Non-OR Ø19[Ø12345689ABCDFGHQR][34]ZX

New/Revised Text in Green ~~deleted~~ Deleted ♀ Females Only ♂ Males Only Coding Clinic
Non-covered Limited Coverage ⊞ Combination (See Appendix E) DRG Non-OR Non-OR Hospital-Acquired Condition

SECTION: Ø MEDICAL AND SURGICAL
BODY SYSTEM: 1 PERIPHERAL NERVOUS SYSTEM
OPERATION: B EXCISION: Cutting out or off, without replacement, a portion of a body part

Body Part	Approach	Device	Qualifier
Ø Cervical Plexus 1 Cervical Nerve 2 Phrenic Nerve 3 Brachial Plexus ⊞ 4 Ulnar Nerve 5 Median Nerve 6 Radial Nerve 8 Thoracic Nerve 9 Lumbar Plexus A Lumbosacral Plexus B Lumbar Nerve C Pudendal Nerve D Femoral Nerve F Sciatic Nerve G Tibial Nerve H Peroneal Nerve K Head and Neck Sympathetic Nerve L Thoracic Sympathetic Nerve ⊞ M Abdominal Sympathetic Nerve N Lumbar Sympathetic Nerve P Sacral Sympathetic Nerve Q Sacral Plexus R Sacral Nerve	Ø Open 3 Percutaneous 4 Percutaneous Endoscopic	Z No Device	X Diagnostic Z No Qualifier

⊞ Ø1B[3L]ØZZ
Non-OR Ø1B[Ø12345689ABCDFGHQR][34]ZX

Coding Clinic: 2Ø17, Q2, P19 – Ø1BLØZZ

SECTION: Ø MEDICAL AND SURGICAL
BODY SYSTEM: 1 PERIPHERAL NERVOUS SYSTEM
OPERATION: C EXTIRPATION: Taking or cutting out solid matter from a body part

Body Part	Approach	Device	Qualifier
Ø Cervical Plexus 1 Cervical Nerve 2 Phrenic Nerve 3 Brachial Plexus 4 Ulnar Nerve 5 Median Nerve 6 Radial Nerve 8 Thoracic Nerve 9 Lumbar Plexus A Lumbosacral Plexus B Lumbar Nerve C Pudendal Nerve D Femoral Nerve F Sciatic Nerve G Tibial Nerve H Peroneal Nerve K Head and Neck Sympathetic Nerve L Thoracic Sympathetic Nerve M Abdominal Sympathetic Nerve N Lumbar Sympathetic Nerve P Sacral Sympathetic Nerve Q Sacral Plexus R Sacral Nerve	Ø Open 3 Percutaneous 4 Percutaneous Endoscopic	Z No Device	Z No Qualifier

SECTION: Ø MEDICAL AND SURGICAL
BODY SYSTEM: 1 PERIPHERAL NERVOUS SYSTEM
OPERATION: D EXTRACTION: Pulling or stripping out or off all or a portion of a body part by the use of force

Body Part	Approach	Device	Qualifier
Ø Cervical Plexus 1 Cervical Nerve 2 Phrenic Nerve 3 Brachial Plexus 4 Ulnar Nerve 5 Median Nerve 6 Radial Nerve 8 Thoracic Nerve 9 Lumbar Plexus A Lumbosacral Plexus B Lumbar Nerve C Pudendal Nerve D Femoral Nerve F Sciatic Nerve G Tibial Nerve H Peroneal Nerve K Head and Neck Sympathetic Nerve L Thoracic Sympathetic Nerve M Abdominal Sympathetic Nerve N Lumbar Sympathetic Nerve P Sacral Sympathetic Nerve Q Sacral Plexus R Sacral Nerve	Ø Open 3 Percutaneous 4 Percutaneous Endoscopic	Z No Device	Z No Qualifier

SECTION: Ø MEDICAL AND SURGICAL
BODY SYSTEM: 1 PERIPHERAL NERVOUS SYSTEM
OPERATION: H INSERTION: Putting in a nonbiological appliance that monitors, assists, performs, or prevents a physiological function but does not physically take the place of a body part

Body Part	Approach	Device	Qualifier
Y Peripheral Nerve ⊞	Ø Open 3 Percutaneous 4 Percutaneous Endoscopic	1 Radioactive Element 2 Monitoring Device M Neurostimulator Lead Y Other Device	Z No Qualifier

⊞ Ø1HY[Ø34][1M]Z

SECTION: Ø MEDICAL AND SURGICAL
BODY SYSTEM: 1 PERIPHERAL NERVOUS SYSTEM
OPERATION: J INSPECTION: Visually and/or manually exploring a body part

Body Part	Approach	Device	Qualifier
Y Peripheral Nerve	Ø Open 3 Percutaneous 4 Percutaneous Endoscopic	Z No Device	Z No Qualifier

Non-OR Ø1JY3ZZ

SECTION: Ø MEDICAL AND SURGICAL
BODY SYSTEM: 1 PERIPHERAL NERVOUS SYSTEM
OPERATION: N RELEASE: Freeing a body part from an abnormal physical constraint by cutting or by the use of force

Body Part	Approach	Device	Qualifier
Ø Cervical Plexus 1 Cervical Nerve 2 Phrenic Nerve 3 Brachial Plexus 4 Ulnar Nerve 5 Median Nerve 6 Radial Nerve 8 Thoracic Nerve 9 Lumbar Plexus A Lumbosacral Plexus B Lumbar Nerve C Pudendal Nerve D Femoral Nerve F Sciatic Nerve G Tibial Nerve H Peroneal Nerve K Head and Neck Sympathetic Nerve L Thoracic Sympathetic Nerve M Abdominal Sympathetic Nerve N Lumbar Sympathetic Nerve P Sacral Sympathetic Nerve Q Sacral Plexus R Sacral Nerve	Ø Open 3 Percutaneous 4 Percutaneous Endoscopic	Z No Device	Z No Qualifier

Coding Clinic: 2Ø16, Q2, P16; 2Ø15, Q2, P34 – Ø1NBØZZ
Coding Clinic: 2Ø16, Q2, P17 – Ø1N1ØZZ
Coding Clinic: 2Ø16, Q2, P23 – Ø1N3ØZZ
Coding Clinic: 2Ø19, Q1, P29; 2Ø18, Q2, P23 – Ø1NBØZZ
Coding Clinic: 2Ø19, Q1, P29 – Ø1NRØZZ

SECTION: Ø MEDICAL AND SURGICAL
BODY SYSTEM: 1 PERIPHERAL NERVOUS SYSTEM
OPERATION: P REMOVAL: Taking out or off a device from a body part

Body Part	Approach	Device	Qualifier
Y Peripheral Nerve	Ø Open 3 Percutaneous 4 Percutaneous Endoscopic	Ø Drainage Device 2 Monitoring Device 7 Autologous Tissue Substitute M Neurostimulator Lead Y Other Device	Z No Qualifier
Y Peripheral Nerve	X External	Ø Drainage Device 2 Monitoring Device M Neurostimulator Lead	Z No Qualifier

Non-OR Ø1PY[3X][Ø2M]Z

SECTION: Ø MEDICAL AND SURGICAL
BODY SYSTEM: 1 PERIPHERAL NERVOUS SYSTEM
OPERATION: Q REPAIR: Restoring, to the extent possible, a body part to its normal anatomic structure and function

Body Part	Approach	Device	Qualifier
Ø Cervical Plexus 1 Cervical Nerve 2 Phrenic Nerve 3 Brachial Plexus 4 Ulnar Nerve 5 Median Nerve 6 Radial Nerve 8 Thoracic Nerve 9 Lumbar Plexus A Lumbosacral Plexus B Lumbar Nerve C Pudendal Nerve D Femoral Nerve F Sciatic Nerve G Tibial Nerve H Peroneal Nerve K Head and Neck Sympathetic Nerve L Thoracic Sympathetic Nerve M Abdominal Sympathetic Nerve N Lumbar Sympathetic Nerve P Sacral Sympathetic Nerve Q Sacral Plexus R Sacral Nerve	Ø Open 3 Percutaneous 4 Percutaneous Endoscopic	Z No Device	Z No Qualifier

SECTION: Ø MEDICAL AND SURGICAL
BODY SYSTEM: 1 PERIPHERAL NERVOUS SYSTEM
OPERATION: R REPLACEMENT: Putting in or on biological or synthetic material that physically takes the place and/or function of all or a portion of a body part

Body Part	Approach	Device	Qualifier
1 Cervical Nerve 2 Phrenic Nerve 4 Ulnar Nerve 5 Median Nerve 6 Radial Nerve 8 Thoracic Nerve B Lumbar Nerve C Pudendal Nerve D Femoral Nerve F Sciatic Nerve G Tibial Nerve H Peroneal Nerve R Sacral Nerve	Ø Open 4 Percutaneous Endoscopic	7 Autologous Tissue Substitute J Synthetic Substitute K Nonautologous Tissue Substitute	Z No Qualifier

SECTION: Ø MEDICAL AND SURGICAL
BODY SYSTEM: 1 PERIPHERAL NERVOUS SYSTEM
OPERATION: S REPOSITION: Moving to its normal location, or other suitable location, all or a portion of a body part

Body Part	Approach	Device	Qualifier
Ø Cervical Plexus 1 Cervical Nerve 2 Phrenic Nerve 3 Brachial Plexus 4 Ulnar Nerve 5 Median Nerve 6 Radial Nerve 8 Thoracic Nerve 9 Lumbar Plexus A Lumbosacral Plexus B Lumbar Nerve C Pudendal Nerve D Femoral Nerve F Sciatic Nerve G Tibial Nerve H Peroneal Nerve Q Sacral Plexus R Sacral Nerve	Ø Open 3 Percutaneous 4 Percutaneous Endoscopic	Z No Device	Z No Qualifier

Coding Clinic: 2Ø21, Q3, P2Ø – Ø1S[3456]ØZZ

SECTION: Ø MEDICAL AND SURGICAL
BODY SYSTEM: 1 PERIPHERAL NERVOUS SYSTEM
OPERATION: U SUPPLEMENT: Putting in or on biological or synthetic material that physically reinforces and/or augments the function of a portion of a body part

Body Part	Approach	Device	Qualifier
1 Cervical Nerve 2 Phrenic Nerve 4 Ulnar Nerve 5 Median Nerve 6 Radial Nerve 8 Thoracic Nerve B Lumbar Nerve C Pudendal Nerve D Femoral Nerve F Sciatic Nerve G Tibial Nerve H Peroneal Nerve R Sacral Nerve	Ø Open 3 Percutaneous 4 Percutaneous Endoscopic	7 Autologous Tissue Substitute J Synthetic Substitute K Nonautologous Tissue Substitute	Z No Qualifier

Coding Clinic: 2Ø17, Q4, P62 – Ø1U5ØKZ
Coding Clinic: 2Ø19, Q3, P33 – Ø1U8ØKZ

SECTION: Ø MEDICAL AND SURGICAL
BODY SYSTEM: 1 PERIPHERAL NERVOUS SYSTEM
OPERATION: W REVISION: Correcting, to the extent possible, a portion of a malfunctioning device or the position of a displaced device

Body Part	Approach	Device	Qualifier
Y Peripheral Nerve	Ø Open 3 Percutaneous 4 Percutaneous Endoscopic	Ø Drainage Device 2 Monitoring Device 7 Autologous Tissue Substitute M Neurostimulator Lead Y Other Device	Z No Qualifier
Y Peripheral Nerve	X External	Ø Drainage Device 2 Monitoring Device 7 Autologous Tissue Substitute M Neurostimulator Lead	Z No Qualifier

Non-OR Ø1WY[ØX][Ø27M]Z

SECTION: Ø MEDICAL AND SURGICAL
BODY SYSTEM: 1 PERIPHERAL NERVOUS SYSTEM
OPERATION: X TRANSFER: Moving, without taking out, all or a portion of a body part to another location to take over the function of all or a portion of a body part

Body Part	Approach	Device	Qualifier
1 Cervical Nerve 2 Phrenic Nerve	Ø Open 4 Percutaneous Endoscopic	Z No Device	1 Cervical Nerve 2 Phrenic Nerve
4 Ulnar Nerve 5 Median Nerve 6 Radial Nerve	Ø Open 4 Percutaneous Endoscopic	Z No Device	4 Ulnar Nerve 5 Median Nerve 6 Radial Nerve
8 Thoracic Nerve	Ø Open 4 Percutaneous Endoscopic	Z No Device	8 Thoracic Nerve
B Lumbar Nerve C Pudendal Nerve	Ø Open 4 Percutaneous Endoscopic	Z No Device	B Lumbar Nerve C Pudendal Nerve
D Femoral Nerve F Sciatic Nerve G Tibial Nerve H Peroneal Nerve	Ø Open 4 Percutaneous Endoscopic	Z No Device	D Femoral Nerve F Sciatic Nerve G Tibial Nerve H Peroneal Nerve

SECTION: Ø MEDICAL AND SURGICAL
BODY SYSTEM: 2 HEART AND GREAT VESSELS
OPERATION: 1 BYPASS: *(on multiple pages)*
Altering the route of passage of the contents of a tubular body part

Body Part	Approach	Device	Qualifier
Ø Coronary Artery, One Artery 1 Coronary Artery, Two Arteries 2 Coronary Artery, Three Arteries 3 Coronary Artery, Four or More Arteries	Ø Open	8 Zooplastic Tissue 9 Autologous Venous Tissue A Autologous Arterial Tissue J Synthetic Substitute K Nonautologous Tissue Substitute	3 Coronary Artery 8 Internal Mammary, Right 9 Internal Mammary, Left C Thoracic Artery F Abdominal Artery W Aorta
Ø Coronary Artery, One Artery 1 Coronary Artery, Two Arteries 2 Coronary Artery, Three Arteries 3 Coronary Artery, Four or More Arteries	Ø Open	Z No Device	3 Coronary Artery 8 Internal Mammary, Right 9 Internal Mammary, Left C Thoracic Artery F Abdominal Artery
Ø Coronary Artery, One Artery 1 Coronary Artery, Two Arteries 2 Coronary Artery, Three Arteries 3 Coronary Artery, Four or More Arteries	3 Percutaneous	4 Drug-eluting Intraluminal Device D Intraluminal Device	4 Coronary Vein
Ø Coronary Artery, One Artery 1 Coronary Artery, Two Arteries 2 Coronary Artery, Three Arteries 3 Coronary Artery, Four or More Arteries	4 Percutaneous Endoscopic	4 Drug-eluting Intraluminal Device D Intraluminal Device	4 Coronary Vein
Ø Coronary Artery, One Artery 1 Coronary Artery, Two Arteries 2 Coronary Artery, Three Arteries 3 Coronary Artery, Four or More Arteries	4 Percutaneous Endoscopic	8 Zooplastic Tissue 9 Autologous Venous Tissue A Autologous Arterial Tissue J Synthetic Substitute K Nonautologous Tissue Substitute	3 Coronary Artery 8 Internal Mammary, Right 9 Internal Mammary, Left C Thoracic Artery F Abdominal Artery W Aorta
Ø Coronary Artery, One Artery 1 Coronary Artery, Two Arteries 2 Coronary Artery, Three Arteries 3 Coronary Artery, Four or More Arteries	4 Percutaneous Endoscopic	Z No Device	3 Coronary Artery 8 Internal Mammary, Right 9 Internal Mammary, Left C Thoracic Artery F Abdominal Artery
6 Atrium, Right	Ø Open 4 Percutaneous Endoscopic	8 Zooplastic Tissue 9 Autologous Venous Tissue A Autologous Arterial Tissue J Synthetic Substitute K Nonautologous Tissue Substitute	P Pulmonary Trunk Q Pulmonary Artery, Right R Pulmonary Artery, Left
6 Atrium, Right	Ø Open 4 Percutaneous Endoscopic	Z No Device	7 Atrium, Left P Pulmonary Trunk Q Pulmonary Artery, Right R Pulmonary Artery, Left
6 Atrium, Right	3 Percutaneous	Z No Device	7 Atrium, Left

Non-OR Ø21[Ø123]4[4D]4
Non-OR Ø21[Ø123]3[4D]4
Ø21[Ø123]Ø[89AJK][389CFW] when reported with Secondary Diagnosis J98.5
Ø21[Ø123]ØZ[389CF] when reported with Secondary Diagnosis J98.5
Ø21[Ø123]4[89AJK][389CFW] when reported with Secondary Diagnosis J98.5
Ø21[Ø123]4Z[389CF] when reported with Secondary Diagnosis J98.5

Coding Clinic: 2Ø15, Q4, P23 P25, Q3, P17 – Ø21KØKP
Coding Clinic: 2Ø16, Q1, P28 – Ø21ØØZ9, Ø212Ø9W
Coding Clinic: 2Ø16, Q4, P81-82, 1Ø2, 1Ø8-1Ø9 – Ø21
Coding Clinic: 2Ø16, Q4, P83 – Ø21ØØAW, Ø211Ø9W
Coding Clinic: 2Ø16, Q4, P84 – Ø21ØØZ9
Coding Clinic: 2Ø16, Q4, P1Ø8 – Ø217ØZU
Coding Clinic: 2Ø16, Q4, P1Ø2 – Ø21WØJQ
Coding Clinic: 2Ø16, Q4, P1Ø3 – Ø21QØJA
Coding Clinic: 2Ø16, Q4, P1Ø7 – Ø21KØKP
Coding Clinic: 2Ø16, Q4, P144 – Ø21VØ9S
Coding Clinic: 2Ø16, Q4, P145 – Ø21VØ8S
Coding Clinic: 2Ø17, Q1, P19 – Ø21KØJP
Coding Clinic: 2Ø17, Q4, P56 – Ø2163Z7
Coding Clinic: 2Ø21, Q3, P22 – Ø21ØØA3

SECTION: Ø MEDICAL AND SURGICAL
BODY SYSTEM: 2 HEART AND GREAT VESSELS
OPERATION: 1 BYPASS: *(continued)*
Altering the route of passage of the contents of a tubular body part

Body Part	Approach	Device	Qualifier
7 Atrium, Left ⊞ V Superior Vena Cava	Ø Open 4 Percutaneous Endoscopic	8 Zooplastic Tissue 9 Autologous Venous Tissue A Autologous Arterial Tissue J Synthetic Substitute K Nonautologous Tissue Substitute Z No Device	P Pulmonary Trunk Q Pulmonary Artery, Right R Pulmonary Artery, Left S Pulmonary Vein, Right T Pulmonary Vein, Left U Pulmonary Vein, Confluence
7 Atrium, Left	3 Percutaneous	J Synthetic Substitute	6 Atrium, Right
K Ventricle, Right L Ventricle, Left	Ø Open 4 Percutaneous Endoscopic	8 Zooplastic Tissue 9 Autologous Venous Tissue A Autologous Arterial Tissue J Synthetic Substitute K Nonautologous Tissue Substitute	P Pulmonary Trunk Q Pulmonary Artery, Right R Pulmonary Artery, Left
K Ventricle, Right L Ventricle, Left	Ø Open 4 Percutaneous Endoscopic	Z No Device	5 Coronary Circulation 8 Internal Mammary, Right 9 Internal Mammary, Left C Thoracic Artery F Abdominal Artery P Pulmonary Trunk Q Pulmonary Artery, Right R Pulmonary Artery, Left W Aorta
P Pulmonary Trunk Q Pulmonary Artery, Right R Pulmonary Artery, Left	Ø Open 4 Percutaneous Endoscopic	8 Zooplastic Tissue 9 Autologous Venous Tissue A Autologous Arterial Tissue J Synthetic Substitute K Nonautologous Tissue Substitute Z No Device	A Innominate Artery B Subclavian D Carotid
V Superior Vena Cava	Ø Open 4 Percutaneous Endoscopic	8 Zooplastic Tissue 9 Autologous Venous Tissue A Autologous Arterial Tissue J Synthetic Substitute K Nonautologous Tissue Substitute Z No Device	P Pulmonary Trunk Q Pulmonary Artery, Right R Pulmonary Artery, Left S Pulmonary Vein, Right T Pulmonary Vein, Left U Pulmonary Vein, Confluence
W Thoracic Aorta, Descending	Ø Open	8 Zooplastic Tissue 9 Autologous Venous Tissue A Autologous Arterial Tissue J Synthetic Substitute K Nonautologous Tissue Substitute	A Innominate Artery B Subclavian D Carotid F Abdominal Artery G Axillary Artery H Brachial Artery P Pulmonary Trunk Q Pulmonary Artery, Right R Pulmonary Artery, Left V Lower Extremity Artery
W Thoracic Aorta, Descending	Ø Open	Z No Device	A Innominate Artery B Subclavian D Carotid P Pulmonary Trunk Q Pulmonary Artery, Right R Pulmonary Artery, Left

Ø217ØZ[PQR]

Coding Clinic: 2018, Q4, P46 – Ø21WØJV
Coding Clinic: 2019, Q3, P31 – Ø21XØJ[B,D]
Coding Clinic: 2019, Q4, P23 – Ø21XØJA
Coding Clinic: 2020, Q1, P25 – Ø21KØJP

SECTION: Ø MEDICAL AND SURGICAL
BODY SYSTEM: 2 HEART AND GREAT VESSELS
OPERATION: 1 BYPASS: *(continued)*
Altering the route of passage of the contents of a tubular body part

Body Part	Approach	Device	Qualifier
W Thoracic Aorta, Descending	4 Percutaneous Endoscopic	8 Zooplastic Tissue 9 Autologous Venous Tissue A Autologous Arterial Tissue J Synthetic Substitute K Nonautologous Tissue Substitute Z No Device	A Innominate Artery B Subclavian D Carotid P Pulmonary Trunk Q Pulmonary Artery, Right R Pulmonary Artery, Left
X Thoracic Aorta, Ascending/Arch	Ø Open 4 Percutaneous Endoscopic	8 Zooplastic Tissue 9 Autologous Venous Tissue A Autologous Arterial Tissue J Synthetic Substitute K Nonautologous Tissue Substitute Z No Device	A Innominate Artery B Subclavian D Carotid P Pulmonary Trunk Q Pulmonary Artery, Right R Pulmonary Artery, Left

SECTION: Ø MEDICAL AND SURGICAL
BODY SYSTEM: 2 HEART AND GREAT VESSELS
OPERATION: 4 CREATION: Putting in or on biological or synthetic material to form a new body part that to the extent possible replicates the anatomic structure or function of an absent body part

Body Part	Approach	Device	Qualifier
F Aortic Valve	Ø Open	7 Autologous Tissue Substitute 8 Zooplastic Tissue J Synthetic Substitute K Nonautologous Tissue Substitute	J Truncal Valve
G Mitral Valve J Tricuspid Valve	Ø Open	7 Autologous Tissue Substitute 8 Zooplastic Tissue J Synthetic Substitute K Nonautologous Tissue Substitute	2 Common Atrioventricular Valve

Coding Clinic: 2Ø16, Q4, P1Ø1-1Ø2, 1Ø6 – Ø24
Coding Clinic: 2Ø16, Q4, P1Ø5 – ØØ2[GJ]Ø[JK]2
Coding Clinic: 2Ø16, Q4, P1Ø7 – Ø24FØ[8J]J

SECTION: Ø MEDICAL AND SURGICAL
BODY SYSTEM: 2 HEART AND GREAT VESSELS
OPERATION: 5 DESTRUCTION: Physical eradication of all or a portion of a body part by the direct use of energy, force, or a destructive agent

Body Part	Approach	Device	Qualifier
4 Coronary Vein 5 Atrial Septum 6 Atrium, Right 7 Atrium, Left 8 Conduction Mechanism 9 Chordae Tendineae D Papillary Muscle F Aortic Valve G Mitral Valve H Pulmonary Valve J Tricuspid Valve K Ventricle, Right L Ventricle, Left M Ventricular Septum N Pericardium P Pulmonary Trunk Q Pulmonary Artery, Right R Pulmonary Artery, Left S Pulmonary Vein, Right T Pulmonary Vein, Left V Superior Vena Cava W Thoracic Aorta, Descending X Thoracic Aorta, Ascending/Arch	Ø Open 3 Percutaneous 4 Percutaneous Endoscopic	Z No Device	Z No Qualifier
7 Atrium, Left	Ø Open 3 Percutaneous 4 Percutaneous Endoscopic	Z No Device	K Left Atrial Appendage Z No Qualifier

DRG Non-OR Ø257[Ø34]ZK

Coding Clinic: 2Ø13, Q2, P39 – Ø25S3ZZ, Ø25T3ZZ
Coding Clinic: 2Ø16, Q2, P18 – Ø25NØZZ
Coding Clinic: 2Ø2Ø, Q1, P33; 2Ø16, Q3, P43 – Ø2583ZZ
Coding Clinic: 2Ø16, Q3, P44 – Ø258ØZZ
Coding Clinic: 2Ø16, Q3, P44 – Ø257ØZK
Coding Clinic: 2Ø16, Q4, P81 – Ø25
Coding Clinic: 2Ø2Ø, Q1, P32 – Ø2584ZZ

New/Revised Text in Green ~~deleted~~ Deleted ♀ Females Only ♂ Males Only Coding Clinic
Non-covered Limited Coverage ⊞ Combination (See Appendix E) DRG Non-OR Non-OR Hospital-Acquired Condition

SECTION: Ø MEDICAL AND SURGICAL
BODY SYSTEM: 2 HEART AND GREAT VESSELS
OPERATION: 7 DILATION: Expanding an orifice or the lumen of a tubular body part

Body Part	Approach	Device	Qualifier
Ø Coronary Artery, One Artery 1 Coronary Artery, Two Arteries 2 Coronary Artery, Three Arteries 3 Coronary Artery, Four or More Arteries	Ø Open 3 Percutaneous 4 Percutaneous Endoscopic	4 Drug-eluting Intraluminal Device 5 Intraluminal Device, Drug-eluting, Two 6 Intraluminal Device, Drug-eluting, Three 7 Intraluminal Device, Drug-eluting, Four or More D Intraluminal Device E Intraluminal Device, Two F Intraluminal Device, Three G Intraluminal Device, Four or More T Radioactive Intraluminal Device Z No Device	6 Bifurcation Z No Qualifier
F Aortic Valve G Mitral Valve H Pulmonary Valve J Tricuspid Valve K Ventricle, Right L Ventricle, Left P Pulmonary Trunk Q Pulmonary Artery, Right S Pulmonary Vein, Right T Pulmonary Vein, Left V Superior Vena Cava W Thoracic Aorta, Descending X Thoracic Aorta, Ascending/Arch	Ø Open 3 Percutaneous 4 Percutaneous Endoscopic	4 Drug-eluting Intraluminal Device D Intraluminal Device Z No Device	Z No Qualifier
R Pulmonary Artery, Left	Ø Open 3 Percutaneous 4 Percutaneous Endoscopic	4 Drug-eluting Intraluminal Device D Intraluminal Device Z No Device	T Ductus Arteriosus Z No Qualifier

Coding Clinic: 2Ø15, Q2, P3-5 – Ø27234Z, Ø27Ø3[4D]Z, Ø27Ø346, Ø27134Z
Coding Clinic: 2Ø15, Q3, P1Ø, P17 – Ø27Ø3ZZ, Ø27QØDZ
Coding Clinic: 2Ø19, Q4, P4Ø; 2Ø15, Q4, P14 – Ø27Ø34Z
Coding Clinic: 2Ø16, Q1, P17 – Ø27HØZZ
Coding Clinic: 2Ø16, Q4, P81-82 – Ø27
Coding Clinic: 2Ø16, Q4, P85 – Ø27Ø3EZ, Ø27136Z
Coding Clinic: 2Ø16, Q4, P86 – Ø27Ø37Z
Coding Clinic: 2Ø16, Q4, P87 – Ø271356
Coding Clinic: 2Ø16, Q4, P88 – Ø27Ø346, Ø27Ø3ZZ
Coding Clinic: 2Ø17, Q4, P33 – Ø27LØZZ

SECTION: Ø MEDICAL AND SURGICAL

BODY SYSTEM: 2 HEART AND GREAT VESSELS

OPERATION: 8 DIVISION: Cutting into a body part, without draining fluids and/or gases from the body part, in order to separate or transect a body part

Body Part	Approach	Device	Qualifier
8 Conduction Mechanism 9 Chordae Tendineae D Papillary Muscle	Ø Open 3 Percutaneous 4 Percutaneous Endoscopic	Z No Device	Z No Qualifier

SECTION: Ø MEDICAL AND SURGICAL

BODY SYSTEM: 2 HEART AND GREAT VESSELS

OPERATION: B EXCISION: Cutting out or off, without replacement, a portion of a body part

Body Part	Approach	Device	Qualifier
4 Coronary Vein 5 Atrial Septum 6 Atrium, Right 8 Conduction Mechanism 9 Chordae Tendineae D Papillary Muscle F Aortic Valve G Mitral Valve H Pulmonary Valve J Tricuspid Valve K Ventricle, Right L Ventricle, Left M Ventricular Septum N Pericardium P Pulmonary Trunk Q Pulmonary Artery, Right R Pulmonary Artery, Left S Pulmonary Vein, Right T Pulmonary Vein, Left V Superior Vena Cava W Thoracic Aorta, Descending X Thoracic Aorta, Ascending/Arch	Ø Open 3 Percutaneous 4 Percutaneous Endoscopic	Z No Device	X Diagnostic Z No Qualifier
7 Atrium, Left	Ø Open 3 Percutaneous 4 Percutaneous Endoscopic	Z No Device	K Left Atrial Appendage X Diagnostic Z No Qualifier

Ø2B[KL][Ø34]ZZ
Ø2BKØZZ
DRG Non-OR Ø2B7[Ø34]ZK
Non-OR Ø2B[45689DFGHJKLM][Ø34]ZX
Non-OR Ø2B7[Ø34]ZX

Coding Clinic: 2Ø15, Q2, P24 – Ø2BGØZZ
Coding Clinic: 2Ø16, Q4, P81 – Ø2B
Coding Clinic: 2Ø19, Q2, P21 – Ø2BNØZZ
Coding Clinic: 2Ø19, Q3, P32 – Ø2BK3ZX

SECTION: Ø MEDICAL AND SURGICAL
BODY SYSTEM: 2 HEART AND GREAT VESSELS
OPERATION: C EXTIRPATION: Taking or cutting out solid matter from a body part

Body Part	Approach	Device	Qualifier
Ø Coronary Artery, One Artery 1 Coronary Artery, Two Arteries 2 Coronary Artery, Three Arteries 3 Coronary Artery, Four or More Arteries	Ø Open 4 Percutaneous Endoscopic	Z No Device	6 Bifurcation Z No Qualifier
Ø Coronary Artery, One Artery 1 Coronary Artery, Two Arteries 2 Coronary Artery, Three Arteries 3 Coronary Artery, Four or More Arteries	3 Percutaneous	Z No Device	6 Bifurcation 7 Orbital Atherectomy Technique Z No Qualifier
4 Coronary Vein 5 Atrial Septum 6 Atrium, Right 7 Atrium, Left 8 Conduction Mechanism 9 Chordae Tendineae D Papillary Muscle F Aortic Valve G Mitral Valve H Pulmonary Valve J Tricuspid Valve K Ventricle, Right L Ventricle, Left M Ventricular Septum N Pericardium P Pulmonary Trunk Q Pulmonary Artery, Right R Pulmonary Artery, Left S Pulmonary Vein, Right T Pulmonary Vein, Left V Superior Vena Cava W Thoracic Aorta, Descending X Thoracic Aorta, Ascending/Arch	Ø Open 3 Percutaneous 4 Percutaneous Endoscopic	Z No Device	Z No Qualifier

Coding Clinic: 2Ø16, Q2, P25 – Ø2CGØZZ

Coding Clinic: 2Ø16, Q4, P81-82, 87 – Ø2C

SECTION: Ø MEDICAL AND SURGICAL
BODY SYSTEM: 2 HEART AND GREAT VESSELS
OPERATION: F FRAGMENTATION: Breaking solid matter in a body part into pieces

Body Part	Approach	Device	Qualifier
Ø Coronary Artery, One Artery 1 Coronary Artery, Two Arteries 2 Coronary Artery, Three Arteries 3 Coronary Artery, Four or More Arteries	3 Percutaneous	Z No Device	Z No Qualifier
N Pericardium	Ø Open 3 Percutaneous 4 Percutaneous Endoscopic X External	Z No Device	Z No Qualifier
P Pulmonary Trunk Q Pulmonary Artery, Right R Pulmonary Artery, Left S Pulmonary Vein, Right T Pulmonary Vein, Left	3 Percutaneous	Z No Device	Ø Ultrasonic Z No Qualifier

Ø2FNXZZ

Non-OR Ø2FNXZZ

SECTION: Ø MEDICAL AND SURGICAL
BODY SYSTEM: 2 HEART AND GREAT VESSELS
OPERATION: H INSERTION: *(on multiple pages)*

Putting in a nonbiological appliance that monitors, assists, performs, or prevents a physiological function but does not physically take the place of a body part

Body Part	Approach	Device	Qualifier
Ø Coronary Artery, One Artery 1 Coronary Artery, Two Arteries 2 Coronary Artery, Three Arteries 3 Coronary Artery, Four or More Arteries	Ø Open 3 Percutaneous 4 Percutaneous Endoscopic	D Intraluminal Device Y Other Device	Z No Qualifier
4 Coronary Vein 6 Atrium, Right 7 Atrium, Left K Ventricle, Right L Ventricle, Left	Ø Open 3 Percutaneous 4 Percutaneous Endoscopic	Ø Monitoring Device, Pressure Sensor 2 Monitoring Device 3 Infusion Device D Intraluminal Device J Cardiac Lead, Pacemaker K Cardiac Lead, Defibrillator M Cardiac Lead N Intracardiac Pacemaker Y Other Device	Z No Qualifier
A Heart	Ø Open 3 Percutaneous 4 Percutaneous Endoscopic	Q Implantable Heart Assist System Y Other Device	Z No Qualifier
A Heart	Ø Open 3 Percutaneous 4 Percutaneous Endoscopic	R Short-term External Heart Assist System	J Intraoperative S Biventricular Z No Qualifier
N Pericardium	Ø Open 3 Percutaneous 4 Percutaneous Endoscopic	Ø Monitoring Device, Pressure Sensor 2 Monitoring Device J Cardiac Lead, Pacemaker K Cardiac Lead, Defibrillator M Cardiac Lead Y Other Device	Z No Qualifier

Ø2HA[34]QZ
Ø2H4[Ø4]KZ
Ø2H43[K]Z
Ø2H[67][Ø34]KZ
Ø2HK[Ø34][Ø2K]Z
Ø2HL[Ø34][KM]Z
Ø2HA[Ø4]R[SZ]
Ø2HA3RS
Ø2HN[Ø34][K]Z
DRG Non-OR Ø2H[467][Ø34][JM]Z
DRG Non-OR Ø2H[67]3JZ
DRG Non-OR Ø2H[KLN][Ø34][JM]Z
DRG Non-OR Ø2HK3[2JM]Z
DRG Non-OR Ø2H[467KL]3DZ
DRG Non-OR Ø2H[PQRSTVW]3DZ
Non-OR Ø2H[467KL]3[23M]Z
Non-OR Ø2HK33Z
Ø2H43[JKM]Z when reported with Secondary Diagnosis K68.11, T81.4XXA, T82.6XXA, or T82.7XXA
Ø2H[6K]33Z when reported with Secondary Diagnosis J95.811
Ø2H[67]3[JM]Z when reported with Secondary Diagnosis K68.11, T81.4XXA, T82.6XXA, or T82.7XXA
Ø2H[KL]3JZ when reported with Secondary Diagnosis K68.11, T81.4XXA, T82.6XXA, or T82.7XXA
Ø2HN[Ø34][JM]Z when reported with Secondary Diagnosis K68.11, T81.4XXA, T82.6XXA, or T82.7XXA

Coding Clinic: 2Ø13, Q3, P18 – Ø2HV33Z
Coding Clinic: 2Ø15, Q2, P32-33 – Ø2HK3DZ, Ø2HV33Z
Coding Clinic: 2Ø15, Q3, P35 – Ø2HP32Z
Coding Clinic: 2Ø17, Q4, P63; 2Ø15, Q4, P14, P28-32 – Ø2HV33Z
Coding Clinic: 2Ø16, Q2, P15 – Ø2H633Z
Coding Clinic: 2Ø17, Q1, P1Ø; 2Ø16, Q4, P81, 95, 137 – Ø2H
Coding Clinic: 2Ø17, Q1, P11-12; 2Ø16, Q4, P139 – Ø2HA3RS
Coding Clinic: 2Ø17, Q2, P25 – Ø2H633Z
Coding Clinic: 2Ø17, Q4, P44-45 – Ø2HA3E[JZ]
Coding Clinic: 2Ø17, Q4, P1Ø5 – Ø2H73DZ
Coding Clinic: 2Ø18, Q2, P19 – Ø2H63KZ
Coding Clinic: 2Ø19, Q1, P24 – Ø2HAØQZ
Coding Clinic: 2Ø19, Q3, P2Ø – Ø2HLØDZ
Coding Clinic: 2Ø19, Q3, P23 – Ø2HL3JZ
Coding Clinic: 2Ø19, Q4, P24 – Ø2H13DZ
Coding Clinic: 2Ø22, Q2, P25 – Ø2HK3JZ

SECTION: Ø MEDICAL AND SURGICAL
BODY SYSTEM: 2 HEART AND GREAT VESSELS
OPERATION: H INSERTION: *(continued)*

Putting in a nonbiological appliance that monitors, assists, performs, or prevents a physiological function but does not physically take the place of a body part

Body Part	Approach	Device	Qualifier
P Pulmonary Trunk Q Pulmonary Artery, Right R Pulmonary Artery, Left S Pulmonary Vein, Right T Pulmonary Vein, Left V Superior Vena Cava ~~W Thoracic Aorta, Descending~~	Ø Open 3 Percutaneous 4 Percutaneous Endoscopic	Ø Monitoring Device, Pressure Sensor 2 Monitoring Device 3 Infusion Device D Intraluminal Device Y Other Device	Z No Qualifier
W Thoracic Aorta, Descending	Ø Open 4 Percutaneous Endoscopic	Ø Monitoring Device, Pressure Sensor 2 Monitoring Device 3 Infusion Device D Intraluminal Device Y Other Device	Z No Qualifier
W Thoracic Aorta,	3 Percutaneous	Ø Monitoring Device, Pressure Sensor 2 Monitoring Device 3 Infusion Device D Intraluminal Device R Short-term External Heart Assist System Y Other Device	Z No Qualifier
X Thoracic Aorta, Ascending/Arch	Ø Open 3 Percutaneous 4 Percutaneous Endoscopic	Ø Monitoring Device, Pressure Sensor 2 Monitoring Device 3 Infusion Device D Intraluminal Device	Z No Qualifier

Non-OR Ø2HP[Ø34][Ø23]Z
Non-OR Ø2H[QR][Ø34][23]Z
Non-OR Ø2H[STV][Ø34]3Z
Non-OR Ø2H[STVW]32Z
Non-OR Ø2HW[Ø34][Ø3]Z
Ø2H[STV][34]3Z when reported with Secondary Diagnosis J95.811

SECTION: Ø MEDICAL AND SURGICAL
BODY SYSTEM: 2 HEART AND GREAT VESSELS
OPERATION: J INSPECTION: Visually and/or manually exploring a body part

Body Part	Approach	Device	Qualifier
A Heart Y Great Vessel	Ø Open 3 Percutaneous 4 Percutaneous Endoscopic	Z No Device	Z No Qualifier

Non-OR Ø2J[AY]3ZZ

Coding Clinic: 2015, Q3, P9 – Ø2JA3ZZ

SECTION: Ø MEDICAL AND SURGICAL
BODY SYSTEM: 2 HEART AND GREAT VESSELS
OPERATION: K MAP: Locating the route of passage of electrical impulses and/or locating functional areas in a body part

Body Part	Approach	Device	Qualifier
8 Conduction Mechanism	Ø Open 3 Percutaneous 4 Percutaneous Endoscopic	Z No Device	Z No Qualifier

DRG Non-OR Ø2K8[Ø34]ZZ

SECTION: 0 MEDICAL AND SURGICAL
BODY SYSTEM: 2 HEART AND GREAT VESSELS
OPERATION: L OCCLUSION: Completely closing an orifice or the lumen of a tubular body part

Body Part	Approach	Device	Qualifier
7 Atrium, Left	0 Open 3 Percutaneous 4 Percutaneous Endoscopic	C Extraluminal Device D Intraluminal Device Z No Device	K Left Atrial Appendage
H Pulmonary Valve P Pulmonary Trunk Q Pulmonary Artery, Right S Pulmonary Vein, Right T Pulmonary Vein, Left V Superior Vena Cava	0 Open 3 Percutaneous 4 Percutaneous Endoscopic	C Extraluminal Device D Intraluminal Device Z No Device	Z No Qualifier
R Pulmonary Artery, Left	0 Open 3 Percutaneous 4 Percutaneous Endoscopic	C Extraluminal Device D Intraluminal Device Z No Device	T Ductus Arteriosus Z No Qualifier
W Thoracic Aorta, Descending	0 Open 3 Percutaneous	D Intraluminal Device	J Temporary

DRG Non-OR 02L7[034][CDZ]K

Coding Clinic: 2015, Q4, P24 – 02LR0ZT

Coding Clinic: 2016, Q2, P26 – 02LS3DZ
Coding Clinic: 2016, Q4, P102, 104 – 02L
Coding Clinic: 2017, Q4, P34 – 02L[QS]3DZ

SECTION: 0 MEDICAL AND SURGICAL
BODY SYSTEM: 2 HEART AND GREAT VESSELS
OPERATION: N RELEASE: Freeing a body part from an abnormal physical constraint by cutting or by the use of force

Body Part	Approach	Device	Qualifier
0 Coronary Artery, One Artery 1 Coronary Artery, Two Arteries 2 Coronary Artery, Three Arteries 3 Coronary Artery, Four or More Arteries 4 Coronary Vein 5 Atrial Septum 6 Atrium, Right 7 Atrium, Left 8 Conduction Mechanism 9 Chordae Tendineae D Papillary Muscle F Aortic Valve G Mitral Valve H Pulmonary Valve J Tricuspid Valve K Ventricle, Right L Ventricle, Left M Ventricular Septum N Pericardium P Pulmonary Trunk Q Pulmonary Artery, Right R Pulmonary Artery, Left S Pulmonary Vein, Right T Pulmonary Vein, Left V Superior Vena Cava W Thoracic Aorta, Descending X Thoracic Aorta, Ascending/Arch	0 Open 3 Percutaneous 4 Percutaneous Endoscopic	Z No Device	Z No Qualifier

Coding Clinic: 2016, Q4, P81 – 02N

Coding Clinic: 2019, Q2, P14, 21 – 02N00ZZ

SECTION: Ø MEDICAL AND SURGICAL
BODY SYSTEM: 2 HEART AND GREAT VESSELS
OPERATION: P REMOVAL: Taking out or off a device from a body part

Body Part	Approach	Device	Qualifier
A Heart	Ø Open 3 Percutaneous 4 Percutaneous Endoscopic	2 Monitoring Device 3 Infusion Device 7 Autologous Tissue Substitute 8 Zooplastic Tissue C Extraluminal Device D Intraluminal Device J Synthetic Substitute K Nonautologous Tissue Substitute M Cardiac Lead N Intracardiac Pacemaker Q Implantable Heart Assist System Y Other Device	Z No Qualifier
A Heart	Ø Open 3 Percutaneous 4 Percutaneous Endoscopic	R Short-term External Heart Assist System	S Biventricular Z No Qualifier
A Heart	X External	2 Monitoring Device 3 Infusion Device D Intraluminal Device M Cardiac Lead	Z No Qualifier
W Thoracic Aorta, Descending	3 Percutaneous	R Short-term External Heart Assist System	Z No Qualifier
Y Great Vessel	Ø Open 3 Percutaneous 4 Percutaneous Endoscopic	2 Monitoring Device 3 Infusion Device 7 Autologous Tissue Substitute 8 Zooplastic Tissue C Extraluminal Device D Intraluminal Device J Synthetic Substitute K Nonautologous Tissue Substitute Y Other Device	Z No Qualifier
Y Great Vessel	X External	2 Monitoring Device 3 Infusion Device D Intraluminal Device	Z No Qualifier

Ø2PA[Ø34]RZ
Ø2PAXMZ
DRG Non-OR Ø2PAXMZ
Non-OR Ø2PAX[23DM]Z
Non-OR Ø2PA3[23D]Z
Non-OR Ø2PY3[23D]Z
Non-OR Ø2PYX[23D]Z
Ø2PA[Ø34]MZ when reported with Secondary Diagnosis K68.11, T81.4XXA, T82.6XXA, or T82.7XXA
Ø2PAXMZ when reported with Secondary Diagnosis K68.11, T81.4XXA, T82.6XXA, or T82.7XXA

Coding Clinic: 2015, Q3, P33 – Ø2PA3MZ
Coding Clinic: 2016, Q2, P15; 2015, Q4, P32 – Ø2PY33Z
Coding Clinic: 2016, Q3, P19 – Ø2PYX3Z
Coding Clinic: 2016, Q4, P95 – Ø2P
Coding Clinic: 2016, Q4, P97 – Ø2PA3NZ
Coding Clinic: 2018, Q4, P54; 2017, Q1, P11-21; 2016, Q4, P139 – Ø2PA3RZ
Coding Clinic: 2017, Q1, P14 – Ø2PAØRZ
Coding Clinic: 2017, Q2, P25 – Ø2PY33Z
Coding Clinic: 2017, Q4, P45, 105 – Ø2PA[DQ]Z
Coding Clinic: 2018, Q4, P85 – Ø2PY3JZ
Coding Clinic: 2019, Q1, P24 – Ø2PAØQZ
Coding Clinic: 2022, Q2, P25 – Ø2PA3MZ

SECTION: Ø MEDICAL AND SURGICAL
BODY SYSTEM: 2 HEART AND GREAT VESSELS
OPERATION: Q REPAIR: Restoring, to the extent possible, a body part to its normal anatomic structure and function

Body Part	Approach	Device	Qualifier
Ø Coronary Artery, One Artery 1 Coronary Artery, Two Arteries 2 Coronary Artery, Three Arteries 3 Coronary Artery, Four or More Arteries 4 Coronary Vein 5 Atrial Septum 6 Atrium, Right 7 Atrium, Left 8 Conduction Mechanism 9 Chordae Tendineae A Heart B Heart, Right C Heart, Left D Papillary Muscle H Pulmonary Valve K Ventricle, Right L Ventricle, Left M Ventricular Septum N Pericardium P Pulmonary Trunk Q Pulmonary Artery, Right R Pulmonary Artery, Left S Pulmonary Vein, Right T Pulmonary Vein, Left V Superior Vena Cava W Thoracic Aorta, Descending X Thoracic Aorta, Ascending/Arch	Ø Open 3 Percutaneous 4 Percutaneous Endoscopic	Z No Device	Z No Qualifier
F Aortic Valve	Ø Open 3 Percutaneous 4 Percutaneous Endoscopic	Z No Device	J Truncal Valve Z No Qualifier
G Mitral Valve	Ø Open 3 Percutaneous 4 Percutaneous Endoscopic	Z No Device	E Atrioventricular Valve, Left Z No Qualifier
J Tricuspid Valve	Ø Open 3 Percutaneous 4 Percutaneous Endoscopic	Z No Device	G Atrioventricular Valve, Right Z No Qualifier

Non-OR Ø2Q[WX][Ø34]ZZ

Coding Clinic: 2015, Q3, P16 – Ø2QWØZZ
Coding Clinic: 2015, Q4, P24 – Ø2Q5ØZZ
Coding Clinic: 2016, Q4, P81, 83, 1Ø2 – Ø2Q
Coding Clinic: 2016, Q4, P1Ø6 – Ø2QGØZE, Ø2QJØZG
Coding Clinic: 2016, Q4, P1Ø7 – Ø2QFØZJ
Coding Clinic: 2017, Q1Ø, P1Ø – Ø2Q[ST]ØZZ
Coding Clinic: 2021, Q3, P27 – Ø2Q[6V]ØZZ
Coding Clinic: 2022, Q1, P4Ø-41 – Ø2QAØZZ

SECTION: Ø MEDICAL AND SURGICAL
BODY SYSTEM: 2 HEART AND GREAT VESSELS
OPERATION: R REPLACEMENT: *(on multiple pages)*

Putting in or on biological or synthetic material that physically takes the place and/or function of all or a portion of a body part

Body Part	Approach	Device	Qualifier
5 Atrial Septum 6 Atrium, Right 7 Atrium, Left 9 Chordae Tendineae D Papillary Muscle K Ventricle, Right L Ventricle, Left M Ventricular Septum N Pericardium P Pulmonary Trunk Q Pulmonary Artery, Right R Pulmonary Artery, Left S Pulmonary Vein, Right T Pulmonary Vein, Left V Superior Vena Cava W Thoracic Aorta, Descending X Thoracic Aorta, Ascending/Arch	Ø Open 4 Percutaneous Endoscopic	7 Autologous Tissue Substitute 8 Zooplastic Tissue J Synthetic Substitute K Nonautologous Tissue Substitute	Z No Qualifier
A Heart	Ø Open	L Biologic with Synthetic Substitute, Autoregulated M Synthetic Substitute, Pneumatic	Z No Qualifier
F Aortic Valve	Ø Open 4 Percutaneous Endoscopic	7 Autologous Tissue Substitute J Synthetic Substitute K Nonautologous Tissue Substitute	Z No Qualifier
F Aortic Valve	Ø Open 4 Percutaneous Endoscopic	8 Zooplastic Tissue	N Rapid Deployment Technique Z No Qualifier
F Aortic Valve	3 Percutaneous	7 Autologous Tissue Substitute J Synthetic Substitute K Nonautologous Tissue Substitute	H Transapical Z No Qualifier
F Aortic Valve	3 Percutaneous	8 Zooplastic Tissue	H Transapical N Rapid Deployment Technique Z No Qualifier
G Mitral Valve J Tricuspid Valve	Ø Open 5 Percutaneous 6 Endoscopic	7 Autologous Tissue Substitute 8 Zooplastic Tissue J Synthetic Substitute K Nonautologous TissueSubstitute	Z No Qualifier
G Mitral Valve J Tricuspid Valve	3 Percutaneous	7 Autologous Tissue Substitute 8 Zooplastic Tissue J Synthetic Substitute K Nonautologous Tissue Substitute	H Transapical Z No Qualifier
H Pulmonary Valve	Ø Open 4 Percutaneous Endoscopic	7 Autologous Tissue Substitute 8 Zooplastic Tissue J Synthetic Substitute K Nonautologous Tissue Substitute	Z No Qualifier

Non-OR Ø2RF[Ø34]8N

Ø2R[KL]ØJZ when combined with ZØØ.6

Ø2R[KL]ØJZ

Coding Clinic: 2Ø16, Q3, P32 – Ø2RJ48Z

Coding Clinic: 2Ø16, Q4, P81 – Ø2R
Coding Clinic: 2Ø17, Q1, P13 – Ø2R[KL]ØJZ
Coding Clinic: 2Ø17, Q4, P56 – Ø2RJ3JZ
Coding Clinic: 2Ø19, Q1, P31 – Ø2RF38Z

SECTION: Ø MEDICAL AND SURGICAL
BODY SYSTEM: 2 HEART AND GREAT VESSELS
OPERATION: R REPLACEMENT: *(continued)*
Putting in or on biological or synthetic material that physically takes the place and/or function of all or a portion of a body part

Body Part	Approach	Device	Qualifier
H Pulmonary Valve	3 Percutaneous	7 Autologous Tissue Substitute 8 Zooplastic Tissue J Synthetic Substitute K Nonautologous Tissue Substitute	H Transapical Z No Qualifier
H Pulmonary Valve	3 Percutaneous	8 Zooplastic Tissue	H Transapical L In Existing Conduit M Native Site Z No Qualifier

Coding Clinic: 2019, Q3, P24 – Ø2RGØ8Z, Ø2RXØJZ
Coding Clinic: 2019, Q4, P24 – Ø2RF3JZ
Coding Clinic: 2020, Q1, P26 – Ø2RXØJZ

SECTION: Ø MEDICAL AND SURGICAL
BODY SYSTEM: 2 HEART AND GREAT VESSELS
OPERATION: S REPOSITION: Moving to its normal location, or other suitable location, all or a portion of a body part

Body Part	Approach	Device	Qualifier
Ø Coronary Artery, One Artery 1 Coronary Artery, Two Arteries P Pulmonary Trunk Q Pulmonary Artery, Right R Pulmonary Artery, Left S Pulmonary Vein, Right T Pulmonary Vein, Left V Superior Vena Cava W Thoracic Aorta, Descending X Thoracic Aorta, Ascending/Arch	Ø Open	Z No Device	Z No Qualifier

Coding Clinic: 2015, Q4, P24 – Ø2S[PW]ØZZ
Coding Clinic: 2016, Q4, P81, 83, 102 – Ø2S
Coding Clinic: 2016, Q4, P1Ø3-1Ø4 – Ø2S[1PX]ØZZ

SECTION: Ø MEDICAL AND SURGICAL
BODY SYSTEM: 2 HEART AND GREAT VESSELS
OPERATION: T RESECTION: Cutting out or off, without replacement, all of a body part

Body Part	Approach	Device	Qualifier
5 Atrial Septum 8 Conduction Mechanism 9 Chordae Tendineae D Papillary Muscle H Pulmonary Valve M Ventricular Septum N Pericardium	Ø Open 3 Percutaneous 4 Percutaneous Endoscopic	Z No Device	Z No Qualifier

SECTION: Ø MEDICAL AND SURGICAL

BODY SYSTEM: 2 HEART AND GREAT VESSELS

OPERATION: U SUPPLEMENT: Putting in or on biological or synthetic material that physically reinforces and/or augments the function of a portion of a body part

Body Part	Approach	Device	Qualifier
Ø Coronary Artery, One Artery 1 Coronary Artery, Two Arteries 2 Coronary Artery, Three Arteries 3 Coronary Artery, Four or More Arteries 5 Atrial Septum 6 Atrium, Right 7 Atrium, Left 9 Chordae Tendineae A Heart D Papillary Muscle H Pulmonary Valve K Ventricle, Right L Ventricle, Left M Ventricular Septum N Pericardium P Pulmonary Trunk Q Pulmonary Artery, Right R Pulmonary Artery, Left S Pulmonary Vein, Right T Pulmonary Vein, Left V Superior Vena Cava W Thoracic Aorta, Descending X Thoracic Aorta, Ascending/Arch	Ø Open 3 Percutaneous 4 Percutaneous Endoscopic	7 Autologous Tissue Substitute 8 Zooplastic Tissue J Synthetic Substitute K Nonautologous Tissue Substitute	Z No Qualifier
F Aortic Valve	Ø Open 3 Percutaneous 4 Percutaneous Endoscopic	7 Autologous Tissue Substitute 8 Zooplastic Tissue J Synthetic Substitute K Nonautologous Tissue Substitute	J Truncal Valve Z No Qualifier
G Mitral Valve	Ø Open 3 Percutaneous 4 Percutaneous Endoscopic	7 Autologous Tissue Substitute 8 Zooplastic Tissue J Synthetic Substitute K Nonautologous Tissue Substitute	E Atrioventricular Valve, Left Z No Qualifier
G Mitral Valve	Ø Open 4 Percutaneous Endoscopic	7 Autologous Tissue Substitute 8 Zooplastic Tissue J Synthetic Substitute K Nonautologous Tissue Substitute	E Atrioventricular Valve, Left Z No Qualifier
G Mitral Valve	3 Percutaneous	7 Autologous Tissue Substitute 8 Zooplastic Tissue K Nonautologous Tissue Substitute	E Atrioventricular Valve, Left Z No Qualifier
G Mitral Valve	3 Percutaneous	J Synthetic Substitute	E Atrioventricular Valve, Left H Transapical Z No Qualifier
J Tricuspid Valve	Ø Open 3 Percutaneous 4 Percutaneous Endoscopic	7 Autologous Tissue Substitute 8 Zooplastic Tissue J Synthetic Substitute K Nonautologous Tissue Substitute	G Atrioventricular Valve, Right Z No Qualifier

DRG Non-OR Ø2U7[34]JZ

Coding Clinic: 2Ø15, Q2, P24 – Ø2UGØJZ
Coding Clinic: 2Ø15, Q3, P17 – Ø2U[QR]ØKZ
Coding Clinic: 2Ø15, Q4, P23-25 – Ø2UFØ8Z, Ø2UMØJZ, Ø2UMØ8Z, Ø2UWØ7Z
Coding Clinic: 2Ø16, Q2, P24 – Ø2U[PR]Ø7Z
Coding Clinic: 2Ø16, Q2, P27 – Ø2UWØJZ
Coding Clinic: 2Ø16, Q4, P81, 1Ø2 – Ø2U
Coding Clinic: 2Ø16, Q4, P1Ø6 – Ø2UGØJE, Ø2UJØKG
Coding Clinic: 2Ø16, Q4, P1Ø7 – Ø2UMØ8Z, Ø2UFØKJ
Coding Clinic: 2Ø17, Q1, P2Ø – Ø2UXØKZ
Coding Clinic: 2Ø17, Q3, P7 - Ø2U[67]Ø7Z
Coding Clinic: 2Ø17, Q4, P36 - Ø2UGØ8Z
Coding Clinic: 2Ø19, Q4, P26 – Ø2UØ3JZ
Coding Clinic: 2Ø2Ø, Q1, P25 – Ø2UPØ8Z
Coding Clinic: 2Ø23, Q2, P21; 2Ø21, Q3, P28 – Ø2UG3JZ
Coding Clinic: 2Ø22, Q1, P38 – Ø2U73JZ, Ø2UAØ8Z

New/Revised Text in Green ~~deleted~~ Deleted ♀ Females Only ♂ Males Only **Coding Clinic**
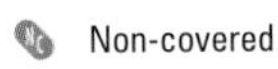 Non-covered 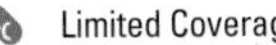 Limited Coverage ⊞ Combination (See Appendix E) DRG Non-OR Non-OR Hospital-Acquired Condition

SECTION: Ø MEDICAL AND SURGICAL
BODY SYSTEM: 2 HEART AND GREAT VESSELS
OPERATION: V RESTRICTION: Partially closing an orifice or the lumen of a tubular body part

Body Part	Approach	Device	Qualifier
A Heart	Ø Open 3 Percutaneous 4 Percutaneous Endoscopic	C Extraluminal Device Z No Device	Z No Qualifier
G Mitral Valve	Ø Open 3 Percutaneous 4 Percutaneous Endoscopic	Z No Device	Z No Qualifier
L Ventricle, Left P Pulmonary Trunk Q Pulmonary Artery, Right S Pulmonary Vein, Right T Pulmonary Vein, Left V Superior Vena Cava	Ø Open 3 Percutaneous 4 Percutaneous Endoscopic	C Extraluminal Device D Intraluminal Device Z No Device	Z No Qualifier
R Pulmonary Artery, Left	Ø Open 3 Percutaneous 4 Percutaneous Endoscopic	C Extraluminal Device D Intraluminal Device Z No Device	T Ductus Arteriosus Z No Qualifier
W Thoracic Aorta, Descending X Thoracic Aorta, Ascending/Arch	Ø Open 3 Percutaneous 4 Percutaneous Endoscopic	C Extraluminal Device D Intraluminal Device E Intraluminal Device, Branched or Fenestrated, One or Two Arteries F Intraluminal Device, Branched or Fenestrated, Three or More Arteries Z No Device	Z No Qualifier

Coding Clinic: 2Ø16, Q4, P81, 89 – Ø2V
Coding Clinic: 2Ø16, Q4, P93 – Ø2VW3DZ
Coding Clinic: 2Ø17, Q4, P36 – Ø2VGØZZ
Coding Clinic: 2Ø2Ø, Q1, P26 – Ø2VWØDZ
Coding Clinic: 2Ø21, Q4, P45 – Ø2VL3DZ

SECTION: Ø MEDICAL AND SURGICAL
BODY SYSTEM: 2 HEART AND GREAT VESSELS
OPERATION: W REVISION: *(on multiple pages)*

Correcting, to the extent possible, a portion of a malfunctioning device or the position of a displaced device

Body Part	Approach	Device	Qualifier
5 Atrial Septum M Ventricular Septum	Ø Open 4 Percutaneous Endoscopic	J Synthetic Substitute	Z No Qualifier
A Heart ⊞	Ø Open 3 Percutaneous 4 Percutaneous Endoscopic	2 Monitoring Device 3 Infusion Device 7 Autologous Tissue Substitute 8 Zooplastic Tissue C Extraluminal Device D Intraluminal Device J Synthetic Substitute K Nonautologous Tissue Substitute M Cardiac Lead N Intracardiac Pacemaker Q Implantable Heart Assist System Y Other Device	Z No Qualifier
A Heart	Ø Open 3 Percutaneous 4 Percutaneous Endoscopic	R Short-term External Heart Assist System	S Biventricular Z No Qualifier
A Heart	X External	2 Monitoring Device 3 Infusion Device 7 Autologous Tissue Substitute 8 Zooplastic Tissue C Extraluminal Device D Intraluminal Device J Synthetic Substitute K Nonautologous Tissue Substitute M Cardiac Lead N Intracardiac Pacemaker Q Implantable Heart Assist System	Z No Qualifier
A Heart	X External	R Short-term External Heart Assist System	S Biventricular Z No Qualifier
F Aortic Valve G Mitral Valve H Pulmonary Valve J Tricuspid Valve	Ø Open 3 Percutaneous 4 Percutaneous Endoscopic	7 Autologous Tissue Substitute 8 Zooplastic Tissue J Synthetic Substitute K Nonautologous Tissue Substitute	Z No Qualifier

⊞ Ø2WA[Ø34][QR]Z
Non-OR Ø2WAX[2378CDJKMQ]Z
Non-OR Ø2WAXRZ
Non-OR Ø2WA3[23D]Z
Ø2WA[Ø34]MZ when reported with Secondary Diagnosis K68.11, T81.4XXA, T82.6XXA, or T82.7XXA
Ø2WA[34]QZ

Coding Clinic: 2Ø15, Q3, P32 – Ø2WA3MZ
Coding Clinic: 2Ø16, Q4, P95 – Ø2W
Coding Clinic: 2Ø16, Q4, P96 – Ø2WA3NZ
Coding Clinic: 2Ø18, Q1, P17 – Ø2WAXRZ

SECTION: Ø MEDICAL AND SURGICAL
BODY SYSTEM: 2 HEART AND GREAT VESSELS
OPERATION: W REVISION: *(continued)*
Correcting, to the extent possible, a portion of a malfunctioning device or the position of a displaced device

Body Part	Approach	Device	Qualifier
W Thoracic Aorta, Descending	3 Percutaneous	R Short-term External Heart Assist System	Z No Qualifier
Y Great Vessel	Ø Open 3 Percutaneous 4 Percutaneous Endoscopic	2 Monitoring Device 3 Infusion Device 7 Autologous Tissue Substitute 8 Zooplastic Tissue C Extraluminal Device D Intraluminal Device J Synthetic Substitute K Nonautologous Tissue Substitute Y Other Device	Z No Qualifier
Y Great Vessel	X External	2 Monitoring Device 3 Infusion Device 7 Autologous Tissue Substitute 8 Zooplastic Tissue C Extraluminal Device D Intraluminal Device J Synthetic Substitute K Nonautologous Tissue Substitute	Z No Qualifier

Non-OR Ø2WY[3X][2378CDJK]Z

SECTION: Ø MEDICAL AND SURGICAL
BODY SYSTEM: 2 HEART AND GREAT VESSELS
OPERATION: Y TRANSPLANTATION: Putting in or on all or a portion of a living body part taken from another individual or animal to physically take the place and/or function of all or a portion of a similar body part

Body Part	Approach	Device	Qualifier
A Heart	Ø Open	Z No Device	Ø Allogeneic 1 Syngeneic 2 Zooplastic

Ø2YAØZ[Ø12]

Coding Clinic: 2013, Q3, P19 – Ø2YAØZØ

SECTION: Ø MEDICAL AND SURGICAL
BODY SYSTEM: 3 UPPER ARTERIES
OPERATION: 1 BYPASS: *(on multiple pages)*
Altering the route of passage of the contents of a tubular body part

Body Part	Approach	Device	Qualifier
2 Innominate Artery	Ø Open	9 Autologous Venous Tissue A Autologous Arterial Tissue J Synthetic Substitute K Nonautologous Tissue Substitute Z No Device	Ø Upper Arm Artery, Right 1 Upper Arm Artery, Left 2 Upper Arm Artery, Bilateral 3 Lower Arm Artery, Right 4 Lower Arm Artery, Left 5 Lower Arm Artery, Bilateral 6 Upper Leg Artery, Right 7 Upper Leg Artery, Left 8 Upper Leg Artery, Bilateral 9 Lower Leg Artery, Right B Lower Leg Artery, Left C Lower Leg Artery, Bilateral D Upper Arm Vein F Lower Arm Vein J Extracranial Artery, Right K Extracranial Artery, Left W Lower Extremity Vein
3 Subclavian Artery, Right 4 Subclavian Artery, Left	Ø Open	9 Autologous Venous Tissue A Autologous Arterial Tissue J Synthetic Substitute K Nonautologous Tissue Substitute Z No Device	Ø Upper Arm Artery, Right 1 Upper Arm Artery, Left 2 Upper Arm Artery, Bilateral 3 Lower Arm Artery, Right 4 Lower Arm Artery, Left 5 Lower Arm Artery, Bilateral 6 Upper Leg Artery, Right 7 Upper Leg Artery, Left 8 Upper Leg Artery, Bilateral 9 Lower Leg Artery, Right B Lower Leg Artery, Left C Lower Leg Artery, Bilateral D Upper Arm Vein F Lower Arm Vein J Extracranial Artery, Right K Extracranial Artery, Left M Pulmonary Artery, Right N Pulmonary Artery, Left W Lower Extremity Vein
5 Axillary Artery, Right 6 Axillary Artery, Left	Ø Open	9 Autologous Venous Tissue A Autologous Arterial Tissue J Synthetic Substitute K Nonautologous Tissue Substitute Z No Device	Ø Upper Arm Artery, Right 1 Upper Arm Artery, Left 2 Upper Arm Artery, Bilateral 3 Lower Arm Artery, Right 4 Lower Arm Artery, Left 5 Lower Arm Artery, Bilateral 6 Upper Leg Artery, Right 7 Upper Leg Artery, Left 8 Upper Leg Artery, Bilateral 9 Lower Leg Artery, Right B Lower Leg Artery, Left C Lower Leg Artery, Bilateral D Upper Arm Vein F Lower Arm Vein J Extracranial Artery, Right K Extracranial Artery, Left T Abdominal Artery V Superior Vena Cava W Lower Extremity Vein

Coding Clinic: 2Ø16, Q3, P38 – Ø318ØJD

SECTION: Ø MEDICAL AND SURGICAL
BODY SYSTEM: 3 UPPER ARTERIES
OPERATION: 1 BYPASS: *(continued)*
Altering the route of passage of the contents of a tubular body part

Body Part	Approach	Device	Qualifier
7 Brachial Artery, Right	Ø Open	9 Autologous Venous Tissue A Autologous Arterial Tissue J Synthetic Substitute K Nonautologous Tissue Substitute Z No Device	Ø Upper Arm Artery, Right 3 Lower Arm Artery, Right D Upper Arm Vein F Lower Arm Vein V Superior Vena Cava W Lower Extremity Vein
7 Brachial Artery, Right	3 Percutaneous	Z No Device	F Lower Arm Vein
8 Brachial Artery, Left	Ø Open	9 Autologous Venous Tissue A Autologous Arterial Tissue J Synthetic Substitute K Nonautologous Tissue Substitute Z No Device	1 Upper Arm Artery, Left 4 Lower Arm Artery, Left D Upper Arm Vein F Lower Arm Vein V Superior Vena Cava W Lower Extremity Vein
8 Brachial Artery, Left	3 Percutaneous	Z No Device	F Lower Arm Vein
9 Ulnar Artery, Right B Radial Artery, Right	Ø Open	9 Autologous Venous Tissue A Autologous Arterial Tissue J Synthetic Substitute K Nonautologous Tissue Substitute Z No Device	3 Lower Arm Artery, Right F Lower Arm Vein
9 Ulnar Artery, Right B Radial Artery, Right	3 Percutaneous	Z No Device	F Lower Arm Vein
A Ulnar Artery, Left C Radial Artery, Left	Ø Open	9 Autologous Venous Tissue A Autologous Arterial Tissue J Synthetic Substitute K Nonautologous Tissue Substitute Z No Device	4 Lower Arm Artery, Left F Lower Arm Vein
A Ulnar Artery, Left C Radial Artery, Left	3 Percutaneous	Z No Device	F Lower Arm Vein
G Intracranial Artery S Temporal Artery, Right T Temporal Artery, Left	Ø Open	9 Autologous Venous Tissue A Autologous Arterial Tissue J Synthetic Substitute K Nonautologous Tissue Substitute Z No Device	G Intracranial Artery
H Common Carotid Artery, Right J Common Carotid Artery, Left	Ø Open	9 Autologous Venous Tissue A Autologous Arterial Tissue J Synthetic Substitute K Nonautologous Tissue Substitute Z No Device	G Intracranial Artery J Extracranial Artery, Right K Extracranial Artery, Left Y Upper Artery
K Internal Carotid Artery, Right L Internal Carotid Artery, Left M External Carotid Artery, Right N External Carotid Artery, Left	Ø Open	9 Autologous Venous Tissue A Autologous Arterial Tissue J Synthetic Substitute K Nonautologous Tissue Substitute Z No Device	J Extracranial Artery, Right K Extracranial Artery, Left

Non-OR Ø31[789ABCGHJ]Ø[9AJKZ][Ø134DFGJK]
Coding Clinic: 2Ø13, Q1, P228 – Ø31CØZF
Coding Clinic: 2Ø17, Q2, P22 – Ø31JØZK
Coding Clinic: 2Ø17, Q4, P65 – Ø31JØJJ
Coding Clinic: 2Ø21, Q3, P15 – Ø317ØKF.

SECTION: Ø MEDICAL AND SURGICAL
BODY SYSTEM: 3 UPPER ARTERIES
OPERATION: 5 DESTRUCTION: Physical eradication of all or a portion of a body part by the direct use of energy, force, or a destructive agent

Body Part	Approach	Device	Qualifier
Ø Internal Mammary Artery, Right 1 Internal Mammary Artery, Left 2 Innominate Artery 3 Subclavian Artery, Right 4 Subclavian Artery, Left 5 Axillary Artery, Right 6 Axillary Artery, Left 7 Brachial Artery, Right 8 Brachial Artery, Left 9 Ulnar Artery, Right A Ulnar Artery, Left B Radial Artery, Right C Radial Artery, Left D Hand Artery, Right F Hand Artery, Left G Intracranial Artery H Common Carotid Artery, Right J Common Carotid Artery, Left K Internal Carotid Artery, Right L Internal Carotid Artery, Left M External Carotid Artery, Right N External Carotid Artery, Left P Vertebral Artery, Right Q Vertebral Artery, Left R Face Artery S Temporal Artery, Right T Temporal Artery, Left U Thyroid Artery, Right V Thyroid Artery, Left Y Upper Artery	Ø Open 3 Percutaneous 4 Percutaneous Endoscopic	Z No Device	Z No Qualifier

SECTION: Ø MEDICAL AND SURGICAL
BODY SYSTEM: 3 UPPER ARTERIES
OPERATION: 7 DILATION: Expanding an orifice or the lumen of a tubular body part

Body Part	Approach	Device	Qualifier
Ø Internal Mammary Artery, Right 1 Internal Mammary Artery, Left 2 Innominate Artery 3 Subclavian Artery, Right 4 Subclavian Artery, Left 5 Axillary Artery, Right 6 Axillary Artery, Left 7 Brachial Artery, Right 8 Brachial Artery, Left 9 Ulnar Artery, Right A Ulnar Artery, Left B Radial Artery, Right C Radial Artery, Left	Ø Open 3 Percutaneous 4 Percutaneous Endoscopic	4 Intraluminal Device, Drug-eluting 5 Intraluminal Device, Drug-eluting, Two 6 Intraluminal Device, Drug-eluting, Three 7 Intraluminal Device, Drug-eluting, Four or More E Intraluminal Device, Two F Intraluminal Device, Three G Intraluminal Device, Four or More	Z No Qualifier
Ø Internal Mammary Artery, Right 1 Internal Mammary Artery, Left 2 Innominate Artery 3 Subclavian Artery, Right 4 Subclavian Artery, Left 5 Axillary Artery, Right 6 Axillary Artery, Left 7 Brachial Artery, Right 8 Brachial Artery, Left 9 Ulnar Artery, Right A Ulnar Artery, Left B Radial Artery, Right C Radial Artery, Left	Ø Open 3 Percutaneous 4 Percutaneous Endoscopic	D Intraluminal Device Z No Device	1 Drug-Coated Balloon Z No Qualifier
D Hand Artery, Right F Hand Artery, Left G Intracranial Artery H Common Carotid Artery, Right J Common Carotid Artery, Left K Internal Carotid Artery, Right L Internal Carotid Artery, Left M External Carotid Artery, Right N External Carotid Artery, Left P Vertebral Artery, Right Q Vertebral Artery, Left R Face Artery S Temporal Artery, Right T Temporal Artery, Left U Thyroid Artery, Right V Thyroid Artery, Left Y Upper Artery	Ø Open 3 Percutaneous 4 Percutaneous Endoscopic	4 Intraluminal Device, Drug-eluting 5 Intraluminal Device, Drug-eluting, Two 6 Intraluminal Device, Drug-eluting, Three 7 Intraluminal Device, Drug-eluting, Four or More D Intraluminal Device E Intraluminal Device, Two F Intraluminal Device, Three G Intraluminal Device, Four or More Z No Device	Z No Qualifier

Ø37G[34]Z[6Z]

Coding Clinic: 2Ø16, Q4, P87 – Ø37
Coding Clinic: 2Ø19, Q3, P3Ø – Ø37K3DZ

SECTION: Ø MEDICAL AND SURGICAL
BODY SYSTEM: 3 UPPER ARTERIES
OPERATION: 9 DRAINAGE: *(on multiple pages)*
Taking or letting out fluids and/or gases from a body part

Body Part	Approach	Device	Qualifier
Ø Internal Mammary Artery, Right 1 Internal Mammary Artery, Left 2 Innominate Artery 3 Subclavian Artery, Right 4 Subclavian Artery, Left 5 Axillary Artery, Right 6 Axillary Artery, Left 7 Brachial Artery, Right 8 Brachial Artery, Left 9 Ulnar Artery, Right A Ulnar Artery, Left B Radial Artery, Right C Radial Artery, Left D Hand Artery, Right F Hand Artery, Left G Intracranial Artery H Common Carotid Artery, Right J Common Carotid Artery, Left K Internal Carotid Artery, Right L Internal Carotid Artery, Left M External Carotid Artery, Right N External Carotid Artery, Left P Vertebral Artery, Right Q Vertebral Artery, Left R Face Artery S Temporal Artery, Right T Temporal Artery, Left U Thyroid Artery, Right V Thyroid Artery, Left Y Upper Artery	Ø Open 3 Percutaneous 4 Percutaneous Endoscopic	Ø Drainage Device	Z No Qualifier

Non-OR Ø39[Ø123456789ABCDFGHJKLMNPQRSTUVY][Ø34]ØZ

SECTION: Ø MEDICAL AND SURGICAL
BODY SYSTEM: 3 UPPER ARTERIES
OPERATION: 9 DRAINAGE: *(continued)*

Taking or letting out fluids and/or gases from a body part

Body Part	Approach	Device	Qualifier
Ø Internal Mammary Artery, Right 1 Internal Mammary Artery, Left 2 Innominate Artery 3 Subclavian Artery, Right 4 Subclavian Artery, Left 5 Axillary Artery, Right 6 Axillary Artery, Left 7 Brachial Artery, Right 8 Brachial Artery, Left 9 Ulnar Artery, Right A Ulnar Artery, Left B Radial Artery, Right C Radial Artery, Left D Hand Artery, Right F Hand Artery, Left G Intracranial Artery H Common Carotid Artery, Right J Common Carotid Artery, Left K Internal Carotid Artery, Right L Internal Carotid Artery, Left M External Carotid Artery, Right N External Carotid Artery, Left P Vertebral Artery, Right Q Vertebral Artery, Left R Face Artery S Temporal Artery, Right T Temporal Artery, Left U Thyroid Artery, Right V Thyroid Artery, Left Y Upper Artery	Ø Open 3 Percutaneous 4 Percutaneous Endoscopic	Z No Device	X Diagnostic Z No Qualifier

Non-OR Ø39[Ø123456789ABCDFGHJKLMNPQRSTUVY][Ø34]Z[3XZ]

SECTION: Ø MEDICAL AND SURGICAL
BODY SYSTEM: 3 UPPER ARTERIES
OPERATION: B EXCISION: Cutting out or off, without replacement, a portion of a body part

Body Part	Approach	Device	Qualifier
Ø Internal Mammary Artery, Right 1 Internal Mammary Artery, Left 2 Innominate Artery 3 Subclavian Artery, Right 4 Subclavian Artery, Left 5 Axillary Artery, Right 6 Axillary Artery, Left 7 Brachial Artery, Right 8 Brachial Artery, Left 9 Ulnar Artery, Right A Ulnar Artery, Left B Radial Artery, Right C Radial Artery, Left D Hand Artery, Right F Hand Artery, Left G Intracranial Artery H Common Carotid Artery, Right J Common Carotid Artery, Left K Internal Carotid Artery, Right L Internal Carotid Artery, Left M External Carotid Artery, Right N External Carotid Artery, Left P Vertebral Artery, Right Q Vertebral Artery, Left R Face Artery S Temporal Artery, Right T Temporal Artery, Left U Thyroid Artery, Right V Thyroid Artery, Left Y Upper Artery	Ø Open 3 Percutaneous 4 Percutaneous Endoscopic	Z No Device	X Diagnostic Z No Qualifier

Coding Clinic: 2Ø16, Q2, P13 – Ø3BNØZZ

SECTION: Ø MEDICAL AND SURGICAL
BODY SYSTEM: 3 UPPER ARTERIES
OPERATION: C EXTIRPATION: Taking or cutting out solid matter from a body part

Body Part	Approach	Device	Qualifier
Ø Internal Mammary Artery, Right 1 Internal Mammary Artery, Left 2 Innominate Artery 3 Subclavian Artery, Right 4 Subclavian Artery, Left 5 Axillary Artery, Right 6 Axillary Artery, Left 7 Brachial Artery, Right 8 Brachial Artery, Left 9 Ulnar Artery, Right A Ulnar Artery, Left B Radial Artery, Right C Radial Artery, Left D Hand Artery, Right F Hand Artery, Left R Face Artery S Temporal Artery, Right T Temporal Artery, Left U Thyroid Artery, Right V Thyroid Artery, Left Y Upper Artery	Ø Open 3 Percutaneous 4 Percutaneous Endoscopic	Z No Device	Z No Qualifier
G Intracranial Artery H Common Carotid Artery, Right J Common Carotid Artery, Left K Internal Carotid Artery, Right L Internal Carotid Artery, Left M External Carotid Artery, Right N External Carotid Artery, Left P Vertebral Artery, Right Q Vertebral Artery, Left	Ø Open 4 Percutaneous Endoscopic	Z No Device	Z No Qualifier
G Intracranial Artery H Common Carotid Artery, Right J Common Carotid Artery, Left K Internal Carotid Artery, Right L Internal Carotid Artery, Left M External Carotid Artery, Right N External Carotid Artery, Left P Vertebral Artery, Right Q Vertebral Artery, Left	3 Percutaneous	Z No Device	7 Stent Retriever Z No Qualifier

Coding Clinic: 2Ø16, Q2, P12 – Ø3CKØZZ
Coding Clinic: 2Ø16, Q4, P87 – Ø3C
Coding Clinic: 2Ø17, Q4, P65 – Ø3CNØZZ
Coding Clinic: 2Ø21, Q2, P13 – Ø3CLØZZ
Coding Clinic: 2Ø22, Q1, P43 – Ø3CG3ZZ

SECTION: Ø MEDICAL AND SURGICAL
BODY SYSTEM: 3 UPPER ARTERIES
OPERATION: F FRAGMENTATION: Breaking solid matter in a body part into pieces

Body Part	Approach	Device	Qualifier
2 Innominate Artery 3 Subclavian Artery, Right 4 Subclavian Artery, Left 5 Axillary Artery, Right 6 Axillary Artery, Left 7 Brachial Artery, Right 8 Brachial Artery, Left 9 Ulnar Artery, Right A Ulnar Artery, Left B Radial Artery, Right C Radial Artery, Left G Intracranial Artery Y Upper Artery	3 Percutaneous	Z No Device	Ø Ultrasonic Z No Qualifier

SECTION: Ø MEDICAL AND SURGICAL
BODY SYSTEM: 3 UPPER ARTERIES
OPERATION: H INSERTION: Putting in a nonbiological appliance that monitors, assists, performs, or prevents a physiological function but does not physically take the place of a body part

Body Part	Approach	Device	Qualifier
Ø Internal Mammary Artery, Right 1 Internal Mammary Artery, Left 2 Innominate Artery 3 Subclavian Artery, Right 4 Subclavian Artery, Left 5 Axillary Artery, Right 6 Axillary Artery, Left 7 Brachial Artery, Right 8 Brachial Artery, Left 9 Ulnar Artery, Right A Ulnar Artery, Left B Radial Artery, Right C Radial Artery, Left D Hand Artery, Right F Hand Artery, Left G Intracranial Artery H Common Carotid Artery, Right J Common Carotid Artery, Left M External Carotid Artery, Right N External Carotid Artery, Left P Vertebral Artery, Right Q Vertebral Artery, Left R Face Artery S Temporal Artery, Right T Temporal Artery, Left U Thyroid Artery, Right V Thyroid Artery, Left	Ø Open 3 Percutaneous 4 Percutaneous Endoscopic	3 Infusion Device D Intraluminal Device	Z No Qualifier
K Internal Carotid Artery, Right L Internal Carotid Artery, Left	Ø Open 3 Percutaneous 4 Percutaneous Endoscopic	3 Infusion Device D Intraluminal Device M Stimulator Lead	Z No Qualifier
Y Upper Artery	Ø Open 3 Percutaneous 4 Percutaneous Endoscopic	2 Monitoring Device 3 Infusion Device D Intraluminal Device Y Other Device	Z No Qualifier

Non-OR Ø3H[Ø123456789ABCDFGHJMNPQRSTUV][Ø34]3Z
Non-OR Ø3H[KL][Ø34]3Z
Non-OR Ø3HY[Ø34]3Z
Non-OR Ø3HY32Z

Coding Clinic: 2Ø16, Q2, P32 – Ø3HY32Z
Coding Clinic: 2Ø2Ø, Q1, P27 – ØHRU7Z

SECTION: Ø MEDICAL AND SURGICAL
BODY SYSTEM: 3 UPPER ARTERIES
OPERATION: J INSPECTION: Visually and/or manually exploring a body part

Body Part	Approach	Device	Qualifier
Y Upper Artery	Ø Open 3 Percutaneous 4 Percutaneous Endoscopic X External	Z No Device	Z No Qualifier

Non-OR Ø3JY[34X]ZZ

Coding Clinic: 2Ø15, Q1, P29 – Ø3JYØZZ
Coding Clinic: 2Ø21, Q1, P17 – Ø3JY3ZZ

SECTION: Ø MEDICAL AND SURGICAL
BODY SYSTEM: 3 UPPER ARTERIES
OPERATION: L OCCLUSION: Completely closing an orifice or the lumen of a tubular body part

Body Part	Approach	Device	Qualifier
Ø Internal Mammary Artery, Right 1 Internal Mammary Artery, Left 2 Innominate Artery 3 Subclavian Artery, Right 4 Subclavian Artery, Left 5 Axillary Artery, Right 6 Axillary Artery, Left 7 Brachial Artery, Right 8 Brachial Artery, Left 9 Ulnar Artery, Right A Ulnar Artery, Left B Radial Artery, Right C Radial Artery, Left D Hand Artery, Right F Hand Artery, Left R Face Artery S Temporal Artery, Right T Temporal Artery, Left U Thyroid Artery, Right V Thyroid Artery, Left Y Upper Artery	Ø Open 3 Percutaneous 4 Percutaneous Endoscopic	C Extraluminal Device D Intraluminal Device Z No Device	Z No Qualifier
G Intracranial Artery H Common Carotid Artery, Right J Common Carotid Artery, Left K Internal Carotid Artery, Right L Internal Carotid Artery, Left M External Carotid Artery, Right N External Carotid Artery, Left P Vertebral Artery, Right Q Vertebral Artery, Left	Ø Open 3 Percutaneous 4 Percutaneous Endoscopic	B Intraluminal Device, Bioactive C Extraluminal Device D Intraluminal Device Z No Device	Z No Qualifier

Coding Clinic: 2Ø16, Q2, P3Ø – Ø3LGØCZ
Coding Clinic: 2Ø21, Q2, P13 – Ø3LLØZZ

SECTION: Ø MEDICAL AND SURGICAL
BODY SYSTEM: 3 UPPER ARTERIES
OPERATION: N RELEASE: Freeing a body part from an abnormal physical constraint by cutting or by the use of force

Body Part	Approach	Device	Qualifier
Ø Internal Mammary Artery, Right 1 Internal Mammary Artery, Left 2 Innominate Artery 3 Subclavian Artery, Right 4 Subclavian Artery, Left 5 Axillary Artery, Right 6 Axillary Artery, Left 7 Brachial Artery, Right 8 Brachial Artery, Left 9 Ulnar Artery, Right A Ulnar Artery, Left B Radial Artery, Right C Radial Artery, Left D Hand Artery, Right F Hand Artery, Left G Intracranial Artery H Common Carotid Artery, Right J Common Carotid Artery, Left K Internal Carotid Artery, Right L Internal Carotid Artery, Left M External Carotid Artery, Right N External Carotid Artery, Left P Vertebral Artery, Right Q Vertebral Artery, Left R Face Artery S Temporal Artery, Right T Temporal Artery, Left U Thyroid Artery, Right V Thyroid Artery, Left Y Upper Artery	Ø Open 3 Percutaneous 4 Percutaneous Endoscopic	Z No Device	Z No Qualifier

SECTION: Ø MEDICAL AND SURGICAL
BODY SYSTEM: 3 UPPER ARTERIES
OPERATION: P REMOVAL: Taking out or off a device from a body part

Body Part	Approach	Device	Qualifier
Y Upper Artery	Ø Open 3 Percutaneous 4 Percutaneous Endoscopic	Ø Drainage Device 2 Monitoring Device 3 Infusion Device 7 Autologous Tissue Substitute C Extraluminal Device D Intraluminal Device J Synthetic Substitute K Nonautologous Tissue Substitute M Stimulator Lead Y Other Device	Z No Qualifier
Y Upper Artery	X External	Ø Drainage Device 2 Monitoring Device 3 Infusion Device D Intraluminal Device M Stimulator Lead	Z No Qualifier

Non-OR Ø3PY3[Ø23D]Z

Non-OR Ø3PYX[Ø23DM]Z

SECTION: Ø MEDICAL AND SURGICAL
BODY SYSTEM: 3 UPPER ARTERIES
OPERATION: Q REPAIR: Restoring, to the extent possible, a body part to its normal anatomic structure and function

Body Part	Approach	Device	Qualifier
Ø Internal Mammary Artery, Right 1 Internal Mammary Artery, Left 2 Innominate Artery 3 Subclavian Artery, Right 4 Subclavian Artery, Left 5 Axillary Artery, Right 6 Axillary Artery, Left 7 Brachial Artery, Right 8 Brachial Artery, Left 9 Ulnar Artery, Right A Ulnar Artery, Left B Radial Artery, Right C Radial Artery, Left D Hand Artery, Right F Hand Artery, Left G Intracranial Artery H Common Carotid Artery, Right J Common Carotid Artery, Left K Internal Carotid Artery, Right L Internal Carotid Artery, Left M External Carotid Artery, Right N External Carotid Artery, Left P Vertebral Artery, Right Q Vertebral Artery, Left R Face Artery S Temporal Artery, Right T Temporal Artery, Left U Thyroid Artery, Right V Thyroid Artery, Left Y Upper Artery	Ø Open 3 Percutaneous 4 Percutaneous Endoscopic	Z No Device	Z No Qualifier

Coding Clinic: 2Ø17, Q1, P32 – Ø3QHØZZ

SECTION: Ø MEDICAL AND SURGICAL
BODY SYSTEM: 3 UPPER ARTERIES
OPERATION: R REPLACEMENT: Putting in or on biological or synthetic material that physically takes the place and/or function of all or a portion of a body part

Body Part	Approach	Device	Qualifier
Ø Internal Mammary Artery, Right 1 Internal Mammary Artery, Left 2 Innominate Artery 3 Subclavian Artery, Right 4 Subclavian Artery, Left 5 Axillary Artery, Right 6 Axillary Artery, Left 7 Brachial Artery, Right 8 Brachial Artery, Left 9 Ulnar Artery, Right A Ulnar Artery, Left B Radial Artery, Right C Radial Artery, Left D Hand Artery, Right F Hand Artery, Left G Intracranial Artery H Common Carotid Artery, Right J Common Carotid Artery, Left K Internal Carotid Artery, Right L Internal Carotid Artery, Left M External Carotid Artery, Right N External Carotid Artery, Left P Vertebral Artery, Right Q Vertebral Artery, Left R Face Artery S Temporal Artery, Right T Temporal Artery, Left U Thyroid Artery, Right V Thyroid Artery, Left Y Upper Artery	Ø Open 4 Percutaneous Endoscopic	7 Autologous Tissue Substitute J Synthetic Substitute K Nonautologous Tissue Substitute	Z No Qualifier

SECTION: Ø MEDICAL AND SURGICAL
BODY SYSTEM: 3 UPPER ARTERIES
OPERATION: S REPOSITION: Moving to its normal location, or other suitable location, all or a portion of a body part

Body Part	Approach	Device	Qualifier
Ø Internal Mammary Artery, Right 1 Internal Mammary Artery, Left 2 Innominate Artery 3 Subclavian Artery, Right 4 Subclavian Artery, Left 5 Axillary Artery, Right 6 Axillary Artery, Left 7 Brachial Artery, Right 8 Brachial Artery, Left 9 Ulnar Artery, Right A Ulnar Artery, Left B Radial Artery, Right C Radial Artery, Left D Hand Artery, Right F Hand Artery, Left G Intracranial Artery H Common Carotid Artery, Right J Common Carotid Artery, Left K Internal Carotid Artery, Right L Internal Carotid Artery, Left M External Carotid Artery, Right N External Carotid Artery, Left P Vertebral Artery, Right Q Vertebral Artery, Left R Face Artery S Temporal Artery, Right T Temporal Artery, Left U Thyroid Artery, Right V Thyroid Artery, Left Y Upper Artery	Ø Open 3 Percutaneous 4 Percutaneous Endoscopic	Z No Device	Z No Qualifier

Coding Clinic: 2Ø15, Q3, P28 – Ø3SSØZZ

SECTION: Ø MEDICAL AND SURGICAL
BODY SYSTEM: 3 UPPER ARTERIES
OPERATION: U SUPPLEMENT: Putting in or on biological or synthetic material that physically reinforces and/or augments the function of a portion of a body part

Body Part	Approach	Device	Qualifier
Ø Internal Mammary Artery, Right 1 Internal Mammary Artery, Left 2 Innominate Artery 3 Subclavian Artery, Right 4 Subclavian Artery, Left 5 Axillary Artery, Right 6 Axillary Artery, Left 7 Brachial Artery, Right 8 Brachial Artery, Left 9 Ulnar Artery, Right A Ulnar Artery, Left B Radial Artery, Right C Radial Artery, Left D Hand Artery, Right F Hand Artery, Left G Intracranial Artery H Common Carotid Artery, Right J Common Carotid Artery, Left K Internal Carotid Artery, Right L Internal Carotid Artery, Left M External Carotid Artery, Right N External Carotid Artery, Left P Vertebral Artery, Right Q Vertebral Artery, Left R Face Artery S Temporal Artery, Right T Temporal Artery, Left U Thyroid Artery, Right V Thyroid Artery, Left Y Upper Artery	Ø Open 3 Percutaneous 4 Percutaneous Endoscopic	7 Autologous Tissue Substitute J Synthetic Substitute K Nonautologous Tissue Substitute	Z No Qualifier

Coding Clinic: 2Ø16, Q2, P12 – Ø3UKØJZ

SECTION: Ø MEDICAL AND SURGICAL
BODY SYSTEM: 3 UPPER ARTERIES
OPERATION: V RESTRICTION: Partially closing an orifice or the lumen of a tubular body part

Body Part	Approach	Device	Qualifier
Ø Internal Mammary Artery, Right 1 Internal Mammary Artery, Left 2 Innominate Artery 3 Subclavian Artery, Right 4 Subclavian Artery, Left 5 Axillary Artery, Right 6 Axillary Artery, Left 7 Brachial Artery, Right 8 Brachial Artery, Left 9 Ulnar Artery, Right A Ulnar Artery, Left B Radial Artery, Right C Radial Artery, Left D Hand Artery, Right F Hand Artery, Left R Face Artery S Temporal Artery, Right T Temporal Artery, Left U Thyroid Artery, Right V Thyroid Artery, Left Y Upper Artery	Ø Open 3 Percutaneous 4 Percutaneous Endoscopic	C Extraluminal Device D Intraluminal Device Z No Device	Z No Qualifier
G Intracranial Artery H Common Carotid Artery, Right J Common Carotid Artery, Left K Internal Carotid Artery, Right L Internal Carotid Artery, Left M External Carotid Artery, Right N External Carotid Artery, Left P Vertebral Artery, Right Q Vertebral Artery, Left	Ø Open 3 Percutaneous 4 Percutaneous Endoscopic	B Intraluminal Device, Bioactive C Extraluminal Device D Intraluminal Device H Intraluminal Device, Flow Diverter Z No Device	Z No Qualifier

Coding Clinic: 2Ø16, Q1, P2Ø – Ø3VG3DZ
Coding Clinic: 2Ø16, Q4, P26 – Ø3VM3DZ
Coding Clinic: 2Ø19, Q1, P22 – Ø3VGØCZ
Coding Clinic: 2Ø23, Q1, P35 – Ø3VK3[DH]Z

SECTION: Ø MEDICAL AND SURGICAL
BODY SYSTEM: 3 UPPER ARTERIES
OPERATION: W REVISION: Correcting, to the extent possible, a portion of a malfunctioning device or the position of a displaced device

Body Part	Approach	Device	Qualifier
Y Upper Artery	Ø Open 3 Percutaneous 4 Percutaneous Endoscopic	Ø Drainage Device 2 Monitoring Device 3 Infusion Device 7 Autologous Tissue Substitute C Extraluminal Device D Intraluminal Device J Synthetic Substitute K Nonautologous Tissue Substitute M Stimulator Lead Y Other Device	Z No Qualifier
Y Upper Artery	X External	Ø Drainage Device 2 Monitoring Device 3 Infusion Device 7 Autologous Tissue Substitute C Extraluminal Device D Intraluminal Device J Synthetic Substitute K Nonautologous Tissue Substitute M Stimulator Lead	Z No Qualifier

Non-OR Ø3WY3[Ø23D]Z
Non-OR Ø3WYX[Ø237CDJKM]Z

Coding Clinic: 2Ø15, Q1, P33 – ØØWY3DZ
Coding Clinic: 2Ø16, Q3, P4Ø – Ø3WYØJZ

New/Revised Text in Green ~~deleted~~ Deleted ♀ Females Only ♂ Males Only Coding Clinic
Non-covered Limited Coverage Combination (See Appendix E) DRG Non-OR Non-OR Hospital-Acquired Condition

SECTION: Ø MEDICAL AND SURGICAL
BODY SYSTEM: 4 LOWER ARTERIES
OPERATION: 1 BYPASS: *(on multiple pages)*
Altering the route of passage of the contents of a tubular body part

Body Part	Approach	Device	Qualifier
Ø Abdominal Aorta C Common Iliac Artery, Right D Common Iliac Artery, Left	Ø Open 4 Percutaneous Endoscopic	9 Autologous Venous Tissue A Autologous Arterial Tissue J Synthetic Substitute K Nonautologous Tissue Substitute Z No Device	Ø Abdominal Aorta 1 Celiac Artery 2 Mesenteric Artery 3 Renal Artery, Right 4 Renal Artery, Left 5 Renal Artery, Bilateral 6 Common Iliac Artery, Right 7 Common Iliac Artery, Left 8 Common Iliac Arteries, Bilateral 9 Internal Iliac Artery, Right B Internal Iliac Artery, Left C Internal Iliac Arteries, Bilateral D External Iliac Artery, Right F External Iliac Artery, Left G External Iliac Arteries, Bilateral H Femoral Artery, Right J Femoral Artery, Left K Femoral Arteries, Bilateral Q Lower Extremity Artery R Lower Artery
3 Hepatic Artery 4 Splenic Artery	Ø Open 4 Percutaneous Endoscopic	9 Autologous Venous Tissue A Autologous Arterial Tissue J Synthetic Substitute K Nonautologous Tissue Substitute Z No Device	3 Renal Artery, Right 4 Renal Artery, Left 5 Renal Artery, Bilateral
E Internal Iliac Artery, Right F Internal Iliac Artery, Left H External Iliac Artery, Right J External Iliac Artery, Left	Ø Open 4 Percutaneous Endoscopic	9 Autologous Venous Tissue A Autologous Arterial Tissue J Synthetic Substitute K Nonautologous Tissue Substitute Z No Device	9 Internal Iliac Artery, Right B Internal Iliac Artery, Left C Internal Iliac Arteries, Bilateral D External Iliac Artery, Right F External Iliac Artery, Left G External Iliac Arteries, Bilateral H Femoral Artery, Right J Femoral Artery, Left K Femoral Arteries, Bilateral P Foot Artery Q Lower Extremity Artery
K Femoral Artery, Right L Femoral Artery, Left	Ø Open 4 Percutaneous Endoscopic	9 Autologous Venous Tissue A Autologous Arterial Tissue J Synthetic Substitute K Nonautologous Tissue Substitute Z No Device	H Femoral Artery, Right J Femoral Artery, Left K Femoral Arteries, Bilateral L Popliteal Artery M Peroneal Artery N Posterior Tibial Artery P Foot Artery Q Lower Extremity Artery S Lower Extremity Vein
K Femoral Artery, Right L Femoral Artery, Left	3 Percutaneous	J Synthetic Substitute	Q Lower Extremity Artery S Lower Extremity Vein
M Popliteal Artery, Right N Popliteal Artery, Left	Ø Open 4 Percutaneous Endoscopic	9 Autologous Venous Tissue A Autologous Arterial Tissue J Synthetic Substitute K Nonautologous Tissue Substitute Z No Device	L Popliteal Artery M Peroneal Artery P Foot Artery Q Lower Extremity Artery S Lower Extremity Vein

Coding Clinic: 2Ø15, Q3, P28 – Ø41ØØZ3, Ø414ØZ4
Coding Clinic: 2Ø16, Q2, P19 – Ø41KØJN
Coding Clinic: 2Ø17, Q3, P6 – Ø41KØ9N, Ø41KØJN
Coding Clinic: 2Ø17, Q3, P16 – Ø41CØJ[25]
Coding Clinic: 2Ø17, Q4, P47 – Ø41[34]ØZ[34]
Coding Clinic: 2Ø22, Q3, P6 – Ø41ØØJH

SECTION: Ø MEDICAL AND SURGICAL
BODY SYSTEM: 4 LOWER ARTERIES
OPERATION: 1 BYPASS: *(continued)*
Altering the route of passage of the contents of a tubular body part

Body Part	Approach	Device	Qualifier
M Popliteal Artery, Right N Popliteal Artery, Left	3 Percutaneous	J Synthetic Substitute	Q Lower Extremity Artery S Lower Extremity Vein
P Anterior Tibial Artery, Right Q Anterior Tibial Artery, Left R Posterior Tibial Artery, Right S Posterior Tibial Artery, Left	Ø Open 3 Percutaneous 4 Percutaneous Endoscopic	J Synthetic Substitute	Q Lower Extremity Artery S Lower Extremity Vein
T Peroneal Artery, Right U Peroneal Artery, Left V Foot Artery, Right W Foot Artery, Left	Ø Open 4 Percutaneous Endoscopic	9 Autologous Venous Tissue A Autologous Arterial Tissue J Synthetic Substitute K Nonautologous Tissue Substitute Z No Device	P Foot Artery Q Lower Extremity Artery S Lower Extremity Vein
T Peroneal Artery, Right U Peroneal Artery, Left V Foot Artery, Right W Foot Artery, Left	3 Percutaneous	J Synthetic Substitute	Q Lower Extremity Artery S Lower Extremity Vein

Coding Clinic: 2Ø17, Q1, P33 – Ø41MØ9P

SECTION: Ø MEDICAL AND SURGICAL
BODY SYSTEM: 4 LOWER ARTERIES
OPERATION: 5 DESTRUCTION: Physical eradication of all or a portion of a body part by the direct use of energy, force, or a destructive agent

Body Part	Approach	Device	Qualifier
Ø Abdominal Aorta 1 Celiac Artery 2 Gastric Artery 3 Hepatic Artery 4 Splenic Artery 5 Superior Mesenteric Artery 6 Colic Artery, Right 7 Colic Artery, Left 8 Colic Artery, Middle 9 Renal Artery, Right A Renal Artery, Left B Inferior Mesenteric Artery C Common Iliac Artery, Right D Common Iliac Artery, Left E Internal Iliac Artery, Right F Internal Iliac Artery, Left H External Iliac Artery, Right J External Iliac Artery, Left K Femoral Artery, Right L Femoral Artery, Left M Popliteal Artery, Right N Popliteal Artery, Left P Anterior Tibial Artery, Right Q Anterior Tibial Artery, Left R Posterior Tibial Artery, Right S Posterior Tibial Artery, Left T Peroneal Artery, Right U Peroneal Artery, Left V Foot Artery, Right W Foot Artery, Left Y Lower Artery	Ø Open 3 Percutaneous 4 Percutaneous Endoscopic	Z No Device	Z No Qualifier

SECTION: Ø MEDICAL AND SURGICAL
BODY SYSTEM: 4 LOWER ARTERIES
OPERATION: 7 DILATION: *(on multiple pages)*
Expanding an orifice or the lumen of a tubular body part

Body Part	Approach	Device	Qualifier
Ø Abdominal Aorta 1 Celiac Artery 2 Gastric Artery 3 Hepatic Artery 4 Splenic Artery 5 Superior Mesenteric Artery 6 Colic Artery, Right 7 Colic Artery, Left 8 Colic Artery, Middle 9 Renal Artery, Right A Renal Artery, Left B Inferior Mesenteric Artery C Common Iliac Artery, Right D Common Iliac Artery, Left E Internal Iliac Artery, Right F Internal Iliac Artery, Left H External Iliac Artery, Right J External Iliac Artery, Left K Femoral Carotid Artery, Right L Femoral Carotid Artery, Left M Popliteal Carotid Artery, Right N Popliteal Carotid Artery, Left P Anterior Tibial Artery, Right Q Anterior Tibial Artery, Left R Posterior Tibial Artery, Right S Posterior Tibial Artery, Left T Peroneal Artery, Right U Peroneal Artery, Left V Foot Artery, Right W Foot Artery, Left Y Lower Artery	Ø Open 3 Percutaneous 4 Percutaneous Endoscopic	4 Intraluminal Device, Drug-eluting D Intraluminal Device Z No Device	1 Drug-Coated Balloon Z No Qualifier

Non-OR Ø47[59A]4DZ

Coding Clinic: 2Ø15, Q4, P7 – Ø47K3D1
Coding Clinic: 2Ø15, Q4, P15 – Ø47K3D1, Ø47L3Z1
Coding Clinic: 2Ø16, Q3, P39 – Ø47C3DZ
Coding Clinic: 2Ø16, Q4, P87 – Ø47
Coding Clinic: 2Ø16, Q4, P89 – Ø47K3Z6

SECTION: Ø MEDICAL AND SURGICAL
BODY SYSTEM: 4 LOWER ARTERIES
OPERATION: 7 DILATION: *(continued)*
Expanding an orifice or the lumen of a tubular body part

Body Part	Approach	Device	Qualifier
Ø Abdominal Aorta 1 Celiac Artery 2 Gastric Artery 3 Hepatic Artery 4 Splenic Artery 5 Superior Mesenteric Artery 6 Colic Artery, Right 7 Colic Artery, Left 8 Colic Artery, Middle 9 Renal Artery, Right A Renal Artery, Left B Inferior Mesenteric Artery C Common Iliac Artery, Right D Common Iliac Artery, Left E Internal Iliac Artery, Right F Internal Iliac Artery, Left H External Iliac Artery, Right J External Iliac Artery, Left K Femoral Carotid Artery, Right L Femoral Carotid Artery, Left M Popliteal Carotid Artery, Right N Popliteal Carotid Artery, Left P Anterior Tibial Artery, Right Q Anterior Tibial Artery, Left R Posterior Tibial Artery, Right S Posterior Tibial Artery, Left T Peroneal Artery, Right U Peroneal Artery, Left V Foot Artery, Right W Foot Artery, Left Y Lower Artery	Ø Open 3 Percutaneous 4 Percutaneous Endoscopic	5 Intraluminal Device, Drug-eluting, Two 6 Intraluminal Device, Drug-eluting, Three 7 Intraluminal Device, Drug-eluting, Four or More E Intraluminal Device, Two F Intraluminal Device, Three G Intraluminal Device, Four or More	Z No Qualifier

SECTION: Ø MEDICAL AND SURGICAL
BODY SYSTEM: 4 LOWER ARTERIES
OPERATION: 9 DRAINAGE: *(on multiple pages)*
Taking or letting out fluids and/or gases from a body part

Body Part	Approach	Device	Qualifier
Ø Abdominal Aorta 1 Celiac Artery 2 Gastric Artery 3 Hepatic Artery 4 Splenic Artery 5 Superior Mesenteric Artery 6 Colic Artery, Right 7 Colic Artery, Left 8 Colic Artery, Middle 9 Renal Artery, Right A Renal Artery, Left B Inferior Mesenteric Artery C Common Iliac Artery, Right D Common Iliac Artery, Left E Internal Iliac Artery, Right F Internal Iliac Artery, Left H External Iliac Artery, Right J External Iliac Artery, Left K Femoral Artery, Right L Femoral Artery, Left M Popliteal Artery, Right N Popliteal Artery, Left P Anterior Tibial Artery, Right Q Anterior Tibial Artery, Left R Posterior Tibial Artery, Right S Posterior Tibial Artery, Left T Peroneal Artery, Right U Peroneal Artery, Left V Foot Artery, Right W Foot Artery, Left Y Lower Artery	Ø Open 3 Percutaneous 4 Percutaneous Endoscopic	Ø Drainage Device	Z No Qualifier

Non-OR Ø49[Ø123456789ABCDEFHJKLMNPQRSTUVWY][Ø34]ØZ

SECTION: Ø MEDICAL AND SURGICAL
BODY SYSTEM: 4 LOWER ARTERIES
OPERATION: 9 DRAINAGE: *(continued)*
Taking or letting out fluids and/or gases from a body part

Body Part	Approach	Device	Qualifier
Ø Abdominal Aorta 1 Celiac Artery 2 Gastric Artery 3 Hepatic Artery 4 Splenic Artery 5 Superior Mesenteric Artery 6 Colic Artery, Right 7 Colic Artery, Left 8 Colic Artery, Middle 9 Renal Artery, Right A Renal Artery, Left B Inferior Mesenteric Artery C Common Iliac Artery, Right D Common Iliac Artery, Left E Internal Iliac Artery, Right F Internal Iliac Artery, Left H External Iliac Artery, Right J External Iliac Artery, Left K Femoral Artery, Right L Femoral Artery, Left M Popliteal Artery, Right N Popliteal Artery, Left P Anterior Tibial Artery, Right Q Anterior Tibial Artery, Left R Posterior Tibial Artery, Right S Posterior Tibial Artery, Left T Peroneal Artery, Right U Peroneal Artery, Left V Foot Artery, Right W Foot Artery, Left Y Lower Artery	Ø Open 3 Percutaneous 4 Percutaneous Endoscopic	Z No Device	X Diagnostic Z No Qualifier

Non-OR Ø49[Ø123456789ABCDEFHJKLMNPQRSTUVWY][Ø34]Z[XZ]

SECTION: Ø MEDICAL AND SURGICAL

BODY SYSTEM: 4 LOWER ARTERIES

OPERATION: B EXCISION: Cutting out or off, without replacement, a portion of a body part

Body Part	Approach	Device	Qualifier
Ø Abdominal Aorta 1 Celiac Artery 2 Gastric Artery 3 Hepatic Artery 4 Splenic Artery 5 Superior Mesenteric Artery 6 Colic Artery, Right 7 Colic Artery, Left 8 Colic Artery, Middle 9 Renal Artery, Right A Renal Artery, Left B Inferior Mesenteric Artery C Common Iliac Artery, Right D Common Iliac Artery, Left E Internal Iliac Artery, Right F Internal Iliac Artery, Left H External Iliac Artery, Right J External Iliac Artery, Left K Femoral Artery, Right L Femoral Artery, Left M Popliteal Artery, Right N Popliteal Artery, Left P Anterior Tibial Artery, Right Q Anterior Tibial Artery, Left R Posterior Tibial Artery, Right S Posterior Tibial Artery, Left T Peroneal Artery, Right U Peroneal Artery, Left V Foot Artery, Right W Foot Artery, Left Y Lower Artery	Ø Open 3 Percutaneous 4 Percutaneous Endoscopic	Z No Device	X Diagnostic Z No Qualifier

SECTION: Ø MEDICAL AND SURGICAL
BODY SYSTEM: 4 LOWER ARTERIES
OPERATION: C EXTIRPATION: Taking or cutting out solid matter from a body part

Body Part	Approach	Device	Qualifier
Ø Abdominal Aorta 1 Celiac Artery 2 Gastric Artery 3 Hepatic Artery 4 Splenic Artery 5 Superior Mesenteric Artery 6 Colic Artery, Right 7 Colic Artery, Left 8 Colic Artery, Middle 9 Renal Artery, Right A Renal Artery, Left B Inferior Mesenteric Artery C Common Iliac Artery, Right D Common Iliac Artery, Left E Internal Iliac Artery, Right F Internal Iliac Artery, Left H External Iliac Artery, Right J External Iliac Artery, Left K Femoral Artery, Right L Femoral Artery, Left M Popliteal Artery, Right N Popliteal Artery, Left P Anterior Tibial Artery, Right Q Anterior Tibial Artery, Left R Posterior Tibial Artery, Right S Posterior Tibial Artery, Left T Peroneal Artery, Right U Peroneal Artery, Left V Foot Artery, Right W Foot Artery, Left Y Lower Artery	Ø Open 3 Percutaneous 4 Percutaneous Endoscopic	Z No Device	Z No Qualifier

Coding Clinic: 2Ø15, Q1, P36 – Ø4CL3ZZ
Coding Clinic: 2Ø21, Q1, P15; 2Ø16, Q1, P31 – Ø4CJØZZ
Coding Clinic: 2Ø16, Q4, P89 – Ø4CK3Z6
Coding Clinic: 2Ø21, Q1, P16 – Ø4CHØZZ

SECTION: Ø MEDICAL AND SURGICAL
BODY SYSTEM: 4 LOWER ARTERIES
OPERATION: F FRAGMENTATION: Breaking solid matter in a body part into pieces

Body Part	Approach	Device	Qualifier
C Common Iliac Artery, Right D Common Iliac Artery, Left E Internal Iliac Artery, Right F Internal Iliac Artery, Left H External Iliac Artery, Right J External Iliac Artery, Left K Femoral Artery, Right L Femoral Artery, Left M Popliteal Artery, Right N Popliteal Artery, Left P Anterior Tibial Artery, Right Q Anterior Tibial Artery, Left R Posterior Tibial Artery, Right S Posterior Tibial Artery, Left T Peroneal Artery, Right U Peroneal Artery, Left Y Lower Artery	3 Percutaneous	Z No Device	Ø Ultrasonic Z No Qualifier

SECTION: Ø MEDICAL AND SURGICAL
BODY SYSTEM: 4 LOWER ARTERIES
OPERATION: H INSERTION: Putting in a nonbiological appliance that monitors, assists, performs, or prevents a physiological function but does not physically take the place of a body part

Body Part	Approach	Device	Qualifier
Ø Abdominal Aorta	Ø Open 3 Percutaneous 4 Percutaneous Endoscopic	2 Monitoring Device 3 Infusion Device D Intraluminal Device	Z No Qualifier
1 Celiac Artery 2 Gastric Artery 3 Hepatic Artery 4 Splenic Artery 5 Superior Mesenteric Artery 6 Colic Artery, Right 7 Colic Artery, Left 8 Colic Artery, Middle 9 Renal Artery, Right A Renal Artery, Left B Inferior Mesenteric Artery C Common Iliac Artery, Right D Common Iliac Artery, Left E Internal Iliac Artery, Right F Internal Iliac Artery, Left H External Iliac Artery, Right J External Iliac Artery, Left K Femoral Artery, Right L Femoral Artery, Left M Popliteal Artery, Right N Popliteal Artery, Left P Anterior Tibial Artery, Right Q Anterior Tibial Artery, Left R Posterior Tibial Artery, Right S Posterior Tibial Artery, Left T Peroneal Artery, Right U Peroneal Artery, Left V Foot Artery, Right W Foot Artery, Left	Ø Open 3 Percutaneous 4 Percutaneous Endoscopic	3 Infusion Device D Intraluminal Device	Z No Qualifier
Y Lower Artery	Ø Open 3 Percutaneous 4 Percutaneous Endoscopic	2 Monitoring Device 3 Infusion Device D Intraluminal Device Y Other Device	Z No Qualifier

DRG Non-OR Ø4HY32Z
Non-OR Ø4HØ[Ø34][23]Z
Non-OR Ø4H[123456789ABCDEFHJKLMNPQRSTUVW][Ø34]3Z
Non-OR Ø4HY[Ø34]3Z

Coding Clinic: 2Ø17, Q1, P21 – Ø4HY32Z
Coding Clinic: 2Ø19, Q1, P23 – Ø4H1[59A]3DZ
Coding Clinic: 2Ø19, Q3, P21 – Ø4HY33Z
Coding Clinic: 2Ø22, Q3, P2Ø – Ø4HØ3DZ

SECTION: Ø MEDICAL AND SURGICAL
BODY SYSTEM: 4 LOWER ARTERIES
OPERATION: J INSPECTION: Visually and/or manually exploring a body part

Body Part	Approach	Device	Qualifier
Y Lower Artery	Ø Open 3 Percutaneous 4 Percutaneous Endoscopic X External	Z No Device	Z No Qualifier

Non-OR Ø4JY[34X]ZZ

Coding Clinic: 2Ø22, Q4, P56 – Ø4JY3ZZ

SECTION: Ø MEDICAL AND SURGICAL
BODY SYSTEM: 4 LOWER ARTERIES
OPERATION: L OCCLUSION: Completely closing an orifice or the lumen of a tubular body part

Body Part	Approach	Device	Qualifier
Ø Abdominal Aorta	~~Ø Open~~ 4 Percutaneous Endoscopic	C Extraluminal Device D Intraluminal Device Z No Device	Z No Qualifier
Ø Abdominal Aorta	Ø Open 3 Percutaneous	C Extraluminal Device Z No Device	Z No Qualifier
Ø Abdominal Aorta	Ø Open 3 Percutaneous	D Intraluminal Device	J Temporary Z No Qualifier
1 Celiac Artery 2 Gastric Artery 3 Hepatic Artery 4 Splenic Artery 5 Superior Mesenteric Artery 6 Colic Artery, Right 7 Colic Artery, Left 8 Colic Artery, Middle 9 Renal Artery, Right A Renal Artery, Left B Inferior Mesenteric Artery C Common Iliac Artery, Right D Common Iliac Artery, Left H External Iliac Artery, Right J External Iliac Artery, Left K Femoral Artery, Right L Femoral Artery, Left M Popliteal Artery, Right N Popliteal Artery, Left P Anterior Tibial Artery, Right Q Anterior Tibial Artery, Left R Posterior Tibial Artery, Right S Posterior Tibial Artery, Left T Peroneal Artery, Right U Peroneal Artery, Left V Foot Artery, Right W Foot Artery, Left Y Lower Artery	Ø Open 3 Percutaneous 4 Percutaneous Endoscopic	C Extraluminal Device D Intraluminal Device Z No Device	Z No Qualifier
E Internal Iliac Artery, Right	Ø Open 3 Percutaneous 4 Percutaneous Endoscopic	C Extraluminal Device D Intraluminal Device Z No Device	T Uterine Artery, Right ♀ V Prostatic Artery, Right ♂ Z No Qualifier
F Internal Iliac Artery, Left	Ø Open 3 Percutaneous 4 Percutaneous Endoscopic	C Extraluminal Device D Intraluminal Device Z No Device	U Uterine Artery, Left ♀ W Prostatic Artery, Left ♂ Z No Qualifier

Non-OR Ø4L23DZ
Non-OR Ø4L[EF][CDZ]V

Coding Clinic: 2Ø15, Q2, P27 – Ø4LE3DT
Coding Clinic: 2Ø18, Q2, P18 – Ø4L[HJ]ØCZ
Coding Clinic: 2Ø22, Q4, P56 – Ø4LE3DV

SECTION: Ø MEDICAL AND SURGICAL
BODY SYSTEM: 4 LOWER ARTERIES
OPERATION: N RELEASE: Freeing a body part from an abnormal physical constraint by cutting or by the use of force

Body Part	Approach	Device	Qualifier
Ø Abdominal Aorta 1 Celiac Artery 2 Gastric Artery 3 Hepatic Artery 4 Splenic Artery 5 Superior Mesenteric Artery 6 Colic Artery, Right 7 Colic Artery, Left 8 Colic Artery, Middle 9 Renal Artery, Right A Renal Artery, Left B Inferior Mesenteric Artery C Common Iliac Artery, Right D Common Iliac Artery, Left E Internal Iliac Artery, Right F Internal Iliac Artery, Left H External Iliac Artery, Right J External Iliac Artery, Left K Femoral Artery, Right L Femoral Artery, Left M Popliteal Artery, Right N Popliteal Artery, Left P Anterior Tibial Artery, Right Q Anterior Tibial Artery, Left R Posterior Tibial Artery, Right S Posterior Tibial Artery, Left T Peroneal Artery, Right U Peroneal Artery, Left V Foot Artery, Right W Foot Artery, Left Y Lower Artery	Ø Open 3 Percutaneous 4 Percutaneous Endoscopic	Z No Device	Z No Qualifier

Coding Clinic: 2Ø15, Q2, P28 – Ø4N1ØZZ

SECTION: Ø MEDICAL AND SURGICAL
BODY SYSTEM: 4 LOWER ARTERIES
OPERATION: P REMOVAL: Taking out or off a device from a body part

Body Part	Approach	Device	Qualifier
Y Lower Artery	Ø Open 3 Percutaneous 4 Percutaneous Endoscopic	Ø Drainage Device 2 Monitoring Device 3 Infusion Device 7 Autologous Tissue Substitute C Extraluminal Device D Intraluminal Device J Synthetic Substitute K Nonautologous Tissue Substitute Y Other Device	Z No Qualifier
Y Lower Artery	X External	Ø Drainage Device 1 Radioactive Element 2 Monitoring Device 3 Infusion Device D Intraluminal Device	Z No Qualifier

Non-OR Ø4PYX[Ø123D]Z

Coding Clinic: 2Ø19, Q3, P21 – Ø4PY33Z

SECTION: Ø MEDICAL AND SURGICAL
BODY SYSTEM: 4 LOWER ARTERIES
OPERATION: Q REPAIR: Restoring, to the extent possible, a body part to its normal anatomic structure and function

Body Part	Approach	Device	Qualifier
Ø Abdominal Aorta 1 Celiac Artery 2 Gastric Artery 3 Hepatic Artery 4 Splenic Artery 5 Superior Mesenteric Artery 6 Colic Artery, Right 7 Colic Artery, Left 8 Colic Artery, Middle 9 Renal Artery, Right A Renal Artery, Left B Inferior Mesenteric Artery C Common Iliac Artery, Right D Common Iliac Artery, Left E Internal Iliac Artery, Right F Internal Iliac Artery, Left H External Iliac Artery, Right J External Iliac Artery, Left K Femoral Artery, Right L Femoral Artery, Left M Popliteal Artery, Right N Popliteal Artery, Left P Anterior Tibial Artery, Right Q Anterior Tibial Artery, Left R Posterior Tibial Artery, Right S Posterior Tibial Artery, Left T Peroneal Artery, Right U Peroneal Artery, Left V Foot Artery, Right W Foot Artery, Left Y Lower Artery	Ø Open 3 Percutaneous 4 Percutaneous Endoscopic	Z No Device	Z No Qualifier

SECTION: Ø MEDICAL AND SURGICAL
BODY SYSTEM: 4 LOWER ARTERIES
OPERATION: R REPLACEMENT: Putting in or on biological or synthetic material that physically takes the place and/or function of all or a portion of a body part

Body Part	Approach	Device	Qualifier
Ø Abdominal Aorta 1 Celiac Artery 2 Gastric Artery 3 Hepatic Artery 4 Splenic Artery 5 Superior Mesenteric Artery 6 Colic Artery, Right 7 Colic Artery, Left 8 Colic Artery, Middle 9 Renal Artery, Right A Renal Artery, Left B Inferior Mesenteric Artery C Common Iliac Artery, Right D Common Iliac Artery, Left E Internal Iliac Artery, Right F Internal Iliac Artery, Left H External Iliac Artery, Right J External Iliac Artery, Left K Femoral Artery, Right L Femoral Artery, Left M Popliteal Artery, Right N Popliteal Artery, Left P Anterior Tibial Artery, Right Q Anterior Tibial Artery, Left R Posterior Tibial Artery, Right S Posterior Tibial Artery, Left T Peroneal Artery, Right U Peroneal Artery, Left V Foot Artery, Right W Foot Artery, Left Y Lower Artery	Ø Open 4 Percutaneous Endoscopic	7 Autologous Tissue Substitute J Synthetic Substitute K Nonautologous Tissue Substitute	Z No Qualifier

Coding Clinic: 2Ø15, Q2, P28 – Ø4R1ØJZ
Coding Clinic: 2Ø22, Q3, P5 – Ø4R[ØD]ØJZ

SECTION: Ø MEDICAL AND SURGICAL
BODY SYSTEM: 4 LOWER ARTERIES
OPERATION: S REPOSITION: Moving to its normal location, or other suitable location, all or a portion of a body part

Body Part	Approach	Device	Qualifier
Ø Abdominal Aorta 1 Celiac Artery 2 Gastric Artery 3 Hepatic Artery 4 Splenic Artery 5 Superior Mesenteric Artery 6 Colic Artery, Right 7 Colic Artery, Left 8 Colic Artery, Middle 9 Renal Artery, Right A Renal Artery, Left B Inferior Mesenteric Artery C Common Iliac Artery, Right D Common Iliac Artery, Left E Internal Iliac Artery, Right F Internal Iliac Artery, Left H External Iliac Artery, Right J External Iliac Artery, Left K Femoral Artery, Right L Femoral Artery, Left M Popliteal Artery, Right N Popliteal Artery, Left P Anterior Tibial Artery, Right Q Anterior Tibial Artery, Left R Posterior Tibial Artery, Right S Posterior Tibial Artery, Left T Peroneal Artery, Right U Peroneal Artery, Left V Foot Artery, Right W Foot Artery, Left Y Lower Artery	Ø Open 3 Percutaneous 4 Percutaneous Endoscopic	Z No Device	Z No Qualifier

SECTION: Ø MEDICAL AND SURGICAL
BODY SYSTEM: 4 LOWER ARTERIES
OPERATION: U SUPPLEMENT: Putting in or on biological or synthetic material that physically reinforces and/or augments the function of a portion of a body part

Body Part	Approach	Device	Qualifier
Ø Abdominal Aorta 1 Celiac Artery 2 Gastric Artery 3 Hepatic Artery 4 Splenic Artery 5 Superior Mesenteric Artery 6 Colic Artery, Right 7 Colic Artery, Left 8 Colic Artery, Middle 9 Renal Artery, Right A Renal Artery, Left B Inferior Mesenteric Artery C Common Iliac Artery, Right D Common Iliac Artery, Left E Internal Iliac Artery, Right F Internal Iliac Artery, Left H External Iliac Artery, Right J External Iliac Artery, Left K Femoral Artery, Right L Femoral Artery, Left M Popliteal Artery, Right N Popliteal Artery, Left P Anterior Tibial Artery, Right Q Anterior Tibial Artery, Left R Posterior Tibial Artery, Right S Posterior Tibial Artery, Left T Peroneal Artery, Right U Peroneal Artery, Left V Foot Artery, Right W Foot Artery, Left Y Lower Artery	Ø Open 3 Percutaneous 4 Percutaneous Endoscopic	7 Autologous Tissue Substitute J Synthetic Substitute K Nonautologous Tissue Substitute	Z No Qualifier

Coding Clinic: 2Ø16, Q1, P31 – Ø4UJØKZ
Coding Clinic: 2Ø16, Q2, P19 – Ø4URØ7Z

SECTION: Ø MEDICAL AND SURGICAL
BODY SYSTEM: 4 LOWER ARTERIES
OPERATION: V RESTRICTION: Partially closing an orifice or the lumen of a tubular body part

Body Part	Approach	Device	Qualifier
Ø Abdominal Aorta	Ø Open 3 Percutaneous 4 Percutaneous Endoscopic	C Extraluminal Device E Intraluminal Device, Branched or Fenestrated, One or Two Arteries F Intraluminal Device, Branched or Fenestrated, Three or More Arteries Z No Device	Z No Qualifier
Ø Abdominal Aorta	Ø Open 3 Percutaneous 4 Percutaneous Endoscopic	D Intraluminal Device	J Temporary Z No Qualifier
1 Celiac Artery 2 Gastric Artery 3 Hepatic Artery 4 Splenic Artery 5 Superior Mesenteric Artery 6 Colic Artery, Right 7 Colic Artery, Left 8 Colic Artery, Middle 9 Renal Artery, Right A Renal Artery, Left B Inferior Mesenteric Artery E Internal Iliac Artery, Right F Internal Iliac Artery, Left H External Iliac Artery, Right J External Iliac Artery, Left K Femoral Artery, Right L Femoral Artery, Left M Popliteal Artery, Right N Popliteal Artery, Left P Anterior Tibial Artery, Right Q Anterior Tibial Artery, Left R Posterior Tibial Artery, Right S Posterior Tibial Artery, Left T Peroneal Artery, Right U Peroneal Artery, Left V Foot Artery, Right W Foot Artery, Left Y Lower Artery	Ø Open 3 Percutaneous 4 Percutaneous Endoscopic	C Extraluminal Device D Intraluminal Device Z No Device	Z No Qualifier
C Common Iliac Artery, Right D Common Iliac Artery, Left	Ø Open 3 Percutaneous 4 Percutaneous Endoscopic	C Extraluminal Device D Intraluminal Device E Intraluminal Device, Branched or Fenestrated, One or Two Arteries F Intraluminal Device, Branched or Fenestrated, Three or More Arteries Z No Device	Z No Qualifier

Non-OR Ø4V[CDY][Ø34][Ø23F]Z

Coding Clinic: 2Ø16, Q3, P39 – Ø4VØ3DZ
Coding Clinic: 2Ø16, Q4, P87, 89-9Ø – Ø4V
Coding Clinic: 2Ø16, Q4, P91 – Ø4VØ3E6
Coding Clinic: 2Ø16, Q4, P93-94 – Ø4VØ3F6
Coding Clinic: 2Ø16, Q4, P94 – Ø4V[CD]3EZ
Coding Clinic: 2Ø19, Q1, P22 – Ø4VØØDZ
Coding Clinic: 2Ø21, Q3, P23 – Ø4V43DZ

SECTION: Ø MEDICAL AND SURGICAL
BODY SYSTEM: 4 LOWER ARTERIES
OPERATION: W REVISION: Correcting, to the extent possible, a portion of a malfunctioning device or the position of a displaced device

Body Part	Approach	Device	Qualifier
Y Lower Artery	Ø Open 3 Percutaneous 4 Percutaneous Endoscopic	Ø Drainage Device 2 Monitoring Device 3 Infusion Device 7 Autologous Tissue Substitute C Extraluminal Device D Intraluminal Device J Synthetic Substitute K Nonautologous Tissue Substitute Y Other Device	Z No Qualifier
Y Lower Artery	X External	Ø Drainage Device 2 Monitoring Device 3 Infusion Device 7 Autologous Tissue Substitute C Extraluminal Device D Intraluminal Device J Synthetic Substitute K Nonautologous Tissue Substitute	Z No Qualifier

DRG Non-OR Ø4WY3[Ø23D]Z *(proposed)*
Non-OR Ø4WYX[Ø237CDJK]Z

Coding Clinic: 2015, Q1, P37 – Ø4WYØ7Z
Coding Clinic: 2019, Q2, P15 – Ø4WYØJZ

SECTION: Ø MEDICAL AND SURGICAL
BODY SYSTEM: 5 UPPER VEINS
OPERATION: 1 BYPASS: Altering the route of passage of the contents of a tubular body part

Body Part	Approach	Device	Qualifier
Ø Azygos Vein 1 Hemiazygos Vein 3 Innominate Vein, Right 4 Innominate Vein, Left 5 Subclavian Vein, Right 6 Subclavian Vein, Left 7 Axillary Vein, Right 8 Axillary Vein, Left 9 Brachial Vein, Right A Brachial Vein, Left B Basilic Vein, Right C Basilic Vein, Left D Cephalic Vein, Right F Cephalic Vein, Left G Hand Vein, Right H Hand Vein, Left L Intracranial Vein M Internal Jugular Vein, Right N Internal Jugular Vein, Left P External Jugular Vein, Right Q External Jugular Vein, Left R Vertebral Vein, Right S Vertebral Vein, Left T Face Vein, Right V Face Vein, Left	Ø Open 4 Percutaneous Endoscopic	7 Autologous Tissue Substitute 9 Autologous Venous Tissue A Autologous Arterial Tissue J Synthetic Substitute K Nonautologous Tissue Substitute Z No Device	Y Upper Vein

Coding Clinic: 2020, Q1, P29 – Ø51Q49Y

SECTION: Ø MEDICAL AND SURGICAL

BODY SYSTEM: 5 UPPER VEINS

OPERATION: 5 DESTRUCTION: Physical eradication of all or a portion of a body part by the direct use of energy, force, or a destructive agent

Body Part	Approach	Device	Qualifier
Ø Azygos Vein 1 Hemiazygos Vein 3 Innominate Vein, Right 4 Innominate Vein, Left 5 Subclavian Vein, Right 6 Subclavian Vein, Left 7 Axillary Vein, Right 8 Axillary Vein, Left 9 Brachial Vein, Right A Brachial Vein, Left B Basilic Vein, Right C Basilic Vein, Left D Cephalic Vein, Right F Cephalic Vein, Left G Hand Vein, Right H Hand Vein, Left L Intracranial Vein M Internal Jugular Vein, Right N Internal Jugular Vein, Left P External Jugular Vein, Right Q External Jugular Vein, Left R Vertebral Vein, Right S Vertebral Vein, Left T Face Vein, Right V Face Vein, Left Y Upper Vein	Ø Open 3 Percutaneous 4 Percutaneous Endoscopic	Z No Device	Z No Qualifier

SECTION: Ø MEDICAL AND SURGICAL
BODY SYSTEM: 5 UPPER VEINS
OPERATION: 7 DILATION: Expanding an orifice or the lumen of a tubular body part

Body Part	Approach	Device	Qualifier
Ø Azygos Vein 1 Hemiazygos Vein G Hand Vein, Right H Hand Vein, Left L Intracranial Vein M Internal Jugular Vein, Right N Internal Jugular Vein, Left P External Jugular Vein, Right Q External Jugular Vein, Left R Vertebral Vein, Right S Vertebral Vein, Left T Face Vein, Right V Face Vein, Left Y Upper Vein	Ø Open 3 Percutaneous 4 Percutaneous Endoscopic	D Intraluminal Device Z No Device	Z No Qualifier
3 Innominate Vein, Right 4 Innominate Vein, Left 5 Subclavian Vein, Right 6 Subclavian Vein, Left 7 Axillary Vein, Right 8 Axillary Vein, Left 9 Brachial Vein, Right A Brachial Vein, Left B Basilic Vein, Right C Basilic Vein, Left D Cephalic Vein, Right F Cephalic Vein, Left	Ø Open 3 Percutaneous 4 Percutaneous Endoscopic	D Intraluminal Device Z No Device	1 Drug-Coated Balloon Z No Qualifier

Ø57L[34]ZZ

SECTION: Ø MEDICAL AND SURGICAL
BODY SYSTEM: 5 UPPER VEINS
OPERATION: 9 DRAINAGE: Taking or letting out fluids and/or gases from a body part

Body Part	Approach	Device	Qualifier
Ø Azygos Vein 1 Hemiazygos Vein 3 Innominate Vein, Right 4 Innominate Vein, Left 5 Subclavian Vein, Right 6 Subclavian Vein, Left 7 Axillary Vein, Right 8 Axillary Vein, Left 9 Brachial Vein, Right A Brachial Vein, Left B Basilic Vein, Right C Basilic Vein, Left D Cephalic Vein, Right F Cephalic Vein, Left G Hand Vein, Right H Hand Vein, Left L Intracranial Vein M Internal Jugular Vein, Right N Internal Jugular Vein, Left P External Jugular Vein, Right Q External Jugular Vein, Left R Vertebral Vein, Right S Vertebral Vein, Left T Face Vein, Right V Face Vein, Left Y Upper Vein	Ø Open 3 Percutaneous 4 Percutaneous Endoscopic	Ø Drainage Device	Z No Qualifier
Ø Azygos Vein 1 Hemiazygos Vein 3 Innominate Vein, Right 4 Innominate Vein, Left 5 Subclavian Vein, Right 6 Subclavian Vein, Left 7 Axillary Vein, Right 8 Axillary Vein, Left 9 Brachial Vein, Right A Brachial Vein, Left B Basilic Vein, Right C Basilic Vein, Left D Cephalic Vein, Right F Cephalic Vein, Left G Hand Vein, Right H Hand Vein, Left L Intracranial Vein M Internal Jugular Vein, Right N Internal Jugular Vein, Left P External Jugular Vein, Right Q External Jugular Vein, Left R Vertebral Vein, Right S Vertebral Vein, Left T Face Vein, Right V Face Vein, Left Y Upper Vein	Ø Open 3 Percutaneous 4 Percutaneous Endoscopic	Z No Device	X Diagnostic Z No Qualifier

Non-OR Ø59[Ø13456789ABCDFGHLMNPQRSTVY][Ø34]ØZ
Non-OR Ø59[Ø13456789ABCDFGHLMNPQRSTVY][Ø34]Z[XZ]

SECTION: Ø MEDICAL AND SURGICAL

BODY SYSTEM: 5 UPPER VEINS

OPERATION: B EXCISION: Cutting out or off, without replacement, a portion of a body part

Body Part	Approach	Device	Qualifier
Ø Azygos Vein 1 Hemiazygos Vein 3 Innominate Vein, Right 4 Innominate Vein, Left 5 Subclavian Vein, Right 6 Subclavian Vein, Left 7 Axillary Vein, Right 8 Axillary Vein, Left 9 Brachial Vein, Right A Brachial Vein, Left B Basilic Vein, Right C Basilic Vein, Left D Cephalic Vein, Right F Cephalic Vein, Left G Hand Vein, Right H Hand Vein, Left L Intracranial Vein M Internal Jugular Vein, Right N Internal Jugular Vein, Left P External Jugular Vein, Right Q External Jugular Vein, Left R Vertebral Vein, Right S Vertebral Vein, Left T Face Vein, Right V Face Vein, Left Y Upper Vein	Ø Open 3 Percutaneous 4 Percutaneous Endoscopic	Z No Device	X Diagnostic Z No Qualifier

Coding Clinic: 2Ø16, Q2, P13-14 – Ø5B[NQ]ØZZ
Coding Clinic: 2Ø21, Q2, P16; 2Ø2Ø, Q1, P24 – Ø5BLØZZ

SECTION: Ø MEDICAL AND SURGICAL
BODY SYSTEM: 5 UPPER VEINS
OPERATION: C EXTIRPATION: Taking or cutting out solid matter from a body part

Body Part	Approach	Device	Qualifier
Ø Azygos Vein 1 Hemiazygos Vein 3 Innominate Vein, Right 4 Innominate Vein, Left 5 Subclavian Vein, Right 6 Subclavian Vein, Left 7 Axillary Vein, Right 8 Axillary Vein, Left 9 Brachial Vein, Right A Brachial Vein, Left B Basilic Vein, Right C Basilic Vein, Left D Cephalic Vein, Right F Cephalic Vein, Left G Hand Vein, Right H Hand Vein, Left L Intracranial Vein M Internal Jugular Vein, Right N Internal Jugular Vein, Left P External Jugular Vein, Right Q External Jugular Vein, Left R Vertebral Vein, Right S Vertebral Vein, Left T Face Vein, Right V Face Vein, Left Y Upper Vein	Ø Open 3 Percutaneous 4 Percutaneous Endoscopic	Z No Device	Z No Qualifier

SECTION: Ø MEDICAL AND SURGICAL
BODY SYSTEM: 5 UPPER VEINS
OPERATION: D EXTRACTION: Pulling or stripping out or off all or a portion of a body part by the use of force

Body Part	Approach	Device	Qualifier
9 Brachial Vein, Right A Brachial Vein, Left B Basilic Vein, Right C Basilic Vein, Left D Cephalic Vein, Right F Cephalic Vein, Left G Hand Vein, Right H Hand Vein, Left Y Upper Vein	Ø Open 3 Percutaneous	Z No Device	Z No Qualifier

SECTION: Ø MEDICAL AND SURGICAL
BODY SYSTEM: 5 UPPER VEINS
OPERATION: F FRAGMENTATION: Breaking solid matter in a body part into pieces

Body Part	Approach	Device	Qualifier
3 Innominate Vein, Right 4 Innominate Vein, Left 5 Subclavian Vein, Right 6 Subclavian Vein, Left 7 Axillary Vein, Right 8 Axillary Vein, Left 9 Brachial Vein, Right A Brachial Vein, Left B Basilic Vein, Right C Basilic Vein, Left D Cephalic Vein, Right F Cephalic Vein, Left Y Upper Vein	3 Percutaneous	Z No Device	Ø Ultrasonic Z No Qualifier

SECTION: Ø MEDICAL AND SURGICAL
BODY SYSTEM: 5 UPPER VEINS
OPERATION: H INSERTION: Putting in a nonbiological appliance that monitors, assists, performs, or prevents a physiological function but does not physically take the place of a body part

Body Part	Approach	Device	Qualifier
Ø Azygos Vein	Ø Open 3 Percutaneous 4 Percutaneous Endoscopic	2 Monitoring Device 3 Infusion Device D Intraluminal Device M Neurostimulator Lead	Z No Qualifier
1 Hemiazygos Vein 5 Subclavian Vein, Right 6 Subclavian Vein, Left 7 Axillary Vein, Right 8 Axillary Vein, Left 9 Brachial Vein, Right A Brachial Vein, Left B Basilic Vein, Right C Basilic Vein, Left D Cephalic Vein, Right F Cephalic Vein, Left G Hand Vein, Right H Hand Vein, Left L Intracranial Vein M Internal Jugular Vein, Right N Internal Jugular Vein, Left P External Jugular Vein, Right Q External Jugular Vein, Left R Vertebral Vein, Right S Vertebral Vein, Left T Face Vein, Right V Face Vein, Left	Ø Open 3 Percutaneous 4 Percutaneous Endoscopic	3 Infusion Device D Intraluminal Device	Z No Qualifier
3 Innominate Vein, Right 4 Innominate Vein, Left	Ø Open 3 Percutaneous 4 Percutaneous Endoscopic	3 Infusion Device D Intraluminal Device M Neurostimulator Lead	Z No Qualifier
Y Upper Vein	Ø Open 3 Percutaneous 4 Percutaneous Endoscopic	2 Monitoring Device 3 Infusion Device D Intraluminal Device Y Other Device	Z No Qualifier

Ø5HØ[Ø34]MZ
Ø5H[34][Ø34]MZ
Non-OR Ø5HØ[Ø34]3Z
Non-OR Ø5H[13789ABCDFGHLRSTV][Ø34]3Z
Non-OR Ø5H[56MNPQ][Ø34]3Z
Non-OR Ø5H[34][Ø34]3Z
Non-OR Ø5HY[Ø34]3Z
Non-OR Ø5HY32Z
Ø5HØ[34]3Z when reported with Secondary Diagnosis J95.811
Ø5H[156][34]3Z when reported with Secondary Diagnosis J95.811
Ø5H[34][34]3Z when reported with Secondary Diagnosis J95.811
Ø5H[MNPQ]33Z when reported with Secondary Diagnosis J95.811

Coding Clinic: 2Ø16, Q4, P98 – Ø5H, Ø5HØ32Z
Coding Clinic: 2Ø16, Q4, P99 – Ø5H43MZ

New/Revised Text in Green ~~deleted~~ Deleted ♀ Females Only ♂ Males Only Coding Clinic
Non-covered Limited Coverage Combination (See Appendix E) DRG Non-OR Non-OR Hospital-Acquired Condition

SECTION: Ø MEDICAL AND SURGICAL
BODY SYSTEM: 5 UPPER VEINS
OPERATION: J INSPECTION: Visually and/or manually exploring a body part

Body Part	Approach	Device	Qualifier
Y Upper Vein	Ø Open 3 Percutaneous 4 Percutaneous Endoscopic X External	Z No Device	Z No Qualifier

Non-OR Ø5JY[3X]ZZ

SECTION: Ø MEDICAL AND SURGICAL
BODY SYSTEM: 5 UPPER VEINS
OPERATION: L OCCLUSION: Completely closing an orifice or the lumen of a tubular body part

Body Part	Approach	Device	Qualifier
Ø Azygos Vein 1 Hemiazygos Vein 3 Innominate Vein, Right 4 Innominate Vein, Left 5 Subclavian Vein, Right 6 Subclavian Vein, Left 7 Axillary Vein, Right 8 Axillary Vein, Left 9 Brachial Vein, Right A Brachial Vein, Left B Basilic Vein, Right C Basilic Vein, Left D Cephalic Vein, Right F Cephalic Vein, Left G Hand Vein, Right H Hand Vein, Left L Intracranial Vein M Internal Jugular Vein, Right N Internal Jugular Vein, Left P External Jugular Vein, Right Q External Jugular Vein, Left R Vertebral Vein, Right S Vertebral Vein, Left T Face Vein, Right V Face Vein, Left Y Upper Vein	Ø Open 3 Percutaneous 4 Percutaneous Endoscopic	C Extraluminal Device D Intraluminal Device Z No Device	Z No Qualifier

SECTION: Ø MEDICAL AND SURGICAL
BODY SYSTEM: 5 UPPER VEINS
OPERATION: N RELEASE: Freeing a body part from an abnormal physical constraint

Body Part	Approach	Device	Qualifier
Ø Azygos Vein 1 Hemiazygos Vein 3 Innominate Vein, Right 4 Innominate Vein, Left 5 Subclavian Vein, Right 6 Subclavian Vein, Left 7 Axillary Vein, Right 8 Axillary Vein, Left 9 Brachial Vein, Right A Brachial Vein, Left B Basilic Vein, Right C Basilic Vein, Left D Cephalic Vein, Right F Cephalic Vein, Left G Hand Vein, Right H Hand Vein, Left L Intracranial Vein M Internal Jugular Vein, Right N Internal Jugular Vein, Left P External Jugular Vein, Right Q External Jugular Vein, Left R Vertebral Vein, Right S Vertebral Vein, Left T Face Vein, Right V Face Vein, Left Y Upper Vein	Ø Open 3 Percutaneous 4 Percutaneous Endoscopic	Z No Device	Z No Qualifier

SECTION: Ø MEDICAL AND SURGICAL
BODY SYSTEM: 5 UPPER VEINS
OPERATION: P REMOVAL: Taking out or off a device from a body part

Body Part	Approach	Device	Qualifier
Ø Azygos Vein	Ø Open 3 Percutaneous 4 Percutaneous Endoscopic X External	2 Monitoring Device M Neurostimulator Lead	Z No Qualifier
3 Innominate Vein, Right 4 Innominate Vein, Left	Ø Open 3 Percutaneous 4 Percutaneous Endoscopic X External	M Neurostimulator Lead	Z No Qualifier
Y Upper Vein	Ø Open 3 Percutaneous 4 Percutaneous Endoscopic	Ø Drainage Device 2 Monitoring Device 3 Infusion Device 7 Autologous Tissue Substitute C Extraluminal Device D Intraluminal Device J Synthetic Substitute K Nonautologous Tissue Substitute Y Other Device	Z No Qualifier
Y Upper Vein	X External	Ø Drainage Device 2 Monitoring Device 3 Infusion Device D Intraluminal Device	Z No Qualifier

Non-OR Ø5PØ[Ø3X]2Z
Non-OR Ø5PY3[Ø23D]Z
Non-OR Ø5PYX[Ø23D]Z

Coding Clinic: 2016, Q4, P98 – Ø5P

SECTION: Ø MEDICAL AND SURGICAL
BODY SYSTEM: 5 UPPER VEINS
OPERATION: Q REPAIR: Restoring, to the extent possible, a body part to its normal anatomic structure and function

Body Part	Approach	Device	Qualifier
Ø Azygos Vein 1 Hemiazygos Vein 3 Innominate Vein, Right 4 Innominate Vein, Left 5 Subclavian Vein, Right 6 Subclavian Vein, Left 7 Axillary Vein, Right 8 Axillary Vein, Left 9 Brachial Vein, Right A Brachial Vein, Left B Basilic Vein, Right C Basilic Vein, Left D Cephalic Vein, Right F Cephalic Vein, Left G Hand Vein, Right H Hand Vein, Left L Intracranial Vein M Internal Jugular Vein, Right N Internal Jugular Vein, Left P External Jugular Vein, Right Q External Jugular Vein, Left R Vertebral Vein, Right S Vertebral Vein, Left T Face Vein, Right V Face Vein, Left Y Upper Vein	Ø Open 3 Percutaneous 4 Percutaneous Endoscopic	Z No Device	Z No Qualifier

Coding Clinic: 2Ø17, Q3, P16 – Ø5Q4ØZZ

SECTION: Ø MEDICAL AND SURGICAL

BODY SYSTEM: 5 UPPER VEINS

OPERATION: R REPLACEMENT: Putting in or on biological or synthetic material that physically takes the place and/or function of all or a portion of a body part

Body Part	Approach	Device	Qualifier
Ø Azygos Vein 1 Hemiazygos Vein 3 Innominate Vein, Right 4 Innominate Vein, Left 5 Subclavian Vein, Right 6 Subclavian Vein, Left 7 Axillary Vein, Right 8 Axillary Vein, Left 9 Brachial Vein, Right A Brachial Vein, Left B Basilic Vein, Right C Basilic Vein, Left D Cephalic Vein, Right F Cephalic Vein, Left G Hand Vein, Right H Hand Vein, Left L Intracranial Vein M Internal Jugular Vein, Right N Internal Jugular Vein, Left P External Jugular Vein, Right Q External Jugular Vein, Left R Vertebral Vein, Right S Vertebral Vein, Left T Face Vein, Right V Face Vein, Left Y Upper Vein	Ø Open 4 Percutaneous Endoscopic	7 Autologous Tissue Substitute J Synthetic Substitute K Nonautologous Tissue Substitute	Z No Qualifier

SECTION: Ø MEDICAL AND SURGICAL
BODY SYSTEM: 5 UPPER VEINS
OPERATION: S REPOSITION: Moving to its normal location, or other suitable location, all or a portion of a body part

Body Part	Approach	Device	Qualifier
Ø Azygos Vein 1 Hemiazygos Vein 3 Innominate Vein, Right 4 Innominate Vein, Left 5 Subclavian Vein, Right 6 Subclavian Vein, Left 7 Axillary Vein, Right 8 Axillary Vein, Left 9 Brachial Vein, Right A Brachial Vein, Left B Basilic Vein, Right C Basilic Vein, Left D Cephalic Vein, Right F Cephalic Vein, Left G Hand Vein, Right H Hand Vein, Left L Intracranial Vein M Internal Jugular Vein, Right N Internal Jugular Vein, Left P External Jugular Vein, Right Q External Jugular Vein, Left R Vertebral Vein, Right S Vertebral Vein, Left T Face Vein, Right V Face Vein, Left Y Upper Vein	Ø Open 3 Percutaneous 4 Percutaneous Endoscopic	Z No Device	Z No Qualifier

SECTION: Ø MEDICAL AND SURGICAL
BODY SYSTEM: 5 UPPER VEINS
OPERATION: U SUPPLEMENT: Putting in or on biological or synthetic material that physically reinforces and/or augments the function of a portion of a body part

Body Part	Approach	Device	Qualifier
Ø Azygos Vein 1 Hemiazygos Vein 3 Innominate Vein, Right 4 Innominate Vein, Left 5 Subclavian Vein, Right 6 Subclavian Vein, Left 7 Axillary Vein, Right 8 Axillary Vein, Left 9 Brachial Vein, Right A Brachial Vein, Left B Basilic Vein, Right C Basilic Vein, Left D Cephalic Vein, Right F Cephalic Vein, Left G Hand Vein, Right H Hand Vein, Left L Intracranial Vein M Internal Jugular Vein, Right N Internal Jugular Vein, Left P External Jugular Vein, Right Q External Jugular Vein, Left R Vertebral Vein, Right S Vertebral Vein, Left T Face Vein, Right V Face Vein, Left Y Upper Vein	Ø Open 3 Percutaneous 4 Percutaneous Endoscopic	7 Autologous Tissue Substitute J Synthetic Substitute K Nonautologous Tissue Substitute	Z No Qualifier

SECTION: Ø MEDICAL AND SURGICAL
BODY SYSTEM: 5 UPPER VEINS
OPERATION: V RESTRICTION: Partially closing an orifice or the lumen of a tubular body part

Body Part	Approach	Device	Qualifier
Ø Azygos Vein 1 Hemiazygos Vein 3 Innominate Vein, Right 4 Innominate Vein, Left 5 Subclavian Vein, Right 6 Subclavian Vein, Left 7 Axillary Vein, Right 8 Axillary Vein, Left 9 Brachial Vein, Right A Brachial Vein, Left B Basilic Vein, Right C Basilic Vein, Left D Cephalic Vein, Right F Cephalic Vein, Left G Hand Vein, Right H Hand Vein, Left L Intracranial Vein M Internal Jugular Vein, Right N Internal Jugular Vein, Left P External Jugular Vein, Right Q External Jugular Vein, Left R Vertebral Vein, Right S Vertebral Vein, Left T Face Vein, Right V Face Vein, Left Y Upper Vein	Ø Open 3 Percutaneous 4 Percutaneous Endoscopic	C Extraluminal Device D Intraluminal Device Z No Device	Z No Qualifier

Ø5W

SECTION: Ø MEDICAL AND SURGICAL
BODY SYSTEM: 5 UPPER VEINS
OPERATION: W REVISION: Correcting, to the extent possible, a portion of a malfunctioning device or the position of a displaced device

Body Part	Approach	Device	Qualifier
Ø Azygos Vein	Ø Open 3 Percutaneous 4 Percutaneous Endoscopic X External	2 Monitoring Device M Neurostimulator Lead	Z No Qualifier
3 Innominate Vein, Right 4 Innominate Vein, Left	Ø Open 3 Percutaneous 4 Percutaneous Endoscopic X External	M Neurostimulator Lead	Z No Qualifier
Y Upper Vein	Ø Open 3 Percutaneous 4 Percutaneous Endoscopic	Ø Drainage Device 2 Monitoring Device 3 Infusion Device 7 Autologous Tissue Substitute C Extraluminal Device D Intraluminal Device J Synthetic Substitute K Nonautologous Tissue Substitute Y Other Device	Z No Qualifier
Y Upper Vein	X External	Ø Drainage Device 2 Monitoring Device 3 Infusion Device 7 Autologous Tissue Substitute C Extraluminal Device D Intraluminal Device J Synthetic Substitute K Nonautologous Tissue Substitute	Z No Qualifier

Non-OR Ø5WY3[Ø23D]Z
Non-OR Ø5WØXMZ
Non-OR Ø5W[34]XMZ
Non-OR Ø5WYX[Ø237CDJK]Z

Coding Clinic: 2016, Q4, P98 – Ø5W

New/Revised Text in Green ~~deleted~~ Deleted ♀ Females Only ♂ Males Only Coding Clinic
Non-covered Limited Coverage Combination (See Appendix E) DRG Non-OR Non-OR Hospital-Acquired Condition

SECTION: Ø MEDICAL AND SURGICAL
BODY SYSTEM: 6 LOWER VEINS
OPERATION: 1 BYPASS: Altering the route of passage of the contents of a tubular body part

Body Part	Approach	Device	Qualifier
Ø Inferior Vena Cava	Ø Open 4 Percutaneous Endoscopic	7 Autologous Tissue Substitute 9 Autologous Venous Tissue A Autologous Arterial Tissue J Synthetic Substitute K Nonautologous Tissue Substitute Z No Device	5 Superior Mesenteric Vein 6 Inferior Mesenteric Vein P Pulmonary Trunk Q Pulmonary Artery, Right R Pulmonary Artery, Left Y Lower Vein
1 Splenic Vein	Ø Open 4 Percutaneous Endoscopic	7 Autologous Tissue Substitute 9 Autologous Venous Tissue A Autologous Arterial Tissue J Synthetic Substitute K Nonautologous Tissue Substitute Z No Device	9 Renal Vein, Right B Renal Vein, Left Y Lower Vein
2 Gastric Vein 3 Esophageal Vein 4 Hepatic Vein 5 Superior Mesenteric Vein 6 Inferior Mesenteric Vein 7 Colic Vein 9 Renal Vein, Right B Renal Vein, Left C Common Iliac Vein, Right D Common Iliac Vein, Left F External Iliac Vein, Right G External Iliac Vein, Left H Hypogastric Vein, Right J Hypogastric Vein, Left M Femoral Vein, Right N Femoral Vein, Left P Saphenous Vein, Right Q Saphenous Vein, Left T Foot Vein, Right V Foot Vein, Left	Ø Open 4 Percutaneous Endoscopic	7 Autologous Tissue Substitute 9 Autologous Venous Tissue A Autologous Arterial Tissue J Synthetic Substitute K Nonautologous Tissue Substitute Z No Device	Y Lower Vein
8 Portal Vein	Ø Open	7 Autologous Tissue Substitute 9 Autologous Venous Tissue A Autologous Arterial Tissue J Synthetic Substitute K Nonautologous Tissue Substitute Z No Device	9 Renal Vein, Right B Renal Vein, Left Y Lower Vein
8 Portal Vein	3 Percutaneous	J Synthetic Substitute	4 Hepatic Vein Y Lower Vein
8 Portal Vein	4 Percutaneous Endoscopic	7 Autologous Tissue Substitute 9 Autologous Venous Tissue A Autologous Arterial Tissue K Nonautologous Tissue Substitute Z No Device	9 Renal Vein, Right B Renal Vein, Left Y Lower Vein
8 Portal Vein	4 Percutaneous Endoscopic	J Synthetic Substitute	4 Hepatic Vein 9 Renal Vein, Right B Renal Vein, Left Y Lower Vein

Coding Clinic: 2Ø17, Q4, P38 – Ø61ØØJP

SECTION: Ø MEDICAL AND SURGICAL
BODY SYSTEM: 6 LOWER VEINS
OPERATION: 5 DESTRUCTION: Physical eradication of all or a portion of a body part by the direct use of energy, force, or a destructive agent

Body Part	Approach	Device	Qualifier
Ø Inferior Vena Cava 1 Splenic Vein 2 Gastric Vein 3 Esophageal Vein 4 Hepatic Vein 5 Superior Mesenteric Vein 6 Inferior Mesenteric Vein 7 Colic Vein 8 Portal Vein 9 Renal Vein, Right B Renal Vein, Left C Common Iliac Vein, Right D Common Iliac Vein, Left F External Iliac Vein, Right G External Iliac Vein, Left H Hypogastric Vein, Right J Hypogastric Vein, Left M Femoral Vein, Right N Femoral Vein, Left P Saphenous Vein, Right Q Saphenous Vein, Left T Foot Vein, Right V Foot Vein, Left	Ø Open 3 Percutaneous 4 Percutaneous Endoscopic	Z No Device	Z No Qualifier
Y Lower Vein	Ø Open 3 Percutaneous 4 Percutaneous Endoscopic	Z No Device	C Hemorrhoidal Plexus Z No Qualifier

SECTION: Ø MEDICAL AND SURGICAL
BODY SYSTEM: 6 LOWER VEINS
OPERATION: 7 DILATION: Expanding an orifice or the lumen of a tubular body part

Body Part	Approach	Device	Qualifier
Ø Inferior Vena Cava 1 Splenic Vein 2 Gastric Vein 3 Esophageal Vein 4 Hepatic Vein 5 Superior Mesenteric Vein 6 Inferior Mesenteric Vein 7 Colic Vein 8 Portal Vein 9 Renal Vein, Right B Renal Vein, Left C Common Iliac Vein, Right D Common Iliac Vein, Left F External Iliac Vein, Right G External Iliac Vein, Left H Hypogastric Vein, Right J Hypogastric Vein, Left M Femoral Vein, Right N Femoral Vein, Left P Saphenous Vein, Right Q Saphenous Vein, Left T Foot Vein, Right V Foot Vein, Left Y Lower Vein	Ø Open 3 Percutaneous 4 Percutaneous Endoscopic	D Intraluminal Device Z No Device	Z No Qualifier

New/Revised Text in Green ~~deleted~~ Deleted ♀ Females Only ♂ Males Only Coding Clinic
Non-covered Limited Coverage Combination (See Appendix E) DRG Non-OR Non-OR Hospital-Acquired Condition

SECTION: Ø MEDICAL AND SURGICAL
BODY SYSTEM: 6 LOWER VEINS
OPERATION: 9 DRAINAGE: Taking or letting out fluids and/or gases from a body part

Body Part	Approach	Device	Qualifier
Ø Inferior Vena Cava 1 Splenic Vein 2 Gastric Vein 3 Esophageal Vein 4 Hepatic Vein 5 Superior Mesenteric Vein 6 Inferior Mesenteric Vein 7 Colic Vein 8 Portal Vein 9 Renal Vein, Right B Renal Vein, Left C Common Iliac Vein, Right D Common Iliac Vein, Left F External Iliac Vein, Right G External Iliac Vein, Left H Hypogastric Vein, Right J Hypogastric Vein, Left M Femoral Vein, Right N Femoral Vein, Left P Saphenous Vein, Right Q Saphenous Vein, Left T Foot Vein, Right V Foot Vein, Left Y Lower Vein	Ø Open 3 Percutaneous 4 Percutaneous Endoscopic	Ø Drainage Device	Z No Qualifier
Ø Inferior Vena Cava 1 Splenic Vein 2 Gastric Vein 3 Esophageal Vein 4 Hepatic Vein 5 Superior Mesenteric Vein 6 Inferior Mesenteric Vein 7 Colic Vein 8 Portal Vein 9 Renal Vein, Right B Renal Vein, Left C Common Iliac Vein, Right D Common Iliac Vein, Left F External Iliac Vein, Right G External Iliac Vein, Left H Hypogastric Vein, Right J Hypogastric Vein, Left M Femoral Vein, Right N Femoral Vein, Left P Saphenous Vein, Right Q Saphenous Vein, Left T Foot Vein, Right V Foot Vein, Left Y Lower Vein	Ø Open 3 Percutaneous 4 Percutaneous Endoscopic	Z No Device	X Diagnostic Z No Qualifier

Non-OR Ø6933ØZ
Non-OR Ø69[Ø12456789BCDFGHJMNPQTVY][Ø34]ØZ
Non-OR Ø6933ZZ
Non-OR Ø69[Ø123456789BCDFGHJMNPQRSTVY][Ø34]Z[XZ]

SECTION: Ø MEDICAL AND SURGICAL
BODY SYSTEM: 6 LOWER VEINS
OPERATION: B EXCISION: Cutting out or off, without replacement, a portion of a body part

Body Part	Approach	Device	Qualifier
Ø Inferior Vena Cava 1 Splenic Vein 2 Gastric Vein 3 Esophageal Vein 4 Hepatic Vein 5 Superior Mesenteric Vein 6 Inferior Mesenteric Vein 7 Colic Vein 8 Portal Vein 9 Renal Vein, Right B Renal Vein, Left C Common Iliac Vein, Right D Common Iliac Vein, Left F External Iliac Vein, Right G External Iliac Vein, Left H Hypogastric Vein, Right J Hypogastric Vein, Left M Femoral Vein, Right N Femoral Vein, Left P Saphenous Vein, Right Q Saphenous Vein, Left T Foot Vein, Right V Foot Vein, Left	Ø Open 3 Percutaneous 4 Percutaneous Endoscopic	Z No Device	X Diagnostic Z No Qualifier
Y Lower Vein	Ø Open 3 Percutaneous 4 Percutaneous Endoscopic	Z No Device	C Hemorrhoidal Plexus X Diagnostic Z No Qualifier

Coding Clinic: 2Ø16, Q1, P28 – Ø6BQ4ZZ
Coding Clinic: 2Ø16, Q2, P19 – Ø6B9ØZZ
Coding Clinic: 2Ø17, Q1, P32 – Ø6BPØZZ
Coding Clinic: 2Ø2Ø, Q1, P29; 2Ø17, Q1, P33 – Ø6BQØZZ
Coding Clinic: 2Ø17, Q3, P6 – Ø6BPØZZ

SECTION: Ø MEDICAL AND SURGICAL
BODY SYSTEM: 6 LOWER VEINS
OPERATION: C EXTIRPATION: Taking or cutting out solid matter from a body part

Body Part	Approach	Device	Qualifier
Ø Inferior Vena Cava 1 Splenic Vein 2 Gastric Vein 3 Esophageal Vein 4 Hepatic Vein 5 Superior Mesenteric Vein 6 Inferior Mesenteric Vein 7 Colic Vein 8 Portal Vein 9 Renal Vein, Right B Renal Vein, Left C Common Iliac Vein, Right D Common Iliac Vein, Left F External Iliac Vein, Right G External Iliac Vein, Left H Hypogastric Vein, Right J Hypogastric Vein, Left M Femoral Vein, Right N Femoral Vein, Left P Saphenous Vein, Right Q Saphenous Vein, Left T Foot Vein, Right V Foot Vein, Left Y Lower Vein	Ø Open 3 Percutaneous 4 Percutaneous Endoscopic	Z No Device	Z No Qualifier

SECTION: Ø MEDICAL AND SURGICAL
BODY SYSTEM: 6 LOWER VEINS
OPERATION: D EXTRACTION: Pulling or stripping out or off all or a portion of a body part by the use of force

Body Part	Approach	Device	Qualifier
M Femoral Vein, Right N Femoral Vein, Left P Saphenous Vein, Right Q Saphenous Vein, Left T Foot Vein, Right V Foot Vein, Left Y Lower Vein	Ø Open 3 Percutaneous 4 Percutaneous Endoscopic	Z No Device	Z No Qualifier

SECTION: Ø MEDICAL AND SURGICAL
BODY SYSTEM: 6 LOWER VEINS
OPERATION: F FRAGMENTATION: Breaking solid matter in a body part into pieces

Body Part	Approach	Device	Qualifier
C Common Iliac Vein, Right D Common Iliac Vein, Left F External Iliac Vein, Right G External Iliac Vein, Left H Hypogastric Vein, Right J Hypogastric Vein, Left M Femoral Vein, Right N Femoral Vein, Left P Saphenous Vein, Right Q Saphenous Vein, Left Y Lower Vein	3 Percutaneous	Z No Device	Ø Ultrasonic Z No Qualifier

SECTION: Ø MEDICAL AND SURGICAL
BODY SYSTEM: 6 LOWER VEINS
OPERATION: H INSERTION: Putting in a nonbiological appliance that monitors, assists, performs, or prevents a physiological function but does not physically take the place of a body part

Body Part	Approach	Device	Qualifier
Ø Inferior Vena Cava	Ø Open 3 Percutaneous	3 Infusion Device	T Via Unbilical Vein Z No Qualifier
Ø Inferior Vena Cava	Ø Open 3 Percutaneous	D Intraluminal Device	Z No Qualifier
Ø Inferior Vena Cava	4 Percutaneous Endoscopic	3 Infusion Device D Intraluminal Device	Z No Qualifier
1 Splenic Vein 2 Gastric Vein 3 Esophageal Vein 4 Hepatic Vein 5 Superior Mesenteric Vein 6 Inferior Mesenteric Vein 7 Colic Vein 8 Portal Vein 9 Renal Vein, Right B Renal Vein, Left C Common Iliac Vein, Right D Common Iliac Vein, Left F External Iliac Vein, Right G External Iliac Vein, Left H Hypogastric Vein, Right J Hypogastric Vein, Left M Femoral Vein, Right N Femoral Vein, Left P Saphenous Vein, Right Q Saphenous Vein, Left T Foot Vein, Right V Foot Vein, Left	Ø Open 3 Percutaneous 4 Percutaneous Endoscopic	3 Infusion Device D Intraluminal Device	Z No Qualifier
Y Lower Vein	Ø Open 3 Percutaneous 4 Percutaneous Endoscopic	2 Monitoring Device 3 Infusion Device D Intraluminal Device Y Other Device	Z No Qualifier

Non-OR Ø6HØ[Ø3]3[DTZ]
Non-OR Ø6HØ43Z
Non-OR Ø6H[123456789BCDFGHJPQTV][Ø34]3Z
Non-OR Ø6H[MN][Ø34]3Z
Non-OR Ø6HY32Z
Non-OR Ø6HY[Ø34]3Z

Coding Clinic: 2Ø13, Q3, P19 – Ø6HØ33Z
Coding Clinic: 2Ø17, Q1, P31 – Ø6HØ33T, Ø6HY33Z
Coding Clinic: 2Ø21, Q3, P19 – Ø6HY33Z

SECTION: Ø MEDICAL AND SURGICAL
BODY SYSTEM: 6 LOWER VEINS
OPERATION: J INSPECTION: Visually and/or manually exploring a body part

Body Part	Approach	Device	Qualifier
Y Lower Vein	Ø Open 3 Percutaneous 4 Percutaneous Endoscopic X External	Z No Device	Z No Qualifier

Non-OR Ø6JY[3X]ZZ

SECTION: Ø MEDICAL AND SURGICAL
BODY SYSTEM: 6 LOWER VEINS
OPERATION: L OCCLUSION: Completely closing an orifice or the lumen of a tubular body part

Body Part	Approach	Device	Qualifier
Ø Inferior Vena Cava 1 Splenic Vein 4 Hepatic Vein 5 Superior Mesenteric Vein 6 Inferior Mesenteric Vein 7 Colic Vein 8 Portal Vein 9 Renal Vein, Right B Renal Vein, Left C Common Iliac Vein, Right D Common Iliac Vein, Left F External Iliac Vein, Right G External Iliac Vein, Left H Hypogastric Vein, Right J Hypogastric Vein, Left M Femoral Vein, Right N Femoral Vein, Left P Saphenous Vein, Right Q Saphenous Vein, Left T Foot Vein, Right V Foot Vein, Left	Ø Open 3 Percutaneous 4 Percutaneous Endoscopic	C Extraluminal Device D Intraluminal Device Z No Device	Z No Qualifier
2 Gastric Vein 3 Esophageal Vein	Ø Open 3 Percutaneous 4 Percutaneous Endoscopic 7 Via Natural or Artificial Opening 8 Via Natural or Artificial Opening Endoscopic	C Extraluminal Device D Intraluminal Device Z No Device	Z No Qualifier
Y Lower Vein	Ø Open 3 Percutaneous 4 Percutaneous Endoscopic 7 Via Natural or Artificial Opening 8 Via Natural or Artificial Opening Endoscopic	C Extraluminal Device D Intraluminal Device Z No Device	C Hemorrhoidal Plexus Z No Qualifier

Non-OR Ø6L3[34][CDZ]Z

Coding Clinic: 2Ø17, Q4, P57 – ØØ6L38CZ
Coding Clinic: 2Ø18, Q2, P19 – Ø6LFØCZ
Coding Clinic: 2Ø21, Q4, P5Ø – Ø6L84CZ

SECTION: Ø MEDICAL AND SURGICAL
BODY SYSTEM: 6 LOWER VEINS
OPERATION: N RELEASE: Freeing a body part from an abnormal physical constraint by cutting or by the use of force

Body Part	Approach	Device	Qualifier
Ø Inferior Vena Cava 1 Splenic Vein 2 Gastric Vein 3 Esophageal Vein 4 Hepatic Vein 5 Superior Mesenteric Vein 6 Inferior Mesenteric Vein 7 Colic Vein 8 Portal Vein 9 Renal Vein, Right B Renal Vein, Left C Common Iliac Vein, Right D Common Iliac Vein, Left F External Iliac Vein, Right G External Iliac Vein, Left H Hypogastric Vein, Right J Hypogastric Vein, Left M Femoral Vein, Right N Femoral Vein, Left P Saphenous Vein, Right Q Saphenous Vein, Left T Foot Vein, Right V Foot Vein, Left Y Lower Vein	Ø Open 3 Percutaneous 4 Percutaneous Endoscopic	Z No Device	Z No Qualifier

SECTION: Ø MEDICAL AND SURGICAL
BODY SYSTEM: 6 LOWER VEINS
OPERATION: P REMOVAL: Taking out or off a device from a body part

Body Part	Approach	Device	Qualifier
Y Lower Vein	Ø Open 3 Percutaneous 4 Percutaneous Endoscopic	Ø Drainage Device 2 Monitoring Device 3 Infusion Device 7 Autologous Tissue Substitute C Extraluminal Device D Intraluminal Device J Synthetic Substitute K Nonautologous Tissue Substitute Y Other Device	Z No Qualifier
Y Lower Vein	X External	Ø Drainage Device 2 Monitoring Device 3 Infusion Device D Intraluminal Device	Z No Qualifier

Non-OR Ø6PY3[Ø23D]Z
Non-OR Ø6PYX[Ø23D]Z

Coding Clinic: 2021, Q3, P19 – Ø6PY33Z

SECTION: Ø MEDICAL AND SURGICAL
BODY SYSTEM: 6 LOWER VEINS
OPERATION: Q REPAIR: Restoring, to the extent possible, a body part to its normal anatomic structure and function

Body Part	Approach	Device	Qualifier
Ø Inferior Vena Cava 1 Splenic Vein 2 Gastric Vein 3 Esophageal Vein 4 Hepatic Vein 5 Superior Mesenteric Vein 6 Inferior Mesenteric Vein 7 Colic Vein 8 Portal Vein 9 Renal Vein, Right B Renal Vein, Left C Common Iliac Vein, Right D Common Iliac Vein, Left F External Iliac Vein, Right G External Iliac Vein, Left H Hypogastric Vein, Right J Hypogastric Vein, Left M Femoral Vein, Right N Femoral Vein, Left P Saphenous Vein, Right Q Saphenous Vein, Left T Foot Vein, Right V Foot Vein, Left Y Lower Vein	Ø Open 3 Percutaneous 4 Percutaneous Endoscopic	Z No Device	Z No Qualifier

SECTION: Ø MEDICAL AND SURGICAL
BODY SYSTEM: 6 LOWER VEINS
OPERATION: R REPLACEMENT: Putting in or on biological or synthetic material that physically takes the place and/or function of all or a portion of a body part

Body Part	Approach	Device	Qualifier
Ø Inferior Vena Cava 1 Splenic Vein 2 Gastric Vein 3 Esophageal Vein 4 Hepatic Vein 5 Superior Mesenteric Vein 6 Inferior Mesenteric Vein 7 Colic Vein 8 Portal Vein 9 Renal Vein, Right B Renal Vein, Left C Common Iliac Vein, Right D Common Iliac Vein, Left F External Iliac Vein, Right G External Iliac Vein, Left H Hypogastric Vein, Right J Hypogastric Vein, Left M Femoral Vein, Right N Femoral Vein, Left P Saphenous Vein, Right Q Saphenous Vein, Left T Foot Vein, Right V Foot Vein, Left Y Lower Vein	Ø Open 4 Percutaneous Endoscopic	7 Autologous Tissue Substitute J Synthetic Substitute K Nonautologous Tissue Substitute	Z No Qualifier

SECTION: Ø MEDICAL AND SURGICAL
BODY SYSTEM: 6 LOWER VEINS
OPERATION: S REPOSITION: Moving to its normal location, or other suitable location, all or a portion of a body part

Body Part	Approach	Device	Qualifier
Ø Inferior Vena Cava 1 Splenic Vein 2 Gastric Vein 3 Esophageal Vein 4 Hepatic Vein 5 Superior Mesenteric Vein 6 Inferior Mesenteric Vein 7 Colic Vein 8 Portal Vein 9 Renal Vein, Right B Renal Vein, Left C Common Iliac Vein, Right D Common Iliac Vein, Left F External Iliac Vein, Right G External Iliac Vein, Left H Hypogastric Vein, Right J Hypogastric Vein, Left M Femoral Vein, Right N Femoral Vein, Left P Saphenous Vein, Right Q Saphenous Vein, Left T Foot Vein, Right V Foot Vein, Left Y Lower Vein	Ø Open 3 Percutaneous 4 Percutaneous Endoscopic	Z No Device	Z No Qualifier

SECTION: Ø MEDICAL AND SURGICAL
BODY SYSTEM: 6 LOWER VEINS
OPERATION: U SUPPLEMENT: Putting in or on biological or synthetic material that physically reinforces and/or augments the function of a portion of a body part

Body Part	Approach	Device	Qualifier
Ø Inferior Vena Cava 1 Splenic Vein 2 Gastric Vein 3 Esophageal Vein 4 Hepatic Vein 5 Superior Mesenteric Vein 6 Inferior Mesenteric Vein 7 Colic Vein 8 Portal Vein 9 Renal Vein, Right B Renal Vein, Left C Common Iliac Vein, Right D Common Iliac Vein, Left F External Iliac Vein, Right G External Iliac Vein, Left H Hypogastric Vein, Right J Hypogastric Vein, Left M Femoral Vein, Right N Femoral Vein, Left P Saphenous Vein, Right Q Saphenous Vein, Left T Foot Vein, Right V Foot Vein, Left Y Lower Vein	Ø Open 3 Percutaneous 4 Percutaneous Endoscopic	7 Autologous Tissue Substitute J Synthetic Substitute K Nonautologous Tissue Substitute	Z No Qualifier

SECTION: Ø MEDICAL AND SURGICAL

BODY SYSTEM: 6 LOWER VEINS

OPERATION: V RESTRICTION: Partially closing an orifice or the lumen of a tubular body part

Body Part	Approach	Device	Qualifier
Ø Inferior Vena Cava 1 Splenic Vein 2 Gastric Vein 3 Esophageal Vein 4 Hepatic Vein 5 Superior Mesenteric Vein 6 Inferior Mesenteric Vein 7 Colic Vein 8 Portal Vein 9 Renal Vein, Right B Renal Vein, Left C Common Iliac Vein, Right D Common Iliac Vein, Left F External Iliac Vein, Right G External Iliac Vein, Left H Hypogastric Vein, Right J Hypogastric Vein, Left M Femoral Vein, Right N Femoral Vein, Left P Saphenous Vein, Right Q Saphenous Vein, Left T Foot Vein, Right V Foot Vein, Left Y Lower Vein	Ø Open 3 Percutaneous 4 Percutaneous Endoscopic	C Extraluminal Device D Intraluminal Device Z No Device	Z No Qualifier

SECTION: Ø MEDICAL AND SURGICAL

BODY SYSTEM: 6 LOWER VEINS

OPERATION: W REVISION: Correcting, to the extent possible, a portion of a malfunctioning device or the position of a displaced device

Body Part	Approach	Device	Qualifier
Y Lower Vein	Ø Open 3 Percutaneous 4 Percutaneous Endoscopic	Ø Drainage Device 2 Monitoring Device 3 Infusion Device 7 Autologous Tissue Substitute C Extraluminal Device D Intraluminal Device J Synthetic Substitute K Nonautologous Tissue Substitute Y Other Device	Z No Qualifier
Y Lower Vein	X External	Ø Drainage Device 2 Monitoring Device 3 Infusion Device 7 Autologous Tissue Substitute C Extraluminal Device D Intraluminal Device J Synthetic Substitute K Nonautologous Tissue Substitute	Z No Qualifier

Non-OR Ø6WY[3X][Ø237CDJK]Z

Coding Clinic: 2Ø18, Q1, P11 – Ø6WY3DZ

SECTION: Ø MEDICAL AND SURGICAL
BODY SYSTEM: 7 LYMPHATIC AND HEMIC SYSTEMS
OPERATION: 2 CHANGE: Taking out or off a device from a body part and putting back an identical or similar device in or on the same body part without cutting or puncturing the skin or a mucous membrane

Body Part	Approach	Device	Qualifier
K Thoracic Duct L Cisterna Chyli M Thymus N Lymphatic P Spleen T Bone Marrow	X External	Ø Drainage Device Y Other Device	Z No Qualifier

Non-OR All Values

Coding Clinic: 2Ø16, Q1, P3Ø – Ø7T5ØZZ

SECTION: Ø MEDICAL AND SURGICAL
BODY SYSTEM: 7 LYMPHATIC AND HEMIC SYSTEMS
OPERATION: 5 DESTRUCTION: Physical eradication of all or a portion of a body part by the direct use of energy, force, or a destructive agent

Body Part	Approach	Device	Qualifier
Ø Lymphatic, Head 1 Lymphatic, Right Neck 2 Lymphatic, Left Neck 3 Lymphatic, Right Upper Extremity 4 Lymphatic, Left Upper Extremity 5 Lymphatic, Right Axillary 6 Lymphatic, Left Axillary 7 Lymphatic, Thorax 8 Lymphatic, Internal Mammary, Right 9 Lymphatic, Internal Mammary, Left B Lymphatic, Mesenteric C Lymphatic, Pelvis D Lymphatic, Aortic F Lymphatic, Right Lower Extremity G Lymphatic, Left Lower Extremity H Lymphatic, Right Inguinal J Lymphatic, Left Inguinal K Thoracic Duct L Cisterna Chyli M Thymus P Spleen	Ø Open 3 Percutaneous 4 Percutaneous Endoscopic	Z No Device	Z No Qualifier

SECTION: Ø MEDICAL AND SURGICAL
BODY SYSTEM: 7 LYMPHATIC AND HEMIC SYSTEMS
OPERATION: 9 DRAINAGE: Taking or letting out fluids and/or gases from a body part

Body Part	Approach	Device	Qualifier
Ø Lymphatic, Head 1 Lymphatic, Right Neck 2 Lymphatic, Left Neck 3 Lymphatic, Right Upper Extremity 4 Lymphatic, Left Upper Extremity 5 Lymphatic, Right Axillary 6 Lymphatic, Left Axillary 7 Lymphatic, Thorax 8 Lymphatic, Internal Mammary, Right 9 Lymphatic, Internal Mammary, Left B Lymphatic, Mesenteric C Lymphatic, Pelvis D Lymphatic, Aortic F Lymphatic, Right Lower Extremity G Lymphatic, Left Lower Extremity H Lymphatic, Right Inguinal J Lymphatic, Left Inguinal K Thoracic Duct L Cisterna Chyli	Ø Open 3 Percutaneous 4 Percutaneous Endoscopic 8 Via Natural or Artificial Opening Endoscopic	Ø Drainage Device	Z No Qualifier
Ø Lymphatic, Head 1 Lymphatic, Right Neck 2 Lymphatic, Left Neck 3 Lymphatic, Right Upper Extremity 4 Lymphatic, Left Upper Extremity 5 Lymphatic, Right Axillary 6 Lymphatic, Left Axillary 7 Lymphatic, Thorax 8 Lymphatic, Internal Mammary, Right 9 Lymphatic, Internal Mammary, Left B Lymphatic, Mesenteric C Lymphatic, Pelvis D Lymphatic, Aortic F Lymphatic, Right Lower Extremity G Lymphatic, Left Lower Extremity H Lymphatic, Right Inguinal J Lymphatic, Left Inguinal K Thoracic Duct L Cisterna Chyli	Ø Open 3 Percutaneous 4 Percutaneous Endoscopic 8 Via Natural or Artificial Opening Endoscopic	Z No Device	X Diagnostic Z No Qualifier
M Thymus P Spleen T Bone Marrow	Ø Open 3 Percutaneous 4 Percutaneous Endoscopic	Ø Drainage Device	Z No Qualifier
M Thymus P Spleen T Bone Marrow	Ø Open 3 Percutaneous 4 Percutaneous Endoscopic	Z No Device	X Diagnostic Z No Qualifier

Non-OR Ø79[123456789BCDEFGHJKL]3ØZ
Non-OR Ø79P[34]ØZ
Non-OR Ø79T[Ø34]ØZ
Non-OR Ø79[123456789BCDEFGHJKL]3ZZ
Non-OR Ø79P[34]Z[XZ]
Non-OR Ø79T[Ø34]Z[XZ]

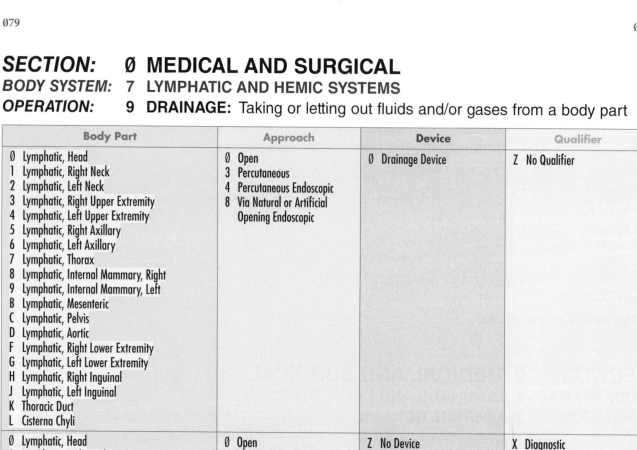

Coding Clinic: 2Ø21, Q4, P48 – Ø79T3ZX

SECTION: Ø MEDICAL AND SURGICAL
BODY SYSTEM: 7 LYMPHATIC AND HEMIC SYSTEMS
OPERATION: B EXCISION: Cutting out or off, without replacement, a portion of a body part

Body Part	Approach	Device	Qualifier
Ø Lymphatic, Head 1 Lymphatic, Right Neck 2 Lymphatic, Left Neck 3 Lymphatic, Right Upper Extremity 4 Lymphatic, Left Upper Extremity 5 Lymphatic, Right Axillary 6 Lymphatic, Left Axillary 7 Lymphatic, Thorax 8 Lymphatic, Internal Mammary, Right 9 Lymphatic, Internal Mammary, Left B Lymphatic, Mesenteric C Lymphatic, Pelvis D Lymphatic, Aortic F Lymphatic, Right Lower Extremity G Lymphatic, Left Lower Extremity H Lymphatic, Right Inguinal ⊞ J Lymphatic, Left Inguinal ⊞ K Thoracic Duct L Cisterna Chyli M Thymus P Spleen	Ø Open 3 Percutaneous 4 Percutaneous Endoscopic	Z No Device	X Diagnostic Z No Qualifier

⊞ Ø7B[HJ][Ø4]ZZ
Non-OR Ø7BP[34]ZX

Coding Clinic: 2Ø19, Q1, P7 – Ø7B[D]ØZZ
Coding Clinic: 2Ø22, Q1, P15 – Ø7B6ØZX

SECTION: Ø MEDICAL AND SURGICAL
BODY SYSTEM: 7 LYMPHATIC AND HEMIC SYSTEMS
OPERATION: C EXTIRPATION: Taking or cutting out solid matter from a body part

Body Part	Approach	Device	Qualifier
Ø Lymphatic, Head 1 Lymphatic, Right Neck 2 Lymphatic, Left Neck 3 Lymphatic, Right Upper Extremity 4 Lymphatic, Left Upper Extremity 5 Lymphatic, Right Axillary 6 Lymphatic, Left Axillary 7 Lymphatic, Thorax 8 Lymphatic, Internal Mammary, Right 9 Lymphatic, Internal Mammary, Left B Lymphatic, Mesenteric C Lymphatic, Pelvis D Lymphatic, Aortic F Lymphatic, Right Lower Extremity G Lymphatic, Left Lower Extremity H Lymphatic, Right Inguinal J Lymphatic, Left Inguinal K Thoracic Duct L Cisterna Chyli M Thymus P Spleen	Ø Open 3 Percutaneous 4 Percutaneous Endoscopic	Z No Device	Z No Qualifier

Non-OR Ø7CP[34]ZZ

SECTION: Ø MEDICAL AND SURGICAL
BODY SYSTEM: 7 LYMPHATIC AND HEMIC SYSTEMS
OPERATION: D EXTRACTION: Pulling or stripping out or off all or a portion of a body part by the use of force

Body Part	Approach	Device	Qualifier
Ø Lymphatic, Head 1 Lymphatic, Right Neck 2 Lymphatic, Left Neck 3 Lymphatic, Right Upper Extremity 4 Lymphatic, Left Upper Extremity 5 Lymphatic, Right Axillary 6 Lymphatic, Left Axillary 7 Lymphatic, Thorax 8 Lymphatic, Internal Mammary, Right 9 Lymphatic, Internal Mammary, Left B Lymphatic, Mesenteric C Lymphatic, Pelvis D Lymphatic, Aortic F Lymphatic, Right Lower Extremity G Lymphatic, Left Lower Extremity H Lymphatic, Right Inguinal J Lymphatic, Left Inguinal K Thoracic Duct L Cisterna Chyli	3 Percutaneous 4 Percutaneous Endoscopic 8 Via Natural or Artificial Opening Endoscopic	Z No Device	X Diagnostic
M Thymus P Spleen	3 Percutaneous 4 Percutaneous Endoscopic	Z No Device	X Diagnostic
Q Bone Marrow, Sternum R Bone Marrow, Iliac S Bone Marrow, Vertebral T Bone Marrow	Ø Open 3 Percutaneous	Z No Device	X Diagnostic Z No Qualifier

Non-OR Ø7D[QRS][Ø3]Z[XZ]

Coding Clinic: 2021, Q4, P48 – Ø7DT3ZX

SECTION: Ø MEDICAL AND SURGICAL
BODY SYSTEM: 7 LYMPHATIC AND HEMIC SYSTEMS
OPERATION: H INSERTION: Putting in a nonbiological appliance that monitors, assists, performs, or prevents a physiological function but does not physically take the place of a body part

Body Part	Approach	Device	Qualifier
K Thoracic Duct L Cisterna Chyli M Thymus N Lymphatic P Spleen T Bone Marrow	Ø Open 3 Percutaneous 4 Percutaneous Endoscopic	1 Radioactive Element 3 Infusion Device Y Other Device	Z No Qualifier

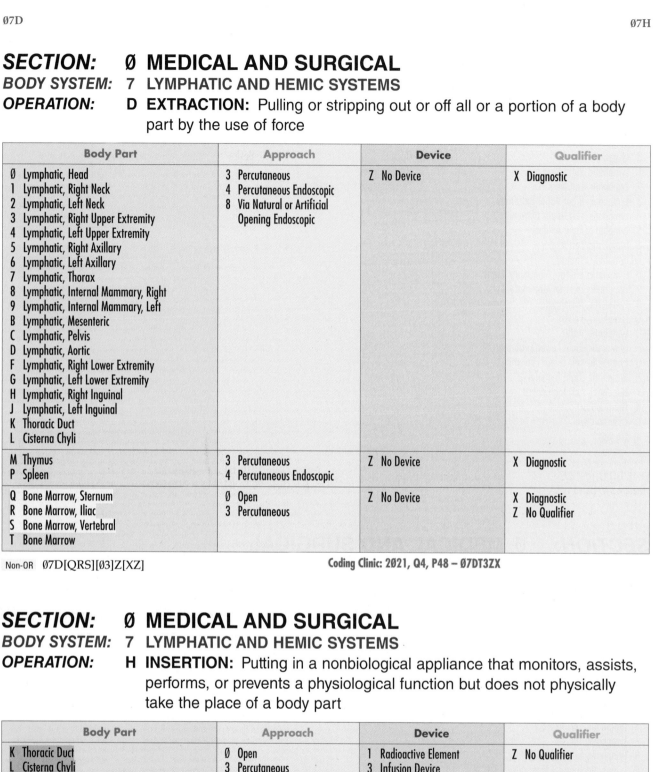

DRG Non-OR Ø7H[KLMNP][Ø34]3Z

SECTION: Ø MEDICAL AND SURGICAL
BODY SYSTEM: 7 LYMPHATIC AND HEMIC SYSTEMS
OPERATION: J INSPECTION: Visually and/or manually exploring a body part

Body Part	Approach	Device	Qualifier
K Thoracic Duct L Cisterna Chyli M Thymus T Bone Marrow	Ø Open 3 Percutaneous 4 Percutaneous Endoscopic	Z No Device	Z No Qualifier
N Lymphatic	Ø Open 3 Percutaneous 4 Percutaneous Endoscopic 8 Via Natural or Artificial Opening Endoscopic X External	Z No Device	Z No Qualifier
P Spleen	Ø Open 3 Percutaneous 4 Percutaneous Endoscopic X External	Z No Device	Z No Qualifier

Non-OR Ø7J[KLM]3ZZ
Non-OR Ø7JN[3X]ZZ
Non-OR Ø7JP[34X]ZZ
Non-OR Ø7JT[Ø34]ZZ

SECTION: Ø MEDICAL AND SURGICAL
BODY SYSTEM: 7 LYMPHATIC AND HEMIC SYSTEMS
OPERATION: L OCCLUSION: Completely closing an orifice or the lumen of a tubular body part

Body Part	Approach	Device	Qualifier
Ø Lymphatic, Head 1 Lymphatic, Right Neck 2 Lymphatic, Left Neck 3 Lymphatic, Right Upper Extremity 4 Lymphatic, Left Upper Extremity 5 Lymphatic, Right Axillary 6 Lymphatic, Left Axillary 7 Lymphatic, Thorax 8 Lymphatic, Internal Mammary, Right 9 Lymphatic, Internal Mammary, Left B Lymphatic, Mesenteric C Lymphatic, Pelvis D Lymphatic, Aortic F Lymphatic, Right Lower Extremity G Lymphatic, Left Lower Extremity H Lymphatic, Right Inguinal J Lymphatic, Left Inguinal K Thoracic Duct L Cisterna Chyli	Ø Open 3 Percutaneous 4 Percutaneous Endoscopic	C Extraluminal Device D Intraluminal Device Z No Device	Z No Qualifier

SECTION: Ø MEDICAL AND SURGICAL
BODY SYSTEM: 7 LYMPHATIC AND HEMIC SYSTEMS
OPERATION: N RELEASE: Freeing a body part from an abnormal physical constraint by cutting or by the use of force

Body Part	Approach	Device	Qualifier
Ø Lymphatic, Head 1 Lymphatic, Right Neck 2 Lymphatic, Left Neck 3 Lymphatic, Right Upper Extremity 4 Lymphatic, Left Upper Extremity 5 Lymphatic, Right Axillary 6 Lymphatic, Left Axillary 7 Lymphatic, Thorax 8 Lymphatic, Internal Mammary, Right 9 Lymphatic, Internal Mammary, Left B Lymphatic, Mesenteric C Lymphatic, Pelvis D Lymphatic, Aortic F Lymphatic, Right Lower Extremity G Lymphatic, Left Lower Extremity H Lymphatic, Right Inguinal J Lymphatic, Left Inguinal K Thoracic Duct L Cisterna Chyli M Thymus P Spleen	Ø Open 3 Percutaneous 4 Percutaneous Endoscopic	Z No Device	Z No Qualifier

SECTION: Ø MEDICAL AND SURGICAL
BODY SYSTEM: 7 LYMPHATIC AND HEMIC SYSTEMS
OPERATION: P REMOVAL: Taking out or off a device from a body part

Body Part	Approach	Device	Qualifier
K Thoracic Duct L Cisterna Chyli N Lymphatic	Ø Open 3 Percutaneous 4 Percutaneous Endoscopic	Ø Drainage Device 3 Infusion Device 7 Autologous Tissue Substitute C Extraluminal Device D Intraluminal Device J Synthetic Substitute K Nonautologous Tissue Substitute Y Other Device	Z No Qualifier
K Thoracic Duct L Cisterna Chyli N Lymphatic	X External	Ø Drainage Device 3 Infusion Device D Intraluminal Device	Z No Qualifier
M Thymus P Spleen	Ø Open 3 Percutaneous 4 Percutaneous Endoscopic	Ø Drainage Device 3 Infusion Device Y Other Device	Z No Qualifier
M Thymus P Spleen	X External	Ø Drainage Device 3 Infusion Device	Z No Qualifier
T Bone Marrow	Ø Open 3 Percutaneous 4 Percutaneous Endoscopic X External	Ø Drainage Device	Z No Qualifier

Non-OR Ø7P[KLN]X[Ø3D]Z Non-OR Ø7P[MP]X[Ø3]Z Non-OR Ø7PT[Ø34X]ØZ

SECTION: Ø MEDICAL AND SURGICAL
BODY SYSTEM: 7 LYMPHATIC AND HEMIC SYSTEMS
OPERATION: Q REPAIR: Restoring, to the extent possible, a body part to its normal anatomic structure and function

Body Part	Approach	Device	Qualifier
Ø Lymphatic, Head 1 Lymphatic, Right Neck 2 Lymphatic, Left Neck 3 Lymphatic, Right Upper Extremity 4 Lymphatic, Left Upper Extremity 5 Lymphatic, Right Axillary 6 Lymphatic, Left Axillary 7 Lymphatic, Thorax 8 Lymphatic, Internal Mammary, Right 9 Lymphatic, Internal Mammary, Left B Lymphatic, Mesenteric C Lymphatic, Pelvis D Lymphatic, Aortic F Lymphatic, Right Lower Extremity G Lymphatic, Left Lower Extremity H Lymphatic, Right Inguinal J Lymphatic, Left Inguinal K Thoracic Duct L Cisterna Chyli	Ø Open 3 Percutaneous 4 Percutaneous Endoscopic 8 Via Natural or Artificial Opening Endoscopic	Z No Device	Z No Qualifier
M Thymus P Spleen	Ø Open 3 Percutaneous 4 Percutaneous Endoscopic	Z No Device	Z No Qualifier

Coding Clinic: 2Ø17, Q1, P34 – Ø7Q6ØZZ

SECTION: Ø MEDICAL AND SURGICAL
BODY SYSTEM: 7 LYMPHATIC AND HEMIC SYSTEMS
OPERATION: S REPOSITION: Moving to its normal location, or other suitable location, all or a portion of a body part

Body Part	Approach	Device	Qualifier
M Thymus P Spleen	Ø Open	Z No Device	Z No Qualifier

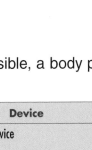

SECTION: Ø MEDICAL AND SURGICAL
BODY SYSTEM: 7 LYMPHATIC AND HEMIC SYSTEMS
OPERATION: T RESECTION: Cutting out or off, without replacement, all of a body part

Body Part	Approach	Device	Qualifier
Ø Lymphatic, Head 1 Lymphatic, Right Neck 2 Lymphatic, Left Neck 3 Lymphatic, Right Upper Extremity 4 Lymphatic, Left Upper Extremity 5 Lymphatic, Right Axillary ⊞ 6 Lymphatic, Left Axillary ⊞ 7 Lymphatic, Thorax ⊞ 8 Lymphatic, Internal Mammary, Right ⊞ 9 Lymphatic, Internal Mammary, Left ⊞ B Lymphatic, Mesenteric C Lymphatic, Pelvis D Lymphatic, Aortic F Lymphatic, Right Lower Extremity G Lymphatic, Left Lower Extremity H Lymphatic, Right Inguinal J Lymphatic, Left Inguinal K Thoracic Duct L Cisterna Chyli M Thymus P Spleen	Ø Open 4 Percutaneous Endoscopic	Z No Device	Z No Qualifier

⊞ Ø7T[56789]ØZZ

Coding Clinic: 2Ø15, Q4, P13 – Ø7TPØZZ
Coding Clinic: 2Ø16, Q2, P13 – Ø7T2ØZZ

SECTION: Ø MEDICAL AND SURGICAL
BODY SYSTEM: 7 LYMPHATIC AND HEMIC SYSTEMS
OPERATION: U SUPPLEMENT: Putting in or on biological or synthetic material that physically reinforces and/or augments the function of a portion of a body part

Body Part	Approach	Device	Qualifier
Ø Lymphatic, Head 1 Lymphatic, Right Neck 2 Lymphatic, Left Neck 3 Lymphatic, Right Upper Extremity 4 Lymphatic, Left Upper Extremity 5 Lymphatic, Right Axillary 6 Lymphatic, Left Axillary 7 Lymphatic, Thorax 8 Lymphatic, Internal Mammary, Right 9 Lymphatic, Internal Mammary, Left B Lymphatic, Mesenteric C Lymphatic, Pelvis D Lymphatic, Aortic F Lymphatic, Right Lower Extremity G Lymphatic, Left Lower Extremity H Lymphatic, Right Inguinal J Lymphatic, Left Inguinal K Thoracic Duct L Cisterna Chyli	Ø Open 4 Percutaneous Endoscopic	7 Autologous Tissue Substitute J Synthetic Substitute K Nonautologous Tissue Substitute	Z No Qualifier

SECTION: Ø MEDICAL AND SURGICAL
BODY SYSTEM: 7 LYMPHATIC AND HEMIC SYSTEMS
OPERATION: V RESTRICTION: Partially closing an orifice or the lumen of a tubular body part

Body Part	Approach	Device	Qualifier
Ø Lymphatic, Head 1 Lymphatic, Right Neck 2 Lymphatic, Left Neck 3 Lymphatic, Right Upper Extremity 4 Lymphatic, Left Upper Extremity 5 Lymphatic, Right Axillary 6 Lymphatic, Left Axillary 7 Lymphatic, Thorax 8 Lymphatic, Internal Mammary, Right 9 Lymphatic, Internal Mammary, Left B Lymphatic, Mesenteric C Lymphatic, Pelvis D Lymphatic, Aortic F Lymphatic, Right Lower Extremity G Lymphatic, Left Lower Extremity H Lymphatic, Right Inguinal J Lymphatic, Left Inguinal K Thoracic Duct L Cisterna Chyli	Ø Open 3 Percutaneous 4 Percutaneous Endoscopic	C Extraluminal Device D Intraluminal Device Z No Device	Z No Qualifier

SECTION: Ø MEDICAL AND SURGICAL
BODY SYSTEM: 7 LYMPHATIC AND HEMIC SYSTEMS
OPERATION: W REVISION: Correcting, to the extent possible, a portion of a malfunctioning device or the position of a displaced device

Body Part	Approach	Device	Qualifier
K Thoracic Duct L Cisterna Chyli N Lymphatic	Ø Open 3 Percutaneous 4 Percutaneous Endoscopic	Ø Drainage Device 3 Infusion Device 7 Autologous Tissue Substitute C Extraluminal Device D Intraluminal Device J Synthetic Substitute K Nonautologous Tissue Substitute Y Other Device	Z No Qualifier
K Thoracic Duct L Cisterna Chyli N Lymphatic	X External	Ø Drainage Device 3 Infusion Device 7 Autologous Tissue Substitute C Extraluminal Device D Intraluminal Device J Synthetic Substitute K Nonautologous Tissue Substitute	Z No Qualifier
M Thymus P Spleen	Ø Open 3 Percutaneous 4 Percutaneous Endoscopic	Ø Drainage Device 3 Infusion Device Y Other Device	Z No Qualifier
M Thymus P Spleen	X External	Ø Drainage Device 3 Infusion Device	Z No Qualifier
T Bone Marrow	Ø Open 3 Percutaneous 4 Percutaneous Endoscopic X External	Ø Drainage Device	Z No Qualifier

Non-OR Ø7W[KLN]X[Ø37CDJK]Z
Non-OR Ø7W[MP]X[Ø3]Z
Non-OR Ø7WT[Ø34X]ØZ

SECTION: Ø MEDICAL AND SURGICAL
BODY SYSTEM: 7 LYMPHATIC AND HEMIC SYSTEMS
OPERATION: Y TRANSPLANTATION: Putting in or on all or a portion of a living body part taken from another individual or animal to physically take the place and/or function of all or a portion of a similar body part

Body Part	Approach	Device	Qualifier
M Thymus P Spleen	Ø Open	Z No Device	Ø Allogeneic 1 Syngeneic 2 Zooplastic

Coding Clinic: 2019, Q3, P29 – Ø7YMØZØ

SECTION: Ø MEDICAL AND SURGICAL
BODY SYSTEM: 8 EYE
OPERATION: Ø **ALTERATION:** Modifying the anatomic structure of a body part without affecting the function of the body part

Body Part	Approach	Device	Qualifier
N Upper Eyelid, Right P Upper Eyelid, Left Q Lower Eyelid, Right R Lower Eyelid, Left	Ø Open 3 Percutaneous X External	7 Autologous Tissue Substitute J Synthetic Substitute K Nonautologous Tissue Substitute Z No Device	Z No Qualifier

Non-OR All Values

SECTION: Ø MEDICAL AND SURGICAL
BODY SYSTEM: 8 EYE
OPERATION: 1 **BYPASS:** Altering the route of passage of the contents of a tubular body part

Body Part	Approach	Device	Qualifier
2 Anterior Chamber, Right 3 Anterior Chamber, Left	3 Percutaneous	J Synthetic Substitute K Nonautologous Tissue Substitute Z No Device	4 Sclera
X Lacrimal Duct, Right Y Lacrimal Duct, Left	Ø Open 3 Percutaneous	J Synthetic Substitute K Nonautologous Tissue Substitute Z No Device	3 Nasal Cavity

Coding Clinic: 2Ø19, Q1, P28 – Ø8133J4

SECTION: Ø MEDICAL AND SURGICAL
BODY SYSTEM: 8 EYE
OPERATION: 2 **CHANGE:** Taking out or off a device from a body part and putting back an identical or similar device in or on the same body part without cutting or puncturing the skin or a mucous membrane

Body Part	Approach	Device	Qualifier
Ø Eye, Right 1 Eye, Left	X External	Ø Drainage Device Y Other Device	Z No Qualifier

Non-OR All Values

SECTION: Ø MEDICAL AND SURGICAL
BODY SYSTEM: 8 EYE
OPERATION: 5 **DESTRUCTION:** Physical eradication of all or a portion of a body part by the direct use of energy, force, or a destructive agent

Body Part	Approach	Device	Qualifier
Ø Eye, Right 1 Eye, Left 6 Sclera, Right 7 Sclera, Left 8 Cornea, Right 9 Cornea, Left S Conjunctiva, Right T Conjunctiva, Left	X External	Z No Device	Z No Qualifier
2 Anterior Chamber, Right 3 Anterior Chamber, Left 4 Vitreous, Right 5 Vitreous, Left C Iris, Right D Iris, Left E Retina, Right F Retina, Left G Retinal Vessel, Right H Retinal Vessel, Left J Lens, Right K Lens, Left	3 Percutaneous	Z No Device	Z No Qualifier
A Choroid, Right B Choroid, Left L Extraocular Muscle, Right M Extraocular Muscle, Left V Lacrimal Gland, Right W Lacrimal Gland, Left	Ø Open 3 Percutaneous	Z No Device	Z No Qualifier
N Upper Eyelid, Right P Upper Eyelid, Left Q Lower Eyelid, Right R Lower Eyelid, Left	Ø Open 3 Percutaneous X External	Z No Device	Z No Qualifier
X Lacrimal Duct, Right Y Lacrimal Duct, Left	Ø Open 3 Percutaneous 7 Via Natural or Artificial Opening 8 Via Natural or Artificial Opening Endoscopic	Z No Device	Z No Qualifier

SECTION: Ø MEDICAL AND SURGICAL
BODY SYSTEM: 8 EYE
OPERATION: 7 **DILATION:** Expanding an orifice or the lumen of a tubular body part

Body Part	Approach	Device	Qualifier
X Lacrimal Duct, Right Y Lacrimal Duct, Left	Ø Open 3 Percutaneous 7 Via Natural or Artificial Opening 8 Via Natural or Artificial Opening Endoscopic	D Intraluminal Device Z No Device	Z No Qualifier

SECTION: Ø MEDICAL AND SURGICAL
BODY SYSTEM: 8 EYE
OPERATION: 9 DRAINAGE: *(on multiple pages)*
Taking or letting out fluids and/or gases from a body part

Body Part	Approach	Device	Qualifier
Ø Eye, Right 1 Eye, Left 6 Sclera, Right 7 Sclera, Left 8 Cornea, Right 9 Cornea, Left S Conjunctiva, Right T Conjunctiva, Left	X External	Ø Drainage Device	Z No Qualifier
Ø Eye, Right 1 Eye, Left 6 Sclera, Right 7 Sclera, Left 8 Cornea, Right 9 Cornea, Left S Conjunctiva, Right T Conjunctiva, Left	X External	Z No Device	X Diagnostic Z No Qualifier
2 Anterior Chamber, Right 3 Anterior Chamber, Left 4 Vitreous, Right 5 Vitreous, Left C Iris, Right D Iris, Left E Retina, Right F Retina, Left G Retinal Vessel, Right H Retinal Vessel, Left J Lens, Right K Lens, Left	3 Percutaneous	Ø Drainage Device	Z No Qualifier
2 Anterior Chamber, Right 3 Anterior Chamber, Left 4 Vitreous, Right 5 Vitreous, Left C Iris, Right D Iris, Left E Retina, Right F Retina, Left G Retinal Vessel, Right H Retinal Vessel, Left J Lens, Right K Lens, Left	3 Percutaneous	Z No Device	X Diagnostic Z No Qualifier
A Choroid, Right B Choroid, Left L Extraocular Muscle, Right M Extraocular Muscle, Left V Lacrimal Gland, Right W Lacrimal Gland, Left	Ø Open 3 Percutaneous	Ø Drainage Device	Z No Qualifier

DRG Non-OR Ø89[Ø16789ST]XZ[XZ] *(proposed)*

Coding Clinic: 2Ø16, Q2, P21 – Ø8923ZZ

SECTION: Ø MEDICAL AND SURGICAL
BODY SYSTEM: 8 EYE
OPERATION: 9 DRAINAGE: *(continued)*
Taking or letting out fluids and/or gases from a body part

Body Part	Approach	Device	Qualifier
A Choroid, Right B Choroid, Left L Extraocular Muscle, Right M Extraocular Muscle, Left V Lacrimal Gland, Right W Lacrimal Gland, Left	Ø Open 3 Percutaneous	Z No Device	X Diagnostic Z No Qualifier
N Upper Eyelid, Right P Upper Eyelid, Left Q Lower Eyelid, Right R Lower Eyelid, Left	Ø Open 3 Percutaneous X External	Ø Drainage Device	Z No Qualifier
N Upper Eyelid, Right P Upper Eyelid, Left Q Lower Eyelid, Right R Lower Eyelid, Left	Ø Open 3 Percutaneous X External	Z No Device	X Diagnostic Z No Qualifier
X Lacrimal Duct, Right Y Lacrimal Duct, Left	Ø Open 3 Percutaneous 7 Via Natural or Artificial Opening 8 Via Natural or Artificial Opening Endoscopic	Ø Drainage Device	Z No Qualifier
X Lacrimal Duct, Right Y Lacrimal Duct, Left	Ø Open 3 Percutaneous 7 Via Natural or Artificial Opening 8 Via Natural or Artificial Opening Endoscopic	Z No Device	X Diagnostic Z No Qualifier

DRG Non-OR Ø89[NPQR]XZX *(proposed)*
Non-OR Ø89[NPQR][Ø3X]ØZ
Non-OR Ø89[NPQR][Ø3X]ZZ

SECTION: Ø MEDICAL AND SURGICAL
BODY SYSTEM: 8 EYE
OPERATION: B EXCISION: Cutting out or off, without replacement, a portion of a body part

Body Part	Approach	Device	Qualifier
Ø Eye, Right 1 Eye, Left N Upper Eyelid, Right P Upper Eyelid, Left Q Lower Eyelid, Right R Lower Eyelid, Left	Ø Open 3 Percutaneous X External	Z No Device	X Diagnostic Z No Qualifier
4 Vitreous, Right 5 Vitreous, Left C Iris, Right D Iris, Left E Retina, Right F Retina, Left J Lens, Right K Lens, Left	3 Percutaneous	Z No Device	X Diagnostic Z No Qualifier
6 Sclera, Right 7 Sclera, Left 8 Cornea, Right 9 Cornea, Left S Conjunctiva, Right T Conjunctiva, Left	X External	Z No Device	X Diagnostic Z No Qualifier
A Choroid, Right B Choroid, Left L Extraocular Muscle, Right M Extraocular Muscle, Left V Lacrimal Gland, Right W Lacrimal Gland, Left	Ø Open 3 Percutaneous	Z No Device	X Diagnostic Z No Qualifier
X Lacrimal Duct, Right Y Lacrimal Duct, Left	Ø Open 3 Percutaneous 7 Via Natural or Artificial Opening 8 Via Natural or Artificial Opening Endoscopic	Z No Device	X Diagnostic Z No Qualifier

SECTION: Ø MEDICAL AND SURGICAL
BODY SYSTEM: 8 EYE
OPERATION: C EXTIRPATION: Taking or cutting out solid matter from a body part

Body Part	Approach	Device	Qualifier
Ø Eye, Right 1 Eye, Left 6 Sclera, Right 7 Sclera, Left 8 Cornea, Right 9 Cornea, Left S Conjunctiva, Right T Conjunctiva, Left	X External	Z No Device	Z No Qualifier
2 Anterior Chamber, Right 3 Anterior Chamber, Left 4 Vitreous, Right 5 Vitreous, Left C Iris, Right D Iris, Left E Retina, Right F Retina, Left G Retinal Vessel, Right H Retinal Vessel, Left J Lens, Right K Lens, Left	3 Percutaneous X External	Z No Device	Z No Qualifier
A Choroid, Right B Choroid, Left L Extraocular Muscle, Right M Extraocular Muscle, Left N Upper Eyelid, Right P Upper Eyelid, Left Q Lower Eyelid, Right R Lower Eyelid, Left V Lacrimal Gland, Right W Lacrimal Gland, Left	Ø Open 3 Percutaneous X External	Z No Device	Z No Qualifier
X Lacrimal Duct, Right Y Lacrimal Duct, Left	Ø Open 3 Percutaneous 7 Via Natural or Artificial Opening 8 Via Natural or Artificial Opening Endoscopic	Z No Device	Z No Qualifier

Non-OR Ø8C[23]XZZ
Non-OR Ø8C[67]XZZ
Non-OR Ø8C[NPQR][Ø3X]ZZ

SECTION: Ø MEDICAL AND SURGICAL
BODY SYSTEM: 8 EYE
OPERATION: D EXTRACTION: Pulling or stripping out or off all or a portion of a body part by the use of force

Body Part	Approach	Device	Qualifier
8 Cornea, Right 9 Cornea, Left	X External	Z No Device	X Diagnostic Z No Qualifier
J Lens, Right K Lens, Left	3 Percutaneous	Z No Device	Z No Qualifier

SECTION: Ø MEDICAL AND SURGICAL
BODY SYSTEM: 8 EYE
OPERATION: F FRAGMENTATION: Breaking solid matter in a body part into pieces

Body Part	Approach	Device	Qualifier
4 Vitreous, Right 5 Vitreous, Left	3 Percutaneous X External	Z No Device	Z No Qualifier

Ø8F[45]XZZ
Non-OR Ø8F[45]XZZ

SECTION: Ø MEDICAL AND SURGICAL
BODY SYSTEM: 8 EYE
OPERATION: H INSERTION: Putting in a nonbiological appliance that monitors, assists, performs, or prevents a physiological function but does not physically take the place of a body part

Body Part	Approach	Device	Qualifier
Ø Eye, Right 1 Eye, Left	Ø Open	5 Epiretinal Visual Prosthesis Y Other Device	Z No Qualifier
Ø Eye, Right 1 Eye, Left	3 Percutaneous	1 Radioactive Element 3 Infusion Device Y Other Device	Z No Qualifier
Ø Eye, Right 1 Eye, Left	7 Via Natural or Artificial Opening 8 Via Natural or Artificial Opening Endoscopic	Y Other Device	Z No Qualifier
Ø Eye, Right 1 Eye, Left	X External	1 Radioactive Element 3 Infusion Device	Z No Qualifier

SECTION: Ø MEDICAL AND SURGICAL
BODY SYSTEM: 8 EYE
OPERATION: J INSPECTION: Visually and/or manually exploring a body part

Body Part	Approach	Device	Qualifier
Ø Eye, Right 1 Eye, Left J Lens, Right K Lens, Left	X External	Z No Device	Z No Qualifier
L Extraocular Muscle, Right M Extraocular Muscle, Left	Ø Open X External	Z No Device	Z No Qualifier

Non-OR Ø8J[Ø1JK]XZZ
Non-OR Ø8J[LM]XZZ

Coding Clinic: 2015, Q1, P36 – Ø8JØXZZ

Ø: M/S 8: EYE F: FRAGMENTATION H: INSERTION J: INSPECTION

New/Revised Text in Green ~~deleted~~ Deleted ♀ Females Only ♂ Males Only Coding Clinic
Non-covered Limited Coverage Combination (See Appendix E) DRG Non-OR Non-OR Hospital-Acquired Condition

SECTION: Ø MEDICAL AND SURGICAL
BODY SYSTEM: 8 EYE
OPERATION: L OCCLUSION: Completely closing an orifice or the lumen of a tubular body part

Body Part	Approach	Device	Qualifier
X Lacrimal Duct, Right Y Lacrimal Duct, Left	Ø Open 3 Percutaneous	C Extraluminal Device D Intraluminal Device Z No Device	Z No Qualifier
X Lacrimal Duct, Right Y Lacrimal Duct, Left	7 Via Natural or Artificial Opening 8 Via Natural or Artificial Opening Endoscopic	D Intraluminal Device Z No Device	Z No Qualifier

SECTION: Ø MEDICAL AND SURGICAL
BODY SYSTEM: 8 EYE
OPERATION: M REATTACHMENT: Putting back in or on all or a portion of a separated body part to its normal location or other suitable location

Body Part	Approach	Device	Qualifier
N Upper Eyelid, Right P Upper Eyelid, Left Q Lower Eyelid, Right R Lower Eyelid, Left	X External	Z No Device	Z No Qualifier

SECTION: Ø MEDICAL AND SURGICAL
BODY SYSTEM: 8 EYE
OPERATION: N RELEASE: Freeing a body part from an abnormal physical constraint by cutting or by the use of force

Body Part	Approach	Device	Qualifier
Ø Eye, Right 1 Eye, Left 6 Sclera, Right 7 Sclera, Left 8 Cornea, Right 9 Cornea, Left S Conjunctiva, Right T Conjunctiva, Left	X External	Z No Device	Z No Qualifier
2 Anterior Chamber, Right 3 Anterior Chamber, Left 4 Vitreous, Right 5 Vitreous, Left C Iris, Right D Iris, Left E Retina, Right F Retina, Left G Retinal Vessel, Right H Retinal Vessel, Left J Lens, Right K Lens, Left	3 Percutaneous	Z No Device	Z No Qualifier
A Choroid, Right B Choroid, Left L Extraocular Muscle, Right M Extraocular Muscle, Left V Lacrimal Gland, Right W Lacrimal Gland, Left	Ø Open 3 Percutaneous	Z No Device	Z No Qualifier
N Upper Eyelid, Right P Upper Eyelid, Left Q Lower Eyelid, Right R Lower Eyelid, Left	Ø Open 3 Percutaneous X External	Z No Device	Z No Qualifier
X Lacrimal Duct, Right Y Lacrimal Duct, Left	Ø Open 3 Percutaneous 7 Via Natural or Artificial Opening 8 Via Natural or Artificial Opening Endoscopic	Z No Device	Z No Qualifier

Coding Clinic: 2Ø15, Q2, P25 – Ø8NC3ZZ

SECTION: Ø MEDICAL AND SURGICAL
BODY SYSTEM: 8 EYE
OPERATION: P REMOVAL: Taking out or off a device from a body part

Body Part	Approach	Device	Qualifier
Ø Eye, Right 1 Eye, Left	Ø Open 3 Percutaneous 7 Via Natural or Artificial Opening 8 Via Natural or Artificial Opening Endoscopic	Ø Drainage Device 1 Radioactive Element 3 Infusion Device 7 Autologous Tissue Substitute C Extraluminal Device D Intraluminal Device J Synthetic Substitute K Nonautologous Tissue Substitute Y Other Device	Z No Qualifier
Ø Eye, Right 1 Eye, Left	X External	Ø Drainage Device 1 Radioactive Element 3 Infusion Device 7 Autologous Tissue Substitute C Extraluminal Device D Intraluminal Device J Synthetic Substitute K Nonautologous Tissue Substitute	Z No Qualifier
J Lens, Right K Lens, Left	3 Percutaneous	J Synthetic Substitute Y Other Device	Z No Qualifier
L Extraocular Muscle, Right M Extraocular Muscle, Left	Ø Open 3 Percutaneous	Ø Drainage Device 7 Autologous Tissue Substitute J Synthetic Substitute K Nonautologous Tissue Substitute Y Other Device	Z No Qualifier

Non-OR Ø8P[Ø1][78][Ø3D]Z
Non-OR Ø8PØX[Ø3CD]Z
Non-OR Ø8P1X[Ø13CD]Z

SECTION: Ø MEDICAL AND SURGICAL
BODY SYSTEM: 8 EYE
OPERATION: Q REPAIR: Restoring, to the extent possible, a body part to its normal anatomic structure and function

Body Part	Approach	Device	Qualifier
Ø Eye, Right 1 Eye, Left 6 Sclera, Right 7 Sclera, Left 8 Cornea, Right 9 Cornea, Left S Conjunctiva, Right T Conjunctiva, Left	X External	Z No Device	Z No Qualifier
2 Anterior Chamber, Right 3 Anterior Chamber, Left 4 Vitreous, Right 5 Vitreous, Left C Iris, Right D Iris, Left E Retina, Right F Retina, Left G Retinal Vessel, Right H Retinal Vessel, Left J Lens, Right K Lens, Left	3 Percutaneous	Z No Device	Z No Qualifier
A Choroid, Right B Choroid, Left L Extraocular Muscle, Right M Extraocular Muscle, Left V Lacrimal Gland, Right W Lacrimal Gland, Left	Ø Open 3 Percutaneous	Z No Device	Z No Qualifier
N Upper Eyelid, Right P Upper Eyelid, Left Q Lower Eyelid, Right R Lower Eyelid, Left	Ø Open 3 Percutaneous X External	Z No Device	Z No Qualifier
X Lacrimal Duct, Right Y Lacrimal Duct, Left	Ø Open 3 Percutaneous 7 Via Natural or Artificial Opening 8 Via Natural or Artificial Opening Endoscopic	Z No Device	Z No Qualifier

Ø8Q[89]XZZ
Non-OR Ø8Q[NPQR][Ø3X]ZZ

SECTION: Ø MEDICAL AND SURGICAL
BODY SYSTEM: 8 EYE
OPERATION: R REPLACEMENT: Putting in or on biological or synthetic material that physically takes the place and/or function of all or a portion of a body part

Body Part	Approach	Device	Qualifier
Ø Eye, Right 1 Eye, Left A Choroid, Right B Choroid, Left	Ø Open 3 Percutaneous	7 Autologous Tissue Substitute J Synthetic Substitute K Nonautologous Tissue Substitute	Z No Qualifier
4 Vitreous, Right 5 Vitreous, Left C Iris, Right D Iris, Left G Retinal Vessel, Right H Retinal Vessel, Left	3 Percutaneous	7 Autologous Tissue Substitute J Synthetic Substitute K Nonautologous Tissue Substitute	Z No Qualifier
6 Sclera, Right 7 Sclera, Left S Conjunctiva, Right T Conjunctiva, Left	X External	7 Autologous Tissue Substitute J Synthetic Substitute K Nonautologous Tissue Substitute	Z No Qualifier
8 Cornea, Right 9 Cornea, Left	3 Percutaneous X External	7 Autologous Tissue Substitute J Synthetic Substitute K Nonautologous Tissue Substitute	Z No Qualifier
J Lens, Right K Lens, Left	3 Percutaneous	Ø Synthetic Substitute, Intraocular Telescope 7 Autologous Tissue Substitute J Synthetic Substitute K Nonautologous Tissue Substitute	Z No Qualifier
N Upper Eyelid, Right P Upper Eyelid, Left Q Lower Eyelid, Right R Lower Eyelid, Left	Ø Open 3 Percutaneous X External	7 Autologous Tissue Substitute J Synthetic Substitute K Nonautologous Tissue Substitute	Z No Qualifier
X Lacrimal Duct, Right Y Lacrimal Duct, Left	Ø Open 3 Percutaneous 7 Via Natural or Artificial Opening 8 Via Natural or Artificial Opening Endoscopic	7 Autologous Tissue Substitute J Synthetic Substitute K Nonautologous Tissue Substitute	Z No Qualifier

Coding Clinic: 2Ø15, Q2, P25-26 – Ø8R8XKZ

SECTION: Ø MEDICAL AND SURGICAL
BODY SYSTEM: 8 EYE
OPERATION: S REPOSITION: Moving to its normal location, or other suitable location, all or a portion of a body part

Body Part	Approach	Device	Qualifier
C Iris, Right D Iris, Left G Retinal Vessel, Right H Retinal Vessel, Left J Lens, Right K Lens, Left	3 Percutaneous	Z No Device	Z No Qualifier
L Extraocular Muscle, Right M Extraocular Muscle, Left V Lacrimal Gland, Right W Lacrimal Gland, Left	Ø Open 3 Percutaneous	Z No Device	Z No Qualifier
N Upper Eyelid, Right P Upper Eyelid, Left Q Lower Eyelid, Right R Lower Eyelid, Left	Ø Open 3 Percutaneous X External	Z No Device	Z No Qualifier
X Lacrimal Duct, Right Y Lacrimal Duct, Left	Ø Open 3 Percutaneous 7 Via Natural or Artificial Opening 8 Via Natural or Artificial Opening Endoscopic	Z No Device	Z No Qualifier

SECTION: Ø MEDICAL AND SURGICAL
BODY SYSTEM: 8 EYE
OPERATION: T RESECTION: Cutting out or off, without replacement, all of a body part

Body Part	Approach	Device	Qualifier
Ø Eye, Right 1 Eye, Left 8 Cornea, Right 9 Cornea, Left	X External	Z No Device	Z No Qualifier
4 Vitreous, Right 5 Vitreous, Left C Iris, Right D Iris, Left J Lens, Right K Lens, Left	3 Percutaneous	Z No Device	Z No Qualifier
L Extraocular Muscle, Right M Extraocular Muscle, Left V Lacrimal Gland, Right W Lacrimal Gland, Left	Ø Open 3 Percutaneous	Z No Device	Z No Qualifier
N Upper Eyelid, Right P Upper Eyelid, Left Q Lower Eyelid, Right R Lower Eyelid, Left	Ø Open X External	Z No Device	Z No Qualifier
X Lacrimal Duct, Right Y Lacrimal Duct, Left	Ø Open 3 Percutaneous 7 Via Natural or Artificial Opening 8 Via Natural or Artificial Opening Endoscopic	Z No Device	Z No Qualifier

Coding Clinic: 2Ø15, Q2, P13 – Ø8T1XZZ, Ø8T[MR]ØZZ

SECTION: Ø MEDICAL AND SURGICAL
BODY SYSTEM: 8 EYE
OPERATION: U SUPPLEMENT: Putting in or on biological or synthetic material that physically reinforces and/or augments the function of a portion of a body part

Body Part	Approach	Device	Qualifier
Ø Eye, Right 1 Eye, Left C Iris, Right D Iris, Left E Retina, Right F Retina, Left G Retinal Vessel, Right H Retinal Vessel, Left L Extraocular Muscle, Right M Extraocular Muscle, Left	Ø Open 3 Percutaneous	7 Autologous Tissue Substitute J Synthetic Substitute K Nonautologous Tissue Substitute	Z No Qualifier
8 Cornea, Right 9 Cornea, Left N Upper Eyelid, Right P Upper Eyelid, Left Q Lower Eyelid, Right R Lower Eyelid, Left	Ø Open 3 Percutaneous X External	7 Autologous Tissue Substitute J Synthetic Substitute K Nonautologous Tissue Substitute	Z No Qualifier
X Lacrimal Duct, Right Y Lacrimal Duct, Left	Ø Open 3 Percutaneous 7 Via Natural or Artificial Opening 8 Via Natural or Artificial Opening Endoscopic	7 Autologous Tissue Substitute J Synthetic Substitute K Nonautologous Tissue Substitute	Z No Qualifier

Ø8U[89][Ø3X]KZ

SECTION: Ø MEDICAL AND SURGICAL
BODY SYSTEM: 8 EYE
OPERATION: V RESTRICTION: Partially closing an orifice or the lumen of a tubular body part

Body Part	Approach	Device	Qualifier
X Lacrimal Duct, Right Y Lacrimal Duct, Left	Ø Open 3 Percutaneous	C Extraluminal Device D Intraluminal Device Z No Device	Z No Qualifier
X Lacrimal Duct, Right Y Lacrimal Duct, Left	7 Via Natural or Artificial Opening 8 Via Natural or Artificial Opening Endoscopic	D Intraluminal Device Z No Device	Z No Qualifier

SECTION: Ø MEDICAL AND SURGICAL
BODY SYSTEM: 8 EYE
OPERATION: W REVISION: Correcting, to the extent possible, a portion of a malfunctioning device or the positon of a displaced device

Body Part	Approach	Device	Qualifier
Ø Eye, Right 1 Eye, Left	Ø Open 3 Percutaneous 7 Via Natural or Artificial Opening 8 Via Natural or Artificial Opening Endoscopic	Ø Drainage Device 3 Infusion Device 7 Autologous Tissue Substitute C Extraluminal Device D Intraluminal Device J Synthetic Substitute K Nonautologous Tissue Substitute Y Other Device	Z No Qualifier
Ø Eye, Right 1 Eye, Left	X External	Ø Drainage Device 3 Infusion Device 7 Autologous Tissue Substitute C Extraluminal Device D Intraluminal Device J Synthetic Substitute K Nonautologous Tissue Substitute	Z No Qualifier
J Lens, Right K Lens, Left	3 Percutaneous	J Synthetic Substitute Y Other Device	Z No Qualifier
J Lens, Right K Lens, Left	X External	J Synthetic Substitute	Z No Qualifier
L Extraocular Muscle, Right M Extraocular Muscle, Left	Ø Open 3 Percutaneous	Ø Drainage Device 7 Autologous Tissue Substitute J Synthetic Substitute K Nonautologous Tissue Substitute Y Other Device	Z No Qualifier

Non-OR Ø8W[Ø1]X[Ø37CDJK]Z
Non-OR Ø8W[JK]XJZ

SECTION: Ø MEDICAL AND SURGICAL
BODY SYSTEM: 8 EYE
OPERATION: X TRANSFER: Moving, without taking out, all or a portion of a body part to another location to take over the function of all or a portion of a body part

Body Part	Approach	Device	Qualifier
L Extraocular Muscle, Right M Extraocular Muscle, Left	Ø Open 3 Percutaneous	Z No Device	Z No Qualifier

SECTION: Ø MEDICAL AND SURGICAL
BODY SYSTEM: 9 EAR, NOSE, SINUS
OPERATION: Ø ALTERATION: Modifying the anatomic structure of a body part without affecting the function of the body part

Body Part	Approach	Device	Qualifier
Ø External Ear, Right 1 External Ear, Left 2 External Ear, Bilateral K Nasal Mucosa and Soft Tissue	Ø Open 3 Percutaneous 4 Percutaneous Endoscopic X External	7 Autologous Tissue Substitute J Synthetic Substitute K Nonautologous Tissue Substitute Z No Device	Z No Qualifier

SECTION: Ø MEDICAL AND SURGICAL
BODY SYSTEM: 9 EAR, NOSE, SINUS
OPERATION: 1 BYPASS: Altering the route of passage of the contents of a tubular body part

Body Part	Approach	Device	Qualifier
D Inner Ear, Right E Inner Ear, Left	Ø Open	7 Autologous Tissue Substitute J Synthetic Substitute K Nonautologous Tissue Substitute Z No Device	Ø Endolymphatic

SECTION: Ø MEDICAL AND SURGICAL
BODY SYSTEM: 9 EAR, NOSE, SINUS
OPERATION: 2 CHANGE: Taking out or off a device from a body part and putting back an identical or similar device in or on the same body part without cutting or puncturing the skin or a mucous membrane

Body Part	Approach	Device	Qualifier
H Ear, Right J Ear, Left K Nasal Mucosa and Soft Tissue Y Sinus	X External	Ø Drainage Device Y Other Device	Z No Qualifier

Non-OR All Values

SECTION: Ø MEDICAL AND SURGICAL
BODY SYSTEM: 9 EAR, NOSE, SINUS
OPERATION: 3 CONTROL: Stopping, or attempting to stop, postprocedural or other acute bleeding

Body Part	Approach	Device	Qualifier
K Nasal Mucosa and Soft Tissue	7 Via Natural or Artificial Opening 8 Via Natural or Artificial Opening Endoscopic	Z No Device	Z No Qualifier

Coding Clinic: 2Ø18, Q4, P38 – Ø93K8ZZ

SECTION: Ø MEDICAL AND SURGICAL
BODY SYSTEM: 9 EAR, NOSE, SINUS
OPERATION: 5 DESTRUCTION: Physical eradication of all or a portion of a body part by the direct use of energy, force, or a destructive agent

Body Part	Approach	Device	Qualifier
Ø External Ear, Right 1 External Ear, Left	Ø Open 3 Percutaneous 4 Percutaneous Endoscopic X External	Z No Device	Z No Qualifier
3 External Auditory Canal, Right 4 External Auditory Canal, Left	Ø Open 3 Percutaneous 4 Percutaneous Endoscopic 7 Via Natural or Artificial Opening 8 Via Natural or Artificial Opening Endoscopic X External	Z No Device	Z No Qualifier
5 Middle Ear, Right 6 Middle Ear, Left 9 Auditory Ossicle, Right A Auditory Ossicle, Left D Inner Ear, Right E Inner Ear, Left	Ø Open 8 Via Natural or Artificial Opening Endoscopic	Z No Device	Z No Qualifier
7 Tympanic Membrane, Right 8 Tympanic Membrane, Left F Eustachian Tube, Right G Eustachian Tube, Left L Nasal Turbinate N Nasopharynx	Ø Open 3 Percutaneous 4 Percutaneous Endoscopic 7 Via Natural or Artificial Opening 8 Via Natural or Artificial Opening Endoscopic	Z No Device	Z No Qualifier
B Mastoid Sinus, Right C Mastoid Sinus, Left M Nasal Septum P Accessory Sinus Q Maxillary Sinus, Right R Maxillary Sinus, Left S Frontal Sinus, Right T Frontal Sinus, Left U Ethmoid Sinus, Right V Ethmoid Sinus, Left W Sphenoid Sinus, Right X Sphenoid Sinus, Left	Ø Open 3 Percutaneous 4 Percutaneous Endoscopic 8 Via Natural or Artificial Opening Endoscopic	Z No Device	Z No Qualifier
K Nasal Mucosa and Soft Tissue	Ø Open 3 Percutaneous 4 Percutaneous Endoscopic 8 Via Natural or Artificial Opening Endoscopic X External	Z No Device	Z No Qualifier

Non-OR Ø95[Ø1][Ø34X]ZZ
Non-OR Ø95[34][Ø3478X]ZZ
Non-OR Ø95[FG][Ø3478]ZZ
Non-OR Ø95M[Ø34]ZZ
Non-OR Ø95K[Ø34X]ZZ

SECTION: Ø MEDICAL AND SURGICAL
BODY SYSTEM: 9 EAR, NOSE, SINUS
OPERATION: 7 DILATION: Expanding an orifice or the lumen of a tubular body part

Body Part	Approach	Device	Qualifier
F Eustachian Tube, Right G Eustachian Tube, Left	Ø Open 7 Via Natural or Artificial Opening 8 Via Natural or Artificial Opening Endoscopic	D Intraluminal Device Z No Device	Z No Qualifier
F Eustachian Tube, Right G Eustachian Tube, Left	3 Percutaneous 4 Percutaneous Endoscopic	Z No Device	Z No Qualifier

Non-OR All Values

SECTION: Ø MEDICAL AND SURGICAL
BODY SYSTEM: 9 EAR, NOSE, SINUS
OPERATION: 8 DIVISION: Cutting into a body part, without draining fluids and/or gases from the body part, in order to separate or transect a body part

Body Part	Approach	Device	Qualifier
L Nasal Turbinate	Ø Open 3 Percutaneous 4 Percutaneous Endoscopic 7 Via Natural or Artificial Opening 8 Via Natural or Artificial Opening Endoscopic	Z No Device	Z No Qualifier

SECTION: Ø MEDICAL AND SURGICAL
BODY SYSTEM: 9 EAR, NOSE, SINUS
OPERATION: 9 DRAINAGE: *(on multiple pages)*
Taking or letting out fluids and/or gases from a body part

Body Part	Approach	Device	Qualifier
Ø External Ear, Right 1 External Ear, Left	Ø Open 3 Percutaneous 4 Percutaneous Endoscopic X External	Ø Drainage Device	Z No Qualifier
Ø External Ear, Right 1 External Ear, Left	Ø Open 3 Percutaneous 4 Percutaneous Endoscopic X External	Z No Device	X Diagnostic Z No Qualifier
3 External Auditory Canal, Right 4 External Auditory Canal, Left K Nasal Mucosa and Soft Tissue	Ø Open 3 Percutaneous 4 Percutaneous Endoscopic 7 Via Natural or Artificial Opening 8 Via Natural or Artificial Opening Endoscopic X External	Ø Drainage Device	Z No Qualifier
3 External Auditory Canal, Right 4 External Auditory Canal, Left K Nasal Mucosa and Soft Tissue	Ø Open 3 Percutaneous 4 Percutaneous Endoscopic 7 Via Natural or Artificial Opening 8 Via Natural or Artificial Opening Endoscopic X External	Z No Device	X Diagnostic Z No Qualifier
5 Middle Ear, Right 6 Middle Ear, Left 9 Auditory Ossicle, Right A Auditory Ossicle, Left D Inner Ear, Right E Inner Ear, Left	Ø Open 7 Via Natural or Artificial Opening 8 Via Natural or Artificial Opening Endoscopic	Ø Drainage Device	Z No Qualifier
5 Middle Ear, Right 6 Middle Ear, Left 9 Auditory Ossicle, Right A Auditory Ossicle, Left D Inner Ear, Right E Inner Ear, Left	Ø Open 7 Via Natural or Artificial Opening 8 Via Natural or Artificial Opening Endoscopic	Z No Device	X Diagnostic Z No Qualifier

Non-OR Ø99[Ø1][Ø34X]ØZ
Non-OR Ø99[Ø1][Ø34X]Z[XZ]
Non-OR Ø99[34][Ø3478X]ØZ
Non-OR Ø99K[Ø34X]ØZ
Non-OR Ø99[34][Ø3478X]Z[XZ]
Non-OR Ø99K[Ø34X]Z[XZ]
Non-OR Ø99[56]ØZZ

SECTION: Ø MEDICAL AND SURGICAL
BODY SYSTEM: 9 EAR, NOSE, SINUS
OPERATION: 9 DRAINAGE: *(continued)*
Taking or letting out fluids and/or gases from a body part

Body Part	Approach	Device	Qualifier
7 Tympanic Membrane, Right 8 Tympanic Membrane, Left B Mastoid Sinus, Right C Mastoid Sinus, Left F Eustachian Tube, Right G Eustachian Tube, Left L Nasal Turbinate M Nasal Septum N Nasopharynx P Accessory Sinus Q Maxillary Sinus, Right R Maxillary Sinus, Left S Frontal Sinus, Right T Frontal Sinus, Left U Ethmoid Sinus, Right V Ethmoid Sinus, Left W Sphenoid Sinus, Right X Sphenoid Sinus, Left	Ø Open 3 Percutaneous 4 Percutaneous Endoscopic 7 Via Natural or Artificial Opening 8 Via Natural or Artificial Opening Endoscopic	Ø Drainage Device	Z No Qualifier
7 Tympanic Membrane, Right 8 Tympanic Membrane, Left B Mastoid Sinus, Right C Mastoid Sinus, Left F Eustachian Tube, Right G Eustachian Tube, Left L Nasal Turbinate M Nasal Septum N Nasopharynx P Accessory Sinus Q Maxillary Sinus, Right R Maxillary Sinus, Left S Frontal Sinus, Right T Frontal Sinus, Left U Ethmoid Sinus, Right V Ethmoid Sinus, Left W Sphenoid Sinus, Right X Sphenoid Sinus, Left	Ø Open 3 Percutaneous 4 Percutaneous Endoscopic 7 Via Natural or Artificial Opening 8 Via Natural or Artificial Opening Endoscopic	Z No Device	X Diagnostic Z No Qualifier

Non-OR Ø99[FGL][Ø3478]ØZ
Non-OR Ø99N3ØZ
Non-OR Ø99[78FG][Ø3478]ZZ
Non-OR Ø99L[Ø3478]Z[XZ]
Non-OR Ø99N[Ø3478]ZX
Non-OR Ø99N3ZZ
Non-OR Ø99[BC]3ØZ
Non-OR Ø99M[Ø34]ØZ
Non-OR Ø99[PQRSTUVWX][34]ØZ
Non-OR Ø99[BC]3ZZ
Non-OR Ø99M[Ø34]Z[XZ]
Non-OR Ø99[PQRSTUVWX][34]Z[XZ]

SECTION: Ø MEDICAL AND SURGICAL
BODY SYSTEM: 9 EAR, NOSE, SINUS
OPERATION: B EXCISION: Cutting out or off, without replacement, a portion of a body part

Body Part	Approach	Device	Qualifier
Ø External Ear, Right 1 External Ear, Left	Ø Open 3 Percutaneous 4 Percutaneous Endoscopic X External	Z No Device	X Diagnostic Z No Qualifier
3 External Auditory Canal, Right 4 External Auditory Canal, Left	Ø Open 3 Percutaneous 4 Percutaneous Endoscopic 7 Via Natural or Artificial Opening 8 Via Natural or Artificial Opening Endoscopic X External	Z No Device	X Diagnostic Z No Qualifier
5 Middle Ear, Right 6 Middle Ear, Left 9 Auditory Ossicle, Right A Auditory Ossicle, Left D Inner Ear, Right E Inner Ear, Left	Ø Open 8 Via Natural or Artificial Opening Endoscopic	Z No Device	X Diagnostic Z No Qualifier
7 Tympanic Membrane, Right 8 Tympanic Membrane, Left F Eustachian Tube, Right G Eustachian Tube, Left L Nasal Turbinate N Nasopharynx	Ø Open 3 Percutaneous 4 Percutaneous Endoscopic 7 Via Natural or Artificial Opening 8 Via Natural or Artificial Opening Endoscopic	Z No Device	X Diagnostic Z No Qualifier
B Mastoid Sinus, Right C Mastoid Sinus, Left M Nasal Septum P Accessory Sinus Q Maxillary Sinus, Right R Maxillary Sinus, Left S Frontal Sinus, Right T Frontal Sinus, Left U Ethmoid Sinus, Right V Ethmoid Sinus, Left W Sphenoid Sinus, Right X Sphenoid Sinus, Left	Ø Open 3 Percutaneous 4 Percutaneous Endoscopic 8 Via Natural or Artificial Opening Endoscopic	Z No Device	X Diagnostic Z No Qualifier
K Nasal Mucosa and Soft Tissue	Ø Open 3 Percutaneous 4 Percutaneous Endoscopic 8 Via Natural or Artificial Opening Endoscopic X External	Z No Device	X Diagnostic Z No Qualifier

Non-OR Ø9B[Ø1][Ø34X]Z[XZ]
Non-OR Ø9B[34][Ø3478X]Z[XZ]
Non-OR Ø9B[FG][Ø3478]Z[XZ]
Non-OR Ø9B[LN][Ø3478]ZX
Non-OR Ø9BM[Ø34]ZX
Non-OR Ø9B[PQRSTUVWX][34]ZX
Non-OR Ø9BK[Ø34X]Z[XZ]

SECTION: Ø MEDICAL AND SURGICAL
BODY SYSTEM: 9 EAR, NOSE, SINUS
OPERATION: C EXTIRPATION: Taking or cutting out solid matter from a body part

Body Part	Approach	Device	Qualifier
Ø External Ear, Right 1 External Ear, Left	Ø Open 3 Percutaneous 4 Percutaneous Endoscopic X External	Z No Device	Z No Qualifier
3 External Auditory Canal, Right 4 External Auditory Canal, Left	Ø Open 3 Percutaneous 4 Percutaneous Endoscopic 7 Via Natural or Artificial Opening 8 Via Natural or Artificial Opening Endoscopic X External	Z No Device	Z No Qualifier
5 Middle Ear, Right 6 Middle Ear, Left 9 Auditory Ossicle, Right A Auditory Ossicle, Left D Inner Ear, Right E Inner Ear, Left	Ø Open 8 Via Natural or Artificial Opening Endoscopic	Z No Device	Z No Qualifier
7 Tympanic Membrane, Right 8 Tympanic Membrane, Left F Eustachian Tube, Right G Eustachian Tube, Left L Nasal Turbinate N Nasopharynx	Ø Open 3 Percutaneous 4 Percutaneous Endoscopic 7 Via Natural or Artificial Opening 8 Via Natural or Artificial Opening Endoscopic	Z No Device	Z No Qualifier
B Mastoid Sinus, Right C Mastoid Sinus, Left M Nasal Septum P Accessory Sinus Q Maxillary Sinus, Right R Maxillary Sinus, Left S Frontal Sinus, Right T Frontal Sinus, Left U Ethmoid Sinus, Right V Ethmoid Sinus, Left W Sphenoid Sinus, Right X Sphenoid Sinus, Left	Ø Open 3 Percutaneous 4 Percutaneous Endoscopic 8 Via Natural or Artificial Opening Endoscopic	Z No Device	Z No Qualifier
K Nasal Mucosa and Soft Tissue	Ø Open 3 Percutaneous 4 Percutaneous Endoscopic 8 Via Natural or Artificial Opening Endoscopic X External	Z No Device	Z No Qualifier

Non-OR Ø9C[Ø1][Ø34X]ZZ
Non-OR Ø9C[34][Ø3478X]ZZ
Non-OR Ø9C[78FGL][Ø3478]ZZ
Non-OR Ø9CM[Ø34]ZZ
Non-OR Ø9BK[Ø34X]ZZ

SECTION: Ø MEDICAL AND SURGICAL
BODY SYSTEM: 9 EAR, NOSE, SINUS
OPERATION: D EXTRACTION: Pulling or stripping out or off all or a portion of a body part by the use of force

Body Part	Approach	Device	Qualifier
7 Tympanic Membrane, Right 8 Tympanic Membrane, Left L Nasal Turbinate	Ø Open 3 Percutaneous 4 Percutaneous Endoscopic 7 Via Natural or Artificial Opening 8 Via Natural or Artificial Opening Endoscopic	Z No Device	Z No Qualifier
9 Auditory Ossicle, Right A Auditory Ossicle, Left	Ø Open	Z No Device	Z No Qualifier
B Mastoid Sinus, Right C Mastoid Sinus, Left M Nasal Septum P Accessory Sinus Q Maxillary Sinus, Right R Maxillary Sinus, Left S Frontal Sinus, Right T Frontal Sinus, Left U Ethmoid Sinus, Right V Ethmoid Sinus, Left W Sphenoid Sinus, Right X Sphenoid Sinus, Left	Ø Open 3 Percutaneous 4 Percutaneous Endoscopic	Z No Device	Z No Qualifier

SECTION: Ø MEDICAL AND SURGICAL
BODY SYSTEM: 9 EAR, NOSE, SINUS
OPERATION: H INSERTION: Putting in a nonbiological appliance that monitors, assists, performs, or prevents a physiological function but does not physically take the place of a body part

Body Part	Approach	Device	Qualifier
D Inner Ear, Right E Inner Ear, Left	Ø Open 3 Percutaneous 4 Percutaneous Endoscopic	1 Radioactive Element 4 Hearing Device, Bone Conduction 5 Hearing Device, Single Channel Cochlear Prosthesis 6 Hearing Device, Multiple Channel Cochlear Prosthesis S Hearing Device	Z No Qualifier
H Ear, Right J Ear, Left K Nasal Mucosa and Soft Tissue Y Sinus	Ø Open 3 Percutaneous 4 Percutaneous Endoscopic 7 Via Natural or Artificial Opening 8 Via Natural or Artificial Opening Endoscopic	1 Radioactive Element Y Other Device	Z No Qualifier
N Nasopharynx	7 Via Natural or Artificial Opening 8 Via Natural or Artificial Opening Endoscopic	1 Radioactive Element B Intraluminal Device, Airway	Z No Qualifier

Non-OR Ø9HN[78]BZ
Coding Clinic: 2022, Q2, P18 – Ø9HK7YZ

SECTION: Ø MEDICAL AND SURGICAL
BODY SYSTEM: 9 EAR, NOSE, SINUS
OPERATION: J INSPECTION: Visually and/or manually exploring a body part

Body Part	Approach	Device	Qualifier
7 Tympanic Membrane, Right 8 Tympanic Membrane, Left H Ear, Right J Ear, Left	Ø Open 3 Percutaneous 4 Percutaneous Endoscopic 7 Via Natural or Artificial Opening 8 Via Natural or Artificial Opening Endoscopic X External	Z No Device	Z No Qualifier
D Inner Ear, Right E Inner Ear, Left K Nasal Mucosa and Soft Tissue Y Sinus	Ø Open 3 Percutaneous 4 Percutaneous Endoscopic 8 Via Natural or Artificial Opening Endoscopic X External	Z No Device	Z No Qualifier

Non-OR Ø9J[78][378X]ZZ
Non-OR Ø9J[HJ][Ø3478X]ZZ
Non-OR Ø9J[DE][3X]ZZ
Non-OR Ø9J[KY][Ø34X]ZZ

SECTION: Ø MEDICAL AND SURGICAL
BODY SYSTEM: 9 EAR, NOSE, SINUS
OPERATION: M REATTACHMENT: Putting back in or on all or a portion of a separated body part to its normal location or other suitable location

Body Part	Approach	Device	Qualifier
Ø External Ear, Right 1 External Ear, Left K Nasal Mucosa and Soft Tissue	X External	Z No Device	Z No Qualifier

SECTION: Ø MEDICAL AND SURGICAL
BODY SYSTEM: 9 EAR, NOSE, SINUS
OPERATION: N RELEASE: Freeing a body part from an abnormal physical constraint

Body Part	Approach	Device	Qualifier
Ø External Ear, Right 1 External Ear, Left	Ø Open 3 Percutaneous 4 Percutaneous Endoscopic X External	Z No Device	Z No Qualifier
3 External Auditory Canal, Right 4 External Auditory Canal, Left	Ø Open 3 Percutaneous 4 Percutaneous Endoscopic 7 Via Natural or Artificial Opening 8 Via Natural or Artificial Opening Endoscopic X External	Z No Device	Z No Qualifier
5 Middle Ear, Right 6 Middle Ear, Left 9 Auditory Ossicle, Right A Auditory Ossicle, Left D Inner Ear, Right E Inner Ear, Left	Ø Open 8 Via Natural or Artificial Opening Endoscopic	Z No Device	Z No Qualifier
7 Tympanic Membrane, Right 8 Tympanic Membrane, Left F Eustachian Tube, Right G Eustachian Tube, Left L Nasal Turbinate N Nasopharynx	Ø Open 3 Percutaneous 4 Percutaneous Endoscopic 7 Via Natural or Artificial Opening 8 Via Natural or Artificial Opening Endoscopic	Z No Device	Z No Qualifier
B Mastoid Sinus, Right C Mastoid Sinus, Left M Nasal Septum P Accessory Sinus Q Maxillary Sinus, Right R Maxillary Sinus, Left S Frontal Sinus, Right T Frontal Sinus, Left U Ethmoid Sinus, Right V Ethmoid Sinus, Left W Sphenoid Sinus, Right X Sphenoid Sinus, Left	Ø Open 3 Percutaneous 4 Percutaneous Endoscopic 8 Via Natural or Artificial Opening Endoscopic	Z No Device	Z No Qualifier
K Nasal Mucosa and Soft Tissue	Ø Open 3 Percutaneous 4 Percutaneous Endoscopic 8 Via Natural or Artificial Opening Endoscopic X External	Z No Device	Z No Qualifier

Non-OR Ø9N[FGL][Ø3478]ZZ
Non-OR Ø9NM[Ø34]ZZ
Non-OR Ø9NK[Ø34X]ZZ

SECTION: Ø MEDICAL AND SURGICAL
BODY SYSTEM: 9 EAR, NOSE, SINUS
OPERATION: P REMOVAL: Taking out or off a device from a body part

Body Part	Approach	Device	Qualifier
7 Tympanic Membrane, Right 8 Tympanic Membrane, Left	Ø Open 7 Via Natural or Artificial Opening 8 Via Natural or Artificial Opening Endoscopic X External	Ø Drainage Device	Z No Qualifier
D Inner Ear, Right E Inner Ear, Left	Ø Open 7 Via Natural or Artificial Opening 8 Via Natural or Artificial Opening Endoscopic	S Hearing Device	Z No Qualifier
H Ear, Right J Ear, Left K Nasal Mucosa and Soft Tissue	Ø Open 3 Percutaneous 4 Percutaneous Endoscopic 7 Via Natural or Artificial Opening 8 Via Natural or Artificial Opening Endoscopic	Ø Drainage Device 7 Autologous Tissue Substitute D Intraluminal Device J Synthetic Substitute K Nonautologous Tissue Substitute Y Other Device	Z No Qualifier
H Ear, Right J Ear, Left K Nasal Mucosa and Soft Tissue	X External	Ø Drainage Device 7 Autologous Tissue Substitute D Intraluminal Device J Synthetic Substitute K Nonautologous Tissue Substitute	Z No Qualifier
Y Sinus	Ø Open 3 Percutaneous 4 Percutaneous Endoscopic	Ø Drainage Device Y Other Device	Z No Qualifier
Y Sinus	7 Via Natural or Artificial Opening 8 Via Natural or Artificial Opening Endoscopic	Y Other Device	Z No Qualifier
Y Sinus	X External	Ø Drainage Device	Z No Qualifier

Non-OR Ø9P[78][Ø78X]ØZ
Non-OR Ø9P[HJ][34][ØJK]Z
Non-OR Ø9P[HJ][78][ØD]Z
Non-OR Ø9P[HJ]X[Ø7DJK]Z
Non-OR Ø9PK[Ø3478][Ø7DJK]Z
Non-OR Ø9PYXØZ
Non-OR Ø9PKX[Ø7DJK]Z

SECTION: Ø MEDICAL AND SURGICAL
BODY SYSTEM: 9 EAR, NOSE, SINUS
OPERATION: Q REPAIR: Restoring, to the extent possible, a body part to its normal anatomic structure and function

Body Part	Approach	Device	Qualifier
Ø External Ear, Right 1 External Ear, Left 2 External Ear, Bilateral	Ø Open 3 Percutaneous 4 Percutaneous Endoscopic X External	Z No Device	Z No Qualifier
3 External Auditory Canal, Right 4 External Auditory Canal, Left F Eustachian Tube, Right G Eustachian Tube, Left	Ø Open 3 Percutaneous 4 Percutaneous Endoscopic 7 Via Natural or Artificial Opening 8 Via Natural or Artificial Opening Endoscopic X External	Z No Device	Z No Qualifier
5 Middle Ear, Right 6 Middle Ear, Left 9 Auditory Ossicle, Right A Auditory Ossicle, Left D Inner Ear, Right E Inner Ear, Left	Ø Open 8 Via Natural or Artificial Opening Endoscopic	Z No Device	Z No Qualifier
7 Tympanic Membrane, Right 8 Tympanic Membrane, Left L Nasal Turbinate N Nasopharynx	Ø Open 3 Percutaneous 4 Percutaneous Endoscopic 7 Via Natural or Artificial Opening 8 Via Natural or Artificial Opening Endoscopic	Z No Device	Z No Qualifier
B Mastoid Sinus, Right C Mastoid Sinus, Left M Nasal Septum P Accessory Sinus Q Maxillary Sinus, Right R Maxillary Sinus, Left S Frontal Sinus, Right T Frontal Sinus, Left U Ethmoid Sinus, Right V Ethmoid Sinus, Left W Sphenoid Sinus, Right X Sphenoid Sinus, Left	Ø Open 3 Percutaneous 4 Percutaneous Endoscopic 8 Via Natural or Artificial Opening Endoscopic	Z No Device	Z No Qualifier
K Nasal Mucosa and Soft Tissue	Ø Open 3 Percutaneous 4 Percutaneous Endoscopic 8 Via Natural or Artificial Opening Endoscopic X External	Z No Device	Z No Qualifier

Non-OR Ø9Q[Ø12]XZZ
Non-OR Ø9Q[34]XZZ
Non-OR Ø9Q[FG][Ø3478X]ZZ

SECTION: Ø MEDICAL AND SURGICAL
BODY SYSTEM: 9 EAR, NOSE, SINUS
OPERATION: R REPLACEMENT: Putting in or on biological or synthetic material that physically takes the place and/or function of all or a portion of a body part

Body Part	Approach	Device	Qualifier
Ø External Ear, Right 1 External Ear, Left 2 External Ear, Bilateral K Nasal Mucosa and Soft Tissue	Ø Open X External	7 Autologous Tissue Substitute J Synthetic Substitute K Nonautologous Tissue Substitute	Z No Qualifier
5 Middle Ear, Right 6 Middle Ear, Left 9 Auditory Ossicle, Right A Auditory Ossicle, Left D Inner Ear, Right E Inner Ear, Left	Ø Open	7 Autologous Tissue Substitute J Synthetic Substitute K Nonautologous Tissue Substitute	Z No Qualifier
7 Tympanic Membrane, Right 8 Tympanic Membrane, Left N Nasopharynx	Ø Open 7 Via Natural or Artificial Opening 8 Via Natural or Artificial Opening Endoscopic	7 Autologous Tissue Substitute J Synthetic Substitute K Nonautologous Tissue Substitute	Z No Qualifier
L Nasal Turbinate	Ø Open 3 Percutaneous 4 Percutaneous Endoscopic 7 Via Natural or Artificial Opening 8 Via Natural or Artificial Opening Endoscopic	7 Autologous Tissue Substitute J Synthetic Substitute K Nonautologous Tissue Substitute	Z No Qualifier
M Nasal Septum	Ø Open 3 Percutaneous 4 Percutaneous Endoscopic	7 Autologous Tissue Substitute J Synthetic Substitute K Nonautologous Tissue Substitute	Z No Qualifier

SECTION: Ø MEDICAL AND SURGICAL
BODY SYSTEM: 9 EAR, NOSE, SINUS
OPERATION: S REPOSITION: Moving to its normal location, or other suitable location, all or a portion of a body part

Body Part	Approach	Device	Qualifier
Ø External Ear, Right 1 External Ear, Left 2 External Ear, Bilateral K Nasal Mucosa and Soft Tissue	Ø Open 4 Percutaneous Endoscopic X External	Z No Device	Z No Qualifier
7 Tympanic Membrane, Right 8 Tympanic Membrane, Left F Eustachian Tube, Right G Eustachian Tube, Left L Nasal Turbinate	Ø Open 4 Percutaneous Endoscopic 7 Via Natural or Artificial Opening 8 Via Natural or Artificial Opening Endoscopic	Z No Device	Z No Qualifier
9 Auditory Ossicle, Right A Auditory Ossicle, Left M Nasal Septum	Ø Open 4 Percutaneous Endoscopic	Z No Device	Z No Qualifier

Non-OR Ø9S[FG][Ø478]ZZ

SECTION: Ø MEDICAL AND SURGICAL
BODY SYSTEM: 9 EAR, NOSE, SINUS
OPERATION: T RESECTION: Cutting out or off, without replacement, all of a body part

Body Part	Approach	Device	Qualifier
Ø External Ear, Right 1 External Ear, Left	Ø Open 4 Percutaneous Endoscopic X External	Z No Device	Z No Qualifier
5 Middle Ear, Right 6 Middle Ear, Left 9 Auditory Ossicle, Right A Auditory Ossicle, Left D Inner Ear, Right E Inner Ear, Left	Ø Open 8 Via Natural or Artificial Opening Endoscopic	Z No Device	Z No Qualifier
7 Tympanic Membrane, Right 8 Tympanic Membrane, Left F Eustachian Tube, Right G Eustachian Tube, Left L Nasal Turbinate N Nasopharynx	Ø Open 4 Percutaneous Endoscopic 7 Via Natural or Artificial Opening 8 Via Natural or Artificial Opening Endoscopic	Z No Device	Z No Qualifier
B Mastoid Sinus, Right C Mastoid Sinus, Left M Nasal Septum P Accessory Sinus Q Maxillary Sinus, Right R Maxillary Sinus, Left S Frontal Sinus, Right T Frontal Sinus, Left U Ethmoid Sinus, Right V Ethmoid Sinus, Left W Sphenoid Sinus, Right X Sphenoid Sinus, Left	Ø Open 4 Percutaneous Endoscopic 8 Via Natural or Artificial Opening Endoscopic	Z No Device	Z No Qualifier
K Nasal Mucosa and Soft Tissue	Ø Open 4 Percutaneous Endoscopic 8 Via Natural or Artificial Opening Endoscopic X External	Z No Device	Z No Qualifier

Non-OR Ø9T[FG][Ø478]ZZ

SECTION: Ø MEDICAL AND SURGICAL
BODY SYSTEM: 9 EAR, NOSE, SINUS
OPERATION: U SUPPLEMENT: Putting in or on biological or synthetic material that physically reinforces and/or augments the function of a portion of a body part

Body Part	Approach	Device	Qualifier
Ø External Ear, Right 1 External Ear, Left 2 External Ear, Bilateral	Ø Open X External	7 Autologous Tissue Substitute J Synthetic Substitute K Nonautologous Tissue Substitute	Z No Qualifier
5 Middle Ear, Right 6 Middle Ear, Left 9 Auditory Ossicle, Right A Auditory Ossicle, Left D Inner Ear, Right E Inner Ear, Left	Ø Open 8 Via Natural or Artificial Opening Endoscopic	7 Autologous Tissue Substitute J Synthetic Substitute K Nonautologous Tissue Substitute	Z No Qualifier
7 Tympanic Membrane, Right 8 Tympanic Membrane, Left N Nasopharynx	Ø Open 7 Via Natural or Artificial Opening 8 Via Natural or Artificial Opening Endoscopic	7 Autologous Tissue Substitute J Synthetic Substitute K Nonautologous Tissue Substitute	Z No Qualifier
B Mastoid Sinus, Right C Mastoid Sinus, Left L Nasal Turbinate P Accessory Sinus Q Maxillary Sinus, Right R Maxillary Sinus, Left S Frontal Sinus, Right T Frontal Sinus, Left U Ethmoid Sinus, Right V Ethmoid Sinus, Left W Sphenoid Sinus, Right X Sphenoid Sinus, Left	Ø Open 3 Percutaneous 4 Percutaneous Endoscopic 7 Via Natural or Artificial Opening 8 Via Natural or Artificial Opening Endoscopic	7 Autologous Tissue Substitute J Synthetic Substitute K Nonautologous Tissue Substitute	Z No Qualifier
K Nasal Mucosa and Soft Tissue	Ø Open 8 Via Natural or Artificial Opening Endoscopic X External	7 Autologous Tissue Substitute J Synthetic Substitute K Nonautologous Tissue Substitute	Z No Qualifier
L Nasal Turbinate	Ø Open 3 Percutaneous 4 Percutaneous Endoscopic 7 Via Natural or Artificial Opening 8 Via Natural or Artificial Opening Endoscopic	7 Autologous Tissue Substitute J Synthetic Substitute K Nonautologous Tissue Substitute	Z No Qualifier
M Nasal Septum	Ø Open 3 Percutaneous 4 Percutaneous Endoscopic 8 Via Natural or Artificial Opening Endoscopic	7 Autologous Tissue Substitute J Synthetic Substitute K Nonautologous Tissue Substitute	Z No Qualifier

SECTION: Ø MEDICAL AND SURGICAL
BODY SYSTEM: 9 EAR, NOSE, SINUS
OPERATION: W REVISION: Correcting, to the extent possible, a portion of a malfunctioning device or the position of a displaced device

Body Part	Approach	Device	Qualifier
7 Tympanic Membrane, Right 8 Tympanic Membrane, Left 9 Auditory Ossicle, Right A Auditory Ossicle, Left	Ø Open 7 Via Natural or Artificial Opening 8 Via Natural or Artificial Opening Endoscopic	7 Autologous Tissue Substitute J Synthetic Substitute K Nonautologous Tissue Substitute	Z No Qualifier
D Inner Ear, Right E Inner Ear, Left	Ø Open 7 Via Natural or Artificial Opening 8 Via Natural or Artificial Opening Endoscopic	S Hearing Device	Z No Qualifier
H Ear, Right J Ear, Left K Nasal Mucosa and Soft Tissue	Ø Open 3 Percutaneous 4 Percutaneous Endoscopic 7 Via Natural or Artificial Opening 8 Via Natural or Artificial Opening Endoscopic	Ø Drainage Device 7 Autologous Tissue Substitute D Intraluminal Device J Synthetic Substitute K Nonautologous Tissue Substitute Y Other Device	Z No Qualifier
H Ear, Right J Ear, Left K Nasal Mucosa and Soft Tissue	X External	Ø Drainage Device 7 Autologous Tissue Substitute D Intraluminal Device J Synthetic Substitute K Nonautologous Tissue Substitute	Z No Qualifier
Y Sinus	Ø Open 3 Percutaneous 4 Percutaneous Endoscopic	Ø Drainage Device Y Other Device	Z No Qualifier
Y Sinus	7 Via Natural or Artificial Opening 8 Via Natural or Artificial Opening Endoscopic	Y Other Device	Z No Qualifier
Y Sinus	X External	Ø Drainage Device	Z No Qualifier

Non-OR Ø9W[HJ][34][JK]Z
Non-OR Ø9W[HJ][78]DZ
Non-OR Ø9W[HJ]X[Ø7DJK]Z
Non-OR Ø9WK[Ø3478][Ø7DJK]Z
Non-OR Ø9WYXØZ
Non-OR Ø9QKX[Ø7DJK]Z

SECTION: Ø MEDICAL AND SURGICAL
BODY SYSTEM: B RESPIRATORY SYSTEM
OPERATION: 1 BYPASS: Altering the route of passage of the contents of a tubular body part

Body Part	Approach	Device	Qualifier
1 Trachea	Ø Open	D Intraluminal Device	6 Esophagus
1 Trachea	Ø Open	F Tracheostomy Device Z No Device	4 Cutaneous
1 Trachea	3 Percutaneous 4 Percutaneous Endoscopic	F Tracheostomy Device Z No Device	4 Cutaneous

DRG Non-OR ØB113[FZ]4
Non-OR ØB11ØD6

SECTION: Ø MEDICAL AND SURGICAL
BODY SYSTEM: B RESPIRATORY SYSTEM
OPERATION: 2 CHANGE: Taking out or off a device from a body part and putting back an identical or similar device in or on the same body part without cutting or puncturing the skin or a mucous membrane

Body Part	Approach	Device	Qualifier
Ø Tracheobronchial Tree K Lung, Right L Lung, Left Q Pleura T Diaphragm	X External	Ø Drainage Device Y Other Device	Z No Qualifier
1 Trachea	X External	Ø Drainage Device E Intraluminal Device, Endotracheal Airway F Tracheostomy Device Y Other Device	Z No Qualifier

Non-OR All Values

SECTION: Ø MEDICAL AND SURGICAL
BODY SYSTEM: B RESPIRATORY SYSTEM
OPERATION: 5 DESTRUCTION: Physical eradication of all or a portion of a body part by the direct use of energy, force, or a destructive agent

Body Part	Approach	Device	Qualifier
1 Trachea 2 Carina 3 Main Bronchus, Right 4 Upper Lobe Bronchus, Right 5 Middle Lobe Bronchus, Right 6 Lower Lobe Bronchus, Right 7 Main Bronchus, Left 8 Upper Lobe Bronchus, Left 9 Lingula Bronchus B Lower Lobe Bronchus, Left	Ø Open 3 Percutaneous 4 Percutaneous Endoscopic 7 Via Natural or Artificial Opening 8 Via Natural or Artificial Opening Endoscopic	Z No Device	Z No Qualifier
C Upper Lung Lobe, Right D Middle Lung Lobe, Right F Lower Lung Lobe, Right G Upper Lung Lobe, Left H Lung Lingula J Lower Lung Lobe, Left K Lung, Right L Lung, Left M Lungs, Bilateral	Ø Open 3 Percutaneous 4 Percutaneous Endoscopic	Z No Device	3 Laser Interstitial Thermal Therapy Z No Qualifier
C Upper Lung Lobe, Right D Middle Lung Lobe, Right F Lower Lung Lobe, Right G Upper Lung Lobe, Left H Lung Lingula J Lower Lung Lobe, Left K Lung, Right L Lung, Left M Lungs, Bilateral	7 Via Natural or Artificial Opening 8 Via Natural or Artificial Opening Endoscopic	Z No Device	Z No Qualifier
N Pleura, Right P Pleura, Left T Diaphragm	Ø Open 3 Percutaneous 4 Percutaneous Endoscopic	Z No Device	Z No Qualifier

Non-OR ØB5[3456789B]4ZZ
Non-OR ØB5[CDFGHJKLM]8ZZ
Non-OR ØB5[CDFGHJKLM][Ø34]Z3

Coding Clinic: 2Ø16, Q2, P18 – ØB5[PS]ØZZ

5: DESTRUCTION
B: RESPIRATORY SYSTEM
Ø: M/S

SECTION: Ø MEDICAL AND SURGICAL
BODY SYSTEM: B RESPIRATORY SYSTEM
OPERATION: 7 DILATION: Expanding an orifice or the lumen of a tubular body part

Body Part	Approach	Device	Qualifier
1 Trachea 2 Carina 3 Main Bronchus, Right 4 Upper Lobe Bronchus, Right 5 Middle Lobe Bronchus, Right 6 Lower Lobe Bronchus, Right 7 Main Bronchus, Left 8 Upper Lobe Bronchus, Left 9 Lingula Bronchus B Lower Lobe Bronchus, Left	Ø Open 3 Percutaneous 4 Percutaneous Endoscopic 7 Via Natural or Artificial Opening 8 Via Natural or Artificial Opening Endoscopic	D Intraluminal Device Z No Device	Z No Qualifier

Non-OR ØB5[3456789B][Ø3478][DZ]Z

SECTION: Ø MEDICAL AND SURGICAL
BODY SYSTEM: B RESPIRATORY SYSTEM
OPERATION: 9 DRAINAGE: *(on multiple pages)*
Taking or letting out fluids and/or gases from a body part

Body Part	Approach	Device	Qualifier
1 Trachea 2 Carina 3 Main Bronchus, Right 4 Upper Lobe Bronchus, Right 5 Middle Lobe Bronchus, Right 6 Lower Lobe Bronchus, Right 7 Main Bronchus, Left 8 Upper Lobe Bronchus, Left 9 Lingula Bronchus B Lower Lobe Bronchus, Left C Upper Lung Lobe, Right D Middle Lung Lobe, Right F Lower Lung Lobe, Right G Upper Lung Lobe, Left H Lung Lingula J Lower Lung Lobe, Left K Lung, Right L Lung, Left M Lungs, Bilateral	Ø Open 3 Percutaneous 4 Percutaneous Endoscopic 7 Via Natural or Artificial Opening 8 Via Natural or Artificial Opening Endoscopic	Ø Drainage Device	Z No Qualifier

Coding Clinic: 2Ø16, Q1, P26 – ØB948ZX, ØB9B8ZX
Coding Clinic: 2Ø16, Q1, P27 – ØB988ZX
Coding Clinic: 2Ø17, Q1, P51 – ØB9[BJ]8ZX
Coding Clinic: 2Ø17, Q3, P15 – ØB9M8ZZ

SECTION: Ø MEDICAL AND SURGICAL
BODY SYSTEM: B RESPIRATORY SYSTEM
OPERATION: 9 DRAINAGE: *(continued)*

Taking or letting out fluids and/or gases from a body part

Body Part	Approach	Device	Qualifier
1 Trachea 2 Carina 3 Main Bronchus, Right 4 Upper Lobe Bronchus, Right 5 Middle Lobe Bronchus, Right 6 Lower Lobe Bronchus, Right 7 Main Bronchus, Left 8 Upper Lobe Bronchus, Left 9 Lingula Bronchus B Lower Lobe Bronchus, Left C Upper Lung Lobe, Right D Middle Lung Lobe, Right F Lower Lung Lobe, Right G Upper Lung Lobe, Left H Lung Lingula J Lower Lung Lobe, Left K Lung, Right L Lung, Left M Lungs, Bilateral	Ø Open 3 Percutaneous 4 Percutaneous Endoscopic 7 Via Natural or Artificial Opening 8 Via Natural or Artificial Opening Endoscopic	Z No Device	X Diagnostic Z No Qualifier
N Pleura, Right P Pleura, Left	Ø Open 3 Percutaneous 4 Percutaneous Endoscopic 8 Via Natural or Artificial Opening Endoscopic	Ø Drainage Device	Z No Qualifier
N Pleura, Right P Pleura, Left	Ø Open 3 Percutaneous 4 Percutaneous Endoscopic 8 Via Natural or Artificial Opening Endoscopic	Z No Device	X Diagnostic Z No Qualifier
T Diaphragm	Ø Open 3 Percutaneous 4 Percutaneous Endoscopic	Ø Drainage	Z No Qualifier
T Diaphragm	Ø Open 3 Percutaneous 4 Percutaneous Endoscopic	Z No Device	X Diagnostic Z No Qualifier

DRG Non-OR ØB9[123456789B][78]ØZ *(proposed)*
DRG Non-OR ØB9[123456789B][78]ZZ *(proposed)*
Non-OR ØB9[123456789B][3478]ZX
Non-OR ØB9[CDFGHJKLM][347]ZX
Non-OR ØB9[NP][Ø3]ØZ
Non-OR ØB9[NP][Ø3]Z[XZ]
Non-OR ØB9[NP]4ZX
Non-OR ØB9T3ZZ

SECTION: Ø MEDICAL AND SURGICAL
BODY SYSTEM: B RESPIRATORY SYSTEM
OPERATION: B EXCISION: Cutting out or off, without replacement, a portion of a body part

Body Part	Approach	Device	Qualifier
1 Trachea 2 Carina 3 Main Bronchus, Right 4 Upper Lobe Bronchus, Right 5 Middle Lobe Bronchus, Right 6 Lower Lobe Bronchus, Right 7 Main Bronchus, Left 8 Upper Lobe Bronchus, Left 9 Lingula Bronchus B Lower Lobe Bronchus, Left C Upper Lung Lobe, Right D Middle Lung Lobe, Right F Lower Lung Lobe, Right G Upper Lung Lobe, Left H Lung Lingula J Lower Lung Lobe, Left K Lung, Right L Lung, Left M Lungs, Bilateral	Ø Open 3 Percutaneous 4 Percutaneous Endoscopic 7 Via Natural or Artificial Opening 8 Via Natural or Artificial Opening Endoscopic	Z No Device	X Diagnostic Z No Qualifier
N Pleura, Right P Pleura, Left	Ø Open 3 Percutaneous 4 Percutaneous Endoscopic 8 Via Natural or Artificial Opening Endoscopic	Z No Device	X Diagnostic Z No Qualifier
T Diaphragm	Ø Open 3 Percutaneous 4 Percutaneous Endoscopic	Z No Device	X Diagnostic Z No Qualifier

Non-OR ØBB[123456789B][3478]ZX
Non-OR ØBB[3456789BM][48]ZZ
Non-OR ØBB[CDFGHJKLM]3ZX
Non-OR ØBB[CDFGHJKL]8ZZ
Non-OR ØBB[NP][Ø3]ZX

Coding Clinic: 2Ø15, Q1, P16 – ØBB1ØZZ
Coding Clinic: 2Ø16, Q1, P26 – ØBB48ZX, ØBBC8ZX
Coding Clinic: 2Ø16, Q1, P27 – ØBB88ZX
Coding Clinic: 2Ø22, Q2, P19 – ØBBG8ZX

SECTION: Ø MEDICAL AND SURGICAL
BODY SYSTEM: B RESPIRATORY SYSTEM
OPERATION: C EXTIRPATION: Taking or cutting out solid matter from a body part

Body Part	Approach	Device	Qualifier
1 Trachea 2 Carina 3 Main Bronchus, Right 4 Upper Lobe Bronchus, Right 5 Middle Lobe Bronchus, Right 6 Lower Lobe Bronchus, Right 7 Main Bronchus, Left 8 Upper Lobe Bronchus, Left 9 Lingula Bronchus B Lower Lobe Bronchus, Left C Upper Lung Lobe, Right D Middle Lung Lobe, Right F Lower Lung Lobe, Right G Upper Lung Lobe, Left H Lung Lingula J Lower Lung Lobe, Left K Lung, Right L Lung, Left M Lungs, Bilateral	Ø Open 3 Percutaneous 4 Percutaneous Endoscopic 7 Via Natural or Artificial Opening 8 Via Natural or Artificial Opening Endoscopic	Z No Device	Z No Qualifier
N Pleura, Right P Pleura, Left T Diaphragm	Ø Open 3 Percutaneous 4 Percutaneous Endoscopic	Z No Device	Z No Qualifier

Non-OR ØBC[123456789B][78]ZZ
Non-OR ØBC[NP][Ø34]ZZ

Coding Clinic: 2Ø17, Q3, P15 – ØBC58ZZ

SECTION: Ø MEDICAL AND SURGICAL
BODY SYSTEM: B RESPIRATORY SYSTEM
OPERATION: D EXTRACTION: Pulling or stripping out or off all or a portion of a body part by the use of force

Body Part	Approach	Device	Qualifier
1 Trachea 2 Carina 3 Main Bronchus, Right 4 Upper Lobe Bronchus, Right 5 Middle Lobe Bronchus, Right 6 Lower Lobe Bronchus, Right 7 Main Bronchus, Left 8 Upper Lobe Bronchus, Left 9 Lingula Bronchus B Lower Lobe Bronchus, Left C Upper Lung Lobe, Right D Middle Lung Lobe, Right F Lower Lung Lobe, Right G Upper Lung Lobe, Left H Lung Lingula J Lower Lung Lobe, Left K Lung, Right L Lung, Left M Lungs, Bilateral	4 Percutaneous Endoscopic 8 Via Natural or Artificial Opening Endoscopic	Z No Device	X Diagnostic
N Pleura, Right P Pleura, Left	Ø Open 3 Percutaneous 4 Percutaneous Endoscopic	Z No Device	X Diagnostic Z No Qualifier

SECTION: Ø MEDICAL AND SURGICAL
BODY SYSTEM: B RESPIRATORY SYSTEM
OPERATION: F FRAGMENTATION: Breaking solid matter in a body part into pieces

Body Part	Approach	Device	Qualifier
1 Trachea 2 Carina 3 Main Bronchus, Right 4 Upper Lobe Bronchus, Right 5 Middle Lobe Bronchus, Right 6 Lower Lobe Bronchus, Right 7 Main Bronchus, Left 8 Upper Lobe Bronchus, Left 9 Lingula Bronchus B Lower Lobe Bronchus, Left	Ø Open 3 Percutaneous 4 Percutaneous Endoscopic 7 Via Natural or Artificial Opening 8 Via Natural or Artificial Opening Endoscopic X External	Z No Device	Z No Qualifier

ØBF[123456789B]XZZ
Non-OR ØBF[123456789B]XZZ

SECTION: Ø MEDICAL AND SURGICAL
BODY SYSTEM: B RESPIRATORY SYSTEM
OPERATION: H INSERTION: *(on multiple pages)*

Putting in a nonbiological appliance that monitors, assists, performs, or prevents a physiological function but does not physically take the place of a body part

Body Part	Approach	Device	Qualifier
Ø Tracheobronchial Tree	Ø Open 3 Percutaneous 4 Percutaneous Endoscopic 7 Via Natural or Artificial Opening 8 Via Natural or Artificial Opening Endoscopic	1 Radioactive Element 2 Monitoring Device 3 Infusion Device D Intraluminal Device Y Other Device	Z No Qualifier
1 Trachea	Ø Open	2 Monitoring Device D Intraluminal Device Y Other Device	Z No Qualifier
1 Trachea	3 Percutaneous	D Intraluminal Device E Intraluminal Device, Endotracheal Airway Y Other Device	Z No Qualifier
1 Trachea	4 Percutaneous Endoscopic	D Intraluminal Device Y Other Device	Z No Qualifier
1 Trachea	7 Via Natural or Artificial Opening 8 Via Natural or Artificial Opening Endoscopic	2 Monitoring Device D Intraluminal Device E Intraluminal Device, Endotracheal Airway Y Other Device	Z No Qualifier

Non-OR ØBHØ[78][23D]Z
Non-OR ØBH13EZ

Coding Clinic: 2Ø19, Q3, P34 – ØBHB8GZ
Coding Clinic: 2Ø22, Q3, P23 – ØBH17EZ

SECTION: Ø MEDICAL AND SURGICAL
BODY SYSTEM: B RESPIRATORY SYSTEM
OPERATION: H INSERTION: *(continued)*

Putting in a nonbiological appliance that monitors, assists, performs, or prevents a physiological function but does not physically take the place of a body part

Body Part	Approach	Device	Qualifier
3 Main Bronchus, Right 4 Upper Lobe Bronchus, Right 5 Middle Lobe Bronchus, Right 6 Lower Lobe Bronchus, Right 7 Main Bronchus, Left 8 Upper Lobe Bronchus, Left 9 Lingula Bronchus B Lower Lobe Bronchus, Left	Ø Open 3 Percutaneous 4 Percutaneous Endoscopic 7 Via Natural or Artificial Opening 8 Via Natural or Artificial Opening Endoscopic	G Endobronchial Device, Endobronchial Valve	Z No Qualifier
K Lung, Right L Lung, Left	Ø Open 3 Percutaneous 4 Percutaneous Endoscopic 7 Via Natural or Artificial Opening 8 Via Natural or Artificial Opening Endoscopic	1 Radioactive Element 2 Monitoring Device 3 Infusion Device Y Other Device	Z No Qualifier
Q Pleura	Ø Open 3 Percutaneous 4 Percutaneous Endoscopic 7 Via Natural or Artificial Opening 8 Via Natural or Artificial Opening Endoscopic	Y Other Device	Z No Qualifier
T Diaphragm	Ø Open 3 Percutaneous 4 Percutaneous Endoscopic	2 Monitoring Device M Diaphragmatic Pacemaker Lead Y Other Device	Z No Qualifier
T Diaphragm	7 Via Natural or Artificial Opening 8 Via Natural or Artificial Opening Endoscopic	Y Other Device	Z No Qualifier

Non-OR ØBH1[78]2Z
Non-OR ØBH1[78]EZ
Non-OR ØBH[3456789B]8GZ
Non-OR ØBH[KL][78][23]Z
DRG Non-OR ØBH[3456789B]8GZ

SECTION: Ø MEDICAL AND SURGICAL
BODY SYSTEM: B RESPIRATORY SYSTEM
OPERATION: J INSPECTION: Visually and/or manually exploring a body part

Body Part	Approach	Device	Qualifier
Ø Tracheobronchial Tree 1 Trachea K Lung, Right L Lung, Left Q Pleura T Diaphragm	Ø Open 3 Percutaneous 4 Percutaneous Endoscopic 7 Via Natural or Artificial Opening 8 Via Natural or Artificial Opening Endoscopic X External	Z No Device	Z No Qualifier

Non-OR ØBJ[ØKL][378X]ZZ
Non-OR ØBJ1[3478X]ZZ
Non-OR ØBJ[QT][378X]ZZ

Coding Clinic: 2015, Q2, P31 – ØBJQ4ZZ

SECTION: Ø **MEDICAL AND SURGICAL**
BODY SYSTEM: B **RESPIRATORY SYSTEM**
OPERATION: L **OCCLUSION:** Completely closing an orifice or the lumen of a tubular body part

Body Part	Approach	Device	Qualifier
1 Trachea 2 Carina 3 Main Bronchus, Right 4 Upper Lobe Bronchus, Right 5 Middle Lobe Bronchus, Right 6 Lower Lobe Bronchus, Right 7 Main Bronchus, Left 8 Upper Lobe Bronchus, Left 9 Lingula Bronchus B Lower Lobe Bronchus, Left	Ø Open 3 Percutaneous 4 Percutaneous Endoscopic	C Extraluminal Device D Intraluminal Device Z No Device	Z No Qualifier
1 Trachea 2 Carina 3 Main Bronchus, Right 4 Upper Lobe Bronchus, Right 5 Middle Lobe Bronchus, Right 6 Lower Lobe Bronchus, Right 7 Main Bronchus, Left 8 Upper Lobe Bronchus, Left 9 Lingula Bronchus B Lower Lobe Bronchus, Left	7 Via Natural or Artificial Opening 8 Via Natural or Artificial Opening Endoscopic	D Intraluminal Device Z No Device	Z No Qualifier

SECTION: Ø **MEDICAL AND SURGICAL**
BODY SYSTEM: B **RESPIRATORY SYSTEM**
OPERATION: M **REATTACHMENT:** Putting back in or on all or a portion of a separated body part to its normal location or other suitable location

Body Part	Approach	Device	Qualifier
1 Trachea 2 Carina 3 Main Bronchus, Right 4 Upper Lobe Bronchus, Right 5 Middle Lobe Bronchus, Right 6 Lower Lobe Bronchus, Right 7 Main Bronchus, Left 8 Upper Lobe Bronchus, Left 9 Lingula Bronchus B Lower Lobe Bronchus, Left C Upper Lung Lobe, Right D Middle Lung Lobe, Right F Lower Lung Lobe, Right G Upper Lung Lobe, Left H Lung Lingula J Lower Lung Lobe, Left K Lung, Right L Lung, Left T Diaphragm	Ø Open	Z No Device	Z No Qualifier

SECTION: Ø **MEDICAL AND SURGICAL**
BODY SYSTEM: B **RESPIRATORY SYSTEM**
OPERATION: N **RELEASE:** Freeing a body part from an abnormal physical constraint by cutting or by the use of force

Body Part	Approach	Device	Qualifier
1 Trachea 2 Carina 3 Main Bronchus, Right 4 Upper Lobe Bronchus, Right 5 Middle Lobe Bronchus, Right 6 Lower Lobe Bronchus, Right 7 Main Bronchus, Left 8 Upper Lobe Bronchus, Left 9 Lingula Bronchus B Lower Lobe Bronchus, Left C Upper Lung Lobe, Right D Middle Lung Lobe, Right F Lower Lung Lobe, Right G Upper Lung Lobe, Left H Lung Lingula J Lower Lung Lobe, Left K Lung, Right L Lung, Left M Lungs, Bilateral	Ø Open 3 Percutaneous 4 Percutaneous Endoscopic 7 Via Natural or Artificial Opening 8 Via Natural or Artificial Opening Endoscopic	Z No Device	Z No Qualifier
N Pleura, Right P Pleura, Left T Diaphragm	Ø Open 3 Percutaneous 4 Percutaneous Endoscopic	Z No Device	Z No Qualifier

Coding Clinic: 2Ø15, Q3, P15 – ØBN1ØZZ
Coding Clinic: 2Ø19, Q2, P21 – ØBNNØZZ

SECTION: Ø **MEDICAL AND SURGICAL**
BODY SYSTEM: B **RESPIRATORY SYSTEM**
OPERATION: P **REMOVAL:** *(on multiple pages)*
Taking out or off a device from a body part

Body Part	Approach	Device	Qualifier
Ø Tracheobronchial Tree	Ø Open 3 Percutaneous 4 Percutaneous Endoscopic 7 Via Natural or Artificial Opening 8 Via Natural or Artificial Opening Endoscopic	Ø Drainage Device 1 Radioactive Element 2 Monitoring Device 3 Infusion Device 7 Autologous Tissue Substitute C Extraluminal Device D Intraluminal Device J Synthetic Substitute K Nonautologous Tissue Substitute Y Other Device	Z No Qualifier
Ø Tracheobronchial Tree	X External	Ø Drainage Device 1 Radioactive Element 2 Monitoring Device 3 Infusion Device D Intraluminal Device	Z No Qualifier

Non-OR ØBPØ[78][Ø23D]Z   Non-OR ØBPØX[Ø123D]Z   Non-OR ØBP1[Ø34]FZ

SECTION: Ø MEDICAL AND SURGICAL
BODY SYSTEM: B RESPIRATORY SYSTEM
OPERATION: P REMOVAL: *(continued)*
Taking out or off a device from a body part

Body Part	Approach	Device	Qualifier
1 Trachea	Ø Open 3 Percutaneous 4 Percutaneous Endoscopic 7 Via Natural or Artificial Opening 8 Via Natural or Artificial Opening Endoscopic	Ø Drainage Device 2 Monitoring Device 7 Autologous Tissue Substitute C Extraluminal Device D Intraluminal Device F Tracheostomy Device J Synthetic Substitute K Nonautologous Tissue Substitute	Z No Qualifier
1 Trachea	X External	Ø Drainage Device 2 Monitoring Device D Intraluminal Device F Tracheostomy Device	Z No Qualifier
K Lung, Right L Lung, Left	Ø Open 3 Percutaneous 4 Percutaneous Endoscopic 7 Via Natural or Artificial Opening 8 Via Natural or Artificial Opening Endoscopic	Ø Drainage Device 1 Radioactive Element 2 Monitoring Device 3 Infusion Device Y Other Device	Z No Qualifier
K Lung, Right L Lung, Left	X External	Ø Drainage Device 1 Radioactive Element 2 Monitoring Device 3 Infusion Device	Z No Qualifier
Q Pleura	Ø Open 3 Percutaneous 4 Percutaneous Endoscopic 7 Via Natural or Artificial Opening 8 Via Natural or Artificial Opening Endoscopic	Ø Drainage Device 1 Radioactive Element 2 Monitoring Device Y Other Device	Z No Qualifier
Q Pleura	X External	Ø Drainage Device 1 Radioactive Element 2 Monitoring Device	Z No Qualifier
T Diaphragm	Ø Open 3 Percutaneous 4 Percutaneous Endoscopic 7 Via Natural or Artificial Opening 8 Via Natural or Artificial Opening Endoscopic	Ø Drainage Device 2 Monitoring Device 7 Autologous Tissue Substitute J Synthetic Substitute K Nonautologous Tissue Substitute M Diaphragmatic Pacemaker Lead Y Other Device	Z No Qualifier
T Diaphragm	X External	Ø Drainage Device 2 Monitoring Device M Diaphragmatic Pacemaker Lead	Z No Qualifier

Non-OR ØBP1[78][Ø2DF]Z
Non-OR ØBP1X[Ø2DF]Z
Non-OR ØBP[KL][78][Ø23]Z
Non-OR ØBP[KL]X[Ø123]Z
Non-OR ØBPQ[Ø3478X][Ø12]Z
Non-OR ØBPQX[Ø12]Z
Non-OR ØBPT[78][Ø2]Z
Non-OR ØBPTX[Ø2M]Z

SECTION: Ø MEDICAL AND SURGICAL
BODY SYSTEM: B RESPIRATORY SYSTEM
OPERATION: Q REPAIR: Restoring, to the extent possible, a body part to its normal anatomic structure and function

Body Part	Approach	Device	Qualifier
1 Trachea 2 Carina 3 Main Bronchus, Right 4 Upper Lobe Bronchus, Right 5 Middle Lobe Bronchus, Right 6 Lower Lobe Bronchus, Right 7 Main Bronchus, Left 8 Upper Lobe Bronchus, Left 9 Lingula Bronchus B Lower Lobe Bronchus, Left C Upper Lung Lobe, Right D Middle Lung Lobe, Right F Lower Lung Lobe, Right G Upper Lung Lobe, Left H Lung Lingula J Lower Lung Lobe, Left K Lung, Right L Lung, Left M Lungs, Bilateral	Ø Open 3 Percutaneous 4 Percutaneous Endoscopic 7 Via Natural or Artificial Opening 8 Via Natural or Artificial Opening Endoscopic	Z No Device	Z No Qualifier
N Pleura, Right P Pleura, Left T Diaphragm	Ø Open 3 Percutaneous 4 Percutaneous Endoscopic	Z No Device	Z No Qualifier

Coding Clinic: 2Ø16, Q2, P23 – ØBQ[RS]ØZZ

SECTION: Ø MEDICAL AND SURGICAL
BODY SYSTEM: B RESPIRATORY SYSTEM
OPERATION: R REPLACEMENT: Putting in or on biological or synthetic material that physically takes the place and/or function of all or a portion of a body part

Body Part	Approach	Device	Qualifier
1 Trachea 2 Carina 3 Main Bronchus, Right 4 Upper Lobe Bronchus, Right 5 Middle Lobe Bronchus, Right 6 Lower Lobe Bronchus, Right 7 Main Bronchus, Left 8 Upper Lobe Bronchus, Left 9 Lingula Bronchus B Lower Lobe Bronchus, Left T Diaphragm	Ø Open 4 Percutaneous Endoscopic	7 Autologous Tissue Substitute J Synthetic Substitute K Nonautologous Tissue Substitute	Z No Qualifier

SECTION: Ø MEDICAL AND SURGICAL
BODY SYSTEM: B RESPIRATORY SYSTEM
OPERATION: S REPOSITION: Moving to its normal location, or other suitable location, all or a portion of a body part

Body Part	Approach	Device	Qualifier
1 Trachea 2 Carina 3 Main Bronchus, Right 4 Upper Lobe Bronchus, Right 5 Middle Lobe Bronchus, Right 6 Lower Lobe Bronchus, Right 7 Main Bronchus, Left 8 Upper Lobe Bronchus, Left 9 Lingula Bronchus B Lower Lobe Bronchus, Left C Upper Lung Lobe, Right D Middle Lung Lobe, Right F Lower Lung Lobe, Right G Upper Lung Lobe, Left H Lung Lingula J Lower Lung Lobe, Left K Lung, Right L Lung, Left T Diaphragm	Ø Open	Z No Device	Z No Qualifier

SECTION: Ø MEDICAL AND SURGICAL
BODY SYSTEM: B RESPIRATORY SYSTEM
OPERATION: T RESECTION: Cutting out or off, without replacement, all of a body part

Body Part	Approach	Device	Qualifier
1 Trachea 2 Carina 3 Main Bronchus, Right 4 Upper Lobe Bronchus, Right 5 Middle Lobe Bronchus, Right 6 Lower Lobe Bronchus, Right 7 Main Bronchus, Left 8 Upper Lobe Bronchus, Left 9 Lingula Bronchus B Lower Lobe Bronchus, Left C Upper Lung Lobe, Right D Middle Lung Lobe, Right F Lower Lung Lobe, Right G Upper Lung Lobe, Left H Lung Lingula J Lower Lung Lobe, Left K Lung, Right L Lung, Left M Lungs, Bilateral T Diaphragm	Ø Open 4 Percutaneous Endoscopic	Z No Device	Z No Qualifier

SECTION: Ø MEDICAL AND SURGICAL
BODY SYSTEM: B RESPIRATORY SYSTEM
OPERATION: U SUPPLEMENT: Putting in or on biological or synthetic material that physically reinforces and/or augments the function of a portion of a body part

Body Part	Approach	Device	Qualifier
1 Trachea 2 Carina 3 Main Bronchus, Right 4 Upper Lobe Bronchus, Right 5 Middle Lobe Bronchus, Right 6 Lower Lobe Bronchus, Right 7 Main Bronchus, Left 8 Upper Lobe Bronchus, Left 9 Lingula Bronchus B Lower Lobe Bronchus, Left	Ø Open 4 Percutaneous Endoscopic 8 Via Natural or Artificial Opening Endoscopic	7 Autologous Tissue Substitute J Synthetic Substitute K Nonautologous Tissue Substitute	Z No Qualifier
T Diaphragm	Ø Open 4 Percutaneous Endoscopic	7 Autologous Tissue Substitute J Synthetic Substitute K Nonautologous Tissue Substitute	Z No Qualifier

Coding Clinic: 2Ø15, Q1, P28 – ØBU3Ø7Z

SECTION: Ø MEDICAL AND SURGICAL
BODY SYSTEM: B RESPIRATORY SYSTEM
OPERATION: V RESTRICTION: Partially closing an orifice or the lumen of a tubular body part

Body Part	Approach	Device	Qualifier
1 Trachea 2 Carina 3 Main Bronchus, Right 4 Upper Lobe Bronchus, Right 5 Middle Lobe Bronchus, Right 6 Lower Lobe Bronchus, Right 7 Main Bronchus, Left 8 Upper Lobe Bronchus, Left 9 Lingula Bronchus B Lower Lobe Bronchus, Left	Ø Open 3 Percutaneous 4 Percutaneous Endoscopic	C Extraluminal Device D Intraluminal Device Z No Device	Z No Qualifier
1 Trachea 2 Carina 3 Main Bronchus, Right 4 Upper Lobe Bronchus, Right 5 Middle Lobe Bronchus, Right 6 Lower Lobe Bronchus, Right 7 Main Bronchus, Left 8 Upper Lobe Bronchus, Left 9 Lingula Bronchus B Lower Lobe Bronchus, Left	7 Via Natural or Artificial Opening 8 Via Natural or Artificial Opening Endoscopic	D Intraluminal Device Z No Device	Z No Qualifier

SECTION: Ø MEDICAL AND SURGICAL
BODY SYSTEM: B RESPIRATORY SYSTEM
OPERATION: W REVISION: *(on multiple pages)*

Correcting, to the extent possible, a portion of a malfunctioning device or the position of a displaced device

Body Part	Approach	Device	Qualifier
Ø Tracheobronchial Tree	Ø Open 3 Percutaneous 4 Percutaneous Endoscopic 7 Via Natural or Artificial Opening 8 Via Natural or Artificial Opening Endoscopic	Ø Drainage Device 2 Monitoring Device 3 Infusion Device 7 Autologous Tissue Substitute C Extraluminal Device D Intraluminal Device J Synthetic Substitute K Nonautologous Tissue Substitute Y Other Device	Z No Qualifier
Ø Tracheobronchial Tree	X External	Ø Drainage Device 2 Monitoring Device 3 Infusion Device 7 Autologous Tissue Substitute C Extraluminal Device D Intraluminal Device J Synthetic Substitute K Nonautologous Tissue Substitute	Z No Qualifier
1 Trachea	Ø Open 3 Percutaneous 4 Percutaneous Endoscopic 7 Via Natural or Artificial Opening 8 Via Natural or Artificial Opening Endoscopic X External	Ø Drainage Device 2 Monitoring Device 7 Autologous Tissue Substitute C Extraluminal Device D Intraluminal Device F Tracheostomy Device J Synthetic Substitute K Nonautologous Tissue Substitute	Z No Qualifier
K Lung, Right L Lung, Left	Ø Open 3 Percutaneous 4 Percutaneous Endoscopic 7 Via Natural or Artificial Opening 8 Via Natural or Artificial Opening Endoscopic	Ø Drainage Device 2 Monitoring Device 3 Infusion Device Y Other Device	Z No Qualifier
K Lung, Right L Lung, Left	X External	Ø Drainage Device 2 Monitoring Device 3 Infusion Device	Z No Qualifier
Q Pleura	Ø Open 3 Percutaneous 4 Percutaneous Endoscopic 7 Via Natural or Artificial Opening 8 Via Natural or Artificial Opening Endoscopic	Ø Drainage Device 2 Monitoring Device Y Other Device	Z No Qualifier
Q Pleura	X External	Ø Drainage Device 2 Monitoring Device	Z No Qualifier

DRG Non-OR ØBWØ[78][23D]Z *(proposed)*
DRG Non-OR ØBWK[78][Ø23D]Z *(proposed)*
DRG Non-OR ØBWL[78][Ø23]Z *(proposed)*

Non-OR ØBWØX[Ø237CDJK]Z
Non-OR ØBW1X[Ø27CDFJK]Z
Non-OR ØBW[KL]X[Ø23]Z
Non-OR ØBWQ[Ø3478][Ø2]Z

SECTION: Ø MEDICAL AND SURGICAL
BODY SYSTEM: B RESPIRATORY SYSTEM
OPERATION: W REVISION: *(continued)*

Correcting, to the extent possible, a portion of a malfunctioning device or the position of a displaced device

Body Part	Approach	Device	Qualifier
T Diaphragm	Ø Open 3 Percutaneous 4 Percutaneous Endoscopic 7 Via Natural or Artificial Opening 8 Via Natural or Artificial Opening Endoscopic	Ø Drainage Device 2 Monitoring Device 7 Autologous Tissue Substitute J Synthetic Substitute K Nonautologous Tissue Substitute M Diaphragmatic Pacemaker Lead Y Other Device	Z No Qualifier
T Diaphragm	X External	Ø Drainage Device 2 Monitoring Device 7 Autologous Tissue Substitute J Synthetic Substitute K Nonautologous Tissue Substitute M Diaphragmatic Pacemaker Lead	Z No Qualifier

Non-OR ØBWQX[Ø2]Z
Non-OR ØBWTX[Ø27JKM]Z

SECTION: Ø MEDICAL AND SURGICAL
BODY SYSTEM: B RESPIRATORY SYSTEM
OPERATION: Y TRANSPLANTATION: Putting in or on all or a portion of a living body part taken from another individual or animal to physically take the place and/or function of all or a portion of a similar body part

Body Part	Approach	Device	Qualifier
C Upper Lung Lobe, Right D Middle Lung Lobe, Right F Lower Lung Lobe, Right G Upper Lung Lobe, Left H Lung Lingula J Lower Lung Lobe, Left K Lung, Right L Lung, Left M Lungs, Bilateral	Ø Open	Z No Device	Ø Allogeneic 1 Syngeneic 2 Zooplastic

All Values

SECTION: Ø MEDICAL AND SURGICAL
BODY SYSTEM: C MOUTH AND THROAT
OPERATION: Ø ALTERATION: Modifying the anatomic structure of a body part without affecting the function of the body part

Body Part	Approach	Device	Qualifier
Ø Upper Lip 1 Lower Lip	X External	7 Autologous Tissue Substitute J Synthetic Substitute K Nonautologous Tissue Substitute Z No Device	Z No Qualifier

SECTION: Ø MEDICAL AND SURGICAL
BODY SYSTEM: C MOUTH AND THROAT
OPERATION: 2 CHANGE: Taking out or off a device from a body part and putting back an identical or similar device in or on the same body part without cutting or puncturing the skin or a mucous membrane

Body Part	Approach	Device	Qualifier
A Salivary Gland S Larynx Y Mouth and Throat	X External	Ø Drainage Device Y Other Device	Z No Qualifier

Non-OR All Values

SECTION: Ø MEDICAL AND SURGICAL
BODY SYSTEM: C MOUTH AND THROAT
OPERATION: 5 DESTRUCTION: *(on multiple pages)*
Physical eradication of all or a portion of a body part by the use of direct energy, force, or a destructive agent

Body Part	Approach	Device	Qualifier
Ø Upper Lip 1 Lower Lip 2 Hard Palate 3 Soft Palate 4 Buccal Mucosa 5 Upper Gingiva 6 Lower Gingiva 7 Tongue N Uvula P Tonsils Q Adenoids	Ø Open 3 Percutaneous X External	Z No Device	Z No Qualifier

Non-OR ØC5[56][Ø3X]ZZ

SECTION: Ø MEDICAL AND SURGICAL
BODY SYSTEM: C MOUTH AND THROAT
OPERATION: 5 DESTRUCTION: *(continued)*

Physical eradication of all or a portion of a body part by the use of direct energy, force, or a destructive agent

Body Part	Approach	Device	Qualifier
8 Parotid Gland, Right 9 Parotid Gland, Left B Parotid Duct, Right C Parotid Duct, Left D Sublingual Gland, Right F Sublingual Gland, Left G Submaxillary Gland, Right H Submaxillary Gland, Left J Minor Salivary Gland	Ø Open 3 Percutaneous	Z No Device	Z No Qualifier
M Pharynx R Epiglottis S Larynx T Vocal Cord, Right V Vocal Cord, Left	Ø Open 3 Percutaneous 4 Percutaneous Endoscopic 7 Via Natural or Artificial Opening 8 Via Natural or Artificial Opening Endoscopic	Z No Device	Z No Qualifier
W Upper Tooth X Lower Tooth	Ø Open X External	Z No Device	Ø Single 1 Multiple 2 All

Non-OR ØC5[WX][ØX]Z[Ø12]

SECTION: Ø MEDICAL AND SURGICAL
BODY SYSTEM: C MOUTH AND THROAT
OPERATION: 7 DILATION: Expanding an orifice or the lumen of a tubular body part

Body Part	Approach	Device	Qualifier
B Parotid Duct, Right C Parotid Duct, Left	Ø Open 3 Percutaneous 7 Via Natural or Artificial Opening	D Intraluminal Device Z No Device	Z No Qualifier
M Pharynx	7 Via Natural or Artificial Opening 8 Via Natural or Artificial Opening Endoscopic	D Intraluminal Device Z No Device	Z No Qualifier
S Larynx	Ø Open 3 Percutaneous 4 Percutaneous Endoscopic 7 Via Natural or Artificial Opening 8 Via Natural or Artificial Opening Endoscopic	D Intraluminal Device Z No Device	Z No Qualifier

Non-OR ØC7[BC][Ø37][DZ]Z
Non-OR ØC7M[78][DZ]Z

SECTION: Ø MEDICAL AND SURGICAL
BODY SYSTEM: C MOUTH AND THROAT
OPERATION: 9 DRAINAGE: *(on multiple pages)*

Taking or letting out fluids and/or gases from a body part

Body Part	Approach	Device	Qualifier
Ø Upper Lip 1 Lower Lip 2 Hard Palate 3 Soft Palate 4 Buccal Mucosa 5 Upper Gingiva 6 Lower Gingiva 7 Tongue N Uvula P Tonsils Q Adenoids	Ø Open 3 Percutaneous X External	Ø Drainage Device	Z No Qualifier
Ø Upper Lip 1 Lower Lip 2 Hard Palate 3 Soft Palate 4 Buccal Mucosa 5 Upper Gingiva 6 Lower Gingiva 7 Tongue N Uvula P Tonsils Q Adenoids	Ø Open 3 Percutaneous X External	Z No Device	X Diagnostic Z No Qualifier
8 Parotid Gland, Right 9 Parotid Gland, Left B Parotid Duct, Right C Parotid Duct, Left D Sublingual Gland, Right F Sublingual Gland, Left G Submaxillary Gland, Right H Submaxillary Gland, Left J Minor Salivary Gland	Ø Open 3 Percutaneous	Ø Drainage Device	Z No Qualifier
8 Parotid Gland, Right 9 Parotid Gland, Left B Parotid Duct, Right C Parotid Duct, Left D Sublingual Gland, Right F Sublingual Gland, Left G Submaxillary Gland, Right H Submaxillary Gland, Left J Minor Salivary Gland	Ø Open 3 Percutaneous	Z No Device	X Diagnostic Z No Qualifier
M Pharynx R Epiglottis S Larynx T Vocal Cord, Right V Vocal Cord, Left	Ø Open 3 Percutaneous 4 Percutaneous Endoscopic 7 Via Natural or Artificial Opening 8 Via Natural or Artificial Opening Endoscopic	Ø Drainage Device	Z No Qualifier

Non-OR ØC9[Ø12347NPQ]3ØZ
Non-OR ØC9[Ø12347NPQ]3ZZ
Non-OR ØC9[56][Ø3X]ØZ
Non-OR ØC9[Ø1456][Ø3X]ZX
Non-OR ØC9[56][Ø3X]ZZ
Non-OR ØC97[3X]ZX
Non-OR ØC9[89BCDFGHJ][Ø3]ØZ
Non-OR ØC9[89BCDFGHJ]3ZX
Non-OR ØC9[89BCDFGHJ][Ø3]ZZ
Non-OR ØC9[MRSTV]3ØZ

SECTION: Ø MEDICAL AND SURGICAL
BODY SYSTEM: C MOUTH AND THROAT
OPERATION: 9 DRAINAGE: *(continued)*
Taking or letting out fluids and/or gases from a body part

Body Part	Approach	Device	Qualifier
M Pharynx R Epiglottis S Larynx T Vocal Cord, Right V Vocal Cord, Left	Ø Open 3 Percutaneous 4 Percutaneous Endoscopic 7 Via Natural or Artificial Opening 8 Via Natural or Artificial Opening Endoscopic	Z No Device	X Diagnostic Z No Qualifier
W Upper Tooth X Lower Tooth	Ø Open X External	Ø Drainage Device Z No Device	Ø Single 1 Multiple 2 All

Non-OR ØC9[MRSTV]3ZZ
Non-OR ØC9M[Ø3478]ZX
Non-OR ØC9[RSTV][3478]ZX
Non-OR ØC9[WX][ØX][ØZ][Ø12]

SECTION: Ø MEDICAL AND SURGICAL
BODY SYSTEM: C MOUTH AND THROAT
OPERATION: B EXCISION: Cutting out or off, without replacement, a portion of a body part

Body Part	Approach	Device	Qualifier
Ø Upper Lip 1 Lower Lip 2 Hard Palate 3 Soft Palate 4 Buccal Mucosa 5 Upper Gingiva 6 Lower Gingiva 7 Tongue N Uvula P Tonsils Q Adenoids	Ø Open 3 Percutaneous X External	Z No Device	X Diagnostic Z No Qualifier
8 Parotid Gland, Right 9 Parotid Gland, Left B Parotid Duct, Right C Parotid Duct, Left D Sublingual Gland, Right F Sublingual Gland, Left G Submaxillary Gland, Right H Submaxillary Gland, Left J Minor Salivary Gland	Ø Open 3 Percutaneous	Z No Device	X Diagnostic Z No Qualifier
M Pharynx R Epiglottis S Larynx T Vocal Cord, Right V Vocal Cord, Left	Ø Open 3 Percutaneous 4 Percutaneous Endoscopic 7 Via Natural or Artificial Opening 8 Via Natural or Artificial Opening Endoscopic	Z No Device	X Diagnostic Z No Qualifier
W Upper Tooth X Lower Tooth	Ø Open X External	Z No Device	Ø Single 1 Multiple 2 All

Non-OR ØCB[Ø1456][Ø3X]ZX
Non-OR ØCB[56][Ø3X]ZZ
Non-OR ØCB7[3X]ZX
Non-OR ØCB[89BCDFGHJ]3ZX
Non-OR ØCBM[Ø3478]ZX
Non-OR ØCB[RSTV][3478]ZX
Non-OR ØCB[WX][ØX]Z[Ø12]

Coding Clinic: 2Ø16, Q2, P2Ø – ØCBM8ZX
Coding Clinic: 2Ø16, Q3, P28 – ØCBM8ZZ

SECTION: Ø MEDICAL AND SURGICAL
BODY SYSTEM: C MOUTH AND THROAT
OPERATION: C EXTIRPATION: Taking or cutting out solid matter from a body part

Body Part	Approach	Device	Qualifier
Ø Upper Lip 1 Lower Lip 2 Hard Palate 3 Soft Palate 4 Buccal Mucosa 5 Upper Gingiva 6 Lower Gingiva 7 Tongue N Uvula P Tonsils Q Adenoids	Ø Open 3 Percutaneous X External	Z No Device	Z No Qualifier
8 Parotid Gland, Right 9 Parotid Gland, Left B Parotid Duct, Right C Parotid Duct, Left D Sublingual Gland, Right F Sublingual Gland, Left G Submaxillary Gland, Right H Submaxillary Gland, Left J Minor Salivary Gland	Ø Open 3 Percutaneous	Z No Device	Z No Qualifier
M Pharynx R Epiglottis S Larynx T Vocal Cord, Right V Vocal Cord, Left	Ø Open 3 Percutaneous 4 Percutaneous Endoscopic 7 Via Natural or Artificial Opening 8 Via Natural or Artificial Opening Endoscopic	Z No Device	Z No Qualifier
W Upper Tooth X Lower Tooth	Ø Open X External	Z No Device	Ø Single 1 Multiple 2 All

Non-OR ØCC[Ø12347NPQ]XZZ
Non-OR ØCC[56][Ø3X]ZZ
Non-OR ØCC[89BCDFGHJ][Ø3]ZZ
Non-OR ØCC[MS][78]ZZ
Non-OR ØCC[WX][ØX]Z[Ø12]

Coding Clinic: 2Ø16, Q2, P2Ø – ØCCH3ZZ

SECTION: Ø MEDICAL AND SURGICAL
BODY SYSTEM: C MOUTH AND THROAT
OPERATION: D EXTRACTION: Pulling or stripping out or off all or a portion of a body part by the use of force

Body Part	Approach	Device	Qualifier
T Vocal Cord, Right V Vocal Cord, Left	Ø Open 3 Percutaneous 4 Percutaneous Endoscopic 7 Via Natural or Artificial Opening 8 Via Natural or Artificial Opening Endoscopic	Z No Device	Z No Qualifier
W Upper Tooth X Lower Tooth	X External	Z No Device	Ø Single 1 Multiple 2 All

Non-OR ØCD[WX]XZ[Ø12]

SECTION: Ø MEDICAL AND SURGICAL
BODY SYSTEM: C MOUTH AND THROAT
OPERATION: F FRAGMENTATION: Breaking solid matter in a body part into pieces

Body Part	Approach	Device	Qualifier
B Parotid Duct, Right C Parotid Duct, Left	Ø Open 3 Percutaneous 7 Via Natural or Artificial Opening X External	Z No Device	Z No Qualifier

ØCF[BC]XZZ

Non-OR All Values

SECTION: Ø MEDICAL AND SURGICAL
BODY SYSTEM: C MOUTH AND THROAT
OPERATION: H INSERTION: Putting in a nonbiological appliance that monitors, assists, performs, or prevents a physiological function but does not physically take the place of a body part

Body Part	Approach	Device	Qualifier
7 Tongue	Ø Open 3 Percutaneous X External	1 Radioactive Element	Z No Qualifier
A Salivary Gland S Larynx	Ø Open 3 Percutaneous 7 Via Natural or Artificial Opening 8 Via Natural or Artificial Opening Endoscopic	1 Radioactive Element Y Other Device	Z No Qualifier
Y Mouth and Throat	Ø Open 3 Percutaneous	1 Radioactive Element Y Other Device	Z No Qualifier
Y Mouth and Throat	7 Via Natural or Artificial Opening 8 Via Natural or Artificial Opening Endoscopic	1 Radioactive Element B Intraluminal Device, Airway Y Other Device	Z No Qualifier

Non-OR ØCHY[78]BZ

SECTION: Ø MEDICAL AND SURGICAL
BODY SYSTEM: C MOUTH AND THROAT
OPERATION: J INSPECTION: Visually and/or manually exploring a body part

Body Part	Approach	Device	Qualifier
A Salivary Gland	Ø Open 3 Percutaneous X External	Z No Device	Z No Qualifier
S Larynx Y Mouth and Throat	Ø Open 3 Percutaneous 4 Percutaneous Endoscopic 7 Via Natural or Artificial Opening 8 Via Natural or Artificial Opening Endoscopic X External	Z No Device	Z No Qualifier

Non-OR All Values

SECTION: Ø MEDICAL AND SURGICAL
BODY SYSTEM: C MOUTH AND THROAT
OPERATION: L OCCLUSION: Completely closing an orifice or the lumen of a tubular body part

Body Part	Approach	Device	Qualifier
B Parotid Duct, Right C Parotid Duct, Left	Ø Open 3 Percutaneous 4 Percutaneous Endoscopic	C Extraluminal Device D Intraluminal Device Z No Device	Z No Qualifier
B Parotid Duct, Right C Parotid Duct, Left	7 Via Natural or Artificial Opening 8 Via Natural or Artificial Opening Endoscopic	D Intraluminal Device Z No Device	Z No Qualifier

SECTION: Ø MEDICAL AND SURGICAL
BODY SYSTEM: C MOUTH AND THROAT
OPERATION: M REATTACHMENT: Putting back in or on all or a portion of a separated body part to its normal location or other suitable location

Body Part	Approach	Device	Qualifier
Ø Upper Lip 1 Lower Lip 3 Soft Palate 7 Tongue N Uvula	Ø Open	Z No Device	Z No Qualifier
W Upper Tooth X Lower Tooth	Ø Open X External	Z No Device	Ø Single 1 Multiple 2 All

Non-OR ØCM[WX][ØX]Z[Ø12]

SECTION: Ø MEDICAL AND SURGICAL
BODY SYSTEM: C MOUTH AND THROAT
OPERATION: N RELEASE: Freeing a body part from an abnormal physical constraint by cutting or by the use of force

Body Part	Approach	Device	Qualifier
Ø Upper Lip 1 Lower Lip 2 Hard Palate 3 Soft Palate 4 Buccal Mucosa 5 Upper Gingiva 6 Lower Gingiva 7 Tongue N Uvula P Tonsils Q Adenoids	Ø Open 3 Percutaneous X External	Z No Device	Z No Qualifier
8 Parotid Gland, Right 9 Parotid Gland, Left B Parotid Duct, Right C Parotid Duct, Left D Sublingual Gland, Right F Sublingual Gland, Left G Submaxillary Gland, Right H Submaxillary Gland, Left J Minor Salivary Gland	Ø Open 3 Percutaneous	Z No Device	Z No Qualifier
M Pharynx R Epiglottis S Larynx T Vocal Cord, Right V Vocal Cord, Left	Ø Open 3 Percutaneous 4 Percutaneous Endoscopic 7 Via Natural or Artificial Opening 8 Via Natural or Artificial Opening Endoscopic	Z No Device	Z No Qualifier
W Upper Tooth X Lower Tooth	Ø Open X External	Z No Device	Ø Single 1 Multiple 2 All

Non-OR ØCN[Ø1567][Ø3X]ZZ
Non-OR ØCN[WX][ØX]Z[Ø12]

SECTION: Ø MEDICAL AND SURGICAL
BODY SYSTEM: C MOUTH AND THROAT
OPERATION: P REMOVAL: Taking out or off a device from a body part

Body Part	Approach	Device	Qualifier
A Salivary Gland	Ø Open 3 Percutaneous	Ø Drainage Device C Extraluminal Device Y Other Device	Z No Qualifier
A Salivary Gland	7 Via Natural or Artificial Opening 8 Via Natural or Artificial Opening Endoscopic	Y Other Device	Z No Qualifier
S Larynx	Ø Open 3 Percutaneous 7 Via Natural or Artificial Opening 8 Via Natural or Artificial Opening Endoscopic	Ø Drainage Device 7 Autologous Tissue Substitute D Intraluminal Device J Synthetic Substitute K Nonautologous Tissue Substitute Y Other Device	Z No Qualifier
S Larynx	X External	Ø Drainage Device 7 Autologous Tissue Substitute D Intraluminal Device J Synthetic Substitute K Nonautologous Tissue Substitute	Z No Qualifier
Y Mouth and Throat	Ø Open 3 Percutaneous 7 Via Natural or Artificial Opening 8 Via Natural or Artificial Opening Endoscopic	Ø Drainage Device 1 Radioactive Element 7 Autologous Tissue Substitute D Intraluminal Device J Synthetic Substitute K Nonautologous Tissue Substitute Y Other Device	Z No Qualifier
Y Mouth and Throat	X External	Ø Drainage Device 1 Radioactive Element 7 Autologous Tissue Substitute D Intraluminal Device J Synthetic Substitute K Nonautologous Tissue Substitute	Z No Qualifier

Non-OR ØCPA[Ø3][ØC]Z
Non-OR ØCPS[78][ØD]Z
Non-OR ØCPSX[Ø7DJK]Z
Non-OR ØCPY[78][ØD]Z
Non-OR ØCPYX[Ø17DJK]Z

SECTION: Ø MEDICAL AND SURGICAL
BODY SYSTEM: C MOUTH AND THROAT
OPERATION: Q REPAIR: Restoring, to the extent possible, a body part to its normal anatomic structure and function

Body Part	Approach	Device	Qualifier
Ø Upper Lip 1 Lower Lip 2 Hard Palate 3 Soft Palate 4 Buccal Mucosa 5 Upper Gingiva 6 Lower Gingiva 7 Tongue N Uvula P Tonsils Q Adenoids	Ø Open 3 Percutaneous X External	Z No Device	Z No Qualifier
8 Parotid Gland, Right 9 Parotid Gland, Left B Parotid Duct, Right C Parotid Duct, Left D Sublingual Gland, Right F Sublingual Gland, Left G Submaxillary Gland, Right H Submaxillary Gland, Left J Minor Salivary Gland	Ø Open 3 Percutaneous	Z No Device	Z No Qualifier
M Pharynx R Epiglottis S Larynx T Vocal Cord, Right V Vocal Cord, Left	Ø Open 3 Percutaneous 4 Percutaneous Endoscopic 7 Via Natural or Artificial Opening 8 Via Natural or Artificial Opening Endoscopic	Z No Device	Z No Qualifier
W Upper Tooth X Lower Tooth	Ø Open X External	Z No Device	Ø Single 1 Multiple 2 All

Non-OR ØCQ[Ø1]XZZ
Non-OR ØCQ[56][Ø3X]ZZ
Non-OR ØCQ[WX][ØX]Z[Ø12]

Coding Clinic: 2017, Q1, P21 – ØCQ5ØZZ

SECTION: Ø MEDICAL AND SURGICAL
BODY SYSTEM: C MOUTH AND THROAT
OPERATION: R REPLACEMENT: Putting in or on biological or synthetic material that physically takes the place and/or function of all or a portion of a body part

Body Part	Approach	Device	Qualifier
Ø Upper Lip 1 Lower Lip 2 Hard Palate 3 Soft Palate 4 Buccal Mucosa 5 Upper Gingiva 6 Lower Gingiva 7 Tongue N Uvula	Ø Open 3 Percutaneous X External	7 Autologous Tissue Substitute J Synthetic Substitute K Nonautologous Tissue Substitute	Z No Qualifier
B Parotid Duct, Right C Parotid Duct, Left	Ø Open 3 Percutaneous	7 Autologous Tissue Substitute J Synthetic Substitute K Nonautologous Tissue Substitute	Z No Qualifier
M Pharynx R Epiglottis S Larynx T Vocal Cord, Right V Vocal Cord, Left	Ø Open 7 Via Natural or Artificial Opening 8 Via Natural or Artificial Opening Endoscopic	7 Autologous Tissue Substitute J Synthetic Substitute K Nonautologous Tissue Substitute	Z No Qualifier
W Upper Tooth X Lower Tooth	Ø Open X External	7 Autologous Tissue Substitute J Synthetic Substitute K Nonautologous Tissue Substitute	Ø Single 1 Multiple 2 All

Non-OR ØCR[WX][ØX][7JK][Ø12]

SECTION: Ø MEDICAL AND SURGICAL
BODY SYSTEM: C MOUTH AND THROAT
OPERATION: S REPOSITION: Moving to its normal location, or other suitable location, all or a portion of a body part

Body Part	Approach	Device	Qualifier
Ø Upper Lip 1 Lower Lip 2 Hard Palate 3 Soft Palate 7 Tongue N Uvula	Ø Open X External	Z No Device	Z No Qualifier
B Parotid Duct, Right C Parotid Duct, Left	Ø Open 3 Percutaneous	Z No Device	Z No Qualifier
R Epiglottis S Larynx T Vocal Cord, Right V Vocal Cord, Left	Ø Open 7 Via Natural or Artificial Opening 8 Via Natural or Artificial Opening Endoscopic	Z No Device	Z No Qualifier
W Upper Tooth X Lower Tooth	Ø Open X External	5 External Fixation Device Z No Device	Ø Single 1 Multiple 2 All

Non-OR 0CS[WX][0X][5Z][012]

Coding Clinic: 2016, Q3, P29 – 0CSR8ZZ
Coding Clinic: 2Ø22, Q2, P24 – ØCS[23]ØZZ

SECTION: Ø MEDICAL AND SURGICAL
BODY SYSTEM: C MOUTH AND THROAT
OPERATION: T RESECTION: Cutting out or off, without replacement, all of a body part

Body Part	Approach	Device	Qualifier
Ø Upper Lip 1 Lower Lip 2 Hard Palate 3 Soft Palate 7 Tongue N Uvula P Tonsils Q Adenoids	Ø Open X External	Z No Device	Z No Qualifier
8 Parotid Gland, Right 9 Parotid Gland, Left B Parotid Duct, Right C Parotid Duct, Left D Sublingual Gland, Right F Sublingual Gland, Left G Submaxillary Gland, Right H Submaxillary Gland, Left J Minor Salivary Gland	Ø Open	Z No Device	Z No Qualifier
M Pharynx R Epiglottis S Larynx T Vocal Cord, Right V Vocal Cord, Left	Ø Open 4 Percutaneous Endoscopic 7 Via Natural or Artificial Opening 8 Via Natural or Artificial Opening Endoscopic	Z No Device	Z No Qualifier
W Upper Tooth X Lower Tooth	Ø Open	Z No Device	Ø Single 1 Multiple 2 All

Non-OR ØCT[WX]ØZ[Ø12]

Coding Clinic: 2Ø16, Q2, P13 – ØCT9ØZZ

SECTION: Ø MEDICAL AND SURGICAL
BODY SYSTEM: C MOUTH AND THROAT
OPERATION: U SUPPLEMENT: Putting in or on biological or synthetic material that physically reinforces and/or augments the function of a portion of a body part

Body Part	Approach	Device	Qualifier
Ø Upper Lip 1 Lower Lip 2 Hard Palate 3 Soft Palate 4 Buccal Mucosa 5 Upper Gingiva 6 Lower Gingiva 7 Tongue N Uvula	Ø Open 3 Percutaneous X External	7 Autologous Tissue Substitute J Synthetic Substitute K Nonautologous Tissue Substitute	Z No Qualifier
M Pharynx R Epiglottis S Larynx T Vocal Cord, Right V Vocal Cord, Left	Ø Open 7 Via Natural or Artificial Opening 8 Via Natural or Artificial Opening Endoscopic	7 Autologous Tissue Substitute J Synthetic Substitute K Nonautologous Tissue Substitute	Z No Qualifier

Non-OR ØCU2[Ø3]JZ

SECTION: Ø MEDICAL AND SURGICAL
BODY SYSTEM: C MOUTH AND THROAT
OPERATION: V RESTRICTION: Partially closing an orifice or the lumen of a tubular body part

Body Part	Approach	Device	Qualifier
B Parotid Duct, Right C Parotid Duct, Left	Ø Open 3 Percutaneous	C Extraluminal Device D Intraluminal Device Z No Device	Z No Qualifier
B Parotid Duct, Right C Parotid Duct, Left	7 Via Natural or Artificial Opening 8 Via Natural or Artificial Opening Endoscopic	D Intraluminal Device Z No Device	Z No Qualifier

SECTION: Ø MEDICAL AND SURGICAL
BODY SYSTEM: C MOUTH AND THROAT
OPERATION: W REVISION: *(on multiple pages)*
Correcting, to the extent possible, a portion of a malfunctioning device or the position of a displaced device

Body Part	Approach	Device	Qualifier
A Salivary Gland	Ø Open 3 Percutaneous	Ø Drainage Device C Extraluminal Device Y Other Device	Z No Qualifier
A Salivary Gland	7 Via Natural or Artificial Opening 8 Via Natural or Artificial Opening Endoscopic	Y Other Device	Z No Qualifier
A Salivary Gland	X External	Ø Drainage Device C Extraluminal Device	Z No Qualifier
S Larynx	Ø Open 3 Percutaneous 7 Via Natural or Artificial Opening 8 Via Natural or Artificial Opening Endoscopic	Ø Drainage Device 7 Autologous Tissue Substitute D Intraluminal Device J Synthetic Substitute K Nonautologous Tissue Substitute Y Other Device	Z No Qualifier
S Larynx	X External	Ø Drainage Device 7 Autologous Tissue Substitute D Intraluminal Device J Synthetic Substitute K Nonautologous Tissue Substitute	Z No Qualifier

Non-OR ØCWA[Ø3X][ØC]Z
Non-OR ØCWSX[Ø7DHJ]Z

SECTION: Ø MEDICAL AND SURGICAL
BODY SYSTEM: C MOUTH AND THROAT
OPERATION: W REVISION: *(continued)*

Correcting, to the extent possible, a portion of a malfunctioning device or the position of a displaced device

Body Part	Approach	Device	Qualifier
Y Mouth and Throat	Ø Open 3 Percutaneous 7 Via Natural or Artificial Opening 8 Via Natural or Artificial Opening Endoscopic	Ø Drainage Device 1 Radioactive Element 7 Autologous Tissue Substitute D Intraluminal Device J Synthetic Substitute K Nonautologous Tissue Substitute Y Other Device	Z No Qualifier
Y Mouth and Throat	X External	Ø Drainage Device 1 Radioactive Element 7 Autologous Tissue Substitute D Intraluminal Device J Synthetic Substitute K Nonautologous Tissue Substitute	Z No Qualifier

Non-OR ØCWYØ7Z
Non-OR ØCWYX[Ø17DJK]Z

SECTION: Ø MEDICAL AND SURGICAL
BODY SYSTEM: C MOUTH AND THROAT
OPERATION: X TRANSFER: Moving, without taking out, all or a portion of a body part to another location to take over the function of all or a portion of a body part

Body Part	Approach	Device	Qualifier
Ø Upper Lip 1 Lower Lip 3 Soft Palate 4 Buccal Mucosa 5 Upper Gingiva 6 Lower Gingiva 7 Tongue	Ø Open X External	Z No Device	Z No Qualifier

New/Revised Text in Green ~~deleted~~ Deleted ♀ Females Only ♂ Males Only Coding Clinic
Non-covered Limited Coverage Combination (See Appendix E) DRG Non-OR Non-OR Hospital-Acquired Condition

SECTION: Ø MEDICAL AND SURGICAL
BODY SYSTEM: D GASTROINTESTINAL SYSTEM
OPERATION: 1 BYPASS: *(on multiple pages)*
Altering the route of passage of the contents of a tubular body part

Body Part	Approach	Device	Qualifier
1 Esophagus, Upper 2 Esophagus, Middle 3 Esophagus, Lower 5 Esophagus	Ø Open 4 Percutaneous Endoscopic 8 Via Natural or Artificial Opening Endoscopic	7 Autologous Tissue Substitute J Synthetic Substitute K Nonautologous Tissue Substitute Z No Device	4 Cutaneous 6 Stomach 9 Duodenum A Jejunum B Ileum
1 Esophagus, Upper 2 Esophagus, Middle 3 Esophagus, Lower 5 Esophagus	3 Percutaneous	J Synthetic Substitute	4 Cutaneous
6 Stomach 9 Duodenum	Ø Open 4 Percutaneous Endoscopic 8 Via Natural or Artificial Opening Endoscopic	7 Autologous Tissue Substitute J Synthetic Substitute K Nonautologous Tissue Substitute Z No Device	4 Cutaneous 9 Duodenum A Jejunum B Ileum L Transverse Colon
6 Stomach 9 Duodenum	3 Percutaneous	J Synthetic Substitute	4 Cutaneous
8 Small Intestine	Ø Open 4 Percutaneous Endoscopic 8 Via Natural or Artificial Opening Endoscopic	7 Autologous Tissue Substitute J Synthetic Substitute K Nonautologous Tissue Substitute Z No Device	4 Cutaneous 8 Small Intestine H Cecum K Ascending Colon L Transverse Colon M Descending Colon N Sigmoid Colon P Rectum Q Anus
A Jejunum	Ø Open 4 Percutaneous Endoscopic 8 Via Natural or Artificial Opening Endoscopic	7 Autologous Tissue Substitute J Synthetic Substitute K Nonautologous Tissue Substitute Z No Device	4 Cutaneous A Jejunum B Ileum H Cecum K Ascending Colon L Transverse Colon M Descending Colon N Sigmoid Colon P Rectum Q Anus
A Jejunum	3 Percutaneous	J Synthetic Substitute	4 Cutaneous
B Ileum	Ø Open 4 Percutaneous Endoscopic 8 Via Natural or Artificial Opening Endoscopic	7 Autologous Tissue Substitute J Synthetic Substitute K Nonautologous Tissue Substitute Z No Device	4 Cutaneous B Ileum H Cecum K Ascending Colon L Transverse Colon M Descending Colon N Sigmoid Colon P Rectum Q Anus
B Ileum	3 Percutaneous	J Synthetic Substitute	4 Cutaneous
E Large Intestine	Ø Open 4 Percutaneous Endoscopic 8 Via Natural or Artificial Opening Endoscopic	7 Autologous Tissue Substitute J Synthetic Substitute K Nonautologous Tissue Substitute Z No Device	4 Cutaneous E Large Intestine P Rectum

Non-OR ØD16[Ø48][7JKZ]4
Non-OR ØD163J4

ØD16[Ø48][7JKZ][9ABL] when reported with Principal Diagnosis E66.Ø1 and Secondary Diagnosis K68.11, K95.Ø1, K95.81, T81.4ØXA,T8141XA, T8142XA, T8143XA, T8144XA, or T8149XA

Coding Clinic: 2Ø16, Q2, P31 – ØD194ZB
Coding Clinic: 2Ø17, Q2, P18 – ØD16ØZA

SECTION: Ø MEDICAL AND SURGICAL
BODY SYSTEM: D GASTROINTESTINAL SYSTEM
OPERATION: 1 BYPASS: *(continued)*
Altering the route of passage of the contents of a tubular body part

Body Part	Approach	Device	Qualifier
H Cecum	Ø Open 4 Percutaneous Endoscopic 8 Via Natural or Artificial Opening Endoscopic	7 Autologous Tissue Substitute J Synthetic Substitute K Nonautologous Tissue Substitute Z No Device	4 Cutaneous H Cecum K Ascending Colon L Transverse Colon M Descending Colon N Sigmoid Colon P Rectum
H Cecum	3 Percutaneous	J Synthetic Substitute	4 Cutaneous
K Ascending Colon	Ø Open 4 Percutaneous Endoscopic 8 Via Natural or Artificial Opening Endoscopic	7 Autologous Tissue Substitute J Synthetic Substitute K Nonautologous Tissue Substitute Z No Device	4 Cutaneous K Ascending Colon L Transverse Colon M Descending Colon N Sigmoid Colon P Rectum
K Ascending Colon	3 Percutaneous	J Synthetic Substitute	4 Cutaneous
L Transverse Colon	Ø Open 4 Percutaneous Endoscopic 8 Via Natural or Artificial Opening Endoscopic	7 Autologous Tissue Substitute J Synthetic Substitute K Nonautologous Tissue Substitute Z No Device	4 Cutaneous L Transverse Colon M Descending Colon N Sigmoid Colon P Rectum
L Transverse Colon	3 Percutaneous	J Synthetic Substitute	4 Cutaneous
M Descending Colon	Ø Open 4 Percutaneous Endoscopic 8 Via Natural or Artificial Opening Endoscopic	7 Autologous Tissue Substitute J Synthetic Substitute K Nonautologous Tissue Substitute Z No Device	4 Cutaneous M Descending Colon N Sigmoid Colon P Rectum
M Descending Colon	3 Percutaneous	J Synthetic Substitute	4 Cutaneous
N Sigmoid Colon	Ø Open 4 Percutaneous Endoscopic 8 Via Natural or Artificial Opening Endoscopic	7 Autologous Tissue Substitute J Synthetic Substitute K Nonautologous Tissue Substitute Z No Device	4 Cutaneous N Sigmoid Colon P Rectum
N Sigmoid Colon	3 Percutaneous	J Synthetic Substitute	4 Cutaneous

SECTION: Ø MEDICAL AND SURGICAL
BODY SYSTEM: D GASTROINTESTINAL SYSTEM
OPERATION: 2 CHANGE: Taking out or off a device from a body part and putting back an identical or similar device in or on the same body part without cutting or puncturing the skin or a mucous membrane

Body Part	Approach	Device	Qualifier
Ø Upper Intestinal Tract D Lower Intestinal Tract	X External	Ø Drainage Device U Feeding Device Y Other Device	Z No Qualifier
U Omentum V Mesentery W Peritoneum	X External	Ø Drainage Device Y Other Device	Z No Qualifier

Non-OR All Values

Coding Clinic: 2Ø19, Q1, P26 – ØD2DXUZ
Coding Clinic: 2Ø22, Q1, P45 – ØD2ØXYZ

SECTION: Ø MEDICAL AND SURGICAL
BODY SYSTEM: D GASTROINTESTINAL SYSTEM
OPERATION: 5 DESTRUCTION: *(on multiple pages)*

Physical eradication of all or a portion of a body part by the direct use of energy, force, or a destructive agent

Body Part	Approach	Device	Qualifier
1 Esophagus, Upper 2 Esophagus, Middle 3 Esophagus, Lower 4 Esophagogastric Junction 5 Esophagus 6 Stomach 7 Stomach, Pylorus 8 Small Intestine 9 Duodenum A Jejunum B Ileum C Ileocecal Valve E Large Intestine F Large Intestine, Right G Large Intestine, Left H Cecum J Appendix K Ascending Colon L Transverse Colon M Descending Colon N Sigmoid Colon P Rectum Q Anus	Ø Open 3 Percutaneous 4 Percutaneous Endoscopic	Z No Device	3 Laser Interstitial Thermal Therapy Z No Qualifier
1 Esophagus, Upper 2 Esophagus, Middle 3 Esophagus, Lower 4 Esophagogastric Junction 5 Esophagus 6 Stomach 7 Stomach, Pylorus 8 Small Intestine 9 Duodenum A Jejunum B Ileum C Ileocecal Valve E Large Intestine F Large Intestine, Right G Large Intestine, Left H Cecum J Appendix K Ascending Colon L Transverse Colon M Descending Colon N Sigmoid Colon P Rectum Q Anus	7 Via Natural or Artificial Opening 8 Via Natural or Artificial Opening Endoscopic	Z No Device	Z No Qualifier

Non-OR ØD5[12345679EFGHKLMN][48]ZZ
Non-OR ØD5P[Ø3478]ZZ
Non-OR ØD5Q[48]ZZ
Non-OR ØD5R4ZZ
Non-OR ØD5[123456789ABCEFGHJKLMNP][Ø34]Z3

Coding Clinic: 2017, Q1, P35 – 0D5W0ZZ

SECTION: Ø MEDICAL AND SURGICAL
BODY SYSTEM: D GASTROINTESTINAL SYSTEM
OPERATION: 5 DESTRUCTION: *(continued)*

Physical eradication of all or a portion of a body part by the direct use of energy, force, or a destructive agent

Body Part	Approach	Device	Qualifier
Q Anus	Ø Open 3 Percutaneous 4 Percutaneous Endoscopic	Z No Device	3 Laser Interstitial Thermal Therapy Z No Qualifier
Q Anus	7 Via Natural or Artificial Opening 8 Via Natural or Artificial Opening Endoscopic X External	Z No Device	Z No Qualifier
R Anal Sphincter U Omentum V Mesentery W Peritoneum	Ø Open 3 Percutaneous 4 Percutaneous Endoscopic	Z No Device	Z No Qualifier

SECTION: Ø MEDICAL AND SURGICAL
BODY SYSTEM: D GASTROINTESTINAL SYSTEM
OPERATION: 7 DILATION: Expanding an orifice or the lumen of a tubular body part

Body Part	Approach	Device	Qualifier
1 Esophagus, Upper 2 Esophagus, Middle 3 Esophagus, Lower 4 Esophagogastric Junction 5 Esophagus 6 Stomach 7 Stomach, Pylorus 8 Small Intestine 9 Duodenum A Jejunum B Ileum C Ileocecal Valve E Large Intestine F Large Intestine, Right G Large Intestine, Left H Cecum K Ascending Colon L Transverse Colon M Descending Colon N Sigmoid Colon P Rectum Q Anus	Ø Open 3 Percutaneous 4 Percutaneous Endoscopic 7 Via Natural or Artificial Opening 8 Via Natural or Artificial Opening Endoscopic	D Intraluminal Device Z No Device	Z No Qualifier

Non-OR ØD7[12345689ABCEFGHKLMNPQ][78][DZ]Z
Non-OR ØD77[478]DZ
Non-OR ØD778ZZ
Non-OR ØD7[89ABCEFGHKLMN][Ø34]DZ

SECTION: Ø MEDICAL AND SURGICAL
BODY SYSTEM: D GASTROINTESTINAL SYSTEM
OPERATION: 8 DIVISION: Cutting into a body part, without draining fluids and/or gases from the body part, in order to separate or transect a body part

Body Part	Approach	Device	Qualifier
4 Esophagogastric Junction 7 Stomach, Pylorus	Ø Open 3 Percutaneous 4 Percutaneous Endoscopic 7 Via Natural or Artificial Opening 8 Via Natural or Artificial Opening Endoscopic	Z No Device	Z No Qualifier
R Anal Sphincter	Ø Open 3 Percutaneous	Z No Device	Z No Qualifier

Coding Clinic: 2Ø17, Q3, P23-24 – ØD8[47]4ZZ
Coding Clinic: 2Ø19, Q2, P16 – ØD874ZZ

SECTION: Ø MEDICAL AND SURGICAL
BODY SYSTEM: D GASTROINTESTINAL SYSTEM
OPERATION: 9 DRAINAGE: *(on multiple pages)* Taking or letting out fluids and/or gases from a body part

Body Part	Approach	Device	Qualifier
1 Esophagus, Upper 2 Esophagus, Middle 3 Esophagus, Lower 4 Esophagogastric Junction 5 Esophagus 6 Stomach 7 Stomach, Pylorus 8 Small Intestine 9 Duodenum A Jejunum B Ileum C Ileocecal Valve E Large Intestine F Large Intestine, Right G Large Intestine, Left H Cecum J Appendix K Ascending Colon L Transverse Colon M Descending Colon N Sigmoid Colon P Rectum	Ø Open 3 Percutaneous 4 Percutaneous Endoscopic 7 Via Natural or Artificial Opening 8 Via Natural or Artificial Opening Endoscopic	Ø Drainage Device	Z No Qualifier

DRG Non-OR ØD9[8ABC]3ØZ
DRG Non-OR ØD9[ABC]3ZZ
Non-OR ØD9[12345679EFGHJKLMNP]3ØZ
Non-OR ØD9[6789ABEFGHKLMNP][78]ØZ
Non-OR ØD9[123456789ABCEFGHKLMNP][3478]ZX
Non-OR ØD9[12345679EFGHJKLMNP]3ZZ

Coding Clinic: 2Ø15, Q2, P29 – ØD967ØZ

SECTION: Ø MEDICAL AND SURGICAL
BODY SYSTEM: D GASTROINTESTINAL SYSTEM
OPERATION: 9 DRAINAGE: *(continued)*
Taking or letting out fluids and/or gases from a body part

Body Part	Approach	Device	Qualifier
1 Esophagus, Upper 2 Esophagus, Middle 3 Esophagus, Lower 4 Esophagogastric Junction 5 Esophagus 6 Stomach 7 Stomach, Pylorus 8 Small Intestine 9 Duodenum A Jejunum B Ileum C Ileocecal Valve E Large Intestine F Large Intestine, Right G Large Intestine, Left H Cecum J Appendix K Ascending Colon L Transverse Colon M Descending Colon N Sigmoid Colon P Rectum	Ø Open 3 Percutaneous 4 Percutaneous Endoscopic 7 Via Natural or Artificial Opening 8 Via Natural or Artificial Opening Endoscopic	Z No Device	X Diagnostic Z No Qualifier
Q Anus	Ø Open 3 Percutaneous 4 Percutaneous Endoscopic 7 Via Natural or Artificial Opening 8 Via Natural or Artificial Opening Endoscopic X External	Ø Drainage Device	Z No Qualifier
Q Anus	Ø Open 3 Percutaneous 4 Percutaneous Endoscopic 7 Via Natural or Artificial Opening 8 Via Natural or Artificial Opening Endoscopic X External	Z No Device	X Diagnostic Z No Qualifier
R Anal Sphincter U Omentum V Mesentery W Peritoneum	Ø Open 3 Percutaneous 4 Percutaneous Endoscopic	Ø Drainage Device	Z No Qualifier
R Anal Sphincter U Omentum V Mesentery W Peritoneum	Ø Open 3 Percutaneous 4 Percutaneous Endoscopic	Z No Device	X Diagnostic Z No Qualifier

DRG Non-OR ØD9[UVW]3ZX *(proposed)*
Non-OR ØD9Q3ØZ
Non-OR ØD9Q[Ø3478X]ZX
Non-OR ØD9Q3ZZ
Non-OR ØD9R3ØZ
Non-OR ØD9R3ZZ
Non-OR ØD9[UVW][34]ØZ
Non-OR ØD9R[Ø34]ZX
Non-OR ØD9[UVW][34]ZZ

SECTION: Ø MEDICAL AND SURGICAL
BODY SYSTEM: D GASTROINTESTINAL SYSTEM
OPERATION: B EXCISION: *(on multiple pages)*
Cutting out or off, without replacement, a portion of a body part

Body Part	Approach	Device	Qualifier
1 Esophagus, Upper 2 Esophagus, Middle 3 Esophagus, Lower 4 Esophagogastric Junction 5 Esophagus 7 Stomach, Pylorus 8 Small Intestine 9 Duodenum A Jejunum B Ileum C Ileocecal Valve E Large Intestine F Large Intestine, Right H Cecum J Appendix K Ascending Colon P Rectum	Ø Open 3 Percutaneous 4 Percutaneous Endoscopic 7 Via Natural or Artificial Opening 8 Via Natural or Artificial Opening Endoscopic	Z No Device	X Diagnostic Z No Qualifier
6 Stomach	Ø Open 3 Percutaneous 4 Percutaneous Endoscopic 7 Via Natural or Artificial Opening 8 Via Natural or Artificial Opening Endoscopic	Z No Device	3 Vertical X Diagnostic Z No Qualifier
G Large Intestine, Left L Transverse Colon M Descending Colon N Sigmoid Colon	Ø Open 3 Percutaneous 4 Percutaneous Endoscopic 7 Via Natural or Artificial Opening 8 Via Natural or Artificial Opening Endoscopic	Z No Device	X Diagnostic Z No Qualifier

Non-OR ØDB[12345789ABCEFHKP][3478]ZX
Non-OR ØDB[123579][48]ZZ
Non-OR ØDB[4EFHKP]8ZZ
Non-OR ØDB6[3478]ZX
Non-OR ØDB6[48]ZZ
Non-OR ØDB[GLMN][3478]ZX
Non-OR ØDB[GLMN]8ZZ

Coding Clinic: 2016, Q1, P22 – ØDBP7ZZ
Coding Clinic: 2016, Q1, P24 – ØDB28ZX
Coding Clinic: 2016, Q2, P31 – ØDB64Z3
Coding Clinic: 2016, Q3, P5-7 – ØDBBØZZ
Coding Clinic: 2017, Q1, P16 – ØDBK8ZZ
Coding Clinic: 2017, Q2, P17 – ØDB6ØZZ
Coding Clinic: 2019, Q1, P5 – ØDB6[A]ØZZ
Coding Clinic: 2019, Q1, P6 – ØDB9ØZZ
Coding Clinic: 2019, Q1, P7 – ØDB6ØZZ
Coding Clinic: 2019, Q1, P27 – ØDBN[P]ØZZ
Coding Clinic: 2019, Q2, P16 – ØDBA4ZZ
Coding Clinic: 2021, Q2, P12 – ØDB8ØZZ
Coding Clinic: 2021, Q3, P29 – ØDBB4ZZ
Coding Clinic: 2023, Q1, P32 – ØDB18ZZ

SECTION: Ø MEDICAL AND SURGICAL
BODY SYSTEM: D GASTROINTESTINAL SYSTEM
OPERATION: B EXCISION: *(continued)* Cutting out or off, without replacement, a portion of a body part

Body Part	Approach	Device	Qualifier
G Large Intestine, Left L Transverse Colon M Descending Colon N Sigmoid Colon	F Via Natural or Artificial Opening With Percutaneous Endoscopic Assistance	Z No Device	Z No Qualifier
Q Anus	Ø Open 3 Percutaneous 4 Percutaneous Endoscopic 7 Via Natural or Artificial Opening 8 Via Natural or Artificial Opening Endoscopic X External	Z No Device	X Diagnostic Z No Qualifier
R Anal Sphincter U Omentum V Mesentery W Peritoneum	Ø Open 3 Percutaneous 4 Percutaneous Endoscopic	Z No Device	X Diagnostic Z No Qualifier

Non-OR ØDBQ[Ø3478X]ZX
Non-OR ØDBR[Ø34]ZX
Non-OR ØDB[UVW][34]ZX

Coding Clinic: 2023, Q2, P24– ØDBQØZZ

SECTION: Ø MEDICAL AND SURGICAL
BODY SYSTEM: D GASTROINTESTINAL SYSTEM
OPERATION: C EXTIRPATION: Taking or cutting out solid matter from a body part

Body Part	Approach	Device	Qualifier
1 Esophagus, Upper 2 Esophagus, Middle 3 Esophagus, Lower 4 Esophagogastric Junction 5 Esophagus 6 Stomach 7 Stomach, Pylorus 8 Small Intestine 9 Duodenum A Jejunum B Ileum C Ileocecal Valve E Large Intestine F Large Intestine, Right G Large Intestine, Left H Cecum J Appendix K Ascending Colon L Transverse Colon M Descending Colon N Sigmoid Colon P Rectum	Ø Open 3 Percutaneous 4 Percutaneous Endoscopic 7 Via Natural or Artificial Opening 8 Via Natural or Artificial Opening Endoscopic	Z No Device	Z No Qualifier
Q Anus	Ø Open 3 Percutaneous 4 Percutaneous Endoscopic 7 Via Natural or Artificial Opening 8 Via Natural or Artificial Opening Endoscopic X External	Z No Device	Z No Qualifier
R Anal Sphincter U Omentum V Mesentery W Peritoneum	Ø Open 3 Percutaneous 4 Percutaneous Endoscopic	Z No Device	Z No Qualifier

Non-OR ØDC[123456789ABCEFGHKLMNP][78]ZZ
Non-OR ØDCQ[78X]ZZ

Ø: M/S D: GASTROINTESTINAL SYSTEM C: EXTIRPATION

SECTION: Ø MEDICAL AND SURGICAL
BODY SYSTEM: D GASTROINTESTINAL SYSTEM
OPERATION: D EXTRACTION: Pulling or stripping out or off all or a portion of a body part by the use of force

Body Part	Approach	Device	Qualifier
1 Esophagus, Upper 2 Esophagus, Middle 3 Esophagus, Lower 4 Esophagogastric Junction 5 Esophagus 6 Stomach 7 Stomach, Pylorus 8 Small Intestine 9 Duodenum A Jejunum B Ileum C Ileocecal Valve E Large Intestine F Large Intestine, Right G Large Intestine, Left H Cecum J Appendix K Ascending Colon L Transverse Colon M Descending Colon N Sigmoid Colon P Rectum	3 Percutaneous 4 Percutaneous Endoscopic 8 Via Natural or Artificial Opening Endoscopic	Z No Device	X Diagnostic
Q Anus	3 Percutaneous 4 Percutaneous Endoscopic 8 Via Natural or Artificial Opening Endoscopic X External	Z No Device	X Diagnostic

Coding Clinic: 2017, Q4, P42 – ØDD68ZX
Coding Clinic: 2021, Q1, P21 – ØDDP8ZX

SECTION: Ø MEDICAL AND SURGICAL
BODY SYSTEM: D GASTROINTESTINAL SYSTEM
OPERATION: F FRAGMENTATION: Breaking solid matter in a body part into pieces

Body Part	Approach	Device	Qualifier
5 Esophagus 6 Stomach 8 Small Intestine 9 Duodenum A Jejunum B Ileum E Large Intestine F Large Intestine, Right G Large Intestine, Left H Cecum J Appendix K Ascending Colon L Transverse Colon M Descending Colon N Sigmoid Colon P Rectum Q Anus	Ø Open 3 Percutaneous 4 Percutaneous Endoscopic 7 Via Natural or Artificial Opening 8 Via Natural or Artificial Opening Endoscopic X External	Z No Device	Z No Qualifier

ØDF[5689ABEFGHJKLMNPQ]XZZ

Non-OR ØDF[5689ABEFGHJKLMNPQ]XZZ

SECTION: Ø MEDICAL AND SURGICAL
BODY SYSTEM: D GASTROINTESTINAL SYSTEM
OPERATION: H INSERTION: *(on multiple pages)*

Putting in a nonbiological appliance that monitors, assists, performs, or prevents a physiological function but does not physically take the place of a body part

Body Part	Approach	Device	Qualifier
Ø Upper Intestinal Tract D Lower Intestinal Tract	Ø Open 3 Percutaneous 4 Percutaneous Endoscopic 7 Via Natural or Artificial Opening 8 Via Natural or Artificial Opening Endoscopic	Y Other Device	Z No Qualifier
1 Esophagus, Upper 2 Esophagus, Middle 3 Esophagus, Lower	7 Via Natural or Artificial Opening	J Magnetic Lengthening Device	Z No Qualifier
5 Esophagus	Ø Open 3 Percutaneous 4 Percutaneous Endoscopic	1 Radioactive Element 2 Monitoring Device 3 Infusion Device D Intraluminal Device U Feeding Device Y Other Device	Z No Qualifier
5 Esophagus	7 Via Natural or Artificial Opening 8 Via Natural or Artificial Opening Endoscopic	1 Radioactive Element 2 Monitoring Device 3 Infusion Device B Airway D Intraluminal Device U Feeding Device Y Other Device	Z No Qualifier
6 Stomach ⊞	Ø Open 3 Percutaneous 4 Percutaneous Endoscopic	1 Radioactive Element 2 Monitoring Device 3 Infusion Device D Intraluminal Device M Stimulator Lead U Feeding Device Y Other Device	Z No Qualifier
6 Stomach	7 Via Natural or Artificial Opening 8 Via Natural or Artificial Opening Endoscopic	1 Radioactive Element 2 Monitoring Device 3 Infusion Device D Intraluminal Device U Feeding Device Y Other Device	Z No Qualifier
8 Small Intestine 9 Duodenum A Jejunum B Ileum	Ø Open 3 Percutaneous 4 Percutaneous Endoscopic 7 Via Natural or Artificial Opening 8 Via Natural or Artificial Opening Endoscopic	1 Radioactive Element 2 Monitoring Device 3 Infusion Device D Intraluminal Device U Feeding Device	Z No Qualifier
E Large Intestine P Rectum	Ø Open 3 Percutaneous 4 Percutaneous Endoscopic 7 Via Natural or Artificial Opening 8 Via Natural or Artificial Opening Endoscopic	1 Radioactive Element D Intraluminal Device	Z No Qualifier

⊞ ØDH6[Ø34][1M]Z
Non-OR ØDH5[Ø34][DU]Z
Non-OR ØDH5[78][23BDU]Z
Non-OR ØDH6[34]UZ
Non-OR ØDH6[78][23U]Z
Non-OR ØDH[89AB][Ø3478][DU]Z
Non-OR ØDH[89AB][78][23]Z
Non-OR ØDHE[Ø3478]DZ
Non-OR ØDHP[Ø3478]DZ

Coding Clinic: 2016, Q2, P5 – ØDH67UZ
Coding Clinic: 2019, Q2, P18 – ØDH68YZ
Coding Clinic: 2022, Q1, P44 – ØDHØ8YZ

SECTION: Ø MEDICAL AND SURGICAL
BODY SYSTEM: D GASTROINTESTINAL SYSTEM
OPERATION: H INSERTION: *(continued)*
Putting in a nonbiological appliance that monitors, assists, performs, or prevents a physiological function but does not physically take the place of a body part

Body Part	Approach	Device	Qualifier
P Rectum	Ø Open 3 Percutaneous 4 Percutaneous Endoscopic 7 Via Natural or Artificial Opening 8 Via Natural or Artificial Opening Endoscopic	1 Radioactive Element D Intraluminal Device	Z No Qualifier
Q Anus	Ø Open 3 Percutaneous 4 Percutaneous Endoscopic	D Intraluminal Device L Artificial Sphincter	Z No Qualifier
Q Anus	7 Via Natural or Artificial Opening 8 Via Natural or Artificial Opening Endoscopic	D Intraluminal Device	Z No Qualifier
R Anal Sphincter	Ø Open 3 Percutaneous 4 Percutaneous Endoscopic	M Stimulator Lead	Z No Qualifier

SECTION: Ø MEDICAL AND SURGICAL
BODY SYSTEM: D GASTROINTESTINAL SYSTEM
OPERATION: J INSPECTION: Visually and/or manually exploring a body part

Body Part	Approach	Device	Qualifier
Ø Upper Intestinal Tract 6 Stomach D Lower Intestinal Tract	Ø Open 3 Percutaneous 4 Percutaneous Endoscopic 7 Via Natural or Artificial Opening 8 Via Natural or Artificial Opening Endoscopic X External	Z No Device	Z No Qualifier
U Omentum V Mesentery W Peritoneum	Ø Open 3 Percutaneous 4 Percutaneous Endoscopic X External	Z No Device	Z No Qualifier

DRG Non-OR ØDJ[UVW]3ZZ
Non-OR ØDJ[Ø6D][378X]ZZ
Non-OR ØDJ[UVW]XZZ

Coding Clinic: 2Ø15, Q3, P25 – ØDJØ8ZZ
Coding Clinic: 2Ø16, Q2, P21 – ØDJØ7ZZ
Coding Clinic: 2Ø17, Q2, P15 – ØDJD8ZZ
Coding Clinic: 2Ø19, Q1, P26 – ØDJDØZZ

SECTION: Ø MEDICAL AND SURGICAL
BODY SYSTEM: D GASTROINTESTINAL SYSTEM
OPERATION: L OCCLUSION: Completely closing an orifice or the lumen of a tubular body part

Body Part	Approach	Device	Qualifier
1 Esophagus, Upper 2 Esophagus, Middle 3 Esophagus, Lower 4 Esophagogastric Junction 5 Esophagus 6 Stomach 7 Stomach, Pylorus 8 Small Intestine 9 Duodenum A Jejunum B Ileum C Ileocecal Valve E Large Intestine F Large Intestine, Right G Large Intestine, Left H Cecum K Ascending Colon L Transverse Colon M Descending Colon N Sigmoid Colon P Rectum	Ø Open 3 Percutaneous 4 Percutaneous Endoscopic	C Extraluminal Device D Intraluminal Device Z No Device	Z No Qualifier
1 Esophagus, Upper 2 Esophagus, Middle 3 Esophagus, Lower 4 Esophagogastric Junction 5 Esophagus 6 Stomach 7 Stomach, Pylorus 8 Small Intestine 9 Duodenum A Jejunum B Ileum C Ileocecal Valve E Large Intestine F Large Intestine, Right G Large Intestine, Left H Cecum K Ascending Colon L Transverse Colon M Descending Colon N Sigmoid Colon P Rectum	7 Via Natural or Artificial Opening 8 Via Natural or Artificial Opening Endoscopic	D Intraluminal Device Z No Device	Z No Qualifier
Q Anus	Ø Open 3 Percutaneous 4 Percutaneous Endoscopic X External	C Extraluminal Device D Intraluminal Device Z No Device	Z No Qualifier
Q Anus	7 Via Natural or Artificial Opening 8 Via Natural or Artificial Opening Endoscopic	D Intraluminal Device Z No Device	Z No Qualifier

Non-OR ØDL[12345][Ø34][CDZ]Z
Non-OR ØDL[12345][78][DZ]Z

SECTION: Ø MEDICAL AND SURGICAL
BODY SYSTEM: D GASTROINTESTINAL SYSTEM
OPERATION: M REATTACHMENT: Putting back in or on all or a portion of a separated body part to its normal location or other suitable location

Body Part	Approach	Device	Qualifier
5 Esophagus 6 Stomach 8 Small Intestine 9 Duodenum A Jejunum B Ileum E Large Intestine F Large Intestine, Right G Large Intestine, Left H Cecum K Ascending Colon L Transverse Colon M Descending Colon N Sigmoid Colon P Rectum	Ø Open 4 Percutaneous Endoscopic	Z No Device	Z No Qualifier

SECTION: Ø MEDICAL AND SURGICAL
BODY SYSTEM: D GASTROINTESTINAL SYSTEM
OPERATION: N RELEASE: Freeing a body part from an abnormal physical constraint by cutting or by the use of force

Body Part	Approach	Device	Qualifier
1 Esophagus, Upper 2 Esophagus, Middle 3 Esophagus, Lower 4 Esophagogastric Junction 5 Esophagus 6 Stomach 7 Stomach, Pylorus 8 Small Intestine 9 Duodenum A Jejunum B Ileum C Ileocecal Valve E Large Intestine F Large Intestine, Right G Large Intestine, Left H Cecum J Appendix K Ascending Colon L Transverse Colon M Descending Colon N Sigmoid Colon P Rectum	Ø Open 3 Percutaneous 4 Percutaneous Endoscopic 7 Via Natural or Artificial Opening 8 Via Natural or Artificial Opening Endoscopic	Z No Device	Z No Qualifier
Q Anus	Ø Open 3 Percutaneous 4 Percutaneous Endoscopic 7 Via Natural or Artificial Opening 8 Via Natural or Artificial Opening Endoscopic X External	Z No Device	Z No Qualifier
R Anal Sphincter U Omentum V Mesentery W Peritoneum	Ø Open 3 Percutaneous 4 Percutaneous Endoscopic	Z No Device	Z No Qualifier

Non-OR ØDN[89ABEFGHKLMN][78]ZZ

Coding Clinic: 2Ø15, Q3, P15-16 – ØDN5ØZZ
Coding Clinic: 2Ø17, Q1, P35 – ØDNWØZZ
Coding Clinic: 2Ø17, Q4, P5Ø – ØDN8ØZZ

SECTION: Ø MEDICAL AND SURGICAL
BODY SYSTEM: D GASTROINTESTINAL SYSTEM
OPERATION: P REMOVAL: *(on multiple pages)*
Taking out or off a device from a body part

Body Part	Approach	Device	Qualifier
Ø Upper Intestinal Tract D Lower Intestinal Tract	Ø Open 3 Percutaneous 4 Percutaneous Endoscopic 7 Via Natural or Artificial Opening 8 Via Natural or Artificial Opening Endoscopic	Ø Drainage Device 2 Monitoring Device 3 Infusion Device 7 Autologous Tissue Substitute C Extraluminal Device D Intraluminal Device J Synthetic Substitute K Nonautologous Tissue Substitute U Feeding Device Y Other Device	Z No Qualifier
Ø Upper Intestinal Tract D Lower Intestinal Tract	X External	Ø Drainage Device 2 Monitoring Device 3 Infusion Device D Intraluminal Device U Feeding Device	Z No Qualifier
5 Esophagus	Ø Open 3 Percutaneous 4 Percutaneous Endoscopic	1 Radioactive Element 2 Monitoring Device 3 Infusion Device U Feeding Device Y Other Device	Z No Qualifier
5 Esophagus	7 Via Natural or Artificial Opening 8 Via Natural or Artificial Opening Endoscopic	1 Radioactive Element D Intraluminal Device Y Other Device	Z No Qualifier
5 Esophagus	X External	1 Radioactive Element 2 Monitoring Device 3 Infusion Device D Intraluminal Device U Feeding Device	Z No Qualifier
6 Stomach	Ø Open 3 Percutaneous 4 Percutaneous Endoscopic	Ø Drainage Device 2 Monitoring Device 3 Infusion Device 7 Autologous Tissue Substitute C Extraluminal Device D Intraluminal Device J Synthetic Substitute K Nonautologous Tissue Substitute M Stimulator Lead U Feeding Device Y Other Device	Z No Qualifier

Non-OR ØDP[ØD][78][Ø23D]Z
Non-OR ØDP[ØD]X[Ø23DU]Z
Non-OR ØDP5[78][1D]Z
Non-OR ØDP5X[123DU]Z

SECTION: Ø MEDICAL AND SURGICAL
BODY SYSTEM: D GASTROINTESTINAL SYSTEM
OPERATION: P REMOVAL: *(continued)*
Taking out or off a device from a body part

Body Part	Approach	Device	Qualifier
6 Stomach	7 Via Natural or Artificial Opening 8 Via Natural or Artificial Opening Endoscopic	Ø Drainage Device 2 Monitoring Device 3 Infusion Device 7 Autologous Tissue Substitute C Extraluminal Device D Intraluminal Device J Synthetic Substitute K Nonautologous Tissue Substitute U Feeding Device Y Other Device	Z No Qualifier
6 Stomach	X External	Ø Drainage Device 2 Monitoring Device 3 Infusion Device D Intraluminal Device U Feeding Device	Z No Qualifier
P Rectum	Ø Open 3 Percutaneous 4 Percutaneous Endoscopic 7 Via Natural or Artificial Opening 8 Via Natural or Artificial Opening Endoscopic X External	1 Radioactive Element	Z No Qualifier
Q Anus	Ø Open 3 Percutaneous 4 Percutaneous Endoscopic 7 Via Natural or Artificial Opening 8 Via Natural or Artificial Opening Endoscopic	L Artificial Sphincter	Z No Qualifier
R Anal Sphincter	Ø Open 3 Percutaneous 4 Percutaneous Endoscopic	M Stimulator Lead	Z No Qualifier
U Omentum V Mesentery W Peritoneum	Ø Open 3 Percutaneous 4 Percutaneous Endoscopic	Ø Drainage Device 1 Radioactive Element 7 Autologous Tissue Substitute J Synthetic Substitute K Nonautologous Tissue Substitute	Z No Qualifier

Non-OR ØDP6[78][Ø23D]Z
Non-OR ØDP6X[Ø23DU]Z
Non-OR ØDPP[78X]1Z

Coding Clinic: 2019, Q2, P19 – ØDP68YZ

SECTION: Ø MEDICAL AND SURGICAL
BODY SYSTEM: D GASTROINTESTINAL SYSTEM
OPERATION: Q REPAIR: Restoring, to the extent possible, a body part to its normal anatomic structure and function

Body Part	Approach	Device	Qualifier
1 Esophagus, Upper 2 Esophagus, Middle 3 Esophagus, Lower 4 Esophagogastric Junction 5 Esophagus 6 Stomach 7 Stomach, Pylorus 8 Small Intestine ⊞ 9 Duodenum ⊞ A Jejunum ⊞ B Ileum ⊞ C Ileocecal Valve E Large Intestine ⊞ F Large Intestine, Right ⊞ G Large Intestine, Left ⊞ H Cecum ⊞ J Appendix K Ascending Colon ⊞ L Transverse Colon ⊞ M Descending Colon ⊞ N Sigmoid Colon ⊞ P Rectum	Ø Open 3 Percutaneous 4 Percutaneous Endoscopic 7 Via Natural or Artificial Opening 8 Via Natural or Artificial Opening Endoscopic	Z No Device	Z No Qualifier
Q Anus	Ø Open 3 Percutaneous 4 Percutaneous Endoscopic 7 Via Natural or Artificial Opening 8 Via Natural or Artificial Opening Endoscopic X External	Z No Device	Z No Qualifier
R Anal Sphincter U Omentum V Mesentery W Peritoneum	Ø Open 3 Percutaneous 4 Percutaneous Endoscopic	Z No Device	Z No Qualifier

⊞ ØDQ[89ABEFGHKLMN]ØZZ
⊞ ØDQW[Ø34]ZZ

Coding Clinic: 2Ø16, Q1, P7-8 – ØDQRØZZ, ØDQPØZZ
Coding Clinic: 2Ø18, Q1, P11 – ØDQV4ZZ
Coding Clinic: 2Ø19, Q2, P16 – ØDQ64ZZ

SECTION: Ø MEDICAL AND SURGICAL
BODY SYSTEM: D GASTROINTESTINAL SYSTEM
OPERATION: R REPLACEMENT: Putting in or on biological or synthetic material that physically takes the place and/or function of all or a portion of a body part

Body Part	Approach	Device	Qualifier
5 Esophagus	Ø Open 4 Percutaneous Endoscopic 7 Via Natural or Artificial Opening 8 Via Natural or Artificial Opening Endoscopic	7 Autologous Tissue Substitute J Synthetic Substitute K Nonautologous Tissue Substitute	Z No Qualifier
R Anal Sphincter U Omentum V Mesentery W Peritoneum	Ø Open 4 Percutaneous Endoscopic	7 Autologous Tissue Substitute J Synthetic Substitute K Nonautologous Tissue Substitute	Z No Qualifier

SECTION: Ø MEDICAL AND SURGICAL
BODY SYSTEM: D GASTROINTESTINAL SYSTEM
OPERATION: S REPOSITION: Moving to its normal location, or other suitable location, all or a portion of a body part

Body Part	Approach	Device	Qualifier
5 Esophagus 6 Stomach 9 Duodenum A Jejunum B Ileum H Cecum K Ascending Colon L Transverse Colon M Descending Colon N Sigmoid Colon P Rectum Q Anus	Ø Open 4 Percutaneous Endoscopic 7 Via Natural or Artificial Opening 8 Via Natural or Artificial Opening Endoscopic X External	Z No Device	Z No Qualifier
8 Small Intestine E Large Intestine	Ø Open 4 Percutaneous Endoscopic 7 Via Natural or Artificial Opening 8 Via Natural or Artificial Opening Endoscopic	Z No Device	Z No Qualifier

Non-OR ØDS[69ABHKLMNP]XZZ

Coding Clinic: 2016, Q3, P5 – ØDSM4ZZ
Coding Clinic: 2017, Q3, P1Ø – ØDS[BK]7ZZ
Coding Clinic: 2019, Q1, P31; 2017, Q3, P18 – ØDSPØZZ
Coding Clinic: 2017, Q4, P5Ø – ØDS[8E]ØZZ

SECTION: Ø MEDICAL AND SURGICAL
BODY SYSTEM: D GASTROINTESTINAL SYSTEM
OPERATION: T RESECTION: Cutting out or off, without replacement, all of a body part

Body Part	Approach	Device	Qualifier
1 Esophagus, Upper 2 Esophagus, Middle 3 Esophagus, Lower 4 Esophagogastric Junction 5 Esophagus 6 Stomach 7 Stomach, Pylorus 8 Small Intestine 9 Duodenum ⊞ A Jejunum B Ileum C Ileocecal Valve E Large Intestine F Large Intestine, Right H Cecum J Appendix K Ascending Colon P Rectum Q Anus	Ø Open 4 Percutaneous Endoscopic 7 Via Natural or Artificial Opening 8 Via Natural or Artificial Opening Endoscopic	Z No Device	Z No Qualifier
G Large Intestine, Left L Transverse Colon M Descending Colon N Sigmoid Colon	Ø Open 4 Percutaneous Endoscopic 7 Via Natural or Artificial Opening 8 Via Natural or Artificial Opening Endoscopic F Via Natural or Artificial Opening With Percutaneous Endoscopic Assistance	Z No Device	Z No Qualifier
R Anal Sphincter U Omentum	Ø Open 4 Percutaneous Endoscopic	Z No Device	Z No Qualifier

⊞ ØDT9ØZZ

Coding Clinic: 2Ø17, Q4, P5Ø – ØDTJØZZ
Coding Clinic: 2Ø19, Q1, P5, 7 – ØDT9ØZZ
Coding Clinic: 2Ø19, Q1, P15 – ØDT3ØZZ

SECTION: Ø MEDICAL AND SURGICAL
BODY SYSTEM: D GASTROINTESTINAL SYSTEM
OPERATION: U SUPPLEMENT: Putting in or on biological or synthetic material that physically reinforces and/or augments the function of a portion of a body part

Body Part	Approach	Device	Qualifier
1 Esophagus, Upper 2 Esophagus, Middle 3 Esophagus, Lower 4 Esophagogastric Junction 5 Esophagus 6 Stomach 7 Stomach, Pylorus 8 Small Intestine 9 Duodenum A Jejunum B Ileum C Ileocecal Valve E Large Intestine F Large Intestine, Right G Large Intestine, Left H Cecum K Ascending Colon L Transverse Colon M Descending Colon N Sigmoid Colon P Rectum	Ø Open 4 Percutaneous Endoscopic 7 Via Natural or Artificial Opening 8 Via Natural or Artificial Opening Endoscopic	7 Autologous Tissue Substitute J Synthetic Substitute K Nonautologous Tissue Substitute	Z No Qualifier
Q Anus	Ø Open 4 Percutaneous Endoscopic 7 Via Natural or Artificial Opening 8 Via Natural or Artificial Opening Endoscopic X External	7 Autologous Tissue Substitute J Synthetic Substitute K Nonautologous Tissue Substitute	Z No Qualifier
R Anal Sphincter U Omentum V Mesentery W Peritoneum	Ø Open 4 Percutaneous Endoscopic	7 Autologous Tissue Substitute J Synthetic Substitute K Nonautologous Tissue Substitute	Z No Qualifier

Coding Clinic: 2Ø19, Q1, P31 – ØDUPØJZ
Coding Clinic: 2Ø21, Q2, P21 – ØDUEØ7Z

SECTION: Ø MEDICAL AND SURGICAL
BODY SYSTEM: D GASTROINTESTINAL SYSTEM
OPERATION: V RESTRICTION: Partially closing an orifice or the lumen of a tubular body part

Body Part	Approach	Device	Qualifier
1 Esophagus, Upper 2 Esophagus, Middle 3 Esophagus, Lower 4 Esophagogastric Junction 5 Esophagus 6 Stomach 7 Stomach, Pylorus 8 Small Intestine 9 Duodenum A Jejunum B Ileum C Ileocecal Valve E Large Intestine F Large Intestine, Right G Large Intestine, Left H Cecum K Ascending Colon L Transverse Colon M Descending Colon N Sigmoid Colon P Rectum	Ø Open 3 Percutaneous 4 Percutaneous Endoscopic	C Extraluminal Device D Intraluminal Device Z No Device	Z No Qualifier
1 Esophagus, Upper 2 Esophagus, Middle 3 Esophagus, Lower 4 Esophagogastric Junction 5 Esophagus 6 Stomach 7 Stomach, Pylorus 8 Small Intestine 9 Duodenum A Jejunum B Ileum C Ileocecal Valve E Large Intestine F Large Intestine, Right G Large Intestine, Left H Cecum K Ascending Colon L Colon M Descending Colon N Sigmoid Colon P Rectum	7 Via Natural or Artificial Opening 8 Via Natural or Artificial Opening Endoscopic	D Intraluminal Device Z No Device	Z No Qualifier
Q Anus	Ø Open 3 Percutaneous 4 Percutaneous Endoscopic X External	C Extraluminal Device D Intraluminal Device Z No Device	Z No Qualifier
Q Anus	7 Via Natural or Artificial Opening 8 Via Natural or Artificial Opening Endoscopic	D Intraluminal Device Z No Device	Z No Qualifier

ØDV6[78]DZ

Non-OR ØDV6[78]DZ

ØDV64CZ when reported with Principal Diagnosis E66.Ø1 and Secondary Diagnosis K68.11, K95.Ø1, K95.81, or T81.4XXA

Coding Clinic: 2Ø16, Q2, P23 – ØDV4ØZZ Coding Clinic: 2Ø17, Q3, P23 – ØDV44ZZ

New/Revised Text in Green ~~deleted~~ Deleted ♀ Females Only ♂ Males Only Coding Clinic
Non-covered Limited Coverage Combination (See Appendix E) DRG Non-OR Non-OR Hospital-Acquired Condition

SECTION: Ø MEDICAL AND SURGICAL
BODY SYSTEM: D GASTROINTESTINAL SYSTEM
OPERATION: W REVISION: *(on multiple pages)*

Correcting, to the extent possible, a portion of a malfunctioning device or the position of a displaced device

Body Part	Approach	Device	Qualifier
Ø Upper Intestinal Tract D Lower Intestinal Tract	Ø Open 3 Percutaneous 4 Percutaneous Endoscopic 7 Via Natural or Artificial Opening 8 Via Natural or Artificial Opening Endoscopic	Ø Drainage Device 2 Monitoring Device 3 Infusion Device 7 Autologous Tissue Substitute C Extraluminal Device D Intraluminal Device J Synthetic Substitute K Nonautologous Tissue Substitute U Feeding Device Y Other Device	Z No Qualifier
Ø Upper Intestinal Tract D Lower Intestinal Tract	X External	Ø Drainage Device 2 Monitoring Device 3 Infusion Device 7 Autologous Tissue Substitute C Extraluminal Device D Intraluminal Device J Synthetic Substitute K Nonautologous Tissue Substitute U Feeding Device	Z No Qualifier
5 Esophagus	Ø Open 3 Percutaneous 4 Percutaneous Endoscopic	Y Other Device	Z No Qualifier
5 Esophagus	7 Via Natural or Artificial Opening 8 Via Natural or Artificial Opening Endoscopic	D Intraluminal Device Y Other Device	Z No Qualifier
5 Esophagus	X External	D Intraluminal Device	Z No Qualifier
6 Stomach	Ø Open 3 Percutaneous 4 Percutaneous Endoscopic	Ø Drainage Device 2 Monitoring Device 3 Infusion Device 7 Autologous Tissue Substitute C Extraluminal Device D Intraluminal Device J Synthetic Substitute K Nonautologous Tissue Substitute M Stimulator Lead U Feeding Device Y Other Device	Z No Qualifier
6 Stomach	7 Via Natural or Artificial Opening 8 Via Natural or Artificial Opening Endoscopic	Ø Drainage Device 2 Monitoring Device 3 Infusion Device 7 Autologous Tissue Substitute C Extraluminal Device D Intraluminal Device J Synthetic Substitute K Nonautologous Tissue Substitute U Feeding Device Y Other Device	Z No Qualifier

Non-OR ØDW[ØD]X[Ø237CDJKU]Z
Non-OR ØDW5XDZ
Non-OR ØDW6X[Ø237CDJKU]Z
Non-OR ØDW[UVW][Ø34]ØZ

Coding Clinic: 2Ø18, Q1, P2Ø – ØDW63CZ

SECTION: Ø MEDICAL AND SURGICAL
BODY SYSTEM: D GASTROINTESTINAL SYSTEM
OPERATION: W REVISION: *(continued)*

Correcting, to the extent possible, a portion of a malfunctioning device or the position of a displaced device

Body Part	Approach	Device	Qualifier
6 Stomach	X External	Ø Drainage Device 2 Monitoring Device 3 Infusion Device 7 Autologous Tissue Substitute C Extraluminal Device D Intraluminal Device J Synthetic Substitute K Nonautologous Tissue Substitute U Feeding Device	Z No Qualifier
8 Small Intestine E Large Intestine	Ø Open 4 Percutaneous Endoscopic 7 Via Natural or Artificial Opening 8 Via Natural or Artificial Opening Endoscopic	7 Autologous Tissue Substitute J Synthetic Substitute K Nonautologous Tissue Substitute	Z No Qualifier
Q Anus	Ø Open 3 Percutaneous 4 Percutaneous Endoscopic 7 Via Natural or Artificial Opening 8 Via Natural or Artificial Opening Endoscopic	L Artificial Sphincter	Z No Qualifier
R Anal Sphincter	Ø Open 3 Percutaneous 4 Percutaneous Endoscopic	M Stimulator Lead	Z No Qualifier
U Omentum V Mesentery W Peritoneum	Ø Open 3 Percutaneous 4 Percutaneous Endoscopic	Ø Drainage Device 7 Autologous Tissue Substitute J Synthetic Substitute K Nonautologous Tissue Substitute	Z No Qualifier

Coding Clinic: 2Ø21, Q1, P2Ø – ØDW8Ø7Z

SECTION: Ø MEDICAL AND SURGICAL
BODY SYSTEM: D GASTROINTESTINAL SYSTEM
OPERATION: X TRANSFER: Moving, without taking out, all or a portion of a body part to another location to take over the function of all or a portion of a body part

Body Part	Approach	Device	Qualifier
6 Stomach	Ø Open 4 Percutaneous Endoscopic	Z No Device	5 Esophagus
8 Small Intestine	Ø Open 4 Percutaneous Endoscopic	Z No Device	5 Esophagus B Bladder C Ureter, Right D Ureter, Left F Ureters, Bilateral
E Large Intestine	Ø Open 4 Percutaneous Endoscopic	Z No Device	5 Esophagus 7 Vagina B Bladder

Coding Clinic: 2017, Q2, P18; 2016, Q2, P24 – ØDX6ØZ5
Coding Clinic: 2019, Q1, P15 – ØDXEØZ5
Coding Clinic: 2019, Q4, P3Ø – ØDXEØZ7A
Coding Clinic: 2022, Q4, P57 – ØDX8ØZB

SECTION: Ø MEDICAL AND SURGICAL
BODY SYSTEM: D GASTROINTESTINAL SYSTEM
OPERATION: Y TRANSPLANTATION: Putting in or on all or a portion of a living body part taken from another individual or animal to physically take the place and/or function of all or a portion of a similar body part

Body Part	Approach	Device	Qualifier
5 Esophagus 6 Stomach 8 Small Intestine E Large Intestine	Ø Open	Z No Device	0 Allogeneic 1 Syngeneic 2 Zooplastic

ØDY[8E]ØZ[Ø12]
Non-OR ØDY5ØZ[Ø12]

ØF

SECTION: Ø **MEDICAL AND SURGICAL**
BODY SYSTEM: F **HEPATOBILIARY SYSTEM AND PANCREAS**
OPERATION: 1 **BYPASS:** Altering the route of passage of the contents of a tubular body part

Body Part	Approach	Device	Qualifier
4 Gallbladder 5 Hepatic Duct, Right 6 Hepatic Duct, Left 7 Hepatic Duct, Common 8 Cystic Duct 9 Common Bile Duct	Ø Open 4 Percutaneous Endoscopic	D Intraluminal Device Z No Device	3 Duodenum 4 Stomach 5 Hepatic Duct, Right 6 Hepatic Duct, Left 7 Hepatic Duct, Caudate 8 Cystic Duct 9 Common Bile Duct B Small Intestine
D Pancreatic Duct F Pancreatic Duct, Accessory G Pancreas	Ø Open 4 Percutaneous Endoscopic	D Intraluminal Device Z No Device	3 Duodenum B Small Intestine C Large Intestine
D Pancreatic Duct	Ø Open 4 Percutaneous Endoscopic	D Intraluminal Device Z No Device	3 Duodenum 4 Stomach B Small Intestine C Large Intestine
D Pancreatic Duct	Ø Open 4 Percutaneous Endoscopic	D Intraluminal Device Z No Device	3 Duodenum 4 Stomach B Small Intestine C Large Intestine
D Pancreatic Duct, Accessory G Pancreas	Ø Open 4 Percutaneous Endoscopic	D Intraluminal Device Z No Device	3 Duodenum B Small Intestine C Large Intestine

SECTION: Ø **MEDICAL AND SURGICAL**
BODY SYSTEM: F **HEPATOBILIARY SYSTEM AND PANCREAS**
OPERATION: 2 **CHANGE:** Taking out or off a device from a body part and putting back an identical or similar device in or on the same body part without cutting or puncturing the skin or a mucous membrane

Body Part	Approach	Device	Qualifier
Ø Liver 4 Gallbladder B Hepatobiliary Duct D Pancreatic Duct G Pancreas	X External	Ø Drainage Device Y Other Device	Z No Qualifier

Non-OR All Values

SECTION: Ø MEDICAL AND SURGICAL
BODY SYSTEM: F HEPATOBILIARY SYSTEM AND PANCREAS
OPERATION: 5 DESTRUCTION: Physical eradication of all or a portion of a body part by the direct use of energy, force, or a destructive agent

Body Part	Approach	Device	Qualifier
Ø Liver 1 Liver, Right Lobe 2 Liver, Left Lobe	Ø Open 3 Percutaneous 4 Percutaneous Endoscopic	Z No Device	3 Laser Interstitial Thermal Therapy F Irreversible Electroporation Z No Qualifier
4 Gallbladder	Ø Open 3 Percutaneous 4 Percutaneous Endoscopic	Z No Device	3 Laser Interstitial Thermal Therapy Z No Qualifier
4 Gallbladder	8 Via Natural or Artificial Opening Endoscopic	Z No Device	Z No Qualifier
5 Hepatic Duct, Right 6 Hepatic Duct, Left 7 Hepatic Duct, Common 8 Cystic Duct 9 Common Bile Duct C Ampulla of Vater D Pancreatic Duct F Pancreatic Duct, Accessory	Ø Open 3 Percutaneous 4 Percutaneous Endoscopic	Z No Device	3 Laser Interstitial Thermal Therapy Z No Qualifier
5 Hepatic Duct, Right 6 Hepatic Duct, Left 7 Hepatic Duct, Common 8 Cystic Duct 9 Common Bile Duct C Ampulla of Vater D Pancreatic Duct F Pancreatic Duct, Accessory	7 Via Natural or Artificial Opening 8 Via Natural or Artificial Opening Endoscopic	Z No Device	Z No Qualifier
G Pancreas	Ø Open 3 Percutaneous 4 Percutaneous Endoscopic	Z No Device	3 Laser Interstitial Thermal Therapy F Irreversible Electroporation Z No Qualifier
G Pancreas	8 Via Natural or Artificial Opening Endoscopic	Z No Device	Z No Qualifier

Non-OR ØF5G4ZZ
Non-OR ØF5[5689CDF][48]ZZ
Non-OR ØF5[56789CDFG]4Z3
Non-OR ØF5[Ø12345679CDFG][Ø34]Z3

Coding Clinic: 2018, Q4, P4Ø – ØF5G4ZF

SECTION: Ø MEDICAL AND SURGICAL
BODY SYSTEM: F HEPATOBILIARY SYSTEM AND PANCREAS
OPERATION: 7 DILATION: Expanding an orifice or the lumen of a tubular body part

Body Part	Approach	Device	Qualifier
5 Hepatic Duct, Right 6 Hepatic Duct, Left 7 Hepatic Duct, Common 8 Cystic Duct 9 Common Bile Duct C Ampulla of Vater D Pancreatic Duct F Pancreatic Duct, Accessory	Ø Open 3 Percutaneous 4 Percutaneous Endoscopic 7 Via Natural or Artificial Opening 8 Via Natural or Artificial Opening Endoscopic	D Intraluminal Device Z No Device	Z No Qualifier

Non-OR ØF7[5689][34][DZ]Z
Non-OR ØF7[5689D][78]DZ
Non-OR ØF7[CF]8DZ
Non-OR ØF7[DF]4[DZ]Z
Non-OR ØF7[5689CDF]8ZZ

Coding Clinic: 2Ø16, Q1, P25 – ØF798DZ, ØF7D8DZ
Coding Clinic: 2Ø16, Q3, P28 – ØF7D8DZ

SECTION: Ø MEDICAL AND SURGICAL
BODY SYSTEM: F HEPATOBILIARY SYSTEM AND PANCREAS
OPERATION: 8 DIVISION: Cutting into a body part, without draining fluids and/or gases from the body part, in order to separate or transect a body part

Body Part	Approach	Device	Qualifier
Ø Liver 1 Liver, Right Lobe 2 Liver, Left Lobe G Pancreas	Ø Open 3 Percutaneous 4 Percutaneous Endoscopic	Z No Device	Z No Qualifier

Coding Clinic: 2Ø21, Q4, P49 – ØF824ZZ

SECTION: Ø MEDICAL AND SURGICAL
BODY SYSTEM: F HEPATOBILIARY SYSTEM AND PANCREAS
OPERATION: 9 DRAINAGE: Taking or letting out fluids and/or gases from a body part

Body Part	Approach	Device	Qualifier
Ø Liver 1 Liver, Right Lobe 2 Liver, Left Lobe	Ø Open 3 Percutaneous 4 Percutaneous Endoscopic	Ø Drainage Device	Z No Qualifier
Ø Liver 1 Liver, Right Lobe 2 Liver, Left Lobe	Ø Open 3 Percutaneous 4 Percutaneous Endoscopic	Z No Device	X Diagnostic Z No Qualifier
4 Gallbladder G Pancreas	Ø Open 3 Percutaneous 4 Percutaneous Endoscopic 8 Via Natural or Artificial Opening Endoscopic	Ø Drainage Device	Z No Qualifier
4 Gallbladder G Pancreas	Ø Open 3 Percutaneous 4 Percutaneous Endoscopic 8 Via Natural or Artificial Opening Endoscopic	Z No Device	X Diagnostic Z No Qualifier
5 Hepatic Duct, Right 6 Hepatic Duct, Left 7 Hepatic Duct, Common 8 Cystic Duct 9 Common Bile Duct C Ampulla of Vater D Pancreatic Duct F Pancreatic Duct, Accessory	Ø Open 3 Percutaneous 4 Percutaneous Endoscopic 7 Via Natural or Artificial Opening 8 Via Natural or Artificial Opening Endoscopic	Ø Drainage Device	Z No Qualifier
5 Hepatic Duct, Right 6 Hepatic Duct, Left 7 Hepatic Duct, Common 8 Cystic Duct 9 Common Bile Duct C Ampulla of Vater D Pancreatic Duct F Pancreatic Duct, Accessory	Ø Open 3 Percutaneous 4 Percutaneous Endoscopic 7 Via Natural or Artificial Opening 8 Via Natural or Artificial Opening Endoscopic	Z No Device	X Diagnostic Z No Qualifier

Non-OR ØF9[Ø12][34]ØZ
Non-OR ØF9[4G]3ØZ
Non-OR ØF944ØZ
Non-OR ØF9G3ZZ
Non-OR ØF9[Ø124][34]Z[XZ]
Non-OR ØF9G[34]ZX
Non-OR ØF9[5689CDF]3ØZ
Non-OR ØF9[9DF]8ØZ
Non-OR ØF9C[48]ØZ
Non-OR ØF9[568][3478]ZX
Non-OR ØF99[3478]Z[XZ]
Non-OR ØF9[CDF][347]ZX
Non-OR ØF9[568CDF]3ZZ
Non-OR ØF994ZZ
Non-OR ØF9C8Z[XZ]
Non-OR ØF9[DF]8ZX

Coding Clinic: 2Ø15, Q1, P32 – ØF963ØZ

SECTION: Ø MEDICAL AND SURGICAL
BODY SYSTEM: F HEPATOBILIARY SYSTEM AND PANCREAS
OPERATION: B EXCISION: Cutting out or off, without replacement, a portion of a body part

Body Part	Approach	Device	Qualifier
Ø Liver 1 Liver, Right Lobe 2 Liver, Left Lobe	Ø Open 3 Percutaneous 4 Percutaneous Endoscopic	Z No Device	X Diagnostic Z No Qualifier
4 Gallbladder G Pancreas	Ø Open 3 Percutaneous 4 Percutaneous Endoscopic 8 Via Natural or Artificial Opening Endoscopic	Z No Device	X Diagnostic Z No Qualifier
5 Hepatic Duct, Right 6 Hepatic Duct, Left 7 Hepatic Duct, Common 8 Cystic Duct 9 Common Bile Duct C Ampulla of Vater D Pancreatic Duct F Pancreatic Duct, Accessory	Ø Open 3 Percutaneous 4 Percutaneous Endoscopic 7 Via Natural or Artificial Opening 8 Via Natural or Artificial Opening Endoscopic	Z No Device	X Diagnostic Z No Qualifier

Non-OR ØFB[Ø12]3ZX
Non-OR ØFB[4G][34]ZX
Non-OR ØFB[5689CDF][3478]ZX
Non-OR ØFB[5689CDF][48]ZZ

Coding Clinic: 2016, Q1, P23, P25 – ØFB98ZX
Coding Clinic: 2016, Q1, P25 – ØFBD8ZX
Coding Clinic: 2016, Q3, P41 – ØFBØØZX
Coding Clinic: 2019, Q1, P5-8 – ØFBG[9]ØZZ

SECTION: Ø MEDICAL AND SURGICAL
BODY SYSTEM: F HEPATOBILIARY SYSTEM AND PANCREAS
OPERATION: C EXTIRPATION: Taking or cutting out solid matter from a body part

Body Part	Approach	Device	Qualifier
Ø Liver 1 Liver, Right Lobe 2 Liver, Left Lobe	Ø Open 3 Percutaneous 4 Percutaneous Endoscopic	Z No Device	Z No Qualifier
4 Gallbladder G Pancreas	Ø Open 3 Percutaneous 4 Percutaneous Endoscopic 8 Via Natural or Artificial Opening Endoscopic	Z No Device	Z No Qualifier
5 Hepatic Duct, Right 6 Hepatic Duct, Left 7 Hepatic Duct, Common 8 Cystic Duct 9 Common Bile Duct C Ampulla of Vater D Pancreatic Duct F Pancreatic Duct, Accessory	Ø Open 3 Percutaneous 4 Percutaneous Endoscopic 7 Via Natural or Artificial Opening 8 Via Natural or Artificial Opening Endoscopic	Z No Device	Z No Qualifier

Non-OR ØFC[5689][3478]ZZ
Non-OR ØFCC[48]ZZ
Non-OR ØFC[DF][348]ZZ

Coding Clinic: 2023, Q2, P23 – ØFCG8ZZ

SECTION: Ø **MEDICAL AND SURGICAL**
BODY SYSTEM: F **HEPATOBILIARY SYSTEM AND PANCREAS**
OPERATION: D **EXTRACTION:** Pulling or stripping out or off all or a portion of a body part by the use of force

Body Part	Approach	Device	Qualifier
Ø Liver 1 Liver, Right Lobe 2 Liver, Left Lobe	3 Percutaneous 4 Percutaneous Endoscopic	Z No Device	X Diagnostic
4 Gallbladder 5 Hepatic Duct, Right 6 Hepatic Duct, Left 7 Hepatic Duct, Common 8 Cystic Duct 9 Common Bile Duct C Ampulla of Vater D Pancreatic Duct F Pancreatic Duct, Accessory G Pancreas	3 Percutaneous 4 Percutaneous Endoscopic 8 Via Natural or Artificial Opening Endoscopic	Z No Device	X Diagnostic

SECTION: Ø **MEDICAL AND SURGICAL**
BODY SYSTEM: F **HEPATOBILIARY SYSTEM AND PANCREAS**
OPERATION: F **FRAGMENTATION:** Breaking solid matter in a body part into pieces

Body Part	Approach	Device	Qualifier
4 Gallbladder 5 Hepatic Duct, Right 6 Hepatic Duct, Left 7 Hepatic Duct, Common 8 Cystic Duct 9 Common Bile Duct C Ampulla of Vater D Pancreatic Duct F Pancreatic Duct, Acessory	Ø Open 3 Percutaneous 4 Percutaneous Endoscopic 7 Via Natural or Artificial Opening 8 Via Natural or Artificial Opening Endoscopic X External	Z No Device	Z No Qualifier

ØFF[45689CDF]XZZ
Non-OR ØFF[45689C][8X]ZZ
Non-OR ØFF[DF]XZZ

SECTION: Ø **MEDICAL AND SURGICAL**
BODY SYSTEM: F **HEPATOBILIARY SYSTEM AND PANCREAS**
OPERATION: H **INSERTION:** Putting in a nonbiological appliance that monitors, assists, performs, or prevents a physiological function but does not physically take the place of a body part

Body Part	Approach	Device	Qualifier
Ø Liver 4 Gallbladder G Pancreas	Ø Open 3 Percutaneous 4 Percutaneous Endoscopic	1 Radioactive Element 2 Monitoring Device 3 Infusion Device Y Other Device	Z No Qualifier
1 Liver, Right Lobe 2 Liver, Left Lobe	Ø Open 3 Percutaneous 4 Percutaneous Endoscopic	2 Monitoring Device 3 Infusion Device	Z No Qualifier
B Hepatobiliary Duct D Pancreatic Duct	Ø Open 3 Percutaneous 4 Percutaneous Endoscopic 7 Via Natural or Artificial Opening 8 Via Natural or Artificial Opening Endoscopic	1 Radioactive Element 2 Monitoring Device 3 Infusion Device D Intraluminal Device Y Other Device	Z No Qualifier

Non-OR ØFH[Ø4G][Ø34]3Z
Non-OR ØFH[12][Ø34]3Z
Non-OR ØFH[BD][78][23]Z
Non-OR ØFH[BD][Ø3478]3Z
Non-OR ØFH[BD]4DZ
Non-OR ØFH[BD]8DZ

Coding Clinic: 2Ø22, Q2, P26 – ØFHØ31Z

SECTION: Ø MEDICAL AND SURGICAL
BODY SYSTEM: F HEPATOBILIARY SYSTEM AND PANCREAS
OPERATION: J INSPECTION: Visually and/or manually exploring a body part

Body Part	Approach	Device	Qualifier
Ø Liver	Ø Open 3 Percutaneous 4 Percutaneous Endoscopic X External	Z No Device	Z No Qualifier
4 Gallbladder G Pancreas	Ø Open 3 Percutaneous 4 Percutaneous Endoscopic 8 Via Natural or Artificial Opening Endoscopic X External	Z No Device	Z No Qualifier
B Hepatobiliary Duct D Pancreatic Duct	Ø Open 3 Percutaneous 4 Percutaneous Endoscopic 7 Via Natural or Artificial Opening 8 Via Natural or Artificial Opening Endoscopic	Z No Device	Z No Qualifier

DRG Non-OR ØFJØ3ZZ
DRG Non-OR ØFJG3ZZ
DRG Non-OR ØFJD[378]ZZ
Non-OR ØFJØXZZ
Non-OR ØFJ[4G]XZZ
Non-OR ØFJ43ZZ
Non-OR ØFJB[378]ZZ

SECTION: Ø MEDICAL AND SURGICAL
BODY SYSTEM: F HEPATOBILIARY SYSTEM AND PANCREAS
OPERATION: L OCCLUSION: Completely closing an orifice or the lumen of a tubular body part

Body Part	Approach	Device	Qualifier
5 Hepatic Duct, Right 6 Hepatic Duct, Left 7 Hepatic Duct, Common 8 Cystic Duct 9 Common Bile Duct C Ampulla of Vater D Pancreatic Duct F Pancreatic Duct, Accessory	Ø Open 3 Percutaneous 4 Percutaneous Endoscopic	C Extraluminal Device D Intraluminal Device Z No Device	Z No Qualifier
5 Hepatic Duct, Right 6 Hepatic Duct, Left 7 Hepatic Duct, Common 8 Cystic Duct 9 Common Bile Duct C Ampulla of Vater D Pancreatic Duct F Pancreatic Duct, Accessory	7 Via Natural or Artificial Opening 8 Via Natural or Artificial Opening Endoscopic	D Intraluminal Device Z No Device	Z No Qualifier

Non-OR ØFL[5689][34][CDZ]Z
Non-OR ØFL[5689][78][DZ]Z

SECTION: Ø **MEDICAL AND SURGICAL**
BODY SYSTEM: F **HEPATOBILIARY SYSTEM AND PANCREAS**
OPERATION: M **REATTACHMENT:** Putting back in or on all or a portion of a separated body part to its normal location or other suitable location

Body Part	Approach	Device	Qualifier
Ø Liver 1 Liver, Right Lobe 2 Liver, Left Lobe 4 Gallbladder 5 Hepatic Duct, Right 6 Hepatic Duct, Left 7 Hepatic Duct, Common 8 Cystic Duct 9 Common Bile Duct C Ampulla of Vater D Pancreatic Duct F Pancreatic Duct, Accessory G Pancreas	Ø Open 4 Percutaneous Endoscopic	Z No Device	Z No Qualifier

Non-OR ØFM[45689]4ZZ

SECTION: Ø **MEDICAL AND SURGICAL**
BODY SYSTEM: F **HEPATOBILIARY SYSTEM AND PANCREAS**
OPERATION: N **RELEASE:** Freeing a body part from an abnormal physical constraint by cutting or by the use of force

Body Part	Approach	Device	Qualifier
Ø Liver 1 Liver, Right Lobe 2 Liver, Left Lobe	Ø Open 3 Percutaneous 4 Percutaneous Endoscopic	Z No Device	Z No Qualifier
4 Gallbladder G Pancreas	Ø Open 3 Percutaneous 4 Percutaneous Endoscopic 8 Via Natural or Artificial Opening Endoscopic	Z No Device	Z No Qualifier
5 Hepatic Duct, Right 6 Hepatic Duct, Left 7 Hepatic Duct, Common 8 Cystic Duct 9 Common Bile Duct C Ampulla of Vater D Pancreatic Duct F Pancreatic Duct, Accessory	Ø Open 3 Percutaneous 4 Percutaneous Endoscopic 7 Via Natural or Artificial Opening 8 Via Natural or Artificial Opening Endoscopic	Z No Device	Z No Qualifier

SECTION: Ø MEDICAL AND SURGICAL
BODY SYSTEM: F HEPATOBILIARY SYSTEM AND PANCREAS
OPERATION: P REMOVAL: Taking out or off a device from a body part

Body Part	Approach	Device	Qualifier
Ø Liver	Ø Open 3 Percutaneous 4 Percutaneous Endoscopic	Ø Drainage Device 2 Monitoring Device 3 Infusion Device Y Other Device	Z No Qualifier
Ø Liver	X External	Ø Drainage Device 2 Monitoring Device 3 Infusion Device	Z No Qualifier
4 Gallbladder G Pancreas	Ø Open 3 Percutaneous 4 Percutaneous Endoscopic	Ø Drainage Device 2 Monitoring Device 3 Infusion Device D Intraluminal Device Y Other Device	Z No Qualifier
4 Gallbladder G Pancreas	X External	Ø Drainage Device 2 Monitoring Device 3 Infusion Device D Intraluminal Device	Z No Qualifier
B Hepatobiliary Duct D Pancreatic Duct	Ø Open 3 Percutaneous 4 Percutaneous Endoscopic 7 Via Natural or Artificial Opening 8 Via Natural or Artificial Opening Endoscopic	Ø Drainage Device 1 Radioactive Element 2 Monitoring Device 3 Infusion Device 7 Autologous Tissue Substitute C Extraluminal Device D Intraluminal Device J Synthetic Substitute K Nonautologous Tissue Substitute Y Other Device	Z No Qualifier
B Hepatobiliary Duct D Pancreatic Duct	X External	Ø Drainage Device 1 Radioactive Element 2 Monitoring Device 3 Infusion Device D Intraluminal Device	Z No Qualifier

Non-OR ØFPØX[Ø23]Z
Non-OR ØFP4X[Ø23D]Z
Non-OR ØFPGX[Ø23]Z
Non-OR ØFP[BD][78][Ø23D]Z
Non-OR ØFP[BD]X[Ø123D]Z

SECTION: Ø MEDICAL AND SURGICAL
BODY SYSTEM: F HEPATOBILIARY SYSTEM AND PANCREAS
OPERATION: Q REPAIR: Restoring, to the extent possible, a body part to its normal anatomic structure and function

Body Part	Approach	Device	Qualifier
Ø Liver 1 Liver, Right Lobe 2 Liver, Left Lobe	Ø Open 3 Percutaneous 4 Percutaneous Endoscopic	Z No Device	Z No Qualifier
4 Gallbladder G Pancreas	Ø Open 3 Percutaneous 4 Percutaneous Endoscopic 8 Via Natural or Artificial Opening Endoscopic	Z No Device	Z No Qualifier
5 Hepatic Duct, Right 6 Hepatic Duct, Left 7 Hepatic Duct, Common 8 Cystic Duct 9 Common Bile Duct C Ampulla of Vater D Pancreatic Duct F Pancreatic Duct, Accessory	Ø Open 3 Percutaneous 4 Percutaneous Endoscopic 7 Via Natural or Artificial Opening 8 Via Natural or Artificial Opening Endoscopic	Z No Device	Z No Qualifier

Coding Clinic: 2Ø16, Q3, P27 – ØFQ9ØZZ

SECTION: Ø MEDICAL AND SURGICAL
BODY SYSTEM: F HEPATOBILIARY SYSTEM AND PANCREAS
OPERATION: R REPLACEMENT: Putting in or on biological or synthetic material that physically takes the place and/or function of all or a portion of a body part

Body Part	Approach	Device	Qualifier
5 Hepatic Duct, Right 6 Hepatic Duct, Left 7 Hepatic Duct, Common 8 Cystic Duct 9 Common Bile Duct C Ampulla of Vater D Pancreatic Duct F Pancreatic Duct, Accessory	Ø Open 4 Percutaneous Endoscopic 8 Via Natural or Artificial Opening Endoscopic	7 Autologous Tissue Substitute J Synthetic Substitute K Nonautologous Tissue Substitute	Z No Qualifier

SECTION: Ø MEDICAL AND SURGICAL
BODY SYSTEM: F HEPATOBILIARY SYSTEM AND PANCREAS
OPERATION: S REPOSITION: Moving to its normal location, or other suitable location, all or a portion of a body part

Body Part	Approach	Device	Qualifier
Ø Liver 4 Gallbladder 5 Hepatic Duct, Right 6 Hepatic Duct, Left 7 Hepatic Duct, Common 8 Cystic Duct 9 Common Bile Duct C Ampulla of Vater D Pancreatic Duct F Pancreatic Duct, Accessory G Pancreas	Ø Open 4 Percutaneous Endoscopic	Z No Device	Z No Qualifier

SECTION: Ø MEDICAL AND SURGICAL
BODY SYSTEM: F HEPATOBILIARY SYSTEM AND PANCREAS
OPERATION: T RESECTION: Cutting out or off, without replacement, all of a body part

Body Part	Approach	Device	Qualifier
Ø Liver 1 Liver, Right Lobe 2 Liver, Left Lobe 4 Gallbladder G Pancreas ⊞	Ø Open 4 Percutaneous Endoscopic	Z No Device	Z No Qualifier
5 Hepatic Duct, Right 6 Hepatic Duct, Left 7 Hepatic Duct, Common 8 Cystic Duct 9 Common Bile Duct C Ampulla of Vater D Pancreatic Duct F Pancreatic Duct, Accessory	Ø Open 4 Percutaneous Endoscopic 7 Via Natural or Artificial Opening 8 Via Natural or Artificial Opening Endoscopic	Z No Device	Z No Qualifier

⊞ ØFTGØZZ
Non-OR ØFT[DF][48]ZZ

Coding Clinic: 2012, Q4, P1ØØ – ØFTØØZZ
Coding Clinic: 2019, Q1, P5 – ØFT4ØZZ
Coding Clinic: 2021, Q4, P49 – ØFT44ZZ

SECTION: Ø **MEDICAL AND SURGICAL**
BODY SYSTEM: F **HEPATOBILIARY SYSTEM AND PANCREAS**
OPERATION: U **SUPPLEMENT:** Putting in or on biological or synthetic material that physically reinforces and/or augments the function of a portion of a body part

Body Part	Approach	Device	Qualifier
5 Hepatic Duct, Right 6 Hepatic Duct, Left 7 Hepatic Duct, Common 8 Cystic Duct 9 Common Bile Duct C Ampulla of Vater D Pancreatic Duct F Pancreatic Duct, Accessory	Ø Open 3 Percutaneous 4 Percutaneous Endoscopic 8 Via Natural or Artificial Opening Endoscopic	7 Autologous Tissue Substitute J Synthetic Substitute K Nonautologous Tissue Substitute	Z No Qualifier

SECTION: Ø **MEDICAL AND SURGICAL**
BODY SYSTEM: F **HEPATOBILIARY SYSTEM AND PANCREAS**
OPERATION: V **RESTRICTION:** Partially closing an orifice or the lumen of a tubular body part

Body Part	Approach	Device	Qualifier
5 Hepatic Duct, Right 6 Hepatic Duct, Left 7 Hepatic Duct, Common 8 Cystic Duct 9 Common Bile Duct C Ampulla of Vater D Pancreatic Duct F Pancreatic Duct, Accessory	Ø Open 3 Percutaneous 4 Percutaneous Endoscopic	C Extraluminal Device D Intraluminal Device Z No Device	Z No Qualifier
5 Hepatic Duct, Right 6 Hepatic Duct, Left 7 Hepatic Duct, Common 8 Cystic Duct 9 Common Bile Duct C Ampulla of Vater D Pancreatic Duct F Pancreatic Duct, Accessory	7 Via Natural or Artificial Opening 8 Via Natural or Artificial Opening Endoscopic	D Intraluminal Device Z No Device	Z No Qualifier

Non-OR ØFV[5689][34][CDZ]Z
Non-OR ØFV[5689][78][DZ]Z

SECTION: Ø **MEDICAL AND SURGICAL**
BODY SYSTEM: F **HEPATOBILIARY SYSTEM AND PANCREAS**
OPERATION: W **REVISION:** Correcting, to the extent possible, a portion of a malfunctioning device or the position of a displaced device

Body Part	Approach	Device	Qualifier
Ø Liver	Ø Open 3 Percutaneous 4 Percutaneous Endoscopic	Ø Drainage Device 2 Monitoring Device 3 Infusion Device Y Other Device	Z No Qualifier
Ø Liver	X External	Ø Drainage Device 2 Monitoring Device 3 Infusion Device	Z No Qualifier
4 Gallbladder G Pancreas	Ø Open 3 Percutaneous 4 Percutaneous Endoscopic	Ø Drainage Device 2 Monitoring Device 3 Infusion Device D Intraluminal Device Y Other Device	Z No Qualifier
4 Gallbladder G Pancreas	X External	Ø Drainage Device 2 Monitoring Device 3 Infusion Device D Intraluminal Device	Z No Qualifier
B Hepatobiliary Duct D Pancreatic Duct	Ø Open 3 Percutaneous 4 Percutaneous Endoscopic 7 Via Natural or Artificial Opening 8 Via Natural or Artificial Opening Endoscopic	Ø Drainage Device 2 Monitoring Device 3 Infusion Device 7 Autologous Tissue Substitute C Extraluminal Device D Intraluminal Device J Synthetic Substitute K Nonautologous Tissue Substitute Y Other Device	Z No Qualifier
B Hepatobiliary Duct D Pancreatic Duct	X External	Ø Drainage Device 2 Monitoring Device 3 Infusion Device 7 Autologous Tissue Substitute C Extraluminal Device D Intraluminal Device J Synthetic Substitute K Nonautologous Tissue Substitute	Z No Qualifier

Non-OR ØFWØX[Ø23]Z
Non-OR ØFW[4G]X[Ø23D]Z
Non-OR ØFW[BD]X[Ø237CDJK]Z

ØFY

SECTION: Ø MEDICAL AND SURGICAL
BODY SYSTEM: F HEPATOBILIARY SYSTEM AND PANCREAS
OPERATION: Y TRANSPLANTATION: Putting in or on all or a portion of a living body part taken from another individual or animal to physically take the place and/or function of all or a portion of a similar body part

Body Part	Approach	Device	Qualifier
Ø Liver G Pancreas ⊞	Ø Open	Z No Device	Ø Allogeneic 1 Syngeneic 2 Zooplastic

ØFYGØZ2

ØFYGØZØ, ØFYGØZ1 alone [without kidney transplant codes (ØTYØØZ[Ø1], ØTY1ØZ[Ø12])], except when ØFYGØZØ or ØFYGØZ1 is combined with at least one principal or secondary diagnosis code from the following list:

E1Ø.1Ø	E1Ø.321	E1Ø.359	E1Ø.44	E1Ø.62Ø	E1Ø.649
E1Ø.11	E1Ø.329	E1Ø.36	E1Ø.49	E1Ø.621	E1Ø.65
E1Ø.21	E1Ø.331	E1Ø.39	E1Ø.51	E1Ø.622	E1Ø.69
E1Ø.22	E1Ø.339	E1Ø.4Ø	E1Ø.52	E1Ø.628	E1Ø.8
E1Ø.29	E1Ø.341	E1Ø.41	E1Ø.59	E1Ø.63Ø	E1Ø.9
E1Ø.311	E1Ø.349	E1Ø.42	E1Ø.61Ø	E1Ø.638	E89.1
E1Ø.319	E1Ø.351	E1Ø.43	E1Ø.618	E1Ø.641	

ØFYØØZ[Ø12]

ØFYGØZ[Ø1]

⊞ ØFYGØZ[Ø12]

Coding Clinic: 2Ø12, Q4, P1ØØ – ØFYØØZØ

SECTION: Ø MEDICAL AND SURGICAL
BODY SYSTEM: G ENDOCRINE SYSTEM
OPERATION: 2 CHANGE: Taking out or off a device from a body part and putting back an identical or similar device in or on the same body part without cutting or puncturing the skin or a mucous membrane

Body Part	Approach	Device	Qualifier
Ø Pituitary Gland 1 Pineal Body 5 Adrenal Gland K Thyroid Gland R Parathyroid Gland S Endocrine Gland	X External	Ø Drainage Device Y Other Device	Z No Qualifier

Non-OR All Values

SECTION: Ø MEDICAL AND SURGICAL
BODY SYSTEM: G ENDOCRINE SYSTEM
OPERATION: 5 DESTRUCTION: Physical eradication of all or a portion of a body part by the direct use of energy, force, or a destructive agent

Body Part	Approach	Device	Qualifier
Ø Pituitary Gland 1 Pineal Body 2 Adrenal Gland, Left 3 Adrenal Gland, Right 4 Adrenal Glands, Bilateral 6 Carotid Body, Left 7 Carotid Body, Right 8 Carotid Bodies, Bilateral 9 Para-aortic Body B Coccygeal Glomus C Glomus Jugulare D Aortic Body F Paraganglion Extremity G Thyroid Gland Lobe, Left H Thyroid Gland Lobe, Right K Thyroid Gland L Superior Parathyroid Gland, Right M Superior Parathyroid Gland, Left N Inferior Parathyroid Gland, Right P Inferior Parathyroid Gland, Left Q Parathyroid Glands, Multiple R Parathyroid Gland	Ø Open 3 Percutaneous 4 Percutaneous Endoscopic	Z No Device	3 Laser Interstitial Thermal Therapy Z No Qualifier

Non-OR All Values

SECTION: Ø MEDICAL AND SURGICAL
BODY SYSTEM: G ENDOCRINE SYSTEM
OPERATION: 8 DIVISION: Cutting into a body part, without draining fluids and/or gases from the body part, in order to separate or transect a body part

Body Part	Approach	Device	Qualifier
Ø Pituitary Gland J Thyroid Gland Isthmus	Ø Open 3 Percutaneous 4 Percutaneous Endoscopic	Z No Device	Z No Qualifier

SECTION: Ø MEDICAL AND SURGICAL
BODY SYSTEM: G ENDOCRINE SYSTEM
OPERATION: 9 DRAINAGE: Taking or letting out fluids and/or gases from a body part

Body Part	Approach	Device	Qualifier
Ø Pituitary Gland 1 Pineal Body 2 Adrenal Gland, Left 3 Adrenal Gland, Right 4 Adrenal Glands, Bilateral 6 Carotid Body, Left 7 Carotid Body, Right 8 Carotid Bodies, Bilateral 9 Para-aortic Body B Coccygeal Glomus C Glomus Jugulare D Aortic Body F Paraganglion Extremity G Thyroid Gland Lobe, Left H Thyroid Gland Lobe, Right K Thyroid Gland L Superior Parathyroid Gland, Right M Superior Parathyroid Gland, Left N Inferior Parathyroid Gland, Right P Inferior Parathyroid Gland, Left Q Parathyroid Glands, Multiple R Parathyroid Gland	Ø Open 3 Percutaneous 4 Percutaneous Endoscopic	Ø Drainage Device	Z No Qualifier
Ø Pituitary Gland 1 Pineal Body 2 Adrenal Gland, Left 3 Adrenal Gland, Right 4 Adrenal Glands, Bilateral 6 Carotid Body, Left 7 Carotid Body, Right 8 Carotid Bodies, Bilateral 9 Para-aortic Body B Coccygeal Glomus C Glomus Jugulare D Aortic Body F Paraganglion Extremity G Thyroid Gland Lobe, Left H Thyroid Gland Lobe, Right K Thyroid Gland L Superior Parathyroid Gland, Right M Superior Parathyroid Gland, Left N Inferior Parathyroid Gland, Right P Inferior Parathyroid Gland, Left Q Parathyroid Glands, Multiple R Parathyroid Gland	Ø Open 3 Percutaneous 4 Percutaneous Endoscopic	Z No Device	X Diagnostic Z No Qualifier

Non-OR ØG9[Ø12346789BCDF]3ØZ
Non-OR ØG9[GHKLMNPQR][34]ØZ
Non-OR ØG9[234GHK][34]ZX
Non-OR ØG9[Ø12346789BCDF]3ZZ
Non-OR ØG9[GHKLMNPQR][34]ZZ

SECTION: Ø MEDICAL AND SURGICAL
BODY SYSTEM: G ENDOCRINE SYSTEM
OPERATION: B EXCISION: Cutting out or off, without replacement, a portion of a body part

Body Part	Approach	Device	Qualifier
Ø Pituitary Gland 1 Pineal Body 2 Adrenal Gland, Left 3 Adrenal Gland, Right 4 Adrenal Glands, Bilateral 6 Carotid Body, Left 7 Carotid Body, Right 8 Carotid Bodies, Bilateral 9 Para-aortic Body B Coccygeal Glomus C Glomus Jugulare D Aortic Body F Paraganglion Extremity G Thyroid Gland Lobe, Left H Thyroid Gland Lobe, Right J Thyroid Gland Isthmus L Superior Parathyroid Gland, Right M Superior Parathyroid Gland, Left N Inferior Parathyroid Gland, Right P Inferior Parathyroid Gland, Left Q Parathyroid Glands, Multiple R Parathyroid Gland	Ø Open 3 Percutaneous 4 Percutaneous Endoscopic	Z No Device	X Diagnostic Z No Qualifier

Non-OR ØGB[234GH][34]ZX

Coding Clinic: 2Ø17, Q2, P2Ø – ØGB[GH]ØZZ
Coding Clinic: 2Ø21, Q2, P7– ØGB9ØZZ

SECTION: Ø MEDICAL AND SURGICAL
BODY SYSTEM: G ENDOCRINE SYSTEM
OPERATION: C EXTIRPATION: Taking or cutting out solid matter from a body part

Body Part	Approach	Device	Qualifier
Ø Pituitary Gland 1 Pineal Body 2 Adrenal Gland, Left 3 Adrenal Gland, Right 4 Adrenal Glands, Bilateral 6 Carotid Body, Left 7 Carotid Body, Right 8 Carotid Bodies, Bilateral 9 Para-aortic Body B Coccygeal Glomus C Glomus Jugulare D Aortic Body F Paraganglion Extremity G Thyroid Gland Lobe, Left H Thyroid Gland Lobe, Right K Thyroid Gland L Superior Parathyroid Gland, Right M Superior Parathyroid Gland, Left N Inferior Parathyroid Gland, Right P Inferior Parathyroid Gland, Left Q Parathyroid Glands, Multiple R Parathyroid Gland	Ø Open 3 Percutaneous 4 Percutaneous Endoscopic	Z No Device	Z No Qualifier

SECTION: Ø MEDICAL AND SURGICAL
BODY SYSTEM: G ENDOCRINE SYSTEM
OPERATION: H INSERTION: Putting in a nonbiological appliance that monitors, assists, performs, or prevents a physiological function but does not physically take the place of a body part

Body Part	Approach	Device	Qualifier
S Endocrine Gland	Ø Open 3 Percutaneous 4 Percutaneous Endoscopic	1 Radioactive Element 2 Monitoring Device 3 Infusion Device Y Other Device	Z No Qualifier

SECTION: Ø MEDICAL AND SURGICAL
BODY SYSTEM: G ENDOCRINE SYSTEM
OPERATION: J INSPECTION: Visually and/or manually exploring a body part

Body Part	Approach	Device	Qualifier
Ø Pituitary Gland 1 Pineal Body 5 Adrenal Gland K Thyroid Gland R Parathyroid Gland S Endocrine Gland	Ø Open 3 Percutaneous 4 Percutaneous Endoscopic	Z No Device	Z No Qualifier

Non-OR ØGJ[Ø15KRS]3ZZ

SECTION: Ø MEDICAL AND SURGICAL
BODY SYSTEM: G ENDOCRINE SYSTEM
OPERATION: M REATTACHMENT: Putting back in or on all or a portion of a separated body part to its normal location or other suitable location

Body Part	Approach	Device	Qualifier
2 Adrenal Gland, Left 3 Adrenal Gland, Right G Thyroid Gland Lobe, Left H Thyroid Gland Lobe, Right L Superior Parathyroid Gland, Right M Superior Parathyroid Gland, Left N Inferior Parathyroid Gland, Right P Inferior Parathyroid Gland, Left Q Parathyroid Glands, Multiple R Parathyroid Gland	Ø Open 4 Percutaneous Endoscopic	Z No Device	Z No Qualifier

SECTION: Ø MEDICAL AND SURGICAL
BODY SYSTEM: G ENDOCRINE SYSTEM
OPERATION: N RELEASE: Freeing a body part from an abnormal physical constraint by cutting or by the use of force

Body Part	Approach	Device	Qualifier
Ø Pituitary Gland 1 Pineal Body 2 Adrenal Gland, Left 3 Adrenal Gland, Right 4 Adrenal Glands, Bilateral 6 Carotid Body, Left 7 Carotid Body, Right 8 Carotid Bodies, Bilateral 9 Para-aortic Body B Coccygeal Glomus C Glomus Jugulare D Aortic Body F Paraganglion Extremity G Thyroid Gland Lobe, Left H Thyroid Gland Lobe, Right K Thyroid Gland L Superior Parathyroid Gland, Right M Superior Parathyroid Gland, Left N Inferior Parathyroid Gland, Right P Inferior Parathyroid Gland, Left Q Parathyroid Glands, Multiple R Parathyroid Gland	Ø Open 3 Percutaneous 4 Percutaneous Endoscopic	Z No Device	Z No Qualifier

SECTION: Ø MEDICAL AND SURGICAL
BODY SYSTEM: G ENDOCRINE SYSTEM
OPERATION: P REMOVAL: Taking out or off a device from a body part

Body Part	Approach	Device	Qualifier
Ø Pituitary Gland 1 Pineal Body 5 Adrenal Gland K Thyroid Gland R Parathyroid Gland	Ø Open 3 Percutaneous 4 Percutaneous Endoscopic X External	Ø Drainage Device	Z No Qualifier
S Endocrine Gland	Ø Open 3 Percutaneous 4 Percutaneous Endoscopic	Ø Drainage Device 2 Monitoring Device 3 Infusion Device Y Other Device	Z No Qualifier
S Endocrine Gland	X External	Ø Drainage Device 2 Monitoring Device 3 Infusion Device	Z No Qualifier

Non-OR ØGP[Ø15KR]XØZ
Non-OR ØGPSX[Ø23]Z

SECTION: Ø MEDICAL AND SURGICAL
BODY SYSTEM: G ENDOCRINE SYSTEM
OPERATION: Q REPAIR: Restoring, to the extent possible, a body part to its normal anatomic structure and function

Body Part	Approach	Device	Qualifier
Ø Pituitary Gland 1 Pineal Body 2 Adrenal Gland, Left 3 Adrenal Gland, Right 4 Adrenal Glands, Bilateral 6 Carotid Body, Left 7 Carotid Body, Right 8 Carotid Bodies, Bilateral 9 Para-aortic Body B Coccygeal Glomus C Glomus Jugulare D Aortic Body F Paraganglion Extremity G Thyroid Gland Lobe, Left H Thyroid Gland Lobe, Right J Thyroid Gland Isthmus K Thyroid Gland L Superior Parathyroid Gland, Right M Superior Parathyroid Gland, Left N Inferior Parathyroid Gland, Right P Inferior Parathyroid Gland, Left Q Parathyroid Glands, Multiple R Parathyroid Gland	Ø Open 3 Percutaneous 4 Percutaneous Endoscopic	Z No Device	Z No Qualifier

SECTION: Ø MEDICAL AND SURGICAL
BODY SYSTEM: G ENDOCRINE SYSTEM
OPERATION: S REPOSITION: Moving to its normal location, or other suitable location, all or a portion of a body part

Body Part	Approach	Device	Qualifier
2 Adrenal Gland, Left 3 Adrenal Gland, Right G Thyroid Gland Lobe, Left H Thyroid Gland Lobe, Right L Superior Parathyroid Gland, Right M Superior Parathyroid Gland, Left N Inferior Parathyroid Gland, Right P Inferior Parathyroid Gland, Left Q Parathyroid Glands, Multiple R Parathyroid Gland	Ø Open 4 Percutaneous Endoscopic	Z No Device	Z No Qualifier

SECTION: Ø MEDICAL AND SURGICAL
BODY SYSTEM: G ENDOCRINE SYSTEM
OPERATION: T RESECTION: Cutting out or off, without replacement, all of a body part

Body Part	Approach	Device	Qualifier
Ø Pituitary Gland 1 Pineal Body 2 Adrenal Gland, Left 3 Adrenal Gland, Right 4 Adrenal Glands, Bilateral 6 Carotid Body, Left 7 Carotid Body, Right 8 Carotid Bodies, Bilateral 9 Para-aortic Body B Coccygeal Glomus C Glomus Jugulare D Aortic Body F Paraganglion Extremity G Thyroid Gland Lobe, Left H Thyroid Gland Lobe, Right J Thyroid Gland Isthmus K Thyroid Gland L Superior Parathyroid Gland, Right M Superior Parathyroid Gland, Left N Inferior Parathyroid Gland, Right P Inferior Parathyroid Gland, Left Q Parathyroid Glands, Multiple R Parathyroid Gland	Ø Open 4 Percutaneous Endoscopic	Z No Device	Z No Qualifier

SECTION: Ø MEDICAL AND SURGICAL
BODY SYSTEM: G ENDOCRINE SYSTEM
OPERATION: W REVISION: Correcting, to the extent possible, a portion of a malfunctioning device or the position of a displaced device

Body Part	Approach	Device	Qualifier
Ø Pituitary Gland 1 Pineal Body 5 Adrenal Gland K Thyroid Gland R Parathyroid Gland	Ø Open 3 Percutaneous 4 Percutaneous Endoscopic X External	Ø Drainage Device	Z No Qualifier
S Endocrine Gland	Ø Open 3 Percutaneous 4 Percutaneous Endoscopic	Ø Drainage Device 2 Monitoring Device 3 Infusion Device Y Other Device	Z No Qualifier
S Endocrine Gland	X External	Ø Drainage Device 2 Monitoring Device 3 Infusion Device	Z No Qualifier

Non-OR ØGW[Ø15KR]XØZ
Non-OR ØGWSX[Ø23]Z

SECTION: Ø MEDICAL AND SURGICAL
BODY SYSTEM: H SKIN AND BREAST
OPERATION: Ø ALTERATION: Modifying the anatomic structure of a body part without affecting the function of the body part

Body Part	Approach	Device	Qualifier
T Breast, Right U Breast, Left V Breast, Bilateral	Ø Open 3 Percutaneous X External	7 Autologous Tissue Substitute J Synthetic Substitute K Nonautologous Tissue Substitute Z No Device	Z No Qualifier

Coding Clinic: 2022, Q1, P15 – ØHØTØZZ

SECTION: Ø MEDICAL AND SURGICAL
BODY SYSTEM: H SKIN AND BREAST
OPERATION: 2 CHANGE: Taking out or off a device from a body part and putting back an identical or similar device in or on the same body part without cutting or puncturing the skin or a mucous membrane

Body Part	Approach	Device	Qualifier
P Skin T Breast, Right U Breast, Left	X External	Ø Drainage Device Y Other Device	Z No Qualifier

Non-OR All Values

SECTION: Ø MEDICAL AND SURGICAL
BODY SYSTEM: H SKIN AND BREAST
OPERATION: 5 DESTRUCTION: Physical eradication of all or a portion of a body part by the direct use of energy, force, or a destructive agent

Body Part	Approach	Device	Qualifier
Ø Skin, Scalp 1 Skin, Face 2 Skin, Right Ear 3 Skin, Left Ear 4 Skin, Neck 5 Skin, Chest 6 Skin, Back 7 Skin, Abdomen 8 Skin, Buttock 9 Skin, Perineum A Skin, Inguinal B Skin, Right Upper Arm C Skin, Left Upper Arm D Skin, Right Lower Arm E Skin, Left Lower Arm F Skin, Right Hand G Skin, Left Hand H Skin, Right Upper Leg J Skin, Left Upper Leg K Skin, Right Lower Leg L Skin, Left Lower Leg M Skin, Right Foot N Skin, Left Foot	X External	Z No Device	D Multiple Z No Qualifier
Q Finger Nail R Toe Nail	X External	Z No Device	Z No Qualifier
T Breast, Right U Breast, Left V Breast, Bilateral	Ø Open 3 Percutaneous	Z No Device	3 Laser Interstitial Thermal Therapy Z No Qualifier
T Breast, Right U Breast, Left V Breast, Bilateral	7 Via Natural or Artificial Opening 8 Via Natural or Artificial Opening Endoscopic	Z No Device	Z No Qualifier
W Nipple, Right X Nipple, Left	Ø Open 3 Percutaneous 7 Via Natural or Artificial Opening 8 Via Natural or Artificial Opening Endoscopic X External	Z No Device	Z No Qualifier

DRG Non-OR ØH5[Ø1456789ABCDEFGHJKLMN]XZ[DZ]
DRG Non-OR ØH5[QR]XZZ
Non-OR ØH5[23]XZ[DZ]
Non-OR ØH5[TUV][Ø3]Z[3Z]

SECTION: Ø MEDICAL AND SURGICAL
BODY SYSTEM: H SKIN AND BREAST
OPERATION: 8 DIVISION: Cutting into a body part, without draining fluids and/or gases from the body part, in order to separate or transect a body part

Body Part	Approach	Device	Qualifier
Ø Skin, Scalp 1 Skin, Face 2 Skin, Right Ear 3 Skin, Left Ear 4 Skin, Neck 5 Skin, Chest 6 Skin, Back 7 Skin, Abdomen 8 Skin, Buttock 9 Skin, Perineum A Skin, Inguinal B Skin, Right Upper Arm C Skin, Left Upper Arm D Skin, Right Lower Arm E Skin, Left Lower Arm F Skin, Right Hand G Skin, Left Hand H Skin, Right Upper Leg J Skin, Left Upper Leg K Skin, Right Lower Leg L Skin, Left Lower Leg M Skin, Right Foot N Skin, Left Foot	X External	Z No Device	Z No Qualifier

DRG Non-OR ØH8[Ø1456789ABCDEFGHJKLMN]XZZ
Non-OR ØH8[23]XZZ

SECTION: Ø MEDICAL AND SURGICAL
BODY SYSTEM: H SKIN AND BREAST
OPERATION: 9 DRAINAGE: *(on multiple pages)*
Taking or letting out fluids and/or gases from a body part

Body Part	Approach	Device	Qualifier
Ø Skin, Scalp 1 Skin, Face 2 Skin, Right Ear 3 Skin, Left Ear 4 Skin, Neck 5 Skin, Chest 6 Skin, Back 7 Skin, Abdomen 8 Skin, Buttock 9 Skin, Perineum A Skin, Inguinal B Skin, Right Upper Arm C Skin, Left Upper Arm D Skin, Right Lower Arm E Skin, Left Lower Arm F Skin, Right Hand G Skin, Left Hand H Skin, Right Upper Leg J Skin, Left Upper Leg K Skin, Right Lower Leg L Skin, Left Lower Leg M Skin, Right Foot N Skin, Left Foot Q Finger Nail R Toe Nail	X External	Ø Drainage Device	Z No Qualifier
Ø Skin, Scalp 1 Skin, Face 2 Skin, Right Ear 3 Skin, Left Ear 4 Skin, Neck 5 Skin, Chest 6 Skin, Back 7 Skin, Abdomen 8 Skin, Buttock 9 Skin, Perineum A Skin, Inguinal B Skin, Right Upper Arm C Skin, Left Upper Arm D Skin, Right Lower Arm E Skin, Left Lower Arm F Skin, Right Hand G Skin, Left Hand H Skin, Right Upper Leg J Skin, Left Upper Leg K Skin, Right Lower Leg L Skin, Left Lower Leg M Skin, Right Foot N Skin, Left Foot Q Finger Nail R Toe Nail	X External	Z No Device	X Diagnostic Z No Qualifier

Non-OR ØH9[Ø12345678ABCDEFGHJKLMNQR]XØZ
Non-OR ØH9[Ø123456789ABCDEFGHJKLMNQR]XZX
Non-OR ØH9[Ø12345678ABCDEFGHJKLMNQR]XZZ

SECTION: Ø MEDICAL AND SURGICAL
BODY SYSTEM: H SKIN AND BREAST
OPERATION: 9 DRAINAGE: *(continued)*
Taking or letting out fluids and/or gases from a body part

Body Part	Approach	Device	Qualifier
T Breast, Right U Breast, Left V Breast, Bilateral	Ø Open 3 Percutaneous 7 Via Natural or Artificial Opening 8 Via Natural or Artificial Opening Endoscopic X External	Ø Drainage Device	Z No Qualifier
T Breast, Right U Breast, Left V Breast, Bilateral	Ø Open 3 Percutaneous 7 Via Natural or Artificial Opening 8 Via Natural or Artificial Opening Endoscopic X External	Z No Device	X Diagnostic Z No Qualifier
W Nipple, Right X Nipple, Left	Ø Open 3 Percutaneous 7 Via Natural or Artificial Opening 8 Via Natural or Artificial Opening Endoscopic X External	Ø Drainage Device	Z No Qualifier
W Nipple, Right X Nipple, Left	Ø Open 3 Percutaneous 7 Via Natural or Artificial Opening 8 Via Natural or Artificial Opening Endoscopic X External	Z No Device	X Diagnostic Z No Qualifier

Non-OR ØH9[TUVWX][Ø378X]ØZ
Non-OR ØH9[TUVWX][378X]ZX
Non-OR ØH9[TUVWX][Ø378X]ZZ

SECTION: Ø MEDICAL AND SURGICAL
BODY SYSTEM: H SKIN AND BREAST
OPERATION: B EXCISION: *(on multiple pages)*
Cutting out or off, without replacement, a portion of a body part

Body Part	Approach	Device	Qualifier
Ø Skin, Scalp 1 Skin, Face 2 Skin, Right Ear 3 Skin, Left Ear 4 Skin, Neck 5 Skin, Chest 6 Skin, Back 7 Skin, Abdomen 8 Skin, Buttock 9 Skin, Perineum A Skin, Inguinal B Skin, Right Upper Arm C Skin, Left Upper Arm D Skin, Right Lower Arm E Skin, Left Lower Arm F Skin, Right Hand G Skin, Left Hand H Skin, Right Upper Leg J Skin, Left Upper Leg K Skin, Right Lower Leg L Skin, Left Lower Leg M Skin, Right Foot N Skin, Left Foot Q Finger Nail R Toe Nail	X External	Z No Device	X Diagnostic Z No Qualifier

DRG Non-OR ØHB9XZZ
DRG Non-OR ØHB[Ø145678ABCDEFGHJKLMN]XZZ
Non-OR ØHB[Ø12456789ABCDEFGHJKLMNQR]XZX
Non-OR ØHB[23QR]XZZ
Coding Clinic: 2Ø16, Q3, P29 – ØHBJXZZ
Coding Clinic: 2Ø2Ø, Q1, P31 – ØHBHXZZ

SECTION: Ø MEDICAL AND SURGICAL
BODY SYSTEM: H SKIN AND BREAST
OPERATION: B EXCISION: *(continued)*
Cutting out or off, without replacement, a portion of a body part

Body Part	Approach	Device	Qualifier
T Breast, Right U Breast, Left V Breast, Bilateral Y Supernumerary Breast	Ø Open 3 Percutaneous 7 Via Natural or Artificial Opening 8 Via Natural or Artificial Opening Endoscopic X External	Z No Device	X Diagnostic Z No Qualifier
W Nipple, Right X Nipple, Left	Ø Open 3 Percutaneous 7 Via Natural or Artificial Opening 8 Via Natural or Artificial Opening Endoscopic X External	Z No Device	X Diagnostic Z No Qualifier

Non-OR ØHB[TUVWXY][378X]ZX

Coding Clinic: 2015, Q3, P3 – ØHB8XZZ
Coding Clinic: 2018, Q1, P15 – ØHBTØZZ
Coding Clinic: 2022, Q1, P14 – ØHBUØZZ

SECTION: Ø MEDICAL AND SURGICAL
BODY SYSTEM: H SKIN AND BREAST
OPERATION: C EXTIRPATION: *(on multiple pages)*
Taking or cutting out solid matter from a body part

Body Part	Approach	Device	Qualifier
Ø Skin, Scalp 1 Skin, Face 2 Skin, Right Ear 3 Skin, Left Ear 4 Skin, Neck 5 Skin, Chest 6 Skin, Back 7 Skin, Abdomen 8 Skin, Buttock 9 Skin, Perineum A Skin, Inguinal B Skin, Right Upper Arm C Skin, Left Upper Arm D Skin, Right Lower Arm E Skin, Left Lower Arm F Skin, Right Hand G Skin, Left Hand H Skin, Right Upper Leg J Skin, Left Upper Leg K Skin, Right Lower Leg L Skin, Left Lower Leg M Skin, Right Foot N Skin, Left Foot Q Finger Nail R Toe Nail	X External	Z No Device	Z No Qualifier
T Breast, Right U Breast, Left V Breast, Bilateral	Ø Open 3 Percutaneous 7 Via Natural or Artificial Opening 8 Via Natural or Artificial Opening Endoscopic X External	Z No Device	Z No Qualifier

Non-OR All Values

SECTION: Ø MEDICAL AND SURGICAL
BODY SYSTEM: H SKIN AND BREAST
OPERATION: C EXTIRPATION: *(continued)*
Taking or cutting out solid matter from a body part

Body Part	Approach	Device	Qualifier
W Nipple, Right X Nipple, Left	Ø Open 3 Percutaneous 7 Via Natural or Artificial Opening 8 Via Natural or Artificial Opening Endoscopic X External	Z No Device	Z No Qualifier

SECTION: Ø MEDICAL AND SURGICAL
BODY SYSTEM: H SKIN AND BREAST
OPERATION: D EXTRACTION: Pulling or stripping out or off all or a portion of a body part by the use of force

Body Part	Approach	Device	Qualifier
Ø Skin, Scalp 1 Skin, Face 2 Skin, Right Ear 3 Skin, Left Ear 4 Skin, Neck 5 Skin, Chest 6 Skin, Back 7 Skin, Abdomen 8 Skin, Buttock 9 Skin, Perineum A Skin, Inguinal B Skin, Right Upper Arm C Skin, Left Upper Arm D Skin, Right Lower Arm E Skin, Left Lower Arm F Skin, Right Hand G Skin, Left Hand H Skin, Right Upper Leg J Skin, Left Upper Leg K Skin, Right Lower Leg L Skin, Left Lower Leg M Skin, Right Foot N Skin, Left Foot Q Finger Nail R Toe Nail S Hair	X External	Z No Device	Z No Qualifier
T Breast, Right U Breast, Left V Breast, Bilateral Y Supernumerary Breast	Ø Open	Z No Device	Z No Qualifier

Non-OR All Values

Coding Clinic: 2Ø15, Q3, P5-6 – ØHD[6H]XZZ

SECTION: Ø MEDICAL AND SURGICAL
BODY SYSTEM: H SKIN AND BREAST
OPERATION: H INSERTION: Putting in a nonbiological appliance that monitors, assists, performs, or prevents a physiological function but does not physically take the place of a body part

Body Part	Approach	Device	Qualifier
P Skin	X External	Y Other Device	Z No Qualifier
T Breast, Right U Breast, Left	Ø Open 3 Percutaneous 7 Via Natural or Artificial Opening 8 Via Natural or Artificial Opening Endoscopic	1 Radioactive Element N Tissue Expander Y Other Device	Z No Qualifier
T Breast, Right U Breast, Left	X External	1 Radioactive Element	Z No Qualifier
V Breast, Bilateral	Ø Open 3 Percutaneous 7 Via Natural or Artificial Opening 8 Via Natural or Artificial Opening Endoscopic	1 Radioactive Element N Tissue Expander	Z No Qualifier
W Nipple, Right X Nipple, Left	Ø Open 3 Percutaneous 7 Via Natural or Artificial Opening 8 Via Natural or Artificial Opening Endoscopic	1 Radioactive Element N Tissue Expander	Z No Qualifier
W Nipple, Right X Nipple, Left	X External	1 Radioactive Element	Z No Qualifier

Coding Clinic: 2017, Q4, P67 – ØHHTØNZ

SECTION: Ø MEDICAL AND SURGICAL
BODY SYSTEM: H SKIN AND BREAST
OPERATION: J INSPECTION: Visually and/or manually exploring a body part

Body Part	Approach	Device	Qualifier
P Skin Q Finger Nail R Toe Nail	X External	Z No Device	Z No Qualifier
T Breast, Right U Breast, Left	Ø Open 3 Percutaneous 7 Via Natural or Artificial Opening 8 Via Natural or Artificial Opening Endoscopic	Z No Device	Z No Qualifier

Non-OR All Values

SECTION: Ø MEDICAL AND SURGICAL
BODY SYSTEM: H SKIN AND BREAST
OPERATION: M REATTACHMENT: Putting back in or on all or a portion of a separated body part to its normal location or other suitable location

Body Part	Approach	Device	Qualifier
Ø Skin, Scalp 1 Skin, Face 2 Skin, Right Ear 3 Skin, Left Ear 4 Skin, Neck 5 Skin, Chest 6 Skin, Back 7 Skin, Abdomen 8 Skin, Buttock 9 Skin, Perineum A Skin, Inguinal B Skin, Right Upper Arm C Skin, Left Upper Arm D Skin, Right Lower Arm E Skin, Left Lower Arm F Skin, Right Hand G Skin, Left Hand H Skin, Right Upper Leg J Skin, Left Upper Leg K Skin, Right Lower Leg L Skin, Left Lower Leg M Skin, Right Foot N Skin, Left Foot T Breast, Right U Breast, Left V Breast, Bilateral W Nipple, Right X Nipple, Left	X External	Z No Device	Z No Qualifier

Non-OR ØHMØXZZ

SECTION: Ø MEDICAL AND SURGICAL
BODY SYSTEM: H SKIN AND BREAST
OPERATION: N RELEASE: Freeing a body part from an abnormal physical constraint by cutting or by the use of force

Body Part	Approach	Device	Qualifier
Ø Skin, Scalp 1 Skin, Face 2 Skin, Right Ear 3 Skin, Left Ear 4 Skin, Neck 5 Skin, Chest 6 Skin, Back 7 Skin, Abdomen 8 Skin, Buttock 9 Skin, Perineum A Skin, Inguinal B Skin, Right Upper Arm C Skin, Left Upper Arm D Skin, Right Lower Arm E Skin, Left Lower Arm F Skin, Right Hand G Skin, Left Hand H Skin, Right Upper Leg J Skin, Left Upper Leg K Skin, Right Lower Leg L Skin, Left Lower Leg M Skin, Right Foot N Skin, Left Foot Q Finger Nail R Toe Nail	X External	Z No Device	Z No Qualifier
T Breast, Right U Breast, Left V Breast, Bilateral	Ø Open 3 Percutaneous 7 Via Natural or Artificial Opening 8 Via Natural or Artificial Opening Endoscopic X External	Z No Device	Z No Qualifier
W Nipple, Right X Nipple, Left	Ø Open 3 Percutaneous 7 Via Natural or Artificial Opening 8 Via Natural or Artificial Opening Endoscopic X External	Z No Device	Z No Qualifier

SECTION: Ø MEDICAL AND SURGICAL
BODY SYSTEM: H SKIN AND BREAST
OPERATION: P REMOVAL: Taking out or off a device from a body part

Body Part	Approach	Device	Qualifier
P Skin	X External	Ø Drainage Device 7 Autologous Tissue Substitute J Synthetic Substitute K Nonautologous Tissue Substitute Y Other Device	Z No Qualifier
Q Finger Nail R Toe Nail	X External	Ø Drainage Device 7 Autologous Tissue Substitute J Synthetic Substitute K Nonautologous Tissue Substitute	Z No Qualifier
S Hair	X External	7 Autologous Tissue Substitute J Synthetic Substitute K Nonautologous Tissue Substitute	Z No Qualifier
T Breast, Right U Breast, Left	Ø Open 3 Percutaneous 7 Via Natural or Artificial Opening 8 Via Natural or Artificial Opening Endoscopic	Ø Drainage Device 1 Radioactive Element 7 Autologous Tissue Substitute J Synthetic Substitute K Nonautologous Tissue Substitute N Tissue Expander Y Other Device	Z No Qualifier

Non-OR ØPHPX[Ø7JK]Z
Non-OR ØHP[QR]X[Ø7JK]Z
Non-OR ØHPSX[7JK]Z
Non-OR ØHP[TU][Ø3][Ø17K]Z
Non-OR ØHP[TU][78][Ø17JKN]Z

Coding Clinic: 2Ø16, Q2, P27 – ØHP[TU]Ø7Z
Coding Clinic: 2Ø22, Q3, P21 – ØHP[TU]ØNZ

SECTION: Ø MEDICAL AND SURGICAL
BODY SYSTEM: H SKIN AND BREAST
OPERATION: Q REPAIR: Restoring, to the extent possible, a body part to its normal anatomic structure and function

Body Part	Approach	Device	Qualifier
Ø Skin, Scalp 1 Skin, Face 2 Skin, Right Ear 3 Skin, Left Ear 4 Skin, Neck 5 Skin, Chest 6 Skin, Back 7 Skin, Abdomen 8 Skin, Buttock 9 Skin, Perineum A Skin, Inguinal B Skin, Right Upper Arm C Skin, Left Upper Arm D Skin, Right Lower Arm E Skin, Left Lower Arm F Skin, Right Hand G Skin, Left Hand H Skin, Right Upper Leg J Skin, Left Upper Leg K Skin, Right Lower Leg L Skin, Left Lower Leg M Skin, Right Foot N Skin, Left Foot Q Finger Nail R Toe Nail	X External	Z No Device	Z No Qualifier
T Breast, Right U Breast, Left V Breast, Bilateral Y Supernumerary Breast	Ø Open 3 Percutaneous 7 Via Natural or Artificial Opening 8 Via Natural or Artificial Opening Endoscopic X External	Z No Device	Z No Qualifier
W Nipple, Right X Nipple, Left	Ø Open 3 Percutaneous 7 Via Natural or Artificial Opening 8 Via Natural or Artificial Opening Endoscopic X External	Z No Device	Z No Qualifier

DRG Non-OR ØHQ9XZZ
Non-OR ØHQ[Ø12345678ABCDEFGHJKLMN]XZZ
Non-OR ØHQ[TUVY]XZZ

Coding Clinic: 2016, Q1, P7 – ØHQ9XZZ

SECTION: Ø MEDICAL AND SURGICAL
BODY SYSTEM: H SKIN AND BREAST
OPERATION: R REPLACEMENT: *(on multiple pages)*

Putting in or on biological or synthetic material that physically takes the place and/or function of all or a portion of a body part

Body Part	Approach	Device	Qualifier
Ø Skin, Scalp 1 Skin, Face 2 Skin, Right Ear 3 Skin, Left Ear 4 Skin, Neck 5 Skin, Chest 6 Skin, Back 7 Skin, Abdomen 8 Skin, Buttock 9 Skin, Perineum A Skin, Inguinal B Skin, Right Upper Arm C Skin, Left Upper Arm D Skin, Right Lower Arm E Skin, Left Lower Arm F Skin, Right Hand G Skin, Left Hand H Skin, Right Upper Leg J Skin, Left Upper Leg K Skin, Right Lower Leg L Skin, Left Lower Leg M Skin, Right Foot N Skin, Left Foot	X External	7 Autologous Tissue Substitute	2 Cell Suspension Technique 3 Full Thickness 4 Partial Thickness
Ø Skin, Scalp 1 Skin, Face 2 Skin, Right Ear 3 Skin, Left Ear 4 Skin, Neck 5 Skin, Chest 6 Skin, Back 7 Skin, Abdomen 8 Skin, Buttock 9 Skin, Perineum A Skin, Inguinal B Skin, Right Upper Arm C Skin, Left Upper Arm D Skin, Right Lower Arm E Skin, Left Lower Arm F Skin, Right Hand G Skin, Left Hand H Skin, Right Upper Leg J Skin, Left Upper Leg K Skin, Right Lower Leg L Skin, Left Lower Leg M Skin, Right Foot N Skin, Left Foot	X External	J Synthetic Substitute	3 Full Thickness 4 Partial Thickness Z No Qualifier

Non-OR ØHRSX7Z

Coding Clinic: 2017, Q1, P36 – ØHRMXK3

SECTION: Ø MEDICAL AND SURGICAL
BODY SYSTEM: H SKIN AND BREAST
OPERATION: R REPLACEMENT: *(continued)*

Putting in or on biological or synthetic material that physically takes the place and/or function of all or a portion of a body part

Body Part	Approach	Device	Qualifier
Ø Skin, Scalp 1 Skin, Face 2 Skin, Right Ear 3 Skin, Left Ear 4 Skin, Neck 5 Skin, Chest 6 Skin, Back 7 Skin, Abdomen 8 Skin, Buttock 9 Skin, Perineum A Skin, Inguinal B Skin, Right Upper Arm C Skin, Left Upper Arm D Skin, Right Lower Arm E Skin, Left Lower Arm F Skin, Right Hand G Skin, Left Hand H Skin, Right Upper Leg J Skin, Left Upper Leg K Skin, Right Lower Leg L Skin, Left Lower Leg M Skin, Right Foot N Skin, Left Foot	X External	K Nonautologous Tissue Substitute	3 Full Thickness 4 Partial Thickness
Q Finger Nail R Toe Nail S Hair	X External	7 Autologous Tissue Substitute J Synthetic Substitute K Nonautologous Tissue Substitute	Z No Qualifier
T Breast, Right U Breast, Left V Breast, Bilateral	Ø Open	7 Autologous Tissue Substitute	5 Latissimus Dorsi Myocutaneous Flap 6 Transverse Rectus Abdominis Myocutaneous Flap 7 Deep Inferior Epigastric Artery Perforator Flap 8 Superficial Inferior Epigastric Artery Flap 9 Gluteal Artery Perforator Flap Z No Qualifier
T Breast, Right U Breast, Left V Breast, Bilateral	Ø Open	J Synthetic Substitute K Nonautologous Tissue Substitute	Z No Qualifier
T Breast, Right ⊞ U Breast, Left ⊞ V Breast, Bilateral ⊞	3 Percutaneous	7 Autologous Tissue Substitute J Synthetic Substitute K Nonautologous Tissue Substitute	Z No Qualifier
W Nipple, Right X Nipple, Left	Ø Open 3 Percutaneous X External	7 Autologous Tissue Substitute J Synthetic Substitute K Nonautologous Tissue Substitute	Z No Qualifier

⊞ ØHR[TUV]37Z

Coding Clinic: 2020, Q1, P27 – ØHRUØ7Z

Coding Clinic: 2022, Q1, P15 – ØHRXØ7Z

SECTION: Ø **MEDICAL AND SURGICAL**
BODY SYSTEM: H **SKIN AND BREAST**
OPERATION: S **REPOSITION:** Moving to its normal location, or other suitable location, all or a portion of a body part

Body Part	Approach	Device	Qualifier
S Hair W Nipple, Right X Nipple, Left	X External	Z No Device	Z No Qualifier
T Breast, Right U Breast, Left V Breast, Bilateral	Ø Open	Z No Device	Z No Qualifier

Non-OR ØHSSXZZ

SECTION: Ø **MEDICAL AND SURGICAL**
BODY SYSTEM: H **SKIN AND BREAST**
OPERATION: T **RESECTION:** Cutting out or off, without replacement, all of a body part

Body Part	Approach	Device	Qualifier
Q Finger Nail R Toe Nail W Nipple, Right X Nipple, Left	X External	Z No Device	Z No Qualifier
T Breast, Right ⊞ U Breast, Left ⊞ V Breast, Bilateral ⊞ Y Supernumerary Breast	Ø Open	Z No Device	Z No Qualifier

⊞ ØHT[TUV]ØZZ
Non-OR ØHT[QR]XZZ

Coding Clinic: 2021, Q2, P16 – ØHTVØZZ

SECTION: Ø MEDICAL AND SURGICAL
BODY SYSTEM: H SKIN AND BREAST
OPERATION: U SUPPLEMENT: Putting in or on biological or synthetic material that physically reinforces and/or augments the function of a portion of a body part

Body Part	Approach	Device	Qualifier
T Breast, Right U Breast, Left V Breast, Bilateral	Ø Open 3 Percutaneous 7 Via Natural of Artificial Opening 8 Via Natural or Artificial Opening Endoscopic	7 Autologous Tissue Substitute J Synthetic Substitute K Nonautologous Tissue Substitute	Z No Qualifier
W Nipple, Right X Nipple, Left	Ø Open 3 Percutaneous 7 Via Natural or Artificial Opening 8 Via Natural or Artificial Opening Endoscopic X External	7 Autologous Tissue Substitute J Synthetic Substitute K Nonautologous Tissue Substitute	Z No Qualifier

SECTION: Ø MEDICAL AND SURGICAL
BODY SYSTEM: H SKIN AND BREAST
OPERATION: W REVISION: Correcting, to the extent possible, a portion of a malfunctioning device or the position of a displaced device

Body Part	Approach	Device	Qualifier
P Skin	X External	Ø Drainage Device 7 Autologous Tissue Substitute J Synthetic Substitute K Nonautologous Tissue Substitute Y Other Device	Z No Qualifier
Q Finger Nail R Toe Nail	X External	Ø Drainage Device 7 Autologous Tissue Substitute J Synthetic Substitute K Nonautologous Tissue Substitute	Z No Qualifier
S Hair	X External	7 Autologous Tissue Substitute J Synthetic Substitute K Nonautologous Tissue Substitute	Z No Qualifier
T Breast, Right U Breast, Left	Ø Open 3 Percutaneous 7 Via Natural or Artificial Opening 8 Via Natural or Artificial Opening Endoscopic	Ø Drainage Device 7 Autologous Tissue Substitute J Synthetic Substitute K Nonautologous Tissue Substitute N Tissue Expander Y Other Device	Z No Qualifier

Non-OR ØHWPX[Ø7JK]Z
Non-OR ØHW[QR]X[Ø7JK]Z
Non-OR ØHWSX[7JK]Z
Non-OR ØHW[TU][Ø3][Ø7KN]Z
Non-OR ØHW[TU][78][Ø7JKN]Z

SECTION: Ø MEDICAL AND SURGICAL
BODY SYSTEM: H SKIN AND BREAST
OPERATION: X TRANSFER: Moving, without taking out, all or a portion of a body part to another location to take over the function of all or a portion of a body part

Body Part	Approach	Device	Qualifier
Ø Skin, Scalp 1 Skin, Face 2 Skin, Right Ear 3 Skin, Left Ear 4 Skin, Neck 5 Skin, Chest 6 Skin, Back 7 Skin, Abdomen 8 Skin, Buttock 9 Skin, Perineum A Skin, Inguinal B Skin, Right Upper Arm C Skin, Left Upper Arm D Skin, Right Lower Arm E Skin, Left Lower Arm F Skin, Right Hand G Skin, Left Hand H Skin, Right Upper Leg J Skin, Left Upper Leg K Skin, Right Lower Leg L Skin, Left Lower Leg M Skin, Right Foot N Skin, Left Foot	X External	Z No Device	Z No Qualifier

Coding Clinic: 2Ø23, Q2, P24,31; 2Ø22, Q3, P14 – ØHX9XZZ

SECTION: Ø MEDICAL AND SURGICAL
BODY SYSTEM: J SUBCUTANEOUS TISSUE AND FASCIA
OPERATION: Ø ALTERATION: Modifying the anatomic structure of a body part without affecting the function of the body part

Body Part	Approach	Device	Qualifier
1 Subcutaneous Tissue and Fascia, Face 4 Subcutaneous Tissue and Fascia, Right Neck 5 Subcutaneous Tissue and Fascia, Left Neck 6 Subcutaneous Tissue and Fascia, Chest 7 Subcutaneous Tissue and Fascia, Back 8 Subcutaneous Tissue and Fascia, Abdomen 9 Subcutaneous Tissue and Fascia, Buttock D Subcutaneous Tissue and Fascia, Right Upper Arm F Subcutaneous Tissue and Fascia, Left Upper Arm G Subcutaneous Tissue and Fascia, Right Lower Arm H Subcutaneous Tissue and Fascia, Left Lower Arm L Subcutaneous Tissue and Fascia, Right Upper Leg M Subcutaneous Tissue and Fascia, Left Upper Leg N Subcutaneous Tissue and Fascia, Right Lower Leg P Subcutaneous Tissue and Fascia, Left Lower Leg	Ø Open 3 Percutaneous	Z No Device	Z No Qualifier

SECTION: Ø MEDICAL AND SURGICAL
BODY SYSTEM: J SUBCUTANEOUS TISSUE AND FASCIA
OPERATION: 2 CHANGE: Taking out or off a device from a body part and putting back an identical or similar device in or on the same body part without cutting or puncturing the skin or a mucous membrane

Body Part	Approach	Device	Qualifier
S Subcutaneous Tissue and Fascia, Head and Neck T Subcutaneous Tissue and Fascia, Trunk V Subcutaneous Tissue and Fascia, Upper Extremity W Subcutaneous Tissue and Fascia, Lower Extremity	X External	Ø Drainage Device Y Other Device	Z No Qualifier

Non-OR All Values

Coding Clinic: 2Ø17, Q2, P25 – ØJ2TXYZ

SECTION: Ø MEDICAL AND SURGICAL
BODY SYSTEM: J SUBCUTANEOUS TISSUE AND FASCIA
OPERATION: 5 DESTRUCTION: Physical eradication of all or a portion of a body part by the direct use of energy, force, or a destructive agent

Body Part	Approach	Device	Qualifier
Ø Subcutaneous Tissue and Fascia, Scalp 1 Subcutaneous Tissue and Fascia, Face 4 Subcutaneous Tissue and Fascia, Right Neck 5 Subcutaneous Tissue and Fascia, Left Neck 6 Subcutaneous Tissue and Fascia, Chest 7 Subcutaneous Tissue and Fascia, Back 8 Subcutaneous Tissue and Fascia, Abdomen 9 Subcutaneous Tissue and Fascia, Buttock B Subcutaneous Tissue and Fascia, Perineum C Subcutaneous Tissue and Fascia, Pelvic Region D Subcutaneous Tissue and Fascia, Right Upper Arm F Subcutaneous Tissue and Fascia, Left Upper Arm G Subcutaneous Tissue and Fascia, Right Lower Arm H Subcutaneous Tissue and Fascia, Left Lower Arm J Subcutaneous Tissue and Fascia, Right Hand K Subcutaneous Tissue and Fascia, Left Hand L Subcutaneous Tissue and Fascia, Right Upper Leg M Subcutaneous Tissue and Fascia, Left Upper Leg N Subcutaneous Tissue and Fascia, Right Lower Leg P Subcutaneous Tissue and Fascia, Left Lower Leg Q Subcutaneous Tissue and Fascia, Right Foot R Subcutaneous Tissue and Fascia, Left Foot	Ø Open 3 Percutaneous	Z No Device	Z No Qualifier

DRG Non-OR All Values

SECTION: Ø MEDICAL AND SURGICAL
BODY SYSTEM: J SUBCUTANEOUS TISSUE AND FASCIA
OPERATION: 8 DIVISION: Cutting into a body part, without draining fluids and/or gases from the body part, in order to separate or transect a body part

Body Part	Approach	Device	Qualifier
Ø Subcutaneous Tissue and Fascia, Scalp 1 Subcutaneous Tissue and Fascia, Face 4 Subcutaneous Tissue and Fascia, Right Neck 5 Subcutaneous Tissue and Fascia, Left Neck 6 Subcutaneous Tissue and Fascia, Chest 7 Subcutaneous Tissue and Fascia, Back 8 Subcutaneous Tissue and Fascia, Abdomen 9 Subcutaneous Tissue and Fascia, Buttock B Subcutaneous Tissue and Fascia, Perineum C Subcutaneous Tissue and Fascia, Pelvic Region D Subcutaneous Tissue and Fascia, Right Upper Arm F Subcutaneous Tissue and Fascia, Left Upper Arm G Subcutaneous Tissue and Fascia, Right Lower Arm H Subcutaneous Tissue and Fascia, Left Lower Arm J Subcutaneous Tissue and Fascia, Right Hand K Subcutaneous Tissue and Fascia, Left Hand L Subcutaneous Tissue and Fascia, Right Upper Leg M Subcutaneous Tissue and Fascia, Left Upper Leg N Subcutaneous Tissue and Fascia, Right Lower Leg P Subcutaneous Tissue and Fascia, Left Lower Leg Q Subcutaneous Tissue and Fascia, Right Foot R Subcutaneous Tissue and Fascia, Left Foot S Subcutaneous Tissue and Fascia, Head and Neck T Subcutaneous Tissue and Fascia, Trunk V Subcutaneous Tissue and Fascia, Upper Extremity W Subcutaneous Tissue and Fascia, Lower Extremity	Ø Open 3 Percutaneous	Z No Device	Z No Qualifier

SECTION: Ø MEDICAL AND SURGICAL
BODY SYSTEM: J SUBCUTANEOUS TISSUE AND FASCIA
OPERATION: 9 DRAINAGE: *(on multiple pages)*
Taking or letting out fluids and/or gases from a body part

Body Part	Approach	Device	Qualifier
Ø Subcutaneous Tissue and Fascia, Scalp 1 Subcutaneous Tissue and Fascia, Face 4 Subcutaneous Tissue and Fascia, Right Neck 5 Subcutaneous Tissue and Fascia, Left Neck 6 Subcutaneous Tissue and Fascia, Chest 7 Subcutaneous Tissue and Fascia, Back 8 Subcutaneous Tissue and Fascia, Abdomen 9 Subcutaneous Tissue and Fascia, Buttock B Subcutaneous Tissue and Fascia, Perineum C Subcutaneous Tissue and Fascia, Pelvic Region D Subcutaneous Tissue and Fascia, Right Upper Arm F Subcutaneous Tissue and Fascia, Left Upper Arm G Subcutaneous Tissue and Fascia, Right Lower Arm H Subcutaneous Tissue and Fascia, Left Lower Arm J Subcutaneous Tissue and Fascia, Right Hand K Subcutaneous Tissue and Fascia, Left Hand L Subcutaneous Tissue and Fascia, Right Upper Leg M Subcutaneous Tissue and Fascia, Left Upper Leg N Subcutaneous Tissue and Fascia, Right Lower Leg P Subcutaneous Tissue and Fascia, Left Lower Leg Q Subcutaneous Tissue and Fascia, Right Foot R Subcutaneous Tissue and Fascia, Left Foot	Ø Open 3 Percutaneous	Ø Drainage Device	Z No Qualifier

DRG Non-OR ØJ9[1]ØØZ
Non-OR ØJ9[1JK]3ØZ
Non-OR ØJ9[Ø456789BCDFGHJKLMNPQR][Ø3]ØZ

SECTION: Ø MEDICAL AND SURGICAL
BODY SYSTEM: J SUBCUTANEOUS TISSUE AND FASCIA
OPERATION: 9 DRAINAGE: *(continued)*
Taking or letting out fluids and/or gases from a body part

Body Part	Approach	Device	Qualifier
Ø Subcutaneous Tissue and Fascia, Scalp 1 Subcutaneous Tissue and Fascia, Face 4 Subcutaneous Tissue and Fascia, Right Neck 5 Subcutaneous Tissue and Fascia, Left Neck 6 Subcutaneous Tissue and Fascia, Chest 7 Subcutaneous Tissue and Fascia, Back 8 Subcutaneous Tissue and Fascia, Abdomen 9 Subcutaneous Tissue and Fascia, Buttock B Subcutaneous Tissue and Fascia, Perineum C Subcutaneous Tissue and Fascia, Pelvic Region D Subcutaneous Tissue and Fascia, Right Upper Arm F Subcutaneous Tissue and Fascia, Left Upper Arm G Subcutaneous Tissue and Fascia, Right Lower Arm H Subcutaneous Tissue and Fascia, Left Lower Arm J Subcutaneous Tissue and Fascia, Right Hand K Subcutaneous Tissue and Fascia, Left Hand L Subcutaneous Tissue and Fascia, Right Upper Leg M Subcutaneous Tissue and Fascia, Left Upper Leg N Subcutaneous Tissue and Fascia, Right Lower Leg P Subcutaneous Tissue and Fascia, Left Lower Leg Q Subcutaneous Tissue and Fascia, Right Foot R Subcutaneous Tissue and Fascia, Left Foot	Ø Open 3 Percutaneous	Z No Device	X Diagnostic Z No Qualifier

DRG Non-OR ØJ9[Ø1456789BCDFGHLMNPQR]ØZZ
Non-OR ØJ9[Ø1456789BCDFGHJKLMNPQR][Ø3]ZX
Non-OR ØJ9[Ø1456789BCDFGHJKLMNPQR]3ZZ

Coding Clinic: 2Ø15, Q3, P24 – ØJ9[6CDFLM]ØZZ

SECTION: Ø MEDICAL AND SURGICAL
BODY SYSTEM: J SUBCUTANEOUS TISSUE AND FASCIA
OPERATION: B EXCISION: Cutting out or off, without replacement, a portion of a body part

Body Part	Approach	Device	Qualifier
Ø Subcutaneous Tissue and Fascia, Scalp 1 Subcutaneous Tissue and Fascia, Face 4 Subcutaneous Tissue and Fascia, Right Neck 5 Subcutaneous Tissue and Fascia, Left Neck 6 Subcutaneous Tissue and Fascia, Chest 7 Subcutaneous Tissue and Fascia, Back 8 Subcutaneous Tissue and Fascia, Abdomen 9 Subcutaneous Tissue and Fascia, Buttock B Subcutaneous Tissue and Fascia, Perineum C Subcutaneous Tissue and Fascia, Pelvic Region D Subcutaneous Tissue and Fascia, Right Upper Arm F Subcutaneous Tissue and Fascia, Left Upper Arm G Subcutaneous Tissue and Fascia, Right Lower Arm H Subcutaneous Tissue and Fascia, Left Lower Arm J Subcutaneous Tissue and Fascia, Right Hand K Subcutaneous Tissue and Fascia, Left Hand L Subcutaneous Tissue and Fascia, Right Upper Leg M Subcutaneous Tissue and Fascia, Left Upper Leg N Subcutaneous Tissue and Fascia, Right Lower Leg P Subcutaneous Tissue and Fascia, Left Lower Leg Q Subcutaneous Tissue and Fascia, Right Foot R Subcutaneous Tissue and Fascia, Left Foot	Ø Open 3 Percutaneous	Z No Device	X Diagnostic Z No Qualifier

DRG Non-OR ØJB[Ø456789BCDFGHLMNPQR]3ZZ
Non-OR ØJB[Ø1456789BCDFGHJKLMNPQR][Ø3]ZX

Coding Clinic: 2Ø15, Q1, P3Ø – ØJBBØZZ
Coding Clinic: 2Ø15, Q2, P13 – ØJBHØZZ
Coding Clinic: 2Ø15, Q3, P7 – ØJB9ØZZ
Coding Clinic: 2Ø23, Q2, P3Ø; 2Ø18, Q1, P7 – ØJB7ØZZ
Coding Clinic: 2Ø19, Q3, P25 – ØJB93ZZ
Coding Clinic: 2Ø2Ø, Q1, P31 – ØJB8ØZZ
Coding Clinic: 2Ø22, Q3, P13 – ØJBLØZZ

SECTION: Ø MEDICAL AND SURGICAL
BODY SYSTEM: J SUBCUTANEOUS TISSUE AND FASCIA
OPERATION: C EXTIRPATION: Taking or cutting out solid matter from a body part

Body Part	Approach	Device	Qualifier
Ø Subcutaneous Tissue and Fascia, Scalp 1 Subcutaneous Tissue and Fascia, Face 4 Subcutaneous Tissue and Fascia, Right Neck 5 Subcutaneous Tissue and Fascia, Left Neck 6 Subcutaneous Tissue and Fascia, Chest 7 Subcutaneous Tissue and Fascia, Back 8 Subcutaneous Tissue and Fascia, Abdomen 9 Subcutaneous Tissue and Fascia, Buttock B Subcutaneous Tissue and Fascia, Perineum C Subcutaneous Tissue and Fascia, Pelvic Region D Subcutaneous Tissue and Fascia, Right Upper Arm F Subcutaneous Tissue and Fascia, Left Upper Arm G Subcutaneous Tissue and Fascia, Right Lower Arm H Subcutaneous Tissue and Fascia, Left Lower Arm J Subcutaneous Tissue and Fascia, Right Hand K Subcutaneous Tissue and Fascia, Left Hand L Subcutaneous Tissue and Fascia, Right Upper Leg M Subcutaneous Tissue and Fascia, Left Upper Leg N Subcutaneous Tissue and Fascia, Right Lower Leg P Subcutaneous Tissue and Fascia, Left Lower Leg Q Subcutaneous Tissue and Fascia, Right Foot R Subcutaneous Tissue and Fascia, Left Foot	Ø Open 3 Percutaneous	Z No Device	Z No Qualifier

Non-OR All Values

Coding Clinic: 2Ø17, Q3, P22 – ØJC8ØZZ

SECTION: Ø MEDICAL AND SURGICAL
BODY SYSTEM: J SUBCUTANEOUS TISSUE AND FASCIA
OPERATION: D EXTRACTION: Pulling or stripping out or off all or a portion of a body part by the use of force

Body Part	Approach	Device	Qualifier
Ø Subcutaneous Tissue and Fascia, Scalp 1 Subcutaneous Tissue and Fascia, Face 4 Subcutaneous Tissue and Fascia, Right Neck 5 Subcutaneous Tissue and Fascia, Left Neck 6 Subcutaneous Tissue and Fascia, Chest ⊞ 7 Subcutaneous Tissue and Fascia, Back ⊞ 8 Subcutaneous Tissue and Fascia, Abdomen ⊞ 9 Subcutaneous Tissue and Fascia, Buttock ⊞ B Subcutaneous Tissue and Fascia, Perineum C Subcutaneous Tissue and Fascia, Pelvic Region D Subcutaneous Tissue and Fascia, Right Upper Arm F Subcutaneous Tissue and Fascia, Left Upper Arm G Subcutaneous Tissue and Fascia, Right Lower Arm H Subcutaneous Tissue and Fascia, Left Lower Arm J Subcutaneous Tissue and Fascia, Right Hand K Subcutaneous Tissue and Fascia, Left Hand L Subcutaneous Tissue and Fascia, Right Upper Leg ⊞ M Subcutaneous Tissue and Fascia, Left Upper Leg ⊞ N Subcutaneous Tissue and Fascia, Right Lower Leg P Subcutaneous Tissue and Fascia, Left Lower Leg Q Subcutaneous Tissue and Fascia, Right Foot R Subcutaneous Tissue and Fascia, Left Foot	Ø Open 3 Percutaneous	Z No Device	Z No Qualifier

⊞ ØJD[6789LM]3ZZ
DRG Non-OR ØJD[Ø1456789BCDFGHJKLMNPQR][Ø3]ZZ

Coding Clinic: 2015, Q1, P23 – ØJDCØZZ
Coding Clinic: 2016, Q1, P4Ø – ØJDLØZZ
Coding Clinic: 2016, Q3, P21-22 – ØJD[7NR]ØZZ
Coding Clinic: 2023, Q1, P36 – ØJDRØZZ

SECTION: Ø MEDICAL AND SURGICAL
BODY SYSTEM: J SUBCUTANEOUS TISSUE AND FASCIA
OPERATION: H INSERTION: *(on multiple pages)*

Putting in a nonbiological appliance that monitors, assists, performs, or prevents a physiological function but does not physically take the place of a body part

Body Part	Approach	Device	Qualifier
Ø Subcutaneous Tissue and Fascia, Scalp 1 Subcutaneous Tissue and Fascia, Face 4 Subcutaneous Tissue and Fascia, Right Neck 5 Subcutaneous Tissue and Fascia, Left Neck 9 Subcutaneous Tissue and Fascia, Buttock B Subcutaneous Tissue and Fascia, Perineum C Subcutaneous Tissue and Fascia, Pelvic Region J Subcutaneous Tissue and Fascia, Right Hand K Subcutaneous Tissue and Fascia, Left Hand Q Subcutaneous Tissue and Fascia, Right Foot R Subcutaneous Tissue and Fascia, Left Foot	Ø Open 3 Percutaneous	N Tissue Expander	Z No Qualifer
6 Subcutaneous Tissue and Fascia, Chest ⊞	Ø Open 3 Percutaneous	Ø Monitoring Device, Hemodynamic 2 Monitoring Device 4 Pacemaker, Single Chamber 5 Pacemaker, Single Chamber Rate Responsive 6 Pacemaker, Dual Chamber 7 Cardiac Resynchronization Pacemaker Pulse Generator 8 Defibrillator Generator 9 Cardiac Resynchronization Defibrillator Pulse Generator A Contractility Modulation Device B Stimulator Generator, Single Array C Stimulator Generator, Single Array Rechargeable D Stimulator Generator, Multiple Array E Stimulator Generator, Multiple Array Rechargeable F Subcutaneous Defibrillator Lead H Contraceptive Device M Stimulator Generator N Tissue Expander P Cardiac Rhythm Related Device V Infusion Device, Pump W Vascular Access Device, Totally Implantable X Vascular Access Device, Tunneled Y Other Device	Z No Qualifier
7 Subcutaneous Tissue and Fascia, Back ⊞	Ø Open 3 Percutaneous	B Stimulator Generator, Single Array C Stimulator Generator, Single Array Rechargeable D Stimulator Generator, Multiple Array E Stimulator Generator, Multiple Array Rechargeable M Stimulator Generator N Tissue Expander V Infusion Device, Pump Y Other Device	Z No Qualifier

ØJH[7][Ø3]MZ
⊞ ØJH[6][Ø3][Ø456789ABCDEF]Z
⊞ ØJH7[3][BCDE]Z
DRG Non-OR ØJH[6][Ø3][4567HPWX]Z
ØJH[6][Ø3][456789P]Z when reported with Secondary Diagnosis K68.11, T81.4XXA, or T82.7XXA, except ØJH63XZ
ØJH63XZ when reported with Secondary Diagnosis J95.811

Coding Clinic: 2Ø15, Q2, P33 – ØJH6ØXZ
Coding Clinic: 2Ø15, Q4, P15 – ØJH63VZ
Coding Clinic: 2Ø17, Q2, P25; 2Ø16, Q2, P16; 2Ø15, Q4, P31-32 – ØJH63XZ
Coding Clinic: 2Ø16, Q4, P99 – ØJH6ØMZ
Coding Clinic: 2Ø17, Q4, P64 – ØJH6ØWZ
Coding Clinic: 2Ø2Ø, Q2, P16 – ØJHS33Z
Coding Clinic: 2Ø2Ø, Q2, P17 – ØØHTØ3Z

SECTION: Ø MEDICAL AND SURGICAL
BODY SYSTEM: J SUBCUTANEOUS TISSUE AND FASCIA
OPERATION: H INSERTION: *(continued)*

Putting in a nonbiological appliance that monitors, assists, performs, or prevents a physiological function but does not physically take the place of a body part

Body Part	Approach	Device	Qualifier
8 Subcutaneous Tissue and Fascia, Abdomen ⊞	Ø Open 3 Percutaneous	Ø Monitoring Device, Hemodynamic 2 Monitoring Device 4 Pacemaker, Single Chamber 5 Pacemaker, Single Chamber Rate Responsive 6 Pacemaker, Dual Chamber 7 Cardiac Resynchronization Pacemaker Pulse Generator 8 Defibrillator Generator 9 Cardiac Resynchronization Defibrillator Pulse Generator A Contractility Modulation Device B Stimulator Generator, Single Array C Stimulator Generator, Single Array Rechargeable D Stimulator Generator, Multiple Array E Stimulator Generator, Multiple Array Rechargeable H Contraceptive Device M Stimulator Generator N Tissue Expander P Cardiac Rhythm Related Device V Infusion Device, Pump W Vascular Access Device, Totally Implantable X Vascular Access Device, Tunneled Y Other Device	Z No Qualifier
D Subcutaneous Tissue and Fascia, Right Upper Arm F Subcutaneous Tissue and Fascia, Left Upper Arm G Subcutaneous Tissue and Fascia, Right Lower Arm H Subcutaneous Tissue and Fascia, Left Lower Arm L Subcutaneous Tissue and Fascia, Right Upper Leg M Subcutaneous Tissue and Fascia, Left Upper Leg N Subcutaneous Tissue and Fascia, Right Lower Leg P Subcutaneous Tissue and Fascia, Left Lower Leg	Ø Open 3 Percutaneous	H Contraceptive Device N Tissue Expander V Infusion Device, Pump W Vascular Access Device, Totally Implantable X Vascular Access Device, Tunneled	Z No Qualifier
S Subcutaneous Tissue and Fascia, Head and Neck V Subcutaneous Tissue and Fascia, Upper Extremity W Subcutaneous Tissue and Fascia, Lower Extremity	Ø Open 3 Percutaneous	1 Radioactive Element 3 Infusion Device Y Other Device	Z No Qualifier
T Subcutaneous Tissue and Fascia, Trunk	Ø Open 3 Percutaneous	1 Radioactive Element 3 Infusion Device V Infusion Device, Pump Y Other Device	Z No Qualifier

ØJH[8][Ø3]MZ
⊞ ØJH8[Ø3][Ø456789ABCDEP]Z
DRG Non-OR ØJH[DFGHLM][Ø3][WX]Z
DRG Non-OR ØJHNØ[WX]Z
DRG Non-OR ØJHN3[HWX]Z
DRG Non-OR ØJHP[Ø3][HWX]Z
DRG Non-OR ØJH[SVW][Ø3]3Z
DRG Non-OR ØJHT[Ø3]3Z
DRG Non-OR ØJH8[Ø3][2456789ABCDEHPWX]Z

Non-OR ØJH[DFGHLM][Ø3]HZ
Non-OR ØJHNØHZ
Non-OR ØJH[SVW][Ø3]3Z
Non-OR ØJHT[Ø3]3Z

ØJH8[Ø3][89]Z

Coding Clinic: 2012, Q4, P1Ø5 – ØJH6Ø8Z & ØJH6ØPZ
Coding Clinic: 2Ø16, Q2, P14 – ØJH8ØWZ
Coding Clinic: 2Ø18, Q4, P43 – ØJHTØYZ

SECTION: Ø MEDICAL AND SURGICAL
BODY SYSTEM: J SUBCUTANEOUS TISSUE AND FASCIA
OPERATION: J INSPECTION: Visually and/or manually exploring a body part

Body Part	Approach	Device	Qualifier
S Subcutaneous Tissue and Fascia, Head and Neck T Subcutaneous Tissue and Fascia, Trunk V Subcutaneous Tissue and Fascia, Upper Extremity W Subcutaneous Tissue and Fascia, Lower Extremity	Ø Open 3 Percutaneous X External	Z No Device	Z No Qualifier

Non-OR All Values

SECTION: Ø MEDICAL AND SURGICAL
BODY SYSTEM: J SUBCUTANEOUS TISSUE AND FASCIA
OPERATION: N RELEASE: Freeing a body part from an abnormal physical constraint by cutting or by the use of force

Body Part	Approach	Device	Qualifier
Ø Subcutaneous Tissue and Fascia, Scalp 1 Subcutaneous Tissue and Fascia, Face 4 Subcutaneous Tissue and Fascia, Right Neck 5 Subcutaneous Tissue and Fascia, Left Neck 6 Subcutaneous Tissue and Fascia, Chest 7 Subcutaneous Tissue and Fascia, Back 8 Subcutaneous Tissue and Fascia, Abdomen 9 Subcutaneous Tissue and Fascia, Buttock B Subcutaneous Tissue and Fascia, Perineum C Subcutaneous Tissue and Fascia, Pelvic Region D Subcutaneous Tissue and Fascia, Right Upper Arm F Subcutaneous Tissue and Fascia, Left Upper Arm G Subcutaneous Tissue and Fascia, Right Lower Arm H Subcutaneous Tissue and Fascia, Left Lower Arm J Subcutaneous Tissue and Fascia, Right Hand K Subcutaneous Tissue and Fascia, Left Hand L Subcutaneous Tissue and Fascia, Right Upper Leg M Subcutaneous Tissue and Fascia, Left Upper Leg N Subcutaneous Tissue and Fascia, Right Lower Leg P Subcutaneous Tissue and Fascia, Left Lower Leg Q Subcutaneous Tissue and Fascia, Right Foot R Subcutaneous Tissue and Fascia, Left Foot	Ø Open 3 Percutaneous X External	Z No Device	Z No Qualifier

Non-OR ØJN[1456789BCDFGHJKLMNPQR]XZZ

Coding Clinic: 2Ø17, Q3, P12 – ØJN[LMNPQR]ØZZ

SECTION: Ø MEDICAL AND SURGICAL
BODY SYSTEM: J SUBCUTANEOUS TISSUE AND FASCIA
OPERATION: P REMOVAL: Taking out or off a device from a body part

Body Part	Approach	Device	Qualifier
S Subcutaneous Tissue and Fascia, Head and Neck	Ø Open 3 Percutaneous	Ø Drainage Device 1 Radioactive Element 3 Infusion Device 7 Autologous Tissue Substitute J Synthetic Substitute K Nonautologous Tissue Substitute N Tissue Expander Y Other Device	Z No Qualifier
S Subcutaneous Tissue and Fascia, Head and Neck	X External	Ø Drainage Device 1 Radioactive Element 3 Infusion Device	Z No Qualifier
T Subcutaneous Tissue and Fascia, Trunk	Ø Open 3 Percutaneous	Ø Drainage Device 1 Radioactive Element 2 Monitoring Device 3 Infusion Device 7 Autologous Tissue Substitute F Subcutaneous Defibrillator H Contraceptive Device J Synthetic Substitute K Nonautologous Tissue Substitute M Stimulator Generator N Tissue Expander P Cardiac Rhythm Related Device V Infusion Device, Pump W Vascular Access Device, Totally Implantable X Vascular Access Device, Tunneled Y Other Device	Z No Qualifier
T Subcutaneous Tissue and Fascia, Trunk	X External	Ø Drainage Device 1 Radioactive Element 2 Monitoring Device 3 Infusion Device H Contraceptive Device V Infusion Device, Pump X Vascular Access Device, Tunneled	Z No Qualifier
V Subcutaneous Tissue and Fascia, Upper Extremity W Subcutaneous Tissue and Fascia, Lower Extremity	Ø Open 3 Percutaneous	Ø Drainage Device 1 Radioactive Element 3 Infusion Device 7 Autologous Tissue Substitute H Contraceptive Device J Synthetic Substitute K Nonautologous Tissue Substitute N Tissue Expander V Infusion Device, Pump W Vascular Access Device, Totally Implantable X Vascular Access Device, Tunneled Y Other Device	Z No Qualifier
V Subcutaneous Tissue and Fascia, Upper Extremity W Subcutaneous Tissue and Fascia, Lower Extremity	X External	Ø Drainage Device 1 Radioactive Element 3 Infusion Device H Contraceptive Device V Infusion Pump X Vascular Access Device, Tunneled	Z No Qualifier

Non-OR ØJPS[Ø3][Ø137JKN]Z
Non-OR ØJPSX[Ø13]Z
Non-OR ØJPT[Ø3][Ø1237HJKMNVWX]Z
Non-OR ØJPTX[Ø123HVX]Z

Non-OR ØJP[VW][Ø3][Ø137HJKNVWX]Z
Non-OR ØJP[VW]X[Ø13HVX]Z
ØJPT[Ø3][FP]Z when reported with Secondary Diagnosis K68.11, T81.4XXA, T82.6XXA, or T82.7XXA

Coding Clinic: 2012, Q4, P1Ø5 – ØJPTØPZ
Coding Clinic: 2016, Q2, P15; 2015, Q4, P32 – ØJPTØXZ
Coding Clinic: 2018, Q4, P86 – ØJPT3JZ

SECTION: Ø MEDICAL AND SURGICAL
BODY SYSTEM: J SUBCUTANEOUS TISSUE AND FASCIA
OPERATION: Q REPAIR: Restoring, to the extent possible, a body part to its normal anatomic structure and function

Body Part	Approach	Device	Qualifier
Ø Subcutaneous Tissue and Fascia, Scalp 1 Subcutaneous Tissue and Fascia, Face 4 Subcutaneous Tissue and Fascia, Right Neck 5 Subcutaneous Tissue and Fascia, Left Neck 6 Subcutaneous Tissue and Fascia, Chest 7 Subcutaneous Tissue and Fascia, Back 8 Subcutaneous Tissue and Fascia, Abdomen 9 Subcutaneous Tissue and Fascia, Buttock B Subcutaneous Tissue and Fascia, Perineum C Subcutaneous Tissue and Fascia, Pelvic Region D Subcutaneous Tissue and Fascia, Right Upper Arm F Subcutaneous Tissue and Fascia, Left Upper Arm G Subcutaneous Tissue and Fascia, Right Lower Arm H Subcutaneous Tissue and Fascia, Left Lower Arm J Subcutaneous Tissue and Fascia, Right Hand K Subcutaneous Tissue and Fascia, Left Hand L Subcutaneous Tissue and Fascia, Right Upper Leg M Subcutaneous Tissue and Fascia, Left Upper Leg N Subcutaneous Tissue and Fascia, Right Lower Leg P Subcutaneous Tissue and Fascia, Left Lower Leg Q Subcutaneous Tissue and Fascia, Right Foot R Subcutaneous Tissue and Fascia, Left Foot	Ø Open 3 Percutaneous	Z No Device	Z No Qualifier

DRG Non-OR ØJQ[Ø1456789BCDFGHJKLMNPQR][Ø3]ZZ
Non-OR ØJQ[Ø1456789BCDFGHJKLMNPQR]3ZZ

Coding Clinic: 2Ø17, Q3, P19 – ØJQCØZZ
Coding Clinic: 2Ø22, Q3, P25 – ØJQ8ØZZ

SECTION: Ø MEDICAL AND SURGICAL
BODY SYSTEM: J SUBCUTANEOUS TISSUE AND FASCIA
OPERATION: R REPLACEMENT: Putting in or on biological or synthetic material that physically takes the place and/or function of all or a portion of a body part

Body Part	Approach	Device	Qualifier
Ø Subcutaneous Tissue and Fascia, Scalp 1 Subcutaneous Tissue and Fascia, Face 4 Subcutaneous Tissue and Fascia, Right Neck 5 Subcutaneous Tissue and Fascia, Left Neck 6 Subcutaneous Tissue and Fascia, Chest 7 Subcutaneous Tissue and Fascia, Back 8 Subcutaneous Tissue and Fascia, Abdomen 9 Subcutaneous Tissue and Fascia, Buttock B Subcutaneous Tissue and Fascia, Perineum C Subcutaneous Tissue and Fascia, Pelvic Region D Subcutaneous Tissue and Fascia, Right Upper Arm F Subcutaneous Tissue and Fascia, Left Upper Arm G Subcutaneous Tissue and Fascia, Right Lower Arm H Subcutaneous Tissue and Fascia, Left Lower Arm J Subcutaneous Tissue and Fascia, Right Hand K Subcutaneous Tissue and Fascia, Left Hand L Subcutaneous Tissue and Fascia, Right Upper Leg M Subcutaneous Tissue and Fascia, Left Upper Leg N Subcutaneous Tissue and Fascia, Right Lower Leg P Subcutaneous Tissue and Fascia, Left Lower Leg Q Subcutaneous Tissue and Fascia, Right Foot R Subcutaneous Tissue and Fascia, Left Foot	Ø Open 3 Percutaneous	7 Autologous Tissue Substitute J Synthetic Substitute K Nonautologous Tissue Substitute	Z No Qualifier

Coding Clinic: 2015, Q2, P13 – ØJR1Ø7Z

SECTION: Ø MEDICAL AND SURGICAL
BODY SYSTEM: J SUBCUTANEOUS TISSUE AND FASCIA
OPERATION: U SUPPLEMENT: Putting in or on biological or synthetic material that physically reinforces and/or augments the function of a portion of a body part

Body Part	Approach	Device	Qualifier
Ø Subcutaneous Tissue and Fascia, Scalp 1 Subcutaneous Tissue and Fascia, Face 4 Subcutaneous Tissue and Fascia, Right Neck 5 Subcutaneous Tissue and Fascia, Left Neck 6 Subcutaneous Tissue and Fascia, Chest 7 Subcutaneous Tissue and Fascia, Back 8 Subcutaneous Tissue and Fascia, Abdomen 9 Subcutaneous Tissue and Fascia, Buttock B Subcutaneous Tissue and Fascia, Perineum C Subcutaneous Tissue and Fascia, Pelvic Region D Subcutaneous Tissue and Fascia, Right Upper Arm F Subcutaneous Tissue and Fascia, Left Upper Arm G Subcutaneous Tissue and Fascia, Right Lower Arm H Subcutaneous Tissue and Fascia, Left Lower Arm J Subcutaneous Tissue and Fascia, Right Hand K Subcutaneous Tissue and Fascia, Left Hand L Subcutaneous Tissue and Fascia, Right Upper Leg M Subcutaneous Tissue and Fascia, Left Upper Leg N Subcutaneous Tissue and Fascia, Right Lower Leg P Subcutaneous Tissue and Fascia, Left Lower Leg Q Subcutaneous Tissue and Fascia, Right Foot R Subcutaneous Tissue and Fascia, Left Foot	Ø Open 3 Percutaneous	7 Autologous Tissue Substitute J Synthetic Substitute K Nonautologous Tissue Substitute	Z No Qualifier

Coding Clinic: 2Ø18, Q1, P7 – ØJU7Ø7Z
Coding Clinic: 2Ø18, Q2, P2Ø – ØJUHØKZ

SECTION: Ø MEDICAL AND SURGICAL
BODY SYSTEM: J SUBCUTANEOUS TISSUE AND FASCIA
OPERATION: W REVISION: *(on multiple pages)*

Correcting, to the extent possible, a portion of a malfunctioning device or the position of a displaced device

Body Part	Approach	Device	Qualifier
S Subcutaneous Tissue and Fascia, Head and Neck	Ø Open 3 Percutaneous	Ø Drainage Device 3 Infusion Device 7 Autologous Tissue Substitute J Synthetic Substitute K Nonautologous Tissue Substitute N Tissue Expander Y Other Device	Z No Qualifier
S Subcutaneous Tissue and Fascia, Head and Neck	X External	Ø Drainage Device 3 Infusion Device 7 Autologous Tissue Substitute J Synthetic Substitute K Nonautologous Tissue Substitute N Tissue Expander	Z No Qualifier
T Subcutaneous Tissue and Fascia, Trunk	Ø Open 3 Percutaneous	Ø Drainage Device 2 Monitoring Device 3 Infusion Device 7 Autologous Tissue Substitute F Subcutaneous Defibrillator H Contraceptive Device J Synthetic Substitute K Nonautologous Tissue Substitute M Stimulator Generator N Tissue Expander P Cardiac Rhythm Related Device V Infusion Device, Pump W Vascular Access Device, Totally Implantable X Vascular Access Device, Tunneled Y Other Device	Z No Qualifier
T Subcutaneous Tissue and Fascia, Trunk	X External	Ø Drainage Device 2 Monitoring Device 3 Infusion Device 7 Autologous Tissue Substitute F Subcutaneous Defibrillator H Contraceptive Device J Synthetic Substitute K Nonautologous Tissue Substitute M Stimulator Generator N Tissue Expander P Cardiac Rhythm Related Device V Infusion Device, Pump W Vascular Access Device, Totally Implantable X Vascular Access Device, Tunneled	Z No Qualifier

DRG Non-OR ØJWS[Ø3][Ø37JKNY]Z
DRG Non-OR ØJWT[Ø3X][Ø37HJKMNVWX]Z
Non-OR ØJWSX[Ø37JKN]Z
Non-OR ØJWTX[Ø237HJKNPVWX]Z
ØJWT[Ø3]PZ when reported with Secondary Diagnosis K68.11, T81.4XXA, T82.6XXA, or T82.7XXA

Coding Clinic: 2Ø12, Q4, P1Ø6 – ØJWTØPZ
Coding Clinic: 2Ø15, Q2, P1Ø – ØJWSØJZ
Coding Clinic: 2Ø15, Q4, P33 – ØJWT33Z
Coding Clinic: 2Ø18, Q1, P9 – ØJWTØJZ
Coding Clinic: 2Ø22, Q3, P25 – ØJWTØ3Z

SECTION: Ø MEDICAL AND SURGICAL
BODY SYSTEM: J SUBCUTANEOUS TISSUE AND FASCIA
OPERATION: W REVISION: *(continued)*

Correcting, to the extent possible, a portion of a malfunctioning device or the position of a displaced device

Body Part	Approach	Device	Qualifier
V Subcutaneous Tissue and Fascia, Upper Extremity W Subcutaneous Tissue and Fascia, Lower Extremity	Ø Open 3 Percutaneous	Ø Drainage Device 3 Infusion Device 7 Autologous Tissue Substitute H Contraceptive Device J Synthetic Substitute K Nonautologous Tissue Substitute N Tissue Expander V Infusion Device, Pump W Vascular Access Device, Totally Implantable X Vascular Access Device, Tunneled Y Other Device	Z No Qualifier
V Subcutaneous Tissue and Fascia, Upper Extremity W Subcutaneous Tissue and Fascia, Lower Extremity	X External	Ø Drainage Device 3 Infusion Device 7 Autologous Tissue Substitute H Contraceptive Device J Synthetic Substitute K Nonautologous Tissue Substitute N Tissue Expander V Infusion Device, Pump W Vascular Access Device, Totally Implantable X Vascular Access Device, Tunneled	Z No Qualifier

DRG Non-OR ØJW[VW][Ø3][Ø37HJKNVWXY]Z
Non-OR ØJW[VW]X[Ø37HJKNVWX]Z

SECTION: Ø MEDICAL AND SURGICAL
BODY SYSTEM: J SUBCUTANEOUS TISSUE AND FASCIA
OPERATION: X TRANSFER: Moving, without taking out, all or a portion of a body part to another location to take over the function of all or a portion of a body part

Body Part	Approach	Device	Qualifier
Ø Subcutaneous Tissue and Fascia, Scalp 1 Subcutaneous Tissue and Fascia, Face 4 Subcutaneous Tissue and Fascia, Right Neck 5 Subcutaneous Tissue and Fascia, Left Neck 6 Subcutaneous Tissue and Fascia, Chest 7 Subcutaneous Tissue and Fascia, Back 8 Subcutaneous Tissue and Fascia, Abdomen 9 Subcutaneous Tissue and Fascia, Buttock B Subcutaneous Tissue and Fascia, Perineum C Subcutaneous Tissue and Fascia, Pelvic Region D Subcutaneous Tissue and Fascia, Right Upper Arm F Subcutaneous Tissue and Fascia, Left Upper Arm G Subcutaneous Tissue and Fascia, Right Lower Arm H Subcutaneous Tissue and Fascia, Left Lower Arm J Subcutaneous Tissue and Fascia, Right Hand K Subcutaneous Tissue and Fascia, Left Hand L Subcutaneous Tissue and Fascia, Right Upper Leg M Subcutaneous Tissue and Fascia, Left Upper Leg N Subcutaneous Tissue and Fascia, Right Lower Leg P Subcutaneous Tissue and Fascia, Left Lower Leg Q Subcutaneous Tissue and Fascia, Right Foot R Subcutaneous Tissue and Fascia, Left Foot	Ø Open 3 Percutaneous	Z No Device	B Skin and Subcutaneous Tissue C Skin, Subcutaneous Tissue and Fascia Z No Qualifier

Coding Clinic: 2018, Q1, P1Ø – ØJXØØZC
Coding Clinic: 2021, Q2, P17 – ØJX6ØZB
Coding Clinic: 2021, Q3, P2Ø – ØJXFØZZ
Coding Clinic: 2022, Q3, P12 – ØJXLØZZ

Ø: M/S J: SUBCUTANEOUS TISSUE AND FASCIA X: TRANSFER

SECTION: Ø MEDICAL AND SURGICAL
BODY SYSTEM: K MUSCLES
OPERATION: 2 CHANGE: Taking out or off a device from a body part and putting back an identical or similar device in or on the same body part without cutting or puncturing the skin or a mucous membrane

Body Part	Approach	Device	Qualifier
X Upper Muscle Y Lower Muscle	X External	Ø Drainage Device Y Other Device	Z No Qualifier

Non-OR All Values

SECTION: Ø MEDICAL AND SURGICAL
BODY SYSTEM: K MUSCLES
OPERATION: 5 DESTRUCTION: Physical eradication of all or a portion of a body part by the direct use of energy, force, or a destructive agent

Body Part	Approach	Device	Qualifier
Ø Head Muscle 1 Facial Muscle 2 Neck Muscle, Right 3 Neck Muscle, Left 4 Tongue, Palate, Pharynx Muscle 5 Shoulder Muscle, Right 6 Shoulder Muscle, Left 7 Upper Arm Muscle, Right 8 Upper Arm Muscle, Left 9 Lower Arm and Wrist Muscle, Right B Lower Arm and Wrist Muscle, Left C Hand Muscle, Right D Hand Muscle, Left F Trunk Muscle, Right G Trunk Muscle, Left H Thorax Muscle, Right J Thorax Muscle, Left K Abdomen Muscle, Right L Abdomen Muscle, Left M Perineum Muscle N Hip Muscle, Right P Hip Muscle, Left Q Upper Leg Muscle, Right R Upper Leg Muscle, Left S Lower Leg Muscle, Right T Lower Leg Muscle, Left V Foot Muscle, Right W Foot Muscle, Left	Ø Open 3 Percutaneous 4 Percutaneous Endoscopic	Z No Device	Z No Qualifier

SECTION: Ø MEDICAL AND SURGICAL
BODY SYSTEM: K MUSCLES
OPERATION: 8 DIVISION: Cutting into a body part, without draining fluids and/or gases from the body part, in order to separate or transect a body part

Body Part	Approach	Device	Qualifier
Ø Head Muscle 1 Facial Muscle 2 Neck Muscle, Right 3 Neck Muscle, Left 5 Shoulder Muscle, Right 6 Shoulder Muscle, Left 7 Upper Arm Muscle, Right 8 Upper Arm Muscle, Left 9 Lower Arm and Wrist Muscle, Right B Lower Arm and Wrist Muscle, Left C Hand Muscle, Right D Hand Muscle, Left F Trunk Muscle, Right G Trunk Muscle, Left H Thorax Muscle, Right J Thorax Muscle, Left K Abdomen Muscle, Right L Abdomen Muscle, Left M Perineum Muscle N Hip Muscle, Right P Hip Muscle, Left Q Upper Leg Muscle, Right R Upper Leg Muscle, Left S Lower Leg Muscle, Right T Lower Leg Muscle, Left V Foot Muscle, Right W Foot Muscle, Left	Ø Open 3 Percutaneous 4 Percutaneous Endoscopic	Z No Device	Z No Qualifier
4 Tongue, Palate, Pharynx Muscle	Ø Open 3 Percutaneous 4 Percutaneous Endoscopic 7 Via Natural or Artificial Opening 8 Via Natural or Artificial Opening Endoscopic	Z No Device	Z No Qualifier

Coding Clinic: 2020, Q2, P25 – ØK844ZZ

SECTION: Ø MEDICAL AND SURGICAL
BODY SYSTEM: K MUSCLES
OPERATION: 9 DRAINAGE: *(on multiple pages)*
Taking or letting out fluids and/or gases from a body part

Body Part	Approach	Device	Qualifier
Ø Head Muscle 1 Facial Muscle 2 Neck Muscle, Right 3 Neck Muscle, Left 4 Tongue, Palate, Pharynx Muscle 5 Shoulder Muscle, Right 6 Shoulder Muscle, Left 7 Upper Arm Muscle, Right 8 Upper Arm Muscle, Left 9 Lower Arm and Wrist Muscle, Right B Lower Arm and Wrist Muscle, Left C Hand Muscle, Right D Hand Muscle, Left F Trunk Muscle, Right G Trunk Muscle, Left H Thorax Muscle, Right J Thorax Muscle, Left K Abdomen Muscle, Right L Abdomen Muscle, Left M Perineum Muscle N Hip Muscle, Right P Hip Muscle, Left Q Upper Leg Muscle, Right R Upper Leg Muscle, Left S Lower Leg Muscle, Right T Lower Leg Muscle, Left V Foot Muscle, Right W Foot Muscle, Left	Ø Open 3 Percutaneous 4 Percutaneous Endoscopic	Ø Drainage Device	Z No Qualifier

Non-OR ØK9[Ø123456789BCDFGHJKLMNPQRSTVW]3ØZ

SECTION: Ø MEDICAL AND SURGICAL
BODY SYSTEM: K MUSCLES
OPERATION: 9 DRAINAGE: *(continued)*
Taking or letting out fluids and/or gases from a body part

Body Part	Approach	Device	Qualifier
Ø Head Muscle 1 Facial Muscle 2 Neck Muscle, Right 3 Neck Muscle, Left 4 Tongue, Palate, Pharynx Muscle 5 Shoulder Muscle, Right 6 Shoulder Muscle, Left 7 Upper Arm Muscle, Right 8 Upper Arm Muscle, Left 9 Lower Arm and Wrist Muscle, Right B Lower Arm and Wrist Muscle, Left C Hand Muscle, Right D Hand Muscle, Left F Trunk Muscle, Right G Trunk Muscle, Left H Thorax Muscle, Right J Thorax Muscle, Left K Abdomen Muscle, Right L Abdomen Muscle, Left M Perineum Muscle N Hip Muscle, Right P Hip Muscle, Left Q Upper Leg Muscle, Right R Upper Leg Muscle, Left S Lower Leg Muscle, Right T Lower Leg Muscle, Left V Foot Muscle, Right W Foot Muscle, Left	Ø Open 3 Percutaneous 4 Percutaneous Endoscopic	Z No Device	X Diagnostic Z No Qualifier

Non-OR ØK9[Ø123456789BFGHJKLMNPQRSTVW]3ZZ
Non-OR ØK9[CD][34]ZZ

SECTION: Ø MEDICAL AND SURGICAL
BODY SYSTEM: K MUSCLES
OPERATION: B EXCISION: Cutting out or off, without replacement, a portion of a body part

Body Part	Approach	Device	Qualifier
Ø Head Muscle 1 Facial Muscle 2 Neck Muscle, Right 3 Neck Muscle, Left 4 Tongue, Palate, Pharynx Muscle 5 Shoulder Muscle, Right 6 Shoulder Muscle, Left 7 Upper Arm Muscle, Right 8 Upper Arm Muscle, Left 9 Lower Arm and Wrist Muscle, Right B Lower Arm and Wrist Muscle, Left C Hand Muscle, Right D Hand Muscle, Left F Trunk Muscle, Right G Trunk Muscle, Left H Thorax Muscle, Right J Thorax Muscle, Left K Abdomen Muscle, Right L Abdomen Muscle, Left M Perineum Muscle N Hip Muscle, Right P Hip Muscle, Left Q Upper Leg Muscle, Right R Upper Leg Muscle, Left S Lower Leg Muscle, Right T Lower Leg Muscle, Left V Foot Muscle, Right W Foot Muscle, Left	Ø Open 3 Percutaneous 4 Percutaneous Endoscopic	Z No Device	X Diagnostic Z No Qualifier

Non-OR ØKB[NP]3Z[XZ]

Coding Clinic: 2016, Q3, P2Ø – ØKB[NP]ØZZ
Coding Clinic: 2019, Q4, P44 – ØKBPØZZ
Coding Clinic: 202Ø, Q1, P28 – ØKBRØZZ
Coding Clinic: 2023, Q1, P33 – ØKB44ZZ

ØKC

SECTION: Ø MEDICAL AND SURGICAL
BODY SYSTEM: K MUSCLES
OPERATION: C EXTIRPATION: Taking or cutting out solid matter from a body part

Body Part	Approach	Device	Qualifier
Ø Head Muscle 1 Facial Muscle 2 Neck Muscle, Right 3 Neck Muscle, Left 4 Tongue, Palate, Pharynx Muscle 5 Shoulder Muscle, Right 6 Shoulder Muscle, Left 7 Upper Arm Muscle, Right 8 Upper Arm Muscle, Left 9 Lower Arm and Wrist Muscle, Right B Lower Arm and Wrist Muscle, Left C Hand Muscle, Right D Hand Muscle, Left F Trunk Muscle, Right G Trunk Muscle, Left H Thorax Muscle, Right J Thorax Muscle, Left K Abdomen Muscle, Right L Abdomen Muscle, Left M Perineum Muscle N Hip Muscle, Right P Hip Muscle, Left Q Upper Leg Muscle, Right R Upper Leg Muscle, Left S Lower Leg Muscle, Right T Lower Leg Muscle, Left V Foot Muscle, Right W Foot Muscle, Left	Ø Open 3 Percutaneous 4 Percutaneous Endoscopic	Z No Device	Z No Qualifier

SECTION: Ø MEDICAL AND SURGICAL
BODY SYSTEM: K MUSCLES
OPERATION: D EXTRACTION: Pulling or stripping out or off all or a portion of a body part by the use of force

Body Part	Approach	Device	Qualifier
Ø Head Muscle 1 Facial Muscle 2 Neck Muscle, Right 3 Neck Muscle, Left 4 Tongue, Palate, Pharynx Muscle 5 Shoulder Muscle, Right 6 Shoulder Muscle, Left 7 Upper Arm Muscle, Right 8 Upper Arm Muscle, Left 9 Lower Arm and Wrist Muscle, Right B Lower Arm and Wrist Muscle, Left C Hand Muscle, Right D Hand Muscle, Left F Trunk Muscle, Right G Trunk Muscle, Left H Thorax Muscle, Right J Thorax Muscle, Left K Abdomen Muscle, Right L Abdomen Muscle, Left M Perineum Muscle N Hip Muscle, Right P Hip Muscle, Left Q Upper Leg Muscle, Right R Upper Leg Muscle, Left S Lower Leg Muscle, Right T Lower Leg Muscle, Left V Foot Muscle, Right W Foot Muscle, Left	Ø Open	Z No Device	Z No Qualifier

Coding Clinic: 2Ø17, Q4, P42 – ØKDSØZZ

SECTION: Ø MEDICAL AND SURGICAL
BODY SYSTEM: K MUSCLES
OPERATION: H INSERTION: Putting in a nonbiological appliance that monitors, assists, performs, or prevents a physiological function but does not physically take the place of a body part

Body Part	Approach	Device	Qualifier
X Upper Muscle Y Lower Muscle	Ø Open 3 Percutaneous 4 Percutaneous Endoscopic	M Stimulator Lead Y Other Device	Z No Qualifier

SECTION: Ø MEDICAL AND SURGICAL
BODY SYSTEM: K MUSCLES
OPERATION: J INSPECTION: Visually and/or manually exploring a body part

Body Part	Approach	Device	Qualifier
X Upper Muscle Y Lower Muscle	Ø Open 3 Percutaneous 4 Percutaneous Endoscopic X External	Z No Device	Z No Qualifier

Non-OR ØKJ[XY][3X]ZZ

SECTION: Ø MEDICAL AND SURGICAL
BODY SYSTEM: K MUSCLES
OPERATION: M REATTACHMENT: Putting back in or on all or a portion of a separated body part to its normal location or other suitable location

Body Part	Approach	Device	Qualifier
Ø Head Muscle 1 Facial Muscle 2 Neck Muscle, Right 3 Neck Muscle, Left 4 Tongue, Palate, Pharynx Muscle 5 Shoulder Muscle, Right 6 Shoulder Muscle, Left 7 Upper Arm Muscle, Right 8 Upper Arm Muscle, Left 9 Lower Arm and Wrist Muscle, Right B Lower Arm and Wrist Muscle, Left C Hand Muscle, Right D Hand Muscle, Left F Trunk Muscle, Right G Trunk Muscle, Left H Thorax Muscle, Right J Thorax Muscle, Left K Abdomen Muscle, Right L Abdomen Muscle, Left M Perineum Muscle N Hip Muscle, Right P Hip Muscle, Left Q Upper Leg Muscle, Right R Upper Leg Muscle, Left S Lower Leg Muscle, Right T Lower Leg Muscle, Left V Foot Muscle, Right W Foot Muscle, Left	Ø Open 4 Percutaneous Endoscopic	Z No Device	Z No Qualifier

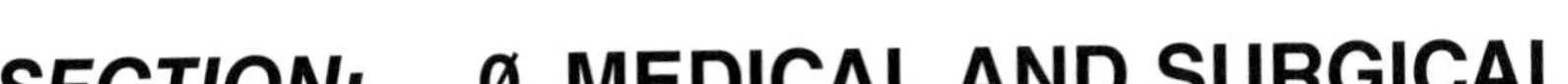

SECTION: Ø MEDICAL AND SURGICAL
BODY SYSTEM: K MUSCLES
OPERATION: N RELEASE: Freeing a body part from an abnormal physical constraint by cutting or by the use of force

Body Part	Approach	Device	Qualifier
Ø Head Muscle 1 Facial Muscle 2 Neck Muscle, Right 3 Neck Muscle, Left 4 Tongue, Palate, Pharynx Muscle 5 Shoulder Muscle, Right 6 Shoulder Muscle, Left 7 Upper Arm Muscle, Right 8 Upper Arm Muscle, Left 9 Lower Arm and Wrist Muscle, Right B Lower Arm and Wrist Muscle, Left C Hand Muscle, Right D Hand Muscle, Left F Trunk Muscle, Right G Trunk Muscle, Left H Thorax Muscle, Right J Thorax Muscle, Left K Abdomen Muscle, Right L Abdomen Muscle, Left M Perineum Muscle N Hip Muscle, Right P Hip Muscle, Left Q Upper Leg Muscle, Right R Upper Leg Muscle, Lefta S Lower Leg Muscle, Right T Lower Leg Muscle, Left V Foot Muscle, Right W Foot Muscle, Left	Ø Open 3 Percutaneous 4 Percutaneous Endoscopic X External	Z No Device	Z No Qualifier

Non-OR ØKN[Ø123456789BCDFGHJKLMNPQRSTVW]XZZ

Coding Clinic: 2Ø15, Q2, P22 – ØKN84ZZ
Coding Clinic: 2Ø17, Q2, P13 – ØKNVØZZ
Coding Clinic: 2Ø17, Q2, P14 – ØKNTØZZ

SECTION: Ø MEDICAL AND SURGICAL
BODY SYSTEM: K MUSCLES
OPERATION: P REMOVAL: Taking out or off a device from a body part

Body Part	Approach	Device	Qualifier
X Upper Muscle Y Lower Muscle	Ø Open 3 Percutaneous 4 Percutaneous Endoscopic	Ø Drainage Device 7 Autologous Tissue Substitute J Synthetic Substitute K Nonautologous Tissue Substitute M Stimulator Lead Y Other Device	Z No Qualifier
X Upper Muscle Y Lower Muscle	X External	Ø Drainage Device M Stimulator Lead	Z No Qualifier

Non-OR ØKP[XY]X[ØM]Z

SECTION: Ø MEDICAL AND SURGICAL
BODY SYSTEM: K MUSCLES
OPERATION: Q REPAIR: Restoring, to the extent possible, a body part to its normal anatomic structure and function

Body Part	Approach	Device	Qualifier
Ø Head Muscle 1 Facial Muscle 2 Neck Muscle, Right 3 Neck Muscle, Left 4 Tongue, Palate, Pharynx Muscle 5 Shoulder Muscle, Right 6 Shoulder Muscle, Left 7 Upper Arm Muscle, Right 8 Upper Arm Muscle, Left 9 Lower Arm and Wrist Muscle, Right B Lower Arm and Wrist Muscle, Left C Hand Muscle, Right D Hand Muscle, Left F Trunk Muscle, Right G Trunk Muscle, Left H Thorax Muscle, Right J Thorax Muscle, Left K Abdomen Muscle, Right L Abdomen Muscle, Left M Perineum Muscle N Hip Muscle, Right P Hip Muscle, Left Q Upper Leg Muscle, Right R Upper Leg Muscle, Left S Lower Leg Muscle, Right T Lower Leg Muscle, Left V Foot Muscle, Right W Foot Muscle, Left	Ø Open 3 Percutaneous 4 Percutaneous Endoscopic	Z No Device	Z No Qualifier

Coding Clinic: 2Ø22, Q3, P14; 2Ø16, Q2, P35, Q1, P7 – ØKQMØZZ

SECTION: Ø MEDICAL AND SURGICAL
BODY SYSTEM: K MUSCLES
OPERATION: R REPLACEMENT: Putting in or on biological or synthetic material that physically takes the place and/or function of all or a portion of a body part

Body Part	Approach	Device	Qualifier
Ø Head Muscle 1 Facial Muscle 2 Neck Muscle, Right 3 Neck Muscle, Left 4 Tongue, Palate, Pharynx Muscle 5 Shoulder Muscle, Right 6 Shoulder Muscle, Left 7 Upper Arm Muscle, Right 8 Upper Arm Muscle, Left 9 Lower Arm and Wrist Muscle, Right B Lower Arm and Wrist Muscle, Left C Hand Muscle, Right D Hand Muscle, Left F Trunk Muscle, Right G Trunk Muscle, Left H Thorax Muscle, Right J Thorax Muscle, Left K Abdomen Muscle, Right L Abdomen Muscle, Left M Perineum Muscle N Hip Muscle, Right P Hip Muscle, Left Q Upper Leg Muscle, Right R Upper Leg Muscle, Left S Lower Leg Muscle, Right T Lower Leg Muscle, Left V Foot Muscle, Right W Foot Muscle, Left	Ø Open 4 Percutaneous Endoscopic	7 Autologous Tissue Substitute J Synthetic Substitute K Nonautologous Tissue Substitute	Z No Qualifier

ØKS

SECTION: Ø MEDICAL AND SURGICAL
BODY SYSTEM: K MUSCLES
OPERATION: S REPOSITION: Moving to its normal location, or other suitable location, all or a portion of a body part

Body Part	Approach	Device	Qualifier
Ø Head Muscle 1 Facial Muscle 2 Neck Muscle, Right 3 Neck Muscle, Left 4 Tongue, Palate, Pharynx Muscle 5 Shoulder Muscle, Right 6 Shoulder Muscle, Left 7 Upper Arm Muscle, Right 8 Upper Arm Muscle, Left 9 Lower Arm and Wrist Muscle, Right B Lower Arm and Wrist Muscle, Left C Hand Muscle, Right D Hand Muscle, Left F Trunk Muscle, Right G Trunk Muscle, Left H Thorax Muscle, Right J Thorax Muscle, Left K Abdomen Muscle, Right L Abdomen Muscle, Left M Perineum Muscle N Hip Muscle, Right P Hip Muscle, Left Q Upper Leg Muscle, Right R Upper Leg Muscle, Left S Lower Leg Muscle, Right T Lower Leg Muscle, Left V Foot Muscle, Right W Foot Muscle, Left	Ø Open 4 Percutaneous Endoscopic	Z No Device	Z No Qualifier

Coding Clinic: 2022, Q3, P12 – ØKSQØZZ

SECTION: Ø MEDICAL AND SURGICAL
BODY SYSTEM: K MUSCLES
OPERATION: T RESECTION: Cutting out or off, without replacement, all of a body part

Body Part	Approach	Device	Qualifier
Ø Head Muscle 1 Facial Muscle 2 Neck Muscle, Right 3 Neck Muscle, Left 4 Tongue, Palate, Pharynx Muscle 5 Shoulder Muscle, Right 6 Shoulder Muscle, Left 7 Upper Arm Muscle, Right 8 Upper Arm Muscle, Left 9 Lower Arm and Wrist Muscle, Right B Lower Arm and Wrist Muscle, Left C Hand Muscle, Right D Hand Muscle, Left F Trunk Muscle, Right G Trunk Muscle, Left H Thorax Muscle, Right ⊞ J Thorax Muscle, Left ⊞ K Abdomen Muscle, Right L Abdomen Muscle, Left M Perineum Muscle N Hip Muscle, Right P Hip Muscle, Left Q Upper Leg Muscle, Right R Upper Leg Muscle, Left S Lower Leg Muscle, Right T Lower Leg Muscle, Left V Foot Muscle, Right W Foot Muscle, Left	Ø Open 4 Percutaneous Endoscopic	Z No Device	Z No Qualifier

⊞ ØKT[HJ]ØZZ

Coding Clinic: 2Ø15, Q1, P38 – ØKTMØZZ
Coding Clinic: 2Ø16, Q2, P13 – ØKT3ØZZ

SECTION: Ø MEDICAL AND SURGICAL
BODY SYSTEM: K MUSCLES
OPERATION: U SUPPLEMENT: Putting in or on biological or synthetic material that physically reinforces and/or augments the function of a portion of a body part

Body Part	Approach	Device	Qualifier
Ø Head Muscle 1 Facial Muscle 2 Neck Muscle, Right 3 Neck Muscle, Left 4 Tongue, Palate, Pharynx Muscle 5 Shoulder Muscle, Right 6 Shoulder Muscle, Left 7 Upper Arm Muscle, Right 8 Upper Arm Muscle, Left 9 Lower Arm and Wrist Muscle, Right B Lower Arm and Wrist Muscle, Left C Hand Muscle, Right D Hand Muscle, Left F Trunk Muscle, Right G Trunk Muscle, Left H Thorax Muscle, Right J Thorax Muscle, Left K Abdomen Muscle, Right L Abdomen Muscle, Left M Perineum Muscle N Hip Muscle, Right P Hip Muscle, Left Q Upper Leg Muscle, Right R Upper Leg Muscle, Left S Lower Leg Muscle, Right T Lower Leg Muscle, Left V Foot Muscle, Right W Foot Muscle, Left	Ø Open 4 Percutaneous Endoscopic	7 Autologous Tissue Substitute J Synthetic Substitute K Nonautologous Tissue Substitute	Z No Qualifier

SECTION: Ø MEDICAL AND SURGICAL
BODY SYSTEM: K MUSCLES
OPERATION: W REVISION: Correcting, to the extent possible, a portion of a malfunctioning device or the position of a displaced device

Body Part	Approach	Device	Qualifier
X Upper Muscle Y Lower Muscle	Ø Open 3 Percutaneous 4 Percutaneous Endoscopic	Ø Drainage Device 7 Autologous Tissue Substitute J Synthetic Substitute K Nonautologous Tissue Substitute M Stimulator Lead Y Other device	Z No Qualifier
X Upper Muscle Y Lower Muscle	X External	Ø Drainage Device 7 Autologous Tissue Substitute J Synthetic Substitute K Nonautologous Tissue Substitute M Stimulator Lead	Z No Qualifier

Non-OR ØKW[XY]X[Ø7JKM]Z

SECTION: Ø MEDICAL AND SURGICAL
BODY SYSTEM: K MUSCLES
OPERATION: X TRANSFER: Moving, without taking out, all or a portion of a body part to another location to take over the function of all or a portion of a body part

Body Part	Approach	Device	Qualifier
Ø Head Muscle 1 Facial Muscle 2 Neck Muscle, Right 3 Neck Muscle, Left 4 Tongue, Palate, Pharynx Muscle 5 Shoulder Muscle, Right 6 Shoulder Muscle, Left 7 Upper Arm Muscle, Right 8 Upper Arm Muscle, Left 9 Lower Arm and Wrist Muscle, Right B Lower Arm and Wrist Muscle, Left C Hand Muscle, Right D Hand Muscle, Left H Thorax Muscle, Right J Thorax Muscle, Left M Perineum Muscle N Hip Muscle, Right P Hip Muscle, Left Q Upper Leg Muscle, Right R Upper Leg Muscle, Left S Lower Leg Muscle, Right T Lower Leg Muscle, Left V Foot Muscle, Right W Foot Muscle, Left	Ø Open 4 Percutaneous Endoscopic	Z No Device	Ø Skin 1 Subcutaneous Tissue 2 Skin and Subcutaneous Tissue Z No Qualifier
F Trunk Muscle, Right G Trunk Muscle, Left	Ø Open 4 Percutaneous Endoscopic	Z No Device	Ø Skin 1 Subcutaneous Tissue 2 Skin and Subcutaneous Tissue 5 Latissimus Dorsi Myocutaneous Flap 7 Deep Inferior Epigastric Artery Perforator Flap 8 Superficial Inferior Epigastric Artery Flap 9 Gluteal Artery Perforator Flap Z No Qualifier
K Abdomen Muscle, Right L Abdomen Muscle, Left	Ø Open 4 Percutaneous Endoscopic	Z No Device	Ø Skin 1 Subcutaneous Tissue 2 Skin and Subcutaneous Tissue 6 Transverse Rectus Abdominis Myocutaneous Flap Z No Qualifier

Coding Clinic: 2Ø15, Q2, P26 – ØKX4ØZ2
Coding Clinic: 2Ø15, Q3, P33 – ØKX1ØZ2
Coding Clinic: 2Ø16, Q3, P3Ø-31 – ØKX[QR]ØZZ
Coding Clinic: 2Ø17, Q4, P67 – ØKXFØZ5

ØL

SECTION: Ø MEDICAL AND SURGICAL
BODY SYSTEM: L TENDONS
OPERATION: 2 CHANGE: Taking out or off a device from a body part and putting back an identical or similar device in or on the same body part without cutting or puncturing the skin or a mucous membrane

Body Part	Approach	Device	Qualifier
X Upper Tendon Y Lower Tendon	X External	Ø Drainage Device Y Other Device	Z No Qualifier

Non-OR All Values

SECTION: Ø MEDICAL AND SURGICAL
BODY SYSTEM: L TENDONS
OPERATION: 5 DESTRUCTION: Physical eradication of all or a portion of a body part by the direct use of energy, force, or a destructive agent

Body Part	Approach	Device	Qualifier
Ø Head and Neck Tendon 1 Shoulder Tendon, Right 2 Shoulder Tendon, Left 3 Upper Arm Tendon, Right 4 Upper Arm Tendon, Left 5 Lower Arm and Wrist Tendon, Right 6 Lower Arm and Wrist Tendon, Left 7 Hand Tendon, Right 8 Hand Tendon, Left 9 Trunk Tendon, Right B Trunk Tendon, Left C Thorax Tendon, Right D Thorax Tendon, Left F Abdomen Tendon, Right G Abdomen Tendon, Left H Perineum Tendon J Hip Tendon, Right K Hip Tendon, Left L Upper Leg Tendon, Right M Upper Leg Tendon, Left N Lower Leg Tendon, Right P Lower Leg Tendon, Left Q Knee Tendon, Right R Knee Tendon, Left S Ankle Tendon, Right T Ankle Tendon, Left V Foot Tendon, Right W Foot Tendon, Left	Ø Open 3 Percutaneous 4 Percutaneous Endoscopic	Z No Device	Z No Qualifier

SECTION: Ø MEDICAL AND SURGICAL
BODY SYSTEM: L TENDONS
OPERATION: 8 DIVISION: Cutting into a body part, without draining fluids and/or gases from the body part, in order to separate or transect a body part

Body Part	Approach	Device	Qualifier
Ø Head and Neck Tendon 1 Shoulder Tendon, Right 2 Shoulder Tendon, Left 3 Upper Arm Tendon, Right 4 Upper Arm Tendon, Left 5 Lower Arm and Wrist Tendon, Right 6 Lower Arm and Wrist Tendon, Left 7 Hand Tendon, Right 8 Hand Tendon, Left 9 Trunk Tendon, Right B Trunk Tendon, Left C Thorax Tendon, Right D Thorax Tendon, Left F Abdomen Tendon, Right G Abdomen Tendon, Left H Perineum Tendon J Hip Tendon, Right K Hip Tendon, Left L Upper Leg Tendon, Right M Upper Leg Tendon, Left N Lower Leg Tendon, Right P Lower Leg Tendon, Left Q Knee Tendon, Right R Knee Tendon, Left S Ankle Tendon, Right T Ankle Tendon, Left V Foot Tendon, Right W Foot Tendon, Left	Ø Open 3 Percutaneous 4 Percutaneous Endoscopic	Z No Device	Z No Qualifier

Coding Clinic: 2Ø16, Q3, P31 – ØL8JØZZ

SECTION: Ø MEDICAL AND SURGICAL
BODY SYSTEM: L TENDONS
OPERATION: 9 DRAINAGE: Taking or letting out fluids and/or gases from a body part

Body Part	Approach	Device	Qualifier
Ø Head and Neck Tendon 1 Shoulder Tendon, Right 2 Shoulder Tendon, Left 3 Upper Arm Tendon, Right 4 Upper Arm Tendon, Left 5 Lower Arm and Wrist Tendon, Right 6 Lower Arm and Wrist Tendon, Left 7 Hand Tendon, Right 8 Hand Tendon, Left 9 Trunk Tendon, Right B Trunk Tendon, Left C Thorax Tendon, Right D Thorax Tendon, Left F Abdomen Tendon, Right G Abdomen Tendon, Left H Perineum Tendon J Hip Tendon, Right K Hip Tendon, Left L Upper Leg Tendon, Right M Upper Leg Tendon, Left N Lower Leg Tendon, Right P Lower Leg Tendon, Left Q Knee Tendon, Right R Knee Tendon, Left S Ankle Tendon, Right T Ankle Tendon, Left V Foot Tendon, Right W Foot Tendon, Left	Ø Open 3 Percutaneous 4 Percutaneous Endoscopic	Ø Drainage Device	Z No Qualifier
Ø Head and Neck Tendon 1 Shoulder Tendon, Right 2 Shoulder Tendon, Left 3 Upper Arm Tendon, Right 4 Upper Arm Tendon, Left 5 Lower Arm and Wrist Tendon, Right 6 Lower Arm and Wrist Tendon, Left 7 Hand Tendon, Right 8 Hand Tendon, Left 9 Trunk Tendon, Right B Trunk Tendon, Left C Thorax Tendon, Right D Thorax Tendon, Left F Abdomen Tendon, Right G Abdomen Tendon, Left H Perineum Tendon J Hip Tendon, Right K Hip Tendon, Left L Upper Leg Tendon, Right M Upper Leg Tendon, Left N Lower Leg Tendon, Right P Lower Leg Tendon, Left Q Knee Tendon, Right R Knee Tendon, Left S Ankle Tendon, Right T Ankle Tendon, Left V Foot Tendon, Right W Foot Tendon, Left	Ø Open 3 Percutaneous 4 Percutaneous Endoscopic	Z No Device	X Diagnostic Z No Qualifier

Non-OR ØL9[Ø123456789BCDFGHJKLMNPQRSTVW]3ØZ
Non-OR ØL9[78][34]ZZ
Non-OR ØL9[Ø1234569BCDFGHJKLMNPQRSTVW]3ZZ

SECTION: Ø MEDICAL AND SURGICAL
BODY SYSTEM: L TENDONS
OPERATION: B EXCISION: Cutting out or off, without replacement, a portion of a body part

Body Part	Approach	Device	Qualifier
Ø Head and Neck Tendon 1 Shoulder Tendon, Right 2 Shoulder Tendon, Left 3 Upper Arm Tendon, Right 4 Upper Arm Tendon, Left 5 Lower Arm and Wrist Tendon, Right 6 Lower Arm and Wrist Tendon, Left 7 Hand Tendon, Right 8 Hand Tendon, Left 9 Trunk Tendon, Right B Trunk Tendon, Left C Thorax Tendon, Right D Thorax Tendon, Left F Abdomen Tendon, Right G Abdomen Tendon, Left H Perineum Tendon J Hip Tendon, Right K Hip Tendon, Left L Upper Leg Tendon, Right M Upper Leg Tendon, Left N Lower Leg Tendon, Right P Lower Leg Tendon, Left Q Knee Tendon, Right R Knee Tendon, Left S Ankle Tendon, Right T Ankle Tendon, Left V Foot Tendon, Right W Foot Tendon, Left	Ø Open 3 Percutaneous 4 Percutaneous Endoscopic	Z No Device	X Diagnostic Z No Qualifier

Coding Clinic: 2Ø15, Q3, P27 – ØLB6ØZZ
Coding Clinic: 2Ø17, Q2, P22 – ØLBLØZZ

SECTION: Ø MEDICAL AND SURGICAL
BODY SYSTEM: L TENDONS
OPERATION: C EXTIRPATION: Taking or cutting out solid matter from a body part

Body Part	Approach	Device	Qualifier
Ø Head and Neck Tendon 1 Shoulder Tendon, Right 2 Shoulder Tendon, Left 3 Upper Arm Tendon, Right 4 Upper Arm Tendon, Left 5 Lower Arm and Wrist Tendon, Right 6 Lower Arm and Wrist Tendon, Left 7 Hand Tendon, Right 8 Hand Tendon, Left 9 Trunk Tendon, Right B Trunk Tendon, Left C Thorax Tendon, Right D Thorax Tendon, Left F Abdomen Tendon, Right G Abdomen Tendon, Left H Perineum Tendon J Hip Tendon, Right K Hip Tendon, Left L Upper Leg Tendon, Right M Upper Leg Tendon, Left N Lower Leg Tendon, Right P Lower Leg Tendon, Left Q Knee Tendon, Right R Knee Tendon, Left S Ankle Tendon, Right T Ankle Tendon, Left V Foot Tendon, Right W Foot Tendon, Left	Ø Open 3 Percutaneous 4 Percutaneous Endoscopic	Z No Device	Z No Qualifier

SECTION: Ø **MEDICAL AND SURGICAL**
BODY SYSTEM: L **TENDONS**
OPERATION: D **EXTRACTION:** Pulling or stripping out or off all or a portion of a body part by the use of force

Body Part	Approach	Device	Qualifier
Ø Head and Neck Tendon 1 Shoulder Tendon, Right 2 Shoulder Tendon, Left 3 Upper Arm Tendon, Right 4 Upper Arm Tendon, Left 5 Lower Arm and Wrist Tendon, Right 6 Lower Arm and Wrist Tendon, Left 7 Hand Tendon, Right 8 Hand Tendon, Left 9 Trunk Tendon, Right B Trunk Tendon, Left C Thorax Tendon, Right D Thorax Tendon, Left F Abdomen Tendon, Right G Abdomen Tendon, Left H Perineum Tendon J Hip Tendon, Right K Hip Tendon, Left L Upper Leg Tendon, Right M Upper Leg Tendon, Left N Lower Leg Tendon, Right P Lower Leg Tendon, Left Q Knee Tendon, Right R Knee Tendon, Left S Ankle Tendon, Right T Ankle Tendon, Left V Foot Tendon, Right W Foot Tendon, Left	Ø Open	Z No Device	Z No Qualifier

SECTION: Ø **MEDICAL AND SURGICAL**
BODY SYSTEM: L **TENDONS**
OPERATION: H **INSERTION:** Putting in a nonbiological appliance that monitors, assists, performs, or prevents a physiological function but does not physically take the place of a body part

Body Part	Approach	Device	Qualifier
X Upper Tendon Y Lower Tendon	Ø Open 3 Percutaneous 4 Percutaneous Endoscopic	Y Other Device	Z No Qualifier

Ø: M/S L: TENDONS D: EXTRACTION H: INSERTION

SECTION: Ø MEDICAL AND SURGICAL
BODY SYSTEM: L TENDONS
OPERATION: J **INSPECTION:** Visually and/or manually exploring a body part

Body Part	Approach	Device	Qualifier
X Upper Tendon Y Lower Tendon	Ø Open 3 Percutaneous 4 Percutaneous Endoscopic X External	Z No Device	Z No Qualifier

Non-OR ØLJ[XY][3X]ZZ

SECTION: Ø MEDICAL AND SURGICAL
BODY SYSTEM: L TENDONS
OPERATION: M **REATTACHMENT:** Putting back in or on all or a portion of a separated body part to its normal location or other suitable location

Body Part	Approach	Device	Qualifier
Ø Head and Neck Tendon 1 Shoulder Tendon, Right 2 Shoulder Tendon, Left 3 Upper Arm Tendon, Right 4 Upper Arm Tendon, Left 5 Lower Arm and Wrist Tendon, Right 6 Lower Arm and Wrist Tendon, Left 7 Hand Tendon, Right 8 Hand Tendon, Left 9 Trunk Tendon, Right B Trunk Tendon, Left C Thorax Tendon, Right D Thorax Tendon, Left F Abdomen Tendon, Right G Abdomen Tendon, Left H Perineum Tendon J Hip Tendon, Right K Hip Tendon, Left L Upper Leg Tendon, Right M Upper Leg Tendon, Left N Lower Leg Tendon, Right P Lower Leg Tendon, Left Q Knee Tendon, Right R Knee Tendon, Left S Ankle Tendon, Right T Ankle Tendon, Left V Foot Tendon, Right W Foot Tendon, Left	Ø Open 4 Percutaneous Endoscopic	Z No Device	Z No Qualifier

SECTION: Ø MEDICAL AND SURGICAL
BODY SYSTEM: L TENDONS
OPERATION: N RELEASE: Freeing a body part from an abnormal physical constraint by cutting or by the use of force

Body Part	Approach	Device	Qualifier
Ø Head and Neck Tendon 1 Shoulder Tendon, Right 2 Shoulder Tendon, Left 3 Upper Arm Tendon, Right 4 Upper Arm Tendon, Left 5 Lower Arm and Wrist Tendon, Right 6 Lower Arm and Wrist Tendon, Left 7 Hand Tendon, Right 8 Hand Tendon, Left 9 Trunk Tendon, Right B Trunk Tendon, Left C Thorax Tendon, Right D Thorax Tendon, Left F Abdomen Tendon, Right G Abdomen Tendon, Left H Perineum Tendon J Hip Tendon, Right K Hip Tendon, Left L Upper Leg Tendon, Right M Upper Leg Tendon, Left N Lower Leg Tendon, Right P Lower Leg Tendon, Left Q Knee Tendon, Right R Knee Tendon, Left S Ankle Tendon, Right T Ankle Tendon, Left V Foot Tendon, Right W Foot Tendon, Left	Ø Open 3 Percutaneous 4 Percutaneous Endoscopic X External	Z No Device	Z No Qualifier

Non-OR ØLN[Ø123456789BCDFGHJKLMNPQRSTVW]XZZ

SECTION: Ø MEDICAL AND SURGICAL
BODY SYSTEM: L TENDONS
OPERATION: P REMOVAL: Taking out or off a device from a body part

Body Part	Approach	Device	Qualifier
X Upper Tendon Y Lower Tendon	Ø Open 3 Percutaneous 4 Percutaneous Endoscopic	Ø Drainage Device 7 Autologous Tissue Substitute J Synthetic Substitute K Nonautologous Tissue Substitute Y Other Device	Z No Qualifier
X Upper Tendon Y Lower Tendon	X External	Ø Drainage Device	Z No Qualifier

Non-OR ØLP[XY]3ØZ
Non-OR ØLP[XY]XØZ

SECTION: Ø MEDICAL AND SURGICAL
BODY SYSTEM: L TENDONS
OPERATION: Q REPAIR: Restoring, to the extent possible, a body part to its normal anatomic structure and function

Body Part	Approach	Device	Qualifier
Ø Head and Neck Tendon 1 Shoulder Tendon, Right 2 Shoulder Tendon, Left 3 Upper Arm Tendon, Right 4 Upper Arm Tendon, Left 5 Lower Arm and Wrist Tendon, Right 6 Lower Arm and Wrist Tendon, Left 7 Hand Tendon, Right 8 Hand Tendon, Left 9 Trunk Tendon, Right B Trunk Tendon, Left C Thorax Tendon, Right D Thorax Tendon, Left F Abdomen Tendon, Right G Abdomen Tendon, Left H Perineum Tendon J Hip Tendon, Right K Hip Tendon, Left L Upper Leg Tendon, Right M Upper Leg Tendon, Left N Lower Leg Tendon, Right P Lower Leg Tendon, Left Q Knee Tendon, Right R Knee Tendon, Left S Ankle Tendon, Right T Ankle Tendon, Left V Foot Tendon, Right W Foot Tendon, Left	Ø Open 3 Percutaneous 4 Percutaneous Endoscopic	Z No Device	Z No Qualifier

Coding Clinic: 2Ø13, Q3, P21 – ØLQ14ZZ
Coding Clinic: 2Ø16, Q3, P33 – ØLQ14ZZ

Ø: M/S L: TENDONS Q: REPAIR

ØLR

SECTION: Ø MEDICAL AND SURGICAL
BODY SYSTEM: L TENDONS
OPERATION: R REPLACEMENT: Putting in or on biological or synthetic material that physically takes the place and/or function of all or a portion of a body part

Body Part	Approach	Device	Qualifier
Ø Head and Neck Tendon 1 Shoulder Tendon, Right 2 Shoulder Tendon, Left 3 Upper Arm Tendon, Right 4 Upper Arm Tendon, Left 5 Lower Arm and Wrist Tendon, Right 6 Lower Arm and Wrist Tendon, Left 7 Hand Tendon, Right 8 Hand Tendon, Left 9 Trunk Tendon, Right B Trunk Tendon, Left C Thorax Tendon, Right D Thorax Tendon, Left F Abdomen Tendon, Right G Abdomen Tendon, Left H Perineum Tendon J Hip Tendon, Right K Hip Tendon, Left L Upper Leg Tendon, Right M Upper Leg Tendon, Left N Lower Leg Tendon, Right P Lower Leg Tendon, Left Q Knee Tendon, Right R Knee Tendon, Left S Ankle Tendon, Right T Ankle Tendon, Left V Foot Tendon, Right W Foot Tendon, Left	Ø Open 4 Percutaneous Endoscopic	7 Autologous Tissue Substitute J Synthetic Substitute K Nonautologous Tissue Substitute	Z No Qualifier

SECTION: Ø MEDICAL AND SURGICAL
BODY SYSTEM: L TENDONS
OPERATION: S REPOSITION: Moving to its normal location, or other suitable location, all or a portion of a body part

Body Part	Approach	Device	Qualifier
Ø Head and Neck Tendon 1 Shoulder Tendon, Right 2 Shoulder Tendon, Left 3 Upper Arm Tendon, Right 4 Upper Arm Tendon, Left 5 Lower Arm and Wrist Tendon, Right 6 Lower Arm and Wrist Tendon, Left 7 Hand Tendon, Right 8 Hand Tendon, Left 9 Trunk Tendon, Right B Trunk Tendon, Left C Thorax Tendon, Right D Thorax Tendon, Left F Abdomen Tendon, Right G Abdomen Tendon, Left H Perineum Tendon J Hip Tendon, Right K Hip Tendon, Left L Upper Leg Tendon, Right M Upper Leg Tendon, Left N Lower Leg Tendon, Right P Lower Leg Tendon, Left Q Knee Tendon, Right R Knee Tendon, Left S Ankle Tendon, Right T Ankle Tendon, Left V Foot Tendon, Right W Foot Tendon, Left	Ø Open 4 Percutaneous Endoscopic	Z No Device	Z No Qualifier

Coding Clinic: 2Ø15, Q3, P15 – ØLS4ØZZ
Coding Clinic: 2Ø16, Q3, P33 – ØLS3ØZZ

SECTION: Ø MEDICAL AND SURGICAL
BODY SYSTEM: L TENDONS
OPERATION: T RESECTION: Cutting out or off, without replacement, all of a body part

Body Part	Approach	Device	Qualifier
Ø Head and Neck Tendon 1 Shoulder Tendon, Right 2 Shoulder Tendon, Left 3 Upper Arm Tendon, Right 4 Upper Arm Tendon, Left 5 Lower Arm and Wrist Tendon, Right 6 Lower Arm and Wrist Tendon, Left 7 Hand Tendon, Right 8 Hand Tendon, Left 9 Trunk Tendon, Right B Trunk Tendon, Left C Thorax Tendon, Right D Thorax Tendon, Left F Abdomen Tendon, Right G Abdomen Tendon, Left H Perineum Tendon J Hip Tendon, Right K Hip Tendon, Left L Upper Leg Tendon, Right M Upper Leg Tendon, Left N Lower Leg Tendon, Right P Lower Leg Tendon, Left Q Knee Tendon, Right R Knee Tendon, Left S Ankle Tendon, Right T Ankle Tendon, Left V Foot Tendon, Right W Foot Tendon, Left	Ø Open 4 Percutaneous Endoscopic	Z No Device	Z No Qualifier

SECTION: Ø MEDICAL AND SURGICAL
BODY SYSTEM: L TENDONS
OPERATION: U SUPPLEMENT: Putting in or on biological or synthetic material that physically reinforces and/or augments the function of a portion of a body part

Body Part	Approach	Device	Qualifier
Ø Head and Neck Tendon 1 Shoulder Tendon, Right 2 Shoulder Tendon, Left 3 Upper Arm Tendon, Right 4 Upper Arm Tendon, Left 5 Lower Arm and Wrist Tendon, Right 6 Lower Arm and Wrist Tendon, Left 7 Hand Tendon, Right 8 Hand Tendon, Left 9 Trunk Tendon, Right B Trunk Tendon, Left C Thorax Tendon, Right D Thorax Tendon, Left F Abdomen Tendon, Right G Abdomen Tendon, Left H Perineum Tendon J Hip Tendon, Right K Hip Tendon, Left L Upper Leg Tendon, Right M Upper Leg Tendon, Left N Lower Leg Tendon, Right P Lower Leg Tendon, Left Q Knee Tendon, Right R Knee Tendon, Left S Ankle Tendon, Right T Ankle Tendon, Left V Foot Tendon, Right W Foot Tendon, Left	Ø Open 4 Percutaneous Endoscopic	7 Autologous Tissue Substitute J Synthetic Substitute K Nonautologous Tissue Substitute	Z No Qualifier

Coding Clinic: 2Ø15, Q2, P11 – ØLU[QM]ØKZ

SECTION: Ø MEDICAL AND SURGICAL
BODY SYSTEM: L TENDONS
OPERATION: W REVISION: Correcting, to the extent possible, a portion of a malfunctioning device or the position of a displaced device

Body Part	Approach	Device	Qualifier
X Upper Tendon Y Lower Tendon	Ø Open 3 Percutaneous 4 Percutaneous Endoscopic	Ø Drainage Device 7 Autologous Tissue Substitute J Synthetic Substitute K Nonautologous Tissue Substitute Y Other Device	Z No Qualifier
X Upper Tendon Y Lower Tendon	X External	Ø Drainage Device 7 Autologous Tissue Substitute J Synthetic Substitute K Nonautologous Tissue Substitute	Z No Qualifier

Non-OR ØLW[XY]X[Ø7JK]Z

SECTION: Ø MEDICAL AND SURGICAL
BODY SYSTEM: L TENDONS
OPERATION: X TRANSFER: Moving, without taking out, all or a portion of a body part to another location to take over the function of all or a portion of a body part

Body Part	Approach	Device	Qualifier
Ø Head and Neck Tendon 1 Shoulder Tendon, Right 2 Shoulder Tendon, Left 3 Upper Arm Tendon, Right 4 Upper Arm Tendon, Left 5 Lower Arm and Wrist Tendon, Right 6 Lower Arm and Wrist Tendon, Left 7 Hand Tendon, Right 8 Hand Tendon, Left 9 Trunk Tendon, Right B Trunk Tendon, Left C Thorax Tendon, Right D Thorax Tendon, Left F Abdomen Tendon, Right G Abdomen Tendon, Left H Perineum Tendon J Hip Tendon, Right K Hip Tendon, Left L Upper Leg Tendon, Right M Upper Leg Tendon, Left N Lower Leg Tendon, Right P Lower Leg Tendon, Left Q Knee Tendon, Right R Knee Tendon, Left S Ankle Tendon, Right T Ankle Tendon, Left V Foot Tendon, Right W Foot Tendon, Left	Ø Open 4 Percutaneous Endoscopic	Z No Device	Z No Qualifier

SECTION: Ø MEDICAL AND SURGICAL
BODY SYSTEM: M BURSAE AND LIGAMENTS
OPERATION: 2 CHANGE: Taking out or off a device from a body part and putting back an identical or similar device in or on the same body part without cutting or puncturing the skin or a mucous membrane

Body Part	Approach	Device	Qualifier
X Upper Bursa and Ligament Y Lower Bursa and Ligament	X External	Ø Drainage Device Y Other Device	Z No Qualifier

Non-OR All Values

SECTION: Ø MEDICAL AND SURGICAL
BODY SYSTEM: M BURSAE AND LIGAMENTS
OPERATION: 5 DESTRUCTION: Physical eradication of all or a portion of a body part by the direct use of energy, force, or a destructive agent

Body Part	Approach	Device	Qualifier
Ø Head and Neck Bursa and Ligament 1 Shoulder Bursa and Ligament, Right 2 Shoulder Bursa and Ligament, Left 3 Elbow Bursa and Ligament, Right 4 Elbow Bursa and Ligament, Left 5 Wrist Bursa and Ligament, Right 6 Wrist Bursa and Ligament, Left 7 Hand Bursa and Ligament, Right 8 Hand Bursa and Ligament, Left 9 Upper Extremity Bursa and Ligament, Right B Upper Extremity Bursa and Ligament, Left C Upper Spine Bursa and Ligament D Lower Spine Bursa and Ligament F Sternum Bursa and Ligament G Rib(s) Bursa and Ligament H Abdomen Bursa and Ligament, Right J Abdomen Bursa and Ligament, Left K Perineum Bursa and Ligament L Hip Bursa and Ligament, Right M Hip Bursa and Ligament, Left N Knee Bursa and Ligament, Right P Knee Bursa and Ligament, Left Q Ankle Bursa and Ligament, Right R Ankle Bursa and Ligament, Left S Foot Bursa and Ligament, Right T Foot Bursa and Ligament, Left V Lower Extremity Bursa and Ligament, Right W Lower Extremity Bursa and Ligament, Left	Ø Open 3 Percutaneous 4 Percutaneous Endoscopic	Z No Device	Z No Qualifier

SECTION: Ø MEDICAL AND SURGICAL
BODY SYSTEM: M BURSAE AND LIGAMENTS
OPERATION: 8 DIVISION: Cutting into a body part, without draining fluids and/or gases from the body part, in order to separate or transect a body part

Body Part	Approach	Device	Qualifier
Ø Head and Neck Bursa and Ligament 1 Shoulder Bursa and Ligament, Right 2 Shoulder Bursa and Ligament, Left 3 Elbow Bursa and Ligament, Right 4 Elbow Bursa and Ligament, Left 5 Wrist Bursa and Ligament, Right 6 Wrist Bursa and Ligament, Left 7 Hand Bursa and Ligament, Right 8 Hand Bursa and Ligament, Left 9 Upper Extremity Bursa and Ligament, Right B Upper Extremity Bursa and Ligament, Left C Upper Spine Bursa and Ligament D Lower Spine Bursa and Ligament F Sternum Bursa and Ligament G Rib(s) Bursa and Ligament H Abdomen Bursa and Ligament, Right J Abdomen Bursa and Ligament, Left K Perineum Bursa and Ligament L Hip Bursa and Ligament, Right M Hip Bursa and Ligament, Left N Knee Bursa and Ligament, Right P Knee Bursa and Ligament, Left Q Ankle Bursa and Ligament, Right R Ankle Bursa and Ligament, Left S Foot Bursa and Ligament, Right T Foot Bursa and Ligament, Left V Lower Extremity Bursa and Ligament, Right W Lower Extremity Bursa and Ligament, Left	Ø Open 3 Percutaneous 4 Percutaneous Endoscopic	Z No Device	Z No Qualifier

ØM9

SECTION: Ø MEDICAL AND SURGICAL
BODY SYSTEM: M BURSAE AND LIGAMENTS
OPERATION: 9 DRAINAGE: Taking or letting out fluids and/or gases from a body part

Body Part	Approach	Device	Qualifier
Ø Head and Neck Bursa and Ligament 1 Shoulder Bursa and Ligament, Right 2 Shoulder Bursa and Ligament, Left 3 Elbow Bursa and Ligament, Right 4 Elbow Bursa and Ligament, Left 5 Wrist Bursa and Ligament, Right 6 Wrist Bursa and Ligament, Left 7 Hand Bursa and Ligament, Right 8 Hand Bursa and Ligament, Left 9 Upper Extremity Bursa and Ligament, Right B Upper Extremity Bursa and Ligament, Left C Upper Spine Bursa and Ligament D Lower Spine Bursa and Ligament F Sternum Bursa and Ligament G Rib(s) Bursa and Ligament H Abdomen Bursa and Ligament, Right J Abdomen Bursa and Ligament, Left K Perineum Bursa and Ligament L Hip Bursa and Ligament, Right M Hip Bursa and Ligament, Left N Knee Bursa and Ligament, Right P Knee Bursa and Ligament, Left Q Ankle Bursa and Ligament, Right R Ankle Bursa and Ligament, Left S Foot Bursa and Ligament, Right T Foot Bursa and Ligament, Left V Lower Extremity Bursa and Ligament, Right W Lower Extremity Bursa and Ligament, Left	Ø Open 3 Percutaneous 4 Percutaneous Endoscopic	Ø Drainage Device	Z No Qualifier
Ø Head and Neck Bursa and Ligament 1 Shoulder Bursa and Ligament, Right 2 Shoulder Bursa and Ligament, Left 3 Elbow Bursa and Ligament, Right 4 Elbow Bursa and Ligament, Left 5 Wrist Bursa and Ligament, Right 6 Wrist Bursa and Ligament, Left 7 Hand Bursa and Ligament, Right 8 Hand Bursa and Ligament, Left 9 Upper Extremity Bursa and Ligament, Right B Upper Extremity Bursa and Ligament, Left C Upper Spine Bursa and Ligament D Lower Spine Bursa and Ligament F Sternum Bursa and Ligament G Rib(s) Bursa and Ligament H Abdomen Bursa and Ligament, Right J Abdomen Bursa and Ligament, Left K Perineum Bursa and Ligament L Hip Bursa and Ligament, Right M Hip Bursa and Ligament, Left N Knee Bursa and Ligament, Right P Knee Bursa and Ligament, Left Q Ankle Bursa and Ligament, Right R Ankle Bursa and Ligament, Left S Foot Bursa and Ligament, Right T Foot Bursa and Ligament, Left V Lower Extremity Bursa and Ligament, Right W Lower Extremity Bursa and Ligament, Left	Ø Open 3 Percutaneous 4 Percutaneous Endoscopic	Z No Device	X Diagnostic Z No Qualifier

Non-OR ØM9[1234789BCDFGHJKLMVW][34]ØZ
Non-OR ØM9[Ø56NPQRST]3ØZ
Non-OR ØM9[Ø12345678CDFGLMNPQRST][Ø34]ZX
Non-OR ØM9[Ø56789BCDFGHJKNPQRSTVW][34]ZZ
Non-OR ØM9[1234LM]3ZZ

SECTION: Ø MEDICAL AND SURGICAL
BODY SYSTEM: M BURSAE AND LIGAMENTS
OPERATION: B EXCISION: Cutting out or off, without replacement, a portion of a body part

Body Part	Approach	Device	Qualifier
Ø Head and Neck Bursa and Ligament 1 Shoulder Bursa and Ligament, Right 2 Shoulder Bursa and Ligament, Left 3 Elbow Bursa and Ligament, Right 4 Elbow Bursa and Ligament, Left 5 Wrist Bursa and Ligament, Right 6 Wrist Bursa and Ligament, Left 7 Hand Bursa and Ligament, Right 8 Hand Bursa and Ligament, Left 9 Upper Extremity Bursa and Ligament, Right B Upper Extremity Bursa and Ligament, Left C Upper Spine Bursa and Ligament D Lower Spine Bursa and Ligament F Sternum Bursa and Ligament G Rib(s) Bursa and Ligament H Abdomen Bursa and Ligament, Right J Abdomen Bursa and Ligament, Left K Perineum Bursa and Ligament L Hip Bursa and Ligament, Right M Hip Bursa and Ligament, Left N Knee Bursa and Ligament, Right P Knee Bursa and Ligament, Left Q Ankle Bursa and Ligament, Right R Ankle Bursa and Ligament, Left S Foot Bursa and Ligament, Right T Foot Bursa and Ligament, Left V Lower Extremity Bursa and Ligament, Right W Lower Extremity Bursa and Ligament, Left	Ø Open 3 Percutaneous 4 Percutaneous Endoscopic	Z No Device	X Diagnostic Z No Qualifier

Non-OR ØMB[Ø12345678BCDFGLMNPQRST][Ø34]ZX
Non-OR ØMB94ZX

SECTION: Ø MEDICAL AND SURGICAL
BODY SYSTEM: M BURSAE AND LIGAMENTS
OPERATION: C EXTIRPATION: Taking or cutting out solid matter from a body part

Body Part	Approach	Device	Qualifier
Ø Head and Neck Bursa and Ligament 1 Shoulder Bursa and Ligament, Right 2 Shoulder Bursa and Ligament, Left 3 Elbow Bursa and Ligament, Right 4 Elbow Bursa and Ligament, Left 5 Wrist Bursa and Ligament, Right 6 Wrist Bursa and Ligament, Left 7 Hand Bursa and Ligament, Right 8 Hand Bursa and Ligament, Left 9 Upper Extremity Bursa and Ligament, Right B Upper Extremity Bursa and Ligament, Left C Upper Spine Bursa and Ligament D Lower Spine Bursa and Ligament F Sternum Bursa and Ligament G Rib(s) Bursa and Ligament H Abdomen Bursa and Ligament, Right J Abdomen Bursa and Ligament, Left K Perineum Bursa and Ligament L Hip Bursa and Ligament, Right M Hip Bursa and Ligament, Left N Knee Bursa and Ligament, Right P Knee Bursa and Ligament, Left Q Ankle Bursa and Ligament, Right R Ankle Bursa and Ligament, Left S Foot Bursa and Ligament, Right T Foot Bursa and Ligament, Left V Lower Extremity Bursa and Ligament, Right W Lower Extremity Bursa and Ligament, Left	Ø Open 3 Percutaneous 4 Percutaneous Endoscopic	Z No Device	Z No Qualifier

SECTION: Ø MEDICAL AND SURGICAL
BODY SYSTEM: M BURSAE AND LIGAMENTS
OPERATION: D EXTRACTION: Pulling or stripping out or off all or a portion of a body part by the use of force

Body Part	Approach	Device	Qualifier
Ø Head and Neck Bursa and Ligament 1 Shoulder Bursa and Ligament, Right 2 Shoulder Bursa and Ligament, Left 3 Elbow Bursa and Ligament, Right 4 Elbow Bursa and Ligament, Left 5 Wrist Bursa and Ligament, Right 6 Wrist Bursa and Ligament, Left 7 Hand Bursa and Ligament, Right 8 Hand Bursa and Ligament, Left 9 Upper Extremity Bursa and Ligament, Right B Upper Extremity Bursa and Ligament, Left C Upper Spine Bursa and Ligament D Lower Spine Bursa and Ligament F Sternum Bursa and Ligament G Rib(s) Bursa and Ligament H Abdomen Bursa and Ligament, Right J Abdomen Bursa and Ligament, Left K Perineum Bursa and Ligament L Hip Bursa and Ligament, Right M Hip Bursa and Ligament, Left N Knee Bursa and Ligament, Right P Knee Bursa and Ligament, Left Q Ankle Bursa and Ligament, Right R Ankle Bursa and Ligament, Left S Foot Bursa and Ligament, Right T Foot Bursa and Ligament, Left V Lower Extremity Bursa and Ligament, Right W Lower Extremity Bursa and Ligament, Left	Ø Open 3 Percutaneous 4 Percutaneous Endoscopic	Z No Device	Z No Qualifier

SECTION: Ø MEDICAL AND SURGICAL
BODY SYSTEM: M BURSAE AND LIGAMENTS
OPERATION: H INSERTION: Putting in a nonbiological appliance that monitors, assists, performs, or prevents a physiological function but does not physically take the place of a body part

Body Part	Approach	Device	Qualifier
X Upper Bursa and Ligament Y Lower Bursa and Ligament	Ø Open 3 Percutaneous 4 Percutaneous Endoscopic	Y Other Device	Z No Qualifier

SECTION: Ø MEDICAL AND SURGICAL
BODY SYSTEM: M BURSAE AND LIGAMENTS
OPERATION: J INSPECTION: Visually and/or manually exploring a body part

Body Part	Approach	Device	Qualifier
X Upper Bursa and Ligament Y Lower Bursa and Ligament	Ø Open 3 Percutaneous 4 Percutaneous Endoscopic X External	Z No Device	Z No Qualifier

Non-OR ØMJ[XY][3X]ZZ

SECTION: Ø MEDICAL AND SURGICAL
BODY SYSTEM: M BURSAE AND LIGAMENTS
OPERATION: M REATTACHMENT: Putting back in or on all or a portion of a separated body part to its normal location or other suitable location

Body Part	Approach	Device	Qualifier
Ø Head and Neck Bursa and Ligament 1 Shoulder Bursa and Ligament, Right 2 Shoulder Bursa and Ligament, Left 3 Elbow Bursa and Ligament, Right 4 Elbow Bursa and Ligament, Left 5 Wrist Bursa and Ligament, Right 6 Wrist Bursa and Ligament, Left 7 Hand Bursa and Ligament, Right 8 Hand Bursa and Ligament, Left 9 Upper Extremity Bursa and Ligament, Right B Upper Extremity Bursa and Ligament, Left C Upper Spine Bursa and Ligament D Lower Spine Bursa and Ligament F Sternum Bursa and Ligament G Rib(s) Bursa and Ligament H Abdomen Bursa and Ligament, Right J Abdomen Bursa and Ligament, Left K Perineum Bursa and Ligament L Hip Bursa and Ligament, Right M Hip Bursa and Ligament, Left N Knee Bursa and Ligament, Right P Knee Bursa and Ligament, Left Q Ankle Bursa and Ligament, Right R Ankle Bursa and Ligament, Left S Foot Bursa and Ligament, Right T Foot Bursa and Ligament, Left V Lower Extremity Bursa and Ligament, Right W Lower Extremity Bursa and Ligament, Left	Ø Open 4 Percutaneous Endoscopic	Z No Device	Z No Qualifier

Coding Clinic: 2Ø13, Q3, P22 – ØMM14ZZ

SECTION: Ø MEDICAL AND SURGICAL
BODY SYSTEM: M BURSAE AND LIGAMENTS
OPERATION: N RELEASE: Freeing a body part from an abnormal physical constraint by cutting or by the use of force

Body Part	Approach	Device	Qualifier
Ø Head and Neck Bursa and Ligament 1 Shoulder Bursa and Ligament, Right 2 Shoulder Bursa and Ligament, Left 3 Elbow Bursa and Ligament, Right 4 Elbow Bursa and Ligament, Left 5 Wrist Bursa and Ligament, Right 6 Wrist Bursa and Ligament, Left 7 Hand Bursa and Ligament, Right 8 Hand Bursa and Ligament, Left 9 Upper Extremity Bursa and Ligament, Right B Upper Extremity Bursa and Ligament, Left C Upper Spine Bursa and Ligament D Lower Spine Bursa and Ligament F Sternum Bursa and Ligament G Rib(s) Bursa and Ligament H Abdomen Bursa and Ligament, Right J Abdomen Bursa and Ligament, Left K Perineum Bursa and Ligament L Hip Bursa and Ligament, Right M Hip Bursa and Ligament, Left N Knee Bursa and Ligament, Right P Knee Bursa and Ligament, Left Q Ankle Bursa and Ligament, Right R Ankle Bursa and Ligament, Left S Foot Bursa and Ligament, Right T Foot Bursa and Ligament, Left V Lower Extremity Bursa and Ligament, Right W Lower Extremity Bursa and Ligament, Left	Ø Open 3 Percutaneous 4 Percutaneous Endoscopic X External	Z No Device	Z No Qualifier

Non-OR ØMN[Ø123456789BCDFGHJKLMNPQRSTVW]XZZ

SECTION: Ø MEDICAL AND SURGICAL
BODY SYSTEM: M BURSAE AND LIGAMENTS
OPERATION: P REMOVAL: Taking out or off a device from a body part

Body Part	Approach	Device	Qualifier
X Upper Bursa and Ligament Y Lower Bursa and Ligament	Ø Open 3 Percutaneous 4 Percutaneous Endoscopic	Ø Drainage Device 7 Autologous Tissue Substitute J Synthetic Substitute K Nonautologous Tissue Substitute Y Other Device	Z No Qualifier
X Upper Bursa and Ligament Y Lower Bursa and Ligament	X External	Ø Drainage Device	Z No Qualifier

Non-OR ØMP[XY]3ØZ
Non-OR ØMP[XY]XØZ

SECTION: Ø MEDICAL AND SURGICAL
BODY SYSTEM: M BURSAE AND LIGAMENTS
OPERATION: Q REPAIR: Restoring, to the extent possible, a body part to its normal anatomic structure and function

Body Part	Approach	Device	Qualifier
Ø Head and Neck Bursa and Ligament 1 Shoulder Bursa and Ligament, Right 2 Shoulder Bursa and Ligament, Left 3 Elbow Bursa and Ligament, Right 4 Elbow Bursa and Ligament, Left 5 Wrist Bursa and Ligament, Right 6 Wrist Bursa and Ligament, Left 7 Hand Bursa and Ligament, Right 8 Hand Bursa and Ligament, Left 9 Upper Extremity Bursa and Ligament, Right B Upper Extremity Bursa and Ligament, Left C Upper Spine Bursa and Ligament D Lower Spine Bursa and Ligament F Sternum Bursa and Ligament G Rib(s) Bursa and Ligament H Abdomen Bursa and Ligament, Right J Abdomen Bursa and Ligament, Left K Perineum Bursa and Ligament L Hip Bursa and Ligament, Right M Hip Bursa and Ligament, Left N Knee Bursa and Ligament, Right P Knee Bursa and Ligament, Left Q Ankle Bursa and Ligament, Right R Ankle Bursa and Ligament, Left S Foot Bursa and Ligament, Right T Foot Bursa and Ligament, Left V Lower Extremity Bursa and Ligament, Right W Lower Extremity Bursa and Ligament, Left	Ø Open 3 Percutaneous 4 Percutaneous Endoscopic	Z No Device	Z No Qualifier

SECTION: Ø MEDICAL AND SURGICAL
BODY SYSTEM: M BURSAE AND LIGAMENTS
OPERATION: R REPLACEMENT: Putting in or on biological or synthetic material that physically takes the place and/or function of all or a portion of a body part

Body Part	Approach	Device	Qualifier
Ø Head and Neck Bursa and Ligament 1 Shoulder Bursa and Ligament, Right 2 Shoulder Bursa and Ligament, Left 3 Elbow Bursa and Ligament, Right 4 Elbow Bursa and Ligament, Left 5 Wrist Bursa and Ligament, Right 6 Wrist Bursa and Ligament, Left 7 Hand Bursa and Ligament, Right 8 Hand Bursa and Ligament, Left 9 Upper Extremity Bursa and Ligament, Right B Upper Extremity Bursa and Ligament, Left C Upper Spine Bursa and Ligament D Lower Spine Bursa and Ligament F Sternum Bursa and Ligament G Rib(s) Bursa and Ligament H Abdomen Bursa and Ligament, Right J Abdomen Bursa and Ligament, Left K Perineum Bursa and Ligament L Hip Bursa and Ligament, Right M Hip Bursa and Ligament, Left N Knee Bursa and Ligament, Right P Knee Bursa and Ligament, Left Q Ankle Bursa and Ligament, Right R Ankle Bursa and Ligament, Left S Foot Bursa and Ligament, Right T Foot Bursa and Ligament, Left V Lower Extremity Bursa and Ligament, Right W Lower Extremity Bursa and Ligament, Left	Ø Open 4 Percutaneous Endoscopic	7 Autologous Tissue Substitute J Synthetic Substitute K Nonautologous Tissue Substitute	Z No Qualifier

SECTION: Ø MEDICAL AND SURGICAL
BODY SYSTEM: M BURSAE AND LIGAMENTS
OPERATION: S REPOSITION: Moving to its normal location, or other suitable location, all or a portion of a body part

Body Part	Approach	Device	Qualifier
Ø Head and Neck Bursa and Ligament 1 Shoulder Bursa and Ligament, Right 2 Shoulder Bursa and Ligament, Left 3 Elbow Bursa and Ligament, Right 4 Elbow Bursa and Ligament, Left 5 Wrist Bursa and Ligament, Right 6 Wrist Bursa and Ligament, Left 7 Hand Bursa and Ligament, Right 8 Hand Bursa and Ligament, Left 9 Upper Extremity Bursa and Ligament, Right B Upper Extremity Bursa and Ligament, Left C Upper Spine Bursa and Ligament D Lower Spine Bursa and Ligament F Sternum Bursa and Ligament G Rib(s) Bursa and Ligament H Abdomen Bursa and Ligament, Right J Abdomen Bursa and Ligament, Left K Perineum Bursa and Ligament L Hip Bursa and Ligament, Right M Hip Bursa and Ligament, Left N Knee Bursa and Ligament, Right P Knee Bursa and Ligament, Left Q Ankle Bursa and Ligament, Right R Ankle Bursa and Ligament, Left S Foot Bursa and Ligament, Right T Foot Bursa and Ligament, Left V Lower Extremity Bursa and Ligament, Right W Lower Extremity Bursa and Ligament, Left	Ø Open 4 Percutaneous Endoscopic	Z No Device	Z No Qualifier

SECTION: Ø MEDICAL AND SURGICAL
BODY SYSTEM: M BURSAE AND LIGAMENTS
OPERATION: T RESECTION: Cutting out or off, without replacement, all of a body part

Body Part	Approach	Device	Qualifier
Ø Head and Neck Bursa and Ligament 1 Shoulder Bursa and Ligament, Right 2 Shoulder Bursa and Ligament, Left 3 Elbow Bursa and Ligament, Right 4 Elbow Bursa and Ligament, Left 5 Wrist Bursa and Ligament, Right 6 Wrist Bursa and Ligament, Left 7 Hand Bursa and Ligament, Right 8 Hand Bursa and Ligament, Left 9 Upper Extremity Bursa and Ligament, Right B Upper Extremity Bursa and Ligament, Left C Upper Spine Bursa and Ligament D Lower Spine Bursa and Ligament F Sternum Bursa and Ligament G Rib(s) Bursa and Ligament H Abdomen Bursa and Ligament, Right J Abdomen Bursa and Ligament, Left K Perineum Bursa and Ligament L Hip Bursa and Ligament, Right M Hip Bursa and Ligament, Left N Knee Bursa and Ligament, Right P Knee Bursa and Ligament, Left Q Ankle Bursa and Ligament, Right R Ankle Bursa and Ligament, Left S Foot Bursa and Ligament, Right T Foot Bursa and Ligament, Left V Lower Extremity Bursa and Ligament, Right W Lower Extremity Bursa and Ligament, Left	Ø Open 4 Percutaneous Endoscopic	Z No Device	Z No Qualifier

SECTION: Ø MEDICAL AND SURGICAL
BODY SYSTEM: M BURSAE AND LIGAMENTS
OPERATION: U SUPPLEMENT: Putting in or on biological or synthetic material that physically reinforces and/or augments the function of a portion of a body part

Body Part	Approach	Device	Qualifier
Ø Head and Neck Bursa and Ligament 1 Shoulder Bursa and Ligament, Right 2 Shoulder Bursa and Ligament, Left 3 Elbow Bursa and Ligament, Right 4 Elbow Bursa and Ligament, Left 5 Wrist Bursa and Ligament, Right 6 Wrist Bursa and Ligament, Left 7 Hand Bursa and Ligament, Right 8 Hand Bursa and Ligament, Left 9 Upper Extremity Bursa and Ligament, Right B Upper Extremity Bursa and Ligament, Left C Upper Spine Bursa and Ligament D Lower Spine Bursa and Ligament F Sternum Bursa and Ligament G Rib(s) Bursa and Ligament H Abdomen Bursa and Ligament, Right J Abdomen Bursa and Ligament, Left K Perineum Bursa and Ligament L Hip Bursa and Ligament, Right M Hip Bursa and Ligament, Left N Knee Bursa and Ligament, Right P Knee Bursa and Ligament, Left Q Ankle Bursa and Ligament, Right R Ankle Bursa and Ligament, Left S Foot Bursa and Ligament, Right T Foot Bursa and Ligament, Left V Lower Extremity Bursa and Ligament, Right W Lower Extremity Bursa and Ligament, Left	Ø Open 4 Percutaneous Endoscopic	7 Autologous Tissue Substitute J Synthetic Substitute K Nonautologous Tissue Substitute	Z No Qualifier

Coding Clinic: 2Ø17, Q2, P22 – ØMUN47Z

SECTION: Ø MEDICAL AND SURGICAL
BODY SYSTEM: M BURSAE AND LIGAMENTS
OPERATION: W REVISION: Correcting, to the extent possible, a portion of a malfunctioning device or the position of a displaced device

Body Part	Approach	Device	Qualifier
X Upper Bursa and Ligament Y Lower Bursa and Ligament	Ø Open 3 Percutaneous 4 Percutaneous Endoscopic	Ø Drainage Device 7 Autologous Tissue Substitute J Synthetic Substitute K Nonautologous Tissue Substitute Y Other Device	Z No Qualifier
X Upper Bursa and Ligament Y Lower Bursa and Ligament	X External	Ø Drainage Device 7 Autologous Tissue Substitute J Synthetic Substitute K Nonautologous Tissue Substitute	Z No Qualifier

Non-OR ØMW[XY]X[Ø7JK]Z

SECTION: Ø MEDICAL AND SURGICAL
BODY SYSTEM: M BURSAE AND LIGAMENTS
OPERATION: X TRANSFER: Moving, without taking out, all or a portion of a body part to another location to take over the function of all or a portion of a body part

Body Part	Approach	Device	Qualifier
Ø Head and Neck Bursa and Ligament 1 Shoulder Bursa and Ligament, Right 2 Shoulder Bursa and Ligament, Left 3 Elbow Bursa and Ligament, Right 4 Elbow Bursa and Ligament, Left 5 Wrist Bursa and Ligament, Right 6 Wrist Bursa and Ligament, Left 7 Hand Bursa and Ligament, Right 8 Hand Bursa and Ligament, Left 9 Upper Extremity Bursa and Ligament, Right B Upper Extremity Bursa and Ligament, Left C Upper Spine Bursa and Ligament D Lower Spine Bursa and Ligament F Sternum Bursa and Ligament G Rib(s) Bursa and Ligament H Abdomen Bursa and Ligament, Right J Abdomen Bursa and Ligament, Left K Perineum Bursa and Ligament L Hip Bursa and Ligament, Right M Hip Bursa and Ligament, Left N Knee Bursa and Ligament, Right P Knee Bursa and Ligament, Left Q Ankle Bursa and Ligament, Right R Ankle Bursa and Ligament, Left S Foot Bursa and Ligament, Right T Foot Bursa and Ligament, Left V Lower Extremity Bursa and Ligament, Right W Lower Extremity Bursa and Ligament, Left	Ø Open 4 Percutaneous Endoscopic	Z No Device	Z No Qualifier

SECTION: Ø MEDICAL AND SURGICAL
BODY SYSTEM: N HEAD AND FACIAL BONES
OPERATION: 2 CHANGE: Taking out or off a device from a body part and putting back an identical or similar device in or on the same body part without cutting or puncturing the skin or a mucous membrane

Body Part	Approach	Device	Qualifier
Ø Skull B Nasal Bone W Facial Bone	X External	Ø Drainage Device Y Other Device	Z No Qualifier

Non-OR All Values

SECTION: Ø MEDICAL AND SURGICAL
BODY SYSTEM: N HEAD AND FACIAL BONES
OPERATION: 5 DESTRUCTION: Physical eradication of all or a portion of a body part by the direct use of energy, force, or a destructive agent

Body Part	Approach	Device	Qualifier
Ø Skull 1 Frontal Bone 3 Parietal Bone, Right 4 Parietal Bone, Left 5 Temporal Bone, Right 6 Temporal Bone, Left 7 Occipital Bone B Nasal Bone C Sphenoid Bone F Ethmoid Bone, Right G Ethmoid Bone, Left H Lacrimal Bone, Right J Lacrimal Bone, Left K Palatine Bone, Right L Palatine Bone, Left M Zygomatic Bone, Right N Zygomatic Bone, Left P Orbit, Right Q Orbit, Left R Maxilla T Mandible, Right V Mandible, Left X Hyoid Bone	Ø Open 3 Percutaneous 4 Percutaneous Endoscopic	Z No Device	Z No Qualifier

SECTION: Ø MEDICAL AND SURGICAL
BODY SYSTEM: N HEAD AND FACIAL BONES
OPERATION: 8 DIVISION: Cutting into a body part, without draining fluids and/or gases from the body part, in order to separate or transect a body part

Body Part	Approach	Device	Qualifier
Ø Skull 1 Frontal Bone 3 Parietal Bone, Right 4 Parietal Bone, Left 5 Temporal Bone, Right 6 Temporal Bone, Left 7 Occipital Bonet B Nasal Bone C Sphenoid Bone F Ethmoid Bone, Right G Ethmoid Bone, Left H Lacrimal Bone, Right J Lacrimal Bone, Left K Palatine Bone, Right L Palatine Bone, Left M Zygomatic Bone, Right N Zygomatic Bone, Left P Orbit, Right Q Orbit, Left R Maxilla T Mandible, Right V Mandible, Left X Hyoid Bone	Ø Open 3 Percutaneous 4 Percutaneous Endoscopic	Z No Device	Z No Qualifier

Non-OR ØN8B[Ø34]ZZ

SECTION: Ø MEDICAL AND SURGICAL
BODY SYSTEM: N HEAD AND FACIAL BONES
OPERATION: 9 DRAINAGE: Taking or letting out fluids and/or gases from a body part

Body Part	Approach	Device	Qualifier
Ø Skull 1 Frontal Bone 3 Parietal Bone, Right 4 Parietal Bone, Left 5 Temporal Bone, Right 6 Temporal Bone, Left 7 Occipital Bone B Nasal Bone C Sphenoid Bone F Ethmoid Bone, Right G Ethmoid Bone, Left H Lacrimal Bone, Right J Lacrimal Bone, Left K Palatine Bone, Right L Palatine Bone, Left M Zygomatic Bone, Right N Zygomatic Bone, Left P Orbit, Right Q Orbit, Left R Maxilla T Mandible, Right V Mandible, Left X Hyoid Bone	Ø Open 3 Percutaneous 4 Percutaneous Endoscopic	Ø Drainage Device	Z No Qualifier
Ø Skull 1 Frontal Bone 3 Parietal Bone, Right 4 Parietal Bone, Left 5 Temporal Bone, Right 6 Temporal Bone, Left 7 Occipital Bone B Nasal Bone C Sphenoid Bone F Ethmoid Bone, Right G Ethmoid Bone, Left H Lacrimal Bone, Right J Lacrimal Bone, Left K Palatine Bone, Right L Palatine Bone, Left M Zygomatic Bone, Right N Zygomatic Bone, Left P Orbit, Right Q Orbit, Left R Maxilla T Mandible, Right V Mandible, Left X Hyoid Bone	Ø Open 3 Percutaneous 4 Percutaneous Endoscopic	Z No Device	X Diagnostic Z No Qualifier

Non-OR ØN9[Ø134567CFGHJKLMNPQX]3ØZ
Non-OR ØN9[BRTV][Ø34]ØZ
Non-OR ØN9[Ø134567CFGHJKLMNPQX]3ZZ
Non-OR ØN9B[Ø34]ZX
Non-OR ØN9[BRTV][Ø34]ZZ

SECTION: Ø MEDICAL AND SURGICAL
BODY SYSTEM: N HEAD AND FACIAL BONES
OPERATION: B EXCISION: Cutting out or off, without replacement, a portion of a body part

Body Part	Approach	Device	Qualifier
Ø Skull 1 Frontal Bone 3 Parietal Bone, Right 4 Parietal Bone, Left 5 Temporal Bone, Right 6 Temporal Bone, Left 7 Occipital Bone B Nasal Bone C Sphenoid Bone F Ethmoid Bone, Right G Ethmoid Bone, Left H Lacrimal Bone, Right J Lacrimal Bone, Left K Palatine Bone, Right L Palatine Bone, Left M Zygomatic Bone, Right N Zygomatic Bone, Left P Orbit, Right Q Orbit, Left R Maxilla T Mandible, Right V Mandible, Left X Hyoid Bone	Ø Open 3 Percutaneous 4 Percutaneous Endoscopic	Z No Device	X Diagnostic Z No Qualifier

Non-OR ØNB[BRTV][Ø34]ZX

Coding Clinic: 2Ø15, Q2, P13 – ØNBQØZZ
Coding Clinic: 2Ø17, Q1, P2Ø – ØNBBØZZ
Coding Clinic: 2Ø22, Q2, P18; 2Ø21, Q1, P21 – ØNBRØZZ
Coding Clinic: 2Ø21, Q3, P2Ø – ØNBXØZZ

New/Revised Text in Green ~~deleted~~ Deleted ♀ Females Only ♂ Males Only Coding Clinic
Non-covered Limited Coverage ⊞ Combination (See Appendix E) DRG Non-OR Non-OR Hospital-Acquired Condition

SECTION: Ø MEDICAL AND SURGICAL
BODY SYSTEM: N HEAD AND FACIAL BONES
OPERATION: C EXTIRPATION: Taking or cutting out solid matter from a body part

Body Part	Approach	Device	Qualifier
1 Frontal Bone 3 Parietal Bone, Right 4 Parietal Bone, Left 5 Temporal Bone, Right 6 Temporal Bone, Left 7 Occipital Bone B Nasal Bone C Sphenoid Bone F Ethmoid Bone, Right G Ethmoid Bone, Left H Lacrimal Bone, Right J Lacrimal Bone, Left K Palatine Bone, Right L Palatine Bone, Left M Zygomatic Bone, Right N Zygomatic Bone, Left P Orbit, Right Q Orbit, Left R Maxilla T Mandible, Right V Mandible, Left X Hyoid Bone	Ø Open 3 Percutaneous 4 Percutaneous Endoscopic	Z No Device	Z No Qualifier

Non-OR ØNC[BRTV][Ø34]ZZ

SECTION: Ø MEDICAL AND SURGICAL
BODY SYSTEM: N HEAD AND FACIAL BONES
OPERATION: D EXTRACTION: Pulling or stripping out or off all or a portion of a body part by the use of force

Body Part	Approach	Device	Qualifier
Ø Skull 1 Frontal Bone 3 Parietal Bone, Right 4 Parietal Bone, Left 5 Temporal Bone, Right 6 Temporal Bone, Left 7 Occipital Bone B Nasal Bone C Sphenoid Bone F Ethmoid Bone, Right G Ethmoid Bone, Left H Lacrimal Bone, Right J Lacrimal Bone, Left K Palatine Bone, Right L Palatine Bone, Left M Zygomatic Bone, Right N Zygomatic Bone, Left P Orbit, Right Q Orbit, Left R Maxilla T Mandible, Right V Mandible, Left X Hyoid Bone	Ø Open	Z No Device	Z No Qualifier

SECTION: Ø MEDICAL AND SURGICAL
BODY SYSTEM: N HEAD AND FACIAL BONES
OPERATION: H INSERTION: Putting in a nonbiological appliance that monitors, assists, performs, or prevents a physiological function but does not physically take the place of a body part

Body Part	Approach	Device	Qualifier
Ø Skull ⊞	Ø Open	3 Infusion Device 4 Internal Fixation Device 5 External Fixation Device M Bone Growth Stimulator N Neurostimulator Generator	Z No Qualifier
Ø Skull	3 Percutaneous 4 Percutaneous Endoscopic	3 Infusion Device 4 Internal Fixation Device 5 External Fixation Device M Bone Growth Stimulator	Z No Qualifier
1 Frontal Bone 3 Parietal Bone, Right 4 Parietal Bone, Left 7 Occipital Bone C Sphenoid Bone F Ethmoid Bone, Right G Ethmoid Bone, Left H Lacrimal Bone, Right J Lacrimal Bone, Left K Palatine Bone, Right L Palatine Bone, Left M Zygomatic Bone, Right N Zygomatic Bone, Left P Orbit, Right Q Orbit, Left X Hyoid Bone	Ø Open 3 Percutaneous 4 Percutaneous Endoscopic	4 Internal Fixation Device	Z No Qualifier
5 Temporal Bone, Right 6 Temporal Bone, Left	Ø Open 3 Percutaneous 4 Percutaneous Endoscopic	4 Internal Fixation Device S Hearing Device	Z No Qualifier
B Nasal Bone	Ø Open 3 Percutaneous 4 Percutaneous Endoscopic	4 Internal Fixation Device M Bone Growth Stimulator	Z No Qualifier
R Maxilla T Mandible, Right V Mandible, Left	Ø Open 3 Percutaneous 4 Percutaneous Endoscopic	4 Internal Fixation Device 5 External Fixation Device	Z No Qualifier
W Facial Bone	Ø Open 3 Percutaneous 4 Percutaneous Endoscopic	M Bone Growth Stimulator	Z No Qualifier

⊞ ØNHØØNZ
Non-OR ØNHØØ5Z
Non-OR ØNHØ[34]5Z
Non-OR ØNHB[Ø34][4M]Z

Coding Clinic: 2015, Q3, P14 – ØNHØØ4Z

SECTION: Ø MEDICAL AND SURGICAL
BODY SYSTEM: N HEAD AND FACIAL BONES
OPERATION: J INSPECTION: Visually and/or manually exploring a body part

Body Part	Approach	Device	Qualifier
Ø Skull B Nasal Bone W Facial Bone	Ø Open 3 Percutaneous 4 Percutaneous Endoscopic X External	Z No Device	Z No Qualifier

Non-OR ØNJ[ØBW][3X]ZZ

SECTION: Ø MEDICAL AND SURGICAL
BODY SYSTEM: N HEAD AND FACIAL BONES
OPERATION: N RELEASE: Freeing a body part from an abnormal physical constraint by cutting or by the use of force

Body Part	Approach	Device	Qualifier
1 Frontal Bone 3 Parietal Bone, Right 4 Parietal Bone, Left 5 Temporal Bone, Right 6 Temporal Bone, Left 7 Occipital Bone B Nasal Bone C Sphenoid Bone F Ethmoid Bone, Right G Ethmoid Bone, Left H Lacrimal Bone, Right J Lacrimal Bone, Left K Palatine Bone, Right L Palatine Bone, Left M Zygomatic Bone, Right N Zygomatic Bone, Left P Orbit, Right Q Orbit, Left R Maxilla T Mandible, Right V Mandible, Left X Hyoid Bone	Ø Open 3 Percutaneous 4 Percutaneous Endoscopic	Z No Device	Z No Qualifier

Non-OR ØNNB[Ø34]ZZ

SECTION: Ø MEDICAL AND SURGICAL
BODY SYSTEM: N HEAD AND FACIAL BONES
OPERATION: P REMOVAL: Taking out or off a device from a body part

Body Part	Approach	Device	Qualifier
Ø Skull	Ø Open	Ø Drainage Device 3 Infusion Device 4 Internal Fixation Device 5 External Fixation Device 7 Autologous Tissue Substitute J Synthetic Substitute K Nonautologous Tissue Substitute M Bone Growth Stimulator N Neurostimulator Generator S Hearing Device	Z No Qualifier
Ø Skull	3 Percutaneous 4 Percutaneous Endoscopic	Ø Drainage Device 3 Infusion Device 4 Internal Fixation Device 5 External Fixation Device 7 Autologous Tissue Substitute J Synthetic Substitute K Nonautologous Tissue Substitute M Bone Growth Stimulator S Hearing Device	Z No Qualifier
Ø Skull	X External	Ø Drainage Device 3 Infusion Device 4 Internal Fixation Device 5 External Fixation Device M Bone Growth Stimulator S Hearing Device	Z No Qualifier
B Nasal Bone W Facial Bone	Ø Open 3 Percutaneous 4 Percutaneous Endoscopic	Ø Drainage Device 4 Internal Fixation Device 7 Autologous Tissue Substitute J Synthetic Substitute K Nonautologous Tissue Substitute M Bone Growth Stimulator	Z No Qualifier
B Nasal Bone W Facial Bone	X External	Ø Drainage Device 4 Internal Fixation Device M Bone Growth Stimulator	Z No Qualifier

Non-OR ØNPØ[34]5Z
Non-OR ØNPØX[Ø5]Z
Non-OR ØNPB[Ø34][Ø47JKM]Z
Non-OR ØNPBX[Ø4M]Z
Non-OR ØNPWX[ØM]Z
Non-OR ØNPØ[Ø34]3Z

Coding Clinic: 2Ø15, Q3, P14 – ØNPØØ4Z
Coding Clinic: 2Ø23, Q1, P32 – ØNPØØ7Z

SECTION: Ø MEDICAL AND SURGICAL
BODY SYSTEM: N HEAD AND FACIAL BONES
OPERATION: Q REPAIR: Restoring, to the extent possible, a body part to its normal anatomic structure and function

Body Part	Approach	Device	Qualifier
Ø Skull 1 Frontal Bone 3 Parietal Bone, Right 4 Parietal Bone, Left 5 Temporal Bone, Right 6 Temporal Bone, Left 7 Occipital Bone B Nasal Bone C Sphenoid Bone F Ethmoid Bone, Right G Ethmoid Bone, Left H Lacrimal Bone, Right J Lacrimal Bone, Left K Palatine Bone, Right L Palatine Bone, Left M Zygomatic Bone, Right N Zygomatic Bone, Left P Orbit, Right Q Orbit, Left R Maxilla T Mandible, Right V Mandible, Left X Hyoid Bone	Ø Open 3 Percutaneous 4 Percutaneous Endoscopic X External	Z No Device	Z No Qualifier

DRG Non-OR ØNQ[Ø12345678BCDFGHJKLMNPQRSTVX]XZZ

Coding Clinic: 2016, Q3, P29 – ØNQSØZZ

SECTION: Ø MEDICAL AND SURGICAL
BODY SYSTEM: N HEAD AND FACIAL BONES
OPERATION: R REPLACEMENT: Putting in or on biological or synthetic material that physically takes the place and/or function of all or a portion of a body part

Body Part	Approach	Device	Qualifier
Ø Skull 1 Frontal Bone 3 Parietal Bone, Right 4 Parietal Bone, Left 5 Temporal Bone, Right 6 Temporal Bone, Left 7 Occipital Bone B Nasal Bone C Sphenoid Bone F Ethmoid Bone, Right G Ethmoid Bone, Left H Lacrimal Bone, Right J Lacrimal Bone, Left K Palatine Bone, Right L Palatine Bone, Left M Zygomatic Bone, Right N Zygomatic Bone, Left P Orbit, Right Q Orbit, Left R Maxilla T Mandible, Right V Mandible, Left X Hyoid Bone	Ø Open 3 Percutaneous 4 Percutaneous Endoscopic	7 Autologous Tissue Substitute J Synthetic Substitute K Nonautologous Tissue Substitute	Z No Qualifier

Coding Clinic: 2017, Q1, P24 – ØNRVØ[7J]Z
Coding Clinic: 2017, Q3, P17 – ØNR8ØJZ
Coding Clinic: 2021, Q1, P22 - ØNRRØJZ
Coding Clinic: 2021, Q3, P3Ø – ØNR5ØJZ

SECTION: Ø MEDICAL AND SURGICAL
BODY SYSTEM: N HEAD AND FACIAL BONES
OPERATION: S REPOSITION: *(on multiple pages)*
Moving to its normal location, or other suitable location, all or a portion of a body part

Body Part	Approach	Device	Qualifier
Ø Skull R Maxilla T Mandible, Right V Mandible, Left	Ø Open 3 Percutaneous 4 Percutaneous Endoscopic	4 Internal Fixation Device 5 External Fixation Device Z No Device	Z No Qualifier
Ø Skull R Maxilla T Mandible, Right V Mandible, Left	X External	Z No Device	Z No Qualifier

Non-OR ØNS[RTV][34][45Z]Z
Non-OR ØNS[RTV]XZZ

Coding Clinic: 2016, Q2, P3Ø; 2015, Q3, P18 – ØNSØØZZ
Coding Clinic: 2017, Q1, P21 – ØNS[RS]ØZZ
Coding Clinic: 2017, Q3, P22 – ØNSØØ4Z

SECTION: Ø MEDICAL AND SURGICAL
BODY SYSTEM: N HEAD AND FACIAL BONES
OPERATION: S REPOSITION: *(continued)*

Moving to its normal location, or other suitable location, all or a portion of a body part

Body Part	Approach	Device	Qualifier
1 Frontal Bone 3 Parietal Bone, Right 4 Parietal Bone, Left 5 Temporal Bone, Right 6 Temporal Bone, Left 7 Occipital Bone B Nasal Bone C Sphenoid Bone F Ethmoid Bone, Right G Ethmoid Bone, Left H Lacrimal Bone, Right J Lacrimal Bone, Left K Palatine Bone, Right L Palatine Bone, Left M Zygomatic Bone, Right N Zygomatic Bone, Left P Orbit, Right Q Orbit, Left X Hyoid Bone	Ø Open 3 Percutaneous 4 Percutaneous Endoscopic	4 Internal Fixation Device Z No Device	Z No Qualifier
1 Frontal Bone 3 Parietal Bone, Right 4 Parietal Bone, Left 5 Temporal Bone, Right 6 Temporal Bone, Left 7 Occipital Bone B Nasal Bone C Sphenoid Bone F Ethmoid Bone, Right G Ethmoid Bone, Left H Lacrimal Bone, Right J Lacrimal Bone, Left K Palatine Bone, Right L Palatine Bone, Left M Zygomatic Bone, Right N Zygomatic Bone, Left P Orbit, Right Q Orbit, Left X Hyoid Bone	X External	Z No Device	Z No Qualifier

Non-OR ØNS[BCFGHJKLMNPQX][34][4Z]Z
Non-OR ØNS[BCFGHJKLMNPQX]XZZ

Coding Clinic: 2Ø13, Q3, P25 – ØNSØØ5Z, ØNS1Ø4Z
Coding Clinic: 2Ø15, Q3, P28 – ØNS5Ø4Z

SECTION: Ø MEDICAL AND SURGICAL
BODY SYSTEM: N HEAD AND FACIAL BONES
OPERATION: T RESECTION: Cutting out or off, without replacement, all of a body part

Body Part	Approach	Device	Qualifier
1 Frontal Bone 3 Parietal Bone, Right 4 Parietal Bone, Left 5 Temporal Bone, Right 6 Temporal Bone, Left 7 Occipital Bone B Nasal Bone C Sphenoid Bone F Ethmoid Bone, Right G Ethmoid Bone, Left H Lacrimal Bone, Right J Lacrimal Bone, Left K Palatine Bone, Right L Palatine Bone, Left M Zygomatic Bone, Right N Zygomatic Bone, Left P Orbit, Right Q Orbit, Left R Maxilla T Mandible, Right V Mandible, Left X Hyoid Bone	Ø Open	Z No Device	Z No Qualifier

SECTION: Ø MEDICAL AND SURGICAL
BODY SYSTEM: N HEAD AND FACIAL BONES
OPERATION: U SUPPLEMENT: Putting in or on biological or synthetic material that physically reinforces and/or augments the function of a portion of a body part

Body Part	Approach	Device	Qualifier
Ø Skull 1 Frontal Bone 3 Parietal Bone, Right 4 Parietal Bone, Left 5 Temporal Bone, Right 6 Temporal Bone, Left 7 Occipital Bone B Nasal Bone C Sphenoid Bone F Ethmoid Bone, Right G Ethmoid Bone, Left H Lacrimal Bone, Right J Lacrimal Bone, Left K Palatine Bone, Right L Palatine Bone, Left M Zygomatic Bone, Right N Zygomatic Bone, Left P Orbit, Right Q Orbit, Left R Maxilla T Mandible, Right V Mandible, Left X Hyoid Bone	Ø Open 3 Percutaneous 4 Percutaneous Endoscopic	7 Autologous Tissue Substitute J Synthetic Substitute K Nonautologous Tissue Substitute	Z No Qualifier

Coding Clinic: 2Ø13, Q3, P25 – ØNUØØJZ
Coding Clinic: 2Ø16, Q3, P29 – ØNURØ7Z
Coding Clinic: 2Ø21, Q1, P22 – ØDUP47Z
Coding Clinic: 2Ø21, Q3, P3Ø – ØNU5ØKZ
Coding Clinic: 2Ø23, Q2, P2Ø – ØNU5ØJZ

SECTION: Ø MEDICAL AND SURGICAL
BODY SYSTEM: N HEAD AND FACIAL BONES
OPERATION: W REVISION: Correcting, to the extent possible, a portion of a malfunctioning device or the position of a displaced device

Body Part	Approach	Device	Qualifier
Ø Skull	Ø Open	Ø Drainage Device 3 Infusion Device 4 Internal Fixation Device 5 External Fixation Device 7 Autologous Tissue Substitute J Synthetic Substitute K Nonautologous Tissue Substitute M Bone Growth Stimulator N Neurostimulator Generator S Hearing Device	Z No Qualifier
Ø Skull	3 Percutaneous 4 Percutaneous Endoscopic X External	Ø Drainage Device 3 Infusion Device 4 Internal Fixation Device 5 External Fixation Device 7 Autologous Tissue Substitute J Synthetic Substitute K Nonautologous Tissue Substitute M Bone Growth Stimulator S Hearing Device	Z No Qualifier
B Nasal Bone W Facial Bone	Ø Open 3 Percutaneous 4 Percutaneous Endoscopic X External	Ø Drainage Device 4 Internal Fixation Device 7 Autologous Tissue Substitute J Synthetic Substitute K Nonautologous Tissue Substitute M Bone Growth Stimulator	Z No Qualifier

Non-OR ØNWØX[Ø457JKMS]Z
Non-OR ØNWB[Ø34X][Ø47JKM]Z
Non-OR ØNWWX[Ø47JKM]Z

Ø: M/S N: HEAD AND FACIAL BONES W: REVISION

SECTION: Ø MEDICAL AND SURGICAL
BODY SYSTEM: P UPPER BONES
OPERATION: 2 CHANGE: Taking out or off a device from a body part and putting back an identical or similar device in or on the same body part without cutting or puncturing the skin or a mucous membrane

Body Part	Approach	Device	Qualifier
Y Upper Bone	X External	Ø Drainage Device Y Other Device	Z No Qualifier

Non-OR All Values

SECTION: Ø MEDICAL AND SURGICAL
BODY SYSTEM: P UPPER BONES
OPERATION: 5 DESTRUCTION: Physical eradication of all or a portion of a body part by the direct use of energy, force, or a destructive agent

Body Part	Approach	Device	Qualifier
Ø Sternum 1 Rib, 1 to 2 2 Rib, 3 or More ~~3 Cervical Vertebra~~ ~~4 Thoracic Vertebra~~ 5 Scapula, Right 6 Scapula, Left 7 Glenoid Cavity, Right 8 Glenoid Cavity, Left 9 Clavicle, Right B Clavicle, Left C Humeral Head, Right D Humeral Head, Left F Humeral Shaft, Right G Humeral Shaft, Left H Radius, Right J Radius, Left K Ulna, Right L Ulna, Left M Carpal, Right N Carpal, Left P Metacarpal, Right Q Metacarpal, Left R Thumb Phalanx, Right S Thumb Phalanx, Left T Finger Phalanx, Right V Finger Phalanx, Left	Ø Open 3 Percutaneous 4 Percutaneous Endoscopic	Z No Device	Z No Qualifier
3 Cervical Vertebra 4 Thoracic Vertebra	Ø Open 3 Percutaneous 4 Percutaneous Endoscopic	Z No Device	3 Laser Interstitial Thermal Z No Qualifier

SECTION: Ø MEDICAL AND SURGICAL
BODY SYSTEM: P UPPER BONES
OPERATION: 8 DIVISION: Cutting into a body part, without draining fluids and/or gases from the body part, in order to separate or transect a body part

Body Part	Approach	Device	Qualifier
Ø Sternum 1 Rib, 1 to 2 2 Rib, 3 or More 3 Cervical Vertebra 4 Thoracic Vertebra 5 Scapula, Right 6 Scapula, Left 7 Glenoid Cavity, Right 8 Glenoid Cavity, Left 9 Clavicle, Right B Clavicle, Left C Humeral Head, Right D Humeral Head, Left F Humeral Shaft, Right G Humeral Shaft, Left H Radius, Right J Radius, Left K Ulna, Right L Ulna, Left M Carpal, Right N Carpal, Left P Metacarpal, Right Q Metacarpal, Left R Thumb Phalanx, Right S Thumb Phalanx, Left T Finger Phalanx, Right V Finger Phalanx, Left	Ø Open 3 Percutaneous 4 Percutaneous Endoscopic	Z No Device	Z No Qualifier

New/Revised Text in Green ~~deleted~~ Deleted ♀ Females Only ♂ Males Only **Coding Clinic**
Non-covered Limited Coverage Combination (See Appendix E) DRG Non-OR Non-OR Hospital-Acquired Condition

SECTION: Ø MEDICAL AND SURGICAL
BODY SYSTEM: P UPPER BONES
OPERATION: 9 DRAINAGE: Taking or letting out fluids and/or gases from a body part

Body Part	Approach	Device	Qualifier
Ø Sternum 1 Rib, 1 to 2 2 Rib, 3 or More 3 Cervical Vertebra 4 Thoracic Vertebra 5 Scapula, Right 6 Scapula, Left 7 Glenoid Cavity, Right 8 Glenoid Cavity, Left 9 Clavicle, Right B Clavicle, Left C Humeral Head, Right D Humeral Head, Left F Humeral Shaft, Right G Humeral Shaft, Left H Radius, Right J Radius, Left K Ulna, Right L Ulna, Left M Carpal, Right N Carpal, Left P Metacarpal, Right Q Metacarpal, Left R Thumb Phalanx, Right S Thumb Phalanx, Left T Finger Phalanx, Right V Finger Phalanx, Left	Ø Open 3 Percutaneous 4 Percutaneous Endoscopic	Ø Drainage Device	Z No Qualifier
Ø Sternum 1 Rib, 1 to 2 2 Rib, 3 or More 3 Cervical Vertebra 4 Thoracic Vertebra 5 Scapula, Right 6 Scapula, Left 7 Glenoid Cavity, Right 8 Glenoid Cavity, Left 9 Clavicle, Right B Clavicle, Left C Humeral Head, Right D Humeral Head, Left F Humeral Shaft, Right G Humeral Shaft, Left H Radius, Right J Radius, Left K Ulna, Right L Ulna, Left M Carpal, Right N Carpal, Left P Metacarpal, Right Q Metacarpal, Left R Thumb Phalanx, Right S Thumb Phalanx, Left T Finger Phalanx, Right V Finger Phalanx, Left	Ø Open 3 Percutaneous 4 Percutaneous Endoscopic	Z No Device	X Diagnostic Z No Qualifier

Non-OR ØP9[Ø123456789BCDFGHJKLMNPQRSTV]3ØZ
Non-OR ØP9[Ø123456789BCDFGHJKLMNPQRSTV]3ZZ

SECTION: Ø MEDICAL AND SURGICAL
BODY SYSTEM: P UPPER BONES
OPERATION: B EXCISION: Cutting out or off, without replacement, a portion of a body part

Body Part	Approach	Device	Qualifier
Ø Sternum 1 Rib, 1 to 2 2 Rib, 3 or More 3 Cervical Vertebra 4 Thoracic Vertebra 5 Scapula, Right 6 Scapula, Left 7 Glenoid Cavity, Right 8 Glenoid Cavity, Left 9 Clavicle, Right B Clavicle, Left C Humeral Head, Right D Humeral Head, Left F Humeral Shaft, Right G Humeral Shaft, Left H Radius, Right J Radius, Left K Ulna, Right L Ulna, Left M Carpal, Right N Carpal, Left P Metacarpal, Right Q Metacarpal, Left R Thumb Phalanx, Right S Thumb Phalanx, Left T Finger Phalanx, Right V Finger Phalanx, Left	Ø Open 3 Percutaneous 4 Percutaneous Endoscopic	Z No Device	X Diagnostic Z No Qualifier

Coding Clinic: 2Ø12, Q4, P1Ø1 – ØPB1ØZZ
Coding Clinic: 2Ø13, Q3, P22 – ØPB54ZZ

SECTION: Ø MEDICAL AND SURGICAL
BODY SYSTEM: P UPPER BONES
OPERATION: C EXTIRPATION: Taking or cutting out solid matter from a body part

Body Part	Approach	Device	Qualifier
Ø Sternum 1 Rib, 1 to 2 2 Rib, 3 or More 3 Cervical Vertebra 4 Thoracic Vertebra 5 Scapula, Right 6 Scapula, Left 7 Glenoid Cavity, Right 8 Glenoid Cavity, Left 9 Clavicle, Right B Clavicle, Left C Humeral Head, Right D Humeral Head, Left F Humeral Shaft, Right G Humeral Shaft, Left H Radius, Right J Radius, Left K Ulna, Right L Ulna, Left M Carpal, Right N Carpal, Left P Metacarpal, Right Q Metacarpal, Left R Thumb Phalanx, Right S Thumb Phalanx, Left T Finger Phalanx, Right V Finger Phalanx, Left	Ø Open 3 Percutaneous 4 Percutaneous Endoscopic	Z No Device	Z No Qualifier

Coding Clinic: 2Ø19, Q3, P19 – ØPCØØZZ
Coding Clinic: 2Ø21, Q3, P16 – ØPC[CD]3ZZ

SECTION: Ø MEDICAL AND SURGICAL
BODY SYSTEM: P UPPER BONES
OPERATION: D EXTRACTION: Pulling or stripping out or off all or a portion of a body part by the use of force

Body Part	Approach	Device	Qualifier
Ø Sternum 1 Rib, 1 to 2 2 Rib, 3 or More 3 Cervical Vertebra 4 Thoracic Vertebra 5 Scapula, Right 6 Scapula, Left 7 Glenoid Cavity, Right 8 Glenoid Cavity, Left 9 Clavicle, Right B Clavicle, Left C Humeral Head, Right D Humeral Head, Left F Humeral Shaft, Right G Humeral Shaft, Left H Radius, Right J Radius, Left K Ulna, Right L Ulna, Left M Carpal, Right N Carpal, Left P Metacarpal, Right Q Metacarpal, Left R Thumb Phalanx, Right S Thumb Phalanx, Left T Finger Phalanx, Right V Finger Phalanx, Left	Ø Open	Z No Device	Z No Qualifier

SECTION: Ø MEDICAL AND SURGICAL
BODY SYSTEM: P UPPER BONES
OPERATION: H INSERTION: Putting in a nonbiological appliance that monitors, assists, performs, or prevents a physiological function but does not physically take the place of a body part

Body Part	Approach	Device	Qualifier
Ø Sternum	Ø Open 3 Percutaneous 4 Percutaneous Endoscopic	Ø Internal Fixation Device, Rigid Plate 4 Internal Fixation Device	Z No Qualifier
1 Rib, 1 to 2 2 Rib, 3 or More 3 Cervical Vertebra 4 Thoracic Vertebra 5 Scapula, Right 6 Scapula, Left 7 Glenoid Cavity, Right 8 Glenoid Cavity, Left 9 Clavicle, Right B Clavicle, Left	Ø Open 3 Percutaneous 4 Percutaneous Endoscopic	4 Internal Fixation Device	Z No Qualifier
C Humeral Head, Right D Humeral Head, Left H Radius, Right J Radius, Left K Ulna, Right L Ulna, Left	Ø Open 3 Percutaneous 4 Percutaneous Endoscopic	4 Internal Fixation Device 5 External Fixation Device 6 Internal Fixation Device, Intramedullary 8 External Fixation Device, Limb Lengthening B External Fixation Device, Monoplanar C External Fixation Device, Ring D External Fixation Device, Hybrid	Z No Qualifier
F Humeral Shaft, Right G Humeral Shaft, Left	Ø Open 3 Percutaneous 4 Percutaneous Endoscopic	4 Internal Fixation Device 5 External Fixation Device 6 Internal Fixation Device, Intramedullary 7 Internal Fixation Device, Intramedullary Limb Lengthening 8 External Fixation Device, Limb Lengthening B External Fixation Device, Monoplanar C External Fixation Device, Ring D External Fixation Device, Hybrid	Z No Qualifier
M Carpal, Right N Carpal, Left P Metacarpal, Right Q Metacarpal, Left R Thumb Phalanx, Right S Thumb Phalanx, Left T Finger Phalanx, Right V Finger Phalanx, Left	Ø Open 3 Percutaneous 4 Percutaneous Endoscopic	4 Internal Fixation Device 5 External Fixation Device	Z No Qualifier
Y Upper Bone	Ø Open 3 Percutaneous 4 Percutaneous Endoscopic	M Bone Growth Stimulator	Z No Qualifier
Y Upper Bone	Ø Open 3 Percutaneous 4 Percutaneous Endoscopic X External	Z No Device	Z No Qualifier

Non-OR ØPH[CDFGHJKL][Ø34]8Z

Coding Clinic: 2018, Q4, P12 – ØPH5Ø4Z
Coding Clinic: 2020, Q1, P30 – ØPHØØØZ

SECTION: Ø MEDICAL AND SURGICAL
BODY SYSTEM: P UPPER BONES
OPERATION: J INSPECTION: Visually and/or manually exploring a body part

Body Part	Approach	Device	Qualifier
Y Upper Bone	Ø Open 3 Percutaneous 4 Percutaneous Endoscopic X External	Z No Device	Z No Qualifier

Non-OR ØPJY[3X]ZZ

SECTION: Ø MEDICAL AND SURGICAL
BODY SYSTEM: P UPPER BONES
OPERATION: N RELEASE: Freeing a body part from an abnormal physical constraint by cutting or by the use of force

Body Part	Approach	Device	Qualifier
Ø Sternum 1 Rib, 1 to 2 2 Rib, 3 or More 3 Cervical Vertebra 4 Thoracic Vertebra 5 Scapula, Right 6 Scapula, Left 7 Glenoid Cavity, Right 8 Glenoid Cavity, Left 9 Clavicle, Right B Clavicle, Left C Humeral Head, Right D Humeral Head, Left F Humeral Shaft, Right G Humeral Shaft, Left H Radius, Right J Radius, Left K Ulna, Right L Ulna, Left M Carpal, Right N Carpal, Left P Metacarpal, Right Q Metacarpal, Left R Thumb Phalanx, Right S Thumb Phalanx, Left T Finger Phalanx, Right V Finger Phalanx, Left	Ø Open 3 Percutaneous 4 Percutaneous Endoscopic	Z No Device	Z No Qualifier

SECTION: Ø MEDICAL AND SURGICAL
BODY SYSTEM: P UPPER BONES
OPERATION: P REMOVAL: *(on multiple pages)*
Taking out or off a device from a body part

Body Part	Approach	Device	Qualifier
Ø Sternum 1 Rib, 1 to 2 2 Rib, 3 or More 3 Cervical Vertebra 4 Thoracic Vertebra 5 Scapula, Right 6 Scapula, Left 7 Glenoid Cavity, Right 8 Glenoid Cavity, Left 9 Clavicle, Right B Clavicle, Left	Ø Open 3 Percutaneous 4 Percutaneous Endoscopic	4 Internal Fixation Device 7 Autologous Tissue Substitute J Synthetic Substitute K Nonautologous Tissue Substitute	Z No Qualifier
Ø Sternum 1 Rib, 1 to 2 2 Rib, 3 or More 3 Cervical Vertebra 4 Thoracic Vertebra 5 Scapula, Right 6 Scapula, Left 7 Glenoid Cavity, Right 8 Glenoid Cavity, Left 9 Clavicle, Right B Clavicle, Left	X External	4 Internal Fixation Device	Z No Qualifier
C Humeral Head, Right D Humeral Head, Left F Humeral Shaft, Right G Humeral Shaft, Left H Radius, Right J Radius, Left K Ulna, Right L Ulna, Left M Carpal, Right N Carpal, Left P Metacarpal, Right Q Metacarpal, Left R Thumb Phalanx, Right S Thumb Phalanx, Left T Finger Phalanx, Right V Finger Phalanx, Left	Ø Open 3 Percutaneous 4 Percutaneous Endoscopic	4 Internal Fixation Device 5 External Fixation Device 7 Autologous Tissue Substitute J Synthetic Substitute K Nonautologous Tissue Substitute	Z No Qualifier

Non-OR ØPP[Ø123456789B]X4Z

SECTION: Ø MEDICAL AND SURGICAL
BODY SYSTEM: P UPPER BONES
OPERATION: P REMOVAL: *(continued)*
Taking out or off a device from a body part

Body Part	Approach	Device	Qualifier
C Humeral Head, Right D Humeral Head, Left F Humeral Shaft, Right G Humeral Shaft, Left H Radius, Right J Radius, Left K Ulna, Right L Ulna, Left M Carpal, Right N Carpal, Left P Metacarpal, Right Q Metacarpal, Left R Thumb Phalanx, Right S Thumb Phalanx, Left T Finger Phalanx, Right V Finger Phalanx, Left	X External	4 Internal Fixation Device 5 External Fixation Device	Z No Qualifier
Y Upper Bone	Ø Open 3 Percutaneous 4 Percutaneous Endoscopic X External	Ø Drainage Device M Bone Growth Stimulator	Z No Qualifier

Non-OR ØPP[CDFGHJKLMNPQRSTV]X[45]Z
Non-OR ØPPY3ØZ
Non-OR ØPPYX[ØM]Z

SECTION: Ø MEDICAL AND SURGICAL
BODY SYSTEM: P UPPER BONES
OPERATION: Q REPAIR: Restoring, to the extent possible, a body part to its normal anatomic structure and function

Body Part	Approach	Device	Qualifier
Ø Sternum 1 Rib, 1 to 2 2 Rib, 3 or More 3 Cervical Vertebra 4 Thoracic Vertebra 5 Scapula, Right 6 Scapula, Left 7 Glenoid Cavity, Right 8 Glenoid Cavity, Left 9 Clavicle, Right B Clavicle, Left C Humeral Head, Right D Humeral Head, Left F Humeral Shaft, Right G Humeral Shaft, Left H Radius, Right J Radius, Left K Ulna, Right L Ulna, Left M Carpal, Right N Carpal, Left P Metacarpal, Right Q Metacarpal, Left R Thumb Phalanx, Right S Thumb Phalanx, Left T Finger Phalanx, Right V Finger Phalanx, Left	Ø Open 3 Percutaneous 4 Percutaneous Endoscopic X External	Z No Device	Z No Qualifier

DRG Non-OR ØPQ[Ø123456789BCDFGHJKLMNPQRSTV]XZZ

Ø: M/S P: UPPER BONES Q: REPAIR

SECTION: Ø MEDICAL AND SURGICAL
BODY SYSTEM: P UPPER BONES
OPERATION: R REPLACEMENT: Putting in or on biological or synthetic material that physically takes the place and/or function of all or a portion of a body part

Body Part	Approach	Device	Qualifier
Ø Sternum 1 Rib, 1 to 2 2 Rib, 3 or More 3 Cervical Vertebra 4 Thoracic Vertebra 5 Scapula, Right 6 Scapula, Left 7 Glenoid Cavity, Right 8 Glenoid Cavity, Left 9 Clavicle, Right B Clavicle, Left C Humeral Head, Right D Humeral Head, Left F Humeral Shaft, Right G Humeral Shaft, Left H Radius, Right J Radius, Left K Ulna, Right L Ulna, Left M Carpal, Right N Carpal, Left P Metacarpal, Right Q Metacarpal, Left R Thumb Phalanx, Right S Thumb Phalanx, Left T Finger Phalanx, Right V Finger Phalanx, Left	Ø Open 3 Percutaneous 4 Percutaneous Endoscopic	7 Autologous Tissue Substitute J Synthetic Substitute K Nonautologous Tissue Substitute	Z No Qualifier

Coding Clinic: 2018, Q4, P92 – ØPRHØJZ

SECTION: Ø MEDICAL AND SURGICAL
BODY SYSTEM: P UPPER BONES
OPERATION: S REPOSITION: *(on multiple pages)*
Moving to its normal location, or other suitable location, all or a portion of a body part

Body Part	Approach	Device	Qualifier
Ø Sternum	Ø Open 3 Percutaneous 4 Percutaneous Endoscopic	Ø Internal Fixation Device, Rigid Plate 4 Internal Fixation Device Z No Device	Z No Qualifier
Ø Sternum	X External	Z No Device	Z No Qualifier
1 Rib, 1 to 2 2 Rib, 3 or More 3 Cervical Vertebra ⊞ 5 Scapula, Right 6 Scapula, Left 7 Glenoid Cavity, Right 8 Glenoid Cavity, Left 9 Clavicle, Right B Clavicle, Left	Ø Open 3 Percutaneous 4 Percutaneous Endoscopic	4 Internal Fixation Device Z No Device	Z No Qualifier

⊞ ØPS3[34]ZZ
Non-OR ØPSØ[34]ZZ
Non-OR ØPSØXZZ

Non-OR ØPS[1256789B][34]ZZ
Coding Clinic: 2015, Q4, P34 – ØPSØØZZ
Coding Clinic: 2016, Q1, P21 – ØPS4XZZ

Coding Clinic: 2017, Q4, P53 – ØPS2Ø4Z
Coding Clinic: 2020, Q1, P33 – ØPS4Ø4Z

New/Revised Text in Green ~~deleted~~ Deleted ♀ Females Only ♂ Males Only Coding Clinic
Non-covered Limited Coverage ⊞ Combination (See Appendix E) DRG Non-OR Non-OR Hospital-Acquired Condition

SECTION: Ø MEDICAL AND SURGICAL
BODY SYSTEM: P UPPER BONES
OPERATION: S REPOSITION: *(on multiple pages)*

Moving to its normal location, or other suitable location, all or a portion of a body part

Body Part	Approach	Device	Qualifier
1 Rib, 1 to 2 2 Rib, 3 or More 3 Cervical Vertebra 5 Scapula, Right 6 Scapula, Left 7 Glenoid Cavity, Right 8 Glenoid Cavity, Left 9 Clavicle, Right B Clavicle, Left	X External	Z No Device	Z No Qualifier
4 Thoracic Vertebra	Ø Open 4 Percutaneous Endoscopic	3 Spinal Stabilization Device, Vertebral Body Tether 4 Internal Fixation Device Z No Device	Z No Qualifier
4 Thoracic Vertebra	3 Percutaneous	4 Internal Fixation Device Z No Device	Z No Qualifier
4 Thoracic Vertebra	X External	Z No Device	Z No Qualifier
C Humeral Head, Right D Humeral Head, Left F Humeral Shaft, Right G Humeral Shaft, Left H Radius, Right J Radius, Left K Ulna, Right L Ulna, Left	Ø Open 3 Percutaneous 4 Percutaneous Endoscopic	4 Internal Fixation Device 5 External Fixation Device 6 Internal Fixation Device, Intramedullary B External Fixation Device, Monoplanar C External Fixation Device, Ring D External Fixation Device, Hybrid Z No Device	Z No Qualifier
C Humeral Head, Right D Humeral Head, Left F Humeral Shaft, Right G Humeral Shaft, Left H Radius, Right J Radius, Left K Ulna, Right L Ulna, Left	X External	Z No Device	Z No Qualifier
M Carpal, Right N Carpal, Left P Metacarpal, Right Q Metacarpal, Left R Thumb Phalanx, Right S Thumb Phalanx, Left T Finger Phalanx, Right V Finger Phalanx, Left	Ø Open 3 Percutaneous 4 Percutaneous Endoscopic	4 Internal Fixation Device 5 External Fixation Device Z No Device	Z No Qualifier

SECTION: Ø MEDICAL AND SURGICAL
BODY SYSTEM: P UPPER BONES
OPERATION: S REPOSITION: *(continued)*
Moving to its normal location, or other suitable location, all or a portion of a body part

Body Part	Approach	Device	Qualifier
M Carpal, Right N Carpal, Left P Metacarpal, Right Q Metacarpal, Left R Thumb Phalanx, Right S Thumb Phalanx, Left T Finger Phalanx, Right V Finger Phalanx, Left	X External	Z No Device	Z No Qualifier

Non-OR ØPS[1256789B]XZZ
Non-OR ØPS[CDFGHJKL][34]ZZ
Non-OR ØPS[CDFGHJKL]XZZ
Non-OR ØPS[MNPQRSTV][34]ZZ
Non-OR ØPS[MNPQRSTV]XZZ

Coding Clinic: 2015, Q2, P35 – ØPS3XZZ

SECTION: Ø MEDICAL AND SURGICAL
BODY SYSTEM: P UPPER BONES
OPERATION: T RESECTION: Cutting out or off, without replacement, all of a body part

Body Part	Approach	Device	Qualifier
Ø Sternum 1 Rib, 1 to 2 2 Rib, 3 or More 5 Scapula, Right 6 Scapula, Left 7 Glenoid Cavity, Right 8 Glenoid Cavity, Left 9 Clavicle, Right B Clavicle, Left C Humeral Head, Right D Humeral Head, Left F Humeral Shaft, Right G Humeral Shaft, Left H Radius, Right J Radius, Left K Ulna, Right L Ulna, Left M Carpal, Right N Carpal, Left P Metacarpal, Right Q Metacarpal, Left R Thumb Phalanx, Right S Thumb Phalanx, Left T Finger Phalanx, Right V Finger Phalanx, Left	Ø Open	Z No Device	Z No Qualifier

Coding Clinic: 2015, Q3, P27 – ØPTNØZZ

SECTION: Ø MEDICAL AND SURGICAL
BODY SYSTEM: P UPPER BONES
OPERATION: U SUPPLEMENT: Putting in or on biological or synthetic material that physically reinforces and/or augments the function of a portion of a body part

Body Part	Approach	Device	Qualifier
Ø Sternum 1 Rib, 1 to 2 2 Rib, 3 or More 3 Cervical Vertebra ⊞ 4 Thoracic Vertebra ⊞ 5 Scapula, Right 6 Scapula, Left 7 Glenoid Cavity, Right 8 Glenoid Cavity, Left 9 Clavicle, Right B Clavicle, Left C Humeral Head, Right D Humeral Head, Left F Humeral Shaft, Right G Humeral Shaft, Left H Radius, Right J Radius, Left K Ulna, Right L Ulna, Left M Carpal, Right N Carpal, Left P Metacarpal, Right Q Metacarpal, Left R Thumb Phalanx, Right S Thumb Phalanx, Left T Finger Phalanx, Right V Finger Phalanx, Left	Ø Open 3 Percutaneous 4 Percutaneous Endoscopic	7 Autologous Tissue Substitute J Synthetic Substitute K Nonautologous Tissue Substitute	Z No Qualifier

⊞ ØPU[34]3JZ

Coding Clinic: 2015, Q2, P2Ø – ØPU3ØKZ
Coding Clinic: 2018, Q4, P12 – ØPU5Ø7Z, ØPU5ØKZ
Coding Clinic: 2021, Q3, P16 – ØPU[CD]3JZ
Coding Clinic: 2023, Q2, P25 – ØPUC47Z

SECTION: Ø MEDICAL AND SURGICAL
BODY SYSTEM: P UPPER BONES
OPERATION: W REVISION: Correcting, to the extent possible, a portion of a malfunctioning device or the position of a displaced device

Body Part	Approach	Device	Qualifier
Ø Sternum 1 Rib, 1 to 2 2 Rib, 3 or More 3 Cervical Vertebra 4 Thoracic Vertebra 5 Scapula, Right 6 Scapula, Left 7 Glenoid Cavity, Right 8 Glenoid Cavity, Left 9 Clavicle, Right B Clavicle, Left	Ø Open 3 Percutaneous 4 Percutaneous Endoscopic X External	4 Internal Fixation Device 7 Autologous Tissue Substitute J Synthetic Substitute K Nonautologous Tissue Substitute	Z No Qualifier
C Humeral Head, Right D Humeral Head, Left F Humeral Shaft, Right G Humeral Shaft, Left H Radius, Right J Radius, Left K Ulna, Right L Ulna, Left M Carpal, Right N Carpal, Left P Metacarpal, Right Q Metacarpal, Left R Thumb Phalanx, Right S Thumb Phalanx, Left T Finger Phalanx, Right V Finger Phalanx, Left	Ø Open 3 Percutaneous 4 Percutaneous Endoscopic X External	4 Internal Fixation Device 5 External Fixation Device 7 Autologous Tissue Substitute J Synthetic Substitute K Nonautologous Tissue Substitute	Z No Qualifier
Y Upper Bone	Ø Open 3 Percutaneous 4 Percutaneous Endoscopic X External	Ø Drainage Device M Bone Growth Stimulator	Z No Qualifier

Non-OR ØPW[Ø123456789B]X[47JK]Z
Non-OR ØPW[CDFGHJKLMNPQRSTV]X[457JK]Z
Non-OR ØPWYX[ØM]Z

SECTION: Ø MEDICAL AND SURGICAL
BODY SYSTEM: Q LOWER BONES
OPERATION: 2 CHANGE: Taking out or off a device from a body part and putting back an identical or similar device in or on the same body part without cutting or puncturing the skin or a mucous membrane

Body Part	Approach	Device	Qualifier
Y Lower Bone	X External	Ø Drainage Device Y Other Device	Z No Qualifier

Non-OR All Values

SECTION: Ø MEDICAL AND SURGICAL
BODY SYSTEM: Q LOWER BONES
OPERATION: 5 DESTRUCTION: Physical eradication of all or a portion of a body part by the direct use of energy, force, or a destructive agent

Body Part	Approach	Device	Qualifier
Ø Lumbar Vertebra 1 Sacrum	Ø Open 3 Percutaneous 4 Percutaneous Endoscopic	Z No Device	3 Laser Interstitial Thermal Therapy Z No Qualifier
~~Ø Lumbar Vertebra~~ ~~1 Sacrum~~ 2 Pelvic Bone, Right 3 Pelvic Bone, Left 4 Acetabulum, Right 5 Acetabulum, Left 6 Upper Femur, Right 7 Upper Femur, Left 8 Femoral Shaft, Right 9 Femoral Shaft, Left B Lower Femur, Right C Lower Femur, Left D Patella, Right F Patella, Left G Tibia, Right H Tibia, Left J Fibula, Right K Fibula, Left L Tarsal, Right M Tarsal, Left N Metatarsal, Right P Metatarsal, Left Q Toe Phalanx, Right R Toe Phalanx, Left S Coccyx	Ø Open 3 Percutaneous 4 Percutaneous Endoscopic	Z No Device	Z No Qualifier

SECTION: Ø MEDICAL AND SURGICAL
BODY SYSTEM: Q LOWER BONES
OPERATION: 8 DIVISION: Cutting into a body part, without draining fluids and/or gases from the body part, in order to separate or transect a body part

Body Part	Approach	Device	Qualifier
Ø Lumbar Vertebra 1 Sacrum 2 Pelvic Bone, Right 3 Pelvic Bone, Left 4 Acetabulum, Right 5 Acetabulum, Left 6 Upper Femur, Right 7 Upper Femur, Left 8 Femoral Shaft, Right 9 Femoral Shaft, Left B Lower Femur, Right C Lower Femur, Left D Patella, Right F Patella, Left G Tibia, Right H Tibia, Left J Fibula, Right K Fibula, Left L Tarsal, Right M Tarsal, Left N Metatarsal, Right P Metatarsal, Left Q Toe Phalanx, Right R Toe Phalanx, Left S Coccyx	Ø Open 3 Percutaneous 4 Percutaneous Endoscopic	Z No Device	Z No Qualifier

Coding Clinic: 2Ø16, Q2, P32 – ØQ83ØZZ

SECTION: Ø MEDICAL AND SURGICAL
BODY SYSTEM: Q LOWER BONES
OPERATION: 9 DRAINAGE: Taking or letting out fluids and/or gases from a body part

Body Part	Approach	Device	Qualifier
Ø Lumbar Vertebra 1 Sacrum 2 Pelvic Bone, Right 3 Pelvic Bone, Left 4 Acetabulum, Right 5 Acetabulum, Left 6 Upper Femur, Right 7 Upper Femur, Left 8 Femoral Shaft, Right 9 Femoral Shaft, Left B Lower Femur, Right C Lower Femur, Left D Patella, Right F Patella, Left G Tibia, Right H Tibia, Left J Fibula, Right K Fibula, Left L Tarsal, Right M Tarsal, Left N Metatarsal, Right P Metatarsal, Left Q Toe Phalanx, Right R Toe Phalanx, Left S Coccyx	Ø Open 3 Percutaneous 4 Percutaneous Endoscopic	Ø Drainage Device	Z No Qualifier
Ø Lumbar Vertebra 1 Sacrum 2 Pelvic Bone, Right 3 Pelvic Bone, Left 4 Acetabulum, Right 5 Acetabulum, Left 6 Upper Femur, Right 7 Upper Femur, Left 8 Femoral Shaft, Right 9 Femoral Shaft, Left B Lower Femur, Right C Lower Femur, Left D Patella, Right F Patella, Left G Tibia, Right H Tibia, Left J Fibula, Right K Fibula, Left L Tarsal, Right M Tarsal, Left N Metatarsal, Right P Metatarsal, Left Q Toe Phalanx, Right R Toe Phalanx, Left S Coccyx	Ø Open 3 Percutaneous 4 Percutaneous Endoscopic	Z No Device	X Diagnostic Z No Qualifier

Non-OR ØQ9[Ø123456789BCDFGHJKLMNPQRS]3ØZ
Non-OR ØQ9[Ø123456789BCDFGHJKLMNPQRS]3ZZ

Coding Clinic: 2022, Q1, P32 – ØQ9[23]3ZX

SECTION: Ø MEDICAL AND SURGICAL
BODY SYSTEM: Q LOWER BONES
OPERATION: B EXCISION: Cutting out or off, without replacement, a portion of a body part

Body Part	Approach	Device	Qualifier
Ø Lumbar Vertebra 1 Sacrum 2 Pelvic Bone, Right 3 Pelvic Bone, Left 4 Acetabulum, Right 5 Acetabulum, Left 6 Upper Femur, Right 7 Upper Femur, Left 8 Femoral Shaft, Right 9 Femoral Shaft, Left B Lower Femur, Right C Lower Femur, Left D Patella, Right F Patella, Left G Tibia, Right H Tibia, Left J Fibula, Right K Fibula, Left L Tarsal, Right M Tarsal, Left Q Toe Phalanx, Right R Toe Phalanx, Left S Coccyx	Ø Open 3 Percutaneous 4 Percutaneous Endoscopic	Z No Device	X Diagnostic Z No Qualifier
N Metatarsal, Right P Metatarsal, Left	Ø Open 3 Percutaneous 4 Percutaneous Endoscopic	Z No Device	2 Sesamoid Bone(s) 1st Toe X Diagnostic Z No Qualifier

Coding Clinic: 2Ø13, Q2, P4Ø – ØQBKØZZ
Coding Clinic: 2Ø15, Q3, P4 – ØQBSØZZ
Coding Clinic: 2Ø17, Q1, P24 – ØQBJØZZ
Coding Clinic: 2Ø19, Q2, P2Ø – ØQB3ØZZ
Coding Clinic: 2Ø2Ø, Q2, P26 – ØQB1ØZZ
Coding Clinic: 2Ø21, Q2, P18 – ØQBNØZZ

SECTION: Ø MEDICAL AND SURGICAL

BODY SYSTEM: Q LOWER BONES

OPERATION: C EXTIRPATION: Taking or cutting out solid matter from a body part

Body Part	Approach	Device	Qualifier
Ø Lumbar Vertebra 1 Sacrum 2 Pelvic Bone, Right 3 Pelvic Bone, Left 4 Acetabulum, Right 5 Acetabulum, Left 6 Upper Femur, Right 7 Upper Femur, Left 8 Femoral Shaft, Right 9 Femoral Shaft, Left B Lower Femur, Right C Lower Femur, Left D Patella, Right F Patella, Left G Tibia, Right H Tibia, Left J Fibula, Right K Fibula, Left L Tarsal, Right M Tarsal, Left N Metatarsal, Right P Metatarsal, Left Q Toe Phalanx, Right R Toe Phalanx, Left S Coccyx	Ø Open 3 Percutaneous 4 Percutaneous Endoscopic	Z No Device	Z No Qualifier

SECTION: Ø MEDICAL AND SURGICAL

BODY SYSTEM: Q LOWER BONES

OPERATION: D EXTRACTION: Pulling or stripping out or off all or a portion of a body part by the use of force

Body Part	Approach	Device	Qualifier
Ø Lumbar Vertebra 1 Sacrum 2 Pelvic Bone, Right 3 Pelvic Bone, Left 4 Acetabulum, Right 5 Acetabulum, Left 6 Upper Femur, Right 7 Upper Femur, Left 8 Femoral Shaft, Right 9 Femoral Shaft, Left B Lower Femur, Right C Lower Femur, Left D Patella, Right F Patella, Left G Tibia, Right H Tibia, Left J Fibula, Right K Fibula, Left L Tarsal, Right M Tarsal, Left N Metatarsal, Right P Metatarsal, Left Q Toe Phalanx, Right R Toe Phalanx, Left S Coccyx	Ø Open	Z No Device	Z No Qualifier

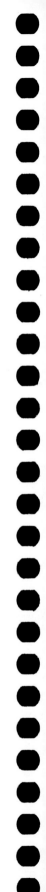

SECTION: Ø MEDICAL AND SURGICAL
BODY SYSTEM: Q LOWER BONES
OPERATION: H INSERTION: Putting in a nonbiological appliance that monitors, assists, performs, or prevents a physiological function but does not physically take the place of a body part

Body Part	Approach	Device	Qualifier
Ø Lumbar Vertebra 1 Sacrum 2 Pelvic Bone, Right 3 Pelvic Bone, Left 4 Acetabulum, Right 5 Acetabulum, Left D Patella, Right F Patella, Left L Tarsal, Right M Tarsal, Left N Metatarsal, Right P Metatarsal, Left Q Toe Phalanx, Right R Toe Phalanx, Left S Coccyx	Ø Open 3 Percutaneous 4 Percutaneous Endoscopic	4 Internal Fixation Device 5 External Fixation Device	Z No Qualifier
6 Upper Femur, Right 7 Upper Femur, Left B Lower Femur, Right C Lower Femur, Left J Fibula, Right K Fibula, Left	Ø Open 3 Percutaneous 4 Percutaneous Endoscopic	4 Internal Fixation Device 5 External Fixation Device 6 Internal Fixation Device, Intramedullary 8 External Fixation Device, Limb Lengthening B External Fixation Device, Monoplanar C External Fixation Device, Ring D External Fixation Device, Hybrid	Z No Qualifier
8 Femoral Shaft, Right 9 Femoral Shaft, Left G Tibia, Right H Tibia, Leftt	Ø Open 3 Percutaneous 4 Percutaneous Endoscopic	4 Internal Fixation Device 5 External Fixation Device 6 Internal Fixation Device, Intramedullary 7 Internal Fixation Device, Intramedullary Limb Lengthening 8 External Fixation Device, Limb Lengthening B External Fixation Device, Monoplanar C External Fixation Device, Ring D External Fixation Device, Hybrid	Z No Qualifier
Y Lower Bone	Ø Open 3 Percutaneous 4 Percutaneous Endoscopic	M Bone Growth Stimulator	Z No Qualifier

Non-OR ØQH[6789BCGHJK][Ø34]8Z

Coding Clinic: 2Ø16, Q3, P35 – ØQH[GJ]Ø4Z
Coding Clinic: 2Ø17, Q1, P22 – ØQH[23]Ø4Z
Coding Clinic: 2Ø22, Q2, P21 – ØQH[HK]38Z

SECTION: Ø MEDICAL AND SURGICAL
BODY SYSTEM: Q LOWER BONES
OPERATION: J **INSPECTION:** Visually and/or manually exploring a body part

Body Part	Approach	Device	Qualifier
Y Lower Bone	Ø Open 3 Percutaneous 4 Percutaneous Endoscopic X External	Z No Device	Z No Qualifier

Non-OR ØQJY[3X]ZZ

SECTION: Ø MEDICAL AND SURGICAL
BODY SYSTEM: Q LOWER BONES
OPERATION: N **RELEASE:** Freeing a body part from an abnormal physical constraint by cutting or by the use of force

Body Part	Approach	Device	Qualifier
Ø Lumbar Vertebra 1 Sacrum 2 Pelvic Bone, Right 3 Pelvic Bone, Left 4 Acetabulum, Right 5 Acetabulum, Left 6 Upper Femur, Right 7 Upper Femur, Left 8 Femoral Shaft, Right 9 Femoral Shaft, Left B Lower Femur, Right C Lower Femur, Left D Patella, Right F Patella, Left G Tibia, Right H Tibia, Left J Fibula, Right K Fibula, Left L Tarsal, Right M Tarsal, Left N Metatarsal, Right P Metatarsal, Left Q Toe Phalanx, Right R Toe Phalanx, Left S Coccyx	Ø Open 3 Percutaneous 4 Percutaneous Endoscopic	Z No Device	Z No Qualifier

SECTION: Ø MEDICAL AND SURGICAL
BODY SYSTEM: Q LOWER BONES
OPERATION: P REMOVAL: *(on multiple pages)*
Taking out or off a device from a body part

Body Part	Approach	Device	Qualifier
Ø Lumbar Vertebra 1 Sacrum 4 Acetabulum, Right 5 Acetabulum, Left S Coccyx	Ø Open 3 Percutaneous 4 Percutaneous Endoscopic	4 Internal Fixation Device 7 Autologous Tissue Substitute J Synthetic Substitute K Nonautologous Tissue Substitute	Z No Qualifier
Ø Lumbar Vertebra 1 Sacrum 4 Acetabulum, Right 5 Acetabulum, Left S Coccyx	X External	4 Internal Fixation Device	Z No Qualifier
Ø Lumbar Vertebra 1 Sacrum 2 Pelvic Bone, Right 3 Pelvic Bone, Left 4 Acetabulum, Right 5 Acetabulum, Left 6 Upper Femur, Right 7 Upper Femur, Left 8 Femoral Shaft, Right 9 Femoral Shaft, Left B Lower Femur, Right C Lower Femur, Left D Patella, Right F Patella, Left G Tibia, Right H Tibia, Left J Fibula, Right K Fibula, Left L Tarsal, Right M Tarsal, Left N Metatarsal, Right P Metatarsal, Left Q Toe Phalanx, Right R Toe Phalanx, Left S Coccyx	Ø Open 3 Percutaneous 4 Percutaneous Endoscopic	4 Internal Fixation Device 5 External Fixation Device 7 Autologous Tissue Substitute J Synthetic Substitute K Nonautologous Tissue Substitute	Z No Qualifier

Non-OR ØQP[Ø145S]X4Z

Coding Clinic: 2Ø15, Q2, P6 – ØQPGØ4Z
Coding Clinic: 2Ø17, Q4, P75 – ØQPØØ4Z
Coding Clinic: 2Ø23, Q1, P34 – ØQP1Ø4Z

SECTION: Ø MEDICAL AND SURGICAL
BODY SYSTEM: Q LOWER BONES
OPERATION: P REMOVAL: *(continued)*
Taking out or off a device from a body part

Body Part	Approach	Device	Qualifier
Ø Lumbar Vertebra 1 Sacrum 2 Pelvic Bone, Right 3 Pelvic Bone, Left 4 Acetabulum, Right 5 Acetabulum, Left 6 Upper Femur, Right 7 Upper Femur, Left 8 Femoral Shaft, Right 9 Femoral Shaft, Left B Lower Femur, Right C Lower Femur, Left D Patella, Right F Patella, Left G Tibia, Right H Tibia, Left J Fibula, Right K Fibula, Left L Tarsal, Right M Tarsal, Left N Metatarsal, Right P Metatarsal, Left Q Toe Phalanx, Right R Toe Phalanx, Left S Coccyx	X External	4 Internal Fixation Device 5 External Fixation Device	Z No Qualifier
Y Lower Bone	Ø Open 3 Percutaneous 4 Percutaneous Endoscopic X External	Ø Drainage Device M Bone Growth Stimulator	Z No Qualifier

Non-OR ØQP[Ø123456789BCDFGHJKLMNPQRS]X[45]Z
Non-OR ØQPY3ØZ
Non-OR ØQPYX[ØM]Z

SECTION: Ø MEDICAL AND SURGICAL
BODY SYSTEM: Q LOWER BONES
OPERATION: Q REPAIR: Restoring, to the extent possible, a body part to its normal anatomic structure and function

Body Part	Approach	Device	Qualifier
Ø Lumbar Vertebra 1 Sacrum 2 Pelvic Bone, Right 3 Pelvic Bone, Left 4 Acetabulum, Right 5 Acetabulum, Left 6 Upper Femur, Right 7 Upper Femur, Left 8 Femoral Shaft, Right 9 Femoral Shaft, Left B Lower Femur, Right C Lower Femur, Left D Patella, Right F Patella, Left G Tibia, Right H Tibia, Left J Fibula, Right K Fibula, Left L Tarsal, Right M Tarsal, Left N Metatarsal, Right P Metatarsal, Left Q Toe Phalanx, Right R Toe Phalanx, Left S Coccyx	Ø Open 3 Percutaneous 4 Percutaneous Endoscopic X External	Z No Device	Z No Qualifier

DRG Non-OR ØQQ[Ø123456789BCDFGHJKLMNPQRS]XZZ

Coding Clinic: 2Ø18, Q1, P15 – ØQQ[23]ØZZ

Ø: M/S Q: LOWER BONES Q: REPAIR

SECTION: Ø MEDICAL AND SURGICAL
BODY SYSTEM: Q LOWER BONES
OPERATION: R REPLACEMENT: Putting in or on biological or synthetic material that physically takes the place and/or function of all or a portion of a body part

Body Part	Approach	Device	Qualifier
Ø Lumbar Vertebra 1 Sacrum 2 Pelvic Bone, Right 3 Pelvic Bone, Left 4 Acetabulum, Right 5 Acetabulum, Left 6 Upper Femur, Right 7 Upper Femur, Left 8 Femoral Shaft, Right 9 Femoral Shaft, Left B Lower Femur, Right C Lower Femur, Left D Patella, Right F Patella, Left G Tibia, Right H Tibia, Left J Fibula, Right K Fibula, Left L Tarsal, Right M Tarsal, Left N Metatarsal, Right P Metatarsal, Left Q Toe Phalanx, Right R Toe Phalanx, Left S Coccyx	Ø Open 3 Percutaneous 4 Percutaneous Endoscopic	7 Autologous Tissue Substitute J Synthetic Substitute K Nonautologous Tissue Substitute	Z No Qualifier

SECTION: Ø MEDICAL AND SURGICAL
BODY SYSTEM: Q LOWER BONES
OPERATION: S REPOSITION: *(on multiple pages)*

Moving to its normal location, or other suitable location, all or a portion of a body part

Body Part	Approach	Device	Qualifier
Ø Lumbar Vertebra	Ø Open 4 Percutaneous Endoscopic	3 Spinal Stabilization Device, Vertebral Body Tether 4 Internal Fixation Device Z No Device	Z No Qualifier
Ø Lumbar Vertebra	3 Percutaneous	4 Internal Fixation Device Z No Device	Z No Qualifier
Ø Lumbar Vertebra	X External	Z No Device	Z No Qualifier
1 Sacrum ⊞ 4 Acetabulum, Right 5 Acetabulum, Left S Coccyx ⊞	Ø Open 3 Percutaneous 4 Percutaneous Endoscopic	4 Internal Fixation Device Z No Device	Z No Qualifier
1 Sacrum 4 Acetabulum, Right 5 Acetabulum, Left S Coccyx	X External	Z No Device	Z No Qualifier
2 Pelvic Bone, Right 3 Pelvic Bone, Left D Patella, Right F Patella, Left L Tarsal, Right M Tarsal, Left Q Toe Phalanx, Right R Toe Phalanx, Left	Ø Open 3 Percutaneous 4 Percutaneous Endoscopic	4 Internal Fixation Device 5 External Fixation Device Z No Device	Z No Qualifier
2 Pelvic Bone, Right 3 Pelvic Bone, Left D Patella, Right F Patella, Left L Tarsal, Right M Tarsal, Left Q Toe Phalanx, Right R Toe Phalanx, Left	X External	Z No Device	Z No Qualifier
6 Upper Femur, Right 7 Upper Femur, Left 8 Femoral Shaft, Right 9 Femoral Shaft, Left B Lower Femur, Right C Lower Femur, Left G Tibia, Right H Tibia, Left J Fibula, Right K Fibula, Left	Ø Open 3 Percutaneous 4 Percutaneous Endoscopic	4 Internal Fixation Device 5 External Fixation Device 6 Internal Fixation Device, Intramedullary B External Fixation Device, Monoplanar C External Fixation Device, Ring D External Fixation Device, Hybrid Z No Device	Z No Qualifier

⊞ ØQS[Ø1S]3ZZ
Non-OR ØQS[45][34]ZZ
Non-OR ØQS[45]XZZ
Non-OR ØQS[23DFLMQR][34]ZZ
Non-OR ØQS[23DFLMQR]XZZ
Non-OR ØQS[6789BCGHJK][34]ZZ

Coding Clinic: 2016, Q3, P35 – ØQS[FH]Ø4Z
Coding Clinic: 2016, Q3, P35 – ØQSKØZZ
Coding Clinic: 2018, Q1, P13 – ØQS[LM]Ø4Z
Coding Clinic: 2019, Q3, P26 – ØQS9Ø4Z
Coding Clinic: 2020, Q1, P34 – ØQSØØ4Z
Coding Clinic: 2022, Q2, P21 – ØQS[HK]3CZ

SECTION: Ø MEDICAL AND SURGICAL
BODY SYSTEM: Q LOWER BONES
OPERATION: S REPOSITION: *(continued)*
Moving to its normal location, or other suitable location, all or a portion of a body part

Body Part	Approach	Device	Qualifier
6 Upper Femur, Right 7 Upper Femur, Left 8 Femoral Shaft, Right 9 Femoral Shaft, Left B Lower Femur, Right C Lower Femur, Left G Tibia, Right H Tibia, Left J Fibula, Right K Fibula, Left	X External	Z No Device	Z No Qualifier
N Metatarsal, Right P Metatarsal, Left	Ø Open 3 Percutaneous 4 Percutaneous Endoscopic	4 Internal Fixation Device 5 External Fixation Device Z No Device	2 Sesamoid Bone(s) 1st Toe Z No Qualifier
N Metatarsal, Right P Metatarsal, Left	X External	Z No Device	2 Sesamoid Bone(s) 1st Toe Z No Qualifier

Non-OR ØQS[6789BCGHJK]XZZ Non-OR ØQS[NP][34]ZZ Non-OR ØQS[NP]XZZ

SECTION: Ø MEDICAL AND SURGICAL
BODY SYSTEM: Q LOWER BONES
OPERATION: T RESECTION: Cutting out or off, without replacement, all of a body part

Body Part	Approach	Device	Qualifier
2 Pelvic Bone, Right 3 Pelvic Bone, Left 4 Acetabulum, Right 5 Acetabulum, Left 6 Upper Femur, Right 7 Upper Femur, Left 8 Femoral Shaft, Right 9 Femoral Shaft, Left B Lower Femur, Right C Lower Femur, Left D Patella, Right F Patella, Left G Tibia, Right H Tibia, Left J Fibula, Right K Fibula, Left L Tarsal, Right M Tarsal, Left N Metatarsal, Right P Metatarsal, Left Q Toe Phalanx, Right R Toe Phalanx, Left S Coccyx	Ø Open	Z No Device	Z No Qualifier

Coding Clinic: 2Ø15, Q3, P26 – ØQT7ØZZ
Coding Clinic: 2Ø16, Q3, P3Ø – ØQT[67]ØZZ

SECTION: Ø MEDICAL AND SURGICAL
BODY SYSTEM: Q LOWER BONES
OPERATION: U SUPPLEMENT: Putting in or on biological or synthetic material that physically reinforces and/or augments the function of a portion of a body part

Body Part	Approach	Device	Qualifier
Ø Lumbar Vertebra ⊞ 1 Sacrum ⊞ 2 Pelvic Bone, Right 3 Pelvic Bone, Left 4 Acetabulum, Right 5 Acetabulum, Left 6 Upper Femur, Right 7 Upper Femur, Left 8 Femoral Shaft, Right 9 Femoral Shaft, Left B Lower Femur, Right C Lower Femur, Left D Patella, Right F Patella, Left G Tibia, Right H Tibia, Left J Fibula, Right K Fibula, Left L Tarsal, Right M Tarsal, Left N Metatarsal, Right P Metatarsal, Left Q Toe Phalanx, Right R Toe Phalanx, Left S Coccyx ⊞	Ø Open 3 Percutaneous 4 Percutaneous Endoscopic	7 Autologous Tissue Substitute J Synthetic Substitute K Nonautologous Tissue Substitute	Z No Qualifier

⊞ ØQU[Ø1S]3JZ

Coding Clinic: 2Ø13, Q2, P36 – ØQU2ØJZ
Coding Clinic: 2Ø15, Q3, P19 – ØQU5ØJZ
Coding Clinic: 2Ø19, Q2, P35 – ØQUØ3JZ
Coding Clinic: 2Ø19, Q3, P26 – ØQU9ØKZ

SECTION: Ø MEDICAL AND SURGICAL
BODY SYSTEM: Q LOWER BONES
OPERATION: W REVISION: Correcting, to the extent possible, a portion of a malfunctioning device or the position of a displaced device

Body Part	Approach	Device	Qualifier
Ø Lumbar Vertebra 1 Sacrum 4 Acetabulum, Right 5 Acetabulum, Left S Coccyx	Ø Open 3 Percutaneous 4 Percutaneous Endoscopic X External	4 Internal Fixation Device 7 Autologous Tissue Substitute J Synthetic Substitute K Nonautologous Tissue Substitute	Z No Qualifier
2 Pelvic Bone, Right 3 Pelvic Bone, Left 6 Upper Femur, Right 7 Upper Femur, Left 8 Femoral Shaft, Right 9 Femoral Shaft, Left B Lower Femur, Right C Lower Femur, Left D Patella, Right F Patella, Left G Tibia, Right H Tibia, Left J Fibula, Right K Fibula, Left L Tarsal, Right M Tarsal, Left N Metatarsal, Right P Metatarsal, Left Q Toe Phalanx, Right R Toe Phalanx, Left	Ø Open 3 Percutaneous 4 Percutaneous Endoscopic X External	4 Internal Fixation Device 5 External Fixation Device 7 Autologous Tissue Substitute J Synthetic Substitute K Nonautologous Tissue Substitute	Z No Qualifier
Y Lower Bone	Ø Open 3 Percutaneous 4 Percutaneous Endoscopic X External	Ø Drainage Device M Bone Growth Stimulator	Z No Qualifier

Non-OR ØQW[Ø145S]X[47JK]Z
Non-OR ØQW[236789BCDFGHJKLMNPQR]X[457JK]Z
Non-OR ØQWYX[ØM]Z

Coding Clinic: 2017, Q4, P75 – ØQWØ34Z

SECTION: Ø MEDICAL AND SURGICAL
BODY SYSTEM: R UPPER JOINTS
OPERATION: 2 CHANGE: Taking out or off a device from a body part and putting back an identical or similar device in or on the same body part without cutting or puncturing the skin or a mucous membrane

Body Part	Approach	Device	Qualifier
Y Upper Joint	X External	Ø Drainage Device Y Other Device	Z No Qualifier

Non-OR All Values

SECTION: Ø MEDICAL AND SURGICAL
BODY SYSTEM: R UPPER JOINTS
OPERATION: 5 DESTRUCTION: Physical eradication of all or a portion of a body part by the direct use of energy, force, or destructive agent

Body Part	Approach	Device	Qualifier
Ø Occipital-cervical Joint 1 Cervical Vertebral Joint 3 Cervical Vertebral Disc 4 Cervicothoracic Vertebral Joint 5 Cervicothoracic Vertebral Disc 6 Thoracic Vertebral Joint 9 Thoracic Vertebral Disc A Thoracolumbar Vertebral Joint B Thoracolumbar Vertebral Disc C Temporomandibular Joint, Right D Temporomandibular Joint, Left E Sternoclavicular Joint, Right F Sternoclavicular Joint, Left G Acromioclavicular Joint, Right H Acromioclavicular Joint, Left J Shoulder Joint, Right K Shoulder Joint, Left L Elbow Joint, Right M Elbow Joint, Left N Wrist Joint, Right P Wrist Joint, Left Q Carpal Joint, Right R Carpal Joint, Left S Carpometacarpal Joint, Right T Carpometacarpal Joint, Left U Metacarpophalangeal Joint, Right V Metacarpophalangeal Joint, Left W Finger Phalangeal Joint, Right X Finger Phalangeal Joint, Left	Ø Open 3 Percutaneous 4 Percutaneous Endoscopic	Z No Device	Z No Qualifier

Non-OR ØR5[359B][34]ZZ

SECTION: Ø MEDICAL AND SURGICAL
BODY SYSTEM: R UPPER JOINTS
OPERATION: 9 DRAINAGE: *(on multiple pages)*
Taking or letting out fluids and/or gases from a body part

Body Part	Approach	Device	Qualifier
Ø Occipital-cervical Joint 1 Cervical Vertebral Joint 3 Cervical Vertebral Disc 4 Cervicothoracic Vertebral Joint 5 Cervicothoracic Vertebral Disc 6 Thoracic Vertebral Joint 9 Thoracic Vertebral Disc A Thoracolumbar Vertebral Joint B Thoracolumbar Vertebral Disc C Temporomandibular Joint, Right D Temporomandibular Joint, Left E Sternoclavicular Joint, Right F Sternoclavicular Joint, Left G Acromioclavicular Joint, Right H Acromioclavicular Joint, Left J Shoulder Joint, Right K Shoulder Joint, Left L Elbow Joint, Right M Elbow Joint, Left N Wrist Joint, Right P Wrist Joint, Left Q Carpal Joint, Right R Carpal Joint, Left S Carpometacarpal Joint, Right T Carpometacarpal Joint, Left U Metacarpophalangeal Joint, Right V Metacarpophalangeal Joint, Left W Finger Phalangeal Joint, Right X Finger Phalangeal Joint, Left	Ø Open 3 Percutaneous 4 Percutaneous Endoscopic	Ø Drainage Device	Z No Qualifier

Non-OR ØR9[CD]3ØZ
Non-OR ØR9[Ø134569ABEFGHJKLMNPQRSTUVWX][34]ØZ

SECTION: Ø MEDICAL AND SURGICAL
BODY SYSTEM: R UPPER JOINTS
OPERATION: 9 DRAINAGE: *(continued)*
Taking or letting out fluids and/or gases from a body part

Body Part	Approach	Device	Qualifier
Ø Occipital-cervical Joint 1 Cervical Vertebral Joint 3 Cervical Vertebral Disc 4 Cervicothoracic Vertebral Joint 5 Cervicothoracic Vertebral Disc 6 Thoracic Vertebral Joint 9 Thoracic Vertebral Disc A Thoracolumbar Vertebral Joint B Thoracolumbar Vertebral Disc C Temporomandibular Joint, Right D Temporomandibular Joint, Left E Sternoclavicular Joint, Right F Sternoclavicular Joint, Left G Acromioclavicular Joint, Right H Acromioclavicular Joint, Left J Shoulder Joint, Right K Shoulder Joint, Left L Elbow Joint, Right M Elbow Joint, Left N Wrist Joint, Right P Wrist Joint, Left Q Carpal Joint, Right R Carpal Joint, Left S Carpometacarpal Joint, Right T Carpometacarpal Joint, Left U Metacarpophalangeal Joint, Right V Metacarpophalangeal Joint, Left W Finger Phalangeal Joint, Right X Finger Phalangeal Joint, Left	Ø Open 3 Percutaneous 4 Percutaneous Endoscopic	Z No Device	X Diagnostic Z No Qualifier

DRG Non-OR ØR9[CD]3ZZ
Non-OR ØR9[Ø134569ABEFGHJKLMNPQRSTUVWX][Ø34]ZX
Non-OR ØR9[Ø134569ABEFGHJKLMNPQRSTUVWX][34]ZZ

SECTION: Ø MEDICAL AND SURGICAL
BODY SYSTEM: R UPPER JOINTS
OPERATION: B EXCISION: Cutting out or off, without replacement, a portion of a body part

Body Part	Approach	Device	Qualifier
Ø Occipital-cervical Joint 1 Cervical Vertebral Joint 3 Cervical Vertebral Disc 4 Cervicothoracic Vertebral Joint 5 Cervicothoracic Vertebral Disc 6 Thoracic Vertebral Joint 9 Thoracic Vertebral Disc A Thoracolumbar Vertebral Joint B Thoracolumbar Vertebral Disc C Temporomandibular Joint, Right D Temporomandibular Joint, Left E Sternoclavicular Joint, Right F Sternoclavicular Joint, Left G Acromioclavicular Joint, Right H Acromioclavicular Joint, Left J Shoulder Joint, Right K Shoulder Joint, Left L Elbow Joint, Right M Elbow Joint, Left N Wrist Joint, Right P Wrist Joint, Left Q Carpal Joint, Right R Carpal Joint, Left S Carpometacarpal Joint, Right T Carpometacarpal Joint, Left U Metacarpophalangeal Joint, Right V Metacarpophalangeal Joint, Left W Finger Phalangeal Joint, Right X Finger Phalangeal Joint, Left	Ø Open 3 Percutaneous 4 Percutaneous Endoscopic	Z No Device	X Diagnostic Z No Qualifier

Non-OR ØRB[Ø134569ABEFGHJKLMNPQRSTUVWX][Ø34]ZX

Ø: M/S R: UPPER JOINTS B: EXCISION

SECTION: Ø MEDICAL AND SURGICAL
BODY SYSTEM: R UPPER JOINTS
OPERATION: C EXTIRPATION: Taking or cutting out solid matter from a body part

Body Part	Approach	Device	Qualifier
Ø Occipital-cervical Joint 1 Cervical Vertebral Joint 3 Cervical Vertebral Disc 4 Cervicothoracic Vertebral Joint 5 Cervicothoracic Vertebral Disc 6 Thoracic Vertebral Joint 9 Thoracic Vertebral Disc A Thoracolumbar Vertebral Joint B Thoracolumbar Vertebral Disc C Temporomandibular Joint, Right D Temporomandibular Joint, Left E Sternoclavicular Joint, Right F Sternoclavicular Joint, Left G Acromioclavicular Joint, Right H Acromioclavicular Joint, Left J Shoulder Joint, Right K Shoulder Joint, Left L Elbow Joint, Right M Elbow Joint, Left N Wrist Joint, Right P Wrist Joint, Left Q Carpal Joint, Right R Carpal Joint, Left S Carpometacarpal Joint, Right T Carpometacarpal Joint, Left U Metacarpophalangeal Joint, Right V Metacarpophalangeal Joint, Left W Finger Phalangeal Joint, Right X Finger Phalangeal Joint, Left	Ø Open 3 Percutaneous 4 Percutaneous Endoscopic	Z No Device	Z No Qualifier

SECTION: Ø MEDICAL AND SURGICAL
BODY SYSTEM: R UPPER JOINTS
OPERATION: G FUSION: Joining together portions of an articular body part, rendering the articular body part immobile

Body Part	Approach	Device	Qualifier
Ø Occipital-cervical Joint 1 Cervical Vertebral Joint 2 Cervical Vertebral Joints, 2 or more 4 Cervicothoracic Vertebral Joint 6 Thoracic Vertebral Joint 7 Thoracic Vertebral Joint, 2 to 7 8 Thoracic Vertebral Joint, 8 or more A Thoracolumbar Vertebral Joint	Ø Open 3 Percutaneous 4 Percutaneous Endoscopic	7 Autologous Tissue Substitute J Synthetic Substitute K Nonautologous Tissue Substitute	Ø Anterior Approach, Anterior Column 1 Posterior Approach, Posterior Column J Posterior Approach, Anterior Column
Ø Occipital-cervical Joint 1 Cervical Vertebral Joint 2 Cervical Vertebral Joints, 2 or more 4 Cervicothoracic Vertebral Joint 6 Thoracic Vertebral Joint 7 Thoracic Vertebral Joints, 2 to 7 8 Thoracic Vertebral Joints, 8 or more A Thoracolumbar Vertebral Joint	Ø Open 3 Percutaneous 4 Percutaneous Endoscopic	A Interbody Fusion Device	Ø Anterior Approach, Anterior Column J Posterior Approach, Anterior Column
C Temporomandibular Joint, Right D Temporomandibular Joint, Left E Sternoclavicular Joint, Right F Sternoclavicular Joint, Left G Acromioclavicular Joint, Right H Acromioclavicular Joint, Left J Shoulder Joint, Right K Shoulder Joint, Left	Ø Open 3 Percutaneous 4 Percutaneous Endoscopic	4 Internal Fixation Device 7 Autologous Tissue Substitute J Synthetic Substitute K Nonautologous Tissue Substitute	Z No Qualifier
L Elbow Joint, Right M Elbow Joint, Left N Wrist Joint, Right P Wrist Joint, Left Q Carpal Joint, Right R Carpal Joint, Left S Carpometacarpal Joint, Right T Carpometacarpal Joint, Left U Metacarpophalangeal Joint, Right V Metacarpophalangeal Joint, Left W Finger Phalangeal Joint, Right X Finger Phalangeal Joint, Left	Ø Open 3 Percutaneous 4 Percutaneous Endoscopic	3 Internal Fixation Device, Sustained Compression 4 Internal Fixation Device 5 External Fixation Device 7 Autologous Tissue Substitute J Synthetic Substitute K Nonautologous Tissue Substitute	Z No Qualifier

ØRG7[Ø34][7JKZ][Ø1J]
ØRG7[Ø34]A[ØJ]
ØRG[Ø124678A][Ø34][7JK][Ø1J] when reported with Secondary Diagnosis K68.11, T81.4XXA, or T84.6ØXA-T84.7XXA
ØRG[Ø124678A][Ø34]A[ØJ] when reported with Secondary Diagnosis K68.11, T81.4XXA, or T84.6ØXA-T84.7XXA
ØRG[EFGHJK][Ø34][47JK]Z when reported with Secondary Diagnosis K68.11, T81.4XXA, or T84.6ØXA-T84.7XXA
ØRG[LM][Ø34][3457JK]Z when reported with Secondary Diagnosis K68.11, T81.4XXA, or T84.6ØXA-T84.7XXA

Coding Clinic: 2Ø13, Q1, P29 – ØRG4ØAØ
Coding Clinic: 2Ø13, Q1, P22 – ØRG7Ø71, ØRGAØ71
Coding Clinic: 2Ø17, Q4, P62 – ØRGWØ4Z
Coding Clinic: 2Ø19, Q2, P19 – ØDG2371
Coding Clinic: 2Ø19, Q3, P28 – ØRG2ØAØ

SECTION: Ø MEDICAL AND SURGICAL
BODY SYSTEM: R UPPER JOINTS
OPERATION: H INSERTION: Putting in a nonbiological appliance that monitors, assists, performs, or prevents a physiological function but does not physically take the place of a body part

Body Part	Approach	Device	Qualifier
Ø Occipital-cervical Joint 1 Cervical Vertebral Joint 4 Cervicothoracic Vertebral Joint 6 Thoracic Vertebral Joint A Thoracolumbar Vertebral Joint	Ø Open 3 Percutaneous 4 Percutaneous Endoscopic	3 Infusion Device 4 Internal Fixation Device 8 Spacer B Spinal Stabilization Device, Interspinous Process C Spinal Stabilization Device, Pedicle-Based D Spinal Stabilization Device, Facet Replacement	Z No Qualifier
3 Cervical Vertebral Disc 5 Cervicothoracic Vertebral Disc 9 Thoracic Vertebral Disc B Thoracolumbar Vertebral Disc	Ø Open 3 Percutaneous 4 Percutaneous Endoscopic	3 Infusion Device	Z No Qualifier
C Temporomandibular Joint, Right D Temporomandibular Joint, Left E Sternoclavicular Joint, Right F Sternoclavicular Joint, Left G Acromioclavicular Joint, Right H Acromioclavicular Joint, Left J Shoulder Joint, Right K Shoulder Joint, Left	Ø Open 3 Percutaneous 4 Percutaneous Endoscopic	3 Infusion Device 4 Internal Fixation Device 8 Spacer	Z No Qualifier
L Elbow Joint, Right M Elbow Joint, Left N Wrist Joint, Right P Wrist Joint, Left Q Carpal Joint, Right R Carpal Joint, Left S Carpometacarpal Joint, Right T Carpometacarpal Joint, Left U Metacarpophalangeal Joint, Right V Metacarpophalangeal Joint, Left W Finger Phalangeal Joint, Right X Finger Phalangeal Joint, Left	Ø Open 3 Percutaneous 4 Percutaneous Endoscopic	3 Infusion Device 4 Internal Fixation Device 5 External Fixation Device 8 Spacer	Z No Qualifier

DRG Non-OR ØRH[Ø146A][34]3Z
DRG Non-OR ØRH[359B][34]3Z
DRG Non-OR ØRH[EFGHJK][34]3Z
DRG Non-OR ØRH[LMNPQRSTUVWX][34]3Z
Non-OR ØRH[Ø146A][Ø34][38]Z
Non-OR ØRH[359B][Ø34]3Z
Non-OR ØRH[CD]33Z
Non-OR ØRH[CD][Ø34]8Z
Non-OR ØRH[EFGHJK][Ø34][38]Z
Non-OR ØRH[LMNPQRSTUVWX][Ø34][38]Z

Coding Clinic: 2016, Q3, P33 – ØRHJØ4ZZ
Coding Clinic: 2017, Q2, P24 – ØRH1Ø4Z

SECTION: Ø MEDICAL AND SURGICAL
BODY SYSTEM: R UPPER JOINTS
OPERATION: J INSPECTION: Visually and/or manually exploring a body part

Body Part	Approach	Device	Qualifier
Ø Occipital-cervical Joint 1 Cervical Vertebral Joint 3 Cervical Vertebral Disc 4 Cervicothoracic Vertebral Joint 5 Cervicothoracic Vertebral Disc 6 Thoracic Vertebral Joint 9 Thoracic Vertebral Disc A Thoracolumbar Vertebral Joint B Thoracolumbar Vertebral Disc C Temporomandibular Joint, Right D Temporomandibular Joint, Left E Sternoclavicular Joint, Right F Sternoclavicular Joint, Left G Acromioclavicular Joint, Right H Acromioclavicular Joint, Left J Shoulder Joint, Right K Shoulder Joint, Left L Elbow Joint, Right M Elbow Joint, Left N Wrist Joint, Right P Wrist Joint, Left Q Carpal Joint, Right R Carpal Joint, Left S Carpometacarpal Joint, Right T Carpometacarpal Joint, Left U Metacarpophalangeal Joint, Right V Metacarpophalangeal Joint, Left W Finger Phalangeal Joint, Right X Finger Phalangeal Joint, Left	Ø Open 3 Percutaneous 4 Percutaneous Endoscopic X External	Z No Device	Z No Qualifier

Non-OR ØRJ[Ø134569ABCDEFGHJKLMNPQRSTUVWX][3X]ZZ

SECTION: Ø MEDICAL AND SURGICAL
BODY SYSTEM: R UPPER JOINTS
OPERATION: N RELEASE: Freeing a body part from an abnormal physical constraint by cutting or by the use of force

Body Part	Approach	Device	Qualifier
Ø Occipital-cervical Joint 1 Cervical Vertebral Joint 3 Cervical Vertebral Disc 4 Cervicothoracic Vertebral Joint 5 Cervicothoracic Vertebral Disc 6 Thoracic Vertebral Joint 9 Thoracic Vertebral Disc A Thoracolumbar Vertebral Joint B Thoracolumbar Vertebral Disc C Temporomandibular Joint, Right D Temporomandibular Joint, Left E Sternoclavicular Joint, Right F Sternoclavicular Joint, Left G Acromioclavicular Joint, Right H Acromioclavicular Joint, Left J Shoulder Joint, Right K Shoulder Joint, Left L Elbow Joint, Right M Elbow Joint, Left N Wrist Joint, Right P Wrist Joint, Left Q Carpal Joint, Right R Carpal Joint, Left S Carpometacarpal Joint, Right T Carpometacarpal Joint, Left U Metacarpophalangeal Joint, Right V Metacarpophalangeal Joint, Left W Finger Phalangeal Joint, Right X Finger Phalangeal Joint, Left	Ø Open 3 Percutaneous 4 Percutaneous Endoscopic X External	Z No Device	Z No Qualifier

Non-OR ØRN[Ø134569ABCDEFGHJKLMNPQRSTUVWX]XZZ

Coding Clinic: 2Ø15, Q2, P23 – ØRNK4ZZ
Coding Clinic: 2Ø16, Q3, P33 – ØRNJ4ZZ

SECTION: Ø MEDICAL AND SURGICAL
BODY SYSTEM: R UPPER JOINTS
OPERATION: P REMOVAL: *(on multiple pages)* Taking out or off a device from a body part

Body Part	Approach	Device	Qualifier
Ø Occipital-cervical Joint 1 Cervical Vertebral Joint 4 Cervicothoracic Vertebral Joint 6 Thoracic Vertebral Joint A Thoracolumbar Vertebral Joint	Ø Open 3 Percutaneous 4 Percutaneous Endoscopic	Ø Drainage Device 3 Infusion Device 4 Internal Fixation Device 7 Autologous Tissue Substitute 8 Spacer A Interbody Fusion Device J Synthetic Substitute K Nonautologous Tissue Substitute	Z No Qualifier
Ø Occipital-cervical Joint 1 Cervical Vertebral Joint 4 Cervicothoracic Vertebral Joint 6 Thoracic Vertebral Joint A Thoracolumbar Vertebral Joint	X External	Ø Drainage Device 3 Infusion Device 4 Internal Fixation Device	Z No Qualifier

DRG Non-OR ØRQ[Ø134569ABEFGHJKLMNPQRSTUVWX]XZZ   Non-OR ØRP[Ø146A][Ø34]8Z
Non-OR ØRP[Ø146A]3[Ø3]Z

SECTION: Ø MEDICAL AND SURGICAL
BODY SYSTEM: R UPPER JOINTS
OPERATION: P REMOVAL: *(continued)*
Taking out or off a device from a body part

Body Part	Approach	Device	Qualifier
3 Cervical Vertebral Disc 5 Cervicothoracic Vertebral Disc 9 Thoracic Vertebral Disc B Thoracolumbar Vertebral Disc	Ø Open 3 Percutaneous 4 Percutaneous Endoscopic	Ø Drainage Device 3 Infusion Device 7 Autologous Tissue Substitute J Synthetic Substitute K Nonautologous Tissue Substitute	Z No Qualifier
3 Cervical Vertebral Disc 5 Cervicothoracic Vertebral Disc 9 Thoracic Vertebral Disc B Thoracolumbar Vertebral Disc	X External	Ø Drainage Device 3 Infusion Device	Z No Qualifier
C Temporomandibular Joint, Right D Temporomandibular Joint, Left E Sternoclavicular Joint, Right F Sternoclavicular Joint, Left G Acromioclavicular Joint, Right H Acromioclavicular Joint, Left	Ø Open 3 Percutaneous 4 Percutaneous Endoscopic	Ø Drainage Device 3 Infusion Device 4 Internal Fixation Device 7 Autologous Tissue Substitute 8 Spacer J Synthetic Substitute K Nonautologous Tissue Substitute	Z No Qualifier
C Temporomandibular Joint, Right D Temporomandibular Joint, Left E Sternoclavicular Joint, Right F Sternoclavicular Joint, Left G Acromioclavicular Joint, Right H Acromioclavicular Joint, Left	X External	Ø Drainage Device 3 Infusion Device 4 Internal Fixation Device	Z No Qualifier
J Shoulder Joint, Right K Shoulder Joint, Left	Ø Open 3 Percutaneous 4 Percutaneous Endoscopic	Ø Drainage Device 3 Infusion Device 4 Internal Fixation Device 7 Autologous Tissue Substitute 8 Spacer K Nonautologous Tissue Substitute	Z No Qualifier
J Shoulder Joint, Right K Shoulder Joint, Left	Ø Open 3 Percutaneous 4 Percutaneous Endoscopic	J Synthetic Substitute	6 Humeral Surface 7 Glenoid Surface Z No Qualifier
J Shoulder Joint, Right K Shoulder Joint, Left	X External	Ø Drainage Device 3 Infusion Device 4 Internal Fixation Device	Z No Qualifier
L Elbow Joint, Right M Elbow Joint, Left N Wrist Joint, Right P Wrist Joint, Left Q Carpal Joint, Right R Carpal Joint, Left S Carpometacarpal Joint, Right T Carpometacarpal Joint, Left U Metacarpophalangeal Joint, Right V Metacarpophalangeal Joint, Left W Finger Phalangeal Joint, Right X Finger Phalangeal Joint, Left	Ø Open 3 Percutaneous 4 Percutaneous Endoscopic	Ø Drainage Device 3 Infusion Device 4 Internal Fixation Device 5 External Fixation Device 7 Autologous Tissue Substitute 8 Spacer J Synthetic Substitute K Nonautologous Tissue Substitute	Z No Qualifier

Non-OR ØRP[Ø146A]X[Ø34]Z
Non-OR ØRP[359B]3[Ø3]Z
Non-OR ØRP[359B]X[Ø3]Z
Non-OR ØRP[CDEFGHJK][Ø34]8Z
Non-OR ØRP[CDEFGHJK]3[Ø3]Z
Non-OR ØRP[CD]X[Ø3]Z
Non-OR ØRP[EFGHJK]X[Ø34]Z
Non-OR ØRP[LMNPQRSTUVWX]3[Ø3]Z
Non-OR ØRP[LMNPQRSTUVWX][Ø34]8Z

SECTION: Ø MEDICAL AND SURGICAL
BODY SYSTEM: R UPPER JOINTS
OPERATION: P REMOVAL: *(continued)*
Taking out or off a device from a body part

Body Part	Approach	Device	Qualifier
L Elbow Joint, Right M Elbow Joint, Left N Wrist Joint, Right P Wrist Joint, Left Q Carpal Joint, Right R Carpal Joint, Left S Carpometacarpal Joint, Right T Carpometacarpal Joint, Left U Metacarpophalangeal Joint, Right V Metacarpophalangeal Joint, Left W Finger Phalangeal Joint, Right X Finger Phalangeal Joint, Left	X External	Ø Drainage Device 3 Infusion Device 4 Internal Fixation Device 5 External Fixation Device	Z No Qualifier

Non-OR ØRP[LMNPQRSTUVWX]X[Ø345]Z

SECTION: Ø MEDICAL AND SURGICAL
BODY SYSTEM: R UPPER JOINTS
OPERATION: Q REPAIR: Restoring, to the extent possible, a body part to its normal anatomic structure and function

Body Part	Approach	Device	Qualifier
Ø Occipital-cervical Joint 1 Cervical Vertebral Joint 3 Cervical Vertebral Disc 4 Cervicothoracic Vertebral Joint 5 Cervicothoracic Vertebral Disc 6 Thoracic Vertebral Joint 9 Thoracic Vertebral Disc A Thoracolumbar Vertebral Joint B Thoracolumbar Vertebral Disc C Temporomandibular Joint, Right D Temporomandibular Joint, Left E Sternoclavicular Joint, Right F Sternoclavicular Joint, Left G Acromioclavicular Joint, Right H Acromioclavicular Joint, Left J Shoulder Joint, Right K Shoulder Joint, Left L Elbow Joint, Right M Elbow Joint, Left N Wrist Joint, Right P Wrist Joint, Left Q Carpal Joint, Right R Carpal Joint, Left S Carpometacarpal Joint, Right T Carpometacarpal Joint, Left U Metacarpophalangeal Joint, Right V Metacarpophalangeal Joint, Left W Finger Phalangeal Joint, Right X Finger Phalangeal Joint, Left	Ø Open 3 Percutaneous 4 Percutaneous Endoscopic X External	Z No Device	Z No Qualifier

DRG Non-OR ØRQ[EFGHJKLM]XZZ
Non-OR ØRQ[CD]XZZ

ØRQ[EFGHJKLM][Ø34X]ZZ when reported with Secondary Diagnosis K68.11, T81.4ØXA-T81.49XA, or T82.7XXA

Coding Clinic: 2016, Q1, P3Ø – ØRQJ4ZZ

SECTION: Ø MEDICAL AND SURGICAL
BODY SYSTEM: R UPPER JOINTS
OPERATION: R REPLACEMENT: Putting in or on biological or synthetic material that physically takes the place and/or function of all or a portion of a body part

Body Part	Approach	Device	Qualifier
Ø Occipital-cervical Joint 1 Cervical Vertebral Joint 3 Cervical Vertebral Disc 4 Cervicothoracic Vertebral Joint 5 Cervicothoracic Vertebral Disc 6 Thoracic Vertebral Joint 9 Thoracic Vertebral Disc A Thoracolumbar Vertebral Joint B Thoracolumbar Vertebral Disc C Temporomandibular Joint, Right D Temporomandibular Joint, Left E Sternoclavicular Joint, Right F Sternoclavicular Joint, Left G Acromioclavicular Joint, Right H Acromioclavicular Joint, Left L Elbow Joint, Right M Elbow Joint, Left N Wrist Joint, Right P Wrist Joint, Left Q Carpal Joint, Right R Carpal Joint, Left S Carpometacarpal Joint, Right T Carpometacarpal Joint, Left U Metacarpophalangeal Joint, Right V Metacarpophalangeal Joint, Left W Finger Phalangeal Joint, Right X Finger Phalangeal Joint, Left	Ø Open	7 Autologous Tissue Substitute J Synthetic Substitute K Nonautologous Tissue Substitute	Z No Qualifier
J Shoulder Joint, Right K Shoulder Joint, Left	Ø Open	Ø Synthetic Substitute, Reverse Ball and Socket 7 Autologous Tissue Substitute K Nonautologous Tissue Substitute	Z No Qualifier
J Shoulder Joint, Right K Shoulder Joint, Left	Ø Open	J Synthetic Substitute	6 Humeral Surface 7 Glenoid Surface Z No Qualifier

Coding Clinic: 2015, Q1, P27 – ØRRJØØZ
Coding Clinic: 2015, Q3, P15 – ØRRKØJ6

SECTION: Ø MEDICAL AND SURGICAL
BODY SYSTEM: R UPPER JOINTS
OPERATION: S REPOSITION: Moving to its normal location, or other suitable location, all or a portion of a body part

Body Part	Approach	Device	Qualifier
Ø Occipital-cervical Joint 1 Cervical Vertebral Joint 4 Cervicothoracic Vertebral Joint 6 Thoracic Vertebral Joint A Thoracolumbar Vertebral Joint C Temporomandibular Joint, Right D Temporomandibular Joint, Left E Sternoclavicular Joint, Right F Sternoclavicular Joint, Left G Acromioclavicular Joint, Right H Acromioclavicular Joint, Left J Shoulder Joint, Right K Shoulder Joint, Left	Ø Open 3 Percutaneous 4 Percutaneous Endoscopic X External	4 Internal Fixation Device Z No Device	Z No Qualifier
L Elbow Joint, Right M Elbow Joint, Left N Wrist Joint, Right P Wrist Joint, Left Q Carpal Joint, Right R Carpal Joint, Left S Carpometacarpal Joint, Right T Carpometacarpal Joint, Left U Metacarpophalangeal Joint, Right V Metacarpophalangeal Joint, Left W Finger Phalangeal Joint, Right X Finger Phalangeal Joint, Left	Ø Open 3 Percutaneous 4 Percutaneous Endoscopic X External	4 Internal Fixation Device 5 External Fixation Device Z No Device	Z No Qualifier

Non-OR ØRS[Ø146ACDEFGHJK][34X][4Z]Z
Non-OR ØRS[LMNPQRSTUVWX][34X][45Z]Z

Coding Clinic: 2Ø15, Q2, P35; 2Ø13, Q2, P39 – ØRS1XZZ
Coding Clinic: 2Ø19, Q3, P27 – ØRSHØ4Z

SECTION: Ø MEDICAL AND SURGICAL
BODY SYSTEM: R UPPER JOINTS
OPERATION: T RESECTION: Cutting out or off, without replacement, all of a body part

Body Part	Approach	Device	Qualifier
3 Cervical Vertebral Disc 4 Cervicothoracic Vertebral Joint 5 Cervicothoracic Vertebral Disc 9 Thoracic Vertebral Disc B Thoracolumbar Vertebral Disc C Temporomandibular Joint, Right D Temporomandibular Joint, Left E Sternoclavicular Joint, Right F Sternoclavicular Joint, Left G Acromioclavicular Joint, Right H Acromioclavicular Joint, Left J Shoulder Joint, Right K Shoulder Joint, Left L Elbow Joint, Right M Elbow Joint, Left N Wrist Joint, Right P Wrist Joint, Left Q Carpal Joint, Right R Carpal Joint, Left S Carpometacarpal Joint, Right T Carpometacarpal Joint, Left U Metacarpophalangeal Joint, Right V Metacarpophalangeal Joint, Left W Finger Phalangeal Joint, Right X Finger Phalangeal Joint, Left	Ø Open	Z No Device	Z No Qualifier

SECTION: Ø MEDICAL AND SURGICAL
BODY SYSTEM: R UPPER JOINTS
OPERATION: U SUPPLEMENT: Putting in or on biological or synthetic material that physically reinforces and/or augments the function of a portion of a body part

Body Part	Approach	Device	Qualifier
Ø Occipital-cervical Joint 1 Cervical Vertebral Joint 3 Cervical Vertebral Disc 4 Cervicothoracic Vertebral Joint 5 Cervicothoracic Vertebral Disc 6 Thoracic Vertebral Joint 9 Thoracic Vertebral Disc A Thoracolumbar Vertebral Joint B Thoracolumbar Vertebral Disc C Temporomandibular Joint, Right D Temporomandibular Joint, Left E Sternoclavicular Joint, Right F Sternoclavicular Joint, Left G Acromioclavicular Joint, Right H Acromioclavicular Joint, Left J Shoulder Joint, Right K Shoulder Joint, Left L Elbow Joint, Right M Elbow Joint, Left N Wrist Joint, Right P Wrist Joint, Left Q Carpal Joint, Right R Carpal Joint, Left S Carpometacarpal Joint, Right T Carpometacarpal Joint, Left U Metacarpophalangeal Joint, Right V Metacarpophalangeal Joint, Left W Finger Phalangeal Joint, Right X Finger Phalangeal Joint, Left	Ø Open 3 Percutaneous 4 Percutaneous Endoscopic	7 Autologous Tissue Substitute J Synthetic Substitute K Nonautologous Tissue Substitute	Z No Qualifier

ØRU[EFGHJKLM][Ø34][7JK]Z when reported with Secondary Diagnosis K68.11, T81.4XXA, or T84.6ØXA-T84.7XXA

Coding Clinic: 2015, Q3, P27 – ØRUTØ7Z
Coding Clinic: 2019, Q3, P27 – ØRUHØKZ

SECTION: Ø MEDICAL AND SURGICAL
BODY SYSTEM: R UPPER JOINTS
OPERATION: W REVISION: Correcting, to the extent possible, a portion of a malfunctioning device or the position of a displaced device

Body Part	Approach	Device	Qualifier
Ø Occipital-cervical Joint 1 Cervical Vertebral Joint 4 Cervicothoracic Vertebral Joint 6 Thoracic Vertebral Joint A Thoracolumbar Vertebral Joint	Ø Open 3 Percutaneous 4 Percutaneous Endoscopic X External	Ø Drainage Device 3 Infusion Device 4 Internal Fixation Device 7 Autologous Tissue Substitute 8 Spacer A Interbody Fusion Device J Synthetic Substitute K Nonautologous Tissue Substitute	Z No Qualifier
3 Cervical Vertebral Disc 5 Cervicothoracic Vertebral Disc 9 Thoracic Vertebral Disc B Thoracolumbar Vertebral Disc	Ø Open 3 Percutaneous 4 Percutaneous Endoscopic X External	Ø Drainage Device 3 Infusion Device 7 Autologous Tissue Substitute J Synthetic Substitute K Nonautologous Tissue Substitute	Z No Qualifier
C Temporomandibular Joint, Right D Temporomandibular Joint, Left E Sternoclavicular Joint, Right F Sternoclavicular Joint, Left G Acromioclavicular Joint, Right H Acromioclavicular Joint, Left	Ø Open 3 Percutaneous 4 Percutaneous Endoscopic X External	Ø Drainage Device 3 Infusion Device 4 Internal Fixation Device 7 Autologous Tissue Substitute 8 Spacer J Synthetic Substitute K Nonautologous Tissue Substitute	Z No Qualifier
J Shoulder Joint, Right K Shoulder Joint, Left	Ø Open 3 Percutaneous 4 Percutaneous Endoscopic X External	Ø Drainage Device 3 Infusion Device 4 Internal Fixation Device 7 Autologous Tissue Substitute 8 Spacer K Nonautologous Tissue Substitute	Z No Qualifier
J Shoulder Joint, Right K Shoulder Joint, Left	Ø Open 3 Percutaneous 4 Percutaneous Endoscopic	J Synthetic Substitute	6 Humeral Surface 7 Glenoid Surface Z No Qualifier
L Elbow Joint, Right M Elbow Joint, Left N Wrist Joint, Right P Wrist Joint, Left Q Carpal Joint, Right R Carpal Joint, Left S Carpometacarpal Joint, Right T Carpometacarpal Joint, Left U Metacarpophalangeal Joint, Right V Metacarpophalangeal Joint, Left W Finger Phalangeal Joint, Right X Finger Phalangeal Joint, Left	Ø Open 3 Percutaneous 4 Percutaneous Endoscopic X External	Ø Drainage Device 3 Infusion Device 4 Internal Fixation Device 5 External Fixation Device 7 Autologous Tissue Substitute 8 Spacer J Synthetic Substitute K Nonautologous Tissue Substitute	Z No Qualifier

Non-OR ØRW[Ø146A]X[Ø3478AJK]Z
Non-OR ØRW[359B]X[Ø37JK]Z
Non-OR ØRW[CDEFGHJK]X[Ø3478JK]Z
Non-OR ØRW[LMNPQRSTUVWX]X[Ø34578JK]Z

SECTION: Ø **MEDICAL AND SURGICAL**
BODY SYSTEM: S **LOWER JOINTS**
OPERATION: 2 **CHANGE:** Taking out or off a device from a body part and putting back an identical or similar device in or on the same body part without cutting or puncturing the skin or a mucous membrane

Body Part	Approach	Device	Qualifier
Y Lower Joint	X External	Ø Drainage Device Y Other Device	Z No Qualifier

Non-OR All Values

SECTION: Ø **MEDICAL AND SURGICAL**
BODY SYSTEM: S **LOWER JOINTS**
OPERATION: 5 **DESTRUCTION:** Physical eradication of all or a portion of a body part by the direct use of energy, force, or destructive agent

Body Part	Approach	Device	Qualifier
Ø Lumbar Vertebral Joint 2 Lumbar Vertebral Disc 3 Lumbosacral Joint 4 Lumbosacral Disc 5 Sacrococcygeal Joint 6 Coccygeal Joint 7 Sacroiliac Joint, Right 8 Sacroiliac Joint, Left 9 Hip Joint, Right B Hip Joint, Left C Knee Joint, Right D Knee Joint, Left F Ankle Joint, Right G Ankle Joint, Left H Tarsal Joint, Right J Tarsal Joint, Left K Tarsometatarsal Joint, Right L Tarsometatarsal Joint, Left M Metatarsal-Phalangeal Joint, Right N Metatarsal-Phalangeal Joint, Left P Toe Phalangeal Joint, Right Q Toe Phalangeal Joint, Left	Ø Open 3 Percutaneous 4 Percutaneous Endoscopic	Z No Device	Z No Qualifier

SECTION: Ø MEDICAL AND SURGICAL
BODY SYSTEM: S LOWER JOINTS
OPERATION: 9 DRAINAGE: Taking or letting out fluids and/or gases from a body part

Body Part	Approach	Device	Qualifier
Ø Lumbar Vertebral Joint 2 Lumbar Vertebral Disc 3 Lumbosacral Joint 4 Lumbosacral Disc 5 Sacrococcygeal Joint 6 Coccygeal Joint 7 Sacroiliac Joint, Right 8 Sacroiliac Joint, Left 9 Hip Joint, Right B Hip Joint, Left C Knee Joint, Right D Knee Joint, Left F Ankle Joint, Right G Ankle Joint, Left H Tarsal Joint, Right J Tarsal Joint, Left K Tarsometatarsal Joint, Right L Tarsometatarsal Joint, Left M Metatarsal-Phalangeal Joint, Right N Metatarsal-Phalangeal Joint, Left P Toe Phalangeal Joint, Right Q Toe Phalangeal Joint, Left	Ø Open 3 Percutaneous 4 Percutaneous Endoscopic	Ø Drainage Device	Z No Qualifier
Ø Lumbar Vertebral Joint 2 Lumbar Vertebral Disc 3 Lumbosacral Joint 4 Lumbosacral Disc 5 Sacrococcygeal Joint 6 Coccygeal Joint 7 Sacroiliac Joint, Right 8 Sacroiliac Joint, Left 9 Hip Joint, Right B Hip Joint, Left C Knee Joint, Right D Knee Joint, Left F Ankle Joint, Right G Ankle Joint, Left H Tarsal Joint, Right J Tarsal Joint, Left K Tarsometatarsal Joint, Right L Tarsometatarsal Joint, Left M Metatarsal-Phalangeal Joint, Right N Metatarsal-Phalangeal Joint, Left P Toe Phalangeal Joint, Right Q Toe Phalangeal Joint, Left	Ø Open 3 Percutaneous 4 Percutaneous Endoscopic	Z No Device	X Diagnostic Z No Qualifier

Non-OR ØS9[Ø23456789BCDFGHJKLMNPQ][34]ØZ
Non-OR ØS9[Ø23456789BCDFGHJKLMNPQ][Ø34]ZX
Non-OR ØS9[Ø23456789BCDFGHJKLMNPQ][34]ZZ

Coding Clinic: 2018, Q2, P17 – ØS9D4ZZ

SECTION: Ø MEDICAL AND SURGICAL
BODY SYSTEM: S LOWER JOINTS
OPERATION: B EXCISION: Cutting out or off, without replacement, a portion of a body part

Body Part	Approach	Device	Qualifier
Ø Lumbar Vertebral Joint 2 Lumbar Vertebral Disc 3 Lumbosacral Joint 4 Lumbosacral Disc 5 Sacrococcygeal Joint 6 Coccygeal Joint 7 Sacroiliac Joint, Right 8 Sacroiliac Joint, Left 9 Hip Joint, Right B Hip Joint, Left C Knee Joint, Right D Knee Joint, Left F Ankle Joint, Right G Ankle Joint, Left H Tarsal Joint, Right J Tarsal Joint, Left K Tarsometatarsal Joint, Right L Tarsometatarsal Joint, Left M Metatarsal-Phalangeal Joint, Right N Metatarsal-Phalangeal Joint, Left P Toe Phalangeal Joint, Right Q Toe Phalangeal Joint, Left	Ø Open 3 Percutaneous 4 Percutaneous Endoscopic	Z No Device	X Diagnostic Z No Qualifier

Non-OR ØSB[Ø23456789BCDFGHJKLMNPQ][Ø34]ZX

Coding Clinic: 2Ø15, Q1, P34 – ØSBD4ZZ
Coding Clinic: 2Ø17, Q4, P76; 2Ø16, Q2, P16 – ØSB2ØZZ
Coding Clinic: 2Ø17, Q4, P76 – ØSB4ØZZ

SECTION: Ø MEDICAL AND SURGICAL
BODY SYSTEM: S LOWER JOINTS
OPERATION: C EXTIRPATION: Taking or cutting out solid matter from a body part

Body Part	Approach	Device	Qualifier
Ø Lumbar Vertebral Joint 2 Lumbar Vertebral Disc 3 Lumbosacral Joint 4 Lumbosacral Disc 5 Sacrococcygeal Joint 6 Coccygeal Joint 7 Sacroiliac Joint, Right 8 Sacroiliac Joint, Left 9 Hip Joint, Right B Hip Joint, Left C Knee Joint, Right D Knee Joint, Left F Ankle Joint, Right G Ankle Joint, Left H Tarsal Joint, Right J Tarsal Joint, Left K Tarsometatarsal Joint, Right L Tarsometatarsal Joint, Left M Metatarsal-Phalangeal Joint, Right N Metatarsal-Phalangeal Joint, Left P Toe Phalangeal Joint, Right Q Toe Phalangeal Joint, Left	Ø Open 3 Percutaneous 4 Percutaneous Endoscopic	Z No Device	Z No Qualifier

SECTION: Ø MEDICAL AND SURGICAL
BODY SYSTEM: S LOWER JOINTS
OPERATION: G FUSION: Joining together portions of an articular body part, rendering the articular body part immobile

Body Part	Approach	Device	Qualifier
Ø Lumbar Vertebral Joint 1 Lumbar Vertebral Joints, 2 or more 3 Lumbosacral Joint	Ø Open 3 Percutaneous 4 Percutaneous Endoscopic	7 Autologous Tissue Substitute J Synthetic Substitute K Nonautologous Tissue Substitute	Ø Anterior Approach, Anterior Column 1 Posterior Approach, Posterior Column J Posterior Approach, Anterior Column
Ø Lumbar Vertebral Joint 1 Lumbar Vertebral Joints, 2 or more 3 Lumbosacral Joint	Ø Open 3 Percutaneous 4 Percutaneous Endoscopic	A Interbody Fusion Device	Ø Anterior Approach, Anterior Column J Posterior Approach, Anterior Column
5 Sacrococcygeal Joint 6 Coccygeal Joint 7 Sacroiliac Joint, Right 8 Sacroiliac Joint, Left	Ø Open 3 Percutaneous 4 Percutaneous Endoscopic	4 Internal Fixation Device 7 Autologous Tissue Substitute J Synthetic Substitute K Nonautologous Tissue Substitute	Z No Qualifier
9 Hip Joint, Right B Hip Joint, Left C Knee Joint, Right D Knee Joint, Left F Ankle Joint, Right G Ankle Joint, Left H Tarsal Joint, Right J Tarsal Joint, Left K Tarsometatarsal Joint, Right L Tarsometatarsal Joint, Left M Metatarsal-Phalangeal Joint, Right N Metatarsal-Phalangeal Joint, Left P Toe Phalangeal Joint, Right Q Toe Phalangeal Joint, Left	Ø Open 3 Percutaneous 4 Percutaneous Endoscopic	3 Internal Fixation Device, Sustained Compression 4 Internal Fixation Device 5 External Fixation Device 7 Autologous Tissue Substitute J Synthetic Substitute K Nonautologous Tissue Substitute	Z No Qualifier

ØSG1[Ø34][7JKZ][Ø1J]
ØSG1[Ø34]A[ØJ]
ØSG[Ø13][Ø34][7JK][Ø1J] when reported with Secondary Diagnosis K68.11, T814XA-T8149XA, or T84.6ØXA-T84.7XXA
ØSG[Ø13][Ø34]A[ØJ] when reported with Secondary Diagnosis K68.11, T814XA-T8149XA, or T84.6ØXA-T84.7XXA
ØSG[78][Ø34][47JK]Z when reported with Secondary Diagnosis K68.11, T814XA-T8149XA, or T84.6ØXA-T84.7XXA

Coding Clinic: 2Ø13, Q3, P26, Q1, P23 – ØSGØØ71
Coding Clinic: 2Ø13, Q3, P26 – ØSGØØAJ
Coding Clinic: 2Ø13, Q2, P4Ø – ØSGGØ4Z, ØSGGØ7Z
Coding Clinic: 2Ø21, Q3, P24 – ØSGJØ[47]Z, ØSGLØ[47]Z
Coding Clinic: 2Ø21, Q3, P25 – ØSGØØK1
Coding Clinic: 2Ø22, Q2, P23 – ØSG834Z
Coding Clinic: 2Ø22, Q3, P22 – ØSGØØAJ
Coding Clinic: 2Ø23, Q2, P26 – ØSG1ØK1

SECTION: Ø MEDICAL AND SURGICAL
BODY SYSTEM: S LOWER JOINTS
OPERATION: H INSERTION: Putting in a nonbiological appliance that monitors, assists, performs, or prevents a physiological function but does not physically take the place of a body part

Body Part	Approach	Device	Qualifier
Ø Lumbar Vertebral Joint 3 Lumbosacral Joint	Ø Open 3 Percutaneous 4 Percutaneous Endoscopic	3 Infusion Device 4 Internal Fixation Device 8 Spacer B Spinal Stabilization Device, Interspinous Process C Spinal Stabilization Device, Pedicle-Based D Spinal Stabilization Device, Facet Replacement	Z No Qualifier
2 Lumbar Vertebral Disc 4 Lumbosacral Disc	Ø Open 3 Percutaneous 4 Percutaneous Endoscopic	3 Infusion Device 8 Spacer	Z No Qualifier
5 Sacrococcygeal Joint 6 Coccygeal Joint 7 Sacroiliac Joint, Right 8 Sacroiliac Joint, Left	Ø Open 3 Percutaneous 4 Percutaneous Endoscopic	3 Infusion Device 4 Internal Fixation Device 8 Spacer	Z No Qualifier
9 Hip Joint, Right B Hip Joint, Left C Knee Joint, Right D Knee Joint, Left F Ankle Joint, Right G Ankle Joint, Left H Tarsal Joint, Right J Tarsal Joint, Left K Tarsometatarsal Joint, Right L Tarsometatarsal Joint, Left M Metatarsal-Phalangeal Joint, Right N Metatarsal-Phalangeal Joint, Left P Toe Phalangeal Joint, Right Q Toe Phalangeal Joint, Left	Ø Open 3 Percutaneous 4 Percutaneous Endoscopic	3 Infusion Device 4 Internal Fixation Device 5 External Fixation Device 8 Spacer	Z No Qualifier

DRG Non-OR ØSH[Ø3][34]3Z
DRG Non-OR ØSH[24][34]3Z
DRG Non-OR ØSH[5678][34]3Z
DRG Non-OR ØSH[9BCDFGHJKLMNPQ][34]3Z
Non-OR ØSH[Ø3]Ø3Z
Non-OR ØSH[Ø3][Ø34]8Z
Non-OR ØSH[24]Ø3Z
Non-OR ØSH[24][Ø34]8Z
Non-OR ØSH[5678]Ø3Z
Non-OR ØSH[5678][Ø34]8Z
Non-OR ØSH[9BCDFGHJKLMNPQ]Ø3Z
Non-OR ØSH[9BCDFGHJKLMNPQ][Ø34]8Z

Coding Clinic: 2Ø21, Q1, P19 - ØSH4Ø8Z
Coding Clinic: 2Ø21, Q3, P25 – ØSHØØBZ

SECTION: Ø MEDICAL AND SURGICAL
BODY SYSTEM: S LOWER JOINTS
OPERATION: J INSPECTION: Visually and/or manually exploring a body part

Body Part	Approach	Device	Qualifier
Ø Lumbar Vertebral Joint 2 Lumbar Vertebral Disc 3 Lumbosacral Joint 4 Lumbosacral Disc 5 Sacrococcygeal Joint 6 Coccygeal Joint 7 Sacroiliac Joint, Right 8 Sacroiliac Joint, Left 9 Hip Joint, Right B Hip Joint, Left C Knee Joint, Right D Knee Joint, Left F Ankle Joint, Right G Ankle Joint, Left H Tarsal Joint, Right J Tarsal Joint, Left K Tarsometatarsal Joint, Right L Tarsometatarsal Joint, Left M Metatarsal-Phalangeal Joint, Right N Metatarsal-Phalangeal Joint, Left P Toe Phalangeal Joint, Right Q Toe Phalangeal Joint, Left	Ø Open 3 Percutaneous 4 Percutaneous Endoscopic X External	Z No Device	Z No Qualifier

Non-OR ØSJ[Ø23456789BCDFGHJKLMNPQ][3X]ZZ

Coding Clinic: 2Ø17, Q1, P5Ø – ØSJG3ZZ

SECTION: Ø MEDICAL AND SURGICAL
BODY SYSTEM: S LOWER JOINTS
OPERATION: N RELEASE: Freeing a body part from an abnormal physical constraint by cutting or by the use of force

Body Part	Approach	Device	Qualifier
Ø Lumbar Vertebral Joint 2 Lumbar Vertebral Disc 3 Lumbosacral Joint 4 Lumbosacral Disc 5 Sacrococcygeal Joint 6 Coccygeal Joint 7 Sacroiliac Joint, Right 8 Sacroiliac Joint, Left 9 Hip Joint, Right B Hip Joint, Left C Knee Joint, Right D Knee Joint, Left F Ankle Joint, Right G Ankle Joint, Left H Tarsal Joint, Right J Tarsal Joint, Left K Tarsometatarsal Joint, Right L Tarsometatarsal Joint, Left M Metatarsal-Phalangeal Joint, Right N Metatarsal-Phalangeal Joint, Left P Toe Phalangeal Joint, Right Q Toe Phalangeal Joint, Left	Ø Open 3 Percutaneous 4 Percutaneous Endoscopic X External	Z No Device	Z No Qualifier

Non-OR ØSN[Ø23456789BCDFGHJKLMNPQ]XZZ

Coding Clinic: 2Ø2Ø, Q2, P27 – ØSNC4ZZ

SECTION: Ø MEDICAL AND SURGICAL
BODY SYSTEM: S LOWER JOINTS
OPERATION: P REMOVAL: (on multiple pages)
Taking out or off a device from a body part

Body Part	Approach	Device	Qualifier
Ø Lumbar Vertebral Joint 3 Lumbosacral Joint	Ø Open 3 Percutaneous 4 Percutaneous Endoscopic	Ø Drainage Device 3 Infusion Device 4 Internal Fixation Device 7 Autologous Tissue Substitute 8 Spacer A Interbody Fusion Device J Synthetic Substitute K Nonautologous Tissue Substitute	Z No Qualifier
Ø Lumbar Vertebral Joint 3 Lumbosacral Joint	X External	Ø Drainage Device 3 Infusion Device 4 Internal Fixation Device	Z No Qualifier
2 Lumbar Vertebral Disc 4 Lumbosacral Disc	Ø Open 3 Percutaneous 4 Percutaneous Endoscopic	Ø Drainage Device 3 Infusion Device 7 Autologous Tissue Substitute J Synthetic Substitute K Nonautologous Tissue Substitute	Z No Qualifier
2 Lumbar Vertebral Disc 4 Lumbosacral Disc	X External	Ø Drainage Device 3 Infusion Device	Z No Qualifier
5 Sacrococcygeal Joint 6 Coccygeal Joint 7 Sacroiliac Joint, Right 8 Sacroiliac Joint, Left	Ø Open 3 Percutaneous 4 Percutaneous Endoscopic	Ø Drainage Device 3 Infusion Device 4 Internal Fixation Device 7 Autologous Tissue Substitute 8 Spacer J Synthetic Substitute K Nonautologous Tissue Substitute	Z No Qualifier
5 Sacrococcygeal Joint 6 Coccygeal Joint 7 Sacroiliac Joint, Right 8 Sacroiliac Joint, Left	X External	Ø Drainage Device 3 Infusion Device 4 Internal Fixation Device	Z No Qualifier
9 Hip Joint, Right ⊞ B Hip Joint, Left ⊞	Ø Open	Ø Drainage Device 3 Infusion Device 4 Internal Fixation Device 5 External Fixation Device 7 Autologous Tissue Substitute 8 Spacer 9 Liner B Resurfacing Device E Articulating Spacer J Synthetic Substitute K Nonautologous Tissue Substitute	Z No Qualifier
9 Hip Joint, Right ⊞ B Hip Joint, Left ⊞	3 Percutaneous 4 Percutaneous Endoscopic	Ø Drainage Device 3 Infusion Device 4 Internal Fixation Device 5 External Fixation Device 7 Autologous Tissue Substitute 8 Spacer J Synthetic Substitute K Nonautologous Tissue Substitute	Z No Qualifier

⊞ ØSP[9B]Ø[89BJ]Z
⊞ ØSP[9B]4[8J]Z
DRG Non-OR ØSP[9B]Ø8Z
DRG Non-OR ØSP[9B]48Z
Non-OR ØSP[Ø3][Ø34]8Z
Non-OR ØSP[Ø3]3[Ø3]Z
Non-OR ØSP[Ø3]X[Ø34]Z
Non-OR ØSP[24]3[Ø3]Z
Non-OR ØSP[24]X[Ø3]Z
Non-OR ØSP[5678][Ø34]8Z
Non-OR ØSP[5678]3[Ø3]Z
Non-OR ØSP[5678]X[Ø34]Z
Non-OR ØSP[9B]3[Ø38]Z

Coding Clinic: 2Ø15, Q2, P2Ø – ØSP9Ø9Z
Coding Clinic: 2Ø16, Q4, P112 – ØSP9Ø9Z

SECTION: Ø MEDICAL AND SURGICAL
BODY SYSTEM: S LOWER JOINTS
OPERATION: P REMOVAL: *(continued)*
Taking out or off a device from a body part

Body Part	Approach	Device	Qualifier
9 Hip Joint, Right B Hip Joint, Left	X External	Ø Drainage Device 3 Infusion Device 4 Internal Fixation Device 5 External Fixation Device	Z No Qualifier
A Hip Joint, Acetabular Surface, Right ⊞ E Hip Joint, Acetabular Surface, Left ⊞ R Hip Joint, Femoral Surface, Right ⊞ S Hip Joint, Femoral Surface, Left ⊞ T Knee Joint, Femoral Surface, Right ⊞ U Knee Joint, Femoral Surface, Left ⊞ V Knee Joint, Tibial Surface, Right ⊞ W Knee Joint, Tibial Surface, Left ⊞	Ø Open 3 Percutaneous 4 Percutaneous Endoscopic	J Synthetic Substitute	Z No Qualifier
C Knee Joint, Right ⊞ D Knee Joint, Left ⊞	Ø Open	Ø Drainage Device 3 Infusion Device 4 Internal Fixation Device 5 External Fixation Device 7 Autologous Tissue Substitute 8 Spacer 9 Liner E Articulating Spacer K Nonautologous Tissue Substitute L Synthetic Substitute, Unicondylar Medial M Synthetic Substitute, Unicondylar Lateral N Synthetic Substitute, Patellofemoral	Z No Qualifier
C Knee Joint, Right ⊞ D Knee Joint, Left ⊞	Ø Open	J Synthetic Substitute	C Patellar Surface Z No Qualifier
C Knee Joint, Right ⊞ D Knee Joint, Left ⊞	3 Percutaneous 4 Percutaneous Endoscopic	Ø Drainage Device 3 Infusion Device 4 Internal Fixation Device 5 External Fixation Device 7 Autologous Tissue Substitute 8 Spacer K Nonautologous Tissue Substitute L Synthetic Substitute, Unicondylar Medial M Synthetic Substitute, Unicondylar Lateral N Synthetic Substitute, Patellofemoral	Z No Qualifier
C Knee Joint, Right ⊞ D Knee Joint, Left ⊞	3 Percutaneous 4 Percutaneous Endoscopic	J Synthetic Substitute	C Patellar Surface Z No Qualifier
C Knee Joint, Right D Knee Joint, Left	X External	Ø Drainage Device 3 Infusion Device 4 Internal Fixation Device 5 External Fixation Device	Z No Qualifier

⊞ ØSP[AERSTUVW][Ø4]JZ
⊞ ØSP[CD]Ø[89]Z
⊞ ØSP[CD]ØJ[CZ]
⊞ ØSP[CD][34]8Z
⊞ ØSP[CD]4J[CZ]

DRG Non-OR ØSP[CD]Ø8Z
DRG Non-OR ØSP[CD][34]8Z
Non-OR ØSP[9B]X[Ø345]Z
Non-OR ØSP[CD]3[Ø3]Z
Non-OR ØSP[CD]X[Ø345]Z

Coding Clinic: 2Ø15, Q2, P18 – ØSPCØJZ
Coding Clinic: 2Ø15, Q2, P2Ø – ØSP9ØJZ
Coding Clinic: 2Ø16, Q4, P112 – ØSPRØJZ
Coding Clinic: 2Ø18, Q2, P16 – ØSPWØJZ
Coding Clinic: 2Ø21, Q3, P26– ØSPDØJZ

SECTION: Ø MEDICAL AND SURGICAL
BODY SYSTEM: S LOWER JOINTS
OPERATION: P REMOVAL: *(continued)*
Taking out or off a device from a body part

Body Part	Approach	Device	Qualifier
F Ankle Joint, Right G Ankle Joint, Left H Tarsal Joint, Right J Tarsal Joint, Left K Tarsometatarsal Joint, Right L Tarsometatarsal Joint, Left M Metatarsal-Phalangeal Joint, Right N Metatarsal-Phalangeal Joint, Left P Toe Phalangeal Joint, Right Q Toe Phalangeal Joint, Left	Ø Open 3 Percutaneous 4 Percutaneous Endoscopic	Ø Drainage Device 3 Infusion Device 4 Internal Fixation Device 5 External Fixation Device 7 Autologous Tissue Substitute 8 Spacer J Synthetic Substitute K Nonautologous Tissue Substitute	Z No Qualifier
F Ankle Joint, Right G Ankle Joint, Left H Tarsal Joint, Right J Tarsal Joint, Left K Tarsometatarsal Joint, Right L Tarsometatarsal Joint, Left M Metatarsal-Phalangeal Joint, Right N Metatarsal-Phalangeal Joint, Left P Toe Phalangeal Joint, Right Q Toe Phalangeal Joint, Left	X External	Ø Drainage Device 3 Infusion Device 4 Internal Fixation Device 5 External Fixation Device	Z No Qualifier

Non-OR ØSP[FGHJKLMNPQ]3[Ø3]Z
Non-OR ØSP[FGHJKLMNPQ][Ø34]8Z
Non-OR ØSP[FGHJKLMNPQ]X[Ø345]Z

Coding Clinic: 2Ø13, Q2, P4Ø – ØSPGØ4Z
Coding Clinic: 2Ø16, Q4, P111 – ØSP
Coding Clinic: 2Ø21, Q1, P18; 2Ø17, Q4, P1Ø8 – ØSPFØJZ

SECTION: Ø MEDICAL AND SURGICAL
BODY SYSTEM: S LOWER JOINTS
OPERATION: Q REPAIR: Restoring, to the extent possible, a body part to its normal anatomic structure and function

Body Part	Approach	Device	Qualifier
Ø Lumbar Vertebral Joint 2 Lumbar Vertebral Disc 3 Lumbosacral Joint 4 Lumbosacral Disc 5 Sacrococcygeal Joint 6 Coccygeal Joint 7 Sacroiliac Joint, Right 8 Sacroiliac Joint, Left 9 Hip Joint, Right B Hip Joint, Left C Knee Joint, Right D Knee Joint, Left F Ankle Joint, Right G Ankle Joint, Left H Tarsal Joint, Right J Tarsal Joint, Left K Tarsometatarsal Joint, Right L Tarsometatarsal Joint, Left M Metatarsal-Phalangeal Joint, Right N Metatarsal-Phalangeal Joint, Left P Toe Phalangeal Joint, Right Q Toe Phalangeal Joint, Left	Ø Open 3 Percutaneous 4 Percutaneous Endoscopic X External	Z No Device	Z No Qualifier

DRG Non-OR ØSQ[Ø23456789BCDFGHJKLMNPQ]XZZ

SECTION: Ø MEDICAL AND SURGICAL
BODY SYSTEM: S LOWER JOINTS
OPERATION: R REPLACEMENT: *(on multiple pages)*

Putting in or on biological or synthetic material that physically takes the place and/or function of all or a portion of a body part

Body Part	Approach	Device	Qualifier
Ø Lumbar Vertebral Joint 2 Lumbar Vertebral Disc 3 Lumbosacral Joint 4 Lumbosacral Disc 5 Sacrococcygeal Joint 6 Coccygeal Joint 7 Sacroiliac Joint, Right 8 Sacroiliac Joint, Left H Tarsal Joint, Right J Tarsal Joint, Left K Tarsometatarsal Joint, Right L Tarsometatarsal Joint, Left M Metatarsal-Phalangeal Joint, Right N Metatarsal-Phalangeal Joint, Left P Toe Phalangeal Joint, Right Q Toe Phalangeal Joint, Left	Ø Open	7 Autologous Tissue Substitute J Synthetic Substitute K Nonautologous Tissue Substitute	Z No Qualifier
9 Hip Joint, Right B Hip Joint, Left	Ø Open	1 Synthetic Substitute, Metal 2 Synthetic Substitute, Metal on Polyethylene 3 Synthetic Substitute, Ceramic 4 Synthetic Substitute, Ceramic on Polyethylene 6 Synthetic Substitute, Oxidized Zirconium on Polyethylene J Synthetic Substitute	9 Cemented A Uncemented Z No Qualifier
9 Hip Joint, Right B Hip Joint, Left	Ø Open	7 Autologous Tissue Substitute E Articulating Spacer K Nonautologous Tissue Substitute	Z No Qualifier
A Hip Joint, Acetabular Surface, Right E Hip Joint, Acetabular Surface, Left	Ø Open	Ø Synthetic Substitute, Polyethylene 1 Synthetic Substitute, Metal 3 Synthetic Substitute, Ceramic J Synthetic Substitute	9 Cemented A Uncemented Z No Qualifier
A Hip Joint, Acetabular Surface, Right E Hip Joint, Acetabular Surface, Left	Ø Open	7 Autologous Tissue Substitute K Nonautologous Tissue Substitute	Z No Qualifier

ØSR[24]Ø[7JK]Z when the beneficiary is over age 6Ø

ØSR[24]ØJZ when beneficiary is over age 6Ø

ØSR[9B]Ø[1234J][9AZ]

ØSR[AE]Ø[Ø13J][9AZ]

ØSR[9B]Ø[1234J][9AZ] when reported with Secondary Diagnosis from I26.Ø2-I26.Ø9, I26.92-I26.99, or I82.4Ø1-I82.4Z9

ØSR[9B]Ø[7K]Z when reported with Secondary Diagnosis from I26.Ø2-I26.Ø9, I26.92-I26.99, or I82.4Ø1-I82.4Z9

ØSR[AE]Ø[Ø13J][9AZ] when reported with Secondary Diagnosis from I26.Ø2-I26.Ø9, I26.92-I26.99, or I82.4Ø1-I82.4Z9

ØSR[AE]Ø[7K]Z when reported with Secondary Diagnosis from I26.Ø2-I26.Ø9, I26.92-I26.99, or I82.4Ø1-I82.4Z9

Coding Clinic: 2Ø16, Q4, P1Ø9 – ØSR
Coding Clinic: 2Ø17, Q4, P39 – ØSRBØ6Z
Coding Clinic: 2Ø22, Q1, P39 – ØSRBØ2A

SECTION: Ø MEDICAL AND SURGICAL
BODY SYSTEM: S LOWER JOINTS
OPERATION: R REPLACEMENT: *(continued)*

Putting in or on biological or synthetic material that physically takes the place and/or function of all or a portion of a body part

Body Part	Approach	Device	Qualifier
C Knee Joint, Right D Knee Joint, Left	Ø Open	6 Synthetic Substitute, Oxidized Zirconium on Polyethylene J Synthetic Substitute L Synthetic Substitute, Unicondylar Medial M Synthetic Substitute, Unicondylar Lateral N Synthetic Substitute, Patellofemoral	9 Cemented A Uncemented Z No Qualifier
C Knee Joint, Right D Knee Joint, Left	Ø Open	7 Autologous Tissue Substitute E Articulating Spacer K Nonautologous Tissue Substitute	Z No Qualifier
F Ankle Joint, Right G Ankle Joint, Left T Knee Joint, Femoral Surface, Right U Knee Joint, Femoral Surface, Left V Knee Joint, Tibial Surface, Right W Knee Joint, Tibial Surface, Left	Ø Open	7 Autologous Tissue Substitute K Nonautologous Tissue Substitute	Z No Qualifier
F Ankle Joint, Right G Ankle Joint, Left T Knee Joint, Femoral Surface, Right U Knee Joint, Femoral Surface, Left V Knee Joint, Tibial Surface, Right W Knee Joint, Tibial Surface, Left	Ø Open	J Synthetic Substitute	9 Cemented A Uncemented Z No Qualifier
R Hip Joint, Femoral Surface, Right S Hip Joint, Femoral Surface, Left	Ø Open	1 Synthetic Substitute, Metal 3 Synthetic Substitute, Ceramic J Synthetic Substitute	9 Cemented A Uncemented Z No Qualifier
R Hip Joint, Femoral Surface, Right S Hip Joint, Femoral Surface, Left	Ø Open	7 Autologous Tissue Substitute K Nonautologous Tissue Substitute	Z No Qualifier

- ØSR[CDTUVW]ØJ[9AZ]
- ØSR[CD]ØL[9AZ]
- ØSR[RS]Ø[13J][9AZ]
- ØSR[CD]Ø[7K]Z when reported with Secondary Diagnosis from I26.Ø2-I26.Ø9, I26.92-I26.99, or I82.4Ø1-I82.4Z9
- ØSR[CD]ØL[9AZ] when reported with Secondary Diagnosis from I26.Ø2-I26.Ø9, I26.92-I26.99, or I82.4Ø1-I82.4Z9
- ØSR[TUVW]Ø[7K]Z when reported with Secondary Diagnosis from I26.Ø2-I26.Ø9, I26.92-I26.99, or I82.4Ø1-I82.4Z9
- ØSR[CD]ØJ[9AZ] when reported with Secondary Diagnosis from I26.Ø2-I26.Ø9, I26.92-I26.99, or I82.4Ø1-I82.4Z9
- ØSR[TUVW]ØJ[9AZ] when reported with Secondary Diagnosis from I26.Ø2-I26.Ø9, I26.92-I26.99, or I82.4Ø1-I82.4Z9
- ØSR[RS]Ø[13J][9AZ] when reported with Secondary Diagnosis from I26.Ø2-I26.Ø9, I26.92-I26.99, or I82.4Ø1-I82.4Z9
- ØSR[RS]Ø[7K]Z when reported with Secondary Diagnosis from I26.Ø2-I26.Ø9, I26.92-I26.99, or I82.4Ø1-I82.4Z9

Coding Clinic: 2015, Q2, P18 – ØSRCØJ9
Coding Clinic: 2015, Q2, P20 – ØSRRØ3A
Coding Clinic: 2015, Q3, P19 – ØSRBØJ9
Coding Clinic: 2016, Q4, P110 – ØSRDØ[JL]Z
Coding Clinic: 2016, Q4, P111 – ØSRRØJ9
Coding Clinic: 2017, Q4, P108 – ØSRFØJA
Coding Clinic: 2018, Q2, P16 – ØSRWØJZ
Coding Clinic: 2021, Q3, P26 – ØSRDØJ9

SECTION: Ø MEDICAL AND SURGICAL
BODY SYSTEM: S LOWER JOINTS
OPERATION: S REPOSITION: Moving to its normal location, or other suitable location, all or a portion of a body part

Body Part	Approach	Device	Qualifier
Ø Lumbar Vertebral Joint 3 Lumbosacral Joint 5 Sacrococcygeal Joint 6 Coccygeal Joint 7 Sacroiliac Joint, Right 8 Sacroiliac Joint, Left	Ø Open 3 Percutaneous 4 Percutaneous Endoscopic X External	4 Internal Fixation Device Z No Device	Z No Qualifier
9 Hip Joint, Right B Hip Joint, Left C Knee Joint, Right D Knee Joint, Left F Ankle Joint, Right G Ankle Joint, Left H Tarsal Joint, Right J Tarsal Joint, Left K Tarsometatarsal Joint, Right L Tarsometatarsal Joint, Left M Metatarsal-Phalangeal Joint, Right N Metatarsal-Phalangeal Joint, Left P Toe Phalangeal Joint, Right Q Toe Phalangeal Joint, Left	Ø Open 3 Percutaneous 4 Percutaneous Endoscopic X External	4 Internal Fixation Device 5 External Fixation Device Z No Device	Z No Qualifier

Non-OR ØSS[Ø35678][34X][4Z]Z
Non-OR ØSS[9BCDFGHJKLMNPQ][34X][45Z]Z

Coding Clinic: 2016, Q2, P32 – ØSSBØ4Z
Coding Clinic: 2022, Q2, P22 – ØSSG35Z
Coding Clinic: 2022, Q3, P27 – ØSS[GJ]35Z

SECTION: Ø MEDICAL AND SURGICAL
BODY SYSTEM: S LOWER JOINTS
OPERATION: T RESECTION: Cutting out or off, without replacement, all of a body part

Body Part	Approach	Device	Qualifier
2 Lumbar Vertebral Disc 4 Lumbosacral Disc 5 Sacrococcygeal Joint 6 Coccygeal Joint 7 Sacroiliac Joint, Right 8 Sacroiliac Joint, Left 9 Hip Joint, Right B Hip Joint, Left C Knee Joint, Right D Knee Joint, Left F Ankle Joint, Right G Ankle Joint, Left H Tarsal Joint, Right J Tarsal Joint, Left K Tarsometatarsal Joint, Right L Tarsometatarsal Joint, Left M Metatarsal-Phalangeal Joint, Right N Metatarsal-Phalangeal Joint, Left P Toe Phalangeal Joint, Right Q Toe Phalangeal Joint, Left	Ø Open	Z No Device	Z No Qualifier

Coding Clinic: 2016, Q1, P20 – ØSTMØZZ

SECTION: Ø MEDICAL AND SURGICAL
BODY SYSTEM: S LOWER JOINTS
OPERATION: U SUPPLEMENT: Putting in or on biological or synthetic material that physically reinforces and/or augments the function of a portion of a body part

Body Part	Approach	Device	Qualifier
Ø Lumbar Vertebral Joint 2 Lumbar Vertebral Disc 3 Lumbosacral Joint 4 Lumbosacral Disc 5 Sacrococcygeal Joint 6 Coccygeal Joint 7 Sacroiliac Joint, Right 8 Sacroiliac Joint, Left F Ankle Joint, Right G Ankle Joint, Left H Tarsal Joint, Right J Tarsal Joint, Left K Tarsometatarsal Joint, Right L Tarsometatarsal Joint, Left M Metatarsal-Phalangeal Joint, Right N Metatarsal-Phalangeal Joint, Left P Toe Phalangeal Joint, Right Q Toe Phalangeal Joint, Left	Ø Open 3 Percutaneous 4 Percutaneous Endoscopic	7 Autologous Tissue Substitute J Synthetic Substitute K Nonautologous Tissue Substitute	Z No Qualifier
9 Hip Joint, Right ⊞ B Hip Joint, Left ⊞	Ø Open	7 Autologous Tissue Substitute 9 Liner B Resurfacing Device J Synthetic Substitute K Nonautologous Tissue Substitute	Z No Qualifier
9 Hip Joint, Right B Hip Joint, Left	3 Percutaneous 4 Percutaneous Endoscopic	7 Autologous Tissue Substitute J Synthetic Substitute K Nonautologous Tissue Substitute	Z No Qualifier
A Hip Joint, Acetabular Surface, Right ⊞ E Hip Joint, Acetabular Surface, Left ⊞ R Hip Joint, Femoral Surface, Right ⊞ S Hip Joint, Femoral Surface, Left ⊞	Ø Open	9 Liner B Resurfacing Device	Z No Qualifier
C Knee Joint, Right D Knee Joint, Left	Ø Open	7 Autologous Tissue Substitute J Synthetic Substitute K Nonautologous Tissue Substitute	Z No Qualifier
C Knee Joint, Right D Knee Joint, Left	Ø Open	9 Liner	C Patellar Surface Z No Qualifier
C Knee Joint, Right D Knee Joint, Left	3 Percutaneous 4 Percutaneous Endoscopic	7 Autologous Tissue Substitute J Synthetic Substitute K Nonautologous Tissue Substitute	Z No Qualifier
T Knee Joint, Femoral Surface, Right U Knee Joint, Femoral Surface, Left V Knee Joint, Tibial Surface, Right ⊞ W Knee Joint, Tibial Surface, Left ⊞	Ø Open	9 Liner	Z No Qualifier

⊞ ØSU[9B]Ø9Z
⊞ ØSU[AERS]Ø9Z
⊞ ØSU[VW]Ø9Z

ØSU[9B]ØBZ when reported with Secondary Diagnosis from I26.Ø2-I26.Ø9, I26.92-I26.99, or I82.4Ø1-I82.4Z9

ØSU[AERS]ØBZ when reported with Secondary Diagnosis from I26.Ø2-I26.Ø9, I26.92-I26.99, or I82.4Ø1-I82.4Z9

Coding Clinic: 2Ø15, Q2, P2Ø – ØSUAØ9Z
Coding Clinic: 2Ø16, Q4, P112 – ØSUAØ9Z
Coding Clinic: 2Ø21, Q1, P18 – ØSUFØJZ
Coding Clinic: 2Ø22, Q1, P47 – ØSUCØ7Z

New/Revised Text in Green ~~deleted~~ Deleted ♀ Females Only ♂ Males Only **Coding Clinic**
Non-covered Limited Coverage ⊞ Combination (See Appendix E) DRG Non-OR Non-OR Hospital-Acquired Condition

SECTION: Ø MEDICAL AND SURGICAL
BODY SYSTEM: S LOWER JOINTS
OPERATION: W REVISION: *(on multiple pages)*

Correcting, to the extent possible, a portion of a malfunctioning device or the position of a displaced device

Body Part	Approach	Device	Qualifier
Ø Lumbar Vertebral Joint 3 Lumbosacral Joint	Ø Open 3 Percutaneous 4 Percutaneous Endoscopic X External	Ø Drainage Device 3 Infusion Device 4 Internal Fixation Device 7 Autologous Tissue Substitute 8 Spacer A Interbody Fusion Device J Synthetic Substitute K Nonautologous Tissue Substitute	Z No Qualifier
2 Lumbar Vertebral Disc 4 Lumbosacral Disc	Ø Open 3 Percutaneous 4 Percutaneous Endoscopic X External	Ø Drainage Device 3 Infusion Device 7 Autologous Tissue Substitute J Synthetic Substitute K Nonautologous Tissue Substitute	Z No Qualifier
5 Sacrococcygeal Joint 6 Coccygeal Joint 7 Sacroiliac Joint, Right 8 Sacroiliac Joint, Left	Ø Open 3 Percutaneous 4 Percutaneous Endoscopic X External	Ø Drainage Device 3 Infusion Device 4 Internal Fixation Device 7 Autologous Tissue Substitute 8 Spacer J Synthetic Substitute K Nonautologous Tissue Substitute	Z No Qualifier
9 Hip Joint, Right B Hip Joint, Left	Ø Open	Ø Drainage Device 3 Infusion Device 4 Internal Fixation Device 5 External Fixation Device 7 Autologous Tissue Substitute 8 Spacer 9 Liner B Resurfacing Device J Synthetic Substitute K Nonautologous Tissue Substitute	Z No Qualifier
9 Hip Joint, Right B Hip Joint, Left	3 Percutaneous 4 Percutaneous Endoscopic X External	Ø Drainage Device 3 Infusion Device 4 Internal Fixation Device 5 External Fixation Device 7 Autologous Tissue Substitute 8 Spacer J Synthetic Substitute K Nonautologous Tissue Substitute	Z No Qualifier

Non-OR ØSW[Ø3]X[Ø3478AJK]Z
Non-OR ØSW[24]X[Ø37JK]Z
Non-OR ØSW[5678]X[Ø3478JK]Z
Non-OR ØSW[9B]X[Ø34578JK]Z

Coding Clinic: 2Ø16, Q4, P111 – ØSW

Ø: M/S S: LOWER JOINTS W: REVISION

SECTION: Ø MEDICAL AND SURGICAL
BODY SYSTEM: S LOWER JOINTS
OPERATION: W REVISION: *(continued)*

Correcting, to the extent possible, a portion of a malfunctioning device or the position of a displaced device

Body Part	Approach	Device	Qualifier
A Hip Joint, Acetabular Surface, Right E Hip Joint, Acetabular Surface, Left R Hip Joint, Femoral Surface, Right S Hip Joint, Femoral Surface, Left T Knee Joint, Femoral Surface, Right U Knee Joint, Femoral Surface, Left V Knee Joint, Tibial Surface, Right W Knee Joint, Tibial Surface, Left	Ø Open 3 Percutaneous 4 Percutaneous Endoscopic X External	J Synthetic Substitute	Z No Qualifier
C Knee Joint, Right D Knee Joint, Left	Ø Open	Ø Drainage Device 3 Infusion Device 4 Internal Fixation Device 5 External Fixation Device 7 Autologous Tissue Substitute 8 Spacer 9 Liner K Nonautologous Tissue Substitute	Z No Qualifier
C Knee Joint, Right D Knee Joint, Left	Ø Open	J Synthetic Substitute	C Patellar Surface Z No Qualifier
C Knee Joint, Right D Knee Joint, Left	3 Percutaneous 4 Percutaneous Endoscopic X External	Ø Drainage Device 3 Infusion Device 4 Internal Fixation Device 5 External Fixation Device 7 Autologous Tissue Substitute 8 Spacer K Nonautologous Tissue Substitute	Z No Qualifier
C Knee Joint, Right D Knee Joint, Left	3 Percutaneous 4 Percutaneous Endoscopic X External	J Synthetic Substitute	C Patellar Surface Z No Qualifier
F Ankle Joint, Right G Ankle Joint, Left H Tarsal Joint, Right J Tarsal Joint, Left K Tarsometatarsal Joint, Right L Tarsometatarsal Joint, Left M Metatarsal-Phalangeal Joint, Right N Metatarsal-Phalangeal Joint, Left P Toe Phalangeal Joint, Right Q Toe Phalangeal Joint, Left	Ø Open 3 Percutaneous 4 Percutaneous Endoscopic X External	Ø Drainage Device 3 Infusion Device 4 Internal Fixation Device 5 External Fixation Device 7 Autologous Tissue Substitute 8 Spacer J Synthetic Substitute K Nonautologous Tissue Substitute	Z No Qualifier

Non-OR ØSW[AERSTUVW]XJZ
Non-OR ØSW[CD]X[Ø34578K]Z
Non-OR ØSW[CD]XJZ
Non-OR ØSW[FGHJKLMNPQ]X[Ø34578JK]Z

Coding Clinic: 2Ø16, Q4, P112 – ØSWWØJZ
Coding Clinic: 2Ø17, Q4, P1Ø7 – ØSWFØJZ

SECTION: Ø MEDICAL AND SURGICAL
BODY SYSTEM: T URINARY SYSTEM
OPERATION: 1 BYPASS: Altering the route of passage of the contents of a tubular body part

Body Part	Approach	Device	Qualifier
3 Kidney Pelvis, Right 4 Kidney Pelvis, Left	Ø Open 4 Percutaneous Endoscopic	7 Autologous Tissue Substitute J Synthetic Substitute K Nonautologous Tissue Substitute Z No Device	3 Kidney Pelvis, Right 4 Kidney Pelvis, Left 6 Ureter, Right 7 Ureter, Left 8 Colon 9 Colocutaneous A Ileum B Bladder C Ileocutaneous D Cutaneous
3 Kidney Pelvis, Right 4 Kidney Pelvis, Left	3 Percutaneous	J Synthetic Substitute	D Cutaneous
6 Ureter, Right 7 Ureter, Left 8 Ureters, Bilateral	Ø Open 4 Percutaneous Endoscopic	7 Autologous Tissue Substitute J Synthetic Substitute K Nonautologous Tissue Substitute Z No Device	6 Ureter, Right 7 Ureter, Left 8 Colon 9 Colocutaneous A Ileum B Bladder C Ileocutaneous D Cutaneous
6 Ureter, Right 7 Ureter, Left 8 Ureters, Bilateral	3 Percutaneous	J Synthetic Substitute	D Cutaneous
B Bladder	Ø Open 4 Percutaneous Endoscopic	7 Autologous Tissue Substitute J Synthetic Substitute K Nonautologous Tissue Substitute Z No Device	9 Colocutaneous C Ileocutaneous D Cutaneous
B Bladder	3 Percutaneous	J Synthetic Substitute	D Cutaneous

Coding Clinic: 2Ø15, Q3, P35 – ØT17ØZB
Coding Clinic: 2Ø17, Q3, P21-22 – ØT1[8B]ØZ[9C]

SECTION: Ø MEDICAL AND SURGICAL
BODY SYSTEM: T URINARY SYSTEM
OPERATION: 2 CHANGE: Taking out or off a device from a body part and putting back an identical or similar device in or on the same body part without cutting or puncturing the skin or a mucous membrane

Body Part	Approach	Device	Qualifier
5 Kidney 9 Ureter B Bladder D Urethra	X External	Ø Drainage Device Y Other Device	Z No Qualifier

Non-OR All Values

SECTION: Ø MEDICAL AND SURGICAL
BODY SYSTEM: T URINARY SYSTEM
OPERATION: 5 DESTRUCTION: Physical eradication of all or a portion of a body part by the direct use of energy, force, or a destructive agent

Body Part	Approach	Device	Qualifier
Ø Kidney, Right 1 Kidney, Left 3 Kidney Pelvis, Right 4 Kidney Pelvis, Left 6 Ureter, Right 7 Ureter, Left B Bladder C Bladder Neck	Ø Open 3 Percutaneous 4 Percutaneous Endoscopic 7 Via Natural or Artificial Opening 8 Via Natural or Artificial Opening Endoscopic	Z No Device	Z No Qualifier
D Urethra	Ø Open 3 Percutaneous 4 Percutaneous Endoscopic 7 Via Natural or Artificial Opening 8 Via Natural or Artificial Opening Endoscopic X External	Z No Device	Z No Qualifier

Non-OR ØT5D[Ø3478X]ZZ

SECTION: Ø MEDICAL AND SURGICAL
BODY SYSTEM: T URINARY SYSTEM
OPERATION: 7 DILATION: Expanding an orifice or the lumen of a tubular body part

Body Part	Approach	Device	Qualifier
3 Kidney Pelvis, Right 4 Kidney Pelvis, Left 6 Ureter, Right 7 Ureter, Left 8 Ureters, Bilateral B Bladder C Bladder Neck D Urethra	Ø Open 3 Percutaneous 4 Percutaneous Endoscopic 7 Via Natural or Artificial Opening 8 Via Natural or Artificial Opening Endoscopic	D Intraluminal Device Z No Device	Z No Qualifier

Non-OR ØT7[67][Ø3478]DZ
Non-OR ØT7[8D][Ø34]DZ
Non-OR ØT7[8D][78][DZ]Z
Non-OR ØT7C[Ø3478][DZ]Z

Coding Clinic: 2Ø16, Q2, P28 – ØT767DZ

SECTION: Ø MEDICAL AND SURGICAL
BODY SYSTEM: T URINARY SYSTEM
OPERATION: 8 DIVISION: Cutting into a body part, without draining fluids and/or gases from the body part, in order to separate or transect a body part

Body Part	Approach	Device	Qualifier
2 Kidneys, Bilateral C Bladder Neck	Ø Open 3 Percutaneous 4 Percutaneous Endoscopic	Z No Device	Z No Qualifier

SECTION: Ø MEDICAL AND SURGICAL
BODY SYSTEM: T URINARY SYSTEM
OPERATION: 9 DRAINAGE: Taking or letting out fluids and/or gases from a body part

Body Part	Approach	Device	Qualifier
Ø Kidney, Right 1 Kidney, Left 3 Kidney Pelvis, Right 4 Kidney Pelvis, Left 6 Ureter, Right 7 Ureter, Left 8 Ureters, Bilateral B Bladder C Bladder Neck	Ø Open 3 Percutaneous 4 Percutaneous Endoscopic 7 Via Natural or Artificial Opening 8 Via Natural or Artificial Opening Endoscopic	Ø Drainage Device	Z No Qualifier
Ø Kidney, Right 1 Kidney, Left 3 Kidney Pelvis, Right 4 Kidney Pelvis, Left 6 Ureter, Right 7 Ureter, Left 8 Ureters, Bilateral B Bladder C Bladder Neck	Ø Open 3 Percutaneous 4 Percutaneous Endoscopic 7 Via Natural or Artificial Opening 8 Via Natural or Artificial Opening Endoscopic	Z No Device	X Diagnostic Z No Qualifier
D Urethra	Ø Open 3 Percutaneous 4 Percutaneous Endoscopic 7 Via Natural or Artificial Opening 8 Via Natural or Artificial Opening Endoscopic X External	Ø Drainage Device	Z No Qualifier
D Urethra	Ø Open 3 Percutaneous 4 Percutaneous Endoscopic 7 Via Natural or Artificial Opening 8 Via Natural or Artificial Opening Endoscopic X External	Z No Device	X Diagnostic Z No Qualifier

DRG Non-OR ØT9[34]3ØZ
Non-OR ØT9[678][Ø3478]ØZ
Non-OR ØT9[678]3ZZ
Non-OR ØT9[BC][3478]ØZ
Non-OR ØT9[Ø134678][3478]ZX
Non-OR ØT9[Ø134][34]ZZ
Non-OR ØT9[BC][3478]ZZ
Non-OR ØT9D[Ø3478X]ZX
Non-OR ØT9D3ØZ
Non-OR ØT9D3ZZ

Coding Clinic: 2017, Q3, P2Ø – ØT968ØZ

SECTION: Ø MEDICAL AND SURGICAL
BODY SYSTEM: T URINARY SYSTEM
OPERATION: B EXCISION: Cutting out or off, without replacement, a portion of a body part

Body Part	Approach	Device	Qualifier
Ø Kidney, Right 1 Kidney, Left 3 Kidney Pelvis, Right 4 Kidney Pelvis, Left 6 Ureter, Right 7 Ureter, Left B Bladder C Bladder Neck	Ø Open 3 Percutaneous 4 Percutaneous Endoscopic 7 Via Natural or Artificial Opening 8 Via Natural or Artificial Opening Endoscopic	Z No Device	X Diagnostic Z No Qualifier
D Urethra	Ø Open 3 Percutaneous 4 Percutaneous Endoscopic 7 Via Natural or Artificial Opening 8 Via Natural or Artificial Opening Endoscopic X External	Z No Device	X Diagnostic Z No Qualifier

Non-OR ØTB[Ø13467][3478]ZX
Non-OR ØTBD[Ø3478X]ZX

Coding Clinic: 2Ø15, Q3, P34 – ØTBD8ZZ
Coding Clinic: 2Ø16, Q1, P19 – ØTBB8ZX

SECTION: Ø MEDICAL AND SURGICAL
BODY SYSTEM: T URINARY SYSTEM
OPERATION: C EXTIRPATION: Taking or cutting out solid matter from a body part

Body Part	Approach	Device	Qualifier
Ø Kidney, Right 1 Kidney, Left 3 Kidney Pelvis, Right 4 Kidney Pelvis, Left 6 Ureter, Right 7 Ureter, Left B Bladder C Bladder Neck	Ø Open 3 Percutaneous 4 Percutaneous Endoscopic 7 Via Natural or Artificial Opening 8 Via Natural or Artificial Opening Endoscopic	Z No Device	Z No Qualifier
D Urethra	Ø Open 3 Percutaneous 4 Percutaneous Endoscopic 7 Via Natural or Artificial Opening 8 Via Natural or Artificial Opening Endoscopic X External	Z No Device	Z No Qualifier

Non-OR ØTC[BC][78]ZZ
Non-OR ØTCD[78X]ZZ

Coding Clinic: 2Ø15, Q2, P8 – ØTC48ZZ
Coding Clinic: 2Ø15, Q2, P9 – ØTC18ZZ, ØTC78ZZ, ØTCB8ZZ, ØTC78DZ
Coding Clinic: 2Ø19, Q3, P4; 2Ø16, Q3, P24 – ØTCB8ZZ

SECTION: Ø MEDICAL AND SURGICAL
BODY SYSTEM: T URINARY SYSTEM
OPERATION: D EXTRACTION: Pulling or stripping out or off all or a portion of a body part by the use of force

Body Part	Approach	Device	Qualifier
Ø Kidney, Right 1 Kidney, Left	Ø Open 3 Percutaneous 4 Percutaneous Endoscopic	Z No Device	Z No Qualifier

SECTION: Ø MEDICAL AND SURGICAL
BODY SYSTEM: T URINARY SYSTEM
OPERATION: F FRAGMENTATION: Breaking solid matter in a body part into pieces

Body Part	Approach	Device	Qualifier
3 Kidney Pelvis, Right 4 Kidney Pelvis, Left 6 Ureter, Right 7 Ureter, Left B Bladder C Bladder Neck D Urethra	Ø Open 3 Percutaneous 4 Percutaneous Endoscopic 7 Via Natural or Artificial Opening 8 Via Natural or Artificial Opening Endoscopic X External	Z No Device	Z No Qualifier

ØTFDXZZ
Non-OR ØTF[34][Ø78]ZZ
Non-OR ØTF[67BC][Ø3478]ZZ
Non-OR ØTFD[Ø3478X]ZZ

SECTION: Ø MEDICAL AND SURGICAL
BODY SYSTEM: T URINARY SYSTEM
OPERATION: H INSERTION: Putting in a nonbiological appliance that monitors, assists, performs, or prevents a physiological function but does not physically take the place of a body part

Body Part	Approach	Device	Qualifier
5 Kidney	Ø Open 3 Percutaneous 4 Percutaneous Endoscopic 7 Via Natural or Artificial Opening 8 Via Natural or Artificial Opening Endoscopic	1 Radioactive Element 2 Monitoring Device 3 Infusion Device Y Other Device	Z No Qualifier
9 Ureter	Ø Open 3 Percutaneous 4 Percutaneous Endoscopic 7 Via Natural or Artificial Opening 8 Via Natural or Artificial Opening Endoscopic	1 Radioactive Element 2 Monitoring Device 3 Infusion Device M Stimulator Lead Y Other Device	Z No Qualifier
B Bladder	Ø Open 3 Percutaneous 4 Percutaneous Endoscopic 7 Via Natural or Artificial Opening 8 Via Natural or Artificial Opening Endoscopic	1 Radioactive Element 2 Monitoring Device 3 Infusion Device L Artificial Sphincter M Stimulator Lead Y Other Device	Z No Qualifier
C Bladder Neck	Ø Open 3 Percutaneous 4 Percutaneous Endoscopic 7 Via Natural or Artificial Opening 8 Via Natural or Artificial Opening Endoscopic	L Artificial Sphincter	Z No Qualifier
D Urethra	Ø Open 3 Percutaneous 4 Percutaneous Endoscopic 7 Via Natural or Artificial Opening 8 Via Natural or Artificial Opening Endoscopic	1 Radioactive Element 2 Monitoring Device 3 Infusion Device L Artificial Sphincter Y Other Device	Z No Qualifier
D Urethra	X External	2 Monitoring Device 3 Infusion Device L Artificial Sphincter	Z No Qualifier

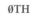

ØTHB[Ø3478]MZ
Non-OR ØTH5[Ø3478]3Z
Non-OR ØTH5[78]2Z
Non-OR ØTH9[Ø3478]3Z
Non-OR ØTH9[78]2Z
Non-OR ØTHB[Ø3478]3Z
Non-OR ØTHB[78]2Z
Non-OR ØTHD[Ø3478]3Z
Non-OR ØTHD[78]2Z
Non-OR ØTHDX3Z

SECTION: Ø MEDICAL AND SURGICAL
BODY SYSTEM: T URINARY SYSTEM
OPERATION: J INSPECTION: Visually and/or manually exploring a body part

Body Part	Approach	Device	Qualifier
5 Kidney 9 Ureter B Bladder D Urethra	Ø Open 3 Percutaneous 4 Percutaneous Endoscopic 7 Via Natural or Artificial Opening 8 Via Natural or Artificial Opening Endoscopic X External	Z No Device	Z No Qualifier

DRG Non-OR ØTJ[5B][37]ZZ
Non-OR ØTJ9[37]ZZ
Non-OR ØTJ[59][48X]ZZ
Non-OR ØTJB[8X]ZZ
Non-OR ØTJD[3478X]ZZ

SECTION: Ø MEDICAL AND SURGICAL
BODY SYSTEM: T URINARY SYSTEM
OPERATION: L OCCLUSION: Completely closing an orifice or the lumen of a tubular body part

Body Part	Approach	Device	Qualifier
3 Kidney Pelvis, Right 4 Kidney Pelvis, Left 6 Ureter, Right 7 Ureter, Left B Bladder C Bladder Neck	Ø Open 3 Percutaneous 4 Percutaneous Endoscopic	C Extraluminal Device D Intraluminal Device Z No Device	Z No Qualifier
3 Kidney Pelvis, Right 4 Kidney Pelvis, Left 6 Ureter, Right 7 Ureter, Left B Bladder C Bladder Neck	7 Via Natural or Artificial Opening 8 Via Natural or Artificial Opening Endoscopic	D Intraluminal Device Z No Device	Z No Qualifier
D Urethra	Ø Open 3 Percutaneous 4 Percutaneous Endoscopic X External	C Extraluminal Device D Intraluminal Device Z No Device	Z No Qualifier
D Urethra	7 Via Natural or Artificial Opening 8 Via Natural or Artificial Opening Endoscopic	D Intraluminal Device Z No Device	Z No Qualifier

SECTION: Ø MEDICAL AND SURGICAL
BODY SYSTEM: T URINARY SYSTEM
OPERATION: M REATTACHMENT: Putting back in or on all or a portion of a separated body part to its normal location or other suitable location

Body Part	Approach	Device	Qualifier
Ø Kidney, Right 1 Kidney, Left 2 Kidneys, Bilateral 3 Kidney Pelvis, Right 4 Kidney Pelvis, Left 6 Ureter, Right 7 Ureter, Left 8 Ureters, Bilateral B Bladder C Bladder Neck D Urethra	Ø Open 4 Percutaneous Endoscopic	Z No Device	Z No Qualifier

SECTION: Ø MEDICAL AND SURGICAL
BODY SYSTEM: T URINARY SYSTEM
OPERATION: N RELEASE: Freeing a body part from an abnormal physical constraint by cutting or by the use of force

Body Part	Approach	Device	Qualifier
Ø Kidney, Right 1 Kidney, Left 3 Kidney Pelvis, Right 4 Kidney Pelvis, Left 6 Ureter, Right 7 Ureter, Left B Bladder C Bladder Neck	Ø Open 3 Percutaneous 4 Percutaneous Endoscopic 7 Via Natural or Artificial Opening 8 Via Natural or Artificial Opening Endoscopic	Z No Device	Z No Qualifier
D Urethra	Ø Open 3 Percutaneous 4 Percutaneous Endoscopic 7 Via Natural or Artificial Opening 8 Via Natural or Artificial Opening Endoscopic X External	Z No Device	Z No Qualifier

SECTION: Ø MEDICAL AND SURGICAL
BODY SYSTEM: T URINARY SYSTEM
OPERATION: P REMOVAL: *(on multiple pages)*
Taking out or off a device from a body part

Body Part	Approach	Device	Qualifier
5 Kidney	Ø Open 3 Percutaneous 4 Percutaneous Endoscopic 7 Via Natural or Artificial Opening 8 Via Natural or Artificial Opening Endoscopic	Ø Drainage Device 2 Monitoring Device 3 Infusion Device 7 Autologous Tissue Substitute C Extraluminal Device D Intraluminal Device J Synthetic Substitute K Nonautologous Tissue Substitute Y Other Device	Z No Qualifier
5 Kidney	X External	Ø Drainage Device 2 Monitoring Device 3 Infusion Device D Intraluminal Device	Z No Qualifier
9 Ureter	Ø Open 3 Percutaneous 4 Percutaneous Endoscopic 7 Via Natural or Artificial Opening 8 Via Natural or Artificial Opening Endoscopic	Ø Drainage Device 2 Monitoring Device 3 Infusion Device 7 Autologous Tissue Substitute C Extraluminal Device D Intraluminal Device J Synthetic Substitute K Nonautologous Tissue Substitute M Stimulator Lead Y Other Device	Z No Qualifier
9 Ureter	X External	Ø Drainage Device 2 Monitoring Device 3 Infusion Device D Intraluminal Device M Stimulator Lead	Z No Qualifier
B Bladder	Ø Open 3 Percutaneous 4 Percutaneous Endoscopic 7 Via Natural or Artificial Opening 8 Via Natural or Artificial Opening Endoscopic	Ø Drainage Device 2 Monitoring Device 3 Infusion Device 7 Autologous Tissue Substitute C Extraluminal Device D Intraluminal Device J Synthetic Substitute K Nonautologous Tissue Substitute L Artificial Sphincter M Stimulator Lead Y Other Device	Z No Qualifier
B Bladder	X External	Ø Drainage Device 2 Monitoring Device 3 Infusion Device D Intraluminal Device L Artificial Sphincter M Stimulator Lead	Z No Qualifier

ØTPB[Ø3478]MZ
Non-OR ØTP5[78][Ø23D]Z
Non-OR ØTP5X[Ø23D]Z
Non-OR ØTP9[78][Ø23D]Z
Non-OR ØTP9X[Ø23D]Z
Non-OR ØTPB[78][Ø23D]Z
Non-OR ØTPBX[Ø23DL]Z

Coding Clinic: 2016, Q2, P28 – Ø2P98DZ

SECTION: Ø MEDICAL AND SURGICAL
BODY SYSTEM: T URINARY SYSTEM
OPERATION: P REMOVAL: *(continued)*
Taking out or off a device from a body part

Body Part	Approach	Device	Qualifier
D Urethra	Ø Open 3 Percutaneous 4 Percutaneous Endoscopic 7 Via Natural or Artificial Opening 8 Via Natural or Artificial Opening Endoscopic	Ø Drainage Device 2 Monitoring Device 3 Infusion Device 7 Autologous Tissue Substitute C Extraluminal Device D Intraluminal Device J Synthetic Substitute K Nonautologous Tissue Substitute L Artificial Sphincter Y Other Device	Z No Qualifier
D Urethra	X External	Ø Drainage Device 2 Monitoring Device 3 Infusion Device D Intraluminal Device L Artificial Sphincter	Z No Qualifier

Non-OR ØTPD[78][Ø23D]Z
Non-OR ØTPDX[Ø23D]Z

SECTION: Ø MEDICAL AND SURGICAL
BODY SYSTEM: T URINARY SYSTEM
OPERATION: Q REPAIR: Restoring, to the extent possible, a body part to its normal anatomic structure and function

Body Part	Approach	Device	Qualifier
Ø Kidney, Right 1 Kidney, Left 3 Kidney Pelvis, Right 4 Kidney Pelvis, Left 6 Ureter, Right 7 Ureter, Left B Bladder ⊞ C Bladder Neck	Ø Open 3 Percutaneous 4 Percutaneous Endoscopic 7 Via Natural or Artificial Opening 8 Via Natural or Artificial Opening Endoscopic	Z No Device	Z No Qualifier
D Urethra	Ø Open 3 Percutaneous 4 Percutaneous Endoscopic 7 Via Natural or Artificial Opening 8 Via Natural or Artificial Opening Endoscopic X External	Z No Device	Z No Qualifier

Non-OR ØTQB[Ø34]ZZ

Coding Clinic: 2Ø17, Q1, P38 – ØTQDØZZ

SECTION: Ø MEDICAL AND SURGICAL
BODY SYSTEM: T URINARY SYSTEM
OPERATION: R REPLACEMENT: Putting in or on biological or synthetic material that physically takes the place and/or function of all or a portion of a body part

Body Part	Approach	Device	Qualifier
3 Kidney Pelvis, Right 4 Kidney Pelvis, Left 6 Ureter, Right 7 Ureter, Left B Bladder C Bladder Neck	Ø Open 4 Percutaneous Endoscopic 7 Via Natural or Artificial Opening 8 Via Natural or Artificial Opening Endoscopic	7 Autologous Tissue Substitute J Synthetic Substitute K Nonautologous Tissue Substitute	Z No Qualifier
D Urethra	Ø Open 4 Percutaneous Endoscopic 7 Via Natural or Artificial Opening 8 Via Natural or Artificial Opening Endoscopic X External	7 Autologous Tissue Substitute J Synthetic Substitute K Nonautologous Tissue Substitute	Z No Qualifier

Coding Clinic: 2Ø17, Q3, P2Ø – ØTRBØ7Z

SECTION: Ø MEDICAL AND SURGICAL
BODY SYSTEM: T URINARY SYSTEM
OPERATION: S REPOSITION: Moving to its normal location, or other suitable location, all or a portion of a body part

Body Part	Approach	Device	Qualifier
Ø Kidney, Right 1 Kidney, Left 2 Kidneys, Bilateral 3 Kidney Pelvis, Right 4 Kidney Pelvis, Left 6 Ureter, Right 7 Ureter, Left 8 Ureters, Bilateral B Bladder C Bladder Neck D Urethra	Ø Open 4 Percutaneous Endoscopic	Z No Device	Z No Qualifier

Coding Clinic: 2Ø16, Q1, P15 – ØTSDØZZ
Coding Clinic: 2Ø19, Q1, P3Ø; 2Ø17, Q1, P37 – ØTS6ØZZ

SECTION: Ø MEDICAL AND SURGICAL
BODY SYSTEM: T URINARY SYSTEM
OPERATION: T RESECTION: Cutting out or off, without replacement, all of a body part

Body Part	Approach	Device	Qualifier
Ø Kidney, Right 1 Kidney, Left 2 Kidneys, Bilateral	Ø Open 4 Percutaneous Endoscopic	Z No Device	Z No Qualifier
3 Kidney Pelvis, Right 4 Kidney Pelvis, Left 6 Ureter, Right 7 Ureter, Left B Bladder ⊞ C Bladder Neck D Urethra ⊞	Ø Open 4 Percutaneous Endoscopic 7 Via Natural or Artificial Opening 8 Via Natural or Artificial Opening Endoscopic	Z No Device	Z No Qualifier

Non-OR ØTTD[Ø478]ZZ
⊞ ØTT[BD]ØZZ

SECTION: Ø MEDICAL AND SURGICAL
BODY SYSTEM: T URINARY SYSTEM
OPERATION: U SUPPLEMENT: Putting in or on biological or synthetic material that physically reinforces and/or augments the function of a portion of a body part

Body Part	Approach	Device	Qualifier
3 Kidney Pelvis, Right 4 Kidney Pelvis, Left 6 Ureter, Right 7 Ureter, Left B Bladder C Bladder Neck	Ø Open 4 Percutaneous Endoscopic 7 Via Natural or Artificial Opening 8 Via Natural or Artificial Opening Endoscopic	7 Autologous Tissue Substitute J Synthetic Substitute K Nonautologous Tissue Substitute	Z No Qualifier
D Urethra	Ø Open 4 Percutaneous Endoscopic 7 Via Natural or Artificial Opening 8 Via Natural or Artificial Opening Endoscopic X External	7 Autologous Tissue Substitute J Synthetic Substitute K Nonautologous Tissue Substitute	Z No Qualifier

Coding Clinic: 2Ø17, Q3, P21 – ØTUBØ7Z

SECTION: Ø MEDICAL AND SURGICAL
BODY SYSTEM: T URINARY SYSTEM
OPERATION: V RESTRICTION: Partially closing an orifice or the lumen of a tubular body part

Body Part	Approach	Device	Qualifier
3 Kidney Pelvis, Right 4 Kidney Pelvis, Left 6 Ureter, Right 7 Ureter, Left B Bladder C Bladder Neck	Ø Open 3 Percutaneous 4 Percutaneous Endoscopic	C Extraluminal Device D Intraluminal Device Z No Device	Z No Qualifier
3 Kidney Pelvis, Right 4 Kidney Pelvis, Left 6 Ureter, Right 7 Ureter, Left B Bladder C Bladder Neck	7 Via Natural or Artificial Opening 8 Via Natural or Artificial Opening Endoscopic	D Intraluminal Device Z No Device	Z No Qualifier
D Urethra	Ø Open 3 Percutaneous 4 Percutaneous Endoscopic	C Extraluminal Device D Intraluminal Device Z No Device	Z No Qualifier
D Urethra	7 Via Natural or Artificial Opening 8 Via Natural or Artificial Opening Endoscopic	D Intraluminal Device Z No Device	Z No Qualifier
D Urethra	X External	Z No Device	Z No Qualifier

Coding Clinic: 2Ø15, Q2, P12 – ØTV[67]8ZZ

SECTION: Ø MEDICAL AND SURGICAL
BODY SYSTEM: T URINARY SYSTEM
OPERATION: W REVISION: *(on multiple pages)*

Correcting, to the extent possible, a portion of a malfunctioning device or the position of a displaced device

Body Part	Approach	Device	Qualifier
5 Kidney	Ø Open 3 Percutaneous 4 Percutaneous Endoscopic 7 Via Natural or Artificial Opening 8 Via Natural or Artificial Opening Endoscopic	Ø Drainage Device 2 Monitoring Device 3 Infusion Device 7 Autologous Tissue Substitute C Extraluminal Device D Intraluminal Device J Synthetic Substitute K Nonautologous Tissue Substitute Y Other Device	Z No Qualifier
5 Kidney	X External	Ø Drainage Device 2 Monitoring Device 3 Infusion Device 7 Autologous Tissue Substitute C Extraluminal Device D Intraluminal Device J Synthetic Substitute K Nonautologous Tissue Substitute	Z No Qualifier
9 Ureter	Ø Open 3 Percutaneous 4 Percutaneous Endoscopic 7 Via Natural or Artificial Opening 8 Via Natural or Artificial Opening Endoscopic	Ø Drainage Device 2 Monitoring Device 3 Infusion Device 7 Autologous Tissue Substitute C Extraluminal Device D Intraluminal Device J Synthetic Substitute K Nonautologous Tissue Substitute M Stimulator Lead Y Other Device	Z No Qualifier
9 Ureter	X External	Ø Drainage Device 2 Monitoring Device 3 Infusion Device 7 Autologous Tissue Substitute C Extraluminal Device D Intraluminal Device J Synthetic Substitute K Nonautologous Tissue Substitute M Stimulator Lead	Z No Qualifier

Non-OR ØTW5X[Ø237CDJK]Z

SECTION: Ø MEDICAL AND SURGICAL
BODY SYSTEM: T URINARY SYSTEM
OPERATION: W REVISION: *(continued)*

Correcting, to the extent possible, a portion of a malfunctioning device or the position of a displaced device

Body Part	Approach	Device	Qualifier
B Bladder	Ø Open 3 Percutaneous 4 Percutaneous Endoscopic 7 Via Natural or Artificial Opening 8 Via Natural or Artificial Opening Endoscopic	Ø Drainage Device 2 Monitoring Device 3 Infusion Device 7 Autologous Tissue Substitute C Extraluminal Device D Intraluminal Device J Synthetic Substitute K Nonautologous Tissue Substitute L Artificial Sphincter M Stimulator Lead Y Other Device	Z No Qualifier
B Bladder	X External	Ø Drainage Device 2 Monitoring Device 3 Infusion Device 7 Autologous Tissue Substitute C Extraluminal Device D Intraluminal Device J Synthetic Substitute K Nonautologous Tissue Substitute L Artificial Sphincter M Stimulator Lead	Z No Qualifier
D Urethra	Ø Open 3 Percutaneous 4 Percutaneous Endoscopic 7 Via Natural or Artificial Opening 8 Via Natural or Artificial Opening Endoscopic	Ø Drainage Device 2 Monitoring Device 3 Infusion Device 7 Autologous Tissue Substitute C Extraluminal Device D Intraluminal Device J Synthetic Substitute K Nonautologous Tissue Substitute L Artificial Sphincter Y Other Device	Z No Qualifier
D Urethra	X External	Ø Drainage Device 2 Monitoring Device 3 Infusion Device 7 Autologous Tissue Substitute C Extraluminal Device D Intraluminal Device J Synthetic Substitute K Nonautologous Tissue Substitute L Artificial Sphincter	Z No Qualifier

Non-OR ØTW9X[Ø237CDJKM]Z
Non-OR ØTWBX[Ø237CDJKLM]Z
Non-OR ØTWDX[Ø237CDJKL]Z

SECTION: Ø MEDICAL AND SURGICAL
BODY SYSTEM: T URINARY SYSTEM
OPERATION: Y TRANSPLANTATION: Putting in or on all or a portion of a living body part taken from another individual or animal to physically take the place and/or function of all or a portion of a similar body part

Body Part	Approach	Device	Qualifier
Ø Kidney, Right 1 Kidney, Left	Ø Open	Z No Device	Ø Allogeneic 1 Syngeneic 2 Zooplastic

ØTY[Ø1]ØZ[Ø12]
ØTY[Ø1]ØZ[Ø12]

SECTION: Ø MEDICAL AND SURGICAL
BODY SYSTEM: U FEMALE REPRODUCTIVE SYSTEM
OPERATION: 1 BYPASS: Altering the route of passage of the contents of a tubular body part

Body Part	Approach	Device	Qualifier
5 Fallopian Tube, Right ♀ 6 Fallopian Tube, Left ♀	Ø Open 4 Percutaneous Endoscopic	7 Autologous Tissue Substitute J Synthetic Substitute K Nonautologous Tissue Substitute Z No Device	5 Fallopian Tube, Right 6 Fallopian Tube, Left 9 Uterus

SECTION: Ø MEDICAL AND SURGICAL
BODY SYSTEM: U FEMALE REPRODUCTIVE SYSTEM
OPERATION: 2 CHANGE: Taking out or off a device from a body part and putting back an identical or similar device in or on the same body part without cutting or puncturing the skin or a mucous membrane

Body Part	Approach	Device	Qualifier
3 Ovary ♀ 8 Fallopian Tube ♀ M Vulva ♀	X External	Ø Drainage Device Y Other Device	Z No Qualifier
D Uterus and Cervix ♀	X External	Ø Drainage Device H Contraceptive Device Y Other Device	Z No Qualifier
H Vagina and Cul-de-sac ♀	X External	Ø Drainage Device G Intraluminal Device, Pessary Y Other Device	Z No Qualifier

Non-OR All Values

SECTION: Ø MEDICAL AND SURGICAL
BODY SYSTEM: U FEMALE REPRODUCTIVE SYSTEM
OPERATION: 5 DESTRUCTION: Physical eradication of all or a portion of a body part by the direct use of energy, force, or a destructive agent

Body Part	Approach	Device	Qualifier
Ø Ovary, Right ♀ 1 Ovary, Left ♀ 2 Ovaries, Bilateral ♀ 4 Uterine Supporting Structure ♀	Ø Open 3 Percutaneous 4 Percutaneous Endoscopic 8 Via Natural or Artificial Opening Endoscopic	Z No Device	Z No Qualifier
5 Fallopian Tube, Right ♀ 6 Fallopian Tube, Left ♀ 7 Fallopian Tubes, Bilateral ♀ 9 Uterus ♀ B Endometrium ♀ C Cervix ♀ F Cul-de-sac ♀	Ø Open 3 Percutaneous 4 Percutaneous Endoscopic 7 Via Natural or Artificial Opening 8 Via Natural or Artificial Opening Endoscopic	Z No Device	Z No Qualifier
G Vagina ♀ K Hymen ♀	Ø Open 3 Percutaneous 4 Percutaneous Endoscopic 7 Via Natural or Artificial Opening 8 Via Natural or Artificial Opening Endoscopic X External	Z No Device	Z No Qualifier
J Clitoris ♀ L Vestibular Gland ♀ M Vulva ♀	Ø Open X External	Z No Device	Z No Qualifier

ØU57[Ø3478]ZZ when Z3Ø.2 is listed as the principal diagnosis

SECTION: Ø MEDICAL AND SURGICAL
BODY SYSTEM: U FEMALE REPRODUCTIVE SYSTEM
OPERATION: 7 DILATION: Expanding an orifice or the lumen of a tubular body part

Body Part	Approach	Device	Qualifier
5 Fallopian Tube, Right ♀ 6 Fallopian Tube, Left ♀ 7 Fallopian Tubes, Bilateral ♀ 9 Uterus ♀ C Cervix ♀ G Vagina ♀	Ø Open 3 Percutaneous 4 Percutaneous Endoscopic 7 Via Natural or Artificial Opening 8 Via Natural or Artificial Opening Endoscopic	D Intraluminal Device Z No Device	Z No Qualifier
K Hymen ♀	Ø Open 3 Percutaneous 4 Percutaneous Endoscopic 7 Via Natural or Artificial Opening 8 Via Natural or Artificial Opening Endoscopic X External	D Intraluminal Device Z No Device	Z No Qualifier

Non-OR ØU7C[Ø3478][DZ]Z
Non-OR ØU7G[78][DZ]Z

Coding Clinic: 2020, Q2, P30 – ØU7C7ZZ

SECTION: Ø MEDICAL AND SURGICAL
BODY SYSTEM: U FEMALE REPRODUCTIVE SYSTEM
OPERATION: 8 DIVISION: Cutting into a body part, without draining fluids and/or gases from the body part, in order to separate or transect a body part

Body Part	Approach	Device	Qualifier
Ø Ovary, Right ♀ 1 Ovary, Left ♀ 2 Ovaries, Bilateral ♀ 4 Uterine Supporting Structure ♀	Ø Open 3 Percutaneous 4 Percutaneous Endoscopic	Z No Device	Z No Qualifier
K Hymen ♀	7 Via Natural or Artificial Opening 8 Via Natural or Artificial Opening Endoscopic X External	Z No Device	Z No Qualifier

Non-OR ØU8K[78X]ZZ

SECTION: Ø MEDICAL AND SURGICAL
BODY SYSTEM: U FEMALE REPRODUCTIVE SYSTEM
OPERATION: 9 DRAINAGE: *(on multiple pages)*
Taking or letting out fluids and/or gases from a body part

Body Part	Approach	Device	Qualifier
Ø Ovary, Right ♀ 1 Ovary, Left ♀ 2 Ovaries, Bilateral ♀	Ø Open 3 Percutaneous 4 Percutaneous Endoscopic 8 Via Natural or Artificial Opening Endoscopic	Ø Drainage Device	Z No Qualifier
Ø Ovary, Right ♀ 1 Ovary, Left ♀ 2 Ovaries, Bilateral ♀	Ø Open 3 Percutaneous 4 Percutaneous Endoscopic 8 Via Natural or Artificial Opening Endoscopic	Z No Device	X Diagnostic Z No Qualifier
Ø Ovary, Right ♀ 1 Ovary, Left ♀ 2 Ovaries, Bilateral ♀	X External	Z No Device	Z No Qualifier
4 Uterine Supporting Structure ♀	Ø Open 3 Percutaneous 4 Percutaneous Endoscopic 8 Via Natural or Artificial Opening Endoscopic	Ø Drainage Device	Z No Qualifier
4 Uterine Supporting Structure ♀	Ø Open 3 Percutaneous 4 Percutaneous Endoscopic 8 Via Natural or Artificial Opening Endoscopic	Z No Device	X Diagnostic Z No Qualifier
5 Fallopian Tube, Right ♀ 6 Fallopian Tube, Left ♀ 7 Fallopian Tubes, Bilateral ♀ 9 Uterus ♀ C Cervix ♀ F Cul-de-sac ♀	Ø Open 3 Percutaneous 4 Percutaneous Endoscopic 7 Via Natural or Artificial Opening 8 Via Natural or Artificial Opening Endoscopic	Ø Drainage Device	Z No Qualifier
5 Fallopian Tube, Right ♀ 6 Fallopian Tube, Left ♀ 7 Fallopian Tubes, Bilateral ♀ 9 Uterus ♀ C Cervix ♀ F Cul-de-sac ♀	Ø Open 3 Percutaneous 4 Percutaneous Endoscopic 7 Via Natural or Artificial Opening 8 Via Natural or Artificial Opening Endoscopic	Z No Device	X Diagnostic Z No Qualifier
G Vagina ♀ K Hymen ♀	Ø Open 3 Percutaneous 4 Percutaneous Endoscopic 7 Via Natural or Artificial Opening 8 Via Natural or Artificial Opening Endoscopic X External	Ø Drainage Device	Z No Qualifier

Non-OR ØU9[Ø12]3ØZ
Non-OR ØU9[Ø12]3ZZ
Non-OR ØU943ØZ
Non-OR ØU943ZZ
Non-OR ØU9[5679C]3ØZ
Non-OR ØU9F[34]ØZ
Non-OR ØU9[567][3478]ZZ
Non-OR ØU9F[34]ZZ
Non-OR ØU9K[Ø3478X]ØZ
Non-OR ØU9K[Ø3478X]ZZ
Non-OR ØU9[9C]3ZZ
Non-OR ØU9G3ØZ
Non-OR ØU9G3ZZ

SECTION: Ø MEDICAL AND SURGICAL
BODY SYSTEM: U FEMALE REPRODUCTIVE SYSTEM
OPERATION: 9 DRAINAGE: *(continued)*
Taking or letting out fluids and/or gases from a body part

Body Part	Approach	Device	Qualifier
G Vagina ♀ K Hymen ♀	Ø Open 3 Percutaneous 4 Percutaneous Endoscopic 7 Via Natural or Artificial Opening 8 Via Natural or Artificial Opening Endoscopic X External	Z No Device	X Diagnostic Z No Qualifier
J Clitoris ♀ L Vestibular Gland ♀ M Vulva ♀	Ø Open X External	Ø Drainage Device	Z No Qualifier
J Clitoris ♀ L Vestibular Gland ♀ M Vulva ♀	Ø Open X External	Z No Device	X Diagnostic Z No Qualifier

Non-OR ØU9L[ØX]ØZ
Non-OR ØU9L[ØX]ZZ

SECTION: Ø MEDICAL AND SURGICAL
BODY SYSTEM: U FEMALE REPRODUCTIVE SYSTEM
OPERATION: B EXCISION: Cutting out or off, without replacement, a portion of a body part

Body Part	Approach	Device	Qualifier
Ø Ovary, Right ♀ 1 Ovary, Left ♀ 2 Ovaries, Bilateral ♀ 4 Uterine Supporting Structure ♀ 5 Fallopian Tube, Right ♀ 6 Fallopian Tube, Left ♀ 7 Fallopian Tubes, Bilateral ♀ 9 Uterus ♀ C Cervix ♀ F Cul-de-sac ♀	Ø Open 3 Percutaneous 4 Percutaneous Endoscopic 7 Via Natural or Artificial Opening 8 Via Natural or Artificial Opening Endoscopic	Z No Device	X Diagnostic Z No Qualifier
G Vagina ♀ K Hymen ♀	Ø Open 3 Percutaneous 4 Percutaneous Endoscopic 7 Via Natural or Artificial Opening 8 Via Natural or Artificial Opening Endoscopic X External	Z No Device	X Diagnostic Z No Qualifier
J Clitoris ♀ L Vestibular Gland ♀ M Vulva ♀	Ø Open X External	Z No Device	X Diagnostic Z No Qualifier

Coding Clinic: 2Ø15, Q3, P31 – ØUB7ØZZ
Coding Clinic: 2Ø15, Q3, P32 – ØUB64ZZ

SECTION: Ø MEDICAL AND SURGICAL
BODY SYSTEM: U FEMALE REPRODUCTIVE SYSTEM
OPERATION: C EXTIRPATION: Taking or cutting out solid matter from a body part

Body Part	Approach	Device	Qualifier
Ø Ovary, Right ♀ 1 Ovary, Left ♀ 2 Ovaries, Bilateral ♀ 4 Uterine Supporting Structure ♀	Ø Open 3 Percutaneous 4 Percutaneous Endoscopic 8 Via Natural or Artificial Opening Endoscopic	Z No Device	Z No Qualifier
5 Fallopian Tube, Right ♀ 6 Fallopian Tube, Left ♀ 7 Fallopian Tubes, Bilateral ♀ 9 Uterus ♀ B Endometrium ♀ C Cervix ♀ F Cul-de-sac ♀	Ø Open 3 Percutaneous 4 Percutaneous Endoscopic 7 Via Natural or Artificial Opening 8 Via Natural or Artificial Opening Endoscopic	Z No Device	Z No Qualifier
G Vagina ♀ K Hymen ♀	Ø Open 3 Percutaneous 4 Percutaneous Endoscopic 7 Via Natural or Artificial Opening 8 Via Natural or Artificial Opening Endoscopic X External	Z No Device	Z No Qualifier
J Clitoris ♀ L Vestibular Gland ♀ M Vulva ♀	Ø Open X External	Z No Device	Z No Qualifier

Non-OR ØUC9[78]ZZ
Non-OR ØUCG[78X]ZZ
Non-OR ØUCK[Ø3478X]ZZ
Non-OR ØUCMXZZ

Coding Clinic: 2Ø13, Q2, P38 – ØUC97ZZ
Coding Clinic: 2Ø15, Q3, P3Ø-31 – ØUCC[78]ZZ

Ø: M/S U: FEMALE REPRODUCTIVE SYSTEM D: EXTRACTION F: FRAGMENTATION

SECTION: Ø **MEDICAL AND SURGICAL**
BODY SYSTEM: U **FEMALE REPRODUCTIVE SYSTEM**
OPERATION: D **EXTRACTION:** Pulling or stripping out or off all or a portion of a body part by the use of force

Body Part	Approach	Device	Qualifier
B Endometrium ♀	7 Via Natural or Artificial Opening 8 Via Natural or Artificial Opening Endoscopic	Z No Device	X Diagnostic Z No Qualifier
N Ova ♀	Ø Open 3 Percutaneous 4 Percutaneous Endoscopic	Z No Device	Z No Qualifier

SECTION: Ø **MEDICAL AND SURGICAL**
BODY SYSTEM: U **FEMALE REPRODUCTIVE SYSTEM**
OPERATION: F **FRAGMENTATION:** Breaking solid matter in a body part into pieces

Body Part	Approach	Device	Qualifier
5 Fallopian Tube, Right ♀ 6 Fallopian Tube, Left ♀ 7 Fallopian Tubes, Bilateral ♀ 9 Uterus ♀	Ø Open 3 Percutaneous 4 Percutaneous Endoscopic 7 Via Natural or Artificial Opening 8 Via Natural or Artificial Opening Endoscopic X External	Z No Device	Z No Qualifier

ØUF[5679]XZZ
Non-OR ØUF[5679]XZZ

New/Revised Text in Green ~~deleted~~ Deleted ♀ Females Only ♂ Males Only Coding Clinic
Non-covered Limited Coverage Combination (See Appendix E) DRG Non-OR Non-OR Hospital-Acquired Condition

SECTION: Ø MEDICAL AND SURGICAL
BODY SYSTEM: U FEMALE REPRODUCTIVE SYSTEM
OPERATION: H INSERTION: Putting in a nonbiological appliance that monitors, assists, performs, or prevents a physiological function but does not physically take the place of a body part

Body Part	Approach	Device	Qualifier
3 Ovary ♀	Ø Open 3 Percutaneous 4 Percutaneous Endoscopic	1 Radioactive Element 3 Infusion Device Y Other Device	Z No Qualifier
3 Ovary ♀	7 Via Natural or Artificial Opening 8 Via Natural or Artificial Opening Endoscopic	1 Radioactive Element Y Other Device	Z No Qualifier
8 Fallopian Tube ♀ D Uterus and Cervix ♀ H Vagina and Cul-de-sac ♀	Ø Open 3 Percutaneous 4 Percutaneous Endoscopic 7 Via Natural or Artificial Opening 8 Via Natural or Artificial Opening Endoscopic	3 Infusion Device Y Other Device	Z No Qualifier
9 Uterus ♀	Ø Open 7 Via Natural or Artificial Opening 8 Via Natural or Artificial Opening Endoscopic	1 Radioactive Element H Contraceptive Device	Z No Qualifier
C Cervix ♀	Ø Open 3 Percutaneous 4 Percutaneous Endoscopic	1 Radioactive Element	Z No Qualifier
C Cervix ♀	7 Via Natural or Artificial Opening 8 Via Natural or Artificial Opening Endoscopic	1 Radioactive Element H Contraceptive Device	Z No Qualifier
F Cul-de-sac ♀	7 Via Natural or Artificial Opening 8 Via Natural or Artificial Opening Endoscopic	G Intraluminal Device, Pessary	Z No Qualifier
G Vagina ♀	Ø Open 3 Percutaneous 4 Percutaneous Endoscopic X External	1 Radioactive Element	Z No Qualifier
G Vagina ♀	7 Via Natural or Artificial Opening 8 Via Natural or Artificial Opening Endoscopic	1 Radioactive Element G Intraluminal Device, Pessary	Z No Qualifier

Non-OR ØUH3[Ø34]3Z
Non-OR ØUH[8D][Ø3478]3Z
Non-OR ØUHH[78]3Z
Non-OR ØUH9[78]HZ
Non-OR ØUHC[78]HZ
Non-OR ØUHF[78]GZ
Non-OR ØUHG[78]GZ

Coding Clinic: 2Ø13, Q2, P34 – ØUH97HZ

SECTION: Ø MEDICAL AND SURGICAL
BODY SYSTEM: U FEMALE REPRODUCTIVE SYSTEM
OPERATION: J INSPECTION: Visually and/or manually exploring a body part

Body Part	Approach	Device	Qualifier
3 Ovary ♀	Ø Open 3 Percutaneous 4 Percutaneous Endoscopic 8 Via Natural or Artificial Opening Endoscopic X External	Z No Device	Z No Qualifier
8 Fallopian Tube ♀ D Uterus and Cervix ♀ H Vagina and Cul-de-sac ♀	Ø Open 3 Percutaneous 4 Percutaneous Endoscopic 7 Via Natural or Artificial Opening 8 Via Natural or Artificial Opening Endoscopic X External	Z No Device	Z No Qualifier
M Vulva ♀	Ø Open X External	Z No Device	Z No Qualifier

Non-OR ØUJ8[378]ZZ
Non-OR ØUJD3ZZ
Non-OR ØUJ3[3X]ZZ
Non-OR ØUJ8XZZ
Non-OR ØUJD[78X]ZZ
Non-OR ØUJH[378X]ZZ
Non-OR ØUJMXZZ

Coding Clinic: 2Ø15, Q1, P34 – ØUJD4ZZ

SECTION: Ø MEDICAL AND SURGICAL
BODY SYSTEM: U FEMALE REPRODUCTIVE SYSTEM
OPERATION: L OCCLUSION: Completely closing an orifice or the lumen of a tubular body part

Body Part	Approach	Device	Qualifier
5 Fallopian Tube, Right ♀ 6 Fallopian Tube, Left ♀ 7 Fallopian Tubes, Bilateral ♀	Ø Open 3 Percutaneous 4 Percutaneous Endoscopic	C Extraluminal Device D Intraluminal Device Z No Device	Z No Qualifier
5 Fallopian Tube, Right ♀ 6 Fallopian Tube, Left ♀ 7 Fallopian Tubes, Bilateral ♀	7 Via Natural or Artificial Opening 8 Via Natural or Artificial Opening Endoscopic	D Intraluminal Device Z No Device	Z No Qualifier
F Cul-de-sac ♀ G Vagina ♀	7 Via Natural or Artificial Opening 8 Via Natural or Artificial Opening Endoscopic	D Intraluminal Device Z No Device	Z No Qualifier

ØUL7[Ø34][CDZ]Z when Z3Ø.2 is listed as the principal diagnosis
ØUL7[78][DZ]Z when Z3Ø.2 is listed as the principal diagnosis

SECTION: Ø MEDICAL AND SURGICAL
BODY SYSTEM: U FEMALE REPRODUCTIVE SYSTEM
OPERATION: M REATTACHMENT: Putting back in or on all or a portion of a separated body part to its normal location or other suitable location

Body Part	Approach	Device	Qualifier
Ø Ovary, Right ♀ 1 Ovary, Left ♀ 2 Ovaries, Bilateral ♀ 4 Uterine Supporting Structure ♀ 5 Fallopian Tube, Right ♀ 6 Fallopian Tube, Left ♀ 7 Fallopian Tubes, Bilateral ♀ 9 Uterus ♀ C Cervix ♀ F Cul-de-sac ♀ G Vagina ♀	Ø Open 4 Percutaneous Endoscopic	Z No Device	Z No Qualifier
J Clitoris ♀ M Vulva ♀	X External	Z No Device	Z No Qualifier
K Hymen ♀	Ø Open 4 Percutaneous Endoscopic X External	Z No Device	Z No Qualifier

SECTION: Ø MEDICAL AND SURGICAL
BODY SYSTEM: U FEMALE REPRODUCTIVE SYSTEM
OPERATION: N RELEASE: Freeing a body part from an abnormal physical constraint by cutting or by the use of force

Body Part	Approach	Device	Qualifier
Ø Ovary, Right ♀ 1 Ovary, Left ♀ 2 Ovaries, Bilateral ♀ 4 Uterine Supporting Structure ♀	Ø Open 3 Percutaneous 4 Percutaneous Endoscopic 8 Via Natural or Artificial Opening Endoscopic	Z No Device	Z No Qualifier
5 Fallopian Tube, Right ♀ 6 Fallopian Tube, Left ♀ 7 Fallopian Tubes, Bilateral ♀ 9 Uterus ♀ C Cervix ♀ F Cul-de-sac ♀	Ø Open 3 Percutaneous 4 Percutaneous Endoscopic 7 Via Natural or Artificial Opening 8 Via Natural or Artificial Opening Endoscopic	Z No Device	Z No Qualifier
G Vagina ♀ K Hymen ♀	Ø Open 3 Percutaneous 4 Percutaneous Endoscopic 7 Via Natural or Artificial Opening 8 Via Natural or Artificial Opening Endoscopic X External	Z No Device	Z No Qualifier
J Clitoris ♀ L Vestibular Gland ♀ M Vulva ♀	Ø Open X External	Z No Device	Z No Qualifier

SECTION: Ø MEDICAL AND SURGICAL
BODY SYSTEM: U FEMALE REPRODUCTIVE SYSTEM
OPERATION: P REMOVAL: *(on multiple pages)*
Taking out or off a device from a body part

Body Part	Approach	Device	Qualifier
3 Ovary ♀	Ø Open 3 Percutaneous 4 Percutaneous Endoscopic	Ø Drainage Device 3 Infusion Device Y Other Device	Z No Qualifier
3 Ovary ♀	7 Via Natural or Artificial Opening 8 Via Natural or Artificial Opening Endoscopic	Y Other Device	Z No Qualifier
3 Ovary ♀	X External	Ø Drainage Device 3 Infusion Device	Z No Qualifier
8 Fallopian Tube ♀	Ø Open 3 Percutaneous 4 Percutaneous Endoscopic 7 Via Natural or Artificial Opening 8 Via Natural or Artificial Opening Endoscopic	Ø Drainage Device 3 Infusion Device 7 Autologous Tissue Substitute C Extraluminal Device D Intraluminal Device J Synthetic Substitute K Nonautologous Tissue Substitute Y Other Device	Z No Qualifier
8 Fallopian Tube ♀	X External	Ø Drainage Device 3 Infusion Device D Intraluminal Device	Z No Qualifier
D Uterus and Cervix ♀	Ø Open 3 Percutaneous 4 Percutaneous Endoscopic 7 Via Natural or Artificial Opening 8 Via Natural or Artificial Opening Endoscopic	Ø Drainage Device 1 Radioactive Element 3 Infusion Device 7 Autologous Tissue Substitute C Extraluminal Device D Intraluminal Device H Contraceptive Device J Synthetic Substitute K Nonautologous Tissue Substitute Y Other Device	Z No Qualifier
D Uterus and Cervix ♀	X External	Ø Drainage Device 3 Infusion Device D Intraluminal Device H Contraceptive Device	Z No Qualifier
H Vagina and Cul-de-sac ♀	Ø Open 3 Percutaneous 4 Percutaneous Endoscopic 7 Via Natural or Artificial Opening 8 Via Natural or Artificial Opening Endoscopic	Ø Drainage Device 1 Radioactive Element 3 Infusion Device 7 Autologous Tissue Substitute D Intraluminal Device J Synthetic Substitute K Nonautologous Tissue Substitute Y Other Device	Z No Qualifier

Non-OR ØUP3X[Ø3]Z
Non-OR ØUP8[78][Ø3D]Z
Non-OR ØUP8X[Ø3D]Z
Non-OR ØUPD[34]CZ
Non-OR ØUPD[78][Ø3CDH]Z
Non-OR ØUPDX[Ø3DH]Z
Non-OR ØUPH[78][Ø3D]Z

Coding Clinic: 2022, Q3, P14 – ØUPH77Z

SECTION: Ø MEDICAL AND SURGICAL
BODY SYSTEM: U FEMALE REPRODUCTIVE SYSTEM
OPERATION: P REMOVAL: *(continued)*
Taking out or off a device from a body part

Body Part	Approach	Device	Qualifier
H Vagina and Cul-de-sac ♀	X External	Ø Drainage Device 1 Radioactive Element 3 Infusion Device D Intraluminal Device	Z No Qualifier
M Vulva ♀	Ø Open	Ø Drainage Device 7 Autologous Tissue Substitute J Synthetic Substitute K Nonautologous Tissue Substitute	Z No Qualifier
M Vulva ♀	X External	Ø Drainage Device	Z No Qualifier

Non-OR ØUPHX[Ø13D]Z
Non-OR ØUPMXØZ

SECTION: Ø MEDICAL AND SURGICAL
BODY SYSTEM: U FEMALE REPRODUCTIVE SYSTEM
OPERATION: Q REPAIR: Restoring, to the extent possible, a body part to its normal anatomic structure and function

Body Part	Approach	Device	Qualifier
Ø Ovary, Right ♀ 1 Ovary, Left ♀ 2 Ovaries, Bilateral ♀ 4 Uterine Supporting Structure ♀	Ø Open 3 Percutaneous 4 Percutaneous Endoscopic 8 Via Natural or Artificial Opening Endoscopic	Z No Device	Z No Qualifier
5 Fallopian Tube, Right ♀ 6 Fallopian Tube, Left ♀ 7 Fallopian Tubes, Bilateral ♀ 9 Uterus ♀ C Cervix ♀ F Cul-de-sac ♀	Ø Open 3 Percutaneous 4 Percutaneous Endoscopic 7 Via Natural or Artificial Opening 8 Via Natural or Artificial Opening Endoscopic	Z No Device	Z No Qualifier
G Vagina ♀ K Hymen ♀	Ø Open 3 Percutaneous 4 Percutaneous Endoscopic 7 Via Natural or Artificial Opening 8 Via Natural or Artificial Opening Endoscopic X External	Z No Device	Z No Qualifier
J Clitoris ♀ L Vestibular Gland ♀ M Vulva ♀	Ø Open X External	Z No Device	Z No Qualifier

SECTION: Ø MEDICAL AND SURGICAL
BODY SYSTEM: U FEMALE REPRODUCTIVE SYSTEM
OPERATION: S REPOSITION: Moving to its normal location, or other suitable location, all or a portion of a body part

Body Part	Approach	Device	Qualifier
Ø Ovary, Right ♀ 1 Ovary, Left ♀ 2 Ovaries, Bilateral ♀ 4 Uterine Supporting Structure ♀ 5 Fallopian Tube, Right ♀ 6 Fallopian Tube, Left ♀ 7 Fallopian Tubes, Bilateral ♀ C Cervix ♀ F Cul-de-sac ♀	Ø Open 4 Percutaneous Endoscopic 8 Via Natural or Artificial Opening Endoscopic	Z No Device	Z No Qualifier
9 Uterus ♀ G Vagina ♀	Ø Open 4 Percutaneous Endoscopic 7 Via Natural or Artificial Opening 8 Via Natural or Artificial Opening Endoscopic X External	Z No Device	Z No Qualifier

Non-OR ØUS9XZZ

Coding Clinic: 2016, Q1, P9 – ØUS9XZZ
Coding Clinic: 2017, Q4, P68 – ØUT9[07]Z[LZ]
Coding Clinic: 2022, Q1, P21 – ØUT[79]ØZZ

SECTION: Ø MEDICAL AND SURGICAL
BODY SYSTEM: U FEMALE REPRODUCTIVE SYSTEM
OPERATION: T RESECTION: Cutting out or off, without replacement, all of a body part

Body Part	Approach	Device	Qualifier
Ø Ovary, Right ♀ 1 Ovary, Left ♀ 2 Ovaries, Bilateral ♀ ⊞ 5 Fallopian Tube, Right ♀ 6 Fallopian Tube, Left ♀ 7 Fallopian Tubes, Bilateral ♀	Ø Open 4 Percutaneous Endoscopic 7 Via Natural or Artificial Opening 8 Via Natural or Artificial Opening Endoscopic F Via Natural or Artificial Opening With Percutaneous Endoscopic Assistance	Z No Device	Z No Qualifier
4 Uterine Supporting Structure ♀ ⊞ C Cervix ♀ ⊞ F Cul-de-sac ♀ G Vagina ♀ ⊞	Ø Open 4 Percutaneous Endoscopic 7 Via Natural or Artificial Opening 8 Via Natural or Artificial Opening Endoscopic	Z No Device	Z No Qualifier
9 Uterus ♀ ⊞	Ø Open 4 Percutaneous Endoscopic 7 Via Natural or Artificial Opening 8 Via Natural or Artificial Opening Endoscopic F Via Natural or Artificial Opening With Percutaneous Endoscopic Assistance	Z No Device	L Supracervical Z No Qualifier
J Clitoris ♀ L Vestibular Gland ♀ M Vulva ♀ ⊞	Ø Open X External	Z No Device	Z No Qualifier
K Hymen ♀	Ø Open 4 Percutaneous Endoscopic 7 Via Natural or Artificial Opening 8 Via Natural or Artificial Opening Endoscopic X External	Z No Device	Z No Qualifier

⊞ ØUT9[Ø478F]ZZ
⊞ ØUT[24CG][Ø478]ZZ
⊞ ØUTM[ØX]ZZ

Coding Clinic: 2013, Q1, P24 – ØUTØØZZ
Coding Clinic: 2015, Q1, P33-34; 2013, Q3, P28 – ØUT9ØZZ, ØUTCØZZ
Coding Clinic: 2015, Q1, P34 – ØUT2ØZZ, ØUT7ØZZ

SECTION: Ø MEDICAL AND SURGICAL
BODY SYSTEM: U FEMALE REPRODUCTIVE SYSTEM
OPERATION: U SUPPLEMENT: Putting in or on biological or synthetic material that physically reinforces and/or augments the function of a portion of a body part

Body Part	Approach	Device	Qualifier
4 Uterine Supporting Structure ♀	Ø Open 4 Percutaneous Endoscopic	7 Autologous Tissue Substitute J Synthetic Substitute K Nonautologous Tissue Substitute	Z No Qualifier
5 Fallopian Tube Right ♀ 6 Fallopian Tube, Left ♀ 7 Fallopian Tubes, Bilateral ♀ F Cul-de-sac ♀	Ø Open 4 Percutaneous Endoscopic 7 Via Natural or Artificial Opening 8 Via Natural or Artificial Opening Endoscopic	7 Autologous Tissue Substitute J Synthetic Substitute K Nonautologous Tissue Substitute	Z No Qualifier
G Vagina ♀ K Hymen ♀	Ø Open 4 Percutaneous Endoscopic 7 Via Natural or Artificial Opening 8 Via Natural or Artificial Opening Endoscopic X External	7 Autologous Tissue Substitute J Synthetic Substitute K Nonautologous Tissue Substitute	Z No Qualifier
J Clitoris ♀ M Vulva ♀	Ø Open X External	7 Autologous Tissue Substitute J Synthetic Substitute K Nonautologous Tissue Substitute	Z No Qualifier

SECTION: Ø MEDICAL AND SURGICAL
BODY SYSTEM: U FEMALE REPRODUCTIVE SYSTEM
OPERATION: V RESTRICTION: Partially closing an orifice or the lumen of a tubular body part

Body Part	Approach	Device	Qualifier
C Cervix ♀	Ø Open 3 Percutaneous 4 Percutaneous Endoscopic	C Extraluminal Device D Intraluminal Device Z No Device	Z No Qualifier
C Cervix ♀	7 Via Natural or Artificial Opening 8 Via Natural or Artificial Opening Endoscopic	D Intraluminal Device Z No Device	Z No Qualifier

Coding Clinic: 2Ø15, Q3, P3Ø – ØUVC7ZZ

SECTION: Ø MEDICAL AND SURGICAL
BODY SYSTEM: U FEMALE REPRODUCTIVE SYSTEM
OPERATION: W REVISION: *(on multiple pages)*

Correcting, to the extent possible, a portion of a malfunctioning device or the position of a displaced device

Body Part	Approach	Device	Qualifier
3 Ovary ♀	Ø Open 3 Percutaneous 4 Percutaneous Endoscopic	Ø Drainage Device 3 Infusion Device Y Other Device	Z No Qualifier
3 Ovary ♀	7 Via Natural or Artificial Opening 8 Via Natural or Artificial Opening Endoscopic	Y Other Device	Z No Qualifier
3 Ovary ♀	X External	Ø Drainage Device 3 Infusion Device	Z No Qualifier
8 Fallopian Tube ♀	Ø Open 3 Percutaneous 4 Percutaneous Endoscopic 7 Via Natural or Artificial Opening 8 Via Natural or Artificial Opening Endoscopic	Ø Drainage Device 3 Infusion Device 7 Autologous Tissue Substitute C Extraluminal Device D Intraluminal Device J Synthetic Substitute K Nonautologous Tissue Substitute Y Other Device	Z No Qualifier
8 Fallopian Tube ♀	X External	Ø Drainage Device 3 Infusion Device 7 Autologous Tissue Substitute C Extraluminal Device D Intraluminal Device J Synthetic Substitute K Nonautologous Tissue Substitute	Z No Qualifier
D Uterus and Cervix ♀	Ø Open 3 Percutaneous 4 Percutaneous Endoscopic 7 Via Natural or Artificial Opening 8 Via Natural or Artificial Opening Endoscopic	Ø Drainage Device 1 Radioactive Element 3 Infusion Device 7 Autologous Tissue Substitute C Extraluminal Device D Intraluminal Device H Contraceptive Device J Synthetic Substitute K Nonautologous Tissue Substitute Y Other Device	Z No Qualifier
D Uterus and Cervix ♀	X External	Ø Drainage Device 3 Infusion Device 7 Autologous Tissue Substitute C Extraluminal Device D Intraluminal Device H Contraceptive Device J Synthetic Substitute K Nonautologous Tissue Substitute	Z No Qualifier
H Vagina and Cul-de-sac ♀	Ø Open 3 Percutaneous 4 Percutaneous Endoscopic 7 Via Natural or Artificial Opening 8 Via Natural or Artificial Opening Endoscopic	Ø Drainage Device 1 Radioactive Element 3 Infusion Device 7 Autologous Tissue Substitute D Intraluminal Device J Synthetic Substitute K Nonautologous Tissue Substitute Y Other Device	Z No Qualifier

Non-OR ØUW3X[Ø3]Z
Non-OR ØUW8X[Ø37CDJK]Z
Non-OR ØUWDX[Ø37CDHJK]Z

SECTION: Ø MEDICAL AND SURGICAL
BODY SYSTEM: U FEMALE REPRODUCTIVE SYSTEM
OPERATION: W REVISION: *(continued)*

Correcting, to the extent possible, a portion of a malfunctioning device or the position of a displaced device

Body Part	Approach	Device	Qualifier
H Vagina and Cul-de-sac ♀	X External	Ø Drainage Device 3 Infusion Device 7 Autologous Tissue Substitute D Intraluminal Device J Synthetic Substitute K Nonautologous Tissue Substitute	Z No Qualifier
M Vulva ♀	Ø Open X External	Ø Drainage Device 7 Autologous Tissue Substitute J Synthetic Substitute K Nonautologous Tissue Substitute	Z No Qualifier

Non-OR ØUWHX[Ø37DJK]Z
Non-OR ØUWMX[Ø7JK]Z

SECTION: Ø MEDICAL AND SURGICAL
BODY SYSTEM: U FEMALE REPRODUCTIVE SYSTEM
OPERATION: Y TRANSPLANTATION: Putting in or on all or a portion of a living body part taken from another individual or animal to physically take the place and/or function of all or a portion of a similar body part

Body Part	Approach	Device	Qualifier
Ø Ovary, Right ♀ 1 Ovary, Left ♀ 9 Uterus ♀	Ø Open	Z No Device	Ø Allogeneic 1 Syngeneic 2 Zooplastic

SECTION: Ø MEDICAL AND SURGICAL
BODY SYSTEM: V MALE REPRODUCTIVE SYSTEM
OPERATION: 1 BYPASS: Altering the route of passage of the contents of a tubular body part

Body Part	Approach	Device	Qualifier
N Vas Deferens, Right ♂ P Vas Deferens, Left ♂ Q Vas Deferens, Bilateral ♂	Ø Open 4 Percutaneous Endoscopic	7 Autologous Tissue Substitute J Synthetic Substitute K Nonautologous Tissue Substitute Z No Device	J Epididymis, Right K Epididymis, Left N Vas Deferens, Right P Vas Deferens, Left

SECTION: Ø MEDICAL AND SURGICAL
BODY SYSTEM: V MALE REPRODUCTIVE SYSTEM
OPERATION: 2 CHANGE: Taking out or off a device from a body part and putting back an identical or similar device in or on the same body part without cutting or puncturing the skin or a mucous membrane

Body Part	Approach	Device	Qualifier
4 Prostate and Seminal Vesicles ♂ 8 Scrotum and Tunica Vaginalis ♂ D Testis ♂ M Epididymis and Spermatic Cord ♂ R Vas Deferens ♂ S Penis ♂	X External	Ø Drainage Device Y Other Device	Z No Qualifier

Non-OR All Values

SECTION: Ø MEDICAL AND SURGICAL
BODY SYSTEM: V MALE REPRODUCTIVE SYSTEM
OPERATION: 5 DESTRUCTION: Physical eradication of all or a portion of a body part by the direct use of energy, force, or a destructive agent

Body Part	Approach	Device	Qualifier
Ø Prostate ♂	Ø Open 3 Percutaneous 4 Percutaneous Endoscopic	Z No Device	3 Laser Interstitial Thermal Therapy Z No Qualifier
Ø Prostate ♂	7 Via Natural or Artificial Opening 8 Via Natural or Artificial Opening Endoscopic	Z No Device	Z No Qualifier
1 Seminal Vesicle, Right ♂ 2 Seminal Vesicle, Left ♂ 3 Seminal Vesicles, Bilateral ♂ 6 Tunica Vaginalis, Right ♂ 7 Tunica Vaginalis, Left ♂ 9 Testis, Right ♂ B Testis, Left ♂ C Testes, Bilateral ♂	Ø Open 3 Percutaneous 4 Percutaneous Endoscopic	Z No Device	Z No Qualifier
5 Scrotum ♂ S Penis ♂ T Prepuce ♂	Ø Open 3 Percutaneous 4 Percutaneous Endoscopic X External	Z No Device	Z No Qualifier
F Spermatic Cord, Right ♂ G Spermatic Cord, Left ♂ H Spermatic Cords, Bilateral ♂ J Epididymis, Right ♂ K Epididymis, Left ♂ L Epididymis, Bilateral ♂ N Vas Deferens, Right ♂ ⓝ P Vas Deferens, Left ♂ ⓝ Q Vas Deferens, Bilateral ♂ ⓝ	Ø Open 3 Percutaneous 4 Percutaneous Endoscopic 8 Via Natural or Artificial Opening Endoscopic	Z No Device	Z No Qualifier

ⓝ ØV5[NPQ][Ø34]ZZ when Z3Ø.2 is listed as the principal diagnosis
Non-OR ØV5[NPQ][Ø34]ZZ
Non-OR ØV55[Ø34X]ZZ
Non-OR ØV5Ø[Ø34]3Z

SECTION: Ø MEDICAL AND SURGICAL
BODY SYSTEM: V MALE REPRODUCTIVE SYSTEM
OPERATION: 7 DILATION: Expanding an orifice or the lumen of a tubular body part

Body Part	Approach	Device	Qualifier
N Vas Deferens, Right ♂ P Vas Deferens, Left ♂ Q Vas Deferens, Bilateral ♂	Ø Open 3 Percutaneous 4 Percutaneous Endoscopic	D Intraluminal Device Z No Device	Z No Qualifier

SECTION: Ø MEDICAL AND SURGICAL
BODY SYSTEM: V MALE REPRODUCTIVE SYSTEM
OPERATION: 9 DRAINAGE: *(on multiple pages)*
Taking or letting out fluids and/or gases from a body part

Body Part	Approach	Device	Qualifier
Ø Prostate ♂	Ø Open 3 Percutaneous 4 Percutaneous Endoscopic 7 Via Natural or Artificial Opening 8 Via Natural or Artificial Opening Endoscopic	Ø Drainage Device	Z No Qualifier
Ø Prostate ♂	Ø Open 3 Percutaneous 4 Percutaneous Endoscopic 7 Via Natural or Artificial Opening 8 Via Natural or Artificial Opening Endoscopic	Z No Device	X Diagnostic Z No Qualifier
1 Seminal Vesicle, Right ♂ 2 Seminal Vesicle, Left ♂ 3 Seminal Vesicles, Bilateral ♂ 6 Tunica Vaginalis, Right ♂ 7 Tunica Vaginalis, Left ♂ 9 Testis, Right ♂ B Testis, Left ♂ C Testes, Bilateral ♂ F Spermatic Cord, Right ♂ G Spermatic Cord, Left ♂ H Spermatic Cords, Bilateral ♂ J Epididymis, Right ♂ K Epididymis, Left ♂ L Epididymis, Bilateral ♂ N Vas Deferens, Right ♂ P Vas Deferens, Left ♂ Q Vas Deferens, Bilateral ♂	Ø Open 3 Percutaneous 4 Percutaneous Endoscopic	Ø Drainage Device	Z No Qualifier
1 Seminal Vesicle, Right ♂ 2 Seminal Vesicle, Left ♂ 3 Seminal Vesicles, Bilateral ♂ 6 Tunica Vaginalis, Right ♂ 7 Tunica Vaginalis, Left ♂ 9 Testis, Right ♂ B Testis, Left ♂ C Testes, Bilateral ♂ F Spermatic Cord, Right ♂ G Spermatic Cord, Left ♂ H Spermatic Cords, Bilateral ♂ J Epididymis, Right ♂ K Epididymis, Left ♂ L Epididymis, Bilateral ♂ N Vas Deferens, Right ♂ P Vas Deferens, Left ♂ Q Vas Deferens, Bilateral ♂	Ø Open 3 Percutaneous 4 Percutaneous Endoscopic	Z No Device	X Diagnostic Z No Qualifier

SECTION: Ø MEDICAL AND SURGICAL
BODY SYSTEM: V MALE REPRODUCTIVE SYSTEM
OPERATION: 9 DRAINAGE: *(continued)*
Taking or letting out fluids and/or gases from a body part

Body Part	Approach	Device	Qualifier
5 Scrotum ♂ S Penis ♂ T Prepuce ♂	Ø Open 3 Percutaneous 4 Percutaneous Endoscopic X External	Ø Drainage Device	Z No Qualifier
5 Scrotum ♂ S Penis ♂ T Prepuce ♂	Ø Open 3 Percutaneous 4 Percutaneous Endoscopic X External	Z No Device	X Diagnostic Z No Qualifier

Non-OR ØV9[ST]3ØZ
Non-OR ØV9[ST]3ZZ
Non-OR ØV95[Ø34X]Z[XZ]

SECTION: Ø MEDICAL AND SURGICAL
BODY SYSTEM: V MALE REPRODUCTIVE SYSTEM
OPERATION: B EXCISION: *(on multiple pages)*
Cutting out or off, without replacement, a portion of a body part

Body Part	Approach	Device	Qualifier
Ø Prostate ♂	Ø Open 3 Percutaneous 4 Percutaneous Endoscopic 7 Via Natural or Artificial Opening 8 Via Natural or Artificial Opening Endoscopic	Z No Device	X Diagnostic Z No Qualifier
1 Seminal Vesicle, Right ♂ 2 Seminal Vesicle, Left ♂ 3 Seminal Vesicles, Bilateral ♂ 6 Tunica Vaginalis, Right ♂ 7 Tunica Vaginalis, Left ♂ 9 Testis, Right ♂ B Testis, Left ♂ C Testes, Bilateral ♂	Ø Open 3 Percutaneous 4 Percutaneous Endoscopic	Z No Device	X Diagnostic Z No Qualifier
5 Scrotum ♂ S Penis ♂ T Prepuce ♂	Ø Open 3 Percutaneous 4 Percutaneous Endoscopic X External	Z No Device	X Diagnostic Z No Qualifier

ØVB[NPQ][Ø34]ZZ when Z3Ø.2 is listed as the principal diagnosis
Non-OR ØVBØ[3478]ZX
Non-OR ØVB[1239BC][34]ZX
Non-OR ØVB[67F][Ø34]ZX
Non-OR ØVB5[Ø34X]Z[XZ]

Coding Clinic: 2Ø16, Q1, P23 – ØVBQ4ZZ

SECTION: Ø MEDICAL AND SURGICAL
BODY SYSTEM: V MALE REPRODUCTIVE SYSTEM
OPERATION: B EXCISION: *(continued)*
Cutting out or off, without replacement, a portion of a body part

Body Part	Approach	Device	Qualifier
F Spermatic Cord, Right ♂ G Spermatic Cord, Left ♂ H Spermatic Cords, Bilateral ♂ J Epididymis, Right ♂ K Epididymis, Left ♂ L Epididymis, Bilateral ♂ N Vas Deferens, Right ♂ P Vas Deferens, Left ♂ Q Vas Deferens, Bilateral ♂	Ø Open 3 Percutaneous 4 Percutaneous Endoscopic 8 Via Natural or Artificial Opening Endoscopic	Z No Device	X Diagnostic Z No Qualifier

Non-OR ØVB[GHJKL][Ø34]ZX
Non-OR ØVB[NPQ][Ø34]Z[XZ]

SECTION: Ø MEDICAL AND SURGICAL
BODY SYSTEM: V MALE REPRODUCTIVE SYSTEM
OPERATION: C EXTIRPATION: Taking or cutting out solid matter from a body part

Body Part	Approach	Device	Qualifier
Ø Prostate ♂	Ø Open 3 Percutaneous 4 Percutaneous Endoscopic 7 Via Natural or Artificial Opening 8 Via Natural or Artificial Opening Endoscopic	Z No Device	Z No Qualifier
1 Seminal Vesicle, Right ♂ 2 Seminal Vesicle, Left ♂ 3 Seminal Vesicles, Bilateral ♂ 6 Tunica Vaginalis, Right ♂ 7 Tunica Vaginalis, Left ♂ 9 Testis, Right ♂ B Testis, Left ♂ C Testes, Bilateral ♂ F Spermatic Cord, Right ♂ G Spermatic Cord, Left ♂ H Spermatic Cords, Bilateral ♂ J Epididymis, Right ♂ K Epididymis, Left ♂ L Epididymis, Bilateral ♂ N Vas Deferens, Right ♂ P Vas Deferens, Left ♂ Q Vas Deferens, Bilateral ♂	Ø Open 3 Percutaneous 4 Percutaneous Endoscopic	Z No Device	Z No Qualifier
5 Scrotum ♂ S Penis ♂ T Prepuce ♂	Ø Open 3 Percutaneous 4 Percutaneous Endoscopic X External	Z No Device	Z No Qualifier

Non-OR ØVC[67NPQ][Ø34]ZZ
Non-OR ØVC5[Ø34X]ZZ
Non-OR ØVCSXZZ

SECTION: Ø MEDICAL AND SURGICAL
BODY SYSTEM: V MALE REPRODUCTIVE SYSTEM
OPERATION: H INSERTION: Putting in a nonbiological appliance that monitors, assists, performs, or prevents a physiological function but does not physically take the place of a body part

Body Part	Approach	Device	Qualifier
Ø Prostate ♂	Ø Open 3 Percutaneous 4 Percutaneous Endoscopic 7 Via Natural or Artificial Opening 8 Via Natural or Artificial Opening Endoscopic	1 Radioactive Element	Z No Qualifier
4 Prostate and Seminal Vesicles ♂ 8 Scrotum and Tunica Vaginalis ♂ M Epididymis and Spermatic Cord ♂ R Vas Deferens ♂	Ø Open 3 Percutaneous 4 Percutaneous Endoscopic 7 Via Natural or Artificial Opening 8 Via Natural or Artificial Opening Endoscopic	3 Infusion Device Y Other Device	Z No Qualifier
D Testis	Ø Open 3 Percutaneous 4 Percutaneous Endoscopic 7 Via Natural or Artificial Opening 8 Via Natural or Artificial Opening Endoscopic	1 Radioactive Element 3 Infusion Device Y Other Device	Z No Qualifier
S Penis ♂	Ø Open 3 Percutaneous 4 Percutaneous Endoscopic	3 Infusion Device Y Other Device	Z No Qualifier
S Penis ♂	7 Via Natural or Artificial Opening 8 Via Natural or Artificial Opening Endoscopic	Y Other Device	Z No Qualifier
S Penis ♂	X External	3 Infusion Device	Z No Qualifier

DRG Non-OR ØVH[48DMR][Ø3478]3Z
DRG Non-OR ØVHS[Ø34]3Z
DRG Non-OR ØVHSX3Z

SECTION: Ø MEDICAL AND SURGICAL
BODY SYSTEM: V MALE REPRODUCTIVE SYSTEM
OPERATION: J INSPECTION: Visually and/or manually exploring a body part

Body Part	Approach	Device	Qualifier
4 Prostate and Seminal Vesicles ♂ 8 Scrotum and Tunica Vaginalis ♂ D Testis ♂ M Epididymis and Spermatic Cord ♂ R Vas Deferens ♂ S Penis ♂	Ø Open 3 Percutaneous 4 Percutaneous Endoscopic X External	Z No Device	Z No Qualifier

Non-OR ØVJ[4DMR][3X]ZZ
Non-OR ØVJ[8S][Ø34X]ZZ

SECTION: Ø MEDICAL AND SURGICAL
BODY SYSTEM: V MALE REPRODUCTIVE SYSTEM
OPERATION: L OCCLUSION: Completely closing an orifice or the lumen of a tubular body part

Body Part	Approach	Device	Qualifier
F Spermatic Cord, Right ♂ G Spermatic Cord, Left ♂ H Spermatic Cords, Bilateral ♂ N Vas Deferens, Right ♂ P Vas Deferens, Left ♂ Q Vas Deferens, Bilateral ♂	Ø Open 3 Percutaneous 4 Percutaneous Endoscopic 8 Via Natural or Artificial Opening Endoscopic	C Extraluminal Device D Intraluminal Device Z No Device	Z No Qualifier

ØVL[FGH][Ø34][CDZ]Z when Z3Ø.2 is listed as the principal diagnosis
ØVL[NPQ][Ø34][CZ]Z when Z3Ø.2 is listed as the principal diagnosis
Non-OR ØVL[FGH][Ø34][CDZ]Z
Non-OR ØVL[NPQ][Ø34][CZ]Z

SECTION: Ø MEDICAL AND SURGICAL
BODY SYSTEM: V MALE REPRODUCTIVE SYSTEM
OPERATION: M REATTACHMENT: Putting back in or on all or a portion of a separated body part to its normal location or other suitable location

Body Part	Approach	Device	Qualifier
5 Scrotum ♂ S Penis ♂	X External	Z No Device	Z No Qualifier
6 Tunica Vaginalis, Right ♂ 7 Tunica Vaginalis, Left ♂ 9 Testis, Right ♂ B Testis, Left ♂ C Testes, Bilateral ♂ F Spermatic Cord, Right ♂ G Spermatic Cord, Left ♂ H Spermatic Cords, Bilateral ♂	Ø Open 4 Percutaneous Endoscopic	Z No Device	Z No Qualifier

SECTION: Ø MEDICAL AND SURGICAL
BODY SYSTEM: V MALE REPRODUCTIVE SYSTEM
OPERATION: N RELEASE: Freeing a body part from an abnormal physical restraint by cutting or by the use of force

Body Part	Approach	Device	Qualifier
Ø Prostate ♂	Ø Open 3 Percutaneous 4 Percutaneous Endoscopic 7 Via Natural or Artificial Opening 8 Via Natural or Artificial Opening Endoscopic	Z No Device	Z No Qualifier
1 Seminal Vesicle, Right ♂ 2 Seminal Vesicle, Left ♂ 3 Seminal Vesicles, Bilateral ♂ 6 Tunica Vaginalis, Right ♂ 7 Tunica Vaginalis, Left ♂ 9 Testis, Right ♂ B Testis, Left ♂ C Testes, Bilateral ♂	Ø Open 3 Percutaneous 4 Percutaneous Endoscopic	Z No Device	Z No Qualifier
5 Scrotum ♂ S Penis ♂ T Prepuce ♂	Ø Open 3 Percutaneous 4 Percutaneous Endoscopic X External	Z No Device	Z No Qualifier
F Spermatic Cord, Right ♂ G Spermatic Cord, Left ♂ H Spermatic Cords, Bilateral ♂ J Epididymis, Right ♂ K Epididymis, Left ♂ L Epididymis, Bilateral ♂ N Vas Deferens, Right ♂ P Vas Deferens, Left ♂ Q Vas Deferens, Bilateral ♂	Ø Open 3 Percutaneous 4 Percutaneous Endoscopic 8 Via Natural or Artificial Opening Endoscopic	Z No Device	Z No Qualifier

Non-OR ØVN[9BC][Ø34]ZZ
Non-OR ØVNT[Ø34X]ZZ

SECTION: Ø MEDICAL AND SURGICAL
BODY SYSTEM: V MALE REPRODUCTIVE SYSTEM
OPERATION: P REMOVAL: Taking out or off a device from a body part

Body Part	Approach	Device	Qualifier
4 Prostate and Seminal Vesicles ♂	Ø Open 3 Percutaneous 4 Percutaneous Endoscopic 7 Via Natural or Artificial Opening 8 Via Natural or Artificial Opening Endoscopic	Ø Drainage Device 1 Radioactive Element 3 Infusion Device 7 Autologous Tissue Substitute J Synthetic Substitute K Nonautologous Tissue Substitute Y Other Device	Z No Qualifier
4 Prostate and Seminal Vesicles ♂	X External	Ø Drainage Device 1 Radioactive Element 3 Infusion Device	Z No Qualifier
8 Scrotum and Tunica Vaginalis ♂ D Testis ♂ S Penis ♂	Ø Open 3 Percutaneous 4 Percutaneous Endoscopic 7 Via Natural or Artificial Opening 8 Via Natural or Artificial Opening Endoscopic	Ø Drainage Device 3 Infusion Device 7 Autologous Tissue Substitute J Synthetic Substitute K Nonautologous Tissue Substitute Y Other Device	Z No Qualifier
8 Scrotum and Tunica Vaginalis ♂ D Testis ♂ S Penis ♂	X External	Ø Drainage Device 3 Infusion Device	Z No Qualifier
M Epididymis and Spermatic Cord ♂	Ø Open 3 Percutaneous 4 Percutaneous Endoscopic 7 Via Natural or Artificial Opening 8 Via Natural or Artificial Opening Endoscopic	Ø Drainage Device 3 Infusion Device 7 Autologous Tissue Substitute C Extraluminal Device J Synthetic Substitute K Nonautologous Tissue Substitute Y Other Device	Z No Qualifier
M Epididymis and Spermatic Cord ♂	X External	Ø Drainage Device 3 Infusion Device	Z No Qualifier
R Vas Deferens ♂	Ø Open 3 Percutaneous 4 Percutaneous Endoscopic 7 Via Natural or Artificial Opening 8 Via Natural or Artificial Opening Endoscopic	Ø Drainage Device 3 Infusion Device 7 Autologous Tissue Substitute C Extraluminal Device D Intraluminal Device J Synthetic Substitute K Nonautologous Tissue Substitute Y Other Device	Z No Qualifier
R Vas Deferens ♂	X External	Ø Drainage Device 3 Infusion Device D Intraluminal Device	Z No Qualifier

Non-OR ØVP4[78][Ø3]Z
Non-OR ØVP4X[Ø13]Z
Non-OR ØVP8[Ø3478][Ø37JK]Z
Non-OR ØVPD[78][Ø3]Z
Non-OR ØVPS[78][Ø3]Z
Non-OR ØVP[8DS]X[Ø3]Z
Non-OR ØVPM[78][Ø3]Z
Non-OR ØVPMX[Ø3]Z
Non-OR ØVPR[Ø3478][Ø37CDJK]Z
Non-OR ØVPR[78]DZ
Non-OR ØVPRX[Ø3D]Z

Coding Clinic: 2016, Q2, P28 – ØVPSØJZ

SECTION: Ø MEDICAL AND SURGICAL
BODY SYSTEM: V MALE REPRODUCTIVE SYSTEM
OPERATION: Q REPAIR: Restoring, to the extent possible, a body part to its normal anatomic structure and function

Body Part	Approach	Device	Qualifier
Ø Prostate ♂	Ø Open 3 Percutaneous 4 Percutaneous Endoscopic 7 Via Natural or Artificial Opening 8 Via Natural or Artificial Opening Endoscopic	Z No Device	Z No Qualifier
1 Seminal Vesicle, Right ♂ 2 Seminal Vesicle, Left ♂ 3 Seminal Vesicles, Bilateral ♂ 6 Tunica Vaginalis, Right ♂ 7 Tunica Vaginalis, Left ♂ 9 Testis, Right ♂ B Testis, Left ♂ C Testes, Bilateral ♂	Ø Open 3 Percutaneous 4 Percutaneous Endoscopic	Z No Device	Z No Qualifier
5 Scrotum ♂ S Penis ♂ T Prepuce ♂	Ø Open 3 Percutaneous 4 Percutaneous Endoscopic X External	Z No Device	Z No Qualifier
F Spermatic Cord, Right ♂ G Spermatic Cord, Left ♂ H Spermatic Cords, Bilateral ♂ J Epididymis, Right ♂ K Epididymis, Left ♂ L Epididymis, Bilateral ♂ N Vas Deferens, Right ♂ P Vas Deferens, Left ♂ Q Vas Deferens, Bilateral ♂	Ø Open 3 Percutaneous 4 Percutaneous Endoscopic 8 Via Natural or Artificial Opening Endoscopic	Z No Device	Z No Qualifier

Non-OR ØVQ[67][Ø34]ZZ
Non-OR ØVQ5[Ø34X]ZZ

SECTION: Ø MEDICAL AND SURGICAL
BODY SYSTEM: V MALE REPRODUCTIVE SYSTEM
OPERATION: R REPLACEMENT: Putting in or on biological or synthetic material that physically takes the place and/or function of all or a portion of a body part

Body Part	Approach	Device	Qualifier
9 Testis, Right ♂ B Testis, Left ♂ C Testis, Bilateral ♂	Ø Open	J Synthetic Substitute	Z No Qualifier

SECTION: Ø MEDICAL AND SURGICAL
BODY SYSTEM: V MALE REPRODUCTIVE SYSTEM
OPERATION: S REPOSITION: Moving to its normal location or other suitable location all or a portion of a body part

Body Part	Approach	Device	Qualifier
9 Testis, Right ♂ B Testis, Left ♂ C Testes, Bilateral ♂ F Spermatic Cord, Right ♂ G Spermatic Cord, Left ♂ H Spermatic Cords, Bilateral ♂	Ø Open 3 Percutaneous 4 Percutaneous Endoscopic 8 Via Natural or Artificial Opening Endoscopic	Z No Device	Z No Qualifier

SECTION: Ø MEDICAL AND SURGICAL
BODY SYSTEM: V MALE REPRODUCTIVE SYSTEM
OPERATION: T RESECTION: Cutting out or off, without replacement, all of a body part

Body Part	Approach	Device	Qualifier
Ø Prostate ♂ ⊞	Ø Open 4 Percutaneous Endoscopic 7 Via Natural or Artificial Opening 8 Via Natural or Artificial Opening Endoscopic	Z No Device	Z No Qualifier
1 Seminal Vesicle, Right ♂ 2 Seminal Vesicle, Left ♂ 3 Seminal Vesicles, Bilateral ♂ ⊞ 6 Tunica Vaginalis, Right ♂ 7 Tunica Vaginalis, Left ♂ 9 Testis, Right ♂ B Testis, Left ♂ C Testes, Bilateral ♂ F Spermatic Cord, Right ♂ G Spermatic Cord, Left ♂ H Spermatic Cords, Bilateral ♂ J Epididymis, Right ♂ K Epididymis, Left ♂ L Epididymis, Bilateral ♂ N Vas Deferens, Right ♂ LC P Vas Deferens, Left ♂ LC Q Vas Deferens, Bilateral ♂ LC	Ø Open 4 Percutaneous Endoscopic	Z No Device	Z No Qualifier
5 Scrotum ♂ S Penis ♂ T Prepuce ♂	Ø Open 4 Percutaneous Endoscopic X External	Z No Device	Z No Qualifier

LC ØVT[NPQ][Ø4]ZZ when Z3Ø.2 is listed as the principal diagnosis
⊞ ØVTØ[Ø478]ZZ
⊞ ØVT3[Ø4]ZZ
Non-OR ØVT[NPQ][Ø4]ZZ
Non-OR ØVT[5T][Ø4X]ZZ

SECTION: Ø MEDICAL AND SURGICAL
BODY SYSTEM: V MALE REPRODUCTIVE SYSTEM
OPERATION: U SUPPLEMENT: Putting in or on biological or synthetic material that physically reinforces and/or augments the function of a portion of a body part

Body Part	Approach	Device	Qualifier
1 Seminal Vesicle, Right ♂ 2 Seminal Vesicle, Left ♂ 3 Seminal Vesicles, Bilateral ♂ 6 Tunica Vaginalis, Right ♂ 7 Tunica Vaginalis, Left ♂ F Spermatic Cord, Right ♂ G Spermatic Cord, Left ♂ H Spermatic Cords, Bilateral ♂ J Epididymis, Right ♂ K Epididymis, Left ♂ L Epididymis, Bilateral ♂ N Vas Deferens, Right ♂ P Vas Deferens, Left ♂ Q Vas Deferens, Bilateral ♂	Ø Open 4 Percutaneous Endoscopic 8 Via Natural or Artificial Opening Endoscopic	7 Autologous Tissue Substitute J Synthetic Substitute K Nonautologous Tissue Substitute	Z No Qualifier
5 Scrotum ♂ S Penis ♂ T Prepuce ♂	Ø Open 4 Percutaneous Endoscopic X External	7 Autologous Tissue Substitute J Synthetic Substitute K Nonautologous Tissue Substitute	Z No Qualifier
9 Testis, Right ♂ B Testis, Left ♂ C Testis, Bilateral ♂	Ø Open	7 Autologous Tissue Substitute J Synthetic Substitute K Nonautologous Tissue Substitute	Z No Qualifier

Non-OR ØVUSX[7JK]Z

Coding Clinic: 2016, Q2, P29; 2015, Q3, P25 – ØVUSØJZ

SECTION: Ø MEDICAL AND SURGICAL
BODY SYSTEM: V MALE REPRODUCTIVE SYSTEM
OPERATION: W REVISION: Correcting, to the extent possible, a portion of a malfunctioning device or the position of a displaced device

Body Part	Approach	Device	Qualifier
4 Prostate and Seminal Vesicles ♂ 8 Scrotum and Tunica Vaginalis ♂ D Testis @ ♂ S Penis @ ♂	Ø Open 3 Percutaneous 4 Percutaneous Endoscopic 7 Via Natural or Artificial Opening 8 Via Natural or Artificial Opening Endoscopic	Ø Drainage Device 3 Infusion Device 7 Autologous Tissue Substitute J Synthetic Substitute K Nonautologous Tissue Substitute Y Other Device	Z No Qualifier
4 Prostate and Seminal Vesicles ♂ 8 Scrotum and Tunica Vaginalis ♂ D Testis ♂ S Penis ♂	X External	Ø Drainage Device 3 Infusion Device 7 Autologous Tissue Substitute J Synthetic Substitute K Nonautologous Tissue Substitute	Z No Qualifier
M Epididymis and Spermatic Cord ♂	Ø Open 3 Percutaneous 4 Percutaneous Endoscopic 7 Via Natural or Artificial Opening 8 Via Natural or Artificial Opening Endoscopic	Ø Drainage Device 3 Infusion Device 7 Autologous Tissue Substitute C Extraluminal Device J Synthetic Substitute K Nonautologous Tissue Substitute Y Other Device	Z No Qualifier
M Epididymis and Spermatic Cord ♂	X External	Ø Drainage Device 3 Infusion Device 7 Autologous Tissue Substitute C Extraluminal Device J Synthetic Substitute K Nonautologous Tissue Substitute	Z No Qualifier
R Vas Deferens ♂	Ø Open 3 Percutaneous 4 Percutaneous Endoscopic 7 Via Natural or Artificial Opening 8 Via Natural or Artificial Opening Endoscopic	Ø Drainage Device 3 Infusion Device 7 Autologous Tissue Substitute C Extraluminal Device D Intraluminal Device J Synthetic Substitute K Nonautologous Tissue Substitute Y Other Device	Z No Qualifier
R Vas Deferens ♂	X External	Ø Drainage Device 3 Infusion Device 7 Autologous Tissue Substitute C Extraluminal Device D Intraluminal Device J Synthetic Substitute K Nonautologous Tissue Substitute	Z No Qualifier

Non-OR ØVW[4DS]X[Ø37JK]Z
Non-OR ØVW8[Ø3478][Ø37JK]Z
Non-OR ØVW8X[Ø37]Z
Non-OR ØVWMX[Ø37CJK]Z
Non-OR ØVWR[Ø3478][Ø37CDJK]Z
Non-OR ØVWRX[Ø37CDJK]Z

SECTION: Ø MEDICAL AND SURGICAL
BODY SYSTEM: V MALE REPRODUCTIVE SYSTEM
OPERATION: X TRANSFER: Moving, without taking out, all or a portion of a body part to another location to take over the function of all or a portion of a body part

Body Part	Approach	Device	Qualifier
T Prepuce ♂	Ø Open X External	Z No Device	D Urethra S Penis

SECTION: Ø MEDICAL AND SURGICAL
BODY SYSTEM: V MALE REPRODUCTIVE SYSTEM
OPERATION: Y TRANSPLANTATION: Putting in or on all or a portion of a living body part taken from another individual or animal to physically take the place and/or function of all or a portion of a similar body part

Body Part	Approach	Device	Qualifier
5 Scrotum S Penis	Ø Open	Z No Device	Ø Allogeneic 1 Syngeneic 2 Zooplastic

Coding Clinic: 2020, Q1, P31 – ØVYSØ7Z

SECTION: Ø MEDICAL AND SURGICAL
BODY SYSTEM: W ANATOMICAL REGIONS, GENERAL
OPERATION: Ø ALTERATION: Modifying the anatomic structure of a body part without affecting the function of the body part

Body Part	Approach	Device	Qualifier
Ø Head 2 Face 4 Upper Jaw 5 Lower Jaw 6 Neck 8 Chest Wall F Abdominal Wall K Upper Back L Lower Back M Perineum, Male ♂ N Perineum, Female ♀	Ø Open 3 Percutaneous 4 Percutaneous Endoscopic	7 Autologous Tissue Substitute J Synthetic Substitute K Nonautologous Tissue Substitute Z No Device	Z No Qualifier

Coding Clinic: 2Ø15, Q1, P31 – ØWØ2ØZZ

SECTION: Ø MEDICAL AND SURGICAL
BODY SYSTEM: W ANATOMICAL REGIONS, GENERAL
OPERATION: 1 BYPASS: Altering the route of passage of the contents of a tubular body part

Body Part	Approach	Device	Qualifier
1 Cranial Cavity	Ø Open	J Synthetic Substitute	9 Pleural Cavity, Right B Pleural Cavity, Left G Peritoneal Cavity J Pelvic Cavity
9 Pleural Cavity, Right B Pleural Cavity, Left J Pelvic Cavity	Ø Open 3 Percutaneous 4 Percutaneous Endoscopic	J Synthetic Substitute	4 Cutaneous 9 Pleural Cavity, Right B Pleural Cavity, Left G Peritoneal Cavity J Pelvic Cavity W Upper Vein Y Lower Vein
G Peritoneal Cavity	Ø Open 3 Percutaneous 4 Percutaneous Endoscopic	J Synthetic Substitute	4 Cutaneous 6 Bladder 9 Pleural Cavity, Right B Pleural Cavity, Left G Peritoneal Cavity J Pelvic Cavity W Upper Vein Y Lower Vein
9 Pleural Cavity, Right B Pleural Cavity, Left G Peritoneal Cavity J Pelvic Cavity	3 Percutaneous	J Synthetic Substitute	4 Cutaneous

Non-OR ØW1[9B][Ø4]J[4GY]
Non-OR ØW1G[Ø4]J[9BGJ]
Non-OR ØW1J[Ø4]J[4Y]
Non-OR ØW1[9BGJ]3J4

Coding Clinic: 2Ø18, Q4, P42 – ØW1G3JW

SECTION: Ø MEDICAL AND SURGICAL
BODY SYSTEM: W ANATOMICAL REGIONS, GENERAL
OPERATION: 2 **CHANGE:** Taking out or off a device from a body part and putting back an identical or similar device in or on the same body part without cutting or puncturing the skin or a mucous membrane

Body Part	Approach	Device	Qualifier
Ø Head 1 Cranial Cavity 2 Face 4 Upper Jaw 5 Lower Jaw 6 Neck 8 Chest Wall 9 Pleural Cavity, Right B Pleural Cavity, Left C Mediastinum D Pericardial Cavity F Abdominal Wall G Peritoneal Cavity H Retroperitoneum J Pelvic Cavity K Upper Back L Lower Back M Perineum, Male ♂ N Perineum, Female ♀	X External	Ø Drainage Device Y Other Device	Z No Qualifier

Non-OR All Values

SECTION: Ø MEDICAL AND SURGICAL
BODY SYSTEM: W ANATOMICAL REGIONS, GENERAL
OPERATION: 3 **CONTROL:** *(on multiple pages)*
Stopping, or attempting to stop, postprocedure or other acute bleeding

Body Part	Approach	Device	Qualifier
Ø Head 1 Cranial Cavity 2 Face 3 Oral Cavity and Throat 4 Upper Jaw 5 Lower Jaw 6 Neck 8 Chest Wall 9 Pleural Cavity, Right B Pleural Cavity, Left C Mediastinum D Pericardial Cavity F Abdominal Wall G Peritoneal Cavity H Retroperitoneum J Pelvic Cavity K Upper Back L Lower Back M Perineum, Male ♂ N Perineum, Female ♀	Ø Open 3 Percutaneous 4 Percutaneous Endoscopic	Z No Device	Z No Qualifier

Ø: M/S W: ANATOMICAL REGIONS, GENERAL 2: CHANGE 3: CONTROL

SECTION: Ø MEDICAL AND SURGICAL
BODY SYSTEM: W ANATOMICAL REGIONS, GENERAL
OPERATION: 3 **CONTROL:** *(continued)*
Stopping, or attempting to stop, postprocedure or other acute bleeding

Body Part	Approach	Device	Qualifier
3 Oral Cavity and Throat	Ø Open 3 Percutaneous 4 Percutaneous Endoscopic 7 Via Natural or Artificial Opening 8 Via Natural or Artificial Opening Endoscopic X External	Z No Device	Z No Qualifier
P Gastrointestinal Tract Q Respiratory Tract R Genitourinary Tract	Ø Open 3 Percutaneous 4 Percutaneous Endoscopic 7 Via Natural or Artificial Opening 8 Via Natural or Artificial Opening Endoscopic	Z No Device	Z No Qualifier

Non-OR ØW3P8ZZ

Coding Clinic: 2Ø18, Q1, P19-2Ø – ØW3[PQ]8ZZ
Coding Clinic: 2Ø23, Q2, P27 – ØW3P8ZZ

SECTION: Ø MEDICAL AND SURGICAL
BODY SYSTEM: W ANATOMICAL REGIONS, GENERAL
OPERATION: 4 **CREATION:** Putting in or on biological or synthetic material to form a new body part that to the extent possible replicates the anatomic structure or function of an absent body part

Body Part	Approach	Device	Qualifier
M Perineum, Male ♂	Ø Open	7 Autologous Tissue Substitute J Synthetic Substitute K Nonautologous Tissue Substitute	Ø Vagina
N Perineum, Female ♀	Ø Open	7 Autologous Tissue Substitute J Synthetic Substitute K Nonautologous Tissue Substitute	1 Penis

Coding Clinic: 2Ø16, Q4, P1Ø1 – ØW4

SECTION: Ø MEDICAL AND SURGICAL
BODY SYSTEM: W ANATOMICAL REGIONS, GENERAL
OPERATION: 8 **DIVISION:** Cutting into a body part, without draining fluids and/or gases from the body part, in order to separate or transect a body part

Body Part	Approach	Device	Qualifier
N Perineum, Female ♀	X External	Z No Device	Z No Qualifier

Non-OR ØW8NXZZ

SECTION: Ø MEDICAL AND SURGICAL
BODY SYSTEM: W ANATOMICAL REGIONS, GENERAL
OPERATION: 9 DRAINAGE: Taking or letting out fluids and/or gases from a body part

Body Part	Approach	Device	Qualifier
Ø Head 1 Cranial Cavity 2 Face 3 Oral Cavity and Throat 4 Upper Jaw 5 Lower Jaw 8 Chest Wall 9 Pleural Cavity, Right B Pleural Cavity, Left C Mediastinum D Pericardial Cavity F Abdominal Wall G Peritoneal Cavity H Retroperitoneum K Upper Back L Lower Back M Perineum, Male ♂ N Perineum, Female ♀	Ø Open 3 Percutaneous 4 Percutaneous Endoscopic	Ø Drainage Device	Z No Qualifier
Ø Head 1 Cranial Cavity 2 Face 3 Oral Cavity and Throat 4 Upper Jaw 5 Lower Jaw 8 Chest Wall 9 Pleural Cavity, Right B Pleural Cavity, Left C Mediastinum D Pericardial Cavity F Abdominal Wall G Peritoneal Cavity H Retroperitoneum K Upper Back L Lower Back M Perineum, Male ♂ N Perineum, Female ♀	Ø Open 3 Percutaneous 4 Percutaneous Endoscopic	Z No Device	X Diagnostic Z No Qualifier
6 Neck J Pelvic Cavity	Ø Open 3 Percutaneous 4 Percutaneous Endoscopic 7 Via Natural or Artificial Opening 8 Via Natural or Artificial Opening Endoscopic	Ø Drainage Device	Z No Qualifier
6 Neck J Pelvic Cavity	Ø Open 3 Percutaneous 4 Percutaneous Endoscopic 7 Via Natural or Artificial Opening 8 Via Natural or Artificial Opening Endoscopic	Z No Device	X Diagnostic Z No Qualifier

DRG Non-OR ØW9H3ØZ
DRG Non-OR ØW9H3ZZ
Non-OR ØW9[Ø8KLM][Ø34]ØZ
Non-OR ØW9[9B][Ø3]ØZ
Non-OR ØW9[1DFG][34]ØZ
Non-OR ØW9J3ØZ
Non-OR ØW9[Ø234568KLMN][Ø34]ZX
Non-OR ØW9G3ZX
Non-OR ØW9[9B][Ø3]ZZ
Non-OR ØW9[Ø8KLM][Ø34]ZZ
Non-OR ØW9[9B][Ø3]ZZ
Non-OR ØW9[1CD][34]ZX
Non-OR ØW9[1DFG][34]ZZ
Non-OR ØW9J3ZZ

Coding Clinic: 2017, Q2, P17 – 0W930ZZ
Coding Clinic: 2017, Q3, P13 – ØW9G3ZZ
Coding Clinic: 2021, Q3, P18,22 – ØW960ZZ
Coding Clinic: 2021, Q3, P27 – ØW9DØZZ
Coding Clinic: 2022, Q4, P57 – ØW968ZZ

SECTION: Ø MEDICAL AND SURGICAL
BODY SYSTEM: W ANATOMICAL REGIONS, GENERAL
OPERATION: B EXCISION: Cutting out or off, without replacement, a portion of a body part

Body Part	Approach	Device	Qualifier
Ø Head 2 Face 3 Oral Cavity and Throat 4 Upper Jaw 5 Lower Jaw 8 Chest Wall K Upper Back L Lower Back M Perineum, Male ♂ N Perineum, Female ♀	Ø Open 3 Percutaneous 4 Percutaneous Endoscopic X External	Z No Device	X Diagnostic Z No Qualifier
6 Neck F Abdominal Wall	Ø Open 3 Percutaneous 4 Percutaneous Endoscopic	Z No Device	X Diagnostic Z No Qualifier
6 Neck F Abdominal Wall	X External	Z No Device	2 Stoma X Diagnostic Z No Qualifier
C Mediastinum H Retroperitoneum	Ø Open 3 Percutaneous 4 Percutaneous Endoscopic	Z No Device	X Diagnostic Z No Qualifier

Non-OR ØWB[Ø2458KLM][Ø34X]ZX
Non-OR ØWB6[Ø34]ZX
Non-OR ØWB6XZX
Non-OR ØWB[CH][34]ZX

Coding Clinic: 2Ø16, Q1, P22 – ØWBF4ZZ
Coding Clinic: 2Ø19, Q1, P27 – ØWBHØZZ
Coding Clinic: 2Ø21, Q3, P21 – ØWB6ØZZ

SECTION: Ø MEDICAL AND SURGICAL
BODY SYSTEM: W ANATOMICAL REGIONS, GENERAL
OPERATION: C EXTIRPATION: Taking or cutting out solid matter from a body part

Body Part	Approach	Device	Qualifier
1 Cranial Cavity 3 Oral Cavity and Throat 9 Pleural Cavity, Right B Pleural Cavity, Left C Mediastinum D Pericardial Cavity G Peritoneal Cavity H Retroperitoneum J Pelvic Cavity	Ø Open 3 Percutaneous 4 Percutaneous Endoscopic X External	Z No Device	Z No Qualifier
4 Upper Jaw 5 Lower Jaw	Ø Open 3 Percutaneous 4 Percutaneous Endoscopic	Z No Device	Z No Qualifier
P Gastrointestinal Tract Q Respiratory Tract R Genitourinary Tract	Ø Open 3 Percutaneous 4 Percutaneous Endoscopic 7 Via Natural or Artificial Opening 8 Via Natural or Artificial Opening Endoscopic X External	Z No Device	Z No Qualifier

Non-OR ØWC[13]XZZ
Non-OR ØWC[9B][Ø34X]ZZ
Non-OR ØWC[CDGJ]XZZ
Non-OR ØWCP[78X]ZZ
Non-OR ØWCQ[Ø34X]ZZ
Non-OR ØWCR[78X]ZZ

Coding Clinic: 2Ø17, Q2, P16 – ØWC3ØZZ
Coding Clinic: 2Ø22, Q1, P43 – ØWC[HJ]ØZZ

SECTION: Ø MEDICAL AND SURGICAL
BODY SYSTEM: W ANATOMICAL REGIONS, GENERAL
OPERATION: F FRAGMENTATION: Breaking solid matter in a body part into pieces

Body Part	Approach	Device	Qualifier
1 Cranial Cavity 3 Oral Cavity and Throat 9 Pleural Cavity, Right B Pleural Cavity, Left C Mediastinum D Pericardial Cavity G Peritoneal Cavity J Pelvic Cavity	Ø Open 3 Percutaneous 4 Percutaneous Endoscopic X External	Z No Device	Z No Qualifier
P Gastrointestinal Tract Q Respiratory Tract R Genitourinary Tract	Ø Open 3 Percutaneous 4 Percutaneous Endoscopic 7 Via Natural or Artificial Opening 8 Via Natural or Artificial Opening Endoscopic X External	Z No Device	Z No Qualifier

ØWF[139BCGJ]XZZ
ØWF[PQ]XZZ
Non-OR ØWF[139BCG]XZZ
Non-OR ØWFJ[Ø34X]ZZ
Non-OR ØWFP[Ø3478X]ZZ
Non-OR ØWFQXZZ
Non-OR ØWFR[Ø3478]ZZ

SECTION: Ø MEDICAL AND SURGICAL
BODY SYSTEM: W ANATOMICAL REGIONS, GENERAL
OPERATION: H INSERTION: Putting in a nonbiological appliance that monitors, assists, performs, or prevents a physiological function but does not physically take the place of a body part

Body Part	Approach	Device	Qualifier
Ø Head 1 Cranial Cavity 2 Face 3 Oral Cavity and Throat 4 Upper Jaw 5 Lower Jaw 6 Neck 8 Chest Wall 9 Pleural Cavity, Right B Pleural Cavity, Left ~~C Mediastinum~~ D Pericardial Cavity F Abdominal Wall G Peritoneal Cavity H Retroperitoneum J Pelvic Cavity K Upper Back L Lower Back M Perineum, Male ♂ N Perineum, Female ♀	Ø Open 3 Percutaneous 4 Percutaneous Endoscopic	1 Radioactive Element 3 Infusion Device Y Other Device	Z No Qualifier
C Mediastinum	Ø Open 3 Percutaneous 4 Percutaneous Endoscopic	1 Radioactive Element 3 Infusion Device G Defibrillator Lead Y Other Device	Z No Qualifier
P Gastrointestinal Tract Q Respiratory Tract R Genitourinary Tract	Ø Open 3 Percutaneous 4 Percutaneous Endoscopic 7 Via Natural or Artificial Opening 8 Via Natural or Artificial Opening Endoscopic	1 Radioactive Element 3 Infusion Device Y Other Device	Z No Qualifier

DRG Non-OR ØWH[Ø2456KLM][Ø34][3Y]Z
Non-OR ØWH1[Ø34]3Z
Non-OR ØWH[89B][Ø34][3Y]Z
Non-OR ØWHPØYZ
Non-OR ØWHP[3478][3Y]Z
Non-OR ØWHQ[Ø78][3Y]Z
Non-OR ØWHR[Ø3478][3Y]Z

Coding Clinic: 2Ø16, Q2, P14 – ØWHG33Z
Coding Clinic: 2Ø17, Q4, P1Ø4 – ØUHD7YZ
Coding Clinic: 2Ø19, Q4, P44 – ØWHJØ1Z
Coding Clinic: 2Ø21, Q2, P14 – ØWHGØ3Z

SECTION: Ø MEDICAL AND SURGICAL
BODY SYSTEM: W ANATOMICAL REGIONS, GENERAL
OPERATION: J INSPECTION: Visually and/or manually exploring a body part

Body Part	Approach	Device	Qualifier
Ø Head 2 Face 3 Oral Cavity and Throat 4 Upper Jaw 5 Lower Jaw 6 Neck 8 Chest Wall F Abdominal Wall K Upper Back L Lower Back M Perineum, Male ♂ N Perineum, Female ♀	Ø Open 3 Percutaneous 4 Percutaneous Endoscopic X External	Z No Device	Z No Qualifier
1 Cranial Cavity 9 Pleural Cavity, Right B Pleural Cavity, Left C Mediastinum D Pericardial Cavity G Peritoneal Cavity H Retroperitoneum J Pelvic Cavity	Ø Open 3 Percutaneous 4 Percutaneous Endoscopic	Z No Device	Z No Qualifier
P Gastrointestinal Tract Q Respiratory Tract R Genitourinary Tract	Ø Open 3 Percutaneous 4 Percutaneous Endoscopic 7 Via Natural or Artificial Opening 8 Via Natural or Artificial Opening Endoscopic	Z No Device	Z No Qualifier

DRG Non-OR ØWJ[Ø245KLM]ØZZ
DRG Non-OR ØWJF3ZZ
DRG Non-OR ØWJM[Ø4]ZZ
DRG Non-OR ØWJ[1GHJ]3ZZ
DRG Non-OR ØWJ[PR][378]ZZ
Non-OR ØWJ[Ø245KL][34X]ZZ
Non-OR ØWJ[68]3ZZ
Non-OR ØWJ3[Ø34X]ZZ
Non-OR ØWJ[68FN]XZZ
Non-OR OWJM[3X]ZZ
Non-OR ØWJ[9BC]3ZZ
Non-OR ØWJD[Ø3]ZZ
Non-OR ØWJQ[378]ZZ
Coding Clinic: 2Ø13, Q2, P37 – ØWJG4ZZ
Coding Clinic: 2Ø21, Q2, P2Ø; 2Ø19, Q1, P5, 25 – ØWJG4ZZ

SECTION: Ø MEDICAL AND SURGICAL
BODY SYSTEM: W ANATOMICAL REGIONS, GENERAL
OPERATION: M REATTACHMENT: Putting back in or on all or a portion of a separated body part to its normal location or other suitable location

Body Part	Approach	Device	Qualifier
2 Face 4 Upper Jaw 5 Lower Jaw 6 Neck 8 Chest Wall F Abdominal Wall K Upper Back L Lower Back M Perineum, Male ♂ N Perineum, Female ♀	Ø Open	Z No Device	Z No Qualifier

SECTION: Ø MEDICAL AND SURGICAL
BODY SYSTEM: W ANATOMICAL REGIONS, GENERAL
OPERATION: P REMOVAL: Taking out or off a device from a body part

Body Part	Approach	Device	Qualifier
Ø Head 2 Face 4 Upper Jaw 5 Lower Jaw 6 Neck 8 Chest Wall ~~C Mediastinum~~ F Abdominal Wall K Upper Back L Lower Back M Perineum, Male ♂ N Perineum, Female ♀	Ø Open 3 Percutaneous 4 Percutaneous Endoscopic X External	Ø Drainage Device 1 Radioactive Element 3 Infusion Device 7 Autologous Tissue Substitute J Synthetic Substitute K Nonautologous Tissue Substitute Y Other Device	Z No Qualifier
1 Cranial Cavity 9 Pleural Cavity, Right B Pleural Cavity, Left G Peritoneal Cavity J Pelvic Cavity	Ø Open 3 Percutaneous 4 Percutaneous Endoscopic	Ø Drainage Device 1 Radioactive Element 3 Infusion Device J Synthetic Substitute Y Other Device	Z No Qualifier
1 Cranial Cavity 9 Pleural Cavity, Right B Pleural Cavity, Left G Peritoneal Cavity J Pelvic Cavity	X External	Ø Drainage Device 1 Radioactive Element 3 Infusion Device	Z No Qualifier
C Mediastinum	Ø Open 3 Percutaneous 4 Percutaneous Endoscopic X External	Ø Drainage Device 1 Radioactive Element 3 Infusion Device 7 Autologous Tissue Substitute G Defibrillator Lead J Synthetic Substitute K Nonautologous Tissue Substitute Y Other Device	Z No Qualifier
D Pericardial Cavity H Retroperitoneum	Ø Open 3 Percutaneous 4 Percutaneous Endoscopic	Ø Drainage Device 1 Radioactive Element 3 Infusion Device Y Other Device	Z No Qualifier
D Pericardial Cavity H Retroperitoneum	X External	Ø Drainage Device 1 Radioactive Element 3 Infusion Device	Z No Qualifier
P Gastrointestinal Tract Q Respiratory Tract R Genitourinary Tract	Ø Open 3 Percutaneous 4 Percutaneous Endoscopic 7 Via Natural or Artificial Opening 8 Via Natural or Artificial Opening Endoscopic X External	1 Radioactive Element 3 Infusion Device Y Other Device	Z No Qualifier

Non-OR OWP[Ø24568KL][Ø34X][Ø137JKY]Z
Non-OR OWPM[Ø34][Ø13JY]Z
Non-OR OWPMX[Ø13Y]Z
Non-OR OWP[CFN]X[Ø137JKY]Z
Non-OR OWP1[Ø34]3Z
Non-OR OWP[9BJ][Ø34][Ø13JY]Z
Non-OR OWP[19BGJ]X[Ø13]Z
Non-OR OWP[DH]X[Ø13]Z
Non-OR OWPP[3478X][13Y]Z
Non-OR ØWPQ73Z
Non-OR OWPQ8[3Y]Z
Non-OR OWPQ[ØX][13Y]Z
Non-OR OWPR[Ø3478X][13Y]Z

New/Revised Text in Green ~~deleted~~ Deleted ♀ Females Only ♂ Males Only Coding Clinic
Non-covered Limited Coverage Combination (See Appendix E) DRG Non-OR Non-OR Hospital-Acquired Condition

SECTION: **Ø MEDICAL AND SURGICAL**
BODY SYSTEM: **W ANATOMICAL REGIONS, GENERAL**
OPERATION: **Q REPAIR:** Restoring, to the extent possible, a body part to its normal anatomic structure and function

Body Part	Approach	Device	Qualifier
Ø Head 2 Face 3 Oral Cavity and Throat 4 Upper Jaw 5 Lower Jaw 8 Chest Wall K Upper Back L Lower Back M Perineum, Male ♂ N Perineum, Female ♀	Ø Open 3 Percutaneous 4 Percutaneous Endoscopic X External	Z No Device	Z No Qualifier
6 Neck F Abdominal Wall	Ø Open 3 Percutaneous 4 Percutaneous Endoscopic	Z No Device	Z No Qualifier
6 Neck F Abdominal Wall ⊞	X External	Z No Device	2 Stoma Z No Qualifier
C Mediastinum	Ø Open 3 Percutaneous 4 Percutaneous Endoscopic	Z No Device	Z No Qualifier

⊞ ØWQFXZ[2Z]
Non-OR ØWQNXZZ

Coding Clinic: 2016, Q3, P6 – ØWQFØZZ
Coding Clinic: 2017, Q3, P9 – ØWQFØZZ

SECTION: **Ø MEDICAL AND SURGICAL**
BODY SYSTEM: **W ANATOMICAL REGIONS, GENERAL**
OPERATION: **U SUPPLEMENT:** Putting in or on biological or synthetic material that physically reinforces and/or augments the function of a portion of a body part

Body Part	Approach	Device	Qualifier
Ø Head 2 Face 4 Upper Jaw 5 Lower Jaw 6 Neck 8 Chest Wall C Mediastinum F Abdominal Wall K Upper Back L Lower Back M Perineum, Male ♂ N Perineum, Female ♀	Ø Open 4 Percutaneous Endoscopic	7 Autologous Tissue Substitute J Synthetic Substitute K Nonautologous Tissue Substitute	Z No Qualifier

Coding Clinic: 2012, Q4, P1Ø1 – ØWU8ØJZ
Coding Clinic: 2016, Q3, P41 – ØWUFØ7Z
Coding Clinic: 2017, Q3, P8 – ØWUFØJZ

SECTION: Ø MEDICAL AND SURGICAL
BODY SYSTEM: W ANATOMICAL REGIONS, GENERAL
OPERATION: W REVISION: Correcting, to the extent possible, a portion of a malfunctioning device or the position of a displaced device

Body Part	Approach	Device	Qualifier
Ø Head 2 Face 4 Upper Jaw 5 Lower Jaw 6 Neck 8 Chest Wall ~~C Mediastinum~~ F Abdominal Wall K Upper Back L Lower Back M Perineum, Male ♂ N Perineum, Female ♀	Ø Open 3 Percutaneous 4 Percutaneous Endoscopic X External	Ø Drainage Device 1 Radioactive Element 3 Infusion Device 7 Autologous Tissue Substitute J Synthetic Substitute K Nonautologous Tissue Substitute Y Other Device	Z No Qualifier
1 Cranial Cavity 9 Pleural Cavity, Right B Pleural Cavity, Left G Peritoneal Cavity J Pelvic Cavity	Ø Open 3 Percutaneous 4 Percutaneous Endoscopic X External	Ø Drainage Device 1 Radioactive Element 3 Infusion Device J Synthetic Substitute Y Other Device	Z No Qualifier
C Mediastinum	Ø Open 3 Percutaneous 4 Percutaneous Endoscopic X External	Ø Drainage Device 1 Radioactive Element 3 Infusion Device 7 Autologous Tissue Substitute G Defibrillator Lead J Synthetic Substitute K Nonautologous Tissue Substitute Y Other Device	Z No Qualifier
D Pericardial Cavity H Retroperitoneum	Ø Open 3 Percutaneous 4 Percutaneous Endoscopic X External	Ø Drainage Device 1 Radioactive Element 3 Infusion Device Y Other Device	Z No Qualifier
P Gastrointestinal Tract Q Respiratory Tract R Genitourinary Tract	Ø Open 3 Percutaneous 4 Percutaneous Endoscopic 7 Via Natural or Artificial Opening 8 Via Natural or Artificial Opening Endoscopic X External	1 Radioactive Element 3 Infusion Device Y Other Device	Z No Qualifier

DRG Non-OR ØWW[Ø2456KL][Ø34][Ø137JKY]Z
DRG Non-OR ØWWM[Ø34][Ø13JY]Z
Non-OR OWW[Ø2456CFKLMN]X[Ø137JKY]Z
Non-OR OWW8[Ø34X][Ø137JKY]Z
Non-OR OWW[1GJ]X[Ø13JY]Z
Non-OR OWW[9B][Ø34X][Ø13JY]Z
Non-OR OWW[DH]X[Ø13Y]Z
Non-OR OWWP[3478X][13Y]Z
Non-OR OWWQ[ØX][13Y]Z
Non-OR OWWR[Ø3478X][13Y]Z

Coding Clinic: 2Ø15, Q2, P1Ø – ØWWG4JZ
Coding Clinic: 2Ø16, Q4, P112 – ØWY

SECTION: Ø MEDICAL AND SURGICAL
BODY SYSTEM: W ANATOMICAL REGIONS, GENERAL
OPERATION: Y TRANSPLANTATION: Putting in or on all or a portion of a living body part taken from another individual or animal to physically take the place and/or function of all or a portion of a similar body part

Body Part	Approach	Device	Qualifier
2 Face	Ø Open	Z No Device	Ø Allogeneic 1 Syngeneic

SECTION: Ø MEDICAL AND SURGICAL
BODY SYSTEM: X ANATOMICAL REGIONS, UPPER EXTREMITIES
OPERATION: Ø ALTERATION: Modifying the anatomic structure of a body part without affecting the function of the body part

Body Part	Approach	Device	Qualifier
2 Shoulder Region, Right 3 Shoulder Region, Left 4 Axilla, Right 5 Axilla, Left 6 Upper Extremity, Right 7 Upper Extremity, Left 8 Upper Arm, Right 9 Upper Arm, Left B Elbow Region, Right C Elbow Region, Left D Lower Arm, Right F Lower Arm, Left G Wrist Region, Right H Wrist Region, Left	Ø Open 3 Percutaneous 4 Percutaneous Endoscopic	7 Autologous Tissue Substitute J Synthetic Substitute K Nonautologous Tissue Substitute Z No Device	Z No Qualifier

SECTION: Ø MEDICAL AND SURGICAL
BODY SYSTEM: X ANATOMICAL REGIONS, UPPER EXTREMITIES
OPERATION: 2 CHANGE: Taking out or off a device from a body part and putting back an identical or similar device in or on the same body part without cutting or puncturing the skin or a mucous membrane

Body Part	Approach	Device	Qualifier
6 Upper Extremity, Right 7 Upper Extremity, Left	X External	Ø Drainage Device Y Other Device	Z No Qualifier

Non-OR All Values

SECTION: Ø MEDICAL AND SURGICAL
BODY SYSTEM: X ANATOMICAL REGIONS, UPPER EXTREMITIES
OPERATION: 3 CONTROL: Stopping, or attempting to stop, postprocedure or other acute bleeding

Body Part	Approach	Device	Qualifier
2 Shoulder Region, Right 3 Shoulder Region, Left 4 Axilla, Right 5 Axilla, Left 6 Upper Extremity, Right 7 Upper Extremity, Left 8 Upper Arm, Right 9 Upper Arm, Left B Elbow Region, Right C Elbow Region, Left D Lower Arm, Right F Lower Arm, Left G Wrist Region, Right H Wrist Region, Left J Hand, Right K Hand, Left	Ø Open 3 Percutaneous 4 Percutaneous Endoscopic	Z No Device	Z No Qualifier

Coding Clinic: 2015, Q1, P35 – ØX37ØZZ   Coding Clinic: 2016, Q4, P99 – ØX3

SECTION: Ø MEDICAL AND SURGICAL
BODY SYSTEM: X ANATOMICAL REGIONS, UPPER EXTREMITIES
OPERATION: 6 DETACHMENT: Cutting off all or a portion of the upper or lower extremities

Body Part	Approach	Device	Qualifier
Ø Forequarter, Right 1 Forequarter, Left 2 Shoulder Region, Right 3 Shoulder Region, Left B Elbow Region, Right C Elbow Region, Left	Ø Open	Z No Device	Z No Qualifier
8 Upper Arm, Right 9 Upper Arm, Left D Lower Arm, Right F Lower Arm, Left	Ø Open	Z No Device	1 High 2 Mid 3 Low
J Hand, Right K Hand, Left	Ø Open	Z No Device	Ø Complete 4 Complete 1st Ray 5 Complete 2nd Ray 6 Complete 3rd Ray 7 Complete 4th Ray 8 Complete 5th Ray 9 Partial 1st Ray B Partial 2nd Ray C Partial 3rd Ray D Partial 4th Ray F Partial 5th Ray
L Thumb, Right M Thumb, Left N Index Finger, Right P Index Finger, Left Q Middle Finger, Right R Middle Finger, Left S Ring Finger, Right T Ring Finger, Left V Little Finger, Right W Little Finger, Left	Ø Open	Z No Device	Ø Complete 1 High 2 Mid 3 Low

Coding Clinic: 2Ø16, Q3, P34 – ØX6[MTW]ØZ1
Coding Clinic: 2Ø17, Q1, P52 – ØX6[MTW]ØZ3
Coding Clinic: 2Ø17, Q2, P19 – ØX6VØZØ

SECTION: Ø MEDICAL AND SURGICAL
BODY SYSTEM: X ANATOMICAL REGIONS, UPPER EXTREMITIES
OPERATION: 9 DRAINAGE: Taking or letting out fluids and/or gases from a body part

Body Part	Approach	Device	Qualifier
2 Shoulder Region, Right 3 Shoulder Region, Left 4 Axilla, Right 5 Axilla, Left 6 Upper Extremity, Right 7 Upper Extremity, Left 8 Upper Arm, Right 9 Upper Arm, Left B Elbow Region, Right C Elbow Region, Left D Lower Arm, Right F Lower Arm, Left G Wrist Region, Right H Wrist Region, Left J Hand, Right K Hand, Left	Ø Open 3 Percutaneous 4 Percutaneous Endoscopic	Ø Drainage Device	Z No Qualifier
2 Shoulder Region, Right 3 Shoulder Region, Left 4 Axilla, Right 5 Axilla, Left 6 Upper Extremity, Right 7 Upper Extremity, Left 8 Upper Arm, Right 9 Upper Arm, Left B Elbow Region, Right C Elbow Region, Left D Lower Arm, Right F Lower Arm, Left G Wrist Region, Right H Wrist Region, Left J Hand, Right K Hand, Left	Ø Open 3 Percutaneous 4 Percutaneous Endoscopic	Z No Device	X Diagnostic Z No Qualifier

Non-OR All Values

SECTION: Ø MEDICAL AND SURGICAL
BODY SYSTEM: X ANATOMICAL REGIONS, UPPER EXTREMITIES
OPERATION: B EXCISION: Cutting out or off, without replacement, a portion of a body part

Body Part	Approach	Device	Qualifier
2 Shoulder Region, Right 3 Shoulder Region, Left 4 Axilla, Right 5 Axilla, Left 6 Upper Extremity, Right 7 Upper Extremity, Left 8 Upper Arm, Right 9 Upper Arm, Left B Elbow Region, Right C Elbow Region, Left D Lower Arm, Right F Lower Arm, Left G Wrist Region, Right H Wrist Region, Left J Hand, Right K Hand, Left	Ø Open 3 Percutaneous 4 Percutaneous Endoscopic	Z No Device	X Diagnostic Z No Qualifier

Non-OR ØXB[23456789BCDFGHJK][Ø34]ZX

SECTION: Ø MEDICAL AND SURGICAL
BODY SYSTEM: X ANATOMICAL REGIONS, UPPER EXTREMITIES
OPERATION: H INSERTION: Putting in a nonbiological appliance that monitors, assists, performs, or prevents a physiological function but does not physically take the place of a body part

Body Part	Approach	Device	Qualifier
2 Shoulder Region, Right 3 Shoulder Region, Left 4 Axilla, Right 5 Axilla, Left 6 Upper Extremity, Right 7 Upper Extremity, Left 8 Upper Arm, Right 9 Upper Arm, Left B Elbow Region, Right C Elbow Region, Left D Lower Arm, Right F Lower Arm, Left G Wrist Region, Right H Wrist Region, Left J Hand, Right K Hand, Left	Ø Open 3 Percutaneous 4 Percutaneous Endoscopic	1 Radioactive Element 3 Infusion Device Y Other Device	Z No Qualifier

DRG Non-OR ØXH[23456789BCDFGHJK][Ø34][3Y]Z

Coding Clinic: 2Ø17, Q2, P21 – ØXH9ØYZ

SECTION: Ø MEDICAL AND SURGICAL
BODY SYSTEM: X ANATOMICAL REGIONS, UPPER EXTREMITIES
OPERATION: J INSPECTION: Visually and/or manually exploring a body part

Body Part	Approach	Device	Qualifier
2 Shoulder Region, Right 3 Shoulder Region, Left 4 Axilla, Right 5 Axilla, Left 6 Upper Extremity, Right 7 Upper Extremity, Left 8 Upper Arm, Right 9 Upper Arm, Left B Elbow Region, Right C Elbow Region, Left D Lower Arm, Right F Lower Arm, Left G Wrist Region, Right H Wrist Region, Left J Hand, Right K Hand, Left	Ø Open 3 Percutaneous 4 Percutaneous Endoscopic X External	Z No Device	Z No Qualifier

DRG Non-OR ØXJ[23456789BCDFGHJK]ØZZ
Non-OR ØXJ[23456789BCDFGH][34X]ZZ
Non-OR ØXJ[JK]3ZZ
Non-OR ØXJ[JK]XZZ

SECTION: Ø MEDICAL AND SURGICAL
BODY SYSTEM: X ANATOMICAL REGIONS, UPPER EXTREMITIES
OPERATION: M REATTACHMENT: Putting back in or on all or a portion of a separated body part to its normal location or other suitable location

Body Part	Approach	Device	Qualifier
Ø Forequarter, Right 1 Forequarter, Left 2 Shoulder Region, Right 3 Shoulder Region, Left 4 Axilla, Right 5 Axilla, Left 6 Upper Extremity, Right 7 Upper Extremity, Left 8 Upper Arm, Right 9 Upper Arm, Left B Elbow Region, Right C Elbow Region, Left D Lower Arm, Right F Lower Arm, Left G Wrist Region, Right H Wrist Region, Left J Hand, Right K Hand, Left L Thumb, Right M Thumb, Left N Index Finger, Right P Index Finger, Left Q Middle Finger, Right R Middle Finger, Left S Ring Finger, Right T Ring Finger, Left V Little Finger, Right W Little Finger, Left	Ø Open	Z No Device	Z No Qualifier

SECTION: Ø MEDICAL AND SURGICAL
BODY SYSTEM: X ANATOMICAL REGIONS, UPPER EXTREMITIES
OPERATION: P REMOVAL: Taking out or off a device from a body part

Body Part	Approach	Device	Qualifier
6 Upper Extremity, Right 7 Upper Extremity, Left	Ø Open 3 Percutaneous 4 Percutaneous Endoscopic X External	Ø Drainage Device 1 Radioactive Element 3 Infusion Device 7 Autologous Tissue Substitute J Synthetic Substitute K Nonautologous Tissue Substitute Y Other Device	Z No Qualifier

Non-OR All Values

Coding Clinic: 2017, Q2, P21 – ØXP7ØYZ

SECTION: Ø MEDICAL AND SURGICAL
BODY SYSTEM: X ANATOMICAL REGIONS, UPPER EXTREMITIES
OPERATION: Q REPAIR: Restoring, to the extent possible, a body part to its normal anatomic structure and function

Body Part	Approach	Device	Qualifier
2 Shoulder Region, Right 3 Shoulder Region, Left 4 Axilla, Right 5 Axilla, Left 6 Upper Extremity, Right 7 Upper Extremity, Left 8 Upper Arm, Right 9 Upper Arm, Left B Elbow Region, Right C Elbow Region, Left D Lower Arm, Right F Lower Arm, Left G Wrist Region, Right H Wrist Region, Left J Hand, Right K Hand, Left L Thumb, Right M Thumb, Left N Index Finger, Right P Index Finger, Left Q Middle Finger, Right R Middle Finger, Left S Ring Finger, Right T Ring Finger, Left V Little Finger, Right W Little Finger, Left	Ø Open 3 Percutaneous 4 Percutaneous Endoscopic X External	Z No Device	Z No Qualifier

SECTION: Ø **MEDICAL AND SURGICAL**
BODY SYSTEM: X **ANATOMICAL REGIONS, UPPER EXTREMITIES**
OPERATION: R **REPLACEMENT:** Putting in or on biological or synthetic material that physically takes the place and/or function of all or a portion of a body part

Body Part	Approach	Device	Qualifier
L Thumb, Right M Thumb, Left	Ø Open 4 Percutaneous Endoscopic	7 Autologous Tissue Substitute	N Toe, Right P Toe, Left

SECTION: Ø **MEDICAL AND SURGICAL**
BODY SYSTEM: X **ANATOMICAL REGIONS, UPPER EXTREMITIES**
OPERATION: U **SUPPLEMENT:** Putting in or on biological or synthetic material that physically reinforces and/or augments the function of a portion of a body part

Body Part	Approach	Device	Qualifier
2 Shoulder Region, Right 3 Shoulder Region, Left 4 Axilla, Right 5 Axilla, Left 6 Upper Extremity, Right 7 Upper Extremity, Left 8 Upper Arm, Right 9 Upper Arm, Left B Elbow Region, Right C Elbow Region, Left D Lower Arm, Right F Lower Arm, Left G Wrist Region, Right H Wrist Region, Left J Hand, Right K Hand, Left L Thumb, Right M Thumb, Left N Index Finger, Right P Index Finger, Left Q Middle Finger, Right R Middle Finger, Left S Ring Finger, Right T Ring Finger, Left V Little Finger, Right W Little Finger, Left	Ø Open 4 Percutaneous Endoscopic	7 Autologous Tissue Substitute J Synthetic Substitute K Nonautologous Tissue Substitute	Z No Qualifier

SECTION: Ø MEDICAL AND SURGICAL
BODY SYSTEM: X ANATOMICAL REGIONS, UPPER EXTREMITIES
OPERATION: W REVISION: Correcting, to the extent possible, a portion of a malfunctioning device or the position of displaced device

Body Part	Approach	Device	Qualifier
6 Upper Extremity, Right 7 Upper Extremity, Left	Ø Open 3 Percutaneous 4 Percutaneous Endoscopic X External	Ø Drainage Device 3 Infusion Device 7 Autologous Tissue Substitute J Synthetic Substitute K Nonautologous Tissue Substitute Y Other Device	Z No Qualifier

DRG Non-OR ØXW[67][Ø34][Ø37JKY]Z
Non-OR ØXW[67]X[Ø37JKY]Z

SECTION: Ø MEDICAL AND SURGICAL
BODY SYSTEM: X ANATOMICAL REGIONS, UPPER EXTREMITIES
OPERATION: X TRANSFER: Moving, without taking out, all or a portion of a body part to another location to take over the function of all or a portion of a body part

Body Part	Approach	Device	Qualifier
N Index Finger, Right	Ø Open	Z No Device	L Thumb, Right
P Index Finger, Left	Ø Open	Z No Device	M Thumb, Left

SECTION: Ø MEDICAL AND SURGICAL
BODY SYSTEM: X ANATOMICAL REGIONS, UPPER EXTREMITIES
OPERATION: Y TRANSPLANTATION: Putting in or on all or a portion of a living body part taken from another individual or animal to physically take the place and/or function of all or a portion of a similar body part

Body Part	Approach	Device	Qualifier
J Hand, Right K Hand, Left	Ø Open	Z No Device	Ø Allogeneic 1 Syngeneic

Coding Clinic: 2016, Q4, P112 – ØXY

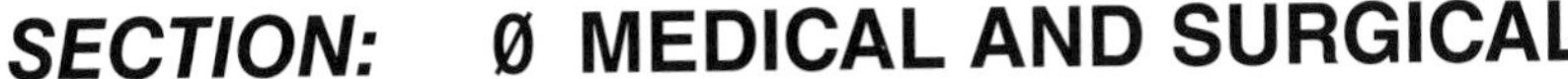

SECTION: Ø MEDICAL AND SURGICAL
BODY SYSTEM: Y ANATOMICAL REGIONS, LOWER EXTREMITIES
OPERATION: Ø ALTERATION: Modifying the anatomic structure of a body part without affecting the function of the body part

Body Part	Approach	Device	Qualifier
Ø Buttock, Right 1 Buttock, Left 9 Lower Extremity, Right B Lower Extremity, Left C Upper Leg, Right D Upper Leg, Left F Knee Region, Right G Knee Region, Left H Lower Leg, Right J Lower Leg, Left K Ankle Region, Right L Ankle Region, Left	Ø Open 3 Percutaneous 4 Percutaneous Endoscopic	7 Autologous Tissue Substitute J Synthetic Substitute K Nonautologous Tissue Substitute Z No Device	Z No Qualifier

SECTION: Ø MEDICAL AND SURGICAL
BODY SYSTEM: Y ANATOMICAL REGIONS, LOWER EXTREMITIES
OPERATION: 2 CHANGE: Taking out or off a device from a body part and putting back an identical or similar device in or on the same body part without cutting or puncturing the skin or a mucous membrane

Body Part	Approach	Device	Qualifier
9 Lower Extremity, Right B Lower Extremity, Left	X External	Ø Drainage Device Y Other Device	Z No Qualifier

Non-OR All Values

SECTION: Ø MEDICAL AND SURGICAL
BODY SYSTEM: Y ANATOMICAL REGIONS, LOWER EXTREMITIES
OPERATION: 3 CONTROL: Stopping, or attempting to stop, postprocedure or other acute bleeding

Body Part	Approach	Device	Qualifier
Ø Buttock, Right 1 Buttock, Left 5 Inguinal Region, Right 6 Inguinal Region, Left 7 Femoral Region, Right 8 Femoral Region, Left 9 Lower Extremity, Right B Lower Extremity, Left C Upper Leg, Right D Upper Leg, Left F Knee Region, Right G Knee Region, Left H Lower Leg, Right J Lower Leg, Left K Ankle Region, Right L Ankle Region, Left M Foot, Right N Foot, Left	Ø Open 3 Percutaneous 4 Percutaneous Endoscopic	Z No Device	Z No Qualifier

Coding Clinic: 2016, Q4, P99 – ØY3

SECTION: Ø MEDICAL AND SURGICAL
BODY SYSTEM: Y ANATOMICAL REGIONS, LOWER EXTREMITIES
OPERATION: 6 DETACHMENT: Cutting off all or a portion of the upper or lower extremities

Body Part	Approach	Device	Qualifier
2 Hindquarter, Right 3 Hindquarter, Left 4 Hindquarter, Bilateral 7 Femoral Region, Right 8 Femoral Region, Left F Knee Region, Right G Knee Region, Left	Ø Open	Z No Device	Z No Qualifier
C Upper Leg, Right D Upper Leg, Left H Lower Leg, Right J Lower Leg, Left	Ø Open	Z No Device	1 High 2 Mid 3 Low
M Foot, Right N Foot, Left	Ø Open	Z No Device	Ø Complete 4 Complete 1st Ray 5 Complete 2nd Ray 6 Complete 3rd Ray 7 Complete 4th Ray 8 Complete 5th Ray 9 Partial 1st Ray B Partial 2nd Ray C Partial 3rd Ray D Partial 4th Ray F Partial 5th Ray
P 1st Toe, Right Q 1st Toe, Left R 2nd Toe, Right S 2nd Toe, Left T 3rd Toe, Right U 3rd Toe, Left V 4th Toe, Right W 4th Toe, Left X 5th Toe, Right Y 5th Toe, Left	Ø Open	Z No Device	Ø Complete 1 High 2 Mid 3 Low

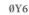

Coding Clinic: 2Ø15, Q1, P28 – ØY6NØZØ
Coding Clinic: 2Ø15, Q2, P29 – ØY6[PQ]ØZ3
Coding Clinic: 2Ø17, Q1, P23 – ØY6NØZØ

SECTION: Ø MEDICAL AND SURGICAL
BODY SYSTEM: Y ANATOMICAL REGIONS, LOWER EXTREMITIES
OPERATION: 9 DRAINAGE: Taking or letting out fluids and/or gases from a body part

Body Part	Approach	Device	Qualifier
Ø Buttock, Right 1 Buttock, Left 5 Inguinal Region, Right 6 Inguinal Region, Left 7 Femoral Region, Right 8 Femoral Region, Left 9 Lower Extremity, Right B Lower Extremity, Left C Upper Leg, Right D Upper Leg, Left F Knee Region, Right G Knee Region, Left H Lower Leg, Right J Lower Leg, Left K Ankle Region, Right L Ankle Region, Left M Foot, Right N Foot, Left	Ø Open 3 Percutaneous 4 Percutaneous Endoscopic	Ø Drainage Device	Z No Qualifier
Ø Buttock, Right 1 Buttock, Left 5 Inguinal Region, Right 6 Inguinal Region, Left 7 Femoral Region, Right 8 Femoral Region, Left 9 Lower Extremity, Right B Lower Extremity, Left C Upper Leg, Right D Upper Leg, Left F Knee Region, Right G Knee Region, Left H Lower Leg, Right J Lower Leg, Left K Ankle Region, Right L Ankle Region, Left M Foot, Right N Foot, Left	Ø Open 3 Percutaneous 4 Percutaneous Endoscopic	Z No Device	X Diagnostic Z No Qualifier

DRG Non-OR ØY9[56]3ØZ
DRG Non-OR ØY9[56]3ZZ
Non-OR ØY9[Ø1789BCDFGHJKLMN][Ø34]ØZ
Non-OR ØY9[Ø1789BCDFGHJKLMN][Ø34]Z[XZ]

Coding Clinic: 2Ø15, Q1, P22-23 – ØY98ØZZ

SECTION: Ø MEDICAL AND SURGICAL
BODY SYSTEM: Y ANATOMICAL REGIONS, LOWER EXTREMITIES
OPERATION: B EXCISION: Cutting out or off, without replacement, a portion of a body part

Body Part	Approach	Device	Qualifier
Ø Buttock, Right 1 Buttock, Left 5 Inguinal Region, Right 6 Inguinal Region, Left 7 Femoral Region, Right 8 Femoral Region, Left 9 Lower Extremity, Right B Lower Extremity, Left C Upper Leg, Right D Upper Leg, Left F Knee Region, Right G Knee Region, Left H Lower Leg, Right J Lower Leg, Left K Ankle Region, Right L Ankle Region, Left M Foot, Right N Foot, Left	Ø Open 3 Percutaneous 4 Percutaneous Endoscopic	Z No Device	X Diagnostic Z No Qualifier

Non-OR ØYB[Ø19BCDFGHJKLMN][Ø34]ZX

SECTION: Ø MEDICAL AND SURGICAL
BODY SYSTEM: Y ANATOMICAL REGIONS, LOWER EXTREMITIES
OPERATION: H INSERTION: Putting in a nonbiological appliance that monitors, assists, performs, or prevents a physiological function but does not physically take the place of a body part

Body Part	Approach	Device	Qualifier
Ø Buttock, Right 1 Buttock, Left 5 Inguinal Region, Right 6 Inguinal Region, Left 7 Femoral Region, Right 8 Femoral Region, Left 9 Lower Extremity, Right B Lower Extremity, Left C Upper Leg, Right D Upper Leg, Left F Knee Region, Right G Knee Region, Left H Lower Leg, Right J Lower Leg, Left K Ankle Region, Right L Ankle Region, Left M Foot, Right N Foot, Left	Ø Open 3 Percutaneous 4 Percutaneous Endoscopic	1 Radioactive Element 3 Infusion Device Y Other Device	Z No Qualifier

DRG Non-OR ØYH[Ø156789BCDFGHJKLMN][Ø34][3Y]Z

Coding Clinic: 2Ø23, Q1, P28-29 – ØYH[CD]ØYZ

SECTION: Ø MEDICAL AND SURGICAL
BODY SYSTEM: Y ANATOMICAL REGIONS, LOWER EXTREMITIES
OPERATION: J INSPECTION: Visually and/or manually exploring a body part

Body Part	Approach	Device	Qualifier
Ø Buttock, Right 1 Buttock, Left 5 Inguinal Region, Right 6 Inguinal Region, Left 7 Femoral Region, Right 8 Femoral Region, Left 9 Lower Extremity, Right A Inguinal Region, Bilateral B Lower Extremity, Left C Upper Leg, Right D Upper Leg, Left E Femoral Region, Bilateral F Knee Region, Right G Knee Region, Left H Lower Leg, Right J Lower Leg, Left K Ankle Region, Right L Ankle Region, Left M Foot, Right N Foot, Left	Ø Open 3 Percutaneous 4 Percutaneous Endoscopic X External	Z No Device	Z No Qualifier

DRG Non-OR ØYJ[Ø19BCDFGHJKLMN]ØZZ
DRG Non-OR ØYJ[567A]3ZZ
DRG Non-OR ØYJ[8E][Ø3]ZZ
Non-OR ØYJ[Ø19BCDFGHJKLMN][34X]ZZ
Non-OR ØYJ[5678AE]XZZ

SECTION: Ø MEDICAL AND SURGICAL
BODY SYSTEM: Y ANATOMICAL REGIONS, LOWER EXTREMITIES
OPERATION: M REATTACHMENT: Putting back in or on all or a portion of a separated body part to its normal location or other suitable location

Body Part	Approach	Device	Qualifier
Ø Buttock, Right 1 Buttock, Left 2 Hindquarter, Right 3 Hindquarter, Left 4 Hindquarter, Bilateral 5 Inguinal Region, Right 6 Inguinal Region, Left 7 Femoral Region, Right 8 Femoral Region, Left 9 Lower Extremity, Right B Lower Extremity, Left C Upper Leg, Right D Upper Leg, Left F Knee Region, Right G Knee Region, Left H Lower Leg, Right J Lower Leg, Left K Ankle Region, Right L Ankle Region, Left M Foot, Right N Foot, Left P 1st Toe, Right Q 1st Toe, Left R 2nd Toe, Right S 2nd Toe, Left T 3rd Toe, Right U 3rd Toe, Left V 4th Toe, Right W 4th Toe, Left X 5th Toe, Right Y 5th Toe, Left	Ø Open	Z No Device	Z No Qualifier

SECTION: Ø MEDICAL AND SURGICAL
BODY SYSTEM: Y ANATOMICAL REGIONS, LOWER EXTREMITIES
OPERATION: P REMOVAL: Taking out or off a device from a body part

Body Part	Approach	Device	Qualifier
9 Lower Extremity, Right B Lower Extremity, Left	Ø Open 3 Percutaneous 4 Percutaneous Endoscopic X External	Ø Drainage Device 1 Radioactive Element 3 Infusion Device 7 Autologous Tissue Substitute J Synthetic Substitute K Nonautologous Tissue Substitute Y Other Device	Z No Qualifier

Non-OR All Values

SECTION: Ø MEDICAL AND SURGICAL
BODY SYSTEM: Y ANATOMICAL REGIONS, LOWER EXTREMITIES
OPERATION: Q REPAIR: Restoring, to the extent possible, a body part to its normal anatomic structure and function

Body Part	Approach	Device	Qualifier
Ø Buttock, Right 1 Buttock, Left 5 Inguinal Region, Right 6 Inguinal Region, Left 7 Femoral Region, Right 8 Femoral Region, Left 9 Lower Extremity, Right A Inguinal Region, Bilateral B Lower Extremity, Left C Upper Leg, Right D Upper Leg, Left E Femoral Region, Bilateral F Knee Region, Right G Knee Region, Left H Lower Leg, Right J Lower Leg, Left K Ankle Region, Right L Ankle Region, Left M Foot, Right N Foot, Left P 1st Toe, Right Q 1st Toe, Left R 2nd Toe, Right S 2nd Toe, Left T 3rd Toe, Right U 3rd Toe, Left V 4th Toe, Right W 4th Toe, Left X 5th Toe, Right Y 5th Toe, Left	Ø Open 3 Percutaneous 4 Percutaneous Endoscopic X External	Z No Device	Z No Qualifier

Non-OR ØYQ[5678AE]XZZ

SECTION: Ø MEDICAL AND SURGICAL
BODY SYSTEM: Y ANATOMICAL REGIONS, LOWER EXTREMITIES
OPERATION: U SUPPLEMENT: Putting in or on biological or synthetic material that physically reinforces and/or augments the function of a portion of a body part

Body Part	Approach	Device	Qualifier
Ø Buttock, Right 1 Buttock, Left 5 Inguinal Region, Right 6 Inguinal Region, Left 7 Femoral Region, Right 8 Femoral Region, Left 9 Lower Extremity, Right A Inguinal Region, Bilateral B Lower Extremity, Left C Upper Leg, Right D Upper Leg, Left E Femoral Region, Bilateral F Knee Region, Right G Knee Region, Left H Lower Leg, Right J Lower Leg, Left K Ankle Region, Right L Ankle Region, Left M Foot, Right N Foot, Left P 1st Toe, Right Q 1st Toe, Left R 2nd Toe, Right S 2nd Toe, Left T 3rd Toe, Right U 3rd Toe, Left V 4th Toe, Right W 4th Toe, Left X 5th Toe, Right Y 5th Toe, Left	Ø Open 4 Percutaneous Endoscopic	7 Autologous Tissue Substitute J Synthetic Substitute K Nonautologous Tissue Substitute	Z No Qualifier

SECTION: Ø MEDICAL AND SURGICAL
BODY SYSTEM: Y ANATOMICAL REGIONS, LOWER EXTREMITIES
OPERATION: W REVISION: Correcting, to the extent possible, a portion of a malfunctioning device or the position of a displaced device

Body Part	Approach	Device	Qualifier
9 Lower Extremity, Right B Lower Extremity, Left	Ø Open 3 Percutaneous 4 Percutaneous Endoscopic X External	Ø Drainage Device 3 Infusion Device 7 Autologous Tissue Substitute J Synthetic Substitute K Nonautologous Tissue Substitute Y Other Device	Z No Qualifier

DRG Non-OR ØYW[9B][Ø34][Ø37JKY]Z
Non-OR ØYW[9B]X[Ø37JKY]Z

ICD-10-PCS Coding Guidelines

Obstetric Section Guidelines (section 1)

C. Obstetrics Section

Products of conception

C1

Procedures performed on the products of conception are coded to the Obstetrics section. Procedures performed on the pregnant female other than the products of conception are coded to the appropriate root operation in the Medical and Surgical section.

Example: Amniocentesis is coded to the products of conception body part in the Obstetrics section. Repair of obstetric urethral laceration is coded to the urethra body part in the Medical and Surgical section.

Procedures following delivery or abortion

C2

Procedures performed following a delivery or abortion for curettage of the endometrium or evacuation of retained products of conception are all coded in the Obstetrics section, to the root operation Extraction and the body part Products of Conception, Retained. Diagnostic or therapeutic dilation and curettage performed during times other than the postpartum or post-abortion period are all coded in the Medical and Surgical section, to the root operation Extraction and the body part Endometrium.

SECTION: 1 **OBSTETRICS**
BODY SYSTEM: Ø **PREGNANCY**
OPERATION: 2 **CHANGE:** Taking out or off a device from a body part and putting back an identical or similar device in or on the same body part without cutting or puncturing the skin or a mucous membrane

Body Part	Approach	Device	Qualifier
Ø Products of Conception ♀	7 Via Natural or Artificial Opening	3 Monitoring Electrode Y Other Device	Z No Qualifier

Non-OR All Values

SECTION: 1 **OBSTETRICS**
BODY SYSTEM: Ø **PREGNANCY**
OPERATION: 9 **DRAINAGE:** Taking or letting out fluids and/or gases from a body part

Body Part	Approach	Device	Qualifier
Ø Products of Conception ♀	Ø Open 3 Percutaneous 4 Percutaneous Endoscopic 7 Via Natural or Artificial Opening 8 Via Natural or Artificial Opening Endoscopic	Z No Device	9 Fetal Blood A Fetal Cerebrospinal Fluid B Fetal Fluid, Other C Amniotic Fluid, Therapeutic D Fluid, Other U Amniotic Fluid, Diagnostic

Non-OR All Values

SECTION: 1 **OBSTETRICS**
BODY SYSTEM: Ø **PREGNANCY**
OPERATION: A **ABORTION:** Artificially terminating a pregnancy

Body Part	Approach	Device	Qualifier
Ø Products of Conception ♀	Ø Open 3 Percutaneous 4 Percutaneous Endoscopic 8 Via Natural or Artificial Opening Endoscopic	Z No Device	Z No Qualifier
Ø Products of Conception ♀	7 Via Natural or Artificial Opening	Z No Device	6 Vacuum W Laminaria X Abortifacient Z No Qualifier

DRG Non-OR 10A07Z6
Non-OR 10A07Z[WX]
Coding Clinic: 2022, Q1, P42 – 10A07ZZ

SECTION: 1 OBSTETRICS
BODY SYSTEM: Ø PREGNANCY
OPERATION: D EXTRACTION: Pulling or stripping out or off all or a portion of a body part by the use of force

Body Part	Approach	Device	Qualifier
Ø Products of Conception ♀	Ø Open	Z No Device	Ø High 1 Low 2 Extraperitoneal
Ø Products of Conception ♀	7 Via Natural or Artificial Opening	Z No Device	3 Low Forceps 4 Mid Forceps 5 High Forceps 6 Vacuum 7 Internal Version 8 Other
1 Products of Conception, Retained ♀	7 Via Natural or Artificial Opening 8 Via Natural or Artificial Opening Endoscopic	Z No Device	9 Manual Z No Qualifier
2 Products of Conception, Ectopic ♀	Ø Open 4 Percutaneous Endoscopic 7 Via Natural or Artificial Opening 8 Via Natural or Artificial Opening Endoscopic	Z No Device	Z No Qualifier

DRG Non-OR 1ØDØ7Z[345678]

Coding Clinic: 2016, Q1, P1Ø – 1ØDØ7Z3

Coding Clinic: 2018, Q4, P51; 2018, Q2, P18 – 1ØDØØZØ

Coding Clinic: 2022, Q1, P19 – 1ØD17ZZ

SECTION: 1 OBSTETRICS
BODY SYSTEM: Ø PREGNANCY
OPERATION: E DELIVERY: Assisting the passage of the products of conception from the genital canal

Body Part	Approach	Device	Qualifier
Ø Products of Conception ♀	X External	Z No Device	Z No Qualifier

DRG Non-OR 1ØEØXZZ

Coding Clinic: 2016, Q2, P34-35 – 1ØEØXZZ

Coding Clinic: 2017, Q3, P5 – 1ØEØXZZ

SECTION: 1 OBSTETRICS
BODY SYSTEM: Ø PREGNANCY
OPERATION: H INSERTION: Putting in a nonbiological appliance that monitors, assists, performs, or prevents a physiological function but does not physically take the place of a body part

Body Part	Approach	Device	Qualifier
Ø Products of Conception ♀	Ø Open 7 Via Natural or Artificial Opening	3 Monitoring Electrode Y Other Device	Z No Qualifier

Non-OR 1ØHØ7[3Y]Z

Coding Clinic: 2013, Q2, P36 – 1ØHØ7YZ

SECTION: 1 OBSTETRICS
BODY SYSTEM: Ø PREGNANCY
OPERATION: J INSPECTION: Visually and/or manually exploring a body part

Body Part	Approach	Device	Qualifier
Ø Products of Conception ♀ 1 Products of Conception, Retained ♀ 2 Products of Conception, Ectopic ♀	Ø Open 3 Percutaneous 4 Percutaneous Endoscopic 7 Via Natural or Artificial Opening 8 Via Natural or Artificial Opening Endoscopic X External	Z No Device	Z No Qualifier

Non-OR All Values

SECTION: 1 OBSTETRICS
BODY SYSTEM: Ø PREGNANCY
OPERATION: P REMOVAL: Taking out or off a device from a body part, region or orifice

Body Part	Approach	Device	Qualifier
Ø Products of Conception ♀	Ø Open 7 Via Natural or Artificial Opening	3 Monitoring Electrode Y Other Device	Z No Qualifier

Non-OR 10P7[3Y]Z

SECTION: 1 OBSTETRICS
BODY SYSTEM: Ø PREGNANCY
OPERATION: Q REPAIR: Restoring, to the extent possible, a body part to its normal anatomic structure and function

Body Part	Approach	Device	Qualifier
Ø Products of Conception ♀	Ø Open 3 Percutaneous 4 Percutaneous Endoscopic 7 Via Natural or Artificial Opening 8 Via Natural or Artificial Opening Endoscopic	Y Other Device Z No Device	E Nervous System F Cardiovascular System G Lymphatics and Hemic H Eye J Ear, Nose, and Sinus K Respiratory System L Mouth and Throat M Gastrointestinal System N Hepatobiliary and Pancreas P Endocrine System Q Skin R Musculoskeletal System S Urinary System T Female Reproductive System V Male Reproductive System Y Other Body System

Coding Clinic: 2021, Q2, P22 – 10Q00ZK

SECTION: 1 OBSTETRICS
BODY SYSTEM: Ø PREGNANCY
OPERATION: S **REPOSITION:** Moving to its normal location or other suitable location all or a portion of a body part

Body Part	Approach	Device	Qualifier
Ø Products of Conception ♀	7 Via Natural or Artificial Opening X External	Z No Device	Z No Qualifier
2 Products of Conception, Ectopic ♀	Ø Open 3 Percutaneous 4 Percutaneous Endoscopic 7 Via Natural or Artificial Opening 8 Via Natural or Artificial Opening Endoscopic	Z No Device	Z No Qualifier

DRG Non-OR 1ØSØ7ZZ
Non-OR 1ØSØXZZ

SECTION: 1 OBSTETRICS
BODY SYSTEM: Ø PREGNANCY
OPERATION: T **RESECTION:** Cutting out or off, without replacement, all of a body part

Body Part	Approach	Device	Qualifier
2 Products of Conception, Ectopic ♀	Ø Open 3 Percutaneous 4 Percutaneous Endoscopic 7 Via Natural or Artificial Opening 8 Via Natural or Artificial Opening Endoscopic	Z No Device	Z No Qualifier

Coding Clinic: 2Ø15, Q3, P32 – 1ØT24ZZ

SECTION: 1 OBSTETRICS
BODY SYSTEM: Ø PREGNANCY
OPERATION: Y **TRANSPLANTATION:** Putting in or on all or a portion of a living body part taken from another individual or animal to physically take the place and/or function of all or a portion of a similar body part

Body Part	Approach	Device	Qualifier
Ø Products of Conception ♀	3 Percutaneous 4 Percutaneous Endoscopic 7 Via Natural or Artificial Opening	Z No Device	E Nervous System F Cardiovascular System G Lymphatics and Hemic H Eye J Ear, Nose, and Sinus K Respiratory System L Mouth and Throat M Gastrointestinal System N Hepatobiliary and Pancreas P Endocrine System Q Skin R Musculoskeletal System S Urinary System T Female Reproductive System V Male Reproductive System Y Other Body System

SECTION: 2 PLACEMENT
BODY SYSTEM: W ANATOMICAL REGIONS
OPERATION: Ø CHANGE: Taking out or off a device from a body part and putting back an identical or similar device in or on the same body part without cutting or puncturing the skin or a mucous membrane

Body Region	Approach	Device	Qualifier
Ø Head 2 Neck 3 Abdominal Wall 4 Chest Wall 5 Back 6 Inguinal Region, Right 7 Inguinal Region, Left 8 Upper Extremity, Right 9 Upper Extremity, Left A Upper Arm, Right B Upper Arm, Left C Lower Arm, Right D Lower Arm, Left E Hand, Right F Hand, Left G Thumb, Right H Thumb, Left J Finger, Right K Finger, Left L Lower Extremity, Right M Lower Extremity, Left N Upper Leg, Right P Upper Leg, Left Q Lower Leg, Right R Lower Leg, Left S Foot, Right T Foot, Left U Toe, Right V Toe, Left	X External	Ø Traction Apparatus 1 Splint 2 Cast 3 Brace 4 Bandage 5 Packing Material 6 Pressure Dressing 7 Intermittent Pressure Device Y Other Device	Z No Qualifier
1 Face	X External	Ø Traction Apparatus 1 Splint 2 Cast 3 Brace 4 Bandage 5 Packing Material 6 Pressure Dressing 7 Intermittent Pressure Device 9 Wire Y Other Device	Z No Qualifier

SECTION: 2 PLACEMENT
BODY SYSTEM: W ANATOMICAL REGIONS
OPERATION: 1 COMPRESSION: Putting pressure on a body region

Body Region	Approach	Device	Qualifier
Ø Head 1 Face 2 Neck 3 Abdominal Wall 4 Chest Wall 5 Back 6 Inguinal Region, Right 7 Inguinal Region, Left 8 Upper Extremity, Right 9 Upper Extremity, Left A Upper Arm, Right B Upper Arm, Left C Lower Arm, Right D Lower Arm, Left E Hand, Right F Hand, Left G Thumb, Right H Thumb, Left J Finger, Right K Finger, Left L Lower Extremity, Right M Lower Extremity, Left N Upper Leg, Right P Upper Leg, Left Q Lower Leg, Right R Lower Leg, Left S Foot, Right T Foot, Left U Toe, Right V Toe, Left	X External	6 Pressure Dressing 7 Intermittent Pressure Device	Z No Qualifier

SECTION: 2 PLACEMENT
BODY SYSTEM: W ANATOMICAL REGIONS
OPERATION: 2 DRESSING: Putting material on a body region for protection

Body Region	Approach	Device	Qualifier
Ø Head 1 Face 2 Neck 3 Abdominal Wall 4 Chest Wall 5 Back 6 Inguinal Region, Right 7 Inguinal Region, Left 8 Upper Extremity, Right 9 Upper Extremity, Left A Upper Arm, Right B Upper Arm, Left C Lower Arm, Right D Lower Arm, Left E Hand, Right F Hand, Left G Thumb, Right H Thumb, Left J Finger, Right K Finger, Left L Lower Extremity, Right M Lower Extremity, Left N Upper Leg, Right P Upper Leg, Left Q Lower Leg, Right R Lower Leg, Left S Foot, Right T Foot, Left U Toe, Right V Toe, Left	X External	4 Bandage	Z No Qualifier

SECTION: 2 PLACEMENT
BODY SYSTEM: W ANATOMICAL REGIONS
OPERATION: 3 IMMOBILIZATION: Limiting or preventing motion of a body region

Body Region	Approach	Device	Qualifier
Ø Head 2 Neck 3 Abdominal Wall 4 Chest Wall 5 Back 6 Inguinal Region, Right 7 Inguinal Region, Left 8 Upper Extremity, Right 9 Upper Extremity, Left A Upper Arm, Right B Upper Arm, Left C Lower Arm, Right D Lower Arm, Left E Hand, Right F Hand, Left G Thumb, Right H Thumb, Left J Finger, Right K Finger, Left L Lower Extremity, Right M Lower Extremity, Left N Upper Leg, Right P Upper Leg, Left Q Lower Leg, Right R Lower Leg, Left S Foot, Right T Foot, Left U Toe, Right V Toe, Left	X External	1 Splint 2 Cast 3 Brace Y Other Device	Z No Qualifier
1 Face	X External	1 Splint 2 Cast 3 Brace 9 Wire Y Other Device	Z No Qualifier

SECTION: 2 PLACEMENT
BODY SYSTEM: W ANATOMICAL REGIONS
OPERATION: 4 PACKING: Putting material in a body region or orifice

Body Region	Approach	Device	Qualifier
Ø Head 1 Face 2 Neck 3 Abdominal Wall 4 Chest Wall 5 Back 6 Inguinal Region, Right 7 Inguinal Region, Left 8 Upper Extremity, Right 9 Upper Extremity, Left A Upper Arm, Right B Upper Arm, Left C Lower Arm, Right D Lower Arm, Left E Hand, Right F Hand, Left G Thumb, Right H Thumb, Left J Finger, Right K Finger, Left L Lower Extremity, Right M Lower Extremity, Left N Upper Leg, Right P Upper Leg, Left Q Lower Leg, Right R Lower Leg, Left S Foot, Right T Foot, Left U Toe, Right V Toe, Left	X External	5 Packing Material	Z No Qualifier

SECTION: 2 PLACEMENT
BODY SYSTEM: W ANATOMICAL REGIONS
OPERATION: 5 REMOVAL: Taking out or off a device from a body part

Body Region	Approach	Device	Qualifier
Ø Head 2 Neck 3 Abdominal Wall 4 Chest Wall 5 Back 6 Inguinal Region, Right 7 Inguinal Region, Left 8 Upper Extremity, Right 9 Upper Extremity, Left A Upper Arm, Right B Upper Arm, Left C Lower Arm, Right D Lower Arm, Left E Hand, Right F Hand, Left G Thumb, Right H Thumb, Left J Finger, Right K Finger, Left L Lower Extremity, Right M Lower Extremity, Left N Upper Leg, Right P Upper Leg, Left Q Lower Leg, Right R Lower Leg, Left S Foot, Right T Foot, Left U Toe, Right V Toe, Left	X External	Ø Traction Apparatus 1 Splint 2 Cast 3 Brace 4 Bandage 5 Packing Material 6 Pressure Dressing 7 Intermittent Pressure Device Y Other Device	Z No Qualifier
1 Face	X External	Ø Traction Apparatus 1 Splint 2 Cast 3 Brace 4 Bandage 5 Packing Material 6 Pressure Dressing 7 Intermittent Pressure Device 9 Wire Y Other Device	Z No Qualifier

SECTION: 2 PLACEMENT

BODY SYSTEM: W ANATOMICAL REGIONS

OPERATION: 6 TRACTION: Exerting a pulling force on a body region in a distal direction

Body Region	Approach	Device	Qualifier
Ø Head 1 Face 2 Neck 3 Abdominal Wall 4 Chest Wall 5 Back 6 Inguinal Region, Right 7 Inguinal Region, Left 8 Upper Extremity, Right 9 Upper Extremity, Left A Upper Arm, Right B Upper Arm, Left C Lower Arm, Right D Lower Arm, Left E Hand, Right F Hand, Left G Thumb, Right H Thumb, Left J Finger, Right K Finger, Left L Lower Extremity, Right M Lower Extremity, Left N Upper Leg, Right P Upper Leg, Left Q Lower Leg, Right R Lower Leg, Left S Foot, Right T Foot, Left U Toe, Right V Toe, Left	X External	Ø Traction Apparatus Z No Device	Z No Qualifier

Coding Clinic: 2015, Q2, P35; 2013, Q2, P39 – 2W60X0Z
Coding Clinic: 2015, Q2, P35 – 2W62X0Z

2: PLACEMENT W: ANATOMICAL REGIONS 6: TRACTION

SECTION: 2 PLACEMENT
BODY SYSTEM: Y ANATOMICAL ORIFICES
OPERATION: Ø **CHANGE:** Taking out or off a device from a body part and putting back an identical or similar device in or on the same body part without cutting or puncturing the skin or a mucous membrane

Body Region	Approach	Device	Qualifier
Ø Mouth and Pharynx 1 Nasal 2 Ear 3 Anorectal 4 Female Genital Tract ♀ 5 Urethra	X External	5 Packing Material	Z No Qualifier

SECTION: 2 PLACEMENT
BODY SYSTEM: Y ANATOMICAL ORIFICES
OPERATION: 4 **PACKING:** Putting material in a body region or orifice

Body Region	Approach	Device	Qualifier
Ø Mouth and Pharynx 1 Nasal 2 Ear 3 Anorectal 4 Female Genital Tract ♀ 5 Urethra	X External	5 Packing Material	Z No Qualifier

Coding Clinic: 2Ø18, Q4, P38; 2Ø17, Q4, P1Ø6 – 2Y41X5Z

SECTION: 2 PLACEMENT
BODY SYSTEM: Y ANATOMICAL ORIFICES
OPERATION: 5 **REMOVAL:** Taking out or off a device from a body part

Body Region	Approach	Device	Qualifier
Ø Mouth and Pharynx 1 Nasal 2 Ear 3 Anorectal 4 Female Genital Tract ♀ 5 Urethra	X External	5 Packing Material	Z No Qualifier

3Ø2

SECTION: 3 ADMINISTRATION
BODY SYSTEM: Ø CIRCULATORY
OPERATION: 2 TRANSFUSION: *(on multiple pages)*
Putting in blood or blood products

Body System / Region	Approach	Substance	Qualifier
3 Peripheral Vein 4 Central Vein	3 Percutaneous	A Stem Cells, Embryonic	Z No Qualifier
3 Peripheral Vein 4 Central Vein	3 Percutaneous	C Hematopoietic Stem/ Progenitor Cells, Genetically Modified	Ø Autologous
3 Peripheral Vein 4 Central Vein	3 Percutaneous	D Pathogen Reduced Cryoprecipitated Fibrinogen Complex	1 Nonautologous
3 Peripheral Vein 4 Central Vein	3 Percutaneous	G Bone Marrow X Stem Cells, Cord Blood Y Stem Cells, Hematopoietic	Ø Autologous 2 Allogeneic, Related 3 Allogeneic, Unrelated 4 Allogeneic, Unspecified
3 Peripheral Vein 4 Central Vein	3 Percutaneous	H Whole Blood J Serum Albumin K Frozen Plasma L Fresh Plasma M Plasma Cryoprecipitate N Red Blood Cells P Frozen Red Cells Q White Cells R Platelets S Globulin T Fibrinogen V Antihemophilic Factors W Factor IX	Ø Autologous 1 Nonautologous
3 Peripheral Vein 4 Central Vein	3 Percutaneous	U Stem Cells, T-cell Depleted Hematopoietic	2 Allogeneic, Related 3 Allogeneic, Unrelated 4 Allogeneic, Unspecified

3Ø2[34][3]AZ is identified as non-covered when a code from the diagnosis list below is present as a principal or secondary diagnosis

C91ØØ	C924Ø	C93ØØ
C92ØØ	C925Ø	C94ØØ
C921Ø	C926Ø	C95ØØ
C9211	C92AØ	

Non-OR 3Ø2[34][Ø3][HJKLMNPQRSTUVWX][Ø1234]

SECTION: 3 ADMINISTRATION
BODY SYSTEM: Ø CIRCULATORY
OPERATION: 2 TRANSFUSION: *(continued)*
Putting in blood or blood products

Body System / Region	Approach	Substance	Qualifier
7 Products of Conception, Circulatory ♀	3 Percutaneous 7 Via Natural or Artificial Opening	H Whole Blood J Serum Albumin K Frozen Plasma L Fresh Plasma M Plasma Cryoprecipitate N Red Blood Cells P Frozen Red Cells Q White Cells R Platelets S Globulin T Fibrinogen V Antihemophilic Factors W Factor IX	1 Nonautologous
8 Vein	3 Percutaneous	B 4-Factor Prothrombin Complex Concentrate	1 Nonautologous
A Bone Marrow	3 Percutaneous	H Whole Blood J Serum Albumin K Frozen Plasma L Fresh Plasma N Red Blood Cells P Frozen Red Cells R Platelets	Ø Autologous 1 Nonautologous

Non-OR 3Ø27[37][HJKLMNPQRSTVW]1
Non-OR 3Ø28[Ø3]B1

Coding Clinic: 2Ø23, Q1, P11 – 3Ø2A3H1

SECTION: 3 **ADMINISTRATION**
BODY SYSTEM: C **INDWELLING DEVICE**
OPERATION: 1 **IRRIGATION:** Putting in or on a cleansing substance

Body System / Region	Approach	Substance	Qualifier
Z None	X External	8 Irrigating Substance	Z No Qualifier

SECTION: 3 **ADMINISTRATION**
BODY SYSTEM: E **PHYSIOLOGICAL SYSTEMS AND ANATOMICAL REGIONS**
OPERATION: Ø **INTRODUCTION:** *(on multiple pages)*
Putting in or on a therapeutic, diagnostic, nutritional, physiological, or prophylactic substance except blood or blood products

Body System / Region	Approach	Substance	Qualifier
Ø Skin and Mucous Membranes	X External	Ø Antineoplastic	5 Other Antineoplastic M Monoclonal Antibody
Ø Skin and Mucous Membranes	X External	2 Anti-infective	8 Oxazolidinones 9 Other Anti-infective
Ø Skin and Mucous Membranes	X External	3 Anti-inflammatory 4 Serum, Toxoid and Vaccine B Anesthetic Agent K Other Diagnostic Substance M Pigment N Analgesics, Hypnotics, Sedatives T Destructive Agent	Z No Qualifier
Ø Skin and Mucous Membranes	X External	G Other Therapeutic Substance	C Other Substance
1 Subcutaneous Tissue	Ø Open	2 Anti-infective	A Anti-Infective Envelope
1 Subcutaneous Tissue	3 Percutaneous	Ø Antineoplastic	5 Other Antineoplastic M Monoclonal Antibody
1 Subcutaneous Tissue	3 Percutaneous	2 Anti-infective	8 Oxazolidinones 9 Other Anti-infective A Anti-Infective Envelope
1 Subcutaneous Tissue	3 Percutaneous	3 Anti-inflammatory 6 Nutritional Substance 7 Electrolytic and Water Balance Substance B Anesthetic Agent H Radioactive Substance K Other Diagnostic Substance N Analgesics, Hypnotics, Sedatives T Destructive Agent	Z No Qualifier
1 Subcutaneous Tissue	3 Percutaneous	4 Serum, Toxoid and Vaccine	Ø Influenza Vaccine Z No Qualifier
1 Subcutaneous Tissue	3 Percutaneous	G Other Therapeutic Substance	C Other Substance
1 Subcutaneous Tissue	3 Percutaneous	V Hormone	G Insulin J Other Hormone
2 Muscle	3 Percutaneous	Ø Antineoplastic	5 Other Antineoplastic M Monoclonal Antibody

SECTION: 3 ADMINISTRATION
BODY SYSTEM: E PHYSIOLOGICAL SYSTEMS AND ANATOMICAL REGIONS
OPERATION: Ø INTRODUCTION: *(continued)*

Putting in or on a therapeutic, diagnostic, nutritional, physiological, or prophylactic substance except blood or blood products

Body System / Region	Approach	Substance	Qualifier
2 Muscle	3 Percutaneous	2 Anti-infective	8 Oxazolidinones 9 Other Anti-infective
2 Muscle	3 Percutaneous	3 Anti-inflammatory 6 Nutritional Substance 7 Electrolytic and Water Balance Substance B Anesthetic Agent H Radioactive Substance K Other Diagnostic Substance N Analgesics, Hypnotics, Sedatives T Destructive Agent	Z No Qualifier
2 Muscle	3 Percutaneous	4 Serum, Toxoid and Vaccine	Ø Influenza Vaccine Z No Qualifier
2 Muscle	3 Percutaneous	G Other Therapeutic Substance	C Other Substance
3 Peripheral Vein	Ø Open	Ø Antineoplastic	2 High-dose Interleukin-2 3 Low-dose Interleukin-2 5 Other Antineoplastic M Monoclonal Antibody P Clofarabine
3 Peripheral Vein	Ø Open	1 Thrombolytic	6 Recombinant Human-activated Protein C 7 Other Thrombolytic
3 Peripheral Vein	Ø Open	2 Anti-infective	8 Oxazolidinones 9 Other Anti-infective
3 Peripheral Vein	Ø Open	3 Anti-inflammatory 4 Serum, Toxoid and Vaccine 6 Nutritional Substance 7 Electrolytic and Water Balance Substance F Intracirculatory Anesthetic H Radioactive Substance K Other Diagnostic Substance N Analgesics, Hypnotics, Sedatives P Platelet Inhibitor R Antiarrhythmic T Destructive Agent X Vasopressor	Z No Qualifier
3 Peripheral Vein	Ø Open	G Other Therapeutic Substance	C Other Substance N Blood Brain Barrier Disruption
3 Peripheral Vein	Ø Open	U Pancreatic Islet Cells	Ø Autologous 1 Nonautologous
3 Peripheral Vein	Ø Open	V Hormone	G Insulin H Human B-type Natriuretic Peptide J Other Hormone
3 Peripheral Vein	Ø Open	W Immunotherapeutic	K Immunostimulator L Immunosuppressive

DRG Non-OR 3EØ3ØØ2
DRG Non-OR 3EØ3Ø17
DRG Non-OR 3EØ3ØU[Ø1]

SECTION: 3 ADMINISTRATION
BODY SYSTEM: E PHYSIOLOGICAL SYSTEMS AND ANATOMICAL REGIONS
OPERATION: Ø INTRODUCTION: *(continued)*

Putting in or on a therapeutic, diagnostic, nutritional, physiological, or prophylactic substance except blood or blood products

Body System / Region	Approach	Substance	Qualifier
3 Peripheral Vein	3 Percutaneous	Ø Antineoplastic	2 High-dose Interleukin-2 3 Low-dose Interleukin-2 5 Other Antineoplastic M Monoclonal Antibody P Clofarabine
3 Peripheral Vein	3 Percutaneous	1 Thrombolytic	6 Recombinant Human-activated Protein C 7 Other Thrombolytic
3 Peripheral Vein	3 Percutaneous	2 Anti-infective	8 Oxazolidinones 9 Other Anti-infective
3 Peripheral Vein	3 Percutaneous	3 Anti-inflammatory 4 Serum, Toxoid and Vaccine 6 Nutritional Substance 7 Electrolytic and Water Balance Substance F Intracirculatory Anesthetic H Radioactive Substance K Other Diagnostic Substance N Analgesics, Hypnotics, Sedatives P Platelet Inhibitor R Antiarrhythmic T Destructive Agent X Vasopressor	Z No Qualifier
3 Peripheral Vein	3 Percutaneous	G Other Therapeutic Substance	C Other Substance N Blood Brain Barrier Disruption Q Glucarpidase R Other Therapeutic Monoclonal Antibody
3 Peripheral Vein	3 Percutaneous	U Pancreatic Islet Cells	Ø Autologous 1 Nonautologous
3 Peripheral Vein	3 Percutaneous	V Hormone	G Insulin H Human B-type Natriuretic Peptide J Other Hormone
3 Peripheral Vein	3 Percutaneous	W Immunotherapeutic	K Immunostimulator L Immunosuppressive
4 Central Vein	Ø Open	Ø Antineoplastic	2 High-dose Interleukin-2 3 Low-dose Interleukin-2 5 Other Antineoplastic M Monoclonal Antibody P Clofarabine
4 Central Vein	Ø Open	1 Thrombolytic	6 Recombinant Human-activated Protein C 7 Other Thrombolytic
4 Central Vein	Ø Open	2 Anti-infective	8 Oxazolidinones 9 Other Anti-infective

DRG Non-OR 3EØ33Ø2
DRG Non-OR 3EØ3317
DRG Non-OR 3EØ33U[Ø1]
DRG Non-OR 3EØ4ØØ2
DRG Non-OR 3EØ417
DRG Non-OR 3EØ33TZ *(proposed)*

SECTION: 3 ADMINISTRATION
BODY SYSTEM: E PHYSIOLOGICAL SYSTEMS AND ANATOMICAL REGIONS
OPERATION: Ø INTRODUCTION: *(continued)*

Putting in or on a therapeutic, diagnostic, nutritional, physiological, or prophylactic substance except blood or blood products

Body System / Region	Approach	Substance	Qualifier
4 Central Vein	Ø Open	3 Anti-inflammatory 4 Serum, Toxoid and Vaccine 6 Nutritional Substance 7 Electrolytic and Water Balance Substance F Intracirculatory Anesthetic H Radioactive Substance K Other Diagnostic Substance N Analgesics, Hypnotics, Sedatives P Platelet Inhibitor R Antiarrhythmic T Destructive Agent X Vasopressor	Z No Qualifier
4 Central Vein	Ø Open	G Other Therapeutic Substance	C Other Substance N Blood Brain Barrier Disruption
4 Central Vein	Ø Open	V Hormone	G Insulin H Human B-type Natriuretic Peptide J Other Hormone
4 Central Vein	Ø Open	W Immunotherapeutic	K Immunostimulator L Immunosuppressive
4 Central Vein	3 Percutaneous	Ø Antineoplastic	2 High-dose Interleukin-2 3 Low-dose Interleukin-2 5 Other Antineoplastic M Monoclonal Antibody P Clofarabine
4 Central Vein	3 Percutaneous	1 Thrombolytic	6 Recombinant Human-activated Protein C 7 Other Thrombolytic
4 Central Vein	3 Percutaneous	2 Anti-infective	8 Oxazolidinones 9 Other Anti-infective
4 Central Vein	3 Percutaneous	3 Anti-inflammatory 4 Serum, Toxoid and Vaccine 6 Nutritional Substance 7 Electrolytic and Water Balance Substance F Intracirculatory Anesthetic H Radioactive Substance K Other Diagnostic Substance N Analgesics, Hypnotics, Sedatives P Platelet Inhibitor R Antiarrhythmic T Destructive Agent X Vasopressor	Z No Qualifier
4 Central Vein	3 Percutaneous	G Other Therapeutic Substance	C Other Substance N Blood Brain Barrier Disruption Q Glucarpidase R Other Therapeutic Monoclonal Antibody
4 Central Vein	3 Percutaneous	V Hormone	G Insulin H Human B-type Natriuretic Peptide J Other Hormone

DRG Non-OR 3EØ43Ø2 DRG Non-OR 3EØ4317 DRG Non-OR 3EØ43TZ *(proposed)*

Coding Clinic: 2Ø22, Q3, P26 – 3EØ43GC

SECTION: 3 ADMINISTRATION
BODY SYSTEM: E PHYSIOLOGICAL SYSTEMS AND ANATOMICAL REGIONS
OPERATION: Ø INTRODUCTION: *(continued)*

Putting in or on a therapeutic, diagnostic, nutritional, physiological, or prophylactic substance except blood or blood products

Body System / Region	Approach	Substance	Qualifier
4 Central Vein	3 Percutaneous	W Immunotherapeutic	K Immunostimulator L Immunosuppressive
5 Peripheral Artery 6 Central Artery	Ø Open 3 Percutaneous	Ø Antineoplastic	2 High-dose Interleukin-2 3 Low-dose Interleukin-2 5 Other Antineoplastic M Monoclonal Antibody P Clofarabine
5 Peripheral Artery 6 Central Artery	Ø Open 3 Percutaneous	1 Thrombolytic	6 Recombinant Human-activated Protein C 7 Other Thrombolytic
5 Peripheral Artery 6 Central Artery	Ø Open 3 Percutaneous	2 Anti-infective	8 Oxazolidinones 9 Other Anti-infective
5 Peripheral Artery 6 Central Artery	Ø Open 3 Percutaneous	3 Anti-inflammatory 4 Serum, Toxoid and Vaccine 6 Nutritional Substance 7 Electrolytic and Water Balance Substance F Intracirculatory Anesthetic H Radioactive Substance K Other Diagnostic Substance N Analgesics, Hypnotics, Sedatives P Platelet Inhibitor R Antiarrhythmic T Destructive Agent X Vasopressor	Z No Qualifier
5 Peripheral Artery 6 Central Artery	Ø Open 3 Percutaneous	G Other Therapeutic Substance	C Other Substance N Blood Brain Barrier Disruption
5 Peripheral Artery 6 Central Artery	Ø Open 3 Percutaneous	V Hormone	G Insulin H Human B-type Natriuretic Peptide J Other Hormone
5 Peripheral Artery 6 Central Artery	Ø Open 3 Percutaneous	W Immunotherapeutic	K Immunostimulator L Immunosuppressive
7 Coronary Artery 8 Heart	Ø Open 3 Percutaneous	1 Thrombolytic	6 Recombinant Human-activated Protein C 7 Other Thrombolytic
7 Coronary Artery 8 Heart	Ø Open 3 Percutaneous	G Other Therapeutic Substance	C Other Substance
7 Coronary Artery 8 Heart	Ø Open 3 Percutaneous	K Other Diagnostic Substance P Platelet Inhibitor	Z No Qualifier
7 Coronary Artery 8 Heart	4 Percutaneous Endoscopic	G Other Therapeutic Substance	C Other Substance
9 Nose	3 Percutaneous 7 Via Natural or Artificial Opening X External	Ø Antineoplastic	5 Other Antineoplastic M Monoclonal Antibody
9 Nose	3 Percutaneous 7 Via Natural or Artificial Opening X External	2 Anti-infective	8 Oxazolidinones 9 Other Anti-infective

DRG Non-OR 3EØ[56][Ø3]Ø2
DRG Non-OR 3EØ[56][Ø3]17
DRG Non-OR 3EØ8[Ø3]17

SECTION: 3 ADMINISTRATION
BODY SYSTEM: E PHYSIOLOGICAL SYSTEMS AND ANATOMICAL REGIONS
OPERATION: Ø INTRODUCTION: *(continued)*

Putting in or on a therapeutic, diagnostic, nutritional, physiological, or prophylactic substance except blood or blood products

Body System / Region	Approach	Substance	Qualifier
9 Nose	3 Percutaneous 7 Via Natural or Artificial Opening X External	3 Anti-inflammatory 4 Serum, Toxoid and Vaccine B Anesthetic Agent H Radioactive Substance K Other Diagnostic Substance N Analgesics, Hypnotics, Sedatives T Destructive Agent	Z No Qualifier
9 Nose	3 Percutaneous 7 Via Natural or Artificial Opening X External	G Other Therapeutic Substance	C Other Substance
A Bone Marrow	3 Percutaneous	Ø Antineoplastic	5 Other Antineoplastic M Monoclonal Antibody
A Bone Marrow	3 Percutaneous	G Other Therapeutic Substance	C Other Substance
B Ear	3 Percutaneous 7 Via Natural or Artificial Opening X External	Ø Antineoplastic	4 Liquid Brachytherapy Radioisotope 5 Other Antineoplastic M Monoclonal Antibody
B Ear	3 Percutaneous 7 Via Natural or Artificial Opening X External	2 Anti-infective	8 Oxazolidinones 9 Other Anti-infective
B Ear	3 Percutaneous 7 Via Natural or Artificial Opening X External	3 Anti-inflammatory B Anesthetic Agent H Radioactive Substance K Other Diagnostic Substance N Analgesics, Hypnotics, Sedatives T Destructive Agent	Z No Qualifier
B Ear	3 Percutaneous 7 Via Natural or Artificial Opening X External	G Other Therapeutic Substance	C Other Substance
C Eye	3 Percutaneous 7 Via Natural or Artificial Opening X External	Ø Antineoplastic	4 Liquid Brachytherapy Radioisotope 5 Other Antineoplastic M Monoclonal Antibody
C Eye	3 Percutaneous 7 Via Natural or Artificial Opening X External	2 Anti-infective	8 Oxazolidinones 9 Other Anti-infective
C Eye	3 Percutaneous 7 Via Natural or Artificial Opening X External	3 Anti-inflammatory B Anesthetic Agent H Radioactive Substance K Other Diagnostic Substance M Pigment N Analgesics, Hypnotics, Sedatives T Destructive Agent	Z No Qualifier
C Eye	3 Percutaneous 7 Via Natural or Artificial Opening X External	G Other Therapeutic Substance	C Other Substance

DRG Non-OR 3EØB329 *(proposed)*
DRG Non-OR 3EØB33Z *(proposed)*
DRG Non-OR 3EØB3[GHKT]C *(proposed)*
DRG Non-OR 3EØB[7X]29 *(proposed)*
DRG Non-OR 3EØB[7X][3BHKT]Z *(proposed)*
DRG Non-OR 3EØB[7X]GC *(proposed)*
DRG Non-OR 3EØC[37X][3BHKMT]Z *(proposed)*
DRG Non-OR 3EØC[37X]GC *(proposed)*
DRG Non-OR 3EØC[37X]SF *(proposed)*
DRG Non-OR 3EØC[7X]29 *(proposed)*

SECTION: 3 ADMINISTRATION
BODY SYSTEM: E PHYSIOLOGICAL SYSTEMS AND ANATOMICAL REGIONS
OPERATION: Ø INTRODUCTION: *(continued)*

Putting in or on a therapeutic, diagnostic, nutritional, physiological, or prophylactic substance except blood or blood products

Body System / Region	Approach	Substance	Qualifier
C Eye	3 Percutaneous 7 Via Natural or Artificial Opening X External	S Gas	F Other Gas
D Mouth and Pharynx	3 Percutaneous 7 Via Natural or Artificial Opening X External	Ø Antineoplastic	4 Liquid Brachytherapy Radioisotope 5 Other Antineoplastic M Monoclonal Antibody
D Mouth and Pharynx	3 Percutaneous 7 Via Natural or Artificial Opening X External	2 Anti-infective	8 Oxazolidinones 9 Other Anti-infective
D Mouth and Pharynx	3 Percutaneous 7 Via Natural or Artificial Opening X External	3 Anti-inflammatory 4 Serum, Toxoid and Vaccine 6 Nutritional Substance 7 Electrolytic and Water Balance Substance B Anesthetic Agent H Radioactive Substance K Other Diagnostic Substance N Analgesics, Hypnotics, Sedatives R Antiarrhythmic T Destructive Agent	Z No Qualifier
D Mouth and Pharynx	3 Percutaneous 7 Via Natural or Artificial Opening X External	G Other Therapeutic Substance	C Other Substance
E Products of Conception ♀ G Upper GI H Lower GI K Genitourinary Tract N Male Reproductive ♂	3 Percutaneous 7 Via Natural or Artificial Opening 8 Via Natural or Artificial Opening Endoscopic	Ø Antineoplastic	4 Liquid Brachytherapy Radioisotope 5 Other Antineoplastic M Monoclonal Antibody
E Products of Conception ♀ G Upper GI H Lower GI K Genitourinary Tract N Male Reproductive ♂	3 Percutaneous 7 Via Natural or Artificial Opening 8 Via Natural or Artificial Opening Endoscopic	2 Anti-infective	8 Oxazolidinones 9 Other Anti-infective
E Products of Conception ♀ G Upper GI H Lower GI K Genitourinary Tract N Male Reproductive ♂	3 Percutaneous 7 Via Natural or Artificial Opening 8 Via Natural or Artificial Opening Endoscopic	3 Anti-inflammatory 6 Nutritional Substance 7 Electrolytic and Water Balance Substance B Anesthetic Agent H Radioactive Substance K Other Diagnostic Substance N Analgesics, Hypnotics, Sedatives T Destructive Agent	Z No Qualifier
E Products of Conception ♀ G Upper GI H Lower GI K Genitourinary Tract N Male Reproductive ♂	3 Percutaneous 7 Via Natural or Artificial Opening 8 Via Natural or Artificial Opening Endoscopic	G Other Therapeutic Substance	C Other Substance

Coding Clinic: 2Ø23, Q2, P34 – 3EØE3KZ

SECTION: 3 ADMINISTRATION
BODY SYSTEM: E PHYSIOLOGICAL SYSTEMS AND ANATOMICAL REGIONS
OPERATION: Ø INTRODUCTION: *(continued)*

Putting in or on a therapeutic, diagnostic, nutritional, physiological, or prophylactic substance except blood or blood products

Body System / Region	Approach	Substance	Qualifier
E Products of Conception ♀ G Upper GI H Lower GI K Genitourinary Tract N Male Reproductive ♂	3 Percutaneous 7 Via Natural or Artificial Opening 8 Via Natural or Artificial Opening Endoscopic	S Gas	F Other Gas
E Products of Conception ♀ G Upper GI H Lower GI K Genitourinary Tract N Male Reproductive ♂	4 Percutaneous Endoscopic	G Other Therapeutic Substance	C Other Substance
F Respiratory Tract	3 Percutaneous 7 Via Natural or Artificial Opening 8 Via Natural or Artificial Opening Endoscopic	Ø Antineoplastic	4 Liquid Brachytherapy Radioisotope 5 Other Antineoplastic M Monoclonal Antibody
F Respiratory Tract	3 Percutaneous 7 Via Natural or Artificial Opening 8 Via Natural or Artificial Opening Endoscopic	2 Anti-infective	8 Oxazolidinones 9 Other Anti-infective
F Respiratory Tract	3 Percutaneous 7 Via Natural or Artificial Opening 8 Via Natural or Artificial Opening Endoscopic	3 Anti-inflammatory 6 Nutritional Substance 7 Electrolytic and Water Balance Substance B Anesthetic Agent H Radioactive Substance K Other Diagnostic Substance N Analgesics, Hypnotics, Sedatives T Destructive Agent	Z No Qualifier
F Respiratory Tract	3 Percutaneous 7 Via Natural or Artificial Opening 8 Via Natural or Artificial Opening Endoscopic	G Other Therapeutic Substance	C Other Substance
F Respiratory Tract	3 Percutaneous 7 Via Natural or Artificial Opening 8 Via Natural or Artificial Opening Endoscopic	S Gas	D Nitric Oxide F Other Gas
F Respiratory Tract	4 Percutaneous Endoscopic	G Other Therapeutic Substance	C Other Substance
J Biliary and Pancreatic Tract	3 Percutaneous 7 Via Natural or Artificial Opening 8 Via Natural or Artificial Opening Endoscopic	Ø Antineoplastic	4 Liquid Brachytherapy Radioisotope 5 Other Antineoplastic M Monoclonal Antibody
J Biliary and Pancreatic Tract	3 Percutaneous 7 Via Natural or Artificial Opening 8 Via Natural or Artificial Opening Endoscopic	2 Anti-infective	8 Oxazolidinones 9 Other Anti-infective
J Biliary and Pancreatic Tract	3 Percutaneous 7 Via Natural or Artificial Opening 8 Via Natural or Artificial Opening Endoscopic	3 Anti-inflammatory 6 Nutritional Substance 7 Electrolytic and Water Balance Substance B Anesthetic Agent H Radioactive Substance K Other Diagnostic Substance N Analgesics, Hypnotics, Sedatives T Destructive Agent	Z No Qualifier

SECTION: 3 ADMINISTRATION
BODY SYSTEM: E PHYSIOLOGICAL SYSTEMS AND ANATOMICAL REGIONS
OPERATION: Ø INTRODUCTION: *(continued)*

Putting in or on a therapeutic, diagnostic, nutritional, physiological, or prophylactic substance except blood or blood products

Body System / Region	Approach	Substance	Qualifier
J Biliary and Pancreatic Tract	3 Percutaneous 7 Via Natural or Artificial Opening 8 Via Natural or Artificial Opening Endoscopic	G Other Therapeutic Substance	C Other Substance
J Biliary and Pancreatic Tract	3 Percutaneous 7 Via Natural or Artificial Opening 8 Via Natural or Artificial Opening Endoscopic	S Gas	F Other Gas
J Biliary and Pancreatic Tract	3 Percutaneous 7 Via Natural or Artificial Opening 8 Via Natural or Artificial Opening Endoscopic	U Pancreatic Islet Cells	Ø Autologous 1 Nonautologous
J Biliary and Pancreatic Tract	4 Percutaneous Endoscopic	G Other Therapeutic Substance	C Other Substance
L Pleural Cavity M Peritoneal Cavity	Ø Open	5 Adhesion Barrier	Z No Qualifier
L Pleural Cavity	3 Percutaneous	Ø Antineoplastic	4 Liquid Brachytherapy Radioisotope 5 Other Antineoplastic M Monoclonal Antibody
L Pleural Cavity	3 Percutaneous	2 Anti-infective	8 Oxazolidinones 9 Other Anti-infective
L Pleural Cavity	3 Percutaneous	3 Anti-inflammatory 5 Adhesion Barrier 6 Nutritional Substance 7 Electrolytic and Water Balance Substance B Anesthetic Agent H Radioactive Substance K Other Diagnostic Substance N Analgesics, Hypnotics, Sedatives T Destructive Agent	Z No Qualifier
L Pleural Cavity	3 Percutaneous	G Other Therapeutic Substance	C Other Substance
L Pleural Cavity	3 Percutaneous	S Gas	F Other Gas
L Pleural Cavity	4 Percutaneous Endoscopic	5 Adhesion Barrier	Z No Qualifier
L Pleural Cavity	4 Percutaneous Endoscopic	G Other Therapeutic Substance	C Other Substance
L Pleural Cavity	7 Via Natural or Artificial Opening	Ø Antineoplastic	4 Liquid Brachytherapy Radioisotope 5 Other Antineoplastic M Monoclonal Antibody
L Pleural Cavity	7 Via Natural or Artificial Opening	S Gas	F Other Gas
M Peritoneal Cavity	Ø Open	5 Adhesion Barrier	Z No Qualifier
M Peritoneal Cavity	3 Percutaneous	Ø Antineoplastic	4 Liquid Brachytherapy Radioisotope 5 Other Antineoplastic M Monoclonal Antibody Y Hyperthermic

DRG Non-OR 3EØJ[378]U[Ø1]

Coding Clinic: 2Ø19, Q4, P37 – 3EØM3ØY

SECTION: 3 ADMINISTRATION
BODY SYSTEM: E PHYSIOLOGICAL SYSTEMS AND ANATOMICAL REGIONS
OPERATION: Ø INTRODUCTION: *(continued)*
Putting in or on a therapeutic, diagnostic, nutritional, physiological, or prophylactic substance except blood or blood products

Body System / Region	Approach	Substance	Qualifier
M Peritoneal Cavity	3 Percutaneous	2 Anti-infective	8 Oxazolidinones 9 Other Anti-infective
M Peritoneal Cavity	3 Percutaneous	3 Anti-inflammatory 5 Adhesion Barrier 6 Nutritional Substance 7 Electrolytic and Water Balance Substance B Anesthetic Agent H Radioactive Substance K Other Diagnostic Substance N Analgesics, Hypnotics, Sedatives T Destructive Agent	Z No Qualifier
M Peritoneal Cavity	3 Percutaneous	G Other Therapeutic Substance	C Other Substance
M Peritoneal Cavity	3 Percutaneous	S Gas	F Other Gas
M Peritoneal Cavity	4 Percutaneous Endoscopic	5 Adhesion Barrier	Z No Qualifier
M Peritoneal Cavity	4 Percutaneous Endoscopic	G Other Therapeutic Substance	C Other Substance
M Peritoneal Cavity	7 Via Natural or Artificial Opening	Ø Antineoplastic	4 Liquid Brachytherapy Radioisotope 5 Other Antineoplastic M Monoclonal Antibody
M Peritoneal Cavity	7 Via Natural or Artificial Opening	S Gas	F Other Gas
P Female Reproductive ♀	Ø Open	5 Adhesion Barrier	Z No Qualifier
P Female Reproductive ♀	3 Percutaneous	Ø Antineoplastic	4 Liquid Brachytherapy Radioisotope 5 Other Antineoplastic M Monoclonal Antibody
P Female Reproductive ♀	3 Percutaneous	2 Anti-infective	8 Oxazolidinones 9 Other Anti-infective
P Female Reproductive ♀	3 Percutaneous	3 Anti-inflammatory 5 Adhesion Barrier 6 Nutritional Substance 7 Electrolytic and Water Balance Substance B Anesthetic Agent H Radioactive Substance K Other Diagnostic Substance L Sperm N Analgesics, Hypnotics, Sedatives T Destructive Agent V Hormone	Z No Qualifier
P Female Reproductive ♀	3 Percutaneous	G Other Therapeutic Substance	C Other Substance
P Female Reproductive ♀	3 Percutaneous	Q Fertilized Ovum	Ø Autologous 1 Nonautologous
P Female Reproductive ♀	3 Percutaneous	S Gas	F Other Gas
P Female Reproductive ♀	4 Percutaneous Endoscopic	5 Adhesion Barrier	Z No Qualifier
P Female Reproductive ♀	4 Percutaneous Endoscopic	G Other Therapeutic Substance	C Other Substance
P Female Reproductive ♀	7 Via Natural or Artificial Opening	Ø Antineoplastic	4 Liquid Brachytherapy Radioisotope 5 Other Antineoplastic M Monoclonal Antibody

Coding Clinic: 2Ø17, Q2, P15; 2Ø15, Q2, P31 – 3EØL3GC

SECTION: 3 ADMINISTRATION
BODY SYSTEM: E PHYSIOLOGICAL SYSTEMS AND ANATOMICAL REGIONS
OPERATION: Ø INTRODUCTION: *(continued)*

Putting in or on a therapeutic, diagnostic, nutritional, physiological, or prophylactic substance except blood or blood products

Body System / Region	Approach	Substance	Qualifier
P Female Reproductive ♀	7 Via Natural or Artificial Opening	2 Anti-infective	8 Oxazolidinones 9 Other Anti-infective
P Female Reproductive ♀	7 Via Natural or Artificial Opening	3 Anti-inflammatory 6 Nutritional Substance 7 Electrolytic and Water Balance Substance B Anesthetic Agent H Radioactive Substance K Other Diagnostic Substance L Sperm N Analgesics, Hypnotics, Sedatives T Destructive Agent V Hormone	Z No Qualifier
P Female Reproductive ♀	7 Via Natural or Artificial Opening	G Other Therapeutic Substance	C Other Substance
P Female Reproductive ♀	7 Via Natural or Artificial Opening	Q Fertilized Ovum	Ø Autologous 1 Nonautologous
P Female Reproductive ♀	7 Via Natural or Artificial Opening	S Gas	F Other Gas
P Female Reproductive ♀	8 Via Natural or Artificial Opening Endoscopic	Ø Antineoplastic	4 Liquid Brachytherapy Radioisotope 5 Other Antineoplastic M Monoclonal Antibody
P Female Reproductive ♀	8 Via Natural or Artificial Opening Endoscopic	2 Anti-infective	8 Oxazolidinones 9 Other Anti-infective
P Female Reproductive ♀	8 Via Natural or Artificial Opening Endoscopic	3 Anti-inflammatory 6 Nutritional Substance 7 Electrolytic and Water Balance Substance B Anesthetic Agent H Radioactive Substance K Other Diagnostic Substance N Analgesics, Hypnotics, Sedatives T Destructive Agent	Z No Qualifier
P Female Reproductive ♀	8 Via Natural or Artificial Opening Endoscopic	G Other Therapeutic Substance	C Other Substance
P Female Reproductive ♀	8 Via Natural or Artificial Opening Endoscopic	S Gas	F Other Gas
Q Cranial Cavity and Brain	Ø Open 3 Percutaneous	Ø Antineoplastic	4 Liquid Brachytherapy Radioisotope 5 Other Antineoplastic M Monoclonal Antibody
Q Cranial Cavity and Brain	Ø Open 3 Percutaneous	2 Anti-infective	8 Oxazolidinones 9 Other Anti-infective
Q Cranial Cavity and Brain	Ø Open 3 Percutaneous	3 Anti-inflammatory 6 Nutritional Substance 7 Electrolytic and Water Balance Substance A Stem Cells, Embryonic B Anesthetic Agent H Radioactive Substance K Other Diagnostic Substance N Analgesics, Hypnotics, Sedatives T Destructive Agent	Z No Qualifier

DRG Non-OR 3EØQ[Ø3]Ø5
DRG Non-OR 3EØP73Z *(proposed)*

Coding Clinic: 2016, Q4, P114 – 3EØQØØ5

SECTION: 3 ADMINISTRATION
BODY SYSTEM: E PHYSIOLOGICAL SYSTEMS AND ANATOMICAL REGIONS
OPERATION: Ø INTRODUCTION: *(continued)*

Putting in or on a therapeutic, diagnostic, nutritional, physiological, or prophylactic substance except blood or blood products

Body System / Region	Approach	Substance	Qualifier
Q Cranial Cavity and Brain	Ø Open 3 Percutaneous	E Stem Cells, Somatic	Ø Autologous 1 Nonautologous
Q Cranial Cavity and Brain	Ø Open 3 Percutaneous	G Other Therapeutic Substance	C Other Substance
Q Cranial Cavity and Brain	Ø Open 3 Percutaneous	S Gas	F Other Gas
Q Cranial Cavity and Brain	7 Via Natural or Artificial Opening	Ø Antineoplastic	4 Liquid Brachytherapy Radioisotope 5 Other Antineoplastic M Monoclonal Antibody
Q Cranial Cavity and Brain	7 Via Natural or Artificial Opening	S Gas	F Other Gas
R Spinal Canal	Ø Open	A Stem Cells, Embryonic	Z No Qualifier
R Spinal Canal	Ø Open	A Stem Cells, Somatic	Ø Autologous 1 Nonautologous
R Spinal Canal	3 Percutaneous	Ø Antineoplastic	2 High-dose Interleukin-2 3 Low-dose Interleukin-2 4 Liquid Brachytherapy Radioisotope 5 Other Antineoplastic M Monoclonal Antibody
R Spinal Canal	3 Percutaneous	2 Anti-infective	8 Oxazolidinones 9 Other Anti-infective
R Spinal Canal	3 Percutaneous	3 Anti-inflammatory 6 Nutritional Substance 7 Electrolytic and Water Balance Substance A Stem Cells, Embryonic B Anesthetic Agent H Radioactive Substance K Other Diagnostic Substance N Analgesics, Hypnotics, Sedatives T Destructive Agent	Z No Qualifier
R Spinal Canal	3 Percutaneous	E Stem Cells, Somatic	Ø Autologous 1 Nonautologous
R Spinal Canal	3 Percutaneous	G Other Therapeutic Substance	C Other Substance
R Spinal Canal	3 Percutaneous	S Gas	F Other Gas
R Spinal Canal	7 Via Natural or Artificial Opening	S Gas	F Other Gas
S Epidural Space	3 Percutaneous	Ø Antineoplastic	2 High-dose Interleukin-2 3 Low-dose Interleukin-2 4 Liquid Brachytherapy Radioisotope 5 Other Antineoplastic M Monoclonal Antibody
S Epidural Space	3 Percutaneous	2 Anti-infective	8 Oxazolidinones 9 Other Anti-infective

DRG Non-OR 3EØQ7Ø5
DRG Non-OR 3EØR3Ø2

SECTION: 3 ADMINISTRATION
BODY SYSTEM: E PHYSIOLOGICAL SYSTEMS AND ANATOMICAL REGIONS
OPERATION: Ø INTRODUCTION: *(continued)*

Putting in or on a therapeutic, diagnostic, nutritional, physiological, or prophylactic substance except blood or blood products

Body System / Region	Approach	Substance	Qualifier
S Epidural Space	3 Percutaneous	3 Anti-inflammatory 6 Nutritional Substance 7 Electrolytic and Water Balance Substance B Anesthetic Agent H Radioactive Substance K Other Diagnostic Substance N Analgesics, Hypnotics, Sedatives T Destructive Agent	Z No Qualifier
S Epidural Space	3 Percutaneous	G Other Therapeutic Substance	C Other Substance
S Epidural Space	3 Percutaneous	S Gas	F Other Gas
S Epidural Space	7 Via Natural or Artificial Opening	S Gas	F Other Gas
T Peripheral Nerves and Plexi X Cranial Nerves	3 Percutaneous	3 Anti-inflammatory B Anesthetic Agent T Destructive Agent	Z No Qualifier
T Peripheral Nerves and Plexi X Cranial Nerves	3 Percutaneous	G Other Therapeutic Substance	C Other Substance
U Joints	Ø Open	2 Anti-infective	8 Oxazolidinones 9 Other Anti-infective
U Joints	Ø Open	G Other Therapeutic Substance	B Recombinant Bone Morphogenetic Protein
U Joints	3 Percutaneous	Ø Antineoplastic	4 Liquid Brachytherapy Radioisotope 5 Other Antineoplastic M Monoclonal Antibody
U Joints	3 Percutaneous	2 Anti-infective	8 Oxazolidinones 9 Other Anti-infective
U Joints	3 Percutaneous	3 Anti-inflammatory 6 Nutritional Substance 7 Electrolytic and Water Balance Substance B Anesthetic Agent H Radioactive Substance K Other Diagnostic Substance N Analgesics, Hypnotics, Sedatives T Destructive Agent	Z No Qualifier
U Joints	3 Percutaneous	G Other Therapeutic Substance	B Recombinant Bone Morphogenetic Protein C Other Substance
U Joints	3 Percutaneous	S Gas	F Other Gas
U Joints	3 Percutaneous Endoscopic	G Other Therapeutic Substance	C Other Substance

DRG Non-OR 3EØS3Ø2

Coding Clinic: 2Ø18, Q1, P8 – 3EØUØGB

3: ADMINISTRATION E: PHYSIOLOGICAL SYSTEMS AND ANATOMICAL REGIONS Ø: INTRODUCTION

SECTION: 3 ADMINISTRATION
BODY SYSTEM: E PHYSIOLOGICAL SYSTEMS AND ANATOMICAL REGIONS
OPERATION: Ø INTRODUCTION: *(continued)*

Putting in or on a therapeutic, diagnostic, nutritional, physiological, or prophylactic substance except blood or blood products

Body System / Region	Approach	Substance	Qualifier
V Bones	Ø Open	G Other Therapeutic Substance	B Recombinant Bone Morphogenetic Protein C Other Substance
V Bones	3 Percutaneous	Ø Antineoplastic	5 Other Antineoplastic M Monoclonal Antibody
V Bones	3 Percutaneous	2 Anti-infective	8 Oxazolidinones 9 Other Anti-infective
V Bones	3 Percutaneous	3 Anti-inflammatory 6 Nutritional Substance 7 Electrolytic and Water Balance Substance B Anesthetic Agent H Radioactive Substance K Other Diagnostic Substance N Analgesics, Hypnotics, Sedatives T Destructive Agent	Z No Qualifier
V Bones	3 Percutaneous	G Other Therapeutic Substance	B Recombinant Bone Morphogenetic Protein C Other Substance
V Bones	4 Percutaneous Endoscopic	G Other Therapeutic Substance	C Other Substance
W Lymphatics	3 Percutaneous	Ø Antineoplastic	5 Other Antineoplastic M Monoclonal Antibody
W Lymphatics	3 Percutaneous	2 Anti-infective	8 Oxazolidinones 9 Other Anti-infective
W Lymphatics	3 Percutaneous	3 Anti-inflammatory 6 Nutritional Substance 7 Electrolytic and Water Balance Substance B Anesthetic Agent H Radioactive Substance K Other Diagnostic Substance N Analgesics, Hypnotics, Sedatives T Destructive Agent	Z No Qualifier
W Lymphatics	3 Percutaneous	G Other Therapeutic Substance	C Other Substance
Y Pericardial Cavity	3 Percutaneous	Ø Antineoplastic	4 Liquid Brachytherapy Radioisotope 5 Other Antineoplastic M Monoclonal Antibody
Y Pericardial Cavity	3 Percutaneous	2 Anti-infective	8 Oxazolidinones 9 Other Anti-infective
Y Pericardial Cavity	3 Percutaneous	3 Anti-inflammatory 6 Nutritional Substance 7 Electrolytic and Water Balance Substance B Anesthetic Agent H Radioactive Substance K Other Diagnostic Substance N Analgesics, Hypnotics, Sedatives T Destructive Agent	Z No Qualifier

Coding Clinic: 2016, Q3, P3Ø – 3EØVØGB

SECTION: 3 ADMINISTRATION
BODY SYSTEM: E PHYSIOLOGICAL SYSTEMS AND ANATOMICAL REGIONS
OPERATION: Ø INTRODUCTION: *(continued)*

Putting in or on a therapeutic, diagnostic, nutritional, physiological, or prophylactic substance except blood or blood products

Body System / Region	Approach	Substance	Qualifier
Y Pericardial Cavity	3 Percutaneous	G Other Therapeutic Substance	C Other Substance
Y Pericardial Cavity	3 Percutaneous	S Gas	F Other Gas
Y Pericardial Cavity	3 Percutaneous Endoscopic	G Other Therapeutic Substance	C Other Substance
Y Pericardial Cavity	7 Via Natural or Artificial Opening	Ø Antineoplastic	4 Liquid Brachytherapy Radioisotope 5 Other Antineoplastic M Monoclonal Antibody
Y Pericardial Cavity	7 Via Natural or Artificial Opening	S Gas	F Other Gas

Coding Clinic: 2Ø13, Q1, P27 – 3EØG8TZ
Coding Clinic: 2Ø15, Q1, P31 – 3EØR3Ø5
Coding Clinic: 2Ø15, Q1, P38 – 3EØ53Ø5

SECTION: 3 ADMINISTRATION
BODY SYSTEM: E PHYSIOLOGICAL SYSTEMS AND ANATOMICAL REGIONS
OPERATION: 1 IRRIGATION: Putting in or on a cleansing substance

Body System / Region	Approach	Substance	Qualifier
Ø Skin and Mucous Membranes C Eye	3 Percutaneous X External	8 Irrigating Substance	X Diagnostic Z No Qualifier
9 Nose B Ear F Respiratory Tract G Upper GI H Lower GI J Biliary and Pancreatic Tract K Genitourinary Tract N Male Reproductive ♂ P Female Reproductive ♀	3 Percutaneous 7 Via Natural or Artificial Opening 8 Via Natural or Artificial Opening Endoscopic	8 Irrigating Substance	X Diagnostic Z No Qualifier
L Pleural Cavity Q Cranial Cavity and Brain R Spinal Canal S Epidural Space Y Pericardial Cavity	3 Percutaneous	8 Irrigating Substance	X Diagnostic Z No Qualifier
M Peritoneal Cavity	3 Percutaneous	8 Irrigating Substance	X Diagnostic Z No Qualifier
M Peritoneal Cavity	3 Percutaneous	9 Dialysate	Z No Qualifier
M Peritoneal Cavity	4 Percutaneous Endoscopic	8 Irrigating Substance	X Diagnostic Z No Qualifier
U Joints	3 Percutaneous 4 Percutaneous Endoscopic	8 Irrigating Substance	X Diagnostic Z No Qualifier

SECTION: 4 MEASUREMENT AND MONITORING
BODY SYSTEM: A PHYSIOLOGICAL SYSTEMS
OPERATION: Ø MEASUREMENT: *(on multiple pages)*

Determining the level of a physiological or physical function at a point in time

Body System	Approach	Function / Device	Qualifier
Ø Central Nervous	Ø Open	2 Conductivity 4 Electrical Activity B Pressure	Z No Qualifier
Ø Central Nervous	3 Percutaneous 7 Via Natural or Artificial Opening 8 Via Natural or Artificial Opening Endoscopic	4 Electrical Activity	Z No Qualifier
Ø Central Nervous	3 Percutaneous 7 Via Natural or Artificial Opening 8 Via Natural or Artificial Opening Endoscopic	B Pressure K Temperature R Saturation	D Intracranial
Ø Central Nervous	X External	2 Conductivity 4 Electrical Activity	Z No Qualifier
1 Peripheral Nervous	Ø Open 3 Percutaneous 7 Via Natural or Artificial Opening 8 Via Natural or Artificial Opening Endoscopic X External	2 Conductivity	9 Sensory B Motor
1 Peripheral Nervous	Ø Open 3 Percutaneous 7 Via Natural or Artificial Opening 8 Via Natural or Artificial Opening Endoscopic X External	4 Electrical Activity	Z No Qualifier
2 Cardiac	Ø Open 3 Percutaneous 7 Via Natural or Artificial Opening 8 Via Natural or Artificial Opening Endoscopic	4 Electrical Activity 9 Output C Rate F Rhythm H Sound P Action Currents	Z No Qualifier
2 Cardiac	Ø Open 3 Percutaneous 7 Via Natural or Artificial Opening 8 Via Natural or Artificial Opening Endoscopic	N Sampling and Pressure	6 Right Heart 7 Left Heart 8 Bilateral
2 Cardiac	X External	4 Electrical Activity	A Guidance Z No Qualifier
2 Cardiac	X External	9 Output C Rate F Rhythm H Sound P Action Currents	Z No Qualifier
2 Cardiac	X External	M Total Activity	4 Stress
3 Arterial	Ø Open 3 Percutaneous	5 Flow J Pulse	1 Peripheral 3 Pulmonary C Coronary
3 Arterial	Ø Open 3 Percutaneous	B Pressure	1 Peripheral 3 Pulmonary C Coronary F Other Thoracic

DRG Non-OR 4AØ2[378]FZ
DRG Non-OR 4AØ2[Ø378]N[678]
Non-OR 4AØ2X4A

Coding Clinic: 2Ø15, Q3, P29 – 4AØ2X4Z
Coding Clinic: 2Ø16, Q3, P37 – 4AØ33BC
Coding Clinic: 2Ø18, Q1, P13 – 4AØ23N8
Coding Clinic: 2Ø19, Q3, P32 – 4AØ23N6
Coding Clinic: 2Ø22, Q1, P46 – 4AØ234Z

SECTION: 4 MEASUREMENT AND MONITORING
BODY SYSTEM: A PHYSIOLOGICAL SYSTEMS
OPERATION: Ø MEASUREMENT: *(continued)*
Determining the level of a physiological or physical function at a point in time

Body System	Approach	Function / Device	Qualifier
3 Arterial	Ø Open 3 Percutaneous	H Sound R Saturation	1 Peripheral
3 Arterial	X External	5 Flow	1 Peripheral D Intracranial
3 Arterial	X External	B Pressure H Sound J Pulse R Saturation	1 Peripheral
4 Venous	Ø Open 3 Percutaneous	5 Flow B Pressure J Pulse	Ø Central 1 Peripheral 2 Portal 3 Pulmonary
4 Venous	Ø Open 3 Percutaneous	R Saturation	1 Peripheral
4 Venous	4 Percutaneous Endoscopic	B Pressure	2 Portal
4 Venous	X External	5 Flow B Pressure J Pulse R Saturation	1 Peripheral
5 Circulatory	X External	L Volume	Z No Qualifier
6 Lymphatic	Ø Open 3 Percutaneous 7 Via Natural or Artificial Opening 8 Via Natural or Artificial Opening Endoscopic	5 Flow B Pressure	Z No Qualifier
7 Visual	X External	Ø Acuity 7 Mobility B Pressure	Z No Qualifier
8 Olfactory	X External	Ø Acuity	Z No Qualifier
9 Respiratory	7 Via Natural or Artificial Opening 8 Via Natural or Artificial Opening Endoscopic X External	1 Capacity 5 Flow C Rate D Resistance L Volume M Total Activity	Z No Qualifier
B Gastrointestinal	7 Via Natural or Artificial Opening 8 Via Natural or Artificial Opening Endoscopic	8 Motility B Pressure G Secretion	Z No Qualifier
C Biliary	3 Percutaneous 4 Percutaneous Endoscopic 7 Via Natural or Artificial Opening 8 Via Natural or Artificial Opening Endoscopic	5 Flow B Pressure	Z No Qualifier
D Urinary	7 Via Natural or Artificial Opening 8 Via Natural or Artificial Opening Endoscopic	3 Contractility 5 Flow B Pressure D Resistance L Volume	Z No Qualifier
F Musculoskeletal	3 Percutaneous	3 Contractility	Z No Qualifier
F Musculoskeletal	3 Percutaneous	B Pressure	E Compartment

SECTION: 4 MEASUREMENT AND MONITORING
BODY SYSTEM: A PHYSIOLOGICAL SYSTEMS
OPERATION: Ø MEASUREMENT: *(continued)*

Determining the level of a physiological or physical function at a point in time

Body System	Approach	Function / Device	Qualifier
F Musculoskeletal	X External	3 Contractility	Z No Qualifier
H Products of Conception, Cardiac ♀	7 Via Natural or Artificial Opening 8 Via Natural or Artificial Opening Endoscopic X External	4 Electrical Activity C Rate F Rhythm H Sound	Z No Qualifier
J Products of Conception, Nervous ♀	7 Via Natural or Artificial Opening 8 Via Natural or Artificial Opening Endoscopic X External	2 Conductivity 4 Electrical Activity B Pressure	Z No Qualifier
Z None	7 Via Natural or Artificial Opening	6 Metabolism K Temperature	Z No Qualifier
Z None	X External	6 Metabolism K Temperature Q Sleep	Z No Qualifier

SECTION: 4 MEASUREMENT AND MONITORING
BODY SYSTEM: A PHYSIOLOGICAL SYSTEMS
OPERATION: 1 MONITORING: *(on multiple pages)*

Determining the level of a physiological or physical function repetitively over a period of time

Body System	Approach	Function / Device	Qualifier
Ø Central Nervous	Ø Open	2 Conductivity B Pressure	Z No Qualifier
Ø Central Nervous	Ø Open	4 Electrical Activity	G Intraoperative Z No Qualifier
Ø Central Nervous	3 Percutaneous 7 Via Natural or Artificial Opening 8 Via Natural or Artificial Opening Endoscopic	4 Electrical Activity	G Intraoperative Z No Qualifier
Ø Central Nervous	3 Percutaneous 7 Via Natural or Artificial Opening 8 Via Natural or Artificial Opening Endoscopic	B Pressure K Temperature R Saturation	D Intracranial
Ø Central Nervous	X External	2 Conductivity	Z No Qualifier
Ø Central Nervous	X External	4 Electrical Activity	G Intraoperative Z No Qualifier
1 Peripheral Nervous	Ø Open 3 Percutaneous 7 Via Natural or Artificial Opening 8 Via Natural or Artificial Opening Endoscopic X External	2 Conductivity	9 Sensory B Motor
1 Peripheral Nervous	Ø Open 3 Percutaneous 7 Via Natural or Artificial Opening 8 Via Natural or Artificial Opening Endoscopic X External	4 Electrical Activity	G Intraoperative Z No Qualifier

Coding Clinic: 2Ø15, Q2, P14 – 4A11X4G
Coding Clinic: 2Ø16, Q2, P29 – 4A1Ø3BD

SECTION: 4 MEASUREMENT AND MONITORING
BODY SYSTEM: A PHYSIOLOGICAL SYSTEMS
OPERATION: 1 MONITORING: *(continued)*

Determining the level of a physiological or physical function repetitively over a period of time

Body System	Approach	Function / Device	Qualifier
2 Cardiac	Ø Open 3 Percutaneous 7 Via Natural or Artificial Opening 8 Via Natural or Artificial Opening Endoscopic	4 Electrical Activity 9 Output C Rate F Rhythm H Sound	Z No Qualifier
2 Cardiac	X External	4 Electrical Activity	5 Ambulatory Z No Qualifier
2 Cardiac	X External	9 Output C Rate F Rhythm H Sound	Z No Qualifier
2 Cardiac	X External	M Total Activity	4 Stress
2 Cardiac	X External	S Vascular Perfusion	H Indocyanine Green Dye
3 Arterial	Ø Open 3 Percutaneous	5 Flow B Pressure J Pulse	1 Peripheral 3 Pulmonary C Coronary
3 Arterial	Ø Open 3 Percutaneous	H Sound R Saturation	1 Peripheral
3 Arterial	X External	5 Flow B Pressure H Sound J Pulse R Saturation	1 Peripheral
4 Venous	Ø Open 3 Percutaneous	5 Flow B Pressure J Pulse	Ø Central 1 Peripheral 2 Portal 3 Pulmonary
4 Venous	Ø Open 3 Percutaneous	R Saturation	Ø Central 2 Portal 3 Pulmonary
4 Venous	X External	5 Flow B Pressure J Pulse	1 Peripheral
6 Lymphatic	Ø Open 3 Percutaneous 7 Via Natural or Artificial Opening 8 Via Natural or Artificial Opening Endoscopic	5 Flow	H Indocyanine Green Dye Z No Qualifier
6 Lymphatic	Ø Open 3 Percutaneous 7 Via Natural or Artificial Opening 8 Via Natural or Artificial Opening Endoscopic	B Pressure	Z No Qualifier

Coding Clinic: 2Ø15, Q3, P35 – 4A1239Z, 4A133B3
Coding Clinic: 2Ø16, Q2, P33 – 4A133[BJ]1

SECTION: 4 MEASUREMENT AND MONITORING
BODY SYSTEM: A PHYSIOLOGICAL SYSTEMS
OPERATION: 1 MONITORING: *(continued)*

Determining the level of a physiological or physical function repetitively over a period of time

Body System	Approach	Function / Device	Qualifier
9 Respiratory	7 Via Natural or Artificial Opening X External	1 Capacity 5 Flow C Rate D Resistance L Volume	Z No Qualifier
B Gastrointestinal	7 Via Natural or Artificial Opening 8 Via Natural or Artificial Opening Endoscopic	8 Motility B Pressure G Secretion	Z No Qualifier
B Gastrointestinal	X External	S Vascular Perfusion	H Indocyanine Green Dye
D Urinary	7 Via Natural or Artificial Opening 8 Via Natural or Artificial Opening Endoscopic	3 Contractility 5 Flow B Pressure D Resistance L Volume	Z No Qualifier
G Skin and Breast	X External	S Vascular Perfusion	H Indocyanine Green Dye
H Products of Conception, Cardiac ♀	7 Via Natural or Artificial Opening 8 Via Natural or Artificial Opening Endoscopic X External	4 Electrical Activity C Rate F Rhythm H Sound	Z No Qualifier
J Products of Conception, Nervous ♀	7 Via Natural or Artificial Opening 8 Via Natural or Artificial Opening Endoscopic X External	2 Conductivity 4 Electrical Activity B Pressure	Z No Qualifier
Z None	7 Via Natural or Artificial Opening	K Temperature	Z No Qualifier
Z None	X External	K Temperature Q Sleep	Z No Qualifier

Coding Clinic: 2015, Q1, P26 – 4A11X4G

SECTION: 4 MEASUREMENT AND MONITORING
BODY SYSTEM: B PHYSIOLOGICAL DEVICES
OPERATION: Ø MEASUREMENT: Determining the level of a physiological or physical function at a point in time

Body System	Approach	Function / Device	Qualifier
Ø Central Nervous	X External	V Stimulator	Z No Qualifier
Ø Central Nervous	X External	W Cerebrospinal Fluid Shunt	Ø Wireless Sensor
1 Peripheral Nervous F Musculoskeletal	X External	V Stimulator	Z No Qualifier
2 Cardiac	X External	S Pacemaker T Defibrillator	Z No Qualifier
9 Respiratory	X External	S Pacemaker	Z No Qualifier

SECTION: 5 EXTRACORPOREAL OR SYSTEMIC ASSISTANCE AND PERFORMANCE

BODY SYSTEM: A PHYSIOLOGICAL SYSTEMS

OPERATION: Ø ASSISTANCE: Taking over a portion of a physiological function by extracorporeal means

Body System	Duration	Function	Qualifier
2 Cardiac	1 Intermittent	1 Output	Ø Balloon Pump 5 Pulsatile Compression 6 Pump D Impeller Pump
2 Cardiac	2 Continuous	1 Output	Ø Balloon Pump 5 Pulsatile Compression 6 Other Pump D Impeller Pump
2 Cardiac	2 Continuous	2 Oxygenation	C Supersaturated
5 Circulatory	1 Intermittent 2 Continuous	2 Oxygenation	1 Hyperbaric
9 Respiratory	2 Continuous	Ø Filtration	Z No Qualifier
9 Respiratory	3 Less than 24 Consecutive Hours 4 24-96 Consecutive Hours 5 Greater than 96 Consecutive Hours	5 Ventilation	7 Continuous Positive Airway Pressure 8 Intermittent Positive Airway Pressure 9 Continuous Negative Airway Pressure A High Nasal Flow/Velocity B Intermittent Negative Airway Pressure Z No Qualifier
9 Respiratory	B Less than 8 Consecutive Hours C 8-24 Consecutive Hours D Greater than 24 Consecutive Hours	5 Ventilation	K Intubated Prone Positioning

Coding Clinic: 2Ø22, Q3, P24; 2Ø21, Q2, P12; 2Ø13, Q3, P19 – 5AØ221Ø
Coding Clinic: 2Ø17, Q1, P1Ø-11, 29; 2Ø16, Q4, P137 – 5AØ
Coding Clinic: 2Ø17, Q1, P11-12; 2Ø16, Q4, P139 – 5AØ221D
Coding Clinic: 2Ø17, Q4, P44-45 – 5AØ221D
Coding Clinic: 2Ø18, Q2, P4-5 – 5AØ221Ø
Coding Clinic: 2Ø2Ø, Q1, P11 – 5AØ9357

SECTION: 5 EXTRACORPOREAL OR SYSTEMIC ASSISTANCE AND PERFORMANCE

BODY SYSTEM: A PHYSIOLOGICAL SYSTEMS

OPERATION: 1 PERFORMANCE: Completely taking over a physiological function by extracorporeal means

Body System	Duration	Function	Qualifier
2 Cardiac	Ø Single	1 Output	2 Manual
2 Cardiac	1 Intermittent	3 Pacing	Z No Qualifier
2 Cardiac	2 Continuous	1 Output	J Automated Z No Qualifier
2 Cardiac	2 Continuous	3 Pacing	Z No Qualifier
5 Circulatory	2 Continuous A Intraoperative	2 Oxygenation	F Membrane, Central G Membrane, Peripheral Veno-arterial H Membrane, Peripheral Veno-venous
9 Respiratory	Ø Single	5 Ventilation	4 Nonmechanical
9 Respiratory	3 Less than 24 Consecutive Hours 4 24-96 Consecutive Hours 5 Greater than 96 Consecutive Hours	5 Ventilation	Z No Qualifier
C Biliary	Ø Single 6 Multiple	Ø Filtration	Z No Qualifier
D Urinary	7 Intermittent, Less than 6 Hours Per Day 8 Prolonged Intermittent, 6-18 Hours Per Day 9 Continuous, Greater than 18 Hours Per Day	Ø Filtration	Z No Qualifier

DRG Non-OR 5A19[345]5Z
DRG Non-OR 5A1522[GH]
DRG Non-OR 5A1D[789]ØZ

NOTE: **5A1955Z** should only be coded on claims when the respiratory ventilation is provided for greater than 4 consecutive days during the length of stay.

Coding Clinic: 2013, Q3, P19 – 5A1223Z
Coding Clinic: 2015, Q4, P23-25; 2013, Q3, P19 – 5A1221Z
Coding Clinic: 2016, Q1, P28 – 5A1221Z
Coding Clinic: 2016, Q1, P29 – 5A1CØØZ, 5A1D6ØZ
Coding Clinic: 2017, Q1, P2Ø – 5A1221Z
Coding Clinic: 2017, Q3, P7 – 5A1221Z
Coding Clinic: 2017, Q4, P72-73 – 51AD[789]ØZ
Coding Clinic: 2018, Q1, P14 – 5A1935Z
Coding Clinic: 2018, Q4, P53-54 – 5A1522H
Coding Clinic: 2018, Q4, P54 – 5A1522G
Coding Clinic: 2019, Q2, P36 – 5A1522F
Coding Clinic: 2019, Q4, P4Ø – 5A15A2G
Coding Clinic: 2022, Q2, P25 – 51A1223Z

SECTION: 5 EXTRACORPOREAL OR SYSTEMIC ASSISTANCE AND PERFORMANCE

BODY SYSTEM: A PHYSIOLOGICAL SYSTEMS

OPERATION: 2 RESTORATION: Returning, or attempting to return, a physiological function to its original state by extracorporeal means

Body System	Duration	Function	Qualifier
2 Cardiac	Ø Single	4 Rhythm	Z No Qualifier

Coding Clinic: 2022, Q1, P46 – 5A22Ø4Z

SECTION: 6 EXTRACORPOREAL OR SYSTEMIC THERAPIES
BODY SYSTEM: A PHYSIOLOGICAL SYSTEMS
OPERATION: Ø **ATMOSPHERIC CONTROL:** Extracorporeal control of atmospheric pressure and composition

Body System	Duration	Qualifier	Qualifier
Z None	Ø Single 1 Multiple	Z No Qualifier	Z No Qualifier

SECTION: 6 EXTRACORPOREAL OR SYSTEMIC THERAPIES
BODY SYSTEM: A PHYSIOLOGICAL SYSTEMS
OPERATION: 1 **DECOMPRESSION:** Extracorporeal elimination of undissolved gas from body fluids

Body System	Duration	Qualifier	Qualifier
5 Circulatory	Ø Single 1 Multiple	Z No Qualifier	Z No Qualifier

SECTION: 6 EXTRACORPOREAL OR SYSTEMIC THERAPIES
BODY SYSTEM: A PHYSIOLOGICAL SYSTEMS
OPERATION: 2 **ELECTROMAGNETIC THERAPY:** Extracorporeal treatment by electromagnetic rays

Body System	Duration	Qualifier	Qualifier
1 Urinary 2 Central Nervous	Ø Single 1 Multiple	Z No Qualifier	Z No Qualifier

SECTION: 6 EXTRACORPOREAL OR SYSTEMIC THERAPIES
BODY SYSTEM: A PHYSIOLOGICAL SYSTEMS
OPERATION: 3 **HYPERTHERMIA:** Extracorporeal raising of body temperature

Body System	Duration	Qualifier	Qualifier
Z None	Ø Single 1 Multiple	Z No Qualifier	Z No Qualifier

SECTION: 6 EXTRACORPOREAL OR SYSTEMIC THERAPIES
BODY SYSTEM: A PHYSIOLOGICAL SYSTEMS
OPERATION: 4 **HYPOTHERMIA:** Extracorporeal lowering of body temperature

Body System	Duration	Qualifier	Qualifier
Z None	Ø Single 1 Multiple	Z No Qualifier	Z No Qualifier

Coding Clinic: 2Ø19, Q2, P18 – 6A4ZØZZ

SECTION: 6 EXTRACORPOREAL OR SYSTEMIC THERAPIES
BODY SYSTEM: A PHYSIOLOGICAL SYSTEMS
OPERATION: 5 PHERESIS: Extracorporeal separation of blood products

Body System	Duration	Qualifier	Qualifier
5 Circulatory	Ø Single 1 Multiple	Z No Qualifier	Ø Erythrocytes 1 Leukocytes 2 Platelets 3 Plasma T Stem Cells, Cord Blood V Stem Cells, Hematopoietic

Coding Clinic: 2Ø22, Q1, P48 – 6A55ØZT

SECTION: 6 EXTRACORPOREAL OR SYSTEMIC THERAPIES
BODY SYSTEM: A PHYSIOLOGICAL SYSTEMS
OPERATION: 6 PHOTOTHERAPY: Extracorporeal treatment by light rays

Body System	Duration	Qualifier	Qualifier
Ø Skin 5 Circulatory	Ø Single 1 Multiple	Z No Qualifier	Z No Qualifier

SECTION: 6 EXTRACORPOREAL OR SYSTEMIC THERAPIES
BODY SYSTEM: A PHYSIOLOGICAL SYSTEMS
OPERATION: 7 ULTRASOUND THERAPY: Extracorporeal treatment by ultrasound

Body System	Duration	Qualifier	Qualifier
5 Circulatory	Ø Single 1 Multiple	Z No Qualifier	4 Head and Neck Vessels 5 Heart 6 Peripheral Vessels 7 Other Vessels Z No Qualifier

SECTION: 6 EXTRACORPOREAL OR SYSTEMIC THERAPIES
BODY SYSTEM: A PHYSIOLOGICAL SYSTEMS
OPERATION: 8 ULTRAVIOLET LIGHT THERAPY: Extracorporeal treatment by ultraviolet light

Body System	Duration	Qualifier	Qualifier
Ø Skin	Ø Single 1 Multiple	Z No Qualifier	Z No Qualifier

SECTION: 6 EXTRACORPOREAL OR SYSTEMIC THERAPIES
BODY SYSTEM: A PHYSIOLOGICAL SYSTEMS
OPERATION: 9 SHOCK WAVE THERAPY: Extracorporeal treatment by shock waves

Body System	Duration	Qualifier	Qualifier
3 Musculoskeletal	Ø Single 1 Multiple	Z No Qualifier	Z No Qualifier

SECTION: 6 EXTRACORPOREAL OR SYSTEMIC THERAPIES
BODY SYSTEM: A PHYSIOLOGICAL SYSTEMS
OPERATION: B PERFUSION: Extracorporeal treatment by diffusion of therapeutic fluid

Body System	Duration	Qualifier	Qualifier
5 Circulatory B Respiratory System F Hepatobiliary System and Pancreas T Urinary System	Ø Single	B Donor Organ	Z No Qualifier

SECTION: 7 OSTEOPATHIC
BODY SYSTEM: W ANATOMICAL REGIONS
OPERATION: Ø TREATMENT: Manual treatment to eliminate or alleviate somatic dysfunction and related disorders

Body Region	Approach	Method	Qualifier
Ø Head 1 Cervical 2 Thoracic 3 Lumbar 4 Sacrum 5 Pelvis 6 Lower Extremities 7 Upper Extremities 8 Rib Cage 9 Abdomen	X External	Ø Articulatory-Raising 1 Fascial Release 2 General Mobilization 3 High Velocity-Low Amplitude 4 Indirect 5 Low Velocity-High Amplitude 6 Lymphatic Pump 7 Muscle Energy-Isometric 8 Muscle Energy-Isotonic 9 Other Method	Z None

SECTION: 8 OTHER PROCEDURES
BODY SYSTEM: C INDWELLING DEVICE
OPERATION: Ø OTHER PROCEDURES: Methodologies which attempt to remediate or cure a disorder or disease

Body Region	Approach	Method	Qualifier
1 Nervous System	X External	6 Collection	J Cerebrospinal Fluid L Other Fluid
2 Circulatory System	X External	6 Collection	K Blood L Other Fluid

SECTION: 8 OTHER PROCEDURES
BODY SYSTEM: E PHYSIOLOGICAL SYSTEMS AND ANATOMICAL REGIONS
OPERATION: Ø OTHER PROCEDURES: *(on multiple pages)* Methodologies which attempt to remediate or cure a disorder or disease

Body Region	Approach	Method	Qualifier
1 Nervous System ~~U Female Reproductive System~~	X External	Y Other Method	7 Examination
2 Circulatory System	3 Percutaneous X External	D Near Infrared Spectroscopy	Z No Qualifier
9 Head and Neck Region	Ø Open	C Robotic Assisted Procedure	Z No Qualifier
9 Head and Neck Region	Ø Open	E Fluorescence Guided Procedure	M Aminolevulinic Acid Z No Qualifier
9 Head and Neck Region	3 Percutaneous 4 Percutaneous Endoscopic 7 Via Natural or Artificial Opening 8 Via Natural or Artificial Opening Endoscopic	C Robotic Assisted Procedure E Fluorescence Guided Procedure	Z No Qualifier
9 Head and Neck Region	X External	B Computer Assisted Procedure	F With Fluoroscopy G With Computerized Tomography H With Magnetic Resonance Imaging Z No Qualifier
9 Head and Neck Region	X External	C Robotic Assisted Procedure	Z No Qualifier
9 Head and Neck Region	X External	Y Other Method	8 Suture Removal
H Integumentary System and Breast	3 Percutaneous	Ø Acupuncture	Ø Anesthesia Z No Qualifier
H Integumentary System and Breast	X External	6 Collection	2 Breast Milk ♀
H Integumentary System and Breast	X External	Y Other Method	9 Piercing

Coding Clinic: 2021, Q2, P2Ø – 8EØ9XBZ

SECTION: 8 OTHER PROCEDURES
BODY SYSTEM: E PHYSIOLOGICAL SYSTEMS AND ANATOMICAL REGIONS
OPERATION: Ø OTHER PROCEDURES: *(continued)*
Methodologies which attempt to remediate or cure a disorder or disease

Body Region	Approach	Method	Qualifier
K Musculoskeletal System	X External	1 Therapeutic Massage	Z No Qualifier
K Musculoskeletal System	X External	Y Other Method	7 Examination
U Female Reproductive System	Ø Open 3 Percutaneous 4 Percutaneous Endoscopic 7 Via Natural or Artificial Opening 8 Via Natural or Artificial Opening Endoscopic	E Fluorescence Guided Procedure	N Pafolacianine
U Female Reproductive System	X External	Y Other Method	7 Examination
V Male Reproductive System ♂	X External	1 Therapeutic Massage	C Prostate D Rectum
V Male Reproductive System ♂	X External	6 Collection	3 Sperm
W Trunk Region	Ø Open 3 Percutaneous 4 Percutaneous Endoscopic 7 Via Natural or Artificial Opening 8 Via Natural or Artificial Opening Endoscopic	C Robotic Assisted Procedure ~~E Fluorescence Guided Procedure~~	Z No Qualifier
W Trunk Region	Ø Open 3 Percutaneous 4 Percutaneous Endoscopic 7 Via Natural or Artificial Opening 8 Via Natural or Artificial Opening Endoscopic	E Fluorescence Guided Procedure	N Pafolacianine Z No Qualifier
W Trunk Region	X External	B Computer Assisted Procedure	F With Fluoroscopy G With Computerized Tomography H With Magnetic Resonance Imaging Z No Qualifier
W Trunk Region	X External	C Robotic Assisted Procedure	Z No Qualifier
W Trunk Region	X External	Y Other Method	8 Suture Removal
X Upper Extremity Y Lower Extremity	Ø Open 3 Percutaneous 4 Percutaneous Endoscopic	C Robotic Assisted Procedure E Fluorescence Guided Procedure	Z No Qualifier
X Upper Extremity Y Lower Extremity	X External	B Computer Assisted Procedure	F With Fluoroscopy G With Computerized Tomography H With Magnetic Resonance Imaging Z No Qualifier
X Upper Extremity Y Lower Extremity	X External	C Robotic Assisted Procedure	Z No Qualifier
X Upper Extremity Y Lower Extremity	X External	Y Other Method	8 Suture Removal
Z None	X External	Y Other Method	1 In Vitro Fertilization 4 Yoga Therapy 5 Meditation 6 Isolation

Coding Clinic: 2Ø19, Q1, P31; 2Ø15, Q1, P34 – 8EØW4CZ
Coding Clinic: 2Ø21, Q4, P5Ø – 8EØW3CZ

9WB

SECTION: 9 CHIROPRACTIC
BODY SYSTEM: W ANATOMICAL REGIONS
OPERATION: B MANIPULATION: Manual procedure that involves a directed thrust to move a joint past the physiological range of motion, without exceeding the anatomical limit

Body Region	Approach	Method	Qualifier
Ø Head 1 Cervical 2 Thoracic 3 Lumbar 4 Sacrum 5 Pelvis 6 Lower Extremities 7 Upper Extremities 8 Rib Cage 9 Abdomen	X External	B Non-Manual C Indirect Visceral D Extra-Articular F Direct Visceral G Long Lever Specific Contact H Short Lever Specific Contact J Long and Short Lever Specific Contact K Mechanically Assisted L Other Method	Z None

SECTION: B IMAGING
BODY SYSTEM: Ø CENTRAL NERVOUS SYSTEM
TYPE: Ø PLAIN RADIOGRAPHY: Planar display of an image developed from the capture of external ionizing radiation on photographic or photoconductive plate

Body Part	Contrast	Qualifier	Qualifier
B Spinal Cord	Ø High Osmolar 1 Low Osmolar Y Other Contrast Z None	Z None	Z None

SECTION: B IMAGING
BODY SYSTEM: Ø CENTRAL NERVOUS SYSTEM
TYPE: 1 FLUOROSCOPY: Single plane or bi-plane real-time display of an image developed from the capture of external ionizing radiation on a fluorescent screen. The image may also be stored by either digital or analog means.

Body Part	Contrast	Qualifier	Qualifier
B Spinal Cord	Ø High Osmolar 1 Low Osmolar Y Other Contrast Z None	Z None	Z None

SECTION: B IMAGING
BODY SYSTEM: Ø CENTRAL NERVOUS SYSTEM
TYPE: 2 COMPUTERIZED TOMOGRAPHY (CT SCAN): Computer-reformatted digital display of multiplanar images developed from the capture of multiple exposures of external ionizing radiation

Body Part	Contrast	Qualifier	Qualifier
Ø Brain 7 Cisterna 8 Cerebral Ventricle(s) 9 Sella Turcica/Pituitary Gland B Spinal Cord	Ø High Osmolar 1 Low Osmolar Y Other Contrast	Ø Unenhanced and Enhanced Z None	Z None
Ø Brain 7 Cisterna 8 Cerebral Ventricle(s) 9 Sella Turcica/Pituitary Gland B Spinal Cord	Z None	Z None	Z None

SECTION: B IMAGING
BODY SYSTEM: Ø CENTRAL NERVOUS SYSTEM
TYPE: 3 MAGNETIC RESONANCE IMAGING (MRI): Computer-reformatted digital display of multiplanar images developed from the capture of radiofrequency signals emitted by nuclei in a body site excited within a magnetic field

Body Part	Contrast	Qualifier	Qualifier
Ø Brain 9 Sella Turcica/Pituitary Gland B Spinal Cord C Acoustic Nerves	Y Other Contrast	Ø Unenhanced and Enhanced Z None	Z None
Ø Brain 9 Sella Turcica/Pituitary Gland B Spinal Cord C Acoustic Nerves	Z None	Z None	Z None

SECTION: B IMAGING
BODY SYSTEM: Ø CENTRAL NERVOUS SYSTEM
TYPE: 4 ULTRASONOGRAPHY: Real-time display of images of anatomy or flow information developed from the capture of reflected and attenuated high-frequency sound waves

Body Part	Contrast	Qualifier	Qualifier
Ø Brain B Spinal Cord	Z None	Z None	Z None

SECTION: B IMAGING
BODY SYSTEM: 2 HEART
TYPE: Ø PLAIN RADIOGRAPHY: Planar display of an image developed from the capture of external ionizing radiation on photographic or photoconductive plate

Body Part	Contrast	Qualifier	Qualifier
Ø Coronary Artery, Single 1 Coronary Arteries, Multiple 2 Coronary Artery Bypass Graft, Single 3 Coronary Artery Bypass Grafts, Multiple 4 Heart, Right 5 Heart, Left 6 Heart, Right and Left 7 Internal Mammary Bypass Graft, Right 8 Internal Mammary Bypass Graft, Left F Bypass Graft, Other	Ø High Osmolar 1 Low Osmolar Y Other Contrast	Z None	Z None

DRG Non-OR B2Ø[Ø1234578F][Ø1Y]ZZ

Coding Clinic: 2Ø18, Q1, P13 – B2151ZZ

SECTION: B IMAGING
BODY SYSTEM: 2 HEART
TYPE: 1 FLUOROSCOPY: Single plane or bi-plane real-time display of an image developed from the capture of external ionizing radiation on a fluorescent screen. The image may also be stored by either digital or analog means.

Body Part	Contrast	Qualifier	Qualifier
Ø Coronary Artery, Single 1 Coronary Arteries, Multiple 2 Coronary Artery Bypass Graft, Single 3 Coronary Artery Bypass Grafts, Multiple	Ø High Osmolar 1 Low Osmolar Y Other Contrast	1 Laser	Ø Intraoperative
Ø Coronary Artery, Single 1 Coronary Arteries, Multiple 2 Coronary Artery Bypass Graft, Single 3 Coronary Artery Bypass Grafts, Multiple	Ø High Osmolar 1 Low Osmolar Y Other Contrast	Z None	Z None
4 Heart, Right 5 Heart, Left 6 Heart, Right and Left 7 Internal Mammary Bypass Graft, Right 8 Internal Mammary Bypass Graft, Left F Bypass Graft, Other	Ø High Osmolar 1 Low Osmolar Y Other Contrast	Z None	Z None

DRG Non-OR B21[Ø123][Ø1Y]ZZ
DRG Non-OR B21[45678F][Ø1Y]ZZ

Coding Clinic: 2Ø16, Q3, P36 – B21

SECTION: B IMAGING
BODY SYSTEM: 2 HEART
TYPE: 2 COMPUTERIZED TOMOGRAPHY (CT SCAN): Computer-reformatted digital display of multiplanar images developed from the capture of multiple exposures of external ionizing radiation

Body Part	Contrast	Qualifier	Qualifier
1 Coronary Arteries, Multiple 3 Coronary Artery Bypass Grafts, Multiple 6 Heart, Right and Left	Ø High Osmolar 1 Low Osmolar Y Other Contrast	Ø Unenhanced and Enhanced Z None	Z None
1 Coronary Arteries, Multiple 3 Coronary Artery Bypass Grafts, Multiple 6 Heart, Right and Left	Z None	2 Intravascular Optical Coherence Z None	Z None

SECTION: B IMAGING
BODY SYSTEM: 2 HEART
TYPE: 3 MAGNETIC RESONANCE IMAGING (MRI): Computer-reformatted digital display of multiplanar images developed from the capture of radiofrequency signals emitted by nuclei in a body site excited within a magnetic field

Body Part	Contrast	Qualifier	Qualifier
1 Coronary Arteries, Multiple 3 Coronary Artery Bypass Grafts, Multiple 6 Heart, Right and Left	Y Other Contrast	Ø Unenhanced and Enhanced Z None	Z None
1 Coronary Arteries, Multiple 3 Coronary Artery Bypass Grafts, Multiple 6 Heart, Right and Left	Z None	Z None	Z None

B24

SECTION: B IMAGING

BODY SYSTEM: 2 HEART

TYPE: 4 ULTRASONOGRAPHY: Real-time display of images of anatomy or flow information developed from the capture of reflected and attenuated high-frequency sound waves

Body Part	Contrast	Qualifier	Qualifier
Ø Coronary Artery, Single 1 Coronary Arteries, Multiple 4 Heart, Right 5 Heart, Left 6 Heart, Right and Left B Heart with Aorta C Pericardium D Pediatric Heart	Y Other Contrast	Z None	Z None
Ø Coronary Artery, Single 1 Coronary Arteries, Multiple 4 Heart, Right 5 Heart, Left 6 Heart, Right and Left B Heart with Aorta C Pericardium D Pediatric Heart	Z None	Z None	3 Intravascular 4 Transesophageal Z None

B3Ø

SECTION: B IMAGING

BODY SYSTEM: 3 UPPER ARTERIES

TYPE: Ø PLAIN RADIOGRAPHY: Planar display of an image developed from the capture of external ionizing radiation on photographic or photoconductive plate

Body Part	Contrast	Qualifier	Qualifier
Ø Thoracic Aorta 1 Brachiocephalic-Subclavian Artery, Right 2 Subclavian Artery, Left 3 Common Carotid Artery, Right 4 Common Carotid Artery, Left 5 Common Carotid Arteries, Bilateral 6 Internal Carotid Artery, Right 7 Internal Carotid Artery, Left 8 Internal Carotid Arteries, Bilateral 9 External Carotid Artery, Right B External Carotid Artery, Left C External Carotid Arteries, Bilateral D Vertebral Artery, Right F Vertebral Artery, Left G Vertebral Arteries, Bilateral H Upper Extremity Arteries, Right J Upper Extremity Arteries, Left K Upper Extremity Arteries, Bilateral L Intercostal and Bronchial Arteries M Spinal Arteries N Upper Arteries, Other P Thoraco-Abdominal Aorta Q Cervico-Cerebral Arch R Intracranial Arteries S Pulmonary Artery, Right T Pulmonary Artery, Left	Ø High Osmolar 1 Low Osmolar Y Other Contrast Z None	Z None	Z None

B31

SECTION: B IMAGING
BODY SYSTEM: 3 UPPER ARTERIES
TYPE: 1 FLUOROSCOPY: *(on multiple pages)*

Single plane or bi-plane real-time display of an image developed from the capture of external ionizing radiation on a fluorescent screen. The image may also be stored by either digital or analog means.

Body Part	Contrast	Qualifier	Qualifier
Ø Thoracic Aorta 1 Brachiocephalic-Subclavian Artery, Right 2 Subclavian Artery, Left 3 Common Carotid Artery, Right 4 Common Carotid Artery, Left 5 Common Carotid Arteries, Bilateral 6 Internal Carotid Artery, Right 7 Internal Carotid Artery, Left 8 Internal Carotid Arteries, Bilateral 9 External Carotid Artery, Right B External Carotid Artery, Left C External Carotid Arteries, Bilateral D Vertebral Artery, Right F Vertebral Artery, Left G Vertebral Arteries, Bilateral H Upper Extremity Arteries, Right J Upper Extremity Arteries, Left K Upper Extremity Arteries, Bilateral L Intercostal and Bronchial Arteries M Spinal Arteries N Upper Arteries, Other P Thoraco-Abdominal Aorta Q Cervico-Cerebral Arch R Intracranial Arteries S Pulmonary Artery, Right T Pulmonary Artery, Left U Pulmonary Trunk	Ø High Osmolar 1 Low Osmolar Y Other Contrast	1 Laser	Ø Intraoperative

SECTION: B IMAGING
BODY SYSTEM: 3 UPPER ARTERIES
TYPE: 1 FLUOROSCOPY: *(continued)*

Single plane or bi-plane real-time display of an image developed from the capture of external ionizing radiation on a fluorescent screen. The image may also be stored by either digital or analog means.

Body Part	Contrast	Qualifier	Qualifier
Ø Thoracic Aorta 1 Brachiocephalic-Subclavian Artery, Right 2 Subclavian Artery, Left 3 Common Carotid Artery, Right 4 Common Carotid Artery, Left 5 Common Carotid Arteries, Bilateral 6 Internal Carotid Artery, Right 7 Internal Carotid Artery, Left 8 Internal Carotid Arteries, Bilateral 9 External Carotid Artery, Right B External Carotid Artery, Left C External Carotid Arteries, Bilateral D Vertebral Artery, Right F Vertebral Artery, Left G Vertebral Arteries, Bilateral H Upper Extremity Arteries, Right J Upper Extremity Arteries, Left K Upper Extremity Arteries, Bilateral L Intercostal and Bronchial Arteries M Spinal Arteries N Upper Arteries, Other P Thoraco-Abdominal Aorta Q Cervico-Cerebral Arch R Intracranial Arteries S Pulmonary Artery, Right T Pulmonary Artery, Left U Pulmonary Trunk	Ø High Osmolar 1 Low Osmolar Y Other Contrast	Z None	Z None

SECTION: B IMAGING
BODY SYSTEM: 3 UPPER ARTERIES
TYPE: 1 FLUOROSCOPY: *(continued)*

Single plane or bi-plane real-time display of an image developed from the capture of external ionizing radiation on a fluorescent screen. The image may also be stored by either digital or analog means.

Body Part	Contrast	Qualifier	Qualifier
Ø Thoracic Aorta 1 Brachiocephalic-Subclavian Artery, Right 2 Subclavian Artery, Left 3 Common Carotid Artery, Right 4 Common Carotid Artery, Left 5 Common Carotid Arteries, Bilateral 6 Internal Carotid Artery, Right 7 Internal Carotid Artery, Left 8 Internal Carotid Arteries, Bilateral 9 External Carotid Artery, Right B External Carotid Artery, Left C External Carotid Arteries, Bilateral D Vertebral Artery, Right F Vertebral Artery, Left G Vertebral Arteries, Bilateral H Upper Extremity Arteries, Right J Upper Extremity Arteries, Left K Upper Extremity Arteries, Bilateral L Intercostal and Bronchial Arteries M Spinal Arteries N Upper Arteries, Other P Thoraco-Abdominal Aorta Q Cervico-Cerebral Arch R Intracranial Arteries S Pulmonary Artery, Right T Pulmonary Artery, Left U Pulmonary Trunk	Z None	Z None	Z None

SECTION: B IMAGING
BODY SYSTEM: 3 UPPER ARTERIES
TYPE: 2 COMPUTERIZED TOMOGRAPHY (CT SCAN): Computer-reformatted digital display of multiplanar images developed from the capture of multiple exposures of external ionizing radiation

Body Part	Contrast	Qualifier	Qualifier
Ø Thoracic Aorta 5 Common Carotid Arteries, Bilateral 8 Internal Carotid Arteries, Bilateral G Vertebral Arteries, Bilateral R Intracranial Arteries S Pulmonary Artery, Right T Pulmonary Artery, Left	Ø High Osmolar 1 Low Osmolar Y Other Contrast	Z None	Z None
Ø Thoracic Aorta 5 Common Carotid Arteries, Bilateral 8 Internal Carotid Arteries, Bilateral G Vertebral Arteries, Bilateral R Intracranial Arteries S Pulmonary Artery, Right T Pulmonary Artery, Left	Z None	2 Intravascular Optical Coherence Z None	Z None

SECTION: B IMAGING

BODY SYSTEM: 3 UPPER ARTERIES

TYPE: 3 MAGNETIC RESONANCE IMAGING (MRI): Computer-reformatted digital display of multiplanar images developed from the capture of radiofrequency signals emitted by nuclei in a body site excited within a magnetic field

Body Part	Contrast	Qualifier	Qualifier
Ø Thoracic Aorta 5 Common Carotid Arteries, Bilateral 8 Internal Carotid Arteries, Bilateral G Vertebral Arteries, Bilateral H Upper Extremity Arteries, Right J Upper Extremity Arteries, Left K Upper Extremity Arteries, Bilateral M Spinal Arteries Q Cervico-Cerebral Arch R Intracranial Arteries	Y Other Contrast	Ø Unenhanced and Enhanced Z None	Z None
Ø Thoracic Aorta 5 Common Carotid Arteries, Bilateral 8 Internal Carotid Arteries, Bilateral G Vertebral Arteries, Bilateral H Upper Extremity Arteries, Right J Upper Extremity Arteries, Left K Upper Extremity Arteries, Bilateral M Spinal Arteries Q Cervico-Cerebral Arch R Intracranial Arteries	Z None	Z None	Z None

SECTION: B IMAGING

BODY SYSTEM: 3 UPPER ARTERIES

TYPE: 4 ULTRASONOGRAPHY: Real-time display of images of anatomy or flow information developed from the capture of reflected and attenuated high-frequency sound waves

Body Part	Contrast	Qualifier	Qualifier
Ø Thoracic Aorta 1 Brachiocephalic-Subclavian Artery, Right 2 Subclavian Artery, Left 3 Common Carotid Artery, Right 4 Common Carotid Artery, Left 5 Common Carotid Arteries, Bilateral 6 Internal Carotid Artery, Right 7 Internal Carotid Artery, Left 8 Internal Carotid Arteries, Bilateral H Upper Extremity Arteries, Right J Upper Extremity Arteries, Left K Upper Extremity Arteries, Bilateral R Intracranial Arteries S Pulmonary Artery, Right T Pulmonary Artery, Left V Ophthalmic Arteries	Z None	Z None	3 Intravascular Z None

New/Revised Text in Green ~~deleted~~ Deleted ♀ Females Only ♂ Males Only Coding Clinic
Non-covered Limited Coverage ⊞ Combination (See Appendix E) DRG Non-OR Non-OR Hospital-Acquired Condition

B4Ø

SECTION: B IMAGING

BODY SYSTEM: 4 LOWER ARTERIES

TYPE: Ø PLAIN RADIOGRAPHY: Planar display of an image developed from the capture of external ionizing radiation on photographic or photoconductive plate

Body Part	Contrast	Qualifier	Qualifier
Ø Abdominal Aorta 2 Hepatic Artery 3 Splenic Arteries 4 Superior Mesenteric Artery 5 Inferior Mesenteric Artery 6 Renal Artery, Right 7 Renal Artery, Left 8 Renal Arteries, Bilateral 9 Lumbar Arteries B Intra-Abdominal Arteries, Other C Pelvic Arteries D Aorta and Bilateral Lower Extremity Arteries F Lower Extremity Arteries, Right G Lower Extremity Arteries, Left J Lower Arteries, Other M Renal Artery Transplant	Ø High Osmolar 1 Low Osmolar Y Other Contrast	Z None	Z None

B41

SECTION: B IMAGING

BODY SYSTEM: 4 LOWER ARTERIES

TYPE: 1 FLUOROSCOPY: Single plane or bi-plane real-time display of an image developed from the capture of external ionizing radiation on a fluorescent screen. The image may also be stored by either digital or analog means.

Body Part	Contrast	Qualifier	Qualifier
Ø Abdominal Aorta 2 Hepatic Artery 3 Splenic Arteries 4 Superior Mesenteric Artery 5 Inferior Mesenteric Artery 6 Renal Artery, Right 7 Renal Artery, Left 8 Renal Arteries, Bilateral 9 Lumbar Arteries B Intra-Abdominal Arteries, Other C Pelvic Arteries D Aorta and Bilateral Lower Extremity Arteries F Lower Extremity Arteries, Right G Lower Extremity Arteries, Left J Lower Arteries, Other	Ø High Osmolar 1 Low Osmolar Y Other Contrast	1 Laser	Ø Intraoperative
Ø Abdominal Aorta 2 Hepatic Artery 3 Splenic Arteries 4 Superior Mesenteric Artery 5 Inferior Mesenteric Artery 6 Renal Artery, Right 7 Renal Artery, Left 8 Renal Arteries, Bilateral 9 Lumbar Arteries B Intra-Abdominal Arteries, Other C Pelvic Arteries D Aorta and Bilateral Lower Extremity Arteries F Lower Extremity Arteries, Right G Lower Extremity Arteries, Left J Lower Arteries, Other	Ø High Osmolar 1 Low Osmolar Y Other Contrast	Z None	Z None
Ø Abdominal Aorta 2 Hepatic Artery 3 Splenic Arteries 4 Superior Mesenteric Artery 5 Inferior Mesenteric Artery 6 Renal Artery, Right 7 Renal Artery, Left 8 Renal Arteries, Bilateral 9 Lumbar Arteries B Intra-Abdominal Arteries, Other C Pelvic Arteries D Aorta and Bilateral Lower Extremity Arteries F Lower Extremity Arteries, Right G Lower Extremity Arteries, Left J Lower Arteries, Other	Z None	Z None	Z None

SECTION: B IMAGING
BODY SYSTEM: 4 LOWER ARTERIES
TYPE: 2 **COMPUTERIZED TOMOGRAPHY (CT SCAN):** Computer-reformatted digital display of multiplanar images developed from the capture of multiple exposures of external ionizing radiation

Body Part	Contrast	Qualifier	Qualifier
Ø Abdominal Aorta 1 Celiac Artery 4 Superior Mesenteric Artery 8 Renal Arteries, Bilateral C Pelvic Arteries F Lower Extremity Arteries, Right G Lower Extremity Arteries, Left H Lower Extremity Arteries, Bilateral M Renal Artery Transplant	Ø High Osmolar 1 Low Osmolar Y Other Contrast	Z None	Z None
Ø Abdominal Aorta 1 Celiac Artery 4 Superior Mesenteric Artery 8 Renal Arteries, Bilateral C Pelvic Arteries F Lower Extremity Arteries, Right G Lower Extremity Arteries, Left H Lower Extremity Arteries, Bilateral M Renal Artery Transplant	Z None	2 Intravascular Optical Coherence Z None	Z None

SECTION: B IMAGING
BODY SYSTEM: 4 LOWER ARTERIES
TYPE: 3 **MAGNETIC RESONANCE IMAGING (MRI):** Computer-reformatted digital display of multiplanar images developed from the capture of radiofrequency signals emitted by nuclei in a body site excited within a magnetic field

Body Part	Contrast	Qualifier	Qualifier
Ø Abdominal Aorta 1 Celiac Artery 4 Superior Mesenteric Artery 8 Renal Arteries, Bilateral C Pelvic Arteries F Lower Extremity Arteries, Right G Lower Extremity Arteries, Left H Lower Extremity Arteries, Bilateral	Y Other Contrast	Ø Unenhanced and Enhanced Z None	Z None
Ø Abdominal Aorta 1 Celiac Artery 4 Superior Mesenteric Artery 8 Renal Arteries, Bilateral C Pelvic Arteries F Lower Extremity Arteries, Right G Lower Extremity Arteries, Left H Lower Extremity Arteries, Bilateral	Z None	Z None	Z None

B44

SECTION: B IMAGING

BODY SYSTEM: 4 LOWER ARTERIES

TYPE: 4 ULTRASONOGRAPHY: Real-time display of images of anatomy or flow information developed from the capture of reflected and attenuated high-frequency sound waves

Body Part	Contrast	Qualifier	Qualifier
Ø Abdominal Aorta 4 Superior Mesenteric Artery 5 Inferior Mesenteric Artery 6 Renal Artery, Right 7 Renal Artery, Left 8 Renal Arteries, Bilateral B Intra-Abdominal Arteries, Other F Lower Extremity Arteries, Right G Lower Extremity Arteries, Left H Lower Extremity Arteries, Bilateral K Celiac and Mesenteric Arteries L Femoral Artery N Penile Arteries ♂	Z None	Z None	3 Intravascular Z None

SECTION: B IMAGING

BODY SYSTEM: 5 VEINS

TYPE: Ø PLAIN RADIOGRAPHY: Planar display of an image developed from the capture of external ionizing radiation on photographic or photoconductive plate

Body Part	Contrast	Qualifier	Qualifier
Ø Epidural Veins 1 Cerebral and Cerebellar Veins 2 Intracranial Sinuses 3 Jugular Veins, Right 4 Jugular Veins, Left 5 Jugular Veins, Bilateral 6 Subclavian Vein, Right 7 Subclavian Vein, Left 8 Superior Vena Cava 9 Inferior Vena Cava B Lower Extremity Veins, Right C Lower Extremity Veins, Left D Lower Extremity Veins, Bilateral F Pelvic (Iliac) Veins, Right G Pelvic (Iliac) Veins, Left H Pelvic (Iliac) Veins, Bilateral J Renal Vein, Right K Renal Vein, Left L Renal Veins, Bilateral M Upper Extremity Veins, Right N Upper Extremity Veins, Left P Upper Extremity Veins, Bilateral Q Pulmonary Vein, Right R Pulmonary Vein, Left S Pulmonary Veins, Bilateral T Portal and Splanchnic Veins V Veins, Other W Dialysis Shunt/Fistula	Ø High Osmolar 1 Low Osmolar Y Other Contrast	Z None	Z None

SECTION: B IMAGING

BODY SYSTEM: 5 VEINS

TYPE: 1 FLUOROSCOPY: Single plane or bi-plane real-time display of an image developed from the capture of external ionizing radiation on a fluorescent screen. The image may also be stored by either digital or analog means.

Body Part	Contrast	Qualifier	Qualifier
Ø Epidural Veins 1 Cerebral and Cerebellar Veins 2 Intracranial Sinuses 3 Jugular Veins, Right 4 Jugular Veins, Left 5 Jugular Veins, Bilateral 6 Subclavian Vein, Right 7 Subclavian Vein, Left 8 Superior Vena Cava 9 Inferior Vena Cava B Lower Extremity Veins, Right C Lower Extremity Veins, Left D Lower Extremity Veins, Bilateral F Pelvic (Iliac) Veins, Right G Pelvic (Iliac) Veins, Left H Pelvic (Iliac) Veins, Bilateral J Renal Vein, Right K Renal Vein, Left L Renal Veins, Bilateral M Upper Extremity Veins, Right N Upper Extremity Veins, Left P Upper Extremity Veins, Bilateral Q Pulmonary Vein, Right R Pulmonary Vein, Left S Pulmonary Veins, Bilateral T Portal and Splanchnic Veins V Veins, Other W Dialysis Shunt/Fistula	Ø High Osmolar 1 Low Osmolar Y Other Contrast Z None	Z None	A Guidance Z None

Coding Clinic: 2Ø15, Q4, P3Ø – B518ZZA

B52

SECTION: B IMAGING
BODY SYSTEM: 5 VEINS
TYPE: 2 COMPUTERIZED TOMOGRAPHY (CT SCAN): Computer-reformatted digital display of multiplanar images developed from the capture of multiple exposures of external ionizing radiation

Body Part	Contrast	Qualifier	Qualifier
2 Intracranial Sinuses 8 Superior Vena Cava 9 Inferior Vena Cava F Pelvic (Iliac) Veins, Right G Pelvic (Iliac) Veins, Left H Pelvic (Iliac) Veins, Bilateral J Renal Vein, Right K Renal Vein, Left L Renal Veins, Bilateral Q Pulmonary Vein, Right R Pulmonary Vein, Left S Pulmonary Veins, Bilateral T Portal and Splanchnic Veins	Ø High Osmolar 1 Low Osmolar Y Other Contrast	Ø Unenhanced and Enhanced Z None	Z None
2 Intracranial Sinuses 8 Superior Vena Cava 9 Inferior Vena Cava F Pelvic (Iliac) Veins, Right G Pelvic (Iliac) Veins, Left H Pelvic (Iliac) Veins, Bilateral J Renal Vein, Right K Renal Vein, Left L Renal Veins, Bilateral Q Pulmonary Vein, Right R Pulmonary Vein, Left S Pulmonary Veins, Bilateral T Portal and Splanchnic Veins	Z None	2 Intravascular Optical Coherence Z None	Z None

SECTION: B IMAGING
BODY SYSTEM: 5 VEINS
TYPE: 3 MAGNETIC RESONANCE IMAGING (MRI): Computer-reformatted digital display of multiplanar images developed from the capture of radiofrequency signals emitted by nuclei in a body site excited within a magnetic field

Body Part	Contrast	Qualifier	Qualifier
1 Cerebral and Cerebellar Veins 2 Intracranial Sinuses 5 Jugular Veins, Bilateral 8 Superior Vena Cava 9 Inferior Vena Cava B Lower Extremity Veins, Right C Lower Extremity Veins, Left D Lower Extremity Veins, Bilateral H Pelvic (Iliac) Veins, Bilateral L Renal Veins, Bilateral M Upper Extremity Veins, Right N Upper Extremity Veins, Left P Upper Extremity Veins, Bilateral S Pulmonary Veins, Bilateral T Portal and Splanchnic Veins V Veins, Other	Y Other Contrast	Ø Unenhanced and Enhanced Z None	Z None
1 Cerebral and Cerebellar Veins 2 Intracranial Sinuses 5 Jugular Veins, Bilateral 8 Superior Vena Cava 9 Inferior Vena Cava B Lower Extremity Veins, Right C Lower Extremity Veins, Left D Lower Extremity Veins, Bilateral H Pelvic (Iliac) Veins, Bilateral L Renal Veins, Bilateral M Upper Extremity Veins, Right N Upper Extremity Veins, Left P Upper Extremity Veins, Bilateral S Pulmonary Veins, Bilateral T Portal and Splanchnic Veins V Veins, Other	Z None	Z None	Z None

SECTION: B IMAGING
BODY SYSTEM: 5 VEINS
TYPE: 4 ULTRASONOGRAPHY: Real-time display of images of anatomy or flow information developed from the capture of reflected and attenuated high-frequency sound waves

Body Part	Contrast	Qualifier	Qualifier
3 Jugular Veins, Right 4 Jugular Veins, Left 6 Subclavian Vein, Right 7 Subclavian Vein, Left 9 Inferior Vena Cava B Lower Extremity Veins, Right C Lower Extremity Veins, Left D Lower Extremity Veins, Bilateral J Renal Vein, Right K Renal Vein, Left L Renal Veins, Bilateral M Upper Extremity Veins, Right N Upper Extremity Veins, Left P Upper Extremity Veins, Bilateral T Portal and Splanchnic Veins	Z None	Z None	3 Intravascular A Guidance Z None

SECTION: B IMAGING

BODY SYSTEM: 7 LYMPHATIC SYSTEM

TYPE: Ø PLAIN RADIOGRAPHY: Planar display of an image developed from the capture of external ionizing radiation on photographic or photoconductive plate

Body Part	Contrast	Qualifier	Qualifier
Ø Abdominal/Retroperitoneal Lymphatics, Unilateral 1 Abdominal/Retroperitoneal Lymphatics, Bilateral 4 Lymphatics, Head and Neck 5 Upper Extremity Lymphatics, Right 6 Upper Extremity Lymphatics, Left 7 Upper Extremity Lymphatics, Bilateral 8 Lower Extremity Lymphatics, Right 9 Lower Extremity Lymphatics, Left B Lower Extremity Lymphatics, Bilateral C Lymphatics, Pelvic	Ø High Osmolar 1 Low Osmolar Y Other Contrast	Z None	Z None

SECTION: B IMAGING
BODY SYSTEM: 8 EYE
TYPE: Ø **PLAIN RADIOGRAPHY:** Planar display of an image developed from the capture of external ionizing radiation on photographic or photoconductive plate

Body Part	Contrast	Qualifier	Qualifier
Ø Lacrimal Duct, Right 1 Lacrimal Duct, Left 2 Lacrimal Ducts, Bilateral	Ø High Osmolar 1 Low Osmolar Y Other Contrast	Z None	Z None
3 Optic Foramina, Right 4 Optic Foramina, Left 5 Eye, Right 6 Eye, Left 7 Eyes, Bilateral	Z None	Z None	Z None

SECTION: B IMAGING
BODY SYSTEM: 8 EYE
TYPE: 2 **COMPUTERIZED TOMOGRAPHY (CT SCAN):** Computer-reformatted digital display of multiplanar images developed from the capture of multiple exposures of external ionizing radiation

Body Part	Contrast	Qualifier	Qualifier
5 Eye, Right 6 Eye, Left 7 Eyes, Bilateral	Ø High Osmolar 1 Low Osmolar Y Other Contrast	Ø Unenhanced and Enhanced Z None	Z None
5 Eye, Right 6 Eye, Left 7 Eyes, Bilateral	Z None	Z None	Z None

SECTION: B IMAGING
BODY SYSTEM: 8 EYE
TYPE: 3 **MAGNETIC RESONANCE IMAGING (MRI):** Computer-reformatted digital display of multiplanar images developed from the capture of radiofrequency signals emitted by nuclei in a body site excited within a magnetic field

Body Part	Contrast	Qualifier	Qualifier
5 Eye, Right 6 Eye, Left 7 Eyes, Bilateral	Y Other Contrast	Ø Unenhanced and Enhanced Z None	Z None
5 Eye, Right 6 Eye, Left 7 Eyes, Bilateral	Z None	Z None	Z None

SECTION: B IMAGING
BODY SYSTEM: 8 EYE
TYPE: 4 **ULTRASONOGRAPHY:** Real-time display of images of anatomy or flow information developed from the capture of reflected and attenuated high-frequency sound waves

Body Part	Contrast	Qualifier	Qualifier
5 Eye, Right 6 Eye, Left 7 Eyes, Bilateral	Z None	Z None	Z None

SECTION: B IMAGING
BODY SYSTEM: 9 EAR, NOSE, MOUTH, AND THROAT
TYPE: Ø PLAIN RADIOGRAPHY: Planar display of an image developed from the capture of external ionizing radiation on photographic or photoconductive plate

Body Part	Contrast	Qualifier	Qualifier
2 Paranasal Sinuses F Nasopharynx/Oropharynx H Mastoids	Z None	Z None	Z None
4 Parotid Gland, Right 5 Parotid Gland, Left 6 Parotid Glands, Bilateral 7 Submandibular Gland, Right 8 Submandibular Gland, Left 9 Submandibular Glands, Bilateral B Salivary Gland, Right C Salivary Gland, Left D Salivary Glands, Bilateral	Ø High Osmolar 1 Low Osmolar Y Other Contrast	Z None	Z None

SECTION: B IMAGING
BODY SYSTEM: 9 EAR, NOSE, MOUTH, AND THROAT
TYPE: 1 FLUOROSCOPY: Single plane or bi-plane real-time display of an image developed from the capture of external ionizing radiation on a fluorescent screen. The image may also be stored by either digital or analog means.

Body Part	Contrast	Qualifier	Qualifier
G Pharynx and Epiglottis J Larynx	Y Other Contrast Z None	Z None	Z None

SECTION: B IMAGING
BODY SYSTEM: 9 EAR, NOSE, MOUTH, AND THROAT
TYPE: 2 COMPUTERIZED TOMOGRAPHY (CT SCAN): Computer-reformatted digital display of multiplanar images developed from the capture of multiple exposures of external ionizing radiation

Body Part	Contrast	Qualifier	Qualifier
Ø Ear 2 Paranasal Sinuses 6 Parotid Glands, Bilateral 9 Submandibular Glands, Bilateral D Salivary Glands, Bilateral F Nasopharynx/Oropharynx J Larynx	Ø High Osmolar 1 Low Osmolar Y Other Contrast	Ø Unenhanced and Enhanced Z None	Z None
Ø Ear 2 Paranasal Sinuses 6 Parotid Glands, Bilateral 9 Submandibular Glands, Bilateral D Salivary Glands, Bilateral F Nasopharynx/Oropharynx J Larynx	Z None	Z None	Z None

SECTION: B IMAGING
BODY SYSTEM: 9 EAR, NOSE, MOUTH, AND THROAT
TYPE: 3 MAGNETIC RESONANCE IMAGING (MRI): Computer-reformatted digital display of multiplanar images developed from the capture of radiofrequency signals emitted by nuclei in a body site excited within a magnetic field

Body Part	Contrast	Qualifier	Qualifier
Ø Ear 2 Paranasal Sinuses 6 Parotid Glands, Bilateral 9 Submandibular Glands, Bilateral D Salivary Glands, Bilateral F Nasopharynx/Oropharynx J Larynx	Y Other Contrast	Ø Unenhanced and Enhanced Z None	Z None
Ø Ear 2 Paranasal Sinuses 6 Parotid Glands, Bilateral 9 Submandibular Glands, Bilateral D Salivary Glands, Bilateral F Nasopharynx/Oropharynx J Larynx	Z None	Z None	Z None

SECTION: B IMAGING
BODY SYSTEM: B RESPIRATORY SYSTEM
TYPE: Ø PLAIN RADIOGRAPHY: Planar display of an image developed from the capture of external ionizing radiation on photographic or photoconductive plate

Body Part	Contrast	Qualifier	Qualifier
7 Tracheobronchial Tree, Right 8 Tracheobronchial Tree, Left 9 Tracheobronchial Trees, Bilateral	Y Other Contrast	Z None	Z None
D Upper Airways	Z None	Z None	Z None

SECTION: B IMAGING
BODY SYSTEM: B RESPIRATORY SYSTEM
TYPE: 1 FLUOROSCOPY: Single plane or bi-plane real-time display of an image developed from the capture of external ionizing radiation on a fluorescent screen. The image may also be stored by either digital or analog means.

Body Part	Contrast	Qualifier	Qualifier
2 Lung, Right 3 Lung, Left 4 Lungs, Bilateral 6 Diaphragm C Mediastinum D Upper Airways	Z None	Z None	Z None
7 Tracheobronchial Tree, Right 8 Tracheobronchial Tree, Left 9 Tracheobronchial Trees, Bilateral	Y Other Contrast	Z None	Z None

SECTION: B IMAGING
BODY SYSTEM: B RESPIRATORY SYSTEM
TYPE: 2 COMPUTERIZED TOMOGRAPHY (CT SCAN): Computer-reformatted digital display of multiplanar images developed from the capture of multiple exposures of external ionizing radiation

Body Part	Contrast	Qualifier	Qualifier
4 Lungs, Bilateral 7 Tracheobronchial Tree, Right 8 Tracheobronchial Tree, Left 9 Tracheobronchial Trees, Bilateral F Trachea/Airways	Ø High Osmolar 1 Low Osmolar Y Other Contrast	Ø Unenhanced and Enhanced Z None	Z None
4 Lungs, Bilateral 7 Tracheobronchial Tree, Right 8 Tracheobronchial Tree, Left 9 Tracheobronchial Trees, Bilateral F Trachea/Airways	Z None	Z None	Z None

SECTION: B IMAGING

BODY SYSTEM: B RESPIRATORY SYSTEM

TYPE: 3 **MAGNETIC RESONANCE IMAGING (MRI):** Computer-reformatted digital display of multiplanar images developed from the capture of radiofrequency signals emitted by nuclei in a body site excited within a magnetic field

Body Part	Contrast	Qualifier	Qualifier
4 Lungs, Bilateral	Z None	3 Hyperpolarized Xenon 129(Xe-129)	Z None
G Lung Apices	Y Other Contrast	Ø Unenhanced and Enhanced Z None	Z None
G Lung Apices	Z None	Z None	Z None

SECTION: B IMAGING

BODY SYSTEM: B RESPIRATORY SYSTEM

TYPE: 4 **ULTRASONOGRAPHY:** Real-time display of images of anatomy or flow information developed from the capture of reflected and attenuated high-frequency sound waves

Body Part	Contrast	Qualifier	Qualifier
B Pleura C Mediastinum	Z None	Z None	Z None

SECTION: B IMAGING
BODY SYSTEM: D GASTROINTESTINAL SYSTEM
TYPE: 1 FLUOROSCOPY: Single plane or bi-plane real-time display of an image developed from the capture of external ionizing radiation on a fluorescent screen. The image may also be stored by either digital or analog means.

Body Part	Contrast	Qualifier	Qualifier
1 Esophagus 2 Stomach 3 Small Bowel 4 Colon 5 Upper GI 6 Upper GI and Small Bowel 9 Duodenum B Mouth/Oropharynx	Y Other Contrast Z None	Z None	Z None

SECTION: B IMAGING
BODY SYSTEM: D GASTROINTESTINAL SYSTEM
TYPE: 2 COMPUTERIZED TOMOGRAPHY (CT SCAN): Computer-reformatted digital display of multiplanar images developed from the capture of multiple exposures of external ionizing radiation

Body Part	Contrast	Qualifier	Qualifier
4 Colon	Ø High Osmolar 1 Low Osmolar Y Other Contrast	Ø Unenhanced and Enhanced Z None	Z None
4 Colon	Z None	Z None	Z None

SECTION: B IMAGING
BODY SYSTEM: D GASTROINTESTINAL SYSTEM
TYPE: 4 ULTRASONOGRAPHY: Real-time display of images of anatomy or flow information developed from the capture of reflected and attenuated high-frequency sound waves

Body Part	Contrast	Qualifier	Qualifier
1 Esophagus 2 Stomach 7 Gastrointestinal Tract 8 Appendix 9 Duodenum C Rectum	Z None	Z None	Z None

SECTION: B IMAGING
BODY SYSTEM: F HEPATOBILIARY SYSTEM AND PANCREAS
TYPE: Ø PLAIN RADIOGRAPHY: Planar display of an image developed from the capture of external ionizing radiation on photographic or photoconductive plate

Body Part	Contrast	Qualifier	Qualifier
Ø Bile Ducts 3 Gallbladder and Bile Ducts C Hepatobiliary System, All	Ø High Osmolar 1 Low Osmolar Y Other Contrast	Z None	Z None

Non-OR BFØ[3C][Ø1Y]ZZ

SECTION: B IMAGING
BODY SYSTEM: F HEPATOBILIARY SYSTEM AND PANCREAS
TYPE: 1 FLUOROSCOPY: Single plane or bi-plane real-time display of an image developed from the capture of external ionizing radiation on a fluorescent screen. The image may also be stored by either digital or analog means.

Body Part	Contrast	Qualifier	Qualifier
Ø Bile Ducts 1 Biliary and Pancreatic Ducts 2 Gallbladder 3 Gallbladder and Bile Ducts 4 Gallbladder, Bile Ducts, and Pancreatic Ducts 8 Pancreatic Ducts	Ø High Osmolar 1 Low Osmolar Y Other Contrast	Z None	Z None
5 Liver	Ø High Osmolar 1 Low Osmolar Y Other Contrast	Z None	Z None
5 Liver	Z None	Z None	A Guidance

SECTION: B IMAGING
BODY SYSTEM: F HEPATOBILIARY SYSTEM AND PANCREAS
TYPE: 2 COMPUTERIZED TOMOGRAPHY (CT SCAN): Computer-reformatted digital display of multiplanar images developed from the capture of multiple exposures of external ionizing radiation

Body Part	Contrast	Qualifier	Qualifier
5 Liver 6 Liver and Spleen 7 Pancreas C Hepatobiliary System, All	Ø High Osmolar 1 Low Osmolar Y Other Contrast	Ø Unenhanced and Enhanced Z None	Z None
5 Liver 6 Liver and Spleen 7 Pancreas C Hepatobiliary System, All	Z None	Z None	Z None

SECTION: B IMAGING
BODY SYSTEM: F HEPATOBILIARY SYSTEM AND PANCREAS
TYPE: 3 MAGNETIC RESONANCE IMAGING (MRI): Computer-reformatted digital display of multiplanar images developed from the capture of radiofrequency signals emitted by nuclei in a body site excited within a magnetic field

Body Part	Contrast	Qualifier	Qualifier
5 Liver 6 Liver and Spleen 7 Pancreas	Y Other Contrast	Ø Unenhanced and Enhanced Z None	Z None
5 Liver 6 Liver and Spleen 7 Pancreas	Z None	Z None	Z None

SECTION: B IMAGING
BODY SYSTEM: F HEPATOBILIARY SYSTEM AND PANCREAS
TYPE: 4 ULTRASONOGRAPHY: Real-time display of images of anatomy or flow information developed from the capture of reflected and attenuated high-frequency sound waves

Body Part	Contrast	Qualifier	Qualifier
Ø Bile Ducts 2 Gallbladder 3 Gallbladder and Bile Ducts 5 Liver 6 Liver and Spleen 7 Pancreas C Hepatobiliary System, All	Z None	Z None	Z None

SECTION: B IMAGING
BODY SYSTEM: F HEPATOBILIARY SYSTEM AND PANCREAS
TYPE: 5 OTHER IMAGING: Other specified modality for visualizing a body part

Body Part	Contrast	Qualifier	Qualifier
Ø Bile Ducts 2 Gallbladder 3 Gallbladder and Bile Ducts 5 Liver 6 Liver and Spleen 7 Pancreas C Hepatobiliary System, All	2 Fluorescing Agent	Ø Indocyanine Green Dye Z None	Ø Intraoperative Z None

SECTION: B IMAGING
BODY SYSTEM: G ENDOCRINE SYSTEM
TYPE: 2 COMPUTERIZED TOMOGRAPHY (CT SCAN): Computer-reformatted digital display of multiplanar images developed from the capture of multiple exposures of external ionizing radiation

Body Part	Contrast	Qualifier	Qualifier
2 Adrenal Glands, Bilateral 3 Parathyroid Glands 4 Thyroid Gland	Ø High Osmolar 1 Low Osmolar Y Other Contrast	Ø Unenhanced and Enhanced Z None	Z None
2 Adrenal Glands, Bilateral 3 Parathyroid Glands 4 Thyroid Gland	Z None	Z None	Z None

SECTION: B IMAGING
BODY SYSTEM: G ENDOCRINE SYSTEM
TYPE: 3 MAGNETIC RESONANCE IMAGING (MRI): Computer-reformatted digital display of multiplanar images developed from the capture of radiofrequency signals emitted by nuclei in a body site excited within a magnetic field

Body Part	Contrast	Qualifier	Qualifier
2 Adrenal Glands, Bilateral 3 Parathyroid Glands 4 Thyroid Gland	Y Other Contrast	Ø Unenhanced and Enhanced Z None	Z None
2 Adrenal Glands, Bilateral 3 Parathyroid Glands 4 Thyroid Gland	Z None	Z None	Z None

SECTION: B IMAGING
BODY SYSTEM: G ENDOCRINE SYSTEM
TYPE: 4 ULTRASONOGRAPHY: Real-time display of images of anatomy or flow information developed from the capture of reflected and attenuated high-frequency sound waves

Body Part	Contrast	Qualifier	Qualifier
Ø Adrenal Gland, Right 1 Adrenal Gland, Left 2 Adrenal Glands, Bilateral 3 Parathyroid Glands 4 Thyroid Gland	Z None	Z None	Z None

SECTION: B IMAGING
BODY SYSTEM: H SKIN, SUBCUTANEOUS TISSUE AND BREAST
TYPE: Ø PLAIN RADIOGRAPHY: Planar display of an image developed from the capture of external ionizing radiation on photographic or photoconductive plate

Body Part	Contrast	Qualifier	Qualifier
Ø Breast, Right 1 Breast, Left 2 Breasts, Bilateral	Z None	Z None	Z None
3 Single Mammary Duct, Right 4 Single Mammary Duct, Left 5 Multiple Mammary Ducts, Right 6 Multiple Mammary Ducts, Left	Ø High Osmolar 1 Low Osmolar Y Other Contrast Z None	Z None	Z None

SECTION: B IMAGING
BODY SYSTEM: H SKIN, SUBCUTANEOUS TISSUE AND BREAST
TYPE: 3 MAGNETIC RESONANCE IMAGING (MRI): Computer-reformatted digital display of multiplanar images developed from the capture of radiofrequency signals emitted by nuclei in a body site excited within a magnetic field

Body Part	Contrast	Qualifier	Qualifier
Ø Breast, Right 1 Breast, Left 2 Breasts, Bilateral D Subcutaneous Tissue, Head/Neck F Subcutaneous Tissue, Upper Extremity G Subcutaneous Tissue, Thorax H Subcutaneous Tissue, Abdomen and Pelvis J Subcutaneous Tissue, Lower Extremity	Y Other Contrast	Ø Unenhanced and Enhanced Z None	Z None
Ø Breast, Right 1 Breast, Left 2 Breasts, Bilateral D Subcutaneous Tissue, Head/Neck F Subcutaneous Tissue, Upper Extremity G Subcutaneous Tissue, Thorax H Subcutaneous Tissue, Abdomen and Pelvis J Subcutaneous Tissue, Lower Extremity	Z None	Z None	Z None

SECTION: B IMAGING

BODY SYSTEM: H SKIN, SUBCUTANEOUS TISSUE AND BREAST

TYPE: 4 ULTRASONOGRAPHY: Real-time display of images of anatomy or flow information developed from the capture of reflected and attenuated high-frequency sound waves

Body Part	Contrast	Qualifier	Qualifier
Ø Breast, Right 1 Breast, Left 2 Breasts, Bilateral 7 Extremity, Upper 8 Extremity, Lower 9 Abdominal Wall B Chest Wall C Head and Neck	Z None	Z None	Z None

SECTION: B IMAGING
BODY SYSTEM: L CONNECTIVE TISSUE
TYPE: 3 MAGNETIC RESONANCE IMAGING (MRI): Computer-reformatted digital display of multiplanar images developed from the capture of radiofrequency signals emitted by nuclei in a body site excited within a magnetic field

Body Part	Contrast	Qualifier	Qualifier
Ø Connective Tissue, Upper Extremity 1 Connective Tissue, Lower Extremity 2 Tendons, Upper Extremity 3 Tendons, Lower Extremity	Y Other Contrast	Ø Unenhanced and Enhanced Z None	Z None
Ø Connective Tissue, Upper Extremity 1 Connective Tissue, Lower Extremity 2 Tendons, Upper Extremity 3 Tendons, Lower Extremity	Z None	Z None	Z None

SECTION: B IMAGING
BODY SYSTEM: L CONNECTIVE TISSUE
TYPE: 4 ULTRASONOGRAPHY: Real-time display of images of anatomy or flow information developed from the capture of reflected and attenuated high-frequency sound waves

Body Part	Contrast	Qualifier	Qualifier
Ø Connective Tissue, Upper Extremity 1 Connective Tissue, Lower Extremity 2 Tendons, Upper Extremity 3 Tendons, Lower Extremity	Z None	Z None	Z None

SECTION: B IMAGING
BODY SYSTEM: N SKULL AND FACIAL BONES
TYPE: Ø PLAIN RADIOGRAPHY: Planar display of an image developed from the capture of external ionizing radiation on photographic or photoconductive plate

Body Part	Contrast	Qualifier	Qualifier
Ø Skull 1 Orbit, Right 2 Orbit, Left 3 Orbits, Bilateral 4 Nasal Bones 5 Facial Bones 6 Mandible B Zygomatic Arch, Right C Zygomatic Arch, Left D Zygomatic Arches, Bilateral G Tooth, Single H Teeth, Multiple J Teeth, All	Z None	Z None	Z None
7 Temporomandibular Joint, Right 8 Temporomandibular Joint, Left 9 Temporomandibular Joints, Bilateral	Ø High Osmolar 1 Low Osmolar Y Other Contrast Z None	Z None	Z None

SECTION: B IMAGING
BODY SYSTEM: N SKULL AND FACIAL BONES
TYPE: 1 FLUOROSCOPY: Single plane or bi-plane real-time display of an image developed from the capture of external ionizing radiation on a fluorescent screen. The image may also be stored by either digital or analog means.

Body Part	Contrast	Qualifier	Qualifier
7 Temporomandibular Joint, Right 8 Temporomandibular Joint, Left 9 Temporomandibular Joints, Bilateral	Ø High Osmolar 1 Low Osmolar Y Other Contrast Z None	Z None	Z None

SECTION: B IMAGING
BODY SYSTEM: N SKULL AND FACIAL BONES
TYPE: 2 **COMPUTERIZED TOMOGRAPHY (CT SCAN):** Computer-reformatted digital display of multiplanar images developed from the capture of multiple exposures of external ionizing radiation

Body Part	Contrast	Qualifier	Qualifier
Ø Skull 3 Orbits, Bilateral 5 Facial Bones 6 Mandible 9 Temporomandibular Joints, Bilateral F Temporal Bones	Ø High Osmolar 1 Low Osmolar Y Other Contrast Z None	Z None	Z None

SECTION: B IMAGING
BODY SYSTEM: N SKULL AND FACIAL BONES
TYPE: 3 **MAGNETIC RESONANCE IMAGING (MRI):** Computer-reformatted digital display of multiplanar images developed from the capture of radiofrequency signals emitted by nuclei in a body site excited within a magnetic field

Body Part	Contrast	Qualifier	Qualifier
9 Temporomandibular Joints, Bilateral	Y Other Contrast Z None	Z None	Z None

SECTION: B IMAGING
BODY SYSTEM: P NON-AXIAL UPPER BONES
TYPE: Ø PLAIN RADIOGRAPHY: Planar display of an image developed from the capture of external ionizing radiation on photographic or photoconductive plate

Body Part	Contrast	Qualifier	Qualifier
Ø Sternoclavicular Joint, Right 1 Sternoclavicular Joint, Left 2 Sternoclavicular Joints, Bilateral 3 Acromioclavicular Joints, Bilateral 4 Clavicle, Right 5 Clavicle, Left 6 Scapula, Right 7 Scapula, Left A Humerus, Right B Humerus, Left E Upper Arm, Right F Upper Arm, Left J Forearm, Right K Forearm, Left N Hand, Right P Hand, Left R Finger(s), Right S Finger(s), Left X Ribs, Right Y Ribs, Left	Z None	Z None	Z None
8 Shoulder, Right 9 Shoulder, Left C Hand/Finger Joint, Right D Hand/Finger Joint, Left G Elbow, Right H Elbow, Left L Wrist, Right M Wrist, Left	Ø High Osmolar 1 Low Osmolar Y Other Contrast Z None	Z None	Z None

SECTION: B IMAGING
BODY SYSTEM: P NON-AXIAL UPPER BONES
TYPE: 1 FLUOROSCOPY: Single plane or bi-plane real-time display of an image developed from the capture of external ionizing radiation on a fluorescent screen. The image may also be stored by either digital or analog means.

Body Part	Contrast	Qualifier	Qualifier
Ø Sternoclavicular Joint, Right 1 Sternoclavicular Joint, Left 2 Sternoclavicular Joints, Bilateral 3 Acromioclavicular Joints, Bilateral 4 Clavicle, Right 5 Clavicle, Left 6 Scapula, Right 7 Scapula, Left A Humerus, Right B Humerus, Left E Upper Arm, Right F Upper Arm, Left J Forearm, Right K Forearm, Left N Hand, Right P Hand, Left R Finger(s), Right S Finger(s), Left X Ribs, Right Y Ribs, Left	Z None	Z None	Z None
8 Shoulder, Right 9 Shoulder, Left L Wrist, Right M Wrist, Left	Ø High Osmolar 1 Low Osmolar Y Other Contrast Z None	Z None	Z None
C Hand/Finger Joint, Right D Hand/Finger Joint, Left G Elbow, Right H Elbow, Left	Ø High Osmolar 1 Low Osmolar Y Other Contrast	Z None	Z None

SECTION: B IMAGING
BODY SYSTEM: P NON-AXIAL UPPER BONES
TYPE: 2 COMPUTERIZED TOMOGRAPHY (CT SCAN): Computer-reformatted digital display of multiplanar images developed from the capture of multiple exposures of external ionizing radiation

Body Part	Contrast	Qualifier	Qualifier
Ø Sternoclavicular Joint, Right 1 Sternoclavicular Joint, Left W Thorax	Ø High Osmolar 1 Low Osmolar Y Other Contrast	Z None	Z None
2 Sternoclavicular Joints, Bilateral 3 Acromioclavicular Joints, Bilateral 4 Clavicle, Right 5 Clavicle, Left 6 Scapula, Right 7 Scapula, Left 8 Shoulder, Right 9 Shoulder, Left A Humerus, Right B Humerus, Left E Upper Arm, Right F Upper Arm, Left G Elbow, Right H Elbow, Left J Forearm, Right K Forearm, Left L Wrist, Right M Wrist, Left N Hand, Right P Hand, Left Q Hands and Wrists, Bilateral R Finger(s), Right S Finger(s), Left T Upper Extremity, Right U Upper Extremity, Left V Upper Extremities, Bilateral X Ribs, Right Y Ribs, Left	Ø High Osmolar 1 Low Osmolar Y Other Contrast Z None	Z None	Z None
C Hand/Finger Joint, Right D Hand/Finger Joint, Left	Z None	Z None	Z None

SECTION: B IMAGING
BODY SYSTEM: P NON-AXIAL UPPER BONES
TYPE: 3 MAGNETIC RESONANCE IMAGING (MRI): Computer-reformatted digital display of multiplanar images developed from the capture of radiofrequency signals emitted by nuclei in a body site excited within a magnetic field

Body Part	Contrast	Qualifier	Qualifier
8 Shoulder, Right 9 Shoulder, Left C Hand/Finger Joint, Right D Hand/Finger Joint, Left E Upper Arm, Right F Upper Arm, Left G Elbow, Right H Elbow, Left J Forearm, Right K Forearm, Left L Wrist, Right M Wrist, Left	Y Other Contrast	Ø Unenhanced and Enhanced Z None	Z None
8 Shoulder, Right 9 Shoulder, Left C Hand/Finger Joint, Right D Hand/Finger Joint, Left E Upper Arm, Right F Upper Arm, Left G Elbow, Right H Elbow, Left J Forearm, Right K Forearm, Left L Wrist, Right M Wrist, Left	Z None	Z None	Z None

SECTION: B IMAGING
BODY SYSTEM: P NON-AXIAL UPPER BONES
TYPE: 4 ULTRASONOGRAPHY: Real-time display of images of anatomy or flow information developed from the capture of reflected and attenuated high-frequency sound waves

Body Part	Contrast	Qualifier	Qualifier
8 Shoulder, Right 9 Shoulder, Left G Elbow, Right H Elbow, Left L Wrist, Right M Wrist, Left N Hand, Right P Hand, Left	Z None	Z None	1 Densitometry Z None

B: IMAGING P: NON-AXIAL UPPER BONES 3: MRI 4: ULTRASONOGRAPHY

SECTION: B IMAGING
BODY SYSTEM: Q NON-AXIAL LOWER BONES
TYPE: Ø PLAIN RADIOGRAPHY: Planar display of an image developed from the capture of external ionizing radiation on photographic or photoconductive plate

Body Part	Contrast	Qualifier	Qualifier
Ø Hip, Right 1 Hip, Left	Ø High Osmolar 1 Low Osmolar Y Other Contrast	Z None	Z None
Ø Hip, Right 1 Hip, Left	Z None	Z None	1 Densitometry Z None
3 Femur, Right 4 Femur, Left	Z None	Z None	1 Densitometry Z None
7 Knee, Right 8 Knee, Left G Ankle, Right H Ankle, Left	Ø High Osmolar 1 Low Osmolar Y Other Contrast Z None	Z None	Z None
D Lower Leg, Right F Lower Leg, Left J Calcaneus, Right K Calcaneus, Left L Foot, Right M Foot, Left P Toe(s), Right Q Toe(s), Left V Patella, Right W Patella, Left	Z None	Z None	Z None
X Foot/Toe Joint, Right Y Foot/Toe Joint, Left	Ø High Osmolar 1 Low Osmolar Y Other Contrast	Z None	Z None

SECTION: B IMAGING
BODY SYSTEM: Q NON-AXIAL LOWER BONES
TYPE: 1 FLUOROSCOPY: Single plane or bi-plane real-time display of an image developed from the capture of external ionizing radiation on a fluorescent screen. The image may also be stored by either digital or analog means.

Body Part	Contrast	Qualifier	Qualifier
Ø Hip, Right 1 Hip, Left 7 Knee, Right 8 Knee, Left G Ankle, Right H Ankle, Left X Foot/Toe Joint, Right Y Foot/Toe Joint, Left	Ø High Osmolar 1 Low Osmolar Y Other Contrast Z None	Z None	Z None
3 Femur, Right 4 Femur, Left D Lower Leg, Right F Lower Leg, Left J Calcaneus, Right K Calcaneus, Left L Foot, Right M Foot, Left P Toe(s), Right Q Toe(s), Left V Patella, Right W Patella, Left	Z None	Z None	Z None

SECTION: B IMAGING

BODY SYSTEM: Q NON-AXIAL LOWER BONES

TYPE: 2 COMPUTERIZED TOMOGRAPHY (CT SCAN): Computer-reformatted digital display of multiplanar images developed from the capture of multiple exposures of external ionizing radiation

Body Part	Contrast	Qualifier	Qualifier
Ø Hip, Right 1 Hip, Left 3 Femur, Right 4 Femur, Left 7 Knee, Right 8 Knee, Left D Lower Leg, Right F Lower Leg, Left G Ankle, Right H Ankle, Left J Calcaneus, Right K Calcaneus, Left L Foot, Right M Foot, Left P Toe(s), Right Q Toe(s), Left R Lower Extremity, Right S Lower Extremity, Left V Patella, Right W Patella, Left X Foot/Toe Joint, Right Y Foot/Toe Joint, Left	Ø High Osmolar 1 Low Osmolar Y Other Contrast Z None	Z None	Z None
B Tibia/Fibula, Right C Tibia/Fibula, Left	Ø High Osmolar 1 Low Osmolar Y Other Contrast	Z None	Z None

SECTION: B IMAGING
BODY SYSTEM: Q NON-AXIAL LOWER BONES
TYPE: 3 MAGNETIC RESONANCE IMAGING (MRI): Computer-reformatted digital display of multiplanar images developed from the capture of radiofrequency signals emitted by nuclei in a body site excited within a magnetic field

Body Part	Contrast	Qualifier	Qualifier
Ø Hip, Right 1 Hip, Left 3 Femur, Right 4 Femur, Left 7 Knee, Right 8 Knee, Left D Lower Leg, Right F Lower Leg, Left G Ankle, Right H Ankle, Left J Calcaneus, Right K Calcaneus, Left L Foot, Right M Foot, Left P Toe(s), Right Q Toe(s), Left V Patella, Right W Patella, Left	Y Other Contrast	Ø Unenhanced and Enhanced Z None	Z None
Ø Hip, Right 1 Hip, Left 3 Femur, Right 4 Femur, Left 7 Knee, Right 8 Knee, Left D Lower Leg, Right F Lower Leg, Left G Ankle, Right H Ankle, Left J Calcaneus, Right K Calcaneus, Left L Foot, Right M Foot, Left P Toe(s), Right Q Toe(s), Left V Patella, Right W Patella, Left	Z None	Z None	Z None

SECTION: B IMAGING
BODY SYSTEM: Q NON-AXIAL LOWER BONES
TYPE: 4 ULTRASONOGRAPHY: Real-time display of images of anatomy or flow information developed from the capture of reflected and attenuated high-frequency sound waves

Body Part	Contrast	Qualifier	Qualifier
Ø Hip, Right 1 Hip, Left 2 Hips, Bilateral 7 Knee, Right 8 Knee, Left 9 Knees, Bilateral	Z None	Z None	Z None

SECTION: B IMAGING
BODY SYSTEM: R AXIAL SKELETON, EXCEPT SKULL AND FACIAL BONES
TYPE: Ø PLAIN RADIOGRAPHY: Planar display of an image developed from the capture of external ionizing radiation on photographic or photoconductive plate

Body Part	Contrast	Qualifier	Qualifier
Ø Cervical Spine 7 Thoracic Spine 9 Lumbar Spine G Whole Spine	Z None	Z None	1 Densitometry Z None
1 Cervical Disc(s) 2 Thoracic Disc(s) 3 Lumbar Disc(s) 4 Cervical Facet Joint(s) 5 Thoracic Facet Joint(s) 6 Lumbar Facet Joint(s) D Sacroiliac Joints	Ø High Osmolar 1 Low Osmolar Y Other Contrast Z None	Z None	Z None
8 Thoracolumbar Joint B Lumbosacral Joint C Pelvis F Sacrum and Coccyx H Sternum	Z None	Z None	Z None

SECTION: B IMAGING
BODY SYSTEM: R AXIAL SKELETON, EXCEPT SKULL AND FACIAL BONES
TYPE: 1 FLUOROSCOPY: Single plane or bi-plane real-time display of an image developed from the capture of external ionizing radiation on a fluorescent screen. The image may also be stored by either digital or analog means.

Body Part	Contrast	Qualifier	Qualifier
Ø Cervical Spine 1 Cervical Disc(s) 2 Thoracic Disc(s) 3 Lumbar Disc(s) 4 Cervical Facet Joint(s) 5 Thoracic Facet Joint(s) 6 Lumbar Facet Joint(s) 7 Thoracic Spine 8 Thoracolumbar Joint 9 Lumbar Spine B Lumbosacral Joint C Pelvis D Sacroiliac Joints F Sacrum and Coccyx G Whole Spine H Sternum	Ø High Osmolar 1 Low Osmolar Y Other Contrast Z None	Z None	Z None

SECTION: B IMAGING
BODY SYSTEM: R AXIAL SKELETON, EXCEPT SKULL AND FACIAL BONES
TYPE: 2 **COMPUTERIZED TOMOGRAPHY (CT SCAN):** Computer-reformatted digital display of multiplanar images developed from the capture of multiple exposures of external ionizing radiation

Body Part	Contrast	Qualifier	Qualifier
Ø Cervical Spine 7 Thoracic Spine 9 Lumbar Spine C Pelvis D Sacroiliac Joints F Sacrum and Coccyx	Ø High Osmolar 1 Low Osmolar Y Other Contrast Z None	Z None	Z None

SECTION: B IMAGING
BODY SYSTEM: R AXIAL SKELETON, EXCEPT SKULL AND FACIAL BONES
TYPE: 3 **MAGNETIC RESONANCE IMAGING (MRI):** Computer-reformatted digital display of multiplanar images developed from the capture of radiofrequency signals emitted by nuclei in a body site excited within a magnetic field

Body Part	Contrast	Qualifier	Qualifier
Ø Cervical Spine 1 Cervical Disc(s) 2 Thoracic Disc(s) 3 Lumbar Disc(s) 7 Thoracic Spine 9 Lumbar Spine C Pelvis F Sacrum and Coccyx	Y Other Contrast	Ø Unenhanced and Enhanced Z None	Z None
Ø Cervical Spine 1 Cervical Disc(s) 2 Thoracic Disc(s) 3 Lumbar Disc(s) 7 Thoracic Spine 9 Lumbar Spine C Pelvis F Sacrum and Coccyx	Z None	Z None	Z None

SECTION: B IMAGING
BODY SYSTEM: R AXIAL SKELETON, EXCEPT SKULL AND FACIAL BONES
TYPE: 4 **ULTRASONOGRAPHY:** Real-time display of images of anatomy or flow information developed from the capture of reflected and attenuated high-frequency sound waves

Body Part	Contrast	Qualifier	Qualifier
Ø Cervical Spine 7 Thoracic Spine 9 Lumbar Spine F Sacrum and Coccyx	Z None	Z None	Z None

SECTION: B IMAGING
BODY SYSTEM: T URINARY SYSTEM
TYPE: Ø PLAIN RADIOGRAPHY: Planar display of an image developed from the capture of external ionizing radiation on photographic or photoconductive plate

Body Part	Contrast	Qualifier	Qualifier
Ø Bladder 1 Kidney, Right 2 Kidney, Left 3 Kidneys, Bilateral 4 Kidneys, Ureters, and Bladder 5 Urethra 6 Ureter, Right 7 Ureter, Left 8 Ureters, Bilateral B Bladder and Urethra C Ileal Diversion Loop	Ø High Osmolar 1 Low Osmolar Y Other Contrast Z None	Z None	Z None

SECTION: B IMAGING
BODY SYSTEM: T URINARY SYSTEM
TYPE: 1 FLUOROSCOPY: Single plane or bi-plane real-time display of an image developed from the capture of external ionizing radiation on a fluorescent screen. The image may also be stored by either digital or analog means.

Body Part	Contrast	Qualifier	Qualifier
Ø Bladder 1 Kidney, Right 2 Kidney, Left 3 Kidneys, Bilateral 4 Kidneys, Ureters, and Bladder 5 Urethra 6 Ureter, Right 7 Ureter, Left B Bladder and Urethra C Ileal Diversion Loop D Kidney, Ureter, and Bladder, Right F Kidney, Ureter, and Bladder, Left G Ileal Loop, Ureters, and Kidneys	Ø High Osmolar 1 Low Osmolar Y Other Contrast Z None	Z None	Z None

SECTION: B IMAGING
BODY SYSTEM: T URINARY SYSTEM
TYPE: 2 COMPUTERIZED TOMOGRAPHY (CT SCAN): Computer-reformatted digital display of multiplanar images developed from the capture of multiple exposures of external ionizing radiation

Body Part	Contrast	Qualifier	Qualifier
Ø Bladder 1 Kidney, Right 2 Kidney, Left 3 Kidneys, Bilateral 9 Kidney Transplant	Ø High Osmolar 1 Low Osmolar Y Other Contrast	Ø Unenhanced and Enhanced Z None	Z None
Ø Bladder 1 Kidney, Right 2 Kidney, Left 3 Kidneys, Bilateral 9 Kidney Transplant	Z None	Z None	Z None

SECTION: B IMAGING
BODY SYSTEM: T URINARY SYSTEM
TYPE: 3 MAGNETIC RESONANCE IMAGING (MRI): Computer-reformatted digital display of multiplanar images developed from the capture of radiofrequency signals emitted by nuclei in a body site excited within a magnetic field

Body Part	Contrast	Qualifier	Qualifier
Ø Bladder 1 Kidney, Right 2 Kidney, Left 3 Kidneys, Bilateral 9 Kidney Transplant	Y Other Contrast	Ø Unenhanced and Enhanced Z None	Z None
Ø Bladder 1 Kidney, Right 2 Kidney, Left 3 Kidneys, Bilateral 9 Kidney Transplant	Z None	Z None	Z None

BT4

SECTION: B IMAGING

BODY SYSTEM: T URINARY SYSTEM

TYPE: 4 ULTRASONOGRAPHY: Real-time display of images of anatomy or flow information developed from the capture of reflected and attenuated high-frequency sound waves

Body Part	Contrast	Qualifier	Qualifier
Ø Bladder 1 Kidney, Right 2 Kidney, Left 3 Kidneys, Bilateral 5 Urethra 6 Ureter, Right 7 Ureter, Left 8 Ureters, Bilateral 9 Kidney Transplant J Kidneys and Bladder	Z None	Z None	Z None

SECTION: B IMAGING
BODY SYSTEM: U FEMALE REPRODUCTIVE SYSTEM
TYPE: Ø PLAIN RADIOGRAPHY: Planar display of an image developed from the capture of external ionizing radiation on photographic or photoconductive plate

Body Part	Contrast	Qualifier	Qualifier
Ø Fallopian Tube, Right♀ 1 Fallopian Tube, Left♀ 2 Fallopian Tubes, Bilateral♀ 6 Uterus♀ 8 Uterus and Fallopian Tubes♀ 9 Vagina♀	Ø High Osmolar 1 Low Osmolar Y Other Contrast	Z None	Z None

SECTION: B IMAGING
BODY SYSTEM: U FEMALE REPRODUCTIVE SYSTEM
TYPE: 1 FLUOROSCOPY: Single plane or bi-plane real-time display of an image developed from the capture of external ionizing radiation on a fluorescent screen. The image may also be stored by either digital or analog means.

Body Part	Contrast	Qualifier	Qualifier
Ø Fallopian Tube, Right♀ 1 Fallopian Tube, Left♀ 2 Fallopian Tubes, Bilateral♀ 6 Uterus♀ 8 Uterus and Fallopian Tubes♀ 9 Vagina♀	Ø High Osmolar 1 Low Osmolar Y Other Contrast Z None	Z None	Z None

SECTION: B IMAGING
BODY SYSTEM: U FEMALE REPRODUCTIVE SYSTEM
TYPE: 3 MAGNETIC RESONANCE IMAGING (MRI): Computer-reformatted digital display of multiplanar images developed from the capture of radiofrequency signals emitted by nuclei in a body site excited within a magnetic field

Body Part	Contrast	Qualifier	Qualifier
3 Ovary, Right ♀ 4 Ovary, Left ♀ 5 Ovaries, Bilateral ♀ 6 Uterus ♀ 9 Vagina ♀ B Pregnant Uterus ♀ C Uterus and Ovaries ♀	Y Other Contrast	Ø Unenhanced and Enhanced Z None	Z None
3 Ovary, Right ♀ 4 Ovary, Left ♀ 5 Ovaries, Bilateral ♀ 6 Uterus ♀ 9 Vagina ♀ B Pregnant Uterus ♀ C Uterus and Ovaries ♀	Z None	Z None	Z None

SECTION: B IMAGING
BODY SYSTEM: U FEMALE REPRODUCTIVE SYSTEM
TYPE: 4 ULTRASONOGRAPHY: Real-time display of images of anatomy or flow information developed from the capture of reflected and attenuated high-frequency sound waves

Body Part	Contrast	Qualifier	Qualifier
Ø Fallopian Tube, Right ♀ 1 Fallopian Tube, Left ♀ 2 Fallopian Tubes, Bilateral ♀ 3 Ovary, Right ♀ 4 Ovary, Left ♀ 5 Ovaries, Bilateral ♀ 6 Uterus ♀ C Uterus and Ovaries ♀	Y Other Contrast Z None	Z None	Z None

SECTION: B **IMAGING**
BODY SYSTEM: V **MALE REPRODUCTIVE SYSTEM**
TYPE: Ø **PLAIN RADIOGRAPHY:** Planar display of an image developed from the capture of external ionizing radiation on photographic or photoconductive plate

Body Part	Contrast	Qualifier	Qualifier
Ø Corpora Cavernosa ♂ 1 Epididymis, Right ♂ 2 Epididymis, Left ♂ 3 Prostate ♂ 5 Testicle, Right ♂ 6 Testicle, Left ♂ 8 Vasa Vasorum ♂	Ø High Osmolar 1 Low Osmolar Y Other Contrast	Z None	Z None

SECTION: B **IMAGING**
BODY SYSTEM: V **MALE REPRODUCTIVE SYSTEM**
TYPE: 1 **FLUOROSCOPY:** Single plane or bi-plane real-time display of an image developed from the capture of external ionizing radiation on a fluorescent screen. The image may also be stored by either digital or analog means.

Body Part	Contrast	Qualifier	Qualifier
Ø Corpora Cavernosa ♂ 8 Vasa Vasorum ♂	Ø High Osmolar 1 Low Osmolar Y Other Contrast Z None	Z None	Z None

SECTION: B IMAGING
BODY SYSTEM: V MALE REPRODUCTIVE SYSTEM
TYPE: 2 **COMPUTERIZED TOMOGRAPHY (CT SCAN):** Computer-reformatted digital display of multiplanar images developed from the capture of multiple exposures of external ionizing radiation

Body Part	Contrast	Qualifier	Qualifier
3 Prostate ♂	Ø High Osmolar 1 Low Osmolar Y Other Contrast	Ø Unenhanced and Enhanced Z None	Z None
3 Prostate ♂	Z None	Z None	Z None

SECTION: B IMAGING
BODY SYSTEM: V MALE REPRODUCTIVE SYSTEM
TYPE: 3 **MAGNETIC RESONANCE IMAGING (MRI):** Computer-reformatted digital display of multiplanar images developed from the capture of radiofrequency signals emitted by nuclei in a body site excited within a magnetic field

Body Part	Contrast	Qualifier	Qualifier
Ø Corpora Cavernosa ♂ 3 Prostate ♂ 4 Scrotum ♂ 5 Testicle, Right ♂ 6 Testicle, Left ♂ 7 Testicles, Bilateral ♂	Y Other Contrast	Ø Unenhanced and Enhanced Z None	Z None
Ø Corpora Cavernosa ♂ 3 Prostate ♂ 4 Scrotum ♂ 5 Testicle, Right ♂ 6 Testicle, Left ♂ 7 Testicles, Bilateral ♂	Z None	Z None	Z None

SECTION: B IMAGING
BODY SYSTEM: V MALE REPRODUCTIVE SYSTEM
TYPE: 4 **ULTRASONOGRAPHY:** Real-time display of images of anatomy or flow information developed from the capture of reflected and attenuated high-frequency sound waves

Body Part	Contrast	Qualifier	Qualifier
4 Scrotum ♂ 9 Prostate and Seminal Vesicles ♂ B Penis ♂	Z None	Z None	Z None

SECTION: B IMAGING
BODY SYSTEM: W ANATOMICAL REGIONS
TYPE: Ø PLAIN RADIOGRAPHY: Planar display of an image developed from the capture of external ionizing radiation on photographic or photoconductive plate

Body Part	Contrast	Qualifier	Qualifier
Ø Abdomen 1 Abdomen and Pelvis 3 Chest B Long Bones, All C Lower Extremity J Upper Extremity K Whole Body L Whole Skeleton M Whole Body, Infant	Z None	Z None	Z None

SECTION: B IMAGING
BODY SYSTEM: W ANATOMICAL REGIONS
TYPE: 1 FLUOROSCOPY: Single plane or bi-plane real-time display of an image developed from the capture of external ionizing radiation on a fluorescent screen. The image may also be stored by either digital or analog means.

Body Part	Contrast	Qualifier	Qualifier
1 Abdomen and Pelvis 9 Head and Neck C Lower Extremity J Upper Extremity	Ø High Osmolar 1 Low Osmolar Y Other Contrast Z None	Z None	Z None

SECTION: B IMAGING
BODY SYSTEM: W ANATOMICAL REGIONS
TYPE: 2 COMPUTERIZED TOMOGRAPHY (CT SCAN): Computer-reformatted digital display of multiplanar images developed from the capture of multiple exposures of external ionizing radiation

Body Part	Contrast	Qualifier	Qualifier
Ø Abdomen 1 Abdomen and Pelvis 4 Chest and Abdomen 5 Chest, Abdomen, and Pelvis 8 Head 9 Head and Neck F Neck G Pelvic Region	Ø High Osmolar 1 Low Osmolar Y Other Contrast	Ø Unenhanced and Enhanced Z None	Z None
Ø Abdomen 1 Abdomen and Pelvis 4 Chest and Abdomen 5 Chest, Abdomen, and Pelvis 8 Head 9 Head and Neck F Neck G Pelvic Region	Z None	Z None	Z None

SECTION: B IMAGING
BODY SYSTEM: W ANATOMICAL REGIONS
TYPE: 3 MAGNETIC RESONANCE IMAGING (MRI): Computer-reformatted digital display of multiplanar images developed from the capture of radiofrequency signals emitted by nuclei in a body site excited within a magnetic field

Body Part	Contrast	Qualifier	Qualifier
Ø Abdomen 8 Head F Neck G Pelvic Region H Retroperitoneum P Brachial Plexus	Y Other Contrast	Ø Unenhanced and Enhanced Z None	Z None
Ø Abdomen 8 Head F Neck G Pelvic Region H Retroperitoneum P Brachial Plexus	Z None	Z None	Z None
3 Chest	Y Other Contrast	Ø Unenhanced and Enhanced Z None	Z None

SECTION: B IMAGING
BODY SYSTEM: W ANATOMICAL REGIONS
TYPE: 4 ULTRASONOGRAPHY: Real-time display of images of anatomy or flow information developed from the capture of reflected and attenuated high-frequency sound waves

Body Part	Contrast	Qualifier	Qualifier
Ø Abdomen 1 Abdomen and Pelvis F Neck G Pelvic Region	Z None	Z None	Z None

SECTION: B IMAGING
BODY SYSTEM: W ANATOMICAL REGIONS
TYPE: 5 OTHER IMAGING: Other specified modality for visualizing a body part

Body Part	Contrast	Qualifier	Qualifier
2 Trunk 9 Head and Neck C Lower Extremity J Upper Extremity	Z None	1 Bacterial Autofluorescence	Z None

SECTION: B IMAGING
BODY SYSTEM: Y FETUS AND OBSTETRICAL
TYPE: 3 MAGNETIC RESONANCE IMAGING (MRI): Computer-reformatted digital display of multiplanar images developed from the capture of radiofrequency signals emitted by nuclei in a body site excited within a magnetic field

Body Part	Contrast	Qualifier	Qualifier
Ø Fetal Head ♀ 1 Fetal Heart ♀ 2 Fetal Thorax ♀ 3 Fetal Abdomen ♀ 4 Fetal Spine ♀ 5 Fetal Extremities ♀ 6 Whole Fetus ♀	Y Other Contrast	Ø Unenhanced and Enhanced Z None	Z None
Ø Fetal Head ♀ 1 Fetal Heart ♀ 2 Fetal Thorax ♀ 3 Fetal Abdomen ♀ 4 Fetal Spine ♀ 5 Fetal Extremities ♀ 6 Whole Fetus ♀	Z None	Z None	Z None

SECTION: B IMAGING
BODY SYSTEM: Y FETUS AND OBSTETRICAL
TYPE: 4 ULTRASONOGRAPHY: Real-time display of images of anatomy or flow information developed from the capture of reflected and attenuated high-frequency sound waves

Body Part	Contrast	Qualifier	Qualifier
7 Fetal Umbilical Cord ♀ 8 Placenta ♀ 9 First Trimester, Single Fetus ♀ B First Trimester, Multiple Gestation ♀ C Second Trimester, Single Fetus ♀ D Second Trimester, Multiple Gestation ♀ F Third Trimester, Single Fetus ♀ G Third Trimester, Multiple Gestation ♀	Z None	Z None	Z None

SECTION: C NUCLEAR MEDICINE
BODY SYSTEM: Ø CENTRAL NERVOUS SYSTEM
TYPE: 1 PLANAR NUCLEAR MEDICINE IMAGING: Introduction of radioactive materials into the body for single plane display of images developed from the capture of radioactive emissions

Body Part	Radionuclide	Qualifier	Qualifier
Ø Brain	1 Technetium 99m (Tc-99m) Y Other Radionuclide	Z None	Z None
5 Cerebrospinal Fluid	D Indium 111 (In-111) Y Other Radionuclide	Z None	Z None
Y Central Nervous System	Y Other Radionuclide	Z None	Z None

SECTION: C NUCLEAR MEDICINE
BODY SYSTEM: Ø CENTRAL NERVOUS SYSTEM
TYPE: 2 TOMOGRAPHIC (TOMO) NUCLEAR MEDICINE IMAGING: Introduction of radioactive materials into the body for three-dimensional display of images developed from the capture of radioactive emissions

Body Part	Radionuclide	Qualifier	Qualifier
Ø Brain	1 Technetium 99m (Tc-99m) F Iodine 123 (I-123) S Thallium 2Ø1 (Tl-2Ø1) Y Other Radionuclide	Z None	Z None
5 Cerebrospinal Fluid	D Indium 111 (In-111) Y Other Radionuclide	Z None	Z None
Y Central Nervous System	Y Other Radionuclide	Z None	Z None

SECTION: C NUCLEAR MEDICINE
BODY SYSTEM: Ø CENTRAL NERVOUS SYSTEM
TYPE: 3 POSITRON EMISSION TOMOGRAPHIC (PET) IMAGING: Introduction of radioactive materials into the body for three-dimensional display of images developed from the simultaneous capture, 180 degrees apart, of radioactive emissions

Body Part	Radionuclide	Qualifier	Qualifier
Ø Brain	B Carbon 11 (C-11) K Fluorine 18 (F-18) M Oxygen 15 (O-15) Y Other Radionuclide	Z None	Z None
Y Central Nervous System	Y Other Radionuclide	Z None	Z None

SECTION: C NUCLEAR MEDICINE
BODY SYSTEM: Ø CENTRAL NERVOUS SYSTEM
TYPE: 5 NONIMAGING NUCLEAR MEDICINE PROBE: Introduction of radioactive materials into the body for the study of distribution and fate of certain substances by the detection of radioactive emissions; or, alternatively, measurement of absorption of radioactive emissions from an external source

Body Part	Radionuclide	Qualifier	Qualifier
Ø Brain	V Xenon 133 (Xe-133) Y Other Radionuclide	Z None	Z None
Y Central Nervous System	Y Other Radionuclide	Z None	Z None

SECTION: C NUCLEAR MEDICINE
BODY SYSTEM: 2 HEART
TYPE: 1 PLANAR NUCLEAR MEDICINE IMAGING: Introduction of radioactive materials into the body for single plane display of images developed from the capture of radioactive emissions

Body Part	Radionuclide	Qualifier	Qualifier
6 Heart, Right and Left	1 Technetium 99m (Tc-99m) Y Other Radionuclide	Z None	Z None
G Myocardium	1 Technetium 99m (Tc-99m) D Indium 111 (In-111) S Thallium 201 (Tl-201) Y Other Radionuclide Z None	Z None	Z None
Y Heart	Y Other Radionuclide	Z None	Z None

SECTION: C NUCLEAR MEDICINE
BODY SYSTEM: 2 HEART
TYPE: 2 TOMOGRAPHIC (TOMO) NUCLEAR MEDICINE IMAGING: Introduction of radioactive materials into the body for three-dimensional display of images developed from the capture of radioactive emissions

Body Part	Radionuclide	Qualifier	Qualifier
6 Heart, Right and Left	1 Technetium 99m (Tc-99m) Y Other Radionuclide	Z None	Z None
G Myocardium	1 Technetium 99m (Tc-99m) D Indium 111 (In-111) K Fluorine 18 (F-18) S Thallium 201 (Tl-201) Y Other Radionuclide Z None	Z None	Z None
Y Heart	Y Other Radionuclide	Z None	Z None

SECTION: C NUCLEAR MEDICINE
BODY SYSTEM: 2 HEART
TYPE: 3 **POSITRON EMISSION TOMOGRAPHIC (PET) IMAGING:** Introduction of radioactive materials into the body for three-dimensional display of images developed from the simultaneous capture, 180 degrees apart, of radioactive emissions

Body Part	Radionuclide	Qualifier	Qualifier
G Myocardium	K Fluorine 18 (F-18) M Oxygen 15 (O-15) Q Rubidium 82 (Rb-82) R Nitrogen 13 (N-13) Y Other Radionuclide	Z None	Z None
Y Heart	Y Other Radionuclide	Z None	Z None

SECTION: C NUCLEAR MEDICINE
BODY SYSTEM: 2 HEART
TYPE: 5 **NONIMAGING NUCLEAR MEDICINE PROBE:** Introduction of radioactive materials into the body for the study of distribution and fate of certain substances by the detection of radioactive emissions; or, alternatively, measurement of absorption of radioactive emissions from an external source

Body Part	Radionuclide	Qualifier	Qualifier
6 Heart, Right and Left	1 Technetium 99m (Tc-99m) Y Other Radionuclide	Z None	Z None
Y Heart	Y Other Radionuclide	Z None	Z None

SECTION: C NUCLEAR MEDICINE

BODY SYSTEM: 5 VEINS

TYPE: 1 PLANAR NUCLEAR MEDICINE IMAGING: Introduction of radioactive materials into the body for single plane display of images developed from the capture of radioactive emissions

Body Part	Radionuclide	Qualifier	Qualifier
B Lower Extremity Veins, Right C Lower Extremity Veins, Left D Lower Extremity Veins, Bilateral N Upper Extremity Veins, Right P Upper Extremity Veins, Left Q Upper Extremity Veins, Bilateral R Central Veins	1 Technetium 99m (Tc-99m) Y Other Radionuclide	Z None	Z None
Y Veins	Y Other Radionuclide	Z None	Z None

SECTION: C NUCLEAR MEDICINE
BODY SYSTEM: 7 LYMPHATIC AND HEMATOLOGIC SYSTEM
TYPE: 1 PLANAR NUCLEAR MEDICINE IMAGING: Introduction of radioactive materials into the body for single plane display of images developed from the capture of radioactive emissions

Body Part	Radionuclide	Qualifier	Qualifier
Ø Bone Marrow	1 Technetium 99m (Tc-99m) D Indium 111 (In-111) Y Other Radionuclide	Z None	Z None
2 Spleen 5 Lymphatics, Head and Neck D Lymphatics, Pelvic J Lymphatics, Head K Lymphatics, Neck L Lymphatics, Upper Chest M Lymphatics, Trunk N Lymphatics, Upper Extremity P Lymphatics, Lower Extremity	1 Technetium 99m (Tc-99m) Y Other Radionuclide	Z None	Z None
3 Blood	D Indium 111 (In-111) Y Other Radionuclide	Z None	Z None
Y Lymphatic and Hematologic System	Y Other Radionuclide	Z None	Z None

SECTION: C NUCLEAR MEDICINE
BODY SYSTEM: 7 LYMPHATIC AND HEMATOLOGIC SYSTEM
TYPE: 2 TOMOGRAPHIC (TOMO) NUCLEAR MEDICINE IMAGING: Introduction of radioactive materials into the body for three-dimensional display of images developed from the capture of radioactive emissions

Body Part	Radionuclide	Qualifier	Qualifier
2 Spleen	1 Technetium 99m (Tc-99m) Y Other Radionuclide	Z None	Z None
Y Lymphatic and Hematologic System	Y Other Radionuclide	Z None	Z None

SECTION: C NUCLEAR MEDICINE
BODY SYSTEM: 7 LYMPHATIC AND HEMATOLOGIC SYSTEM
TYPE: 5 NONIMAGING NUCLEAR MEDICINE PROBE: Introduction of radioactive materials into the body for the study of distribution and fate of certain substances by the detection of radioactive emissions; or, alternatively, measurement of absorption of radioactive emissions from an external source

Body Part	Radionuclide	Qualifier	Qualifier
5 Lymphatics, Head and Neck D Lymphatics, Pelvic J Lymphatics, Head K Lymphatics, Neck L Lymphatics, Upper Chest M Lymphatics, Trunk N Lymphatics, Upper Extremity P Lymphatics, Lower Extremity	1 Technetium 99m (Tc-99m) Y Other Radionuclide	Z None	Z None
Y Lymphatic and Hematologic System	Y Other Radionuclide	Z None	Z None

SECTION: C NUCLEAR MEDICINE
BODY SYSTEM: 7 LYMPHATIC AND HEMATOLOGIC SYSTEM
TYPE: 6 NONIMAGING NUCLEAR MEDICINE ASSAY: Introduction of radioactive materials into the body for the study of body fluids and blood elements, by the detection of radioactive emissions

Body Part	Radionuclide	Qualifier	Qualifier
3 Blood	1 Technetium 99m (Tc-99m) 7 Cobalt 58 (Co-58) C Cobalt 57 (Co-57) D Indium 111 (In-111) H Iodine 125 (I-125) W Chromium (Cr-51) Y Other Radionuclide	Z None	Z None
Y Lymphatic and Hematologic System	Y Other Radionuclide	Z None	Z None

SECTION: C NUCLEAR MEDICINE

BODY SYSTEM: 8 EYE

TYPE: 1 PLANAR NUCLEAR MEDICINE IMAGING: Introduction of radioactive materials into the body for single plane display of images developed from the capture of radioactive emissions

Body Part	Radionuclide	Qualifier	Qualifier
9 Lacrimal Ducts, Bilateral	1 Technetium 99m (Tc-99m) Y Other Radionuclide	Z None	Z None
Y Eye	Y Other Radionuclide	Z None	Z None

SECTION: C NUCLEAR MEDICINE

BODY SYSTEM: 9 EAR, NOSE, MOUTH, AND THROAT

TYPE: 1 PLANAR NUCLEAR MEDICINE IMAGING: Introduction of radioactive materials into the body for single plane display of images developed from the capture of radioactive emissions

Body Part	Radionuclide	Qualifier	Qualifier
B Salivary Glands, Bilateral	1 Technetium 99m (Tc-99m) Y Other Radionuclide	Z None	Z None
Y Ear, Nose, Mouth, and Throat	Y Other Radionuclide	Z None	Z None

SECTION: C NUCLEAR MEDICINE
BODY SYSTEM: B RESPIRATORY SYSTEM
TYPE: 1 PLANAR NUCLEAR MEDICINE IMAGING: Introduction of radioactive materials into the body for single plane display of images developed from the capture of radioactive emissions

Body Part	Radionuclide	Qualifier	Qualifier
2 Lungs and Bronchi	1 Technetium 99m (Tc-99m) 9 Krypton (Kr-81m) T Xenon 127 (Xe-127) V Xenon 133 (Xe-133) Y Other Radionuclide	Z None	Z None
Y Respiratory System	Y Other Radionuclide	Z None	Z None

SECTION: C NUCLEAR MEDICINE
BODY SYSTEM: B RESPIRATORY SYSTEM
TYPE: 2 TOMOGRAPHIC (TOMO) NUCLEAR MEDICINE IMAGING: Introduction of radioactive materials into the body for three-dimensional display of images developed from the capture of radioactive emissions

Body Part	Radionuclide	Qualifier	Qualifier
2 Lungs and Bronchi	1 Technetium 99m (Tc-99m) 9 Krypton (Kr-81m) Y Other Radionuclide	Z None	Z None
Y Respiratory System	Y Other Radionuclide	Z None	Z None

SECTION: C NUCLEAR MEDICINE
BODY SYSTEM: B RESPIRATORY SYSTEM
TYPE: 3 POSITRON EMISSION TOMOGRAPHIC (PET) IMAGING: Introduction of radioactive materials into the body for three-dimensional display of images developed from the simultaneous capture, 180 degrees apart, of radioactive emissions

Body Part	Radionuclide	Qualifier	Qualifier
2 Lungs and Bronchi	K Fluorine 18 (F-18) Y Other Radionuclide	Z None	Z None
Y Respiratory System	Y Other Radionuclide	Z None	Z None

SECTION: C NUCLEAR MEDICINE
BODY SYSTEM: D GASTROINTESTINAL SYSTEM
TYPE: 1 PLANAR NUCLEAR MEDICINE IMAGING: Introduction of radioactive materials into the body for single plane display of images developed from the capture of radioactive emissions

Body Part	Radionuclide	Qualifier	Qualifier
5 Upper Gastrointestinal Tract 7 Gastrointestinal Tract	1 Technetium 99m (Tc-99m) D Indium 111 (In-111) Y Other Radionuclide	Z None	Z None
Y Digestive System	Y Other Radionuclide	Z None	Z None

SECTION: C NUCLEAR MEDICINE
BODY SYSTEM: D GASTROINTESTINAL SYSTEM
TYPE: 2 TOMOGRAPHIC (TOMO) NUCLEAR MEDICINE IMAGING: Introduction of radioactive materials into the body for three-dimensional display of images developed from the capture of radioactive emissions

Body Part	Radionuclide	Qualifier	Qualifier
7 Gastrointestinal Tract	1 Technetium 99m (Tc-99m) D Indium 111 (In-111) Y Other Radionuclide	Z None	Z None
Y Digestive System	Y Other Radionuclide	Z None	Z None

New/Revised Text in Green ~~deleted~~ Deleted ♀ Females Only ♂ Males Only Coding Clinic
Non-covered Limited Coverage Combination (See Appendix E) DRG Non-OR Non-OR Hospital-Acquired Condition

SECTION: C NUCLEAR MEDICINE
BODY SYSTEM: F HEPATOBILIARY SYSTEM AND PANCREAS
TYPE: 1 PLANAR NUCLEAR MEDICINE IMAGING: Introduction of radioactive materials into the body for single plane display of images developed from the capture of radioactive emissions

Body Part	Radionuclide	Qualifier	Qualifier
4 Gallbladder 5 Liver 6 Liver and Spleen C Hepatobiliary System, All	1 Technetium 99m (Tc-99m) Y Other Radionuclide	Z None	Z None
Y Hepatobiliary System and Pancreas	Y Other Radionuclide	Z None	Z None

SECTION: C NUCLEAR MEDICINE
BODY SYSTEM: F HEPATOBILIARY SYSTEM AND PANCREAS
TYPE: 2 TOMOGRAPHIC (TOMO) NUCLEAR MEDICINE IMAGING: Introduction of radioactive materials into the body for three-dimensional display of images developed from the capture of radioactive emissions

Body Part	Radionuclide	Qualifier	Qualifier
4 Gallbladder 5 Liver 6 Liver and Spleen	1 Technetium 99m (Tc-99m) Y Other Radionuclide	Z None	Z None
Y Hepatobiliary System and Pancreas	Y Other Radionuclide	Z None	Z None

SECTION: C NUCLEAR MEDICINE
BODY SYSTEM: G ENDOCRINE SYSTEM
TYPE: 1 PLANAR NUCLEAR MEDICINE IMAGING: Introduction of radioactive materials into the body for single plane display of images developed from the capture of radioactive emissions

Body Part	Radionuclide	Qualifier	Qualifier
1 Parathyroid Glands	1 Technetium 99m (Tc-99m) S Thallium 201 (Tl-201) Y Other Radionuclide	Z None	Z None
2 Thyroid Gland	1 Technetium 99m (Tc-99m) F Iodine 123 (I-123) G Iodine 131 (I-131) Y Other Radionuclide	Z None	Z None
4 Adrenal Glands, Bilateral	G Iodine 131 (I-131) Y Other Radionuclide	Z None	Z None
Y Endocrine System	Y Other Radionuclide	Z None	Z None

SECTION: C NUCLEAR MEDICINE
BODY SYSTEM: G ENDOCRINE SYSTEM
TYPE: 2 TOMOGRAPHIC (TOMO) NUCLEAR MEDICINE IMAGING: Introduction of radioactive materials into the body for three-dimensional display of images developed from the capture of radioactive emissions

Body Part	Radionuclide	Qualifier	Qualifier
1 Parathyroid Glands	1 Technetium 99m (Tc-99m) S Thallium 201 (Tl-201) Y Other Radionuclide	Z None	Z None
Y Endocrine System	Y Other Radionuclide	Z None	Z None

SECTION: C NUCLEAR MEDICINE
BODY SYSTEM: G ENDOCRINE SYSTEM
TYPE: 4 NONIMAGING NUCLEAR MEDICINE UPTAKE: Introduction of radioactive materials into the body for measurements of organ function, from the detection of radioactive emissions

Body Part	Radionuclide	Qualifier	Qualifier
2 Thyroid Gland	1 Technetium 99m (Tc-99m) F Iodine 123 (I-123) G Iodine 131 (I-131) Y Other Radionuclide	Z None	Z None
Y Endocrine System	Y Other Radionuclide	Z None	Z None

SECTION: C NUCLEAR MEDICINE
BODY SYSTEM: H SKIN, SUBCUTANEOUS TISSUE AND BREAST
TYPE: 1 **PLANAR NUCLEAR MEDICINE IMAGING:** Introduction of radioactive materials into the body for single plane display of images developed from the capture of radioactive emissions

Body Part	Radionuclide	Qualifier	Qualifier
0 Breast, Right 1 Breast, Left 2 Breasts, Bilateral	1 Technetium 99m (Tc-99m) S Thallium 201 (Tl-201) Y Other Radionuclide	Z None	Z None
Y Skin, Subcutaneous Tissue, and Breast	Y Other Radionuclide	Z None	Z None

SECTION: C NUCLEAR MEDICINE
BODY SYSTEM: H SKIN, SUBCUTANEOUS TISSUE AND BREAST
TYPE: 2 **TOMOGRAPHIC (TOMO) NUCLEAR MEDICINE IMAGING:** Introduction of radioactive materials into the body for three-dimensional display of images developed from the capture of radioactive emissions

Body Part	Radionuclide	Qualifier	Qualifier
0 Breast, Right 1 Breast, Left 2 Breasts, Bilateral	1 Technetium 99m (Tc-99m) S Thallium 201 (Tl-201) Y Other Radionuclide	Z None	Z None
Y Skin, Subcutaneous Tissue, and Breast	Y Other Radionuclide	Z None	Z None

SECTION: C NUCLEAR MEDICINE
BODY SYSTEM: P MUSCULOSKELETAL SYSTEM
TYPE: 1 PLANAR NUCLEAR MEDICINE IMAGING: Introduction of radioactive materials into the body for single plane display of images developed from the capture of radioactive emissions

Body Part	Radionuclide	Qualifier	Qualifier
1 Skull 4 Thorax 5 Spine 6 Pelvis 7 Spine and Pelvis 8 Upper Extremity, Right 9 Upper Extremity, Left B Upper Extremities, Bilateral C Lower Extremity, Right D Lower Extremity, Left F Lower Extremities, Bilateral Z Musculoskeletal System, All	1 Technetium 99m (Tc-99m) Y Other Radionuclide	Z None	Z None
Y Musculoskeletal System, Other	Y Other Radionuclide	Z None	Z None

SECTION: C NUCLEAR MEDICINE
BODY SYSTEM: P MUSCULOSKELETAL SYSTEM
TYPE: 2 TOMOGRAPHIC (TOMO) NUCLEAR MEDICINE IMAGING: Introduction of radioactive materials into the body for three-dimensional display of images developed from the capture of radioactive emissions

Body Part	Radionuclide	Qualifier	Qualifier
1 Skull 2 Cervical Spine 3 Skull and Cervical Spine 4 Thorax 6 Pelvis 7 Spine and Pelvis 8 Upper Extremity, Right 9 Upper Extremity, Left B Upper Extremities, Bilateral C Lower Extremity, Right D Lower Extremity, Left F Lower Extremities, Bilateral G Thoracic Spine H Lumbar Spine J Thoracolumbar Spine	1 Technetium 99m (Tc-99m) Y Other Radionuclide	Z None	Z None
Y Musculoskeletal System, Other	Y Other Radionuclide	Z None	Z None

SECTION: C NUCLEAR MEDICINE
BODY SYSTEM: P MUSCULOSKELETAL SYSTEM
TYPE: 5 NONIMAGING NUCLEAR MEDICINE PROBE: Introduction of radioactive materials into the body for the study of distribution and fate of certain substances by the detection of radioactive emissions; or, alternatively, measurement of absorption of radioactive emissions from an external source

Body Part	Radionuclide	Qualifier	Qualifier
5 Spine N Upper Extremities P Lower Extremities	Z None	Z None	Z None
Y Musculoskeletal System, Other	Y Other Radionuclide	Z None	Z None

SECTION: C NUCLEAR MEDICINE
BODY SYSTEM: T URINARY SYSTEM
TYPE: 1 **PLANAR NUCLEAR MEDICINE IMAGING:** Introduction of radioactive materials into the body for single plane display of images developed from the capture of radioactive emissions

Body Part	Radionuclide	Qualifier	Qualifier
3 Kidneys, Ureters, and Bladder	1 Technetium 99m (Tc-99m) F Iodine 123 (I-123) G Iodine 131 (I-131) Y Other Radionuclide	Z None	Z None
H Bladder and Ureters	1 Technetium 99m (Tc-99m) Y Other Radionuclide	Z None	Z None
Y Urinary System	Y Other Radionuclide	Z None	Z None

SECTION: C NUCLEAR MEDICINE
BODY SYSTEM: T URINARY SYSTEM
TYPE: 2 **TOMOGRAPHIC (TOMO) NUCLEAR MEDICINE IMAGING:** Introduction of radioactive materials into the body for three-dimensional display of images developed from the capture of radioactive emissions

Body Part	Radionuclide	Qualifier	Qualifier
3 Kidneys, Ureters, and Bladder	1 Technetium 99m (Tc-99m) Y Other Radionuclide	Z None	Z None
Y Urinary System	Y Other Radionuclide	Z None	Z None

SECTION: C NUCLEAR MEDICINE
BODY SYSTEM: T URINARY SYSTEM
TYPE: 6 **NONIMAGING NUCLEAR MEDICINE ASSAY:** Introduction of radioactive materials into the body for the study of body fluids and blood elements, by the detection of radioactive emissions

Body Part	Radionuclide	Qualifier	Qualifier
3 Kidneys, Ureters, and Bladder	1 Technetium 99m (Tc-99m) F Iodine 123 (I-123) G Iodine 131 (I-131) H Iodine 125 (I-125) Y Other Radionuclide	Z None	Z None
Y Urinary System	Y Other Radionuclide	Z None	Z None

SECTION: C NUCLEAR MEDICINE
BODY SYSTEM: V MALE REPRODUCTIVE SYSTEM
TYPE: 1 PLANAR NUCLEAR MEDICINE IMAGING: Introduction of radioactive materials into the body for single plane display of images developed from the capture of radioactive emissions

Body Part	Radionuclide	Qualifier	Qualifier
9 Testicles, Bilateral ♂	1 Technetium 99m (Tc-99m) Y Other Radionuclide	Z None	Z None
Y Male Reproductive System ♂	Y Other Radionuclide	Z None	Z None

SECTION: C NUCLEAR MEDICINE
BODY SYSTEM: W ANATOMICAL REGIONS
TYPE: 1 PLANAR NUCLEAR MEDICINE IMAGING: Introduction of radioactive materials into the body for single plane display of images developed from the capture of radioactive emissions

Body Part	Radionuclide	Qualifier	Qualifier
Ø Abdomen 1 Abdomen and Pelvis 4 Chest and Abdomen 6 Chest and Neck B Head and Neck D Lower Extremity J Pelvic Region M Upper Extremity N Whole Body	1 Technetium 99m (Tc-99m) D Indium 111 (In-111) F Iodine 123 (I-123) G Iodine 131 (I-131) L Gallium 67 (Ga-67) S Thallium 2Ø1 (Tl-2Ø1) Y Other Radionuclide	Z None	Z None
3 Chest	1 Technetium 99m (Tc-99m) D Indium 111 (In-111) F Iodine 123 (I-123) G Iodine 131 (I-131) K Fluorine 18 (F-18) L Gallium 67 (Ga-67) S Thallium 2Ø1 (Tl-2Ø1) Y Other Radionuclide	Z None	Z None
Y Anatomical Regions, Multiple	Y Other Radionuclide	Z None	Z None
Z Anatomical Region, Other	Z None	Z None	Z None

SECTION: C NUCLEAR MEDICINE
BODY SYSTEM: W ANATOMICAL REGIONS
TYPE: 2 TOMOGRAPHIC (TOMO) NUCLEAR MEDICINE IMAGING: Introduction of radioactive materials into the body for three-dimensional display of images developed from the capture of radioactive emissions

Body Part	Radionuclide	Qualifier	Qualifier
Ø Abdomen 1 Abdomen and Pelvis 3 Chest 4 Chest and Abdomen 6 Chest and Neck B Head and Neck D Lower Extremity J Pelvic Region M Upper Extremity	1 Technetium 99m (Tc-99m) D Indium 111 (In-111) F Iodine 123 (I-123) G Iodine 131 (I-131) K Fluorine 18 (F-18) L Gallium 67 (Ga-67) S Thallium 2Ø1 (Tl-2Ø1) Y Other Radionuclide	Z None	Z None
Y Anatomical Regions, Multiple	Y Other Radionuclide	Z None	Z None

SECTION: C NUCLEAR MEDICINE
BODY SYSTEM: W ANATOMICAL REGIONS
TYPE: 3 **POSITRON EMISSION TOMOGRAPHIC (PET) IMAGING:** Introduction of radioactive materials into the body for three-dimensional display of images developed from the simultaneous capture, 180 degrees apart, of radioactive emissions

Body Part	Radionuclide	Qualifier	Qualifier
N Whole Body	Y Other Radionuclide	Z None	Z None

SECTION: C NUCLEAR MEDICINE
BODY SYSTEM: W ANATOMICAL REGIONS
TYPE: 5 **NONIMAGING NUCLEAR MEDICINE PROBE:** Introduction of radioactive materials into the body for the study of distribution and fate of certain substances by the detection of radioactive emissions; or, alternatively, measurement of absorption of radioactive emissions from an external source

Body Part	Radionuclide	Qualifier	Qualifier
Ø Abdomen 1 Abdomen and Pelvis 3 Chest 4 Chest and Abdomen 6 Chest and Neck B Head and Neck D Lower Extremity J Pelvic Region M Upper Extremity	1 Technetium 99m (Tc-99m) D Indium 111 (In-111) Y Other Radionuclide	Z None	Z None

SECTION: C NUCLEAR MEDICINE
BODY SYSTEM: W ANATOMICAL REGIONS
TYPE: 7 **SYSTEMIC NUCLEAR MEDICINE THERAPY:** Introduction of unsealed radioactive materials into the body for treatment

Body Part	Radionuclide	Qualifier	Qualifier
Ø Abdomen 3 Chest	N Phosphorus 32 (P-32) Y Other Radionuclide	Z None	Z None
G Thyroid	G Iodine 131 (I-131) Y Other Radionuclide	Z None	Z None
N Whole Body	8 Samarium 153 (Sm-153) G Iodine 131 (I-131) N Phosphorus 32 (P-32) P Strontium 89 (Sr-89) Y Other Radionuclide	Z None	Z None
Y Anatomical Regions, Multiple	Y Other Radionuclide	Z None	Z None

SECTION: D RADIATION THERAPY
BODY SYSTEM: Ø CENTRAL AND PERIPHERAL NERVOUS SYSTEM
MODALITY: Ø BEAM RADIATION

Treatment Site	Modality Qualifier	Isotope	Qualifier
Ø Brain 1 Brain Stem 6 Spinal Cord 7 Peripheral Nerve	Ø Photons <1 MeV 1 Photons 1 - 1Ø MeV 2 Photons >1Ø MeV 4 Heavy Particles (Protons,Ions) 5 Neutrons 6 Neutron Capture	Z None	Z None
Ø Brain 1 Brain Stem 6 Spinal Cord 7 Peripheral Nerve	3 Electrons	Z None	Ø Intraoperative Z None

SECTION: D RADIATION THERAPY
BODY SYSTEM: Ø CENTRAL AND PERIPHERAL NERVOUS SYSTEM
MODALITY: 1 BRACHYTHERAPY

Treatment Site	Modality Qualifier	Isotope	Qualifier
Ø Brain 1 Brain Stem 6 Spinal Cord 7 Peripheral Nerve	9 High Dose Rate (HDR)	7 Cesium 137 (Cs-137) 8 Iridium 192 (Ir-192) 9 Iodine 125 (I-125) B Palladium 1Ø3 (Pd-1Ø3) C Californium 252 (Cf-252) Y Other Isotope	Z None
Ø Brain 1 Brain Stem 6 Spinal Cord 7 Peripheral Nerve	B Low Dose Rate (LDR)	6 Cesium 131 (Cs-131) 7 Cesium 137 (Cs-137) 8 Iridium 192 (Ir-192) 9 Iodine 125 (I-125) C Californium 252 (Cf-252) Y Other Isotope	Z None
Ø Brain 1 Brain Stem 6 Spinal Cord 7 Peripheral Nerve	B Low Dose Rate (LDR)	B Palladium 1Ø3 (Pd-1Ø3)	1 Unidirectional Source Z None

SECTION: D RADIATION THERAPY
BODY SYSTEM: Ø CENTRAL AND PERIPHERAL NERVOUS SYSTEM
MODALITY: 2 STEREOTACTIC RADIOSURGERY

Treatment Site	Modality Qualifier	Isotope	Qualifier
Ø Brain 1 Brain Stem 6 Spinal Cord 7 Peripheral Nerve	D Stereotactic Other Photon Radiosurgery H Stereotactic Particulate Radiosurgery J Stereotactic Gamma Beam Radiosurgery	Z None	Z None

DRG Non-OR DØ2[Ø167][DJ]ZZ

SECTION: D RADIATION THERAPY
BODY SYSTEM: Ø CENTRAL AND PERIPHERAL NERVOUS SYSTEM
MODALITY: Y OTHER RADIATION

Treatment Site	Modality Qualifier	Isotope	Qualifier
Ø Brain 1 Brain Stem 6 Spinal Cord 7 Peripheral Nerve	7 Contact Radiation 8 Hyperthermia C Intraoperative Radiation Therapy (IORT) F Plaque Radiation	Z None	Z None

SECTION: D RADIATION THERAPY
BODY SYSTEM: 7 LYMPHATIC AND HEMATOLOGIC SYSTEM
MODALITY: Ø BEAM RADIATION

Treatment Site	Modality Qualifier	Isotope	Qualifier
Ø Bone Marrow 1 Thymus 2 Spleen 3 Lymphatics, Neck 4 Lymphatics, Axillary 5 Lymphatics, Thorax 6 Lymphatics, Abdomen 7 Lymphatics, Pelvis 8 Lymphatics, Inguinal	Ø Photons <1 MeV 1 Photons 1 - 1Ø MeV 2 Photons >1Ø MeV 4 Heavy Particles (Protons, Ions) 5 Neutrons 6 Neutron Capture	Z None	Z None
Ø Bone Marrow 1 Thymus 2 Spleen 3 Lymphatics, Neck 4 Lymphatics, Axillary 5 Lymphatics, Thorax 6 Lymphatics, Abdomen 7 Lymphatics, Pelvis 8 Lymphatics, Inguinal	3 Electrons	Z None	Ø Intraoperative Z None

SECTION: D RADIATION THERAPY
BODY SYSTEM: 7 LYMPHATIC AND HEMATOLOGIC SYSTEM
MODALITY: 1 BRACHYTHERAPY

Treatment Site	Modality Qualifier	Isotope	Qualifier
Ø Bone Marrow 1 Thymus 2 Spleen 3 Lymphatics, Neck 4 Lymphatics, Axillary 5 Lymphatics, Thorax 6 Lymphatics, Abdomen 7 Lymphatics, Pelvis 8 Lymphatics, Inguinal	9 High Dose Rate (HDR)	7 Cesium 137 (Cs-137) 8 Iridium 192 (Ir-192) 9 Iodine 125 (I-125) B Palladium 1Ø3 (Pd-1Ø3) C Californium 252 (Cf-252) Y Other Isotope	Z None
Ø Bone Marrow 1 Thymus 2 Spleen 3 Lymphatics, Neck 4 Lymphatics, Axillary 5 Lymphatics, Thorax 6 Lymphatics, Abdomen 7 Lymphatics, Pelvis 8 Lymphatics, Inguinal	B Low Dose Rate (LDR)	6 Cesium 131 (Cs-131) 7 Cesium 137 (Cs-137) 8 Iridium 192 (Ir-192) 9 Iodine 125 (I-125) C Californium 252 (Cf-252) Y Other Isotope	Z None
Ø Bone Marrow 1 Thymus 2 Spleen 3 Lymphatics, Neck 4 Lymphatics, Axillary 5 Lymphatics, Thorax 6 Lymphatics, Abdomen 7 Lymphatics, Pelvis 8 Lymphatics, Inguinal	B Low Dose Rate (LDR)	B Palladium 1Ø3 (Pd-1Ø3)	1 Unidirectional Source Z None

SECTION: D RADIATION THERAPY
BODY SYSTEM: 7 LYMPHATIC AND HEMATOLOGIC SYSTEM
MODALITY: 2 STEREOTACTIC RADIOSURGERY

Treatment Site	Modality Qualifier	Isotope	Qualifier
Ø Bone Marrow 1 Thymus 2 Spleen 3 Lymphatics, Neck 4 Lymphatics, Axillary 5 Lymphatics, Thorax 6 Lymphatics, Abdomen 7 Lymphatics, Pelvis 8 Lymphatics, Inguinal	D Stereotactic Other Photon Radiosurgery H Stereotactic Particulate Radiosurgery J Stereotactic Gamma Beam Radiosurgery	Z None	Z None

DRG Non-OR All Values

SECTION: D RADIATION THERAPY
BODY SYSTEM: 7 LYMPHATIC AND HEMATOLOGIC SYSTEM
MODALITY: Y OTHER RADIATION

Treatment Site	Modality Qualifier	Isotope	Qualifier
Ø Bone Marrow 1 Thymus 2 Spleen 3 Lymphatics, Neck 4 Lymphatics, Axillary 5 Lymphatics, Thorax 6 Lymphatics, Abdomen 7 Lymphatics, Pelvis 8 Lymphatics, Inguinal	8 Hyperthermia F Plaque Radiation	Z None	Z None

SECTION: D RADIATION THERAPY
BODY SYSTEM: 8 EYE
MODALITY: 0 BEAM RADIATION

Treatment Site	Modality Qualifier	Isotope	Qualifier
0 Eye	0 Photons <1 MeV 1 Photons 1 - 10 MeV 2 Photons >10 MeV 4 Heavy Particles (Protons, Ions) 5 Neutrons 6 Neutron Capture	Z None	Z None
0 Eye	3 Electrons	Z None	0 Intraoperative Z None

SECTION: D RADIATION THERAPY
BODY SYSTEM: 8 EYE
MODALITY: 1 BRACHYTHERAPY

Treatment Site	Modality Qualifier	Isotope	Qualifier
0 Eye	9 High Dose Rate (HDR)	7 Cesium 137 (Cs-137) 8 Iridium 192 (Ir-192) 9 Iodine 125 (I-125) B Palladium 103 (Pd-103) C Californium 252 (Cf-252) Y Other Isotope	Z None
0 Eye	B Low Dose Rate (LDR)	6 Cesium 131 (Cs-131) 7 Cesium 137 (Cs-137) 8 Iridium 192 (Ir-192) 9 Iodine 125 (I-125) C Californium 252 (Cf-252) Y Other Isotope	Z None
0 Eye	B Low Dose Rate (LDR)	B Palladium 103 (Pd-103)	1 Unidirectional Source Z None

SECTION: D RADIATION THERAPY
BODY SYSTEM: 8 EYE
MODALITY: 2 STEREOTACTIC RADIOSURGERY

Treatment Site	Modality Qualifier	Isotope	Qualifier
0 Eye	D Stereotactic Other Photon Radiosurgery H Stereotactic Particulate Radiosurgery J Stereotactic Gamma Beam Radiosurgery	Z None	Z None

DRG Non-OR All Values

SECTION: D RADIATION THERAPY
BODY SYSTEM: 8 EYE
MODALITY: Y OTHER RADIATION

Treatment Site	Modality Qualifier	Isotope	Qualifier
0 Eye	7 Contact Radiation 8 Hyperthermia F Plaque Radiation	Z None	Z None

SECTION: D RADIATION THERAPY
BODY SYSTEM: 9 EAR, NOSE, MOUTH, AND THROAT
MODALITY: Ø BEAM RADIATION

Treatment Site	Modality Qualifier	Isotope	Qualifier
Ø Ear 1 Nose 3 Hypopharynx 4 Mouth 5 Tongue 6 Salivary Glands 7 Sinuses 8 Hard Palate 9 Soft Palate B Larynx D Nasopharynx F Oropharynx	Ø Photons <1 MeV 1 Photons 1 - 1Ø MeV 2 Photons >1Ø MeV 4 Heavy Particles (Protons, Ions) 5 Neutrons 6 Neutron Capture	Z None	Z None
Ø Ear 1 Nose 3 Hypopharynx 4 Mouth 5 Tongue 6 Salivary Glands 7 Sinuses 8 Hard Palate 9 Soft Palate B Larynx D Nasopharynx F Oropharynx	3 Electrons	Z None	Ø Intraoperative Z None

SECTION: D RADIATION THERAPY
BODY SYSTEM: 9 EAR, NOSE, MOUTH, AND THROAT
MODALITY: 1 BRACHYTHERAPY *(on multiple pages)*

Treatment Site	Modality Qualifier	Isotope	Qualifier
Ø Ear 1 Nose 3 Hypopharynx 4 Mouth 5 Tongue 6 Salivary Glands 7 Sinuses 8 Hard Palate 9 Soft Palate B Larynx D Nasopharynx F Oropharynx	9 High Dose Rate (HDR)	7 Cesium 137 (Cs-137) 8 Iridium 192 (Ir-192) 9 Iodine 125 (I-125) B Palladium 1Ø3 (Pd-1Ø3) C Californium 252 (Cf-252) Y Other Isotope	Z None
Ø Ear 1 Nose 3 Hypopharynx 4 Mouth 5 Tongue 6 Salivary Glands 7 Sinuses 8 Hard Palate 9 Soft Palate B Larynx D Nasopharynx F Oropharynx	B Low Dose Rate (LDR)	6 Cesium 131 (Cs-131) 7 Cesium 137 (Cs-137) 8 Iridium 192 (Ir-192) 9 Iodine 125 (I-125) C Californium 252 (Cf-252) Y Other Isotope	Z None

SECTION: D RADIATION THERAPY
BODY SYSTEM: 9 EAR, NOSE, MOUTH, AND THROAT
MODALITY: 1 BRACHYTHERAPY *(continued)*

Ø Ear 1 Nose 3 Hypopharynx 4 Mouth 5 Tongue 6 Salivary Glands 7 Sinuses 8 Hard Palate 9 Soft Palate B Larynx D Nasopharynx F Oropharynx	B Low Dose Rate (LDR)	B Palladium 1Ø3 (Pd-1Ø3)	1 Unidirectional Source Z None

SECTION: D RADIATION THERAPY
BODY SYSTEM: 9 EAR, NOSE, MOUTH, AND THROAT
MODALITY: 2 STEREOTACTIC RADIOSURGERY

Treatment Site	Modality Qualifier	Isotope	Qualifier
Ø Ear 1 Nose 4 Mouth 5 Tongue 6 Salivary Glands 7 Sinuses 8 Hard Palate 9 Soft Palate B Larynx C Pharynx D Nasopharynx	D Stereotactic Other Photon Radiosurgery H Stereotactic Particulate Radiosurgery J Stereotactic Gamma Beam Radiosurgery	Z None	Z None

DRG Non-OR All Values

SECTION: D RADIATION THERAPY
BODY SYSTEM: 9 EAR, NOSE, MOUTH, AND THROAT
MODALITY: Y OTHER RADIATION

Treatment Site	Modality Qualifier	Isotope	Qualifier
Ø Ear 1 Nose 5 Tongue 6 Salivary Glands 7 Sinuses 8 Hard Palate 9 Soft Palate	7 Contact Radiation 8 Hyperthermia F Plaque Radiation	Z None	Z None
3 Hypopharynx F Oropharynx	7 Contact Radiation 8 Hyperthermia	Z None	Z None
4 Mouth B Larynx D Nasopharynx	7 Contact Radiation 8 Hyperthermia C Intraoperative Radiation Therapy (IORT) F Plaque Radiation	Z None	Z None
C Pharynx	C Intraoperative Radiation Therapy (IORT) F Plaque Radiation	Z None	Z None

SECTION: D RADIATION THERAPY
BODY SYSTEM: B RESPIRATORY SYSTEM
MODALITY: 0 BEAM RADIATION

Treatment Site	Modality Qualifier	Isotope	Qualifier
0 Trachea 1 Bronchus 2 Lung 5 Pleura 6 Mediastinum 7 Chest Wall 8 Diaphragm	0 Photons <1 MeV 1 Photons 1 - 10 MeV 2 Photons >10 MeV 4 Heavy Particles (Protons, Ions) 5 Neutrons 6 Neutron Capture	Z None	Z None
0 Trachea 1 Bronchus 2 Lung 5 Pleura 6 Mediastinum 7 Chest Wall 8 Diaphragm	3 Electrons	Z None	0 Intraoperative Z None

SECTION: D RADIATION THERAPY
BODY SYSTEM: B RESPIRATORY SYSTEM
MODALITY: 1 BRACHYTHERAPY

Treatment Site	Modality Qualifier	Isotope	Qualifier
0 Trachea 1 Bronchus 2 Lung 5 Pleura 6 Mediastinum 7 Chest Wall 8 Diaphragm	9 High Dose Rate (HDR)	7 Cesium 137 (Cs-137) 8 Iridium 192 (Ir-192) 9 Iodine 125 (I-125) B Palladium 103 (Pd-103) C Californium 252 (Cf-252) Y Other Isotope	Z None
0 Trachea 1 Bronchus 2 Lung 5 Pleura 6 Mediastinum 7 Chest Wall 8 Diaphragm	B Low Dose Rate (LDR)	6 Cesium 131 (Cs-131) 7 Cesium 137 (Cs-137) 8 Iridium 192 (Ir-192) 9 Iodine 125 (I-125) C Californium 252 (Cf-252) Y Other Isotope	Z None
0 Trachea 1 Bronchus 2 Lung 5 Pleura 6 Mediastinum 7 Chest Wall 8 Diaphragm	B Low Dose Rate (LDR)	B Palladium 103 (Pd-103)	1 Unidirectional Source Z None

SECTION: D RADIATION THERAPY
BODY SYSTEM: B RESPIRATORY SYSTEM
MODALITY: 2 STEREOTACTIC RADIOSURGERY

Treatment Site	Modality Qualifier	Isotope	Qualifier
Ø Trachea 1 Bronchus 2 Lung 5 Pleura 6 Mediastinum 7 Chest Wall 8 Diaphragm	D Stereotactic Other Photon Radiosurgery H Stereotactic Particulate Radiosurgery J Stereotactic Gamma Beam Radiosurgery	Z None	Z None

DRG Non-OR DB2[125678][DJ]ZZ

SECTION: D RADIATION THERAPY
BODY SYSTEM: B RESPIRATORY SYSTEM
MODALITY: Y OTHER RADIATION

Treatment Site	Modality Qualifier	Isotope	Qualifier
Ø Trachea 1 Bronchus 2 Lung 5 Pleura 6 Mediastinum 7 Chest Wall 8 Diaphragm	7 Contact Radiation 8 Hyperthermia F Plaque Radiation	Z None	Z None

SECTION: D RADIATION THERAPY
BODY SYSTEM: D GASTROINTESTINAL SYSTEM
MODALITY: Ø BEAM RADIATION

Treatment Site	Modality Qualifier	Isotope	Qualifier
Ø Esophagus 1 Stomach 2 Duodenum 3 Jejunum 4 Ileum 5 Colon 7 Rectum	Ø Photons <1 MeV 1 Photons 1 - 1Ø MeV 2 Photons >1Ø MeV 4 Heavy Particles (Protons, Ions) 5 Neutrons 6 Neutron Capture	Z None	Z None
Ø Esophagus 1 Stomach 2 Duodenum 3 Jejunum 4 Ileum 5 Colon 7 Rectum	3 Electrons	Z None	Ø Intraoperative Z None

SECTION: D RADIATION THERAPY
BODY SYSTEM: D GASTROINTESTINAL SYSTEM
MODALITY: 1 BRACHYTHERAPY

Treatment Site	Modality Qualifier	Isotope	Qualifier
Ø Esophagus 1 Stomach 2 Duodenum 3 Jejunum 4 Ileum 5 Colon 7 Rectum	9 High Dose Rate (HDR)	7 Cesium 137 (Cs-137) 8 Iridium 192 (Ir-192) 9 Iodine 125 (I-125) B Palladium 1Ø3 (Pd-1Ø3) C Californium 252 (Cf-252) Y Other Isotope	Z None
Ø Esophagus 1 Stomach 2 Duodenum 3 Jejunum 4 Ileum 5 Colon 7 Rectum	B Low Dose Rate (LDR)	6 Cesium 131 (Cs-131) 7 Cesium 137 (Cs-137) 8 Iridium 192 (Ir-192) 9 Iodine 125 (I-125) C Californium 252 (Cf-252) Y Other Isotope	Z None
Ø Esophagus 1 Stomach 2 Duodenum 3 Jejunum 4 Ileum 5 Colon 7 Rectum	B Low Dose Rate (LDR)	B Palladium 1Ø3 (Pd-1Ø3)	1 Unidirectional Source Z None

SECTION: D RADIATION THERAPY
BODY SYSTEM: D GASTROINTESTINAL SYSTEM
MODALITY: 2 STEREOTACTIC RADIOSURGERY

Treatment Site	Modality Qualifier	Isotope	Qualifier
Ø Esophagus 1 Stomach 2 Duodenum 3 Jejunum 4 Ileum 5 Colon 7 Rectum	D Stereotactic Other Photon Radiosurgery H Stereotactic Particulate Radiosurgery J Stereotactic Gamma Beam Radiosurgery	Z None	Z None

DRG Non-OR All Values

SECTION: D RADIATION THERAPY
BODY SYSTEM: D GASTROINTESTINAL SYSTEM
MODALITY: Y OTHER RADIATION

Treatment Site	Modality Qualifier	Isotope	Qualifier
Ø Esophagus	7 Contact Radiation 8 Hyperthermia F Plaque Radiation	Z None	Z None
1 Stomach 2 Duodenum 3 Jejunum 4 Ileum 5 Colon 7 Rectum	7 Contact Radiation 8 Hyperthermia C Intraoperative Radiation Therapy (IORT) F Plaque Radiation	Z None	Z None
8 Anus	C Intraoperative Radiation Therapy (IORT) F Plaque Radiation	Z None	Z None

SECTION: D RADIATION THERAPY
BODY SYSTEM: F HEPATOBILIARY SYSTEM AND PANCREAS
MODALITY: Ø BEAM RADIATION

Treatment Site	Modality Qualifier	Isotope	Qualifier
Ø Liver 1 Gallbladder 2 Bile Ducts 3 Pancreas	Ø Photons <1 MeV 1 Photons 1 - 1Ø MeV 2 Photons >1Ø MeV 4 Heavy Particles (Protons, Ions) 5 Neutrons 6 Neutron Capture	Z None	Z None
Ø Liver 1 Gallbladder 2 Bile Ducts 3 Pancreas	3 Electrons	Z None	Ø Intraoperative Z None

SECTION: D RADIATION THERAPY
BODY SYSTEM: F HEPATOBILIARY SYSTEM AND PANCREAS
MODALITY: 1 BRACHYTHERAPY

Treatment Site	Modality Qualifier	Isotope	Qualifier
Ø Liver 1 Gallbladder 2 Bile Ducts 3 Pancreas	9 High Dose Rate (HDR)	7 Cesium 137 (Cs-137) 8 Iridium 192 (Ir-192) 9 Iodine 125 (I-125) B Palladium 1Ø3 (Pd-1Ø3) C Californium 252 (Cf-252) Y Other Isotope	Z None
Ø Liver 1 Gallbladder 2 Bile Ducts 3 Pancreas	B Low Dose Rate (LDR)	6 Cesium 131 (Cs-131) 7 Cesium 137 (Cs-137) 8 Iridium 192 (Ir-192) 9 Iodine 125 (I-125) C Californium 252 (Cf-252) Y Other Isotope	Z None
Ø Liver 1 Gallbladder 2 Bile Ducts 3 Pancreas	B Low Dose Rate (LDR)	B Palladium 1Ø3 (Pd-1Ø3)	1 Unidirectional Source Z None

Coding Clinic: 2Ø22, Q2, P26 – DF1ØBYZ

SECTION: D RADIATION THERAPY
BODY SYSTEM: F HEPATOBILIARY SYSTEM AND PANCREAS
MODALITY: 2 STEREOTACTIC RADIOSURGERY

Treatment Site	Modality Qualifier	Isotope	Qualifier
Ø Liver 1 Gallbladder 2 Bile Ducts 3 Pancreas	D Stereotactic Other Photon Radiosurgery H Stereotactic Particulate Radiosurgery J Stereotactic Gamma Beam Radiosurgery	Z None	Z None

DRG Non-OR All Values

SECTION: D RADIATION THERAPY
BODY SYSTEM: F HEPATOBILIARY SYSTEM AND PANCREAS
MODALITY: Y OTHER RADIATION

Treatment Site	Modality Qualifier	Isotope	Qualifier
Ø Liver 1 Gallbladder 2 Bile Ducts 3 Pancreas	7 Contact Radiation 8 Hyperthermia C Intraoperative Radiation Therapy (IORT) F Plaque Radiation	Z None	Z None

SECTION: D RADIATION THERAPY
BODY SYSTEM: G ENDOCRINE SYSTEM
MODALITY: Ø BEAM RADIATION

Treatment Site	Modality Qualifier	Isotope	Qualifier
Ø Pituitary Gland 1 Pineal Body 2 Adrenal Glands 4 Parathyroid Glands 5 Thyroid	Ø Photons <1 MeV 1 Photons 1 - 1Ø MeV 2 Photons >1Ø MeV 5 Neutrons 6 Neutron Capture	Z None	Z None
Ø Pituitary Gland 1 Pineal Body 2 Adrenal Glands 4 Parathyroid Glands 5 Thyroid	3 Electrons	Z None	Ø Intraoperative Z None

SECTION: D RADIATION THERAPY
BODY SYSTEM: G ENDOCRINE SYSTEM
MODALITY: 1 BRACHYTHERAPY

Treatment Site	Modality Qualifier	Isotope	Qualifier
Ø Pituitary Gland 1 Pineal Body 2 Adrenal Glands 4 Parathyroid Glands 5 Thyroid	9 High Dose Rate (HDR)	7 Cesium 137 (Cs-137) 8 Iridium 192 (Ir-192) 9 Iodine 125 (I-125) B Palladium 1Ø3 (Pd-1Ø3) C Californium 252 (Cf-252) Y Other Isotope	Z None
Ø Pituitary Gland 1 Pineal Body 2 Adrenal Glands 4 Parathyroid Glands 5 Thyroid	B Low Dose Rate (LDR)	6 Cesium 131 (Cs-131) 7 Cesium 137 (Cs-137) 8 Iridium 192 (Ir-192) 9 Iodine 125 (I-125) C Californium 252 (Cf-252) Y Other Isotope	Z None
Ø Pituitary Gland 1 Pineal Body 2 Adrenal Glands 4 Parathyroid Glands 5 Thyroid	B Low Dose Rate (LDR)	B Palladium 1Ø3 (Pd-1Ø3)	1 Unidirectional Source Z None

SECTION: D RADIATION THERAPY
BODY SYSTEM: G ENDOCRINE SYSTEM
MODALITY: 2 STEREOTACTIC RADIOSURGERY

Treatment Site	Modality Qualifier	Isotope	Qualifier
Ø Pituitary Gland 1 Pineal Body 2 Adrenal Glands 4 Parathyroid Glands 5 Thyroid	D Stereotactic Other Photon Radiosurgery H Stereotactic Particulate Radiosurgery J Stereotactic Gamma Beam Radiosurgery	Z None	Z None

DRG Non-OR All Values

SECTION: D RADIATION THERAPY
BODY SYSTEM: G ENDOCRINE SYSTEM
MODALITY: Y OTHER RADIATION

Treatment Site	Modality Qualifier	Isotope	Qualifier
Ø Pituitary Gland 1 Pineal Body 2 Adrenal Glands 4 Parathyroid Glands 5 Thyroid	7 Contact Radiation 8 Hyperthermia F Plaque Radiation	Z None	Z None

SECTION: D RADIATION THERAPY
BODY SYSTEM: H SKIN
MODALITY: Ø BEAM RADIATION

Treatment Site	Modality Qualifier	Isotope	Qualifier
2 Skin, Face 3 Skin, Neck 4 Skin, Arm 6 Skin, Chest 7 Skin, Back 8 Skin, Abdomen 9 Skin, Buttock B Skin, Leg	Ø Photons <1 MeV 1 Photons 1 - 1Ø MeV 2 Photons >1Ø MeV 4 Heavy Particles (Protons, Ions) 5 Neutrons 6 Neutron Capture	Z None	Z None
2 Skin, Face 3 Skin, Neck 4 Skin, Arm 6 Skin, Chest 7 Skin, Back 8 Skin, Abdomen 9 Skin, Buttock B Skin, Leg	3 Electrons	Z None	Ø Intraoperative Z None

SECTION: D RADIATION THERAPY
BODY SYSTEM: H SKIN
MODALITY: Y OTHER RADIATION

Treatment Site	Modality Qualifier	Isotope	Qualifier
2 Skin, Face 3 Skin, Neck 4 Skin, Arm 6 Skin, Chest 7 Skin, Back 8 Skin, Abdomen 9 Skin, Buttock B Skin, Leg	7 Contact Radiation 8 Hyperthermia F Plaque Radiation	Z None	Z None
5 Skin, Hand C Skin, Foot	F Plaque Radiation	Z None	Z None

SECTION: D RADIATION THERAPY
BODY SYSTEM: M BREAST
MODALITY: Ø BEAM RADIATION

Treatment Site	Modality Qualifier	Isotope	Qualifier
Ø Breast, Left 1 Breast, Right	Ø Photons <1 MeV 1 Photons 1 - 1Ø MeV 2 Photons >1Ø MeV 4 Heavy Particles (Protons, Ions) 5 Neutrons 6 Neutron Capture	Z None	Z None
Ø Breast, Left 1 Breast, Right	3 Electrons	Z None	Ø Intraoperative Z None

SECTION: D RADIATION THERAPY
BODY SYSTEM: M BREAST
MODALITY: 1 BRACHYTHERAPY

Treatment Site	Modality Qualifier	Isotope	Qualifier
Ø Breast, Left 1 Breast, Right	9 High Dose Rate (HDR)	7 Cesium 137 (Cs-137) 8 Iridium 192 (Ir-192) 9 Iodine 125 (I-125) B Palladium 1Ø3 (Pd-1Ø3) C Californium 252 (Cf-252) Y Other Isotope	Z None
Ø Breast, Left 1 Breast, Right	B Low Dose Rate (LDR)	6 Cesium 131 (Cs-131) 7 Cesium 137 (Cs-137) 8 Iridium 192 (Ir-192) 9 Iodine 125 (I-125) C Californium 252 (Cf-252) Y Other Isotope	Z None
Ø Breast, Left 1 Breast, Right	B Low Dose Rate (LDR)	B Palladium 1Ø3 (Pd-1Ø3)	1 Unidirectional Source Z None

SECTION: D RADIATION THERAPY
BODY SYSTEM: M BREAST
MODALITY: 2 STEREOTACTIC RADIOSURGERY

Treatment Site	Modality Qualifier	Isotope	Qualifier
Ø Breast, Left 1 Breast, Right	D Stereotactic Other Photon Radiosurgery H Stereotactic Particulate Radiosurgery J Stereotactic Gamma Beam Radiosurgery	Z None	Z None

DRG Non-OR All Values

SECTION: D RADIATION THERAPY
BODY SYSTEM: M BREAST
MODALITY: Y OTHER RADIATION

Treatment Site	Modality Qualifier	Isotope	Qualifier
Ø Breast, Left 1 Breast, Right	7 Contact Radiation 8 Hyperthermia F Plaque Radiation	Z None	Z None

SECTION: D RADIATION THERAPY
BODY SYSTEM: P MUSCULOSKELETAL SYSTEM
MODALITY: Ø BEAM RADIATION

Treatment Site	Modality Qualifier	Isotope	Qualifier
Ø Skull 2 Maxilla 3 Mandible 4 Sternum 5 Rib(s) 6 Humerus 7 Radius/Ulna 8 Pelvic Bones 9 Femur B Tibia/Fibula C Other Bone	Ø Photons <1 MeV 1 Photons 1 - 1Ø MeV 2 Photons >1Ø MeV 4 Heavy Particles (Protons, Ions) 5 Neutrons 6 Neutron Capture	Z None	Z None
Ø Skull 2 Maxilla 3 Mandible 4 Sternum 5 Rib(s) 6 Humerus 7 Radius/Ulna 8 Pelvic Bones 9 Femur B Tibia/Fibula C Other Bone	3 Electrons	Z None	Ø Intraoperative Z None

SECTION: D RADIATION THERAPY
BODY SYSTEM: P MUSCULOSKELETAL SYSTEM
MODALITY: Y OTHER RADIATION

Treatment Site	Modality Qualifier	Isotope	Qualifier
Ø Skull 2 Maxilla 3 Mandible 4 Sternum 5 Rib(s) 6 Humerus 7 Radius/Ulna 8 Pelvic Bones 9 Femur B Tibia/Fibula C Other Bone	7 Contact Radiation 8 Hyperthermia F Plaque Radiation	Z None	Z None

SECTION: D RADIATION THERAPY
BODY SYSTEM: T URINARY SYSTEM
MODALITY: Ø BEAM RADIATION

Treatment Site	Modality Qualifier	Isotope	Qualifier
Ø Kidney 1 Ureter 2 Bladder 3 Urethra	Ø Photons <1 MeV 1 Photons 1 - 1Ø MeV 2 Photons >1Ø MeV 4 Heavy Particles (Protons, Ions) 5 Neutrons 6 Neutron Capture	Z None	Z None
Ø Kidney 1 Ureter 2 Bladder 3 Urethra	3 Electrons	Z None	Ø Intraoperative Z None

SECTION: D RADIATION THERAPY
BODY SYSTEM: T URINARY SYSTEM
MODALITY: 1 BRACHYTHERAPY

Treatment Site	Modality Qualifier	Isotope	Qualifier
Ø Kidney 1 Ureter 2 Bladder 3 Urethra	9 High Dose Rate (HDR)	7 Cesium 137 (Cs-137) 8 Iridium 192 (Ir-192) 9 Iodine 125 (I-125) B Palladium 1Ø3 (Pd-1Ø3) C Californium 252 (Cf-252) Y Other Isotope	Z None
Ø Kidney 1 Ureter 2 Bladder 3 Urethra	B Low Dose Rate (LDR)	6 Cesium 131 (Cs-131) 7 Cesium 137 (Cs-137) 8 Iridium 192 (Ir-192) 9 Iodine 125 (I-125) C Californium 252 (Cf-252) Y Other Isotope	Z None
Ø Kidney 1 Ureter 2 Bladder 3 Urethra	B Low Dose Rate (LDR)	B Palladium 1Ø3 (Pd-1Ø3)	1 Unidirectional Source Z None

SECTION: D RADIATION THERAPY
BODY SYSTEM: T URINARY SYSTEM
MODALITY: 2 STEREOTACTIC RADIOSURGERY

Treatment Site	Modality Qualifier	Isotope	Qualifier
Ø Kidney 1 Ureter 2 Bladder 3 Urethra	D Stereotactic Other Photon Radiosurgery H Stereotactic Particulate Radiosurgery J Stereotactic Gamma Beam Radiosurgery	Z None	Z None

DRG Non-OR All Values

SECTION: D RADIATION THERAPY
BODY SYSTEM: T URINARY SYSTEM
MODALITY: Y OTHER RADIATION

Treatment Site	Modality Qualifier	Isotope	Qualifier
Ø Kidney 1 Ureter 2 Bladder 3 Urethra	7 Contact Radiation 8 Hyperthermia C Intraoperative Radiation Therapy (IORT) F Plaque Radiation	Z None	Z None

SECTION: D RADIATION THERAPY
BODY SYSTEM: U FEMALE REPRODUCTIVE SYSTEM
MODALITY: Ø BEAM RADIATION

Treatment Site	Modality Qualifier	Isotope	Qualifier
Ø Ovary♀ 1 Cervix♀ 2 Uterus♀	Ø Photons <1 MeV 1 Photons 1 - 1Ø MeV 2 Photons >1Ø MeV 4 Heavy Particles (Protons, Ions) 5 Neutrons 6 Neutron Capture	Z None	Z None
Ø Ovary♀ 1 Cervix♀ 2 Uterus♀	3 Electrons	Z None	Ø Intraoperative Z None

SECTION: D RADIATION THERAPY
BODY SYSTEM: U FEMALE REPRODUCTIVE SYSTEM
MODALITY: 1 BRACHYTHERAPY

Treatment Site	Modality Qualifier	Isotope	Qualifier
Ø Ovary♀ 1 Cervix♀ 2 Uterus♀	9 High Dose Rate (HDR)	7 Cesium 137 (Cs-137) 8 Iridium 192 (Ir-192) 9 Iodine 125 (I-125) B Palladium 1Ø3 (Pd-1Ø3) C Californium 252 (Cf-252) Y Other Isotope	Z None
Ø Ovary ♀ 1 Cervix♀ 2 Uterus♀	B Low Dose Rate (LDR)	6 Cesium 131 (Cs-131) 7 Cesium 137 (Cs-137) 8 Iridium 192 (Ir-192) 9 Iodine 125 (I-125) C Californium 252 (Cf-252) Y Other Isotope	Z None
Ø Ovary ♀ 1 Cervix♀ 2 Uterus♀	B Low Dose Rate (LDR)	B Palladium 1Ø3 (Pd-1Ø3)	1 Unidirectional Source Z None

Coding Clinic: 2Ø17, Q4, P1Ø4 – DU11B7Z

SECTION: D RADIATION THERAPY
BODY SYSTEM: U FEMALE REPRODUCTIVE SYSTEM
MODALITY: 2 STEREOTACTIC RADIOSURGERY

Treatment Site	Modality Qualifier	Isotope	Qualifier
Ø Ovary ♀ 1 Cervix ♀ 2 Uterus ♀	D Stereotactic Other Photon Radiosurgery H Stereotactic Particulate Radiosurgery J Stereotactic Gamma Beam Radiosurgery	Z None	Z None

DRG Non-OR All Values

SECTION: D RADIATION THERAPY
BODY SYSTEM: U FEMALE REPRODUCTIVE SYSTEM
MODALITY: Y OTHER RADIATION

Treatment Site	Modality Qualifier	Isotope	Qualifier
Ø Ovary ♀ 1 Cervix ♀ 2 Uterus ♀	7 Contact Radiation 8 Hyperthermia C Intraoperative Radiation Therapy (IORT) F Plaque Radiation	Z None	Z None

SECTION: D RADIATION THERAPY
BODY SYSTEM: V MALE REPRODUCTIVE SYSTEM
MODALITY: Ø BEAM RADIATION

Treatment Site	Modality Qualifier	Isotope	Qualifier
Ø Prostate ♂ 1 Testis ♂	Ø Photons <1 MeV 1 Photons 1 - 1Ø MeV 2 Photons >1Ø MeV 4 Heavy Particles (Protons, Ions) 5 Neutrons 6 Neutron Capture	Z None	Z None
Ø Prostate ♂ 1 Testis ♂	3 Electrons	Z None	Ø Intraoperative Z None

SECTION: D RADIATION THERAPY
BODY SYSTEM: V MALE REPRODUCTIVE SYSTEM
MODALITY: 1 BRACHYTHERAPY

Treatment Site	Modality Qualifier	Isotope	Qualifier
Ø Prostate ♂ 1 Testis ♂	9 High Dose Rate (HDR)	7 Cesium 137 (Cs-137) 8 Iridium 192 (Ir-192) 9 Iodine 125 (I-125) B Palladium 1Ø3 (Pd-1Ø3) C Californium 252 (Cf-252) Y Other Isotope	Z None
Ø Prostate ♂ 1 Testis ♂	B Low Dose Rate (LDR)	6 Cesium 131 (Cs-131) 7 Cesium 137 (Cs-137) 8 Iridium 192 (Ir-192) 9 Iodine 125 (I-125) C Californium 252 (Cf-252) Y Other Isotope	Z None
Ø Prostate ♂ 1 Testis ♂	B Low Dose Rate (LDR)	B Palladium 1Ø3 (Pd-1Ø3)	1 Unidirectional Source Z None

SECTION: D RADIATION THERAPY
BODY SYSTEM: V MALE REPRODUCTIVE SYSTEM
MODALITY: 2 STEREOTACTIC RADIOSURGERY

Treatment Site	Modality Qualifier	Isotope	Qualifier
Ø Prostate ♂ 1 Testis ♂	D Stereotactic Other Photon Radiosurgery H Stereotactic Particulate Radiosurgery J Stereotactic Gamma Beam Radiosurgery	Z None	Z None

DRG Non-OR All Values

SECTION: D RADIATION THERAPY
BODY SYSTEM: V MALE REPRODUCTIVE SYSTEM
MODALITY: Y OTHER RADIATION

Treatment Site	Modality Qualifier	Isotope	Qualifier
Ø Prostate ♂	7 Contact Radiation 8 Hyperthermia C Intraoperative Radiation Therapy (IORT) F Plaque Radiation	Z None	Z None
1 Testis ♂	7 Contact Radiation 8 Hyperthermia F Plaque Radiation	Z None	Z None

SECTION: D RADIATION THERAPY
BODY SYSTEM: W ANATOMICAL REGIONS
MODALITY: Ø BEAM RADIATION

Treatment Site	Modality Qualifier	Isotope	Qualifier
1 Head and Neck 2 Chest 3 Abdomen 4 Hemibody 5 Whole Body 6 Pelvic Region	Ø Photons <1 MeV 1 Photons 1 - 1Ø MeV 2 Photons >1Ø MeV 4 Heavy Particles (Protons, Ions) 5 Neutrons 6 Neutron Capture	Z None	Z None
1 Head and Neck 2 Chest 3 Abdomen 4 Hemibody 5 Whole Body 6 Pelvic Region	3 Electrons	Z None	Ø Intraoperative Z None

SECTION: D RADIATION THERAPY
BODY SYSTEM: W ANATOMICAL REGIONS
MODALITY: 1 BRACHYTHERAPY

Treatment Site	Modality Qualifier	Isotope	Qualifier
Ø Cranial Cavity K Upper Back L Lower Back P Gastrointestinal Tract Q Respiratory Tract R Genitourinary Tract X Upper Extremity Y Lower Extremity	B Low Dose Rate (LDR)	B Palladium 1Ø3 (Pd-1Ø3)	1 Unidirectional Source Z None
1 Head and Neck 2 Chest 3 Abdomen 6 Pelvic Region	9 High Dose Rate (HDR)	7 Cesium 137 (Cs-137) 8 Iridium 192 (Ir-192) 9 Iodine 125 (I-125) B Palladium 1Ø3 (Pd-1Ø3) C Californium 252 (Cf-252) Y Other Isotope	Z None
1 Head and Neck 2 Chest 3 Abdomen 6 Pelvic Region	B Low Dose Rate (LDR)	6 Cesium 131 (Cs-131) 7 Cesium 137 (Cs-137) 8 Iridium 192 (Ir-192) 9 Iodine 125 (I-125) C Californium 252 (Cf-252) Y Other Isotope	Z None
1 Head and Neck 2 Chest 3 Abdomen 6 Pelvic Region	B Low Dose Rate (LDR)	B Palladium 1Ø3 (Pd-1Ø3)	1 Unidirectional Source Z None

Coding Clinic: 2Ø19, Q4, P44 – DW16BB1

SECTION: D RADIATION THERAPY
BODY SYSTEM: W ANATOMICAL REGIONS
MODALITY: 2 STEREOTACTIC RADIOSURGERY

Treatment Site	Modality Qualifier	Isotope	Qualifier
1 Head and Neck 2 Chest 3 Abdomen 6 Pelvic Region	D Stereotactic Other Photon Radiosurgery H Stereotactic Particulate Radiosurgery J Stereotactic Gamma Beam Radiosurgery	Z None	Z None

DRG Non-OR All Values

SECTION: D RADIATION THERAPY
BODY SYSTEM: W ANATOMICAL REGIONS
MODALITY: Y OTHER RADIATION

Treatment Site	Modality Qualifier	Isotope	Qualifier
1 Head and Neck 2 Chest 3 Abdomen 4 Hemibody 6 Pelvic Region	7 Contact Radiation 8 Hyperthermia F Plaque Radiation	Z None	Z None
5 Whole Body	7 Contact Radiation 8 Hyperthermia F Plaque Radiation	Z None	Z None
5 Whole Body	G Isotope Administration	D Iodine 131 (I-131) F Phosphorus 32 (P-32) G Strontium 89 (Sr-89) H Strontium 90 (Sr-90) Y Other Isotope	Z None

SECTION: F PHYSICAL REHABILITATION AND DIAGNOSTIC AUDIOLOGY
SECTION QUALIFIER: Ø REHABILITATION
TYPE: Ø SPEECH ASSESSMENT: *(on multiple pages)*
Measurement of speech and related functions

Body System – Body Region	Type Qualifier	Equipment	Qualifier
3 Neurological System - Whole Body	G Communicative/Cognitive Integration Skills	K Audiovisual M Augmentative/Alternative Communication P Computer Y Other Equipment Z None	Z None
Z None	Ø Filtered Speech 3 Staggered Spondaic Word Q Performance Intensity Phonetically Balanced Speech Discrimination R Brief Tone Stimuli S Distorted Speech T Dichotic Stimuli V Temporal Ordering of Stimuli W Masking Patterns	1 Audiometer 2 Sound Field/Booth K Audiovisual Z None	Z None
Z None	1 Speech Threshold 2 Speech/Word Recognition	1 Audiometer 2 Sound Field/Booth 9 Cochlear Implant K Audiovisual Z None	Z None
Z None	4 Sensorineural Acuity Level	1 Audiometer 2 Sound Field/Booth Z None	Z None
Z None	5 Synthetic Sentence Identification	1 Audiometer 2 Sound Field/Booth 9 Cochlear Implant K Audiovisual	Z None
Z None	6 Speech and/or Language Screening 7 Nonspoken Language 8 Receptive/Expressive Language C Aphasia G Communicative/Cognitive Integration Skills L Augmentative/Alternative Communication System	K Audiovisual M Augmentative/Alternative Communication P Computer Y Other Equipment Z None	Z None
Z None	9 Articulation/Phonology	K Audiovisual P Computer Q Speech Analysis Y Other Equipment Z None	Z None
Z None	B Motor Speech	K Audiovisual N Biosensory Feedback P Computer Q Speech Analysis T Aerodynamic Function Y Other Equipment Z None	Z None

DRG Non-OR All Values

SECTION: F PHYSICAL REHABILITATION AND DIAGNOSTIC AUDIOLOGY
SECTION QUALIFIER: Ø REHABILITATION
TYPE: Ø SPEECH ASSESSMENT: *(continued)*
Measurement of speech and related functions

Body System – Body Region	Type Qualifier	Equipment	Qualifier
Z None	D Fluency	K Audiovisual N Biosensory Feedback P Computer Q Speech Analysis S Voice Analysis T Aerodynamic Function Y Other Equipment Z None	Z None
Z None	F Voice	K Audiovisual N Biosensory Feedback P Computer S Voice Analysis T Aerodynamic Function Y Other Equipment Z None	Z None
Z None	H Bedside Swallowing and Oral Function P Oral Peripheral Mechanism	Y Other Equipment Z None	Z None
Z None	J Instrumental Swallowing and Oral Function	T Aerodynamic Function W Swallowing Y Other Equipment	Z None
Z None	K Orofacial Myofunctional	K Audiovisual P Computer Y Other Equipment Z None	Z None
Z None	M Voice Prosthetic	K Audiovisual P Computer S Voice Analysis V Speech Prosthesis Y Other Equipment Z None	Z None
Z None	N Non-invasive Instrumental Status	N Biosensory Feedback P Computer Q Speech Analysis S Voice Analysis T Aerodynamic Function Y Other Equipment	Z None
Z None	X Other Specified Central Auditory Processing	Z None	Z None

DRG Non-OR All Values

SECTION: F PHYSICAL REHABILITATION AND DIAGNOSTIC AUDIOLOGY
SECTION QUALIFIER: Ø REHABILITATION
TYPE: 1 MOTOR AND/OR NERVE FUNCTION ASSESSMENT: *(on multiple pages)*

Measurement of motor, nerve, and related functions

Body System – Body Region	Type Qualifier	Equipment	Qualifier
Ø Neurological System - Head and Neck 1 Neurological System - Upper Back/Upper Extremity 2 Neurological System - Lower Back/Lower Extremity 3 Neurological System - Whole Body	Ø Muscle Performance	E Orthosis F Assistive, Adaptive, Supportive or Protective U Prosthesis Y Other Equipment Z None	Z None
Ø Neurological System - Head and Neck 1 Neurological System - Upper Back/Upper Extremity 2 Neurological System - Lower Back/Lower Extremity 3 Neurological System - Whole Body	1 Integumentary Integrity 3 Coordination/Dexterity 4 Motor Function G Reflex Integrity	Z None	Z None
Ø Neurological System - Head and Neck 1 Neurological System - Upper Back/Upper Extremity 2 Neurological System - Lower Back/Lower Extremity 3 Neurological System - Whole Body	5 Range of Motion and Joint Integrity 6 Sensory Awareness/ Processing/Integrity	Y Other Equipment Z None	Z None
D Integumentary System - Head and Neck F Integumentary System - Upper Back/Upper Extremity G Integumentary System - Lower Back/Lower Extremity H Integumentary System - Whole Body J Musculoskeletal System - Head and Neck K Musculoskeletal System - Upper Back/Upper Extremity L Musculoskeletal System - Lower Back/Lower Extremity M Musculoskeletal System - Whole Body	Ø Muscle Performance	E Orthosis F Assistive, Adaptive, Supportive or Protective U Prosthesis Y Other Equipment Z None	Z None
D Integumentary System - Head and Neck F Integumentary System - Upper Back/Upper Extremity G Integumentary System - Lower Back/Lower Extremity H Integumentary System - Whole Body J Musculoskeletal System - Head and Neck K Musculoskeletal System - Upper Back/Upper Extremity L Musculoskeletal System - Lower Back/Lower Extremity M Musculoskeletal System - Whole Body	1 Integumentary Integrity	Z None	Z None
D Integumentary System - Head and Neck F Integumentary System - Upper Back/Upper Extremity G Integumentary System - Lower Back/Lower Extremity H Integumentary System - Whole Body J Musculoskeletal System - Head and Neck K Musculoskeletal System - Upper Back/Upper Extremity L Musculoskeletal System - Lower Back/Lower Extremity M Musculoskeletal System - Whole Body	5 Range of Motion and Joint Integrity 6 Sensory Awareness/ Processing/Integrity	Y Other Equipment Z None	Z None

DRG Non-OR All Values

SECTION: F PHYSICAL REHABILITATION AND DIAGNOSTIC AUDIOLOGY

SECTION QUALIFIER: Ø REHABILITATION

TYPE: 1 MOTOR AND/OR NERVE FUNCTION ASSESSMENT: *(continued)*

Measurement of motor, nerve, and related functions

Body System – Body Region	Type Qualifier	Equipment	Qualifier
N Genitourinary System	Ø Muscle Performance	E Orthosis F Assistive, Adaptive, Supportive or Protective U Prosthesis Y Other Equipment Z None	Z None
Z None	2 Visual Motor Integration	K Audiovisual M Augmentative/Alternative Communication N Biosensory Feedback P Computer Q Speech Analysis S Voice Analysis Y Other Equipment Z None	Z None
Z None	7 Facial Nerve Function	7 Electrophysiologic	Z None
Z None	9 Somatosensory Evoked Potentials	J Somatosensory	Z None
Z None	B Bed Mobility C Transfer F Wheelchair Mobility	E Orthosis F Assistive, Adaptive, Supportive or Protective U Prosthesis Z None	Z None
Z None	D Gait and/or Balance	E Orthosis F Assistive, Adaptive, Supportive or Protective U Prosthesis Y Other Equipment Z None	Z None

DRG Non-OR All Values

SECTION: F PHYSICAL REHABILITATION AND DIAGNOSTIC AUDIOLOGY

SECTION QUALIFIER: Ø REHABILITATION

TYPE: 2 ACTIVITIES OF DAILY LIVING ASSESSMENT: *(on multiple pages)*

Measurement of functional level for activities of daily living

Body System – Body Region	Type Qualifier	Equipment	Qualifier
Ø Neurological System - Head and Neck	9 Cranial Nerve Integrity D Neuromotor Development	Y Other Equipment Z None	Z None
1 Neurological System - Upper Back/Upper Extremity 2 Neurological System - Lower Back/Lower Extremity 3 Neurological System - Whole Body	D Neuromotor Development	Y Other Equipment Z None	Z None
4 Circulatory System - Head and Neck 5 Circulatory System - Upper Back/Upper Extremity 6 Circulatory System - Lower Back/Lower Extremity 8 Respiratory System - Head and Neck 9 Respiratory System - Upper Back/Upper Extremity B Respiratory System - Lower Back/Lower Extremity	G Ventilation, Respiration and Circulation	C Mechanical G Aerobic Endurance and Conditioning Y Other Equipment Z None	Z None
7 Circulatory System - Whole Body C Respiratory System - Whole Body	7 Aerobic Capacity and Endurance	E Orthosis G Aerobic Endurance and Conditioning U Prosthesis Y Other Equipment Z None	Z None
7 Circulatory System - Whole Body C Respiratory System - Whole Body	G Ventilation, Respiration and Circulation	C Mechanical G Aerobic Endurance and Conditioning Y Other Equipment Z None	Z None

DRG Non-OR All Values

SECTION: F PHYSICAL REHABILITATION AND DIAGNOSTIC AUDIOLOGY

SECTION QUALIFIER: Ø REHABILITATION

TYPE: 2 ACTIVITIES OF DAILY LIVING ASSESSMENT: *(continued)*

Measurement of functional level for activities of daily living

Body System – Body Region	Type Qualifier	Equipment	Qualifier
Z None	Ø Bathing/Showering 1 Dressing 3 Grooming/Personal Hygiene 4 Home Management	E Orthosis F Assistive, Adaptive, Supportive or Protective U Prosthesis Z None	Z None
Z None	2 Feeding/Eating 8 Anthropometric Characteristics F Pain	Y Other Equipment Z None	Z None
Z None	5 Perceptual Processing	K Audiovisual M Augmentative/Alternative Communication N Biosensory Feedback P Computer Q Speech Analysis S Voice Analysis Y Other Equipment Z None	Z None
Z None	6 Psychosocial Skills	Z None	Z None
Z None	B Environmental, Home and Work Barriers C Ergonomics and Body Mechanics	E Orthosis F Assistive, Adaptive, Supportive or Protective U Prosthesis Y Other Equipment Z None	Z None
Z None	H Vocational Activities and Functional Community or Work Reintegration Skills	E Orthosis F Assistive, Adaptive, Supportive or Protective G Aerobic Endurance and Conditioning U Prosthesis Y Other Equipment Z None	Z None

DRG Non-OR All Values

SECTION: F PHYSICAL REHABILITATION AND DIAGNOSTIC AUDIOLOGY

SECTION QUALIFIER: 0 REHABILITATION

TYPE: 6 SPEECH TREATMENT: *(on multiple pages)*

Application of techniques to improve, augment, or compensate for speech and related functional impairment

Body System – Body Region	Type Qualifier	Equipment	Qualifier
3 Neurological System - Whole Body	6 Communicative/Cognitive Integration Skills	K Audiovisual M Augmentative/Alternative Communication P Computer Y Other Equipment Z None	Z None
Z None	0 Nonspoken Language 3 Aphasia 6 Communicative/Cognitive Integration Skills	K Audiovisual M Augmentative/Alternative Communication P Computer Y Other Equipment Z None	Z None
Z None	1 Speech-Language Pathology and Related Disorders Counseling 2 Speech-Language Pathology and Related Disorders Prevention	K Audiovisual Z None	Z None
Z None	4 Articulation/Phonology	K Audiovisual P Computer Q Speech Analysis T Aerodynamic Function Y Other Equipment Z None	Z None
Z None	5 Aural Rehabilitation	K Audiovisual L Assistive Listening M Augmentative/Alternative Communication N Biosensory Feedback P Computer Q Speech Analysis S Voice Analysis Y Other Equipment Z None	Z None
Z None	7 Fluency	4 Electroacoustic Immitance/ Acoustic Reflex K Audiovisual N Biosensory Feedback Q Speech Analysis S Voice Analysis T Aerodynamic Function Y Other Equipment Z None	Z None

DRG Non-OR All Values

SECTION: F PHYSICAL REHABILITATION AND DIAGNOSTIC AUDIOLOGY

SECTION QUALIFIER: Ø REHABILITATION

TYPE: 6 SPEECH TREATMENT: *(continued)*

Application of techniques to improve, augment, or compensate for speech and related functional impairment

Body System – Body Region	Type Qualifier	Equipment	Qualifier
Z None	8 Motor Speech	K Audiovisual N Biosensory Feedback P Computer Q Speech Analysis S Voice Analysis T Aerodynamic Function Y Other Equipment Z None	Z None
Z None	9 Orofacial Myofunctional	K Audiovisual P Computer Y Other Equipment Z None	Z None
Z None	B Receptive/Expressive Language	K Audiovisual L Assistive Listening M Augmentative/Alternative Communication P Computer Y Other Equipment Z None	Z None
Z None	C Voice	K Audiovisual N Biosensory Feedback P Computer S Voice Analysis T Aerodynamic Function V Speech Prosthesis Y Other Equipment Z None	Z None
Z None	D Swallowing Dysfunction	M Augmentative/Alternative Communication T Aerodynamic Function V Speech Prosthesis Y Other Equipment Z None	Z None

DRG Non-OR All Values

SECTION: F PHYSICAL REHABILITATION AND DIAGNOSTIC AUDIOLOGY

SECTION QUALIFIER: Ø REHABILITATION

TYPE: 7 MOTOR TREATMENT: *(on multiple pages)*

Exercise or activities to increase or facilitate motor function

Body System – Body Region	Type Qualifier	Equipment	Qualifier
Ø Neurological System - Head and Neck 1 Neurological System - Upper Back/Upper Extremity 2 Neurological System - Lower Back/Lower Extremity 3 Neurological System - Whole Body D Integumentary System - Head and Neck F Integumentary System - Upper Back/Upper Extremity G Integumentary System - Lower Back/Lower Extremity H Integumentary System - Whole Body J Musculoskeletal System - Head and Neck K Musculoskeletal System - Upper Back/Upper Extremity L Musculoskeletal System - Lower Back/Lower Extremity M Musculoskeletal System - Whole Body	Ø Range of Motion and Joint Mobility 1 Muscle Performance 2 Coordination/Dexterity 3 Motor Function	E Orthosis F Assistive, Adaptive, Supportive or Protective U Prosthesis Y Other Equipment Z None	Z None
Ø Neurological System - Head and Neck 1 Neurological System - Upper Back/Upper Extremity 2 Neurological System - Lower Back/Lower Extremity 3 Neurological System - Whole Body D Integumentary System - Head and Neck F Integumentary System - Upper Back/Upper Extremity G Integumentary System - Lower Back/Lower Extremity H Integumentary System - Whole Body J Musculoskeletal System - Head and Neck K Musculoskeletal System - Upper Back/Upper Extremity L Musculoskeletal System - Lower Back/Lower Extremity M Musculoskeletal System - Whole Body	6 Therapeutic Exercise	B Physical Agents C Mechanical D Electrotherapeutic E Orthosis F Assistive, Adaptive, Supportive or Protective G Aerobic Endurance and Conditioning H Mechanical or Electromechanical U Prosthesis Y Other Equipment Z None	Z None
Ø Neurological System - Head and Neck 1 Neurological System - Upper Back/Upper Extremity 2 Neurological System - Lower Back/Lower Extremity 3 Neurological System - Whole Body D Integumentary System - Head and Neck F Integumentary System - Upper Back/Upper Extremity G Integumentary System - Lower Back/Lower Extremity H Integumentary System - Whole Body J Musculoskeletal System - Head and Neck K Musculoskeletal System - Upper Back/Upper Extremity L Musculoskeletal System - Lower Back/Lower Extremity M Musculoskeletal System - Whole Body	7 Manual Therapy Techniques	Z None	Z None

DRG Non-OR All Values

SECTION: F PHYSICAL REHABILITATION AND DIAGNOSTIC AUDIOLOGY

SECTION QUALIFIER: Ø REHABILITATION

TYPE: 7 MOTOR TREATMENT: *(continued)*

Exercise or activities to increase or facilitate motor function

Body System – Body Region	Type Qualifier	Equipment	Qualifier
4 Circulatory System - Head and Neck 5 Circulatory System - Upper Back/Upper Extremity 6 Circulatory System - Lower Back/Lower Extremity 7 Circulatory System - Whole Body 8 Respiratory System - Head and Neck 9 Respiratory System - Upper Back/Upper Extremity B Respiratory System - Lower Back/Lower Extremity C Respiratory System - Whole Body	6 Therapeutic Exercise	B Physical Agents C Mechanical D Electrotherapeutic E Orthosis F Assistive, Adaptive, Supportive or Protective G Aerobic Endurance and Conditioning H Mechanical or Electromechanical U Prosthesis Y Other Equipment Z None	Z None
N Genitourinary System	1 Muscle Performance	E Orthosis F Assistive, Adaptive, Supportive or Protective U Prosthesis Y Other Equipment Z None	Z None
N Genitourinary System	6 Therapeutic Exercise	B Physical Agents C Mechanical D Electrotherapeutic E Orthosis F Assistive, Adaptive, Supportive or Protective G Aerobic Endurance and Conditioning H Mechanical or Electromechanical U Prosthesis Y Other Equipment Z None	Z None
Z None	4 Wheelchair Mobility	D Electrotherapeutic E Orthosis F Assistive, Adaptive, Supportive or Protective U Prosthesis Y Other Equipment Z None	Z None
Z None	5 Bed Mobility	C Mechanical E Orthosis F Assistive, Adaptive, Supportive or Protective U Prosthesis Y Other Equipment Z None	Z None
Z None	8 Transfer Training	C Mechanical D Electrotherapeutic E Orthosis F Assistive, Adaptive, Supportive or Protective U Prosthesis Y Other Equipment Z None	Z None
Z None	9 Gait Training/Functional Ambulation	C Mechanical D Electrotherapeutic E Orthosis F Assistive, Adaptive, Supportive or Protective G Aerobic Endurance and Conditioning U Prosthesis Y Other Equipment Z None	Z None

DRG Non-OR All Values

SECTION: F PHYSICAL REHABILITATION AND DIAGNOSTIC AUDIOLOGY

SECTION QUALIFIER: Ø REHABILITATION

TYPE: 8 ACTIVITIES OF DAILY LIVING TREATMENT: Exercise or activities to facilitate functional competence for activities of daily living

Body System – Body Region	Type Qualifier	Equipment	Qualifier
D Integumentary System - Head and Neck F Integumentary System - Upper Back/Upper Extremity G Integumentary System - Lower Back/Lower Extremity H Integumentary System - Whole Body J Musculoskeletal System - Head and Neck K Musculoskeletal System - Upper Back/Upper Extremity L Musculoskeletal System - Lower Back/Lower Extremity M Musculoskeletal System - Whole Body	5 Wound Management	B Physical Agents C Mechanical D Electrotherapeutic E Orthosis F Assistive, Adaptive, Supportive or Protective U Prosthesis Y Other Equipment Z None	Z None
Z None	Ø Bathing/Showering Techniques 1 Dressing Techniques 2 Grooming/Personal Hygiene	E Orthosis F Assistive, Adaptive, Supportive or Protective U Prosthesis Y Other Equipment Z None	Z None
Z None	3 Feeding/Eating	C Mechanical D Electrotherapeutic E Orthosis F Assistive, Adaptive, Supportive or Protective U Prosthesis Y Other Equipment Z None	Z None
Z None	4 Home Management	D Electrotherapeutic E Orthosis F Assistive, Adaptive, Supportive or Protective U Prosthesis Y Other Equipment Z None	Z None
Z None	6 Psychosocial Skills	Z None	Z None
Z None	7 Vocational Activities and Functional Community or Work Reintegration Skills	B Physical Agents C Mechanical D Electrotherapeutic E Orthosis F Assistive, Adaptive, Supportive or Protective G Aerobic Endurance and Conditioning U Prosthesis Y Other Equipment Z None	Z None

DRG Non-OR All Values

SECTION: F **PHYSICAL REHABILITATION AND DIAGNOSTIC AUDIOLOGY**
SECTION QUALIFIER: Ø **REHABILITATION**
TYPE: 9 **HEARING TREATMENT:** Application of techniques to improve, augment, or compensate for hearing and related functional impairment

Body System – Body Region	Type Qualifier	Equipment	Qualifier
Z None	Ø Hearing and Related Disorders Counseling 1 Hearing and Related Disorders Prevention	K Audiovisual Z None	Z None
Z None	2 Auditory Processing	K Audiovisual L Assistive Listening P Computer Y Other Equipment Z None	Z None
Z None	3 Cerumen Management	X Cerumen Management Z None	Z None

DRG Non-OR All Values

SECTION: F **PHYSICAL REHABILITATION AND DIAGNOSTIC AUDIOLOGY**
SECTION QUALIFIER: Ø **REHABILITATION**
TYPE: B **COCHLEAR IMPLANT TREATMENT:** Application of techniques to improve the communication abilities of individuals with cochlear implant

Body System – Body Region	Type Qualifier	Equipment	Qualifier
Z None	Ø Cochlear Implant Rehabilitation	1 Audiometer 2 Sound Field/Booth 9 Cochlear Implant K Audiovisual P Computer Y Other Equipment	Z None

DRG Non-OR All Values

SECTION: F PHYSICAL REHABILITATION AND DIAGNOSTIC AUDIOLOGY

SECTION QUALIFIER: Ø **REHABILITATION**

TYPE: C **VESTIBULAR TREATMENT:** Application of techniques to improve, augment, or compensate for vestibular and related functional impairment

Body System – Body Region	Type Qualifier	Equipment	Qualifier
3 Neurological System - Whole Body H Integumentary System - Whole Body M Musculoskeletal System - Whole Body	3 Postural Control	E Orthosis F Assistive, Adaptive, Supportive or Protective U Prosthesis Y Other Equipment Z None	Z None
Z None	Ø Vestibular	8 Vestibular/Balance Z None	Z None
Z None	1 Perceptual Processing 2 Visual Motor Integration	K Audiovisual L Assistive Listening N Biosensory Feedback P Computer Q Speech Analysis S Voice Analysis T Aerodynamic Function Y Other Equipment Z None	Z None

DRG Non-OR All Values

SECTION: F PHYSICAL REHABILITATION AND DIAGNOSTIC AUDIOLOGY

SECTION QUALIFIER: Ø **REHABILITATION**

TYPE: D **DEVICE FITTING:** Fitting of a device designed to facilitate or support achievement of a higher level of function

Body System – Body Region	Type Qualifier	Equipment	Qualifier
Z None	Ø Tinnitus Masker	5 Hearing Aid Selection/Fitting/Test Z None	Z None
Z None	1 Monaural Hearing Aid 2 Binaural Hearing Aid 5 Assistive Listening Device	1 Audiometer 2 Sound Field/Booth 5 Hearing Aid Selection/Fitting/Test K Audiovisual L Assistive Listening Z None	Z None
Z None	3 Augmentative/Alternative Communication System	M Augmentative/Alternative Communication	Z None
Z None	4 Voice Prosthetic	S Voice Analysis V Speech Prosthesis	Z None
Z None	6 Dynamic Orthosis 7 Static Orthosis 8 Prosthesis 9 Assistive, Adaptive, Supportive or Protective Devices	E Orthosis F Assistive, Adaptive, Supportive or Protective U Prosthesis Z None	Z None

DRG Non-OR FØDZØ[5Z]Z
DRG Non-OR FØDZ[125][125KLZ]Z
DRG Non-OR FØDZ3MZ
DRG Non-OR FØDZ4[SV]Z
DRG Non-OR FØDZ[67][EFUZ]Z
DRG Non-OR FØDZ8[EFU]Z

SECTION: F PHYSICAL REHABILITATION AND DIAGNOSTIC AUDIOLOGY

SECTION QUALIFIER: Ø REHABILITATION

TYPE: F CAREGIVER TRAINING: Training in activities to support patient's optimal level of function

Body System – Body Region	Type Qualifier	Equipment	Qualifier
Z None	Ø Bathing/Showering Technique 1 Dressing 2 Feeding and Eating 3 Grooming/Personal Hygiene 4 Bed Mobility 5 Transfer 6 Wheelchair Mobility 7 Therapeutic Exercise 8 Airway Clearance Techniques 9 Wound Management B Vocational Activities and Functional Community or Work Reintegration Skills C Gait Training/Functional Ambulation D Application, Proper Use and Care Devices F Application, Proper Use and Care of Orthoses G Application, Proper Use and Care of Prosthesis H Home Management	E Orthosis F Assistive, Adaptive, Supportive or Protective U Prosthesis Z None	Z None
Z None	J Communication Skills	K Audiovisual L Assistive Listening M Augmentative/Alternative Communication P Computer Z None	Z None

DRG Non-OR All Values

SECTION: F PHYSICAL REHABILITATION AND DIAGNOSTIC AUDIOLOGY

SECTION QUALIFIER: 1 DIAGNOSTIC AUDIOLOGY

TYPE: 3 HEARING ASSESSMENT: Measurement of hearing and related functions

Body System – Body Region	Type Qualifier	Equipment	Qualifier
Z None	Ø Hearing Screening	Ø Occupational Hearing 1 Audiometer 2 Sound Field/Booth 3 Tympanometer 8 Vestibular/Balance 9 Cochlear Implant Z None	Z None
Z None	1 Pure Tone Audiometry, Air 2 Pure Tone Audiometry, Air and Bone	Ø Occupational Hearing 1 Audiometer 2 Sound Field/Booth Z None	Z None
Z None	3 Bekesy Audiometry 6 Visual Reinforcement Audiometry 9 Short Increment Sensitivity Index B Stenger C Pure Tone Stenger	1 Audiometer 2 Sound Field/Booth Z None	Z None
Z None	4 Conditioned Play Audiometry 5 Select Picture Audiometry	1 Audiometer 2 Sound Field/Booth K Audiovisual Z None	Z None
Z None	7 Alternate Binaural or Monaural Loudness Balance	1 Audiometer K Audiovisual Z None	Z None
Z None	8 Tone Decay D Tympanometry F Eustachian Tube Function G Acoustic Reflex Patterns H Acoustic Reflex Threshold J Acoustic Reflex Decay	3 Tympanometer 4 Electroacoustic Immitance/ Acoustic Reflex Z None	Z None
Z None	K Electrocochleography L Auditory Evoked Potentials	7 Electrophysiologic Z None	Z None
Z None	M Evoked Otoacoustic Emissions, Screening N Evoked Otoacoustic Emissions, Diagnostic	6 Otoacoustic Emission (OAE) Z None	Z None
Z None	P Aural Rehabilitation Status	1 Audiometer 2 Sound Field/Booth 4 Electroacoustic Immitance/ Acoustic Reflex 9 Cochlear Implant K Audiovisual L Assistive Listening P Computer Z None	Z None
Z None	Q Auditory Processing	K Audiovisual P Computer Y Other Equipment Z None	Z None

SECTION: F PHYSICAL REHABILITATION AND DIAGNOSTIC AUDIOLOGY

SECTION QUALIFIER: 1 DIAGNOSTIC AUDIOLOGY

TYPE: 4 HEARING AID ASSESSMENT: Measurement of the appropriateness and/or effectiveness of a hearing device

Body System – Body Region	Type Qualifier	Equipment	Qualifier
Z None	Ø Cochlear Implant	1 Audiometer 2 Sound Field/Booth 3 Tympanometer 4 Electroacoustic Immitance/ Acoustic Reflex 5 Hearing Aid Selection/ Fitting/Test 7 Electrophysiologic 9 Cochlear Implant K Audiovisual L Assistive Listening P Computer Y Other Equipment Z None	Z None
Z None	1 Ear Canal Probe Microphone 6 Binaural Electroacoustic Hearing Aid Check 8 Monaural Electroacoustic Hearing Aid Check	5 Hearing Aid Selection/ Fitting/Test Z None	Z None
Z None	2 Monaural Hearing Aid 3 Binaural Hearing Aid	1 Audiometer 2 Sound Field/Booth 3 Tympanometer 4 Electroacoustic Immitance/ Acoustic Reflex 5 Hearing Aid Selection/ Fitting/Test K Audiovisual L Assistive Listening P Computer Z None	Z None
Z None	4 Assistive Listening System/ Device Selection	1 Audiometer 2 Sound Field/Booth 3 Tympanometer 4 Electroacoustic Immitance/ Acoustic Reflex K Audiovisual L Assistive Listening Z None	Z None
Z None	5 Sensory Aids	1 Audiometer 2 Sound Field/Booth 3 Tympanometer 4 Electroacoustic Immitance/ Acoustic Reflex 5 Hearing Aid Selection/ Fitting/Test K Audiovisual L Assistive Listening Z None	Z None
Z None	7 Ear Protector Attentuation	Ø Occupational Hearing Z None	Z None

SECTION: F PHYSICAL REHABILITATION AND DIAGNOSTIC AUDIOLOGY

SECTION QUALIFIER: 1 DIAGNOSTIC AUDIOLOGY

TYPE: 5 VESTIBULAR ASSESSMENT: Measurement of the vestibular system and related functions

Body System – Body Region	Type Qualifier	Equipment	Qualifier
Z None	Ø Bithermal, Binaural Caloric Irrigation 1 Bithermal, Monaural Caloric Irrigation 2 Unithermal Binaural Screen 3 Oscillating Tracking 4 Sinusoidal Vertical Axis Rotational 5 Dix-Hallpike Dynamic 6 Computerized Dynamic Posturography	8 Vestibular/Balance Z None	Z None
Z None	7 Tinnitus Masker	5 Hearing Aid Selection/ Fitting/Test Z None	Z None

SECTION: **G MENTAL HEALTH**
SECTION QUALIFIER: Z NONE
TYPE: 1 **PSYCHOLOGICAL TESTS:** The administration and interpretation of standardized psychological tests and measurement instruments for the assessment of psychological function

Qualifier	Qualifier	Qualifier	Qualifier
Ø Developmental 1 Personality and Behavioral 2 Intellectual and Psychoeducational 3 Neuropsychological 4 Neurobehavioral and Cognitive Status	Z None	Z None	Z None

SECTION: **G MENTAL HEALTH**
SECTION QUALIFIER: Z NONE
TYPE: 2 **CRISIS INTERVENTION:** Treatment of a traumatized, acutely disturbed or distressed individual for the purpose of short-term stabilization

Qualifier	Qualifier	Qualifier	Qualifier
Z None	Z None	Z None	Z None

SECTION: **G MENTAL HEALTH**
SECTION QUALIFIER: Z NONE
TYPE: 3 **MEDICATION MANAGEMENT:** Monitoring and adjusting the use of medications for the treatment of a mental health disorder

Qualifier	Qualifier	Qualifier	Qualifier
Z None	Z None	Z None	Z None

SECTION: **G MENTAL HEALTH**
SECTION QUALIFIER: Z NONE
TYPE: 5 **INDIVIDUAL PSYCHOTHERAPY:** Treatment of an individual with a mental health disorder by behavioral, cognitive, psychoanalytic, psychodynamic or psychophysiological means to improve functioning or well-being

Qualifier	Qualifier	Qualifier	Qualifier
Ø Interactive 1 Behavioral 2 Cognitive 3 Interpersonal 4 Psychoanalysis 5 Psychodynamic 6 Supportive 8 Cognitive-Behavioral 9 Psychophysiological	Z None	Z None	Z None

SECTION: **G MENTAL HEALTH**
SECTION QUALIFIER: Z NONE
TYPE: **6 COUNSELING:** The application of psychological methods to treat an individual with normal developmental issues and psychological problems in order to increase function, improve well-being, alleviate distress, maladjustment or resolve crises

Qualifier	Qualifier	Qualifier	Qualifier
Ø Educational 1 Vocational 3 Other Counseling	Z None	Z None	Z None

SECTION: **G MENTAL HEALTH**
SECTION QUALIFIER: Z NONE
TYPE: **7 FAMILY PSYCHOTHERAPY:** Treatment that includes one or more family members of an individual with a mental health disorder by behavioral, cognitive, psychoanalytic, psychodynamic or psychophysiological means to improve functioning or well-being

Qualifier	Qualifier	Qualifier	Qualifier
2 Other Family Psychotherapy	Z None	Z None	Z None

SECTION: **G MENTAL HEALTH**
SECTION QUALIFIER: Z NONE
TYPE: **B ELECTROCONVULSIVE THERAPY:** The application of controlled electrical voltages to treat a mental health disorder

Qualifier	Qualifier	Qualifier	Qualifier
Ø Unilateral-Single Seizure 1 Unilateral-Multiple Seizure 2 Bilateral-Single Seizure 3 Bilateral-Multiple Seizure 4 Other Electroconvulsive Therapy	Z None	Z None	Z None

SECTION: **G MENTAL HEALTH**
SECTION QUALIFIER: Z NONE
TYPE: **C BIOFEEDBACK:** Provision of information from the monitoring and regulating of physiological processes in conjunction with cognitive-behavioral techniques to improve patient functioning or well-being

Qualifier	Qualifier	Qualifier	Qualifier
9 Other Biofeedback	Z None	Z None	Z None

SECTION: G **MENTAL HEALTH**
SECTION QUALIFIER: Z NONE
TYPE: F **HYPNOSIS:** Induction of a state of heightened suggestibility by auditory, visual, and tactile techniques to elicit an emotional or behavioral response

Qualifier	Qualifier	Qualifier	Qualifier
Z None	Z None	Z None	Z None

SECTION: G **MENTAL HEALTH**
SECTION QUALIFIER: Z NONE
TYPE: G **NARCOSYNTHESIS:** Administration of intravenous barbiturates in order to release suppressed or repressed thoughts

Qualifier	Qualifier	Qualifier	Qualifier
Z None	Z None	Z None	Z None

SECTION: G **MENTAL HEALTH**
SECTION QUALIFIER: Z NONE
TYPE: H **GROUP PSYCHOTHERAPY:** Treatment of two or more individuals with a mental health disorder by behavioral, cognitive, psychoanalytic, psychodynamic, or psychophysiological means to improve functioning or well-being

Qualifier	Qualifier	Qualifier	Qualifier
Z None	Z None	Z None	Z None

SECTION: G **MENTAL HEALTH**
SECTION QUALIFIER: Z NONE
TYPE: J **LIGHT THERAPY:** Application of specialized light treatments to improve functioning or well-being

Qualifier	Qualifier	Qualifier	Qualifier
Z None	Z None	Z None	Z None

SECTION: H SUBSTANCE ABUSE TREATMENT
SECTION QUALIFIER: Z NONE
TYPE: 2 **DETOXIFICATION SERVICES:** Detoxification from alcohol and/or drugs

Qualifier	Qualifier	Qualifier	Qualifier
Z None	Z None	Z None	Z None

Coding Clinic: 2020, Q1, P22 – HZ2ZZZZ

SECTION: H SUBSTANCE ABUSE TREATMENT
SECTION QUALIFIER: Z NONE
TYPE: 3 **INDIVIDUAL COUNSELING:** The application of psychological methods to treat an individual with addictive behavior

Qualifier	Qualifier	Qualifier	Qualifier
Ø Cognitive 1 Behavioral 2 Cognitive-Behavioral 3 12-Step 4 Interpersonal 5 Vocational 6 Psychoeducation 7 Motivational Enhancement 8 Confrontational 9 Continuing Care B Spiritual C Pre/Post-Test Infectious Disease	Z None	Z None	Z None

DRG Non-OR HZ3[Ø123456789B]ZZZ

SECTION: H SUBSTANCE ABUSE TREATMENT
SECTION QUALIFIER: Z NONE
TYPE: 4 **GROUP COUNSELING:** The application of psychological methods to treat two or more individuals with addictive behavior

Qualifier	Qualifier	Qualifier	Qualifier
Ø Cognitive 1 Behavioral 2 Cognitive-Behavioral 3 12-Step 4 Interpersonal 5 Vocational 6 Psychoeducation 7 Motivational Enhancement 8 Confrontational 9 Continuing Care B Spiritual C Pre/Post-Test Infectious Disease	Z None	Z None	Z None

DRG Non-OR HZ4[Ø123456789B]ZZZ

SECTION: H SUBSTANCE ABUSE TREATMENT
SECTION QUALIFIER: Z NONE
TYPE: 5 INDIVIDUAL PSYCHOTHERAPY: Treatment of an individual with addictive behavior by behavioral, cognitive, psychoanalytic, psychodynamic, or psychophysiological means

Qualifier	Qualifier	Qualifier	Qualifier
Ø Cognitive 1 Behavioral 2 Cognitive-Behavioral 3 12-Step 4 Interpersonal 5 Interactive 6 Psychoeducation 7 Motivational Enhancement 8 Confrontational 9 Supportive B Psychoanalysis C Psychodynamic D Psychophysiological	Z None	Z None	Z None

DRG Non-OR All Values

SECTION: H SUBSTANCE ABUSE TREATMENT
SECTION QUALIFIER: Z NONE
TYPE: 6 FAMILY COUNSELING: The application of psychological methods that includes one or more family members to treat an individual with addictive behavior

Qualifier	Qualifier	Qualifier	Qualifier
3 Other Family Counseling	Z None	Z None	Z None

SECTION: H SUBSTANCE ABUSE TREATMENT
SECTION QUALIFIER: Z NONE
TYPE: 8 MEDICATION MANAGEMENT: Monitoring and adjusting the use of replacement medications for the treatment of addiction

Qualifier	Qualifier	Qualifier	Qualifier
Ø Nicotine Replacement 1 Methadone Maintenance 2 Levo-alpha-acetyl-methadol (LAAM) 3 Antabuse 4 Naltrexone 5 Naloxone 6 Clonidine 7 Bupropion 8 Psychiatric Medication 9 Other Replacement Medication	Z None	Z None	Z None

SECTION: H SUBSTANCE ABUSE TREATMENT
SECTION QUALIFIER: Z NONE
TYPE: 9 PHARMACOTHERAPY: The use of replacement medications for the treatment of addiction

Qualifier	Qualifier	Qualifier	Qualifier
Ø Nicotine Replacement 1 Methadone Maintenance 2 Levo-alpha-acetyl-methadol (LAAM) 3 Antabuse 4 Naltrexone 5 Naloxone 6 Clonidine 7 Bupropion 8 Psychiatric Medication 9 Other Replacement Medication	Z None	Z None	Z None

New/Revised Text in Green ~~deleted~~ Deleted ♀ Females Only ♂ Males Only Coding Clinic
Non-covered Limited Coverage Combination (See Appendix E) DRG Non-OR Non-OR Hospital-Acquired Condition

ICD-10-PCS Coding Guidelines

New Technology Section Guidelines (section X)

D. New Technology Section

General guidelines

D1

Section X codes are standalone codes. They are not supplemental codes. Section X codes fully represent the specific procedure described in the code title, and do not require any additional codes from other sections of ICD-10-PCS. When section X contains a code title which describes a specific new technology procedure, only that X code is reported for the procedure. There is no need to report a broader, non-specific code in another section of ICD-10-PCS.

Example: XW04321 Introduction of Ceftazidime-Avibactam Anti-infective into Central Vein, Percutaneous Approach, New Technology Group 1, can be coded to indicate that Ceftazidime-Avibactam Anti-infective was administered via a central vein. A separate code from table 3E0 in the Administration section of ICD-10-PCS is not coded in addition to this code.

Selection of Principal Procedure

The following instructions should be applied in the selection of principal procedure and clarification on the importance of the relation to the principal diagnosis when more than one procedure is performed:

1. Procedure performed for definitive treatment of both principal diagnosis and secondary diagnosis
   a. Sequence procedure performed for definitive treatment most related to principal diagnosis as principal procedure.
2. Procedure performed for definitive treatment and diagnostic procedures performed for both principal diagnosis and secondary diagnosis
   a. Sequence procedure performed for definitive treatment most related to principal diagnosis as principal procedure.
3. A diagnostic procedure was performed for the principal diagnosis and a procedure is performed for definitive treatment of a secondary diagnosis
   a. Sequence diagnostic procedure as principal procedure, since the procedure most related to the principal diagnosis takes precedence.
4. No procedures performed that are related to principal diagnosis; procedures performed for definitive treatment and diagnostic procedures were performed for secondary diagnosis
   a. Sequence procedure performed for definitive treatment of secondary diagnosis as principal procedure, since there are no procedures (definitive or nondefinitive treatment) related to principal diagnosis.

SECTION: X NEW TECHNOLOGY
BODY SYSTEM: Ø NERVOUS SYSTEM
OPERATION: 5 **DESTRUCTION:** Physical eradication of all or a portion of a body part by the direct use of energy, force, or a destructive agent

Body Part	Approach	Device / Substance / Technology	Qualifier
1 Renal Sympathetic Nerve(s)	3 Percutaneous	2 Ultrasound Ablation	9 New Technology Group 9

SECTION: X NEW TECHNOLOGY
BODY SYSTEM: Ø NERVOUS SYSTEM
OPERATION: H **INSERTION:** Putting in a nonbiological appliance that monitors, assists, performs, or prevents a physiological function but does not physically take the place of a body part

Body Part	Approach	Device / Substance / Technology	Qualifier
K Sphenopalatine Ganglion	3 Percutaneous	Q Neurostimulator Lead	8 New Technology Group 8
Q Vagus Nerve ⊞	3 Percutaneous	R Neurostimulator Lead with Paired Stimulation System	8 New Technology Group 8

Non-OR XØHQ3R8 Non-OR XØHK3Q3 Coding Clinic: 2022, Q4, P64 – XØHK3Q8

SECTION: X NEW TECHNOLOGY
BODY SYSTEM: Ø NERVOUS SYSTEM
OPERATION: Z **OTHER PROCEDURES:** Methodologies which attempt to remediate or cure a disorder or disease

Body Part	Approach	Device / Substance / Technology	Qualifier
Ø Prefrontal Cortex	X External	1 Computer-assisted Transcranial Magnetic Stimulation	8 New Technology Group 8

SECTION: X NEW TECHNOLOGY
BODY SYSTEM: 2 CARDIOVASCULAR SYSTEM
OPERATION: 7 **DILATION:** Expanding an orifice or the lumen of a tubular body part

Body Part	Approach	Device / Substance / Technology	Qualifier
H Femoral Artery, Right J Femoral Artery, Left K Popliteal Artery, Proximal Right L Popliteal Artery, Proximal Left M Popliteal Artery, Distal Right N Popliteal Artery, Distal Left P Anterior Tibial Artery, Right Q Anterior Tibial Artery, Left R Posterior Tibial Artery, Right S Posterior Tibial Artery, Left T Peroneal Artery, Right U Peroneal Artery, Left	3 Percutaneous	8 Intraluminal Device, Sustained Release Drug-eluting 9 Intraluminal Device, Sustained Release Drug-eluting, Two B Intraluminal Device, Sustained Release Drug-eluting, Three C Intraluminal Device, Sustained Release Drug-eluting, Four or More	5 New Technology Group 5

SECTION: X NEW TECHNOLOGY
BODY SYSTEM: 2 CARDIOVASCULAR SYSTEM
OPERATION: A ASSISTANCE: Taking over a portion of a physiological function by extracorporeal means

Body Part	Approach	Device / Substance / Technology	Qualifier
5 Innominate Artery and Left Common Carotid Artery	3 Percutaneous	1 Cerebral Embolic Filtration, Dual Filter	2 New Technology Group 2
6 Aortic Arch	3 Percutaneous	2 Cerebral Embolic Filtration, Single Deflection Filter	5 New Technology Group 5
7 Coronary Sinus	3 Percutaneous	5 Intermittent Coronary Sinus Occlusion	8 New Technology Group 8
H Common Carotid Artery, Right J Common Carotid Artery, Left	3 Percutaneous	3 Cerebral Embolic Filtration, Extracorporeal Flow Reversal Circuit	6 New Technology Group 6

Coding Clinic: 2016, Q4, P115 – X2A Coding Clinic: 2021, Q1, P16-17 – X2A5312 DRG Non-OR X2A7358

SECTION: X NEW TECHNOLOGY
BODY SYSTEM: 2 CARDIOVASCULAR SYSTEM
OPERATION: C EXTIRPATION: Taking or cutting out solid matter from a body part

Body Part	Approach	Device / Substance / Technology	Qualifier
P Abdominal Aorta Q Upper Extremity Vein, Right R Upper Extremity Vein, Left S Lower Extremity Artery, Right T Lower Extremity Artery, Left U Lower Extremity Vein, Right V Lower Extremity Vein, Left Y Great Vessel	3 Percutaneous	7 Computer-aided Mechanical Aspiration	7 New Technology Group 7

SECTION: X NEW TECHNOLOGY
BODY SYSTEM: 2 CARDIOVASCULAR SYSTEM
OPERATION: H INSERTION: Putting in a nonbiological appliance that monitors, assists, performs, or prevents a physiological function but does not physically take the place of a body part

Body Part	Approach	Device / Substance / Technology	Qualifier
Ø Inferior Vena Cava 1 Superior Vena Cava	3 Percutaneous	R Intraluminal Device, Bioprosthetic Valve	9 New Technology Group 9
2 Femoral Vein, Right 3 Femoral Vein, Left	Ø Open	R Intraluminal Device, Bioprosthetic Valve	9 New Technology Group 9
6 Atrium, Right K Ventricle, Right	3 Percutaneous	V Intracardiac Pacemaker, Dual-Chamber	9 New Technology Group 9
L Axillary Artery, Right M Axillary Artery, Left X Thoracic Aorta, Ascending	Ø Open	F Conduit to Short-term External Heart Assist System	9 New Technology Group 9

SECTION: X NEW TECHNOLOGY
BODY SYSTEM: 2 CARDIOVASCULAR SYSTEM
OPERATION: J **INSPECTION:** Visually and/or manually exploring a body part

Body Part	Approach	Device / Substance / Technology	Qualifier
A Heart	X External	4 Transthoracic Echocardiography, Computer-aided Guidance	7 New Technology Group 7

SECTION: X NEW TECHNOLOGY
BODY SYSTEM: 2 CARDIOVASCULAR SYSTEM
OPERATION: K **BYPASS:** Altering the route of passage of the contents of a tubular body part

Body Part	Approach	Device / Substance / Technology	Qualifier
B Radial Artery, Right C Radial Artery, Left	3 Percutaneous	1 Thermal Resistance Energy	7 New Technology Group 7
H Femoral Artery, Right J Femoral Artery, Left	3 Percutaneous	D Conduit through Femoral Vein to Superficial Femoral Artery E Conduit through Femoral Vein to Popliteal Artery	9 New Technology Group 9

SECTION: X NEW TECHNOLOGY
BODY SYSTEM: 2 CARDIOVASCULAR SYSTEM
OPERATION: R **REPLACEMENT:** Putting in or on biological or synthetic material that physically takes the place and/or function of all or a portion of a body part

Body Part	Approach	Device / Substance / Technology	Qualifier
X Thoracic Aorta, Arch	Ø Open	N Branched Synthetic Substitute with Intraluminal Device	7 New Technology Group 7

Coding Clinic: 2Ø16, Q4, P116 – X2R

SECTION: X NEW TECHNOLOGY
BODY SYSTEM: 2 CARDIOVASCULAR SYSTEM
OPERATION: U **SUPPLEMENT:** Putting in or on biological or synthetic material that physically reinforces and/or augments the function of a portion of a body part

Body Part	Approach	Device / Substance / Technology	Qualifier
4 Coronary Artery/Arteries	Ø Open	7 Vein Graft Extraluminal Support Device(s)	9 New Technology Group 9
Q Upper Extremity Vein, Right R Upper Extremity Vein, Left	Ø Open	P Synthetic Substitute, Extraluminal Support Device	9 New Technology Group 9

SECTION: X NEW TECHNOLOGY
BODY SYSTEM: 2 CARDIOVASCULAR SYSTEM
OPERATION: V RESTRICTION: Partially closing an orifice or the lumen of a tubular body part

Body Part	Approach	Device / Substance / Technology	Qualifier
7 Coronary Sinus	3 Percutaneous	Q Reduction Device	7 New Technology Group 7
W Thoracic Aorta, Descending	Ø Open	N Branched Synthetic Substitute with Intraluminal Device	7 New Technology Group 7

SECTION: X NEW TECHNOLOGY
BODY SYSTEM: D GASTROINTESTINAL SYSTEM
OPERATION: 2 MONITORING: Determining the level of a psysiological or physical function repetitively over a period of time

Body Part	Approach	Device / Substance / Technology	Qualifier
G Upper GI H Lower GI	4 Percutaneous Endoscopic 8 Via Natural or Artificial Opening Endoscopic	V Oxygen Saturation	7 New Technology Group 7

SECTION: X NEW TECHNOLOGY
BODY SYSTEM: D GASTROINTESTINAL SYSTEM
OPERATION: P IRRIGATION: Putting in or on a cleansing substance

Body Part	Approach	Device / Substance / Technology	Qualifier
H Lower GI	8 Via Natural or Artificial Opening Endoscopic	K Intraoperative Single-use Oversleeve	7 New Technology Group 7

SECTION: X NEW TECHNOLOGY
BODY SYSTEM: F HEPATOBILIARY SYSTEM AND PANCREAS
OPERATION: 5 DESTRUCTION: Physical eradication of all or a portion of a body part by the direct use of energy, force, or a destruction agent

Body Part	Approach	Device / Substance / Technology	Qualifier
Ø Liver 1 Liver, Right Lobe 2 Liver, Left Lobe	X External	Ø Ultrasound-guided Cavitation	8 New Technology Group 8

DRG Non-OR XF5[012]X08
Non-OR XF5[Ø12]XØ8

SECTION: X NEW TECHNOLOGY
BODY SYSTEM: F HEPATOBILIARY SYSTEM AND PANCREAS
OPERATION: J **INSPECTION:** Visually and/or manually exploring a body part

Body Part	Approach	Device / Substance / Technology	Qualifier
B Hepatobiliary Duct D Pancreatic Duck	8 Via Natural or Artificial Opening Endoscopic	A Single-use Duodenoscope	7 New Technology Group 7

SECTION: X NEW TECHNOLOGY
BODY SYSTEM: H SKIN, SUBCUTANEOUS TISSUE, FASCIA AND BREAST
OPERATION: R **REPLACEMENT:** Putting in or on biological or synthetic material that physically takes the place and/or function of all or a portion of a body part

Body Part	Approach	Device / Substance / Technology	Qualifier
P Skin	X External	F Bioengineered Allogeneic Construct	7 New Technology Group 7

SECTION: X NEW TECHNOLOGY
BODY SYSTEM: K MUSCLES, TENDONS, BURSAE AND LIGAMENTS
OPERATION: Ø **INTRODUCTION:** Putting in or on a therapeutic, diagnostic, nutritional, physiological, or prophylactic substance except blood or blood products

Body Part	Approach	Device / Substance / Technology	Qualifier

SECTION: X NEW TECHNOLOGY
BODY SYSTEM: K MUSCLES, TENDONS, BURSAE AND LIGAMENTS
OPERATION: U **SUPPLEMENT:** Putting in or on biological or synthetic material that physically reinforces and/or augments the function of a portion of a body part

Body Part	Approach	Device / Substance / Technology	Qualifier
C Upper Spine Bursa and Ligament D Lower Spine Bursa and Ligament	Ø Open	6 Posterior Vertebral Tether	8 New Technology Group 8

Non-OR XKU[CD]Ø68

SECTION: X NEW TECHNOLOGY
BODY SYSTEM: N BONES
OPERATION: H **INSERTION:** Putting in a nonbiological appliance that monitors, assists, performs, or prevents a physiological function by does not physically take the place of a body part

Body Part	Approach	Device / Substance / Technology	Qualifier
6 Pelvic Bone, Right 7 Pelvic Bone, Left	Ø Open 3 Percutaneous	5 Internal Fixation Device with Tulip Connector	8 New Technology Group 8
G Tibia, Right H Tibia, Left	Ø Open	F Tibial Extension with Motion Sensors	9 New Technology Group 9

Non-OR XNH[67][Ø3]58

SECTION: X NEW TECHNOLOGY
BODY SYSTEM: N BONES
OPERATION: R REPLACEMENT: Putting in or on biological or synthetic material that physically takes the place and/or function of all or a portion of a body part

Body Part	Approach	Device / Substance / Technology	Qualifier
8 Skull	Ø Open	D Synthetic Substitute, Ultrasound Penetrable	9 New Technology Group 9
L Tarsal, Right M Tarsal, Left	Ø Open	9 Synthetic Substitute, Talar Prosthesis	9 New Technology Group 9

SECTION: X NEW TECHNOLOGY
BODY SYSTEM: N BONES
OPERATION: S REPOSITION: Moving to its normal location, or other suitable location, all or a portion of a body part

Body Part	Approach	Device / Substance / Technology	Qualifier
Ø Lumbar Vertebra	Ø Open	3 Magnetically Controlled Growth Rod(s)	2 New Technology Group 2
Ø Lumbar Vertebra	Ø Open	C Posterior (Dynamic) Distraction Device	7 New Technology Group 7
Ø Lumbar Vertebra	3 Percutaneous	3 Magnetically Controlled Growth Rod(s)	2 New Technology Group 2
Ø Lumbar Vertebra	3 Percutaneous	C Posterior (Dynamic) Distraction Device	7 New Technology Group 7
3 Cervical Vertebra	Ø Open 3 Percutaneous	3 Magnetically Controlled Growth Rod(s)	2 New Technology Group 2
4 Thoracic Vertebra	Ø Open	3 Magnetically Controlled Growth Rod(s)	2 New Technology Group 2
4 Thoracic Vertebra	Ø Open	C Posterior (Dynamic) Distraction Device	7 New Technology Group 7
4 Thoracic Vertebra	3 Percutaneous	3 Magnetically Controlled Growth Rod(s)	2 New Technology Group 2
4 Thoracic Vertebra	3 Percutaneous	C Posterior (Dynamic) Distraction Device	7 New Technology Group 7

Coding Clinic: 2Ø16, Q4, P117 – XNS

Coding Clinic: 2Ø17, Q4, P75 – XNSØØ32

SECTION: X NEW TECHNOLOGY
BODY SYSTEM: N BONES
OPERATION: U SUPPLEMENT: Putting in or on biological or synthetic material that physically reinforces and/or augments the function of a portion of a body part

Body Part	Approach	Device / Substance / Technology	Qualifier
Ø Lumbar Vertebra 4 Thoracic Vertebra	3 Percutaneous	5 Synthetic Substitute, Mechanically Expandable (Paired)	6 New Technology Group 6

SECTION: X NEW TECHNOLOGY
BODY SYSTEM: R JOINTS
OPERATION: 2 MONITORING: Determining the level of a physiological or physical function repetitively over a period of time

Body Part	Approach	Device / Substance / Technology	Qualifier

SECTION: X NEW TECHNOLOGY
BODY SYSTEM: R JOINTS
OPERATION: G FUSION: *(on multiple pages)*

Joining together portions of an articular body part rendering the articular body part immobile

Body Part	Approach	Device / Substance / Technology	Qualifier
Ø Occipital-cervical Joint	Ø Open	9 Interbody Fusion Device, Nanotextured Surface	2 New Technology Group 2
Ø Occipital-cervical Joint	Ø Open	F Interbody Fusion Device, Radiolucent Porous	3 New Technology Group 3
1 Cervical Vertebral Joint	Ø Open	9 Interbody Fusion Device, Nanotextured Surface	2 New Technology Group 2
1 Cervical Vertebral Joint	Ø Open	F Interbody Fusion Device, Radiolucent Porous	3 New Technology Group 3
2 Cervical Vertebral Joints, 2 or more	Ø Open	9 Interbody Fusion Device, Nanotextured Surface	2 New Technology Group 2
2 Cervical Vertebral Joints, 2 or more	Ø Open	F Interbody Fusion Device, Radiolucent Porous	3 New Technology Group 3
4 Cervicothoracic Vertebral Joint	Ø Open	9 Interbody Fusion Device, Nanotextured Surface	2 New Technology Group 2
4 Cervicothoracic Vertebral Joint	Ø Open	F Interbody Fusion Device, Radiolucent Porous	3 New Technology Group 3
6 Thoracic Vertebral Joint	Ø Open	9 Interbody Fusion Device, Nanotextured Surface	2 New Technology Group 2
6 Thoracic Vertebral Joint	Ø Open	F Interbody Fusion Device, Radiolucent Porous	3 New Technology Group 3
7 Thoracic Vertebral Joints, 2 to 7	Ø Open	9 Interbody Fusion Device, Nanotextured Surface	2 New Technology Group 2
7 Thoracic Vertebral Joints, 2 to 7	Ø Open	F Interbody Fusion Device, Radiolucent Porous	3 New Technology Group 3
8 Thoracic Vertebral Joints, 8 or more	Ø Open	9 Interbody Fusion Device, Nanotextured Surface	2 New Technology Group 2
8 Thoracic Vertebral Joints, 8 or more	Ø Open	F Interbody Fusion Device, Radiolucent Porous	3 New Technology Group 3
A Thoracolumbar Vertebral Joint	Ø Open	9 Interbody Fusion Device, Nanotextured Surface	2 New Technology Group 2
A Thoracolumbar Vertebral Joint	Ø Open	F Interbody Fusion Device, Radiolucent Porous	3 New Technology Group 3
A Thoracolumbar Vertebral Joint B Lumbar Vertebral Joint C Lumbar Vertebral Joints, 2 or more D Lumbosacral Joint	Ø Open 3 Percutaneous 4 Percutaneous Endoscopic	R Interbody Fusion Device, Custom-Made Anatomically Designed	7 New Technology Group 7
B Lumbar Vertebral Joint	Ø Open	9 Interbody Fusion Device, Nanotextured Surface	2 New Technology Group 2
B Lumbar Vertebral Joint	Ø Open	F Interbody Fusion Device, Radiolucent Porous	3 New Technology Group 3
B Lumbar Vertebral Joint	Ø Open 3 Percutaneous 4 Percutaneous Endoscopic	R Interbody Fusion Device, Customizable	7 New Technology Group 7
C Lumbar Vertebral, Joints, 2 or more	Ø Open	9 Interbody Fusion Device, Nanotextured Surface	2 New Technology Group 2
C Lumbar Vertebral Joints, 2 or more	Ø Open	F Interbody Fusion Device, Radiolucent Porous	3 New Technology Group 3
C Lumbar Vertebral Joints, 2 or more	Ø Open 3 Percutaneous 4 Percutaneous Endoscopic	R Interbody Fusion Device, Customizable	7 New Technology Group 7

XRGC[Ø34]R7

XRGAØR7 when reported with Secondary Diagnosis K68.11, T81.4ØXA-T81.49XA, or T82.7XXA
XRGA3R7 when reported with Secondary Diagnosis K68.11, T81.4ØXA-T81.49XA, or T82.7XXA
XRGA4R7 when reported with Secondary Diagnosis K68.11, T81.4ØXA-T81.49XA, or T82.7XXA
XRGBØR7 when reported with Secondary Diagnosis K68.11, T81.4ØXA-T81.49XA, or T82.7XXA
XRGB3R7 when reported with Secondary Diagnosis K68.11, T81.4ØXA-T81.49XA, or T82.7XXA
XRGB4R7 when reported with Secondary Diagnosis K68.11, T81.4ØXA-T81.49XA, or T82.7XXA
XRGCØR7 when reported with Secondary Diagnosis K68.11, T81.4ØXA-T81.49XA, or T82.7XXA
XRGC3R7 when reported with Secondary Diagnosis K68.11, T81.4ØXA-T81.49XA, or T82.7XXA
XRGC4R7 when reported with Secondary Diagnosis K68.11, T81.4ØXA-T81.49XA, or T82.7XXA

SECTION: X NEW TECHNOLOGY
BODY SYSTEM: R JOINTS
OPERATION: G FUSION: *(continued)*
Joining together portions of an articular body part rendering the articular body part immobile

Body Part	Approach	Device / Substance / Technology	Qualifier
D Lumbosacral Joint	Ø Open	9 Interbody Fusion Device, Nanotextured Surface	2 New Technology Group 2
D Lumbosacral Joint	Ø Open	F Interbody Fusion Device, Radiolucent Porous	3 New Technology Group 3
D Lumbosacral Joint	Ø Open 3 Percutaneous 4 Percutaneous Endoscopic	R Interbody Fusion Device, Customizable	7 New Technology Group 7
E Sacroiliac Joint, Right F Sacroiliac Joint, Left	Ø Open 3 Percutaneous	5 Internal Fixation Device with Tulip Connector	8 New Technology Group 8
J Ankle Joint, Right K Ankle Joint, Left L Tarsal Joint, Right M Tarsal Joint, Left	Ø Open	B Internal Fixation Device, Open-truss Design	9 New Technology Group 9

XRGCØ92 when reported with Secondary Diagnosis K68.11, T81.4ØXA-T81.49XA, or T82.7XXA
XRGDØ92 when reported with Secondary Diagnosis K68.11, T81.4ØXA-T81.49XA, or T82.7XXA
XRGDØR7 when reported with Secondary Diagnosis K68.11, T81.4ØXA-T81.49XA, or T82.7XXA
XRGD3R7 when reported with Secondary Diagnosis K68.11, T81.4ØXA-T81.49XA, or T82.7XXA
XRGD4R7 when reported with Secondary Diagnosis K68.11, T81.4ØXA-T81.49XA, or T82.7XXA

Non-OR XRG[EF][Ø3]58

Coding Clinic: 2Ø17, Q4, P76 – XRG[BD]F3

SECTION: X NEW TECHNOLOGY
BODY SYSTEM: R JOINTS
OPERATION: H **INSERTION:** Putting in a nonbiological appliance that monitors, assists, performs, or prevents a physiological function but does not physically take the place of a body part

Body Part	Approach	Device / Substance / Technology	Qualifier
B Lumbar Vertebral Joint D Lumbosacral Joint	Ø Open	1 Posterior Spinal Motion Preservation Device	8 New Technology Group 8

Non-OR XRH[BD]Ø18

SECTION: X NEW TECHNOLOGY
BODY SYSTEM: R JOINTS
OPERATION: R **REPLACEMENT:** Putting in or on biological or synthetic material that physically takes the place and/or function of all or a portion of a body part

Body Part	Approach	Device / Substance / Technology	Qualifier
G Knee Joint, Right H Knee Joint, Left	Ø Open	L Synthetic Substitute, Lateral Meniscus M Synthetic Substitute, Medial Meniscus	8 New Technology Group 8

XRR[GH]Ø[LM]8

Non-OR XRR[GH]Ø[LM]8

XRR[GH]Ø[LM]8 when reported with Secondary Diagnosis from I26.Ø2-I26.Ø9, I26.92-I26.99, or I82.4Ø1-I82.4Z9

SECTION: X NEW TECHNOLOGY
BODY SYSTEM: T URINARY SYSTEM
OPERATION: 2 MONITORING: Determining the level of a physiological or physical function repetitively over a period of time

Body Part	Approach	Device / Substance / Technology	Qualifier
5 Kidney	X External	E Fluorescent Pyrazine	5 New Technology Group 5

SECTION: X NEW TECHNOLOGY
BODY SYSTEM: V MALE REPRODUCTIVE SYSTEM
OPERATION: 5 DESTRUCTION: Physical eradication of all or a portion of a body part by the direct use of energy, force, or a destructive agent

Body Part	Approach	Device / Substance / Technology	Qualifier
~~Ø Prostate~~	~~8 Via Natural or Artificial Opening Endoscopic~~	~~A Robotic Waterjet Ablation~~	~~4 New Technology Group 4~~

SECTION: X NEW TECHNOLOGY
BODY SYSTEM: W ANATOMICAL REGIONS
OPERATION: Ø INTRODUCTION: *(on multiple pages)*
Putting in or on a therapeutic, diagnostic, nutritional, physiological, or prophylactic substance except blood or blood products

Body Part	Approach	Device / Substance / Technology	Qualifier
Ø Skin	X External	2 Anacaulase-bcdb	7 New Technology Group 7
1 Subcutaneous Tissue	3 Percutaneous	1 Daratumumab and Hyaluronidase-fihj 4 Teclistamab Antineoplastic	8 New Technology Group 8
1 Subcutaneous Tissue	3 Percutaneous	9 Satralizumab-mwge	7 New Technology Group 7
1 Subcutaneous Tissue	3 Percutaneous	F Other New Technology Therapeutic Substance	5 New Technology Group 5
1 Subcutaneous Tissue	3 Percutaneous	G REGN-COV2 Monoclonal Antibody H Other New Technology Monoclonal Antibody K Leronlimab Monoclonal Antibody	6 New Technology Group 6
~~1 Subcutaneous Tissue~~	~~3 Percutaneous~~	~~H Other New Technology Monoclonal Antibody~~ ~~K Leronlimab Monoclonal Antibody~~ ~~S COVID-19 Vaccine Dose 1~~ ~~T COVID-19 Vaccine Dose 2~~ ~~U COVID-19 Vaccine Dose~~	~~6 New Technology Group 6~~
1 Subcutaneous Tissue	3 Percutaneous	L Elranatamab Antineoplastic	9 New Technology Group 9
1 Subcutaneous Tissue	3 Percutaneous	S COVID-19 Vaccine Dose 1	6 New Technology Group 6
1 Subcutaneous Tissue	3 Percutaneous	S Epcoritamab Monoclonal Antibody	9 New Technology Group 9
1 Subcutaneous Tissue	3 Percutaneous	T COVID-19 Vaccine Dose 2 U COVID-19 Vaccine	6 New Technology Group 6
1 Subcutaneous Tissue	3 Percutaneous	V COVID-19 Vaccine Dose 3	7 New Technology Group 7
1 Subcutaneous Tissue	3 Percutaneous	W Caplacizumab	5 New Technology Group 5
1 Subcutaneous Tissue	3 Percutaneous	W COVID-19 Vaccine Booster	7 New Technology Group 7
1 Subcutaneous Tissue	X External	2 Anacaulase-bcdb	7 New Technology Group 7
2 Muscle	Ø Open	D Engineered Allogeneic Thymus Tissue	8 New Technology Group 8
2 Muscle	3 Percutaneous	S COVID-19 Vaccine Dose 1 T COVID-19 Vaccine Dose 2 U COVID-19 Vaccine Dose	6 New Technology Group 6

New/Revised Text in Green ~~deleted~~ Deleted ♀ Females Only ♂ Males Only Coding Clinic
Non-covered Limited Coverage ⊞ Combination (See Appendix E) DRG Non-OR Non-OR Hospital-Acquired Condition

SECTION: X **NEW TECHNOLOGY**
BODY SYSTEM: W **ANATOMICAL REGIONS**
OPERATION: Ø **INTRODUCTION:** *(continued)*
Putting in or on a therapeutic, diagnostic, nutritional, physiological, or prophylactic substance except blood or blood products

Body Part	Approach	Device / Substance / Technology	Qualifier
2 Muscle	3 Percutaneous	V COVID-19 Vaccine Dose 3 W COVID-19 Vaccine Booster X Tixagevimab and Cilgavimab Monoclonal Antibody Y Other New Technology Monoclonal Antibody	7 New Technology Group 7
3 Peripheral Vein	3 Percutaneous	Ø Brexanolone	6 New Technology Group 6
3 Peripheral Vein	3 Percutaneous	Ø Spesolimab Monoclonal Antibody	8 New Technology Group 8
3 Peripheral Vein	3 Percutaneous	2 Nerinitide 3 Durvalumab Antineoplastic	6 New Technology Group 6
3 Peripheral Vein	3 Percutaneous	5 Narsoplimab Monoclonal Antibody	7 New Technology Group 7
3 Peripheral Vein	3 Percutaneous	5 Mosunetuzumab Antineoplastic	8 New Technology Group 8
3 Peripheral Vein	3 Percutaneous	6 Lefamulin Anti-infective	6 New Technology Group 6
3 Peripheral Vein	3 Percutaneous	6 Afamitresgene Autoleucel Immunotherapy	8 New Technology Group 8
3 Peripheral Vein	3 Percutaneous	6 Terlipressin	7 New Technology Group 7
3 Peripheral Vein	3 Percutaneous	7 Coagulation Factor Xa, Inactivated	2 New Technology Group 2
3 Peripheral Vein	3 Percutaneous	7 Trilaciclib	7 New Technology Group 7
3 Peripheral Vein	3 Percutaneous	7 Tabelecleucel Immunotherapy	8 New Technology Group 8
3 Peripheral Vein	3 Percutaneous	8 Lurbinectedin	7 New Technology Group 7
3 Peripheral Vein	3 Percutaneous	8 Treosulfan	8 New Technology Group 8
3 Peripheral Vein	3 Percutaneous	9 Inebilzumab-cdon	8 New Technology Group 8
3 Peripheral Vein	3 Percutaneous	A Cefiderocol Anti-infective	6 New Technology Group 6
3 Peripheral Vein	3 Percutaneous	A Ciltacabtagene Autoleucel	7 New Technology Group 7
3 Peripheral Vein	3 Percutaneous	B Cytarabine and Daunorubicin Liposome Antineoplastic	3 New Technology Group 3
3 Peripheral Vein	3 Percutaneous	B Omadacycline Anti-infective	6 New Technology Group 6
3 Peripheral Vein	3 Percutaneous	B Amivantamab Monoclonal Antibody	7 New Technology Group 7
3 Peripheral Vein	3 Percutaneous	C Eculizumab	6 New Technology Group 6
3 Peripheral Vein	3 Percutaneous	C Engineered Chimeric Antigen Receptor T-cell Immunotherapy, Autologous	7 New Technology Group 7
3 Peripheral Vein	3 Percutaneous	D Atezolizumab Antineoplastic	6 New Technology Group 6
3 Peripheral Vein	3 Percutaneous	E Remdesivir Anti-infective	5 New Technology Group 5
3 Peripheral Vein	3 Percutaneous	E Etesevimab Monoclonal Antibody	6 New Technology Group 6
3 Peripheral Vein	3 Percutaneous	F Other New Technology Therapeutic Substance	3 New Technology Group 3
3 Peripheral Vein	3 Percutaneous	F Other New Technology Therapeutic Substance	5 New Technology Group 5
3 Peripheral Vein	3 Percutaneous	F Bamlanivimab Monoclonal Antibody	6 New Technology Group 6
3 Peripheral Vein	3 Percutaneous	G Plazomicin Anti-infective	4 New Technology Group 4
3 Peripheral Vein	3 Percutaneous	G Sarilumab	5 New Technology Group 5
3 Peripheral Vein	3 Percutaneous	G REGN-COV2 Monoclonal Antibody	6 New Technology Group 6
3 Peripheral Vein	3 Percutaneous	G Engineered Chimeric Antigen Receptor T-cell Immunotherapy, Allogeneic	7 New Technology Group 7
3 Peripheral Vein	3 Percutaneous	H Synthetic Human Angiotensin II	4 New Technology Group 4
3 Peripheral Vein	3 Percutaneous	H Tocilizumab	5 New Technology Group 5

DRG Non-OR XW0[34]3C3
DRG Non-OR XW033[6AGHJK][78]

Coding Clinic: 2015, Q4, P13, P15 – XWØ4331, XWØ4351
Coding Clinic: 2021, Q4, P111 – XWØ33F5

SECTION: X NEW TECHNOLOGY
BODY SYSTEM: W ANATOMICAL REGIONS
OPERATION: Ø INTRODUCTION: *(continued)*
Putting in or on a therapeutic, diagnostic, nutritional, physiological, or prophylactic substance except blood or blood products

Body Part	Approach	Device / Substance / Technology	Qualifier
3 Peripheral Vein	3 Percutaneous	H Other New Technology Monoclonal Antibody	6 New Technology Group 6
3 Peripheral Vein	3 Percutaneous	H Axicabtagene Ciloleucel Immunotherapy J Tisagenlecleucel Immunotherapy	7 New Technology Group 7
3 Peripheral Vein	3 Percutaneous	K Fosfomycin Anti-infective	5 New Technology Group 5
3 Peripheral Vein	3 Percutaneous	K Idecabtagene Vicleucel Immunotherapy	7 New Technology Group 7
3 Peripheral Vein	3 Percutaneous	K Sulbactam-Durlobactam	9 New Technology Group 9
3 Peripheral Vein	3 Percutaneous	L CD24Fc Immunomodulator	6 New Technology Group 6
3 Peripheral Vein	3 Percutaneous	L Lifileucel Immunotherapy M Brexucabtagene Autoleucel Immunotherapy	7 New Technology Group 7
3 Peripheral Vein	3 Percutaneous	N Meropenem-vaborbactam Anti-infective	5 New Technology Group 5
3 Peripheral Vein	3 Percutaneous	N Lisocabtagene Maraleucel Immuntherapy	7 New Technology Group 7
3 Peripheral Vein	3 Percutaneous	P Glofitamab Antineoplastic	9 New Technology Group 9
3 Peripheral Vein	3 Percutaneous	Q Tagraxofusp-erzs Antineoplastic	5 New Technology Group 5
3 Peripheral Vein	3 Percutaneous	Q Posoleucel R Rezafungin	9 New Technology Group 9
3 Peripheral Vein	3 Percutaneous	~~Q Tagraxofusp-erzs Antineoplastic~~ S Iobenguane I-131 Antineoplastic U Imipenem-cilastatin-relebactam Anti-infective W Caplacizumab	5 New Technology Group 5
4 Central Vein	3 Percutaneous	Ø Brexanolone	6 New Technology Group 6
4 Central Vein	3 Percutaneous	Ø Brexanolone	6 New Technology Group 6
4 Central Vein	3 Percutaneous	2 Nerinitide 3 Durvalumab Antineoplastic	6 New Technology Group 6
4 Central Vein	3 Percutaneous	5 Narsoplimab Monoclonal Antibody	7 New Technology Group 7
4 Central Vein	3 Percutaneous	5 Mosunetuzumab Antineoplastic	8 New Technology Group 8
4 Central Vein	3 Percutaneous	6 Lefamulin Anti-infective	6 New Technology Group 6
4 Central Vein	3 Percutaneous	6 Terlipressin	7 New Technology Group 7
4 Central Vein	3 Percutaneous	6 Afamitresgene Autoleucel Immunotherapy	8 New Technology Group 8
4 Central Vein	3 Percutaneous	7 Coagulation Factor Xa, Inactivated	2 New Technology Group 2
4 Central Vein	3 Percutaneous	7 Trilaciclib	7 New Technology Group 7
4 Central Vein	3 Percutaneous	7 Tabelecleuce Immunotherapy	8 New Technology Group 8
4 Central Vein	3 Percutaneous	8 Lurbinectedin	7 New Technology Group 7
4 Central Vein	3 Percutaneous	8 Treosulfan	8 New Technology Group 8
4 Central Vein	3 Percutaneous	9 Ceftolozane/Tazobactam Anti-infective	6 New Technology Group 6
4 Central Vein	3 Percutaneous	9 Inebilizumab-cdon	8 New Technology Group 8
4 Central Vein	3 Percutaneous	A Cefiderocol Anti-infective	6 New Technology Group 6
4 Central Vein	3 Percutaneous	A Ciltacabtagene Autoleucel	7 New Technology Group 7
4 Central Vein	3 Percutaneous	B Cytarabine and Daunorubicin Liposome Antineoplastic	3 New Technology Group 3
4 Central Vein	3 Percutaneous	B Omadacycline Anti-infective	6 New Technology Group 6
4 Central Vein	3 Percutaneous	B Amivantamab Monoclonal Antibody	7 New Technology Group 7
4 Central Vein	3 Percutaneous	C Eculizumab	6 New Technology Group 6

New/Revised Text in Green ~~deleted~~ Deleted ♀ Females Only ♂ Males Only Coding Clinic
Non-covered Limited Coverage Combination (See Appendix E) DRG Non-OR Non-OR Hospital-Acquired Condition

SECTION: X NEW TECHNOLOGY
BODY SYSTEM: W ANATOMICAL REGIONS
OPERATION: Ø INTRODUCTION: *(continued)*

Putting in or on a therapeutic, diagnostic, nutritional, physiological, or prophylactic substance except blood or blood products

Body Part	Approach	Device / Substance / Technology	Qualifier
4 Central Vein	3 Percutaneous	C Engineered Autologous Chimeric Antigen Receptor T-cell Immunotherapy, Autologous	7 New Technology Group 7
4 Central Vein	3 Percutaneous	D Atezolizumab Antineoplastic	6 New Technology Group 6
4 Central Vein	3 Percutaneous	E Remdesivir Anti-infective	5 New Technology Group 5
4 Central Vein	3 Percutaneous	E Eteseviman Monoclonal Antibody	6 New Technology Group 6
4 Central Vein	3 Percutaneous	F Other New Technology Therapeutic Substance	3 New Technology Group 3
4 Central Vein	3 Percutaneous	F Other New Technology Therapeutic Substance	5 New Technology Group 5
4 Central Vein	3 Percutaneous	F Bamlanivimab Monoclonal Antibody	6 New Technology Group 6
4 Central Vein	3 Percutaneous	G Plazomicin Anti-infective	4 New Technology Group 4
4 Central Vein	3 Percutaneous	G Sarilumab	5 New Technology Group 5
4 Central Vein	3 Percutaneous	G REGN-COV2 Monoclonal Antibody	6 New Technology Group 6
4 Central Vein	3 Percutaneous	G Engineered Chimeric Antigen Receptor T-cell Immunotherapy, Allogeneic	7 New Technology Group 7
4 Central Vein	3 Percutaneous	H Synthetic Human Angiotensin II	4 New Technology Group 4
4 Central Vein	3 Percutaneous	H Tocilizumab	5 New Technology Group 5
4 Central Vein	3 Percutaneous	H Other New Technology Monoclonal Antibody	6 New Technology Group 6
4 Central Vein	3 Percutaneous	H Axicabtagene Ciloleucel Immunotherapy J Tisagenlecleucel Immunotherapy	7 New Technology Group 7
4 Central Vein	3 Percutaneous	K Fosfomycin Anti-infective	5 New Technology Group 5
4 Central Vein	3 Percutaneous	K Idecabtagene Vicleucel Immunotherapy	7 New Technology Group 7
4 Central Vein	3 Percutaneous	K Sulbactam-Durlobactam	9 New Technology Group 9
4 Central Vein	3 Percutaneous	L CD24Fc Immunomodulator	6 New Technology Group 6
4 Central Vein	3 Percutaneous	L Lifileucel Immunotherapy M Brexucabtagene Autoleucel Immunotherapy	7 New Technology Group 7
4 Central Vein	3 Percutaneous	N Meropenem-vaborbactam Anti-infective	5 New Technology Group 5
4 Central Vein	3 Percutaneous	N Lisocabtagene Maraleucel Immuntherapy	7 New Technology Group 7
4 Central Vein	3 Percutaneous	P Glofitamab Antineoplastic	9 New Technology Group 9
4 Central Vein	3 Percutaneous	Q Tagraxofusp-erzs Antineoplastic	5 New Technology Group 5
4 Central Vein	3 Percutaneous	Q Posoleucel R Rezafungin	9 New Technology Group 9
4 Central Vein	3 Percutaneous	~~Q Tagraxofusp-erzs Antineoplastic~~ S Iobenguane I-131 Antineoplastic U Imipenem-cilastatin-relebactam Anti-infective W Caplacizumab	5 New Technology Group 5
5 Peripheral Artery	3 Percutaneous	T Melphalan Hydrochloride Antineoplastic	9 New Technology Group 9
9 Nose	7 Via Natural or Artificial Opening	M Esketamine Hydrochloride	5 New Technology Group 5
D Mouth and Pharynx	X External	3 Maribavir Anti-infective	8 New Technology Group 8
D Mouth and Pharynx	X External	6 Lefamulin Anti-infective	6 New Technology Group 6
D Mouth and Pharynx	X External	8 Uridine Triacetate	2 New Technology Group 2

DRG Non-OR XW043[567ACGHJKLMN][7]

Coding Clinic: 2021, Q4, P111 – XWØ43F5

SECTION: **X NEW TECHNOLOGY**
BODY SYSTEM: **W ANATOMICAL REGIONS**
OPERATION: **Ø INTRODUCTION:** *(continued)*
Putting in or on a therapeutic, diagnostic, nutritional, physiological, or prophylactic substance except blood or blood products

Body Part	Approach	Device / Substance / Technology	Qualifier
D Mouth and Pharynx	X External	F Other New Technology Therapeutic Substance J Apalutamide Antineoplastic ~~L Erdafitinib Antineoplastic~~	5 New Technology Group 5
D Mouth and Pharynx	X External	J Quizartinib Antineoplastic	9 New Technology Group 9
D Mouth and Pharynx	X External	K Sabizabulin	8 New Technology Group 8
D Mouth and Pharynx	X External	L Erdafitinib Antineoplastic	5 New Technology Group 5
D Mouth and Pharynx	X External	M Baricitinib	6 New Technology Group 6
D Mouth and Pharynx	X External	N SER-109	9 New Technology Group 9
D Mouth and Pharynx	X External	R Venetoclax Antineoplastic	5 New Technology Group 5
D Mouth and Pharynx	X External	R Fostamatinib	7 New Technology Group 7
D Mouth and Pharynx	X External	T Ruxolitinib V Gilteritinib Antineoplastic	5 New Technology Group 5
G Upper GI	7 Via Natural or Artificial Opening	3 Maribavir Anti-infective K Sabizabulin	8 New Technology Group 8
G Upper GI	7 Via Natural or Artificial Opening	M Baricitinib	6 New Technology Group 6
G Upper GI	7 Via Natural or Artificial Opening	R Fostamatinib	7 New Technology Group 7
~~G Upper GI~~ ~~H Lower GI~~	~~7 Via Natural or Artificial Opening~~	~~M Baricitinib~~	~~6 New Technology Group 6~~
G Upper GI ~~H Lower GI~~	8 Via Natural or Artificial Opening Endoscopic	8 Mineral-based Topical Hemostatic Agent	6 New Technology Group 6
H Lower GI	7 Via Natural or Artificial Opening	3 Maribavir Anti-infective K Sabizabulin	8 New Technology Group 8
H Lower GI	7 Via Natural or Artificial Opening	M Baricitinib	6 New Technology Group 6
H Lower GI	7 Via Natural or Artificial Opening	R Fostamatinib	7 New Technology Group 7
H Lower GI	7 Via Natural or Artificial Opening	X Broad Consortium Microbiota-based Live Biotherapeutic Suspension	8 New Technology Group 8
H Lower GI	8 Via Natural or Artificial Opening Endoscopic	8 Mineral-based Topical Hemostatic Agent	6 New Technology Group 6
Q Cranial Cavity and Brain	3 Percutaneous	1 Eladocagene exuparvovec	6 New Technology Group 6
V Bones	Ø Open	P Antibiotic-eluting Bone Void Filler	7 New Technology Group 7

Coding Clinic: 2021, Q4, P111 – XWØDXF5
Coding Clinic: 2023, Q2, P27 – XWØG886

New/Revised Text in Green ~~deleted~~ Deleted ♀ Females Only ♂ Males Only **Coding Clinic**
Non-covered Limited Coverage Combination (See Appendix E) DRG Non-OR Non-OR Hospital-Acquired Condition

SECTION: X **NEW TECHNOLOGY**
BODY SYSTEM: W **ANATOMICAL REGIONS**
OPERATION: 1 **TRANSFUSION:** Putting in blood or blood products

Body Part	Approach	Device / Substance / Technology	Qualifier
3 Peripheral Vein	3 Percutaneous	2 Plasma, Convalescent (Nonautologous)	5 New Technology Group 5
3 Peripheral Vein	3 Percutaneous	B Betibeglogene Autotemcel C Omidubicel	8 New Technology Group 8
3 Peripheral Vein	3 Percutaneous	D High-Dose Intravenous Immune Globulin E Hyperinmmune Globulin	7 New Technology Group 7
3 Peripheral Vein	3 Percutaneous	F OTL-103 G OTL-200	8 New Technology Group 8
3 Peripheral Vein	3 Percutaneous	H Lovotibeglogene Autotemcel	9 New Technology Group 9
3 Peripheral Vein	3 Percutaneous	J Exagamglogene Autotemcel	8 New Technology Group 8
4 Central Vein	3 Percutaneous	2 Plasma, Convalescent (Nonautologous)	5 New Technology Group 5
4 Central Vein	3 Percutaneous	B Betibeglogene Autotemcel C Omidubicel	8 New Technology Group 8
4 Central Vein	3 Percutaneous	D High-Dose Intravenous Immune Globulin E Hyperinmmune Globulin	7 New Technology Group 7
4 Central Vein	3 Percutaneous	F OTL-103 G OTL-200	8 New Technology Group 8
4 Central Vein	3 Percutaneous	H Lovotibeglogene Autotemcel	9 New Technology Group 9
4 Central Vein	3 Percutaneous	J Exagamglogene Autotemcel	8 New Technology Group 8

DRG Non-OR XW1[34]3[BCFG]8

SECTION: X **NEW TECHNOLOGY**
BODY SYSTEM: W **ANATOMICAL REGIONS**
OPERATION: 2 **TRANSFUSION:** Putting in blood or blood products

Body Part	Approach	Device / Substance / Technology	Qualifier

DRG Non-OR ~~XW2[34][47]6~~

SECTION: X **NEW TECHNOLOGY**
BODY SYSTEM: W **ANATOMICAL REGIONS**
OPERATION: H **INSERTION:** Putting in a nonbiological appliance that monitors, assists, performs, or prevents a physiological function but does not physically take the place of a body part

Body Part	Approach	Device / Substance / Technology	Qualifier
D Mouth and Pharynx	7 Via Natural or Artificial Opening	Q Neurostimulator Lead	7 New Technology Group 7

SECTION: X NEW TECHNOLOGY
BODY SYSTEM: X PHYSIOLOGICAL SYSTEMS
OPERATION: 2 MONITORING: Determining the level of a physiological or physical function repetitively over a period of time

Body Part	Approach	Device / Substance / Technology	Qualifier
Ø Central Nervous	X External	8 Brain Electrical Activity, Computer-aided Detection and Notification	9 New Technology Group 9
F Musculoskeletal	3 Percutaneous	W Muscle Compartment Pressure, Micro-Electro-Mechanical System	9 New Technology Group 9

SECTION: X NEW TECHNOLOGY
BODY SYSTEM: X PHYSIOLOGICAL SYSTEMS
OPERATION: E MEASUREMENT: Determining the level of a physiological or physical function at a point in time

Body Part	Approach	Device / Substance / Technology	Qualifier
Ø Central Nervous	X External	Ø Intracranial Vascular Activity, Computer-aided Assessment	7 New Technology Group 7
Ø Central Nervous	X External	4 Brain Electrical Activity, Computer-aided Semiologic Analysis	8 New Technology Group 8
2 Cardiac	X External	1 Output, Computer-aided Assessment	9 New Technology Group 9
3 Arterial	X External	2 Pulmonary Artery Flow, Computer-aided Triage and Notification	7 New Technology Group 7
3 Arterial	X External	5 Coronary Artery Flow, Quantitative Flow Ratio Analysis 6 Coronary Artery Flow, Computer-aided Valve Modeling and Notification	8 New Technology Group 8
5 Circulatory	X External	3 Infection, Whole Blood Reverse Transcription and Quantitative Real-time Polymerase Chain Reaction	8 New Technology Group 8
5 Circulatory	X External	M Infection, Whole Blood Nucleic Acid-base Microbial Detection	5 New Technology Group 5
5 Circulatory	X External	N Infection, Positive Blood Culture Fluorescence Hybridization for Organism Identification, Concentration and Susceptibility	6 New Technology Group 6
5 Circulatory	X External	R Infection, Mechanical Initial Specimen Diversion Technique Using Active Negative Pressure T Intracranial Arterial Flow, Whole Blood mRNA V Infection, Serum/Plasma Nanoparticle Fluorescence SARS-CoV-2 Antibody Detection	7 New Technology Group 7
5 Circulatory	X External	Y Infection, Other Positive Blood/Isolated Colonies Bimodal Phenotypic Susceptibility Technology	9 New Technology Group 9
9 Nose	7 Via Natural or Artificial Opening	U Infection, Nasopharyngeal Fluid SARS-CoV-2 Polymerase Chain Reaction	7 New Technology Group 7
B Respiratory	X External	Q Infection, Lower Respiratory Fluid Nucleic Acid-base Microbial Detection	6 New Technology Group 6

SECTION: X NEW TECHNOLOGY
BODY SYSTEM: Y EXTRACORPOREAL
OPERATION: Ø INTRODUCTION: Putting in or on a therapeutic, diagnostic, nutritional, physiological, or prophylactic substance except blood or blood products

Body Part	Approach	Device / Substance / Technology	Qualifier
V Vein Graft	X External	8 Endothelial Damage Inhibitor	3 New Technology Group 3
Y Extracorporeal	X External	2 Taurolidine Anti-infective and Heparin Anticoagulant	8 New Technology Group 8
Y Extracorporeal	X External	3 Nafamostat Anticoagulant	7 New Technology Group 7

INDEX

INDEX TO PROCEDURES

3

3f (Aortic) Bioprosthesis valve *use* Zooplastic Tissue in Heart and Great Vessels

A

Abdominal aortic plexus *use* Abdominal Sympathetic Nerve
Abdominal cavity *use* Peritoneal Cavity
Abdominal esophagus *use* Esophagus, Lower
Abdominohysterectomy *see* Resection, Uterus 0UT9
Abdominoplasty
- *see* Alteration, Abdominal Wall, 0W0F
- *see* Repair, Abdominal Wall, 0WQF
- *see* Supplement, Abdominal Wall, 0WUF

Abductor hallucis muscle
- *use* Foot Muscle, Right
- *use* Foot Muscle, Left

ABECMA® *use* Idecabtagene Vicleucel Immunotherapy
AbioCor® Total Replacement Heart *use* Synthetic Substitute
Ablation
- *see* Control bleeding in
- *see* Destruction

Abortion
- Products of Conception 10A0
- Abortifacient 10A07ZX
- Laminaria 10A07ZW
- Vacuum 10A07Z6

Abrasion *see* Extraction
Absolute Pro Vascular (OTW) Self-Expanding Stent System *use* Intraluminal Device
Accelerate PhenoTest™ BC XXE5XN6
Accessory cephalic vein
- *use* Cephalic Vein, Right
- *use* Cephalic Vein, Left

Accessory obturator nerve *use* Lumbar Plexus
Accessory phrenic nerve *use* Phrenic Nerve
Accessory spleen *use* Spleen
Acculink (RX) Carotid Stent System *use* Intraluminal Device
Acellular Hydrated Dermis *use* Nonautologous Tissue Substitute
Acetabular cup *use* Liner in Lower Joints
Acetabulectomy
- *see* Excision, Lower Bones 0QB
- *see* Resection, Lower Bones 0QT

Acetabulofemoral joint
- *use* Hip Joint, Right
- *use* Hip Joint, Left

Acetabuloplasty
- *see* Repair, Lower Bones 0QQ
- *see* Replacement, Lower Bones 0QR
- *see* Supplement, Lower Bones 0QU

Achilles tendon
- *use* Lower Leg Tendon, Right
- *use* Lower Leg Tendon, Left

Achillorrhaphy *use* Repair, Tendons 0LQ
Achillotenotomy, achillotomy
- *see* Division, Tendons 0L8
- *see* Drainage, Tendons 0L9

Acoustic Pulse Thrombolysis *see* Fragmentation, Artery
Acromioclavicular ligament
- *use* Shoulder Bursa and Ligament, Right
- *use* Shoulder Bursa and Ligament, Left

Acromion (process)
- *use* Scapula, Right
- *use* Scapula, Left

Acromionectomy
- *see* Excision, Upper Joints 0RB
- *see* Resection, Upper Joints 0RT

Acromioplasty
- *see* Repair, Upper Joints 0RQ
- *see* Replacement, Upper Joints 0RR
- *see* Supplement, Upper Joints 0RU

ACTEMRA® *use* Tocilzumab
Activa PC neurostimulator *use* Stimulator Generator, Multiple Array in 0JH
Activa RC neurostimulator *use* Stimulator Generator, Multiple Array Rechargeable in 0JH
Activa SC neurostimulator *use* Stimulator Generator, Single Array in 0JH
Activities of Daily Living Assessment F02
Activities of Daily Living Treatment F08
ACUITY™ Steerable Lead
- *use* Cardiac Lead, Pacemaker in 02H
- *use* Cardiac Lead, Defibrillator in O2H

Acupuncture
- Breast
  - Anesthesia 8E0H300
  - No Qualifier 8E0H30Z
- Integumentary System
  - Anesthesia 8E0H300
  - No Qualifier 8E0H30Z

Adductor brevis muscle
- *use* Upper Leg Muscle, Right
- *use* Upper Leg Muscle, Left

Adductor hallucis muscle
- *use* Foot Muscle, Right
- *use* Foot Muscle, Left

Adductor longus muscle
- *use* Upper Leg Muscle, Right
- *use* Upper Leg Muscle, Left

Adductor magnus muscle
- *use* Upper Leg Muscle, Right
- *use* Upper Leg Muscle, Left

Adenohypophysis *use* Pituitary Gland
Adenoidectomy
- *see* Excision, Adenoids 0CBQ
- *see* Resection, Adenoids 0CTQ

Adenoidotomy *see* Drainage, Adenoids 0C9Q
Adhesiolysis *see* Release
Administration
- Blood products *see* Transfusion
- Other substance *see* Introduction of substance in or on

Adrenalectomy
- *see* Excision, Endocrine System 0GB
- *see* Resection, Endocrine System 0GT

Adrenalorrhaphy *see* Repair, Endocrine System 0GQ
Adrenalotomy *see* Drainage, Endocrine System 0G9
Advancement
- *see* Reposition
- *see* Transfer

Advisa (MRI) *use* Pacemaker, Dual Chamber in 0JH
afami-cel *use* Afamitresgene Autoleucel Immunotherapy
Afamitresgene Autoleucel Immunotherapy XW0
AFX® Endovascular AAA System *use* Intraluminal Device
Aidoc briefcase for PE (pulmonary embolism) XXE3X27
AIGISRx Antibacterial Envelope *use* Anti-Infective Envelope
Alar ligament of axis *use* Head and Neck Bursa and Ligament
Alfapump® system *use* Other Device
Alimentation *see* Introduction of substance in or on
ALPPS (Associating liver partition and portal vein ligation)
- *see* Division, Hepatobiliary System and Pancreas 0F8
- *see* Resection, Hepatobiliary System and Pancreas 0FT

Alteration
- Abdominal Wall 0W0F
- Ankle Region
  - Left 0Y0L
  - Right 0Y0K

Alteration *(Continued)*
- Arm
  - Lower
    - Left 0X0F
    - Right 0X0D
  - Upper
    - Left 0X09
    - Right 0X08
- Axilla
  - Left 0X05
  - Right 0X04
- Back
  - Lower 0W0L
  - Upper 0W0K
- Breast
  - Bilateral 0H0V
  - Left 0H0U
  - Right 0H0T
- Buttock
  - Left 0Y01
  - Right 0Y00
- Chest Wall 0W08
- Ear
  - Bilateral 0902
  - Left 0901
  - Right 0900
- Elbow Region
  - Left 0X0C
  - Right 0X0B
- Extremity
  - Lower
    - Left 0Y0B
    - Right 0Y09
  - Upper
    - Left 0X07
    - Right 0X06
- Eyelid
  - Lower
    - Left 080R
    - Right 080Q
  - Upper
    - Left 080P
    - Right 080N
- Face 0W02
- Head 0W00
- Jaw
  - Lower 0W05
  - Upper 0W04
- Knee Region
  - Left 0Y0G
  - Right 0Y0F
- Leg
  - Lower
    - Left 0Y0J
    - Right 0Y0H
  - Upper
    - Left 0Y0D
    - Right 0Y0C
- Lip
  - Lower 0C01X
  - Upper 0C00X
- Nasal Mucosa and Soft Tissue 090K
- Neck 0W06
- Perineum
  - Female 0W0N
  - Male 0W0M
- Shoulder Region
  - Left 0X03
  - Right 0X02
- Subcutaneous Tissue and Fascia
  - Abdomen 0J08
  - Back 0J07
  - Buttock 0J09
  - Chest 0J06
  - Face 0J01
  - Lower Arm
    - Left 0J0H
    - Right 0J0G
  - Lower Leg
    - Left 0J0P
    - Right 0J0N

Alteration *(Continued)*
Subcutaneous Tissue and Fascia *(Continued)*
Neck
Left 0J05
Right 0J04
Upper Arm
Left 0J0F
Right 0J0D
Upper Leg
Left 0J0M
Right 0J0L
Alteration
Wrist Region
Left 0X0H
Right 0X0G
Alveolar process of mandible *use* Maxilla
Alveolar process of maxilla
use Maxilla, Right
use Maxilla, Left
Alveolectomy
see Excision, Head and Facial Bones 0NB
see Resection, Head and Facial Bones 0NT
Alveoloplasty
see Repair, Head and Facial Bones 0NQ
see Replacement, Head and Facial Bones 0NR
see Supplement, Head and Facial Bones 0NU
Alveolotomy
see Division, Head and Facial Bones 0N8
see Drainage, Head and Facial Bones 0N9
Ambulatory cardiac monitoring 4A12X45
Amivantamab monoclonal antibody XW0
Amniocentesis *see* Drainage, Products of Conception 1090
Amnioinfusion *see* Introduction of substance in or on, Products of Conception 3E0E
Amnioscopy 10J08ZZ
Amniotomy *see* Drainage, Products of Conception 1090
AMPLATZER® Muscular VSD Occluder *use* Synthetic Substitute
Amputation *see* Detachment
AMS 800® Urinary Control System *use* Artificial Sphincter in Urinary System
▶ **Anacaulase-bcdb** XW0
Anal orifice *use* Anus
Analog radiography *see* Plain Radiography
Analog radiology *see* Plain Radiography
Anastomosis *see* Bypass
Anatomical snuffbox
use Lower Arm and Wrist Muscle, Right
use Lower Arm and Wrist Muscle, Left
Andexanet Alfa, Factor Xa Inhibitor Reversal Agent *use* Coagulation Factor Xa, Inactivated
Andexxa *use* Coagulation Factor Xa, Inactivated
AneuRx® AAA Advantage® *use* Intraluminal Device
Angiectomy
see Excision, Heart and Great Vessels 02B
see Excision, Upper Arteries 03B
see Excision, Lower Arteries 04B
see Excision, Upper Veins 05B
see Excision, Lower Veins 06B
Angiocardiography
Combined right and left heart *see* Fluoroscopy, Heart, Right and Left B216
Left Heart *see* Fluoroscopy, Heart, Left B215
Right Heart *see* Fluoroscopy, Heart, Right B214
SPY system intravascular fluorescence *see* Monitoring, Physiological Systems 4A1
Angiography
see Computerized Tomography (CT Scan), Artery
see Fluoroscopy, Artery
see Magnetic Resonance Imaging (MRI), Artery
see Plain Radiography, Artery
Angioplasty
see Dilation, Heart and Great Vessels 027
see Repair, Heart and Great Vessels 02Q

Angioplasty *(Continued)*
see Replacement, Heart and Great Vessels 02R
see Supplement, Heart and Great Vessels 02U
see Dilation, Upper Arteries 037
see Repair, Upper Arteries 03Q
see Replacement, Upper Arteries 03R
see Supplement, Upper Arteries 03U
see Dilation, Lower Arteries 047
see Repair, Lower Arteries 04Q
see Replacement, Lower Arteries 04R
see Supplement, Lower Arteries 04U
Angiorrhaphy
see Repair, Heart and Great Vessels 02Q
see Repair, Upper Arteries 03Q
see Repair, Lower Arteries 04Q
Angioscopy
02JY4ZZ
03JY4ZZ
04JY4ZZ
➡ **Angiotensin II** *use* Vasopressor
Angiotripsy
see Occlusion, Upper Arteries 03L
see Occlusion, Lower Arteries 04L
Angular artery *use* Face Artery
Angular vein
use Face Vein, Right
use Face Vein, Left
▶ **Ankle Truss System™ (ATS)** *use* Internal Fixation Device, Open-truss Design in New Technology
Annular ligament
use Elbow Bursa and Ligament, Right
use Elbow Bursa and Ligament, Left
Annuloplasty
see Repair, Heart and Great Vessels 02Q
see Supplement, Heart and Great Vessels 02U
Annuloplasty ring *use* Synthetic Substitute
Anoplasty
see Repair, Anus 0DQQ
see Supplement, Anus 0DUQ
Anorectal junction *use* Rectum
Anoscopy 0DJD8ZZ
Ansa cervicalis *use* Cervical Plexus
Antabuse therapy HZ93ZZZ
Antebrachial fascia
use Subcutaneous Tissue and Fascia, Right Lower Arm
use Subcutaneous Tissue and Fascia, Left Lower Arm
Anterior (pectoral) lymph node
use Lymphatic, Right Axillary
use Lymphatic, Left Axillary
Anterior cerebral artery *use* Intracranial Artery
Anterior cerebral vein *use* Intracranial Vein
Anterior choroidal artery *use* Intracranial Artery
Anterior circumflex humeral artery
use Axillary Artery, Right
use Axillary Artery, Left
Anterior communicating artery *use* Intracranial Artery
Anterior cruciate ligament (ACL)
use Knee Bursa and Ligament, Right
use Knee Bursa and Ligament, Left
Anterior crural nerve *use* Femoral Nerve
Anterior facial vein
use Face Vein, Right
use Face Vein, Left
Anterior intercostal artery
use Internal Mammary Artery, Right
use Internal Mammary Artery, Left
Anterior interosseous nerve *use* Median Nerve
Anterior lateral malleolar artery
use Anterior Tibial Artery, Right
use Anterior Tibial Artery, Left
Anterior lingual gland *use* Minor Salivary Gland
Anterior medial malleolar artery
use Anterior Tibial Artery, Right
use Anterior Tibial Artery, Left

Anterior spinal artery
use Vertebral Artery, Right
use Vertebral Artery, Left
Anterior tibial recurrent artery
use Anterior Tibial Artery, Right
use Anterior Tibial Artery, Left
Anterior ulnar recurrent artery
use Ulnar Artery, Right
use Ulnar Artery, Left
Anterior vagal trunk *use* Vagus Nerve
Anterior vertebral muscle
use Neck Muscle, Right
use Neck Muscle, Left
Antibacterial Envelope (TYRX) (AIGISRx) *use* Anti-Infective Envelope
Antibiotic-eluting bone void filler XW0V0P7
Antigen-free air conditioning *see* Atmospheric Control, Physiological Systems 6A0
Antihelix
use External Ear, Right
use External Ear, Left
use External Ear, Bilateral
Antimicrobial envelope *use* Anti-Infective Envelope
Anti-SARS-CoV-2 hyperimmune globulin *use* Hyperimmune Globulin
Antitragus
use External Ear, Right
use External Ear, Left
use External Ear, Bilateral
Antrostomy *see* Drainage, Ear, Nose, Sinus 099
Antrotomy *see* Drainage, Ear, Nose, Sinus 099
Antrum of Highmore
use Maxillary Sinus, Right
use Maxillary Sinus, Left
Aortic annulus *use* Aortic Valve
Aortic arch *use* Thoracic Aorta, Ascending/Arch
Aortic intercostal artery *use* Upper Artery
▶ **Aortix™ System** *use* Short-term External Heart Assist System in Heart and Great Vessels
Aortography
see Plain Radiography, Upper Arteries B30
see Fluoroscopy, Upper Arteries B31
see Plain Radiography, Lower Arteries B40
see Fluoroscopy, Lower Arteries B41
Aortoplasty
see Repair, Aorta, Thoracic, Descending 02QW
see Repair, Aorta, Thoracic, Ascending/Arch 02QX
see Replacement, Aorta, Thoracic, Descending 02RW
see Replacement, Aorta, Thoracic, Ascending/Arch 02RX
see Supplement, Aorta, Thoracic, Descending 02UW
see Supplement, Aorta, Thoracic, Ascending/Arch 02UX
see Repair, Aorta, Abdominal 04Q0
see Replacement, Aorta, Abdominal 04R0
see Supplement, Aorta, Abdominal 04U0
Apalutamide Antineoplastic XW0DXJ5
Apical (subclavicular) lymph node
use Lymphatic, Axillary, Right
use Lymphatic, Axillary, Left
ApiFix® Minimally Invasive Deformity Correction (MID-C) system *use* Posterior (Dynamic)Distraction Device in New Technology
Apneustic center *use* Pons
Appendectomy
see Excision, Appendix 0DBJ
see Resection, Appendix 0DTJ
▶ **Appendiceal orifice** *use* Appendix
Appendicolysis *see* Release, Appendix 0DNJ
Appendicotomy *see* Drainage, Appendix 0D9J
Application *see* Introduction of substance in or on
➡ **Aprevo™** *use* Interbody Fusion Device, Custom-Made Anatomically Designed in New Technology

▶ New ➡ Revised ~~deleted~~ Deleted

A

Atlantoaxial joint *use* Cervical Vertebral Joint
Atmospheric Control 6A0Z
AtriClip LAA Exclusion System *use* Extraluminal Device **Atrioseptoplasty**
see Repair, Heart and Great Vessels 02Q
see Replacement, Heart and Great Vessels 02R
see Supplement, Heart and Great Vessels 02U
Atrioventricular node *use* Conduction Mechanism
Atrium dextrum cordis *use* Atrium, Right
Atrium pulmonale *use* Atrium, Left
Attain Ability® lead
use Cardiac Lead, Pacemaker in 02H
use Cardiac Lead, Defibrillator in 02H
Attain StarFix® (OTW) lead
use Cardiac Lead, Pacemaker in 02H
use Cardiac Lead, Defibrillator in O2H
Audiology, diagnostic
see Hearing Assessment, Diagnostic Audiology F13
see Hearing Aid Assessment, Diagnostic Audiology F14
see Vestibular Assessment, Diagnostic Audiology F15
Audiometry *see* Hearing Assessment, Diagnostic Audiology F13
Auditory tube
use Eustachian Tube, Right
use Eustachian Tube, Left
Auerbach's (myenteric) plexus *use* Nerve, Abdominal Sympathetic
Auricle
use External Ear, Right
use External Ear, Left
use External Ear, Bilateral
Auricularis muscle *use* Head Muscle
Autograft *use* Autologous Tissue Substitute
AutoLITT® System *see* Destruction
Autologous artery graft
use Autologous Arterial Tissue in Heart and Great Vessels
use Autologous Arterial Tissue in Upper Arteries
use Autologous Arterial Tissue in Lower Arteries
use Autologous Arterial Tissue in Upper Veins
use Autologous Arterial Tissue in Lower Veins
Autologous vein graft
use Autologous Venous Tissue in Heart and Great Vessels
use Autologous Venous Tissue in Upper Arteries
use Autologous Venous Tissue in Lower Arteries
use Autologous Venous Tissue in Upper Veins
use Autologous Venous Tissue in Lower Veins
Automated chest compression (ACC) 5A1221J
AutoPulse® resuscitation system 5A1221J
Autotransfusion *see* Transfusion
Autotransplant
Adrenal tissue *see* Reposition, Endocrine System 0GS
Kidney
see Reposition, Urinary System 0TS
Pancreatic tissue *see* Reposition, Pancreas 0FSG
Autotransplant *(Continued)*
Parathyroid tissue *see* Reposition, Endocrine System 0GS
Thyroid tissue *see* Reposition, Endocrine System 0GS
Tooth *see* Reattachment, Mouth and Throat 0CM
▶ **Aveir™ AR, as dual chamber** *use* Intracardiac Pacemaker, Dual-Chamber in New Technology
▶ **Aveir™ DR, dual chamber** *use* Intracardiac Pacemaker, Dual-Chamber in New Technology
▶ **Aveir™ VR, as single chamber** *use* Intracardiac Pacemaker in Heart and Great Vessels
Avulsion *see* Extraction
AVYCAZ® (ceftazidime-avibactam) *use* Other Anti-infective
Axial Lumbar Interbody Fusion System *use* Interbody Fusion Device in Lower Joints
AxiaLIF® System *use* Interbody Fusion Device in Lower Joints
Axicabtagene Ciloleucel *use* Axicabtagene Ciloleucel Immunotherapy
Axicabtagene Ciloleucel Immunotherapy XW0
Axillary fascia
use Subcutaneous Tissue and Fascia, Right Upper Arm
use Subcutaneous Tissue and Fascia, Left Upper Arm
Axillary nerve *use* Brachial Plexus
AZEDRA *use* Iobenguane I-131 Antineoplastic

B

BAK/C® Interbody Cervical Fusion System *use* Interbody Fusion Device in Upper Joints
BAL (bronchial alveolar lavage), diagnostic *see* Drainage, Respiratory System 0B9
Balanoplasty
see Repair, Penis 0VQS
see Supplement, Penis 0VUS
Balloon atrial septostomy (BAS) 02163Z7
Balloon Pump
Continuous, Output 5A02210
Intermittent, Output 5A02110
Bamlanivimab monoclonal antibody XW0
Bandage, Elastic *see* Compression
Banding
see Occlusion
see Restriction
Banding, esophageal varices *see* Occlusion, Vein, Esophageal 06L3
Banding, laparoscopic (adjustable) gastric
Surgical correction *see* Revision of device in, Stomach 0DW6
Initial procedure 0DV64CZ
Bard® Composix® (E/X) (LP) mesh *use* Synthetic Substitute
Bard® Composix® Kugel® patch *use* Synthetic Substitute
Bard® Dulex™ mesh *use* Synthetic Substitute
Bard® Ventralex™ hernia patch *use* Synthetic Substitute
Baricitinib XW0
Barium swallow *see* Fluoroscopy, Gastrointestinal System BD1
Baroreflex Activation Therapy® (BAT®)
use Stimulator Generator in Subcutaneous Tissue and Fascia
use Stimulator Lead in Upper Arteries
Barricaid® Annular Closure Device (ACD) *use* Synthetic Substitute
Bartholin's (greater vestibular) gland *use* Vestibular Gland
Basal (internal) cerebral vein *use* Intracranial Vein
Basal metabolic rate (BMR) *see* Measurement, Physiological Systems 4A0Z
Basal nuclei *use* Basal Ganglia
Base of Tongue *use* Pharynx
Basilar artery *use* Intracranial Artery
Basis pontis *use* Pons
Beam Radiation
Abdomen DW03
Intraoperative DW033Z0
Adrenal Gland DG02
Intraoperative DG023Z0
Bile Ducts DF02
Intraoperative DF023Z0
Bladder DT02
Intraoperative DT023Z0
Bone
Other DP0C
Intraoperative DP0C3Z0
Bone Marrow D700
Intraoperative D7003Z0
Brain D000
Intraoperative D0003Z0
Brain Stem D001
Intraoperative D0013Z0
Breast
Left DM00
Intraoperative DM003Z0
Right DM01
Intraoperative DM013Z0
Bronchus DB01
Intraoperative DB013Z0
Cervix DU01
Intraoperative DU013Z0
Chest DW02
Intraoperative DW023Z0
Chest Wall DB07
Intraoperative DB073Z0

Beam Radiation *(Continued)*
Colon DD05
Intraoperative DD053Z0
Diaphragm DB08
Intraoperative DB083Z0
Duodenum DD02
Intraoperative DD023Z0
Ear D900
Intraoperative D9003Z0
Esophagus DD00
Intraoperative DD003Z0
Eye D800
Intraoperative D8003Z0
Femur DP09
Intraoperative DP093Z0
Fibula DP0B
Intraoperative DP0B3Z0
Gallbladder DF01
Intraoperative DF013Z0
Gland
Adrenal DG02
Intraoperative DG023Z0
Parathyroid DG04
Intraoperative DG043Z0
Pituitary DG00
Intraoperative DG003Z0
Thyroid DG05
Intraoperative DG053Z0
Glands
Salivary D906
Intraoperative D9063Z0
Head and Neck DW01
Intraoperative DW013Z0
Hemibody DW04
Intraoperative DW043Z0
Humerus DP06
Intraoperative DP063Z0
Hypopharynx D903
Intraoperative D9033Z0
Ileum DD04
Intraoperative DD043Z0
Jejunum DD03
Intraoperative DD033Z0
Kidney DT00
Intraoperative DT003Z0
Larynx D90B
Intraoperative D90B3Z0
Liver DF00
Intraoperative DF003Z0
Lung DB02
Intraoperative DB023Z0
Lymphatics
Abdomen D706
Intraoperative D7063Z0
Axillary D704
Intraoperative D7043Z0
Inguinal D708
Intraoperative D7083Z0
Neck D703
Intraoperative D7033Z0
Pelvis D707
Intraoperative D7073Z0
Thorax D705
Intraoperative D7053Z0
Mandible DP03
Intraoperative DP033Z0
Maxilla DP02
Intraoperative DP023Z0
Mediastinum DB06
Intraoperative DB063Z0
Mouth D904
Intraoperative D9043Z0
Nasopharynx D90D
Intraoperative D90D3Z0
Neck and Head DW01
Intraoperative DW013Z0
Nerve
Peripheral D007
Intraoperative D0073Z0
Nose D901
Intraoperative D9013Z0
Oropharynx D90F
Intraoperative D90F3Z0

Beam Radiation *(Continued)*
Ovary DU00
Intraoperative DU003Z0
Palate
Hard D908
Intraoperative D9083Z0
Soft D909
Intraoperative D9093Z0
Pancreas DF03
Intraoperative DF033Z0
Parathyroid Gland DG04
Intraoperative DG043Z0
Pelvic Bones DP08
Intraoperative DP083Z0
Pelvic Region DW06
Intraoperative DW063Z0
Pineal Body DG01
Intraoperative DG013Z0
Pituitary Gland DG00
Intraoperative DG003Z0
Pleura DB05
Intraoperative DB053Z0
Prostate DV00
Intraoperative DV003Z0
Radius DP07
Intraoperative DP073Z0
Rectum DD07
Intraoperative DD073Z0
Rib DP05
Intraoperative DP053Z0
Sinuses D907
Intraoperative D9073Z0
Skin
Abdomen DH08
Intraoperative DH083Z0
Arm DH04
Intraoperative DH043Z0
Back DH07
Intraoperative DH073Z0
Buttock DH09
Intraoperative DH093Z0
Chest DH06
Intraoperative DH063Z0
Face DH02
Intraoperative DH023Z0
Leg DH0B
Intraoperative DH0B3Z0
Neck DH03
Intraoperative DH033Z0
Skull DP00
Intraoperative DP003Z0
Spinal Cord D006
Intraoperative D0063Z0
Spleen D702
Intraoperative D7023Z0
Sternum DP04
Intraoperative DP043Z0
Stomach DD01
Intraoperative DD013Z0
Testis DV01
Intraoperative DV013Z0
Thymus D701
Intraoperative D7013Z0
Thyroid Gland DG05
Intraoperative DG053Z0
Tibia DP0B
Intraoperative DP0B3Z0
Tongue D905
Intraoperative D9053Z0
Trachea DB00
Intraoperative DB003Z0
Ulna DP07
Intraoperative DP073Z0
Ureter DT01
Intraoperative DT013Z0
Urethra DT03
Intraoperative DT033Z0
Uterus DU02
Intraoperative DU023Z0
Whole Body DW05
Intraoperative DW053Z0

Bedside swallow F00ZJWZ
Berlin Heart Ventricular Assist Device *use* Implantable Heart Assist System in Heart and Great Vessels
beti-cel *use* Betibeglogene Autotemcel
Betibeglogene Autotemcel XW1
Bezlotoxumab infusion *see* Introduction with qualifier Other Therapeutic Monoclonal Antibody
Biceps brachii muscle
  use Upper Arm Muscle, Right
  use Upper Arm Muscle, Left
Biceps femoris muscle
  use Upper Leg Muscle, Right
  use Upper Leg Muscle, Left
Bicipital aponeurosis
  use Subcutaneous Tissue and Fascia, Right Lower Arm
  use Subcutaneous Tissue and Fascia, Left Lower Arm
Bicuspid valve *use* Mitral Valve
Bill light therapy *see* Phototherapy, Skin 6A60
Bioactive embolization coil(s) *use* Intraluminal Device, Bioactive in Upper Arteries
Bioengineered allogeneic construct, skin XHRPXF7
Biofeedback GZC9ZZZ
BioFire® Film Array® Pneumonia Panel XXEBXQ6
Biopsy
  see Drainage with qualifier Diagnostic
  see Excision with qualifier Diagnostic
  see Extraction with qualifier Diagnostic
BiPAP *see* Assistance, Respiratory 5A09
Bisection *see* Division
Biventricular external heart assist system *use* Short-term External Heart Assist System in Heart and Great Vessels
Blepharectomy
  see Excision, Eye 08B
  see Resection, Eye 08T
Blepharoplasty
  see Repair, Eye 08Q
  see Replacement, Eye 08R
  see Reposition, Eye 08S
  see Supplement, Eye 08U
Blepharorrhaphy *see* Repair, Eye 08Q
Blepharotomy *see* Drainage, Eye 089
Blinatumomab *use* Other Antineoplastic
BLINCYTO® (blinatumomab) *use* Other Antineoplastic
Block, Nerve, anesthetic injection 3E0T3BZ
Blood glucose monitoring system *use* Monitoring Device
Blood pressure *see* Measurement, Arterial 4A03
BMR (basal metabolic rate) *see* Measurement, Physiological Systems 4A0Z
Body of femur
  use Femoral Shaft, Right
  use Femoral Shaft, Left
Body of fibula
  use Fibula, Right
  use Fibula, Left
Bone anchored hearing device
  use Hearing Device, Bone Conduction in 09H
  use Hearing Device, in Head and Facial Bones
Bone bank bone graft *use* Nonautologous Tissue Substitute
Bone Growth Stimulator
  Insertion of device in
    Bone
      Facial 0NHW
      Lower 0QHY
      Nasal 0NHB
      Upper 0PHY
    Skull 0NH0
  Removal of device from
    Bone
      Facial 0NPW
      Lower 0QPY
      Nasal 0NPB
      Upper 0PPY
    Skull 0NP0
Bone Growth Stimulator *(Continued)*
  Revision of device in
    Bone
      Facial 0NWW
      Lower 0QWY
      Nasal 0NWB
      Upper 0PWY
    Skull 0NW0
Bone marrow transplant *see* Transfusion, Circulatory 302
Bone morphogenetic protein 2 (BMP 2) *use* Recombinant Bone Morphogenetic Protein
Bone screw (interlocking) (lag) (pedicle) (recessed)
  use Internal Fixation Device in Head and Facial Bones
  use Internal Fixation Device in Upper Bones
  use Internal Fixation Device in Lower Bones
Bony labyrinth
  use Inner Ear, Right
  use Inner Ear, Left
Bony orbit
  use Orbit, Right
  use Orbit, Left
Bony vestibule
  use Inner Ear, Right
  use Inner Ear, Left
Botallo's duct *use* Pulmonary Artery, Left
Bovine pericardial valve *use* Zooplastic Tissue in Heart and Great Vessels
Bovine pericardium graft *use* Zooplastic Tissue in Heart and Great Vessels
BP (blood pressure) *see* Measurement, Arterial 4A03
Brachial (lateral) lymph node
  use Lymphatic, Axillary Right
  use Lymphatic, Axillary Left
Brachialis muscle
  use Upper Arm Muscle, Right
  use Upper Arm Muscle, Left
Brachiocephalic artery *use* Innominate Artery
Brachiocephalic trunk *use* Innominate Artery
Brachiocephalic vein
  use Innominate Vein, Right
  use Innominate Vein, Left
Brachioradialis muscle
  use Lower Arm and Wrist Muscle, Right
  use Lower Arm and Wrist Muscle, Left
Brachytherapy
  Abdomen DW13
  Adrenal Gland DG12
  Back
    Lower DW1LBB
    Upper DW1KBB
  Bile Ducts DF12
  Bladder DT12
  Bone Marrow D710
  Brain D010
  Brain Stem D011
  Breast
    Left DM10
    Right DM11
  Bronchus DB11
  Cervix DU11
  Chest DW12
  Chest Wall DB17
  Colon DD15
  Cranial Cavity DW10BB
  Diaphragm DB18
  Duodenum DD12
  Ear D910
  Esophagus DD10
  Extremity
    Lower DW1YBB
    Upper DW1XBB
  Eye D810
  Gallbladder DF11
  Gastrointestinal Tract DW1PBB
  Genitourinary Tract DW1RBB
  Gland
    Adrenal DG12
    Parathyroid DG14
Brachytherapy *(Continued)*
  Gland *(Continued)*
    Pituitary DG10
    Thyroid DG15
  Glands, Salivary D916
  Head and Neck DW11
  Hypopharynx D913
  Ileum DD14
  Jejunum DD13
  Kidney DT10
  Larynx D91B
  Liver DF10
  Lung DB12
  Lymphatics
    Abdomen D716
    Axillary D714
    Inguinal D718
    Neck D713
    Pelvis D717
    Thorax D715
  Mediastinum DB16
  Mouth D914
  Nasopharynx D91D
  Neck and Head DW11
  Nerve, Peripheral D017
  Nose D911
  Oropharynx D91F
  Ovary DU10
  Palate
    Hard D918
    Soft D919
  Pancreas DF13
  Parathyroid Gland DG14
  Pelvic Region DW16
  Pineal Body DG11
  Pituitary Gland DG10
  Pleura DB15
  Prostate DV10
  Rectum DD17
  Respiratory Tract DW1QBB
  Sinuses D917
  Spinal Cord D016
  Spleen D712
  Stomach DD11
  Testis DV11
  Thymus D711
  Thyroid Gland DG15
  Tongue D915
  Trachea DB10
  Ureter DT11
  Urethra DT13
  Uterus DU12
Brachytherapy, CivaSheet®
  see Brachytherapy with qualifier Unidirectional Source
  see Insertion with device Radioactive Element
Brachytherapy seeds *use* Radioactive Element
~~Brain Electrical Activity, Computer-aided Semiologic Analysis XXE0X48~~
▶Brain Electrical Activity
  ▶Computer-aided Detection and Notification XX20X89
  ▶Computer-aided Semiologic Analysis XXE0X48
Broad Consortium Microbiota-based Live Biotherapeutic Suspension XW0H7X8
Breast procedures, skin only *use* Skin, Chest
Brexanolone XW0
Brexucabtagene Autoleucel *use* Brexucatagene Autoleucel Immunotherapy
Brexucabtagene Autoleucel Immunotherapy XW0
Broad ligament *use* Uterine Supporting Structure
➡Bromelain-enriched proteolytic enzyme *use* Anacaulase-bcdb
Bronchial artery *use* Upper Artery
Bronchography
  see Plain Radiography, Respiratory System BB0
  see Fluoroscopy, Respiratory System BB1
Bronchoplasty
  see Repair, Respiratory System 0BQ
  see Supplement, Respiratory System 0BU

▶ New ➡ Revised ~~deleted~~ Deleted

Bronchorrhaphy *see* Repair, Respiratory System 0BQ
Bronchoscopy 0BJ08ZZ
Bronchotomy *see* Drainage, Respiratory System 0B9
Bronchus Intermedius *use* Main Bronchus, Right
BRYAN® Cervical Disc System *use* Synthetic Substitute
Buccal gland *use* Buccal Mucosa
Buccinator lymph node *use* Lymphatic, Head
Buccinator muscle *use* Facial Muscle
Buckling, scleral with implant *see* Supplement, Eye 08U
Bulbospongiosus muscle *use* Perineum Muscle
Bulbourethral (Cowper's) gland *use* Urethra
Bundle of His *use* Conduction Mechanism
Bundle of Kent *use* Conduction Mechanism
Bunionectomy *see* Excision, Lower Bones 0QB
Bursectomy
 see Excision, Bursae and Ligaments 0MB
 see Resection, Bursae and Ligaments 0MT
Bursocentesis *see* Drainage, Bursae and Ligaments 0M9
Bursography
 see Plain Radiography, Non-Axial Upper Bones BP0
 see Plain Radiography, Non-Axial Lower Bones BQ0
Bursotomy
 see Division, Bursae and Ligaments 0M8
 see Drainage, Bursae and Ligaments 0M9
BVS 5000 Ventricular Assist Device *use* Short-term External Heart Assist System in Heart and Great Vessels
Bypass
 Anterior Chamber
  Left 08133
  Right 08123
 Aorta
  Abdominal 0410
  Thoracic
   Ascending/Arch 021X
   Descending 021W
 Artery
  Anterior Tibial
   Left 041Q
   Right 041P
  Axillary
   Left 03160
   Right 03150
  Brachial
   Left 0318
   Right 0317
  Common Carotid
   Left 031J0
   Right 031H0
  Common Iliac
   Left 041D
   Right 041C
  Coronary
   Four or More Arteries 0213
   One Artery 0210
   Three Arteries 0212
   Two Arteries 0211
  External Carotid
   Left 031N0
   Right 031M0
  External Iliac
   Left 041J
   Right 041H
  Femoral
   Left 041L
   Right 041K
  Foot
   Left 041W
   Right 041V
  Hepatic 0413
  Innominate 03120
  Internal Carotid
   Left 031L0
   Right 031K0
  Internal Iliac
   Left 041F
   Right 041E

Bypass *(Continued)*
 Artery *(Continued)*
  Intracranial 031G0
  Peroneal
   Left 041U
   Right 041T
  Popliteal
   Left 041N
   Right 041M
  Posterior Tibial
   Left 041S
   Right 041R
  Pulmonary
   Left 021R
   Right 021Q
  Pulmonary Trunk 021P
  Radial
   Left 031C
   Right 031B
  Splenic 0414
  Subclavian
   Left 03140
   Right 03130
  Temporal
   Left 031T0
   Right 031S0
  Ulnar
   Left 031A
   Right 0319
 Atrium
  Left 0217
  Right 0216
 Bladder 0T1B
 Cavity, Cranial 0W110J
 Cecum 0D1H
 Cerebral Ventricle 0016
 Colon
  Ascending 0D1K
  Descending 0D1M
  Sigmoid 0D1N
  Transverse 0D1L
 ▶Conduit through Femoral Vein to Popliteal Artery X2K
 ▶Conduit through Femoral Vein to Superficial Femoral Artery X2K
 Duct
  Common Bile 0F19
  Cystic 0F18
  Hepatic
   Common 0F17
   Left 0F16
   Right 0F15
  Lacrimal
   Left 081Y
   Right 081X
  Pancreatic 0F1D
   Accessory 0F1F
 Duodenum 0D19
 Ear
  Left 091E0
  Right 091D0
 Esophagus 0D15
  Lower 0D13
  Middle 0D12
  Upper 0D11
 Fallopian Tube
  Left 0U16
  Right 0U15
 Gallbladder 0F14
 Ileum 0D1B
 Intestine
  Large 0D1E
  Small 0D1E
 Jejunum 0D1A
 Kidney Pelvis
  Left 0T14
  Right 0T13
 Pancreas 0F1G
 Pelvic Cavity 0W1J
 Peritoneal Cavity 0W1G
 Pleural Cavity
  Left 0W1B
  Right 0W19

Bypass *(Continued)*
 Spinal Canal 001U
 Stomach 0D16
 Trachea 0B11
 Ureter
  Left 0T17
  Right 0T16
 Vein Ureters, Bilateral 0T18
 Vas Deferens
  Bilateral 0V1Q
  Left 0V1P
  Right 0V1N
  Axillary
   Left 0518
   Right 0517
  Azygos 0510
  Basilic
   Left 051C
   Right 051B
  Brachial
   Left 051A
   Right 0519
  Cephalic
   Left 051F
   Right 051D
  Colic 0617
  Common Iliac
   Left 061D
   Right 061C
  Esophageal 0613
  External Iliac
   Left 061G
   Right 061F
  External Jugular
   Left 051Q
   Right 051P
  Face
   Left 051V
   Right 051T
  Femoral
   Left 061N
   Right 061M
  Foot
   Left 061V
   Right 061T
  Gastric 0612
  Hand
   Left 051H
   Right 051G
  Hemiazygos 0511
  Hepatic 0614
  Hypogastric
   Left 061J
   Right 061H
  Inferior Mesenteric 0616
  Innominate
   Left 0514
   Right 0513
  Internal Jugular
   Left 051N
   Right 051M
  Intracranial 051L
  Portal 0618
  Renal
   Left 061B
   Right 0619
  Saphenous
   Left 061Q
   Right 061P
  Splenic 0611
  Subclavian
   Left 0516
   Right 0515
  Superior Mesenteric 0615
  Vertebral
   Left 051S
   Right 051R
 Vena Cava
  Inferior 0610
  Superior 021V
 Ventricle
  Left 021L
  Right 021K
Bypass, cardiopulmonary 5A1221Z

C

Caesarean section *see* Extraction, Products of Conception 10D0
Calcaneocuboid joint
- *use* Tarsal Joint, Right
- *use* Tarsal Joint, Left

Calcaneocuboid ligament
- *use* Foot Bursa and Ligament, Right
- *use* Foot Bursa and Ligament, Left

Calcaneofibular ligament
- *use* Ankle Bursa and Ligament, Right
- *use* Ankle Bursa and Ligament, Left

Calcaneus
- *use* Tarsal, Right
- *use* Tarsal, Left

Cannulation
- *see* Bypass
- *see* Dilation
- *see* Drainage
- *see* Irrigation

Canthorrhaphy *see* Repair, Eye 08Q
Canthotomy *see* Release, Eye 08N
▶Canturio™ te (Tibial Extension) *use* Tibial Extension with Motion Sensors in New Technology
Capitate bone
- *use* Carpal, Right
- *use* Carpal, Left

Caplacizumab XW0
Capsulectomy, lens *see* Excision, Eye 08B
Capsulorrhaphy, joint
- *see* Repair, Upper Joints 0RQ
- *see* Repair, Lower Joints 0SQ

Caption guidance system X2JAX47
Cardia *use* Esophagogastric Junction
Cardiac contractility modulation lead *use* Cardiac Lead in Heart and Great Vessels
Cardiac event recorder *use* Monitoring Device
Cardiac Lead
- Defibrillator
  - Atrium
    - Left 02H7
    - Right 02H6
  - Pericardium 02HN
  - Vein, Coronary 02H4
  - Ventricle
    - Left 02HL
    - Right 02HK
- Insertion of device in
  - Atrium
    - Left 02H7
    - Right 02H6
  - Pericardium 02HN
  - Vein, Coronary 02H4
  - Ventricle
    - Left 02HL
    - Right 02HK
- Pacemaker
  - Atrium
    - Left 02H7
    - Right 02H6
  - Pericardium 02HN
  - Vein, Coronary 02H4
  - Ventricle
    - Left 02HL
    - Right 02HK
- Removal of device from, Heart 02PA
- Revision of device in, Heart 02WA

Cardiac plexus *use* Nerve, Thoracic Sympathetic
Cardiac Resynchronization Defibrillator Pulse Generator
- Abdomen 0JH8
- Chest 0JH6

Cardiac Resynchronization Pacemaker Pulse Generator
- Abdomen 0JH8
- Chest 0JH6

Cardiac resynchronization therapy (CRT) lead
- *use* Cardiac Lead, Pacemaker in O2H
- *use* Cardiac Lead, Defibrillator in 02H

Cardiac Rhythm Related Device
- Insertion of device in
- Abdomen 0JH8
- Chest 0JH6
- Removal of device from, Subcutaneous Tissue and Fascia, Trunk 0JPT
- Revision of device in, Subcutaneous Tissue and Fascia, Trunk 0JWT

Cardiocentesis *see* Drainage, Pericardial Cavity 0W9D
Cardioesophageal junction *use* Esophagogastric Junction
Cardiolysis *see* Release, Heart and Great Vessels 02N
CardioMEMS® pressure sensor *use* Monitoring Device, Pressure Sensor in 02H
Cardiomyotomy *see* Division, Esophagogastric Junction 0D84
Cardioplegia *see* Introduction of substance in or on, Heart 3E08
Cardiorrhaphy *see* Repair, Heart and Great Vessels 02Q
Cardioversion 5A2204Z
Caregiver Training F0FZ
Carmat total artificial heart (TAH) *use* Biologic with Synthetic Substitute, Autoregulated Electrohydraulic in 02R
Caroticotympanic artery
- *use* Internal Carotid Artery, Right
- *use* Internal Carotid Artery, Left

Carotid (artery) sinus (baroreceptor) lead *use* Stimulator Lead in Upper Arteries
Carotid glomus
- *use* Carotid Body, Left
- *use* Carotid Body, Right
- *use* Carotid Bodies, Bilateral

Carotid sinus
- *use* Internal Carotid Artery, Right
- *use* Internal Carotid Artery, Left

Carotid sinus nerve *use* Glossopharyngeal Nerve
Carotid WALLSTENT® Monorail® Endoprosthesis *use* Intraluminal Device
Carpectomy
- *see* Excision, Upper Bones 0PB
- *see* Resection, Upper Bones 0PT

Carpometacarpal ligament
- *use* Hand Bursa and Ligament, Right
- *use* Hand Bursa and Ligament, Left

CARVYKTI™ *use* Ciltacabtagene Autoleucel
Casirivimab (REGN10933) and Imdevimab (REGN10987) *use* REGN-COV2 Monoclonal Antibody
Casting *see* Immobilization
CAT scan *see* Computerized Tomography (CT Scan)
Catheterization
- *see* Dilation
- *see* Drainage
- *see* Insertion of device in
- *see* Irrigation
- Heart *see* Measurement, Cardiac 4A02
- Umbilical vein, for infusion 06H033T

Cauda equina *use* Lumbar Spinal Cord
Cauterization
- *see* Destruction
- *see* Repair

Cavernous plexus *use* Head and Neck Sympathetic Nerve
Cavoatrial junction *use* Superior Vena Cava
CBMA (Concentrated Bone Marrow Aspirate) *use* Other Substance
CBMA (Concentrated Bone Marrow Aspirate) injection *see* Introduction of substance in or on, Muscle 3E02
CD24Fc Immunomodulator XW0
Cecectomy
- *see* Excision, Cecum 0DBH
- *see* Resection, Cecum 0DTH

Cecocolostomy
- *see* Bypass, Gastrointestinal System 0D1
- *see* Drainage, Gastrointestinal System 0D9

Cecopexy
- *see* Repair, Cecum 0DQH
- *see* Reposition, Cecum 0DSH

Cecoplication *see* Restriction, Cecum 0DVH
Cecorrhaphy *see* Repair, Cecum 0DQH
Cecostomy
- *see* Bypass, Cecum 0D1H
- *see* Drainage, Cecum 0D9H

Cecotomy *see* Drainage, Cecum 0D9H
Cefiderocol Anti-infective XW0
Ceftazidime-avibactam *use* Other Anti-infective
Ceftolozane/Tazobactam Anti-infective XW0
Celiac (solar) plexus *use* Abdominal Sympathetic Nerve
Celiac ganglion *use* Abdominal Sympathetic Nerve
Celiac lymph node *use* Lymphatic, Aortic
Celiac trunk *use* Celiac Artery
Central axillary lymph node
- *use* Lymphatic, Right Axillary
- *use* Lymphatic, Left Axillary

Central venous pressure *see* Measurement, Venous 4A04
Centrimag® Blood Pump *use* Short-term External Heart Assist System in Heart and Great Vessels
Cephalogram BN00ZZZ
CERAMENT® G *use* Antibiotic-eluting Bone Void Filler
Ceramic on ceramic bearing surface *use* Synthetic Substitute, Ceramic in 0SR
Cerclage *see* Restriction
Cerebral aqueduct (Sylvius) *use* Cerebral Ventricle
Cerebral Embolic Filtration
- Duel Filter X2A5312
- Extracorporeal Flow Reversal Circuit X2A
- Single Deflection Filter X2A6325

Cerebrum *use* Brain
▶Ceribell® Monitor XX20X89
Cervical esophagus *use* Esophagus, Upper
Cervical facet joint
- *use* Cervical Vertebral Joint
- *use* Cervical Vertebral Joint, 2 or more

Cervical ganglion *use* Head and Neck Sympathetic Nerve
Cervical interspinous ligament *use* Head and Neck Bursa and Ligament
Cervical intertransverse ligament *use* Head and Neck Bursa and Ligament
Cervical ligamentum flavum *use* Head and Neck Bursa and Ligament
Cervical lymph node
- *use* Lymphatic, Right Neck
- *use* Lymphatic, Left Neck

Cervicectomy
- *see* Excision, Cervix 0UBC
- *see* Resection, Cervix 0UTC

Cervicothoracic facet joint *use* Cervicothoracic Vertebral Joint
Cesarean section *see* Extraction, Products of Conception 10D0
Cesium-131 Collagen Implant *use* Radioactive Element, Cesium-131 Collagen Implant in 00H
Change device in
- Abdominal Wall 0W2FX
- Back
  - Lower 0W2LX
  - Upper 0W2KX
- Bladder 0T2BX
- Bone
  - Facial 0N2WX
  - Lower 0Q2YX
  - Nasal 0N2BX
  - Upper 0P2YX
- Bone Marrow 072TX
- Brain 0020X
- Breast
  - Left 0H2UX
  - Right 0H2TX

C

▶ New ➡ Revised ~~deleted~~ Deleted

Change device in *(Continued)*
Bursa and Ligament
Lower 0M2YX
Upper 0M2XX
Cavity, Cranial 0W21X
Chest Wall 0W28X
Cisterna Chyli 072LX
Diaphragm 0B2TX
Duct
Hepatobiliary 0F2BX
Pancreatic 0F2DX
Ear
Left 092JX
Right 092HX
Epididymis and Spermatic Cord 0V2MX
Extremity
Lower
Left 0Y2BX
Right 0Y29X
Upper
Left 0X27X
Right 0X26X
Eye
Left 0821X
Right 0820X
Face 0W22X
Fallopian Tube 0U28X
Gallbladder 0F24X
Gland
Adrenal 0G25X
Endocrine 0G2SX
Pituitary 0G20X
Salivary 0C2AX
Head 0W20X
Intestinal Tract
Lower Intestinal Tract 0D2DXUZ
Upper Intestinal Tract 0D20XUZ
Jaw
Lower 0W25X
Upper 0W24X
Joint
Lower 0S2YX
Upper 0R2YX
Kidney 0T25X
Larynx 0C2SX
Liver 0F20X
Lung
Left 0B2LX
Right 0B2KX
Lymphatic 072NX
Thoracic Duct 072KX
Mediastinum 0W2CX
Mesentery 0D2VX
Mouth and Throat 0C2YX
Muscle
Lower 0K2YX
Upper 0K2XX
Nasal Mucosa and Soft Tissue 092KX
Neck 0W26X
Nerve
Cranial 002EX
Peripheral 012YX
Omentum 0D2UX
Ovary 0U23X
Pancreas 0F2GX
Parathyroid Gland 0G2RX
Pelvic Cavity 0W2JX
Penis 0V2SX
Pericardial Cavity 0W2DX
Perineum
Female 0W2NX
Male 0W2MX
Peritoneal Cavity 0W2GX
Peritoneum 0D2WX
Pineal Body 0G21X
Pleura 0B2QX
Pleural Cavity
Left 0W2BX
Right 0W29X
Products of Conception 10207
Prostate and Seminal Vesicles 0V24X

Change device in *(Continued)*
Retroperitoneum 0W2HX
Scrotum and Tunica Vaginalis 0V28X
Sinus 092YX
Skin 0H2PX
Skull 0N20X
Spinal Canal 002UX
Spleen 072PX
Subcutaneous Tissue and Fascia
Head and Neck 0J2SX
Lower Extremity 0J2WX
Trunk 0J2TX
Upper Extremity 0J2VX
Tendon
Lower 0L2YX
Upper 0L2XX
Testis 0V2DX
Thymus 072MX
Thyroid Gland 0G2KX
Trachea 0B21
Tracheobronchial Tree 0B20X
Ureter 0T29X
Urethra 0T2DX
Uterus and Cervix 0U2DXHZ
Vagina and Cul-de-sac 0U2HXGZ
Vas Deferens 0V2RX
Vulva 0U2MX
Change device in or on
Abdominal Wall 2W03X
Anorectal 2Y03X5Z
Arm
Lower
Left 2W0DX
Right 2W0CX
Upper
Left 2W0BX
Right 2W0AX
Back 2W05X
Chest Wall 2W04X
Ear 2Y02X5Z
Extremity
Lower
Left 2W0MX
Right 2W0LX
Upper
Left 2W09X
Right 2W08X
Face 2W01X
Finger
Left 2W0KX
Right 2W0JX
Foot
Left 2W0TX
Right 2W0SX
Genital Tract, Female 2Y04X5Z
Hand
Left 2W0FX
Right 2W0EX
Head 2W00X
Inguinal Region
Left 2W07X
Right 2W06X
Leg
Lower
Left 2W0RX
Right 2W0QX
Upper
Left 2W0PX
Right 2W0NX
Mouth and Pharynx 2Y00X5Z
Nasal 2Y01X5Z
Neck 2W02X
Thumb
Left 2W0HX
Right 2W0GX
Toe
Left 2W0VX
Right 2W0UX
Urethra 2Y05X5Z
Chemoembolization *see* Introduction of substance in or on

Chemosurgery, Skin 3E00XTZ
Chemothalamectomy *see* Destruction, Thalamus 0059
Chemotherapy, Infusion for cancer *see* Introduction of substance in or on
Chest compression (CPR), external
Manual 5A12012
Mechanical 5A1221J
Chest x-ray *see* Plain Radiography, Chest BW03
▶ Chin *use* Subcutaneous Tissue and Fascia, Face
Chiropractic Manipulation
Abdomen 9WB9X
Cervical 9WB1X
Extremities
Lower 9WB6X
Upper 9WB7X
Head 9WB0X
Lumbar 9WB3X
Pelvis 9WB5X
Rib Cage 9WB8X
Sacrum 9WB4X
Thoracic 9WB2X
Choana *use* Nasopharynx
Cholangiogram
see Plain Radiography, Hepatobiliary System and Pancreas BF0
see Fluoroscopy, Hepatobiliary System and Pancreas BF1
Cholecystectomy
see Excision, Gallbladder 0FB4
see Resection, Gallbladder 0FT4
Cholecystojejunostomy
see Bypass, Hepatobiliary System and Pancreas 0F1
see Drainage, Hepatobiliary System and Pancreas 0F9
Cholecystopexy
see Repair, Gallbladder 0FQ4
see Reposition, Gallbladder 0FS4
Cholecystoscopy 0FJ44ZZ
Cholecystostomy
see Bypass, Gallbladder 0F14
see Drainage, Gallbladder 0F94
Cholecystotomy *see* Drainage, Gallbladder 0F94
Choledochectomy
see Excision, Hepatobiliary System and Pancreas 0FB
see Resection, Hepatobiliary System and Pancreas 0FT
Choledocholithotomy *see* Extirpation, Duct, Common Bile 0FC9
Choledochoplasty
see Repair, Hepatobiliary System and Pancreas 0FQ
see Replacement, Hepatobiliary System and Pancreas 0FR
see Supplement, Hepatobiliary System and Pancreas 0FU
Choledochoscopy 0FJB8ZZ
Choledochotomy *see* Drainage, Hepatobiliary System and Pancreas 0F9
Cholelithotomy *see* Extirpation, Hepatobiliary System and Pancreas 0FC
Chondrectomy
see Excision, Upper Joints 0RB
see Excision, Lower Joints 0SB
Knee *see* Excision, Lower Joints 0SB
Semilunar cartilage *see* Excision, Lower Joints 0SB
Chondroglossus muscle *use* Tongue, Palate, Pharynx Muscle
Chorda tympani *use* Facial Nerve
Chordotomy *see* Division, Central Nervous System and Cranial Nerves 008
Choroid plexus *use* Cerebral Ventricle
Choroidectomy
see Excision, Eye 08B
see Resection, Eye 08T
Ciliary body
use Eye, Right
use Eye, Left

▶ New ➡ Revised ~~deleted~~ Deleted

Ciliary ganglion *use* Head and Neck Sympathetic Nerve
Cilta-cel *use* Ciltacabtagene Autoleucel
Ciltacabtagene autoleucel XW0
Circle of Willis *use* Intracranial Artery
Circumcision 0VTTXZZ
Circumflex iliac artery
  use Femoral Artery, Right
  use Femoral Artery, Left
CivaSheet® *use* Radioactive Element
CivaSheet® Bradytherapy
  see Bradytherapy with qualifier Unidirectional Source
  see Insertion with device Radioactive Element
Clamp and rod internal fixation system (CRIF)
  use Internal Fixation Device in Upper Bones
  use Internal Fixation Device in Lower Bones
Clamping *see* Occlusion
Claustrum *use* Basal Ganglia
Claviculectomy
  see Excision, Upper Bones 0PB
  see Resection, Upper Bones 0PT
Claviculotomy
  see Division, Upper Bones 0P8
  see Drainage, Upper Bones 0P9
Clipping, aneurysm
  see Occlusion using Extraluminal Device
  see Restriction using Extraluminal Device
Clitorectomy, clitoridectomy
  see Excision, Clitoris 0UBJ
  see Resection, Clitoris 0UTJ
Clolar *use* Clofarabine
Closure
  see Occlusion
  see Repair
Clysis *see* Introduction of substance in or on
Coagulation *see* Destruction
Coagulation Factor Xa, Inactivated XW0
Coagulation Factor Xa, (Recombinant) Inactivated
  use Coagulation Factor Xa, Inactivated
COALESCE® radiolucent interbody fusion device
  use Interbody Fusion Device in Upper Joints
  use Interbody Fusion Device in Lower Joints
CoAxia NeuroFlo catheter *use* Intraluminal Device
Cobalt/chromium head and polyethylene socket *use* Synthetic Substitute, Metal on Polyethylene in 0SR
Cobalt/chromium head and socket *use* Synthetic Substitute, Metal in 0SR
Coccygeal body *use* Coccygeal Glomus
Coccygeus muscle
  use Trunk Muscle, Right
  use Trunk Muscle, Left
Cochlea
  use Inner Ear, Right
  use Inner Ear, Left
Cochlear implant (CI), multiple channel (electrode) *use* Hearing Device, Multiple Channel Cochlear Prosthesis in 09H
Cochlear implant (CI), single channel (electrode) *use* Hearing Device, Single Channel Cochlear Prosthesis in 09H
Cochlear Implant Treatment F0BZ0
Cochlear nerve *use* Acoustic Nerve
COGNIS® CRT-D *use* Cardiac Resynchronization Defibrillator Pulse Generator in 0JH
COHERE® radiolucent interbody fusion device
  use Interbody Fusion Device in Upper Joints
  use Interbody Fusion Device in Lower Joints
Colectomy
  see Excision, Gastrointestinal System 0DB
  see Resection, Gastrointestinal System 0DT
Collapse *see* Occlusion
Collection from
  Breast, Breast Milk 8E0HX62
  Indwelling Device
    Circulatory System
      Blood 8C02X6K
      Other Fluid 8C02X6L
    Nervous System
      Cerebrospinal Fluid 8C01X6J
      Other Fluid 8C01X6L
  Integumentary System, Breast Milk 8E0HX62
  Reproductive System, Male, Sperm 8E0VX63
Colocentesis *see* Drainage, Gastrointestinal System 0D9
Colofixation
  see Repair, Gastrointestinal System 0DQ
  see Reposition, Gastrointestinal System 0DS
Cololysis *see* Release, Gastrointestinal System 0DN
Colonic Z-Stent® *use* Intraluminal Device
Colonoscopy 0DJD8ZZ
Colopexy
  see Repair, Gastrointestinal System 0DQ
  see Reposition, Gastrointestinal System 0DS
Coloplication *see* Restriction, Gastrointestinal System 0DV
Coloproctectomy
  see Excision, Gastrointestinal System 0DB
  see Resection, Gastrointestinal System 0DT
Coloproctostomy
  see Bypass, Gastrointestinal System 0D1
  see Drainage, Gastrointestinal System 0D9
Colopuncture *see* Drainage, Gastrointestinal System 0D9
Colorrhaphy *see* Repair, Gastrointestinal System 0DQ
Colostomy
  see Bypass, Gastrointestinal System 0D1
  see Drainage, Gastrointestinal System 0D9
Colpectomy
  see Excision, Vagina 0UBG
  see Resection, Vagina 0UTG
Colpocentesis *see* Drainage, Vagina 0U9G
Colpopexy
  see Repair, Vagina 0UQG
  see Reposition, Vagina 0USG
Colpoplasty
  see Repair, Vagina 0UQG
  see Supplement, Vagina 0UUG
Colporrhaphy *see* Repair, Vagina 0UQG
Colposcopy 0UJH8ZZ
Columella *use* Nasal Mucosa and Soft Tissue
▶**COMIRNATY®**
  ▶*use* COVID-19 Vaccine Dose 1
  ▶*use* COVID-19 Vaccine Dose 2
  ▶*use* COVID-19 Vaccine
  ▶*use* COVID-19 Vaccine Dose 3
  ▶*use* COVID-19 Vaccine Booster
Common digital vein
  use Foot Vein, Right
  use Foot Vein, Left
Common facial vein
  use Face Vein, Right
  use Face Vein, Left
Common fibular nerve *use* Peroneal Nerve
Common hepatic artery *use* Hepatic Artery
Common iliac (subaortic) lymph node *use* Lymphatic, Pelvis
Common interosseous artery
  use Ulnar Artery, Right
  use Ulnar Artery, Left
Common peroneal nerve *use* Peroneal Nerve
Complete (SE) stent *use* Intraluminal Device
Compression *see* Restriction
  Abdominal Wall 2W13X
  Arm
    Lower
      Left 2W1DX
      Right 2W1CX
    Upper
      Left 2W1BX
      Right 2W1AX
Compression *(Continued)*
  Back 2W15X
  Chest Wall 2W14X
  Extremity
    Lower
      Left 2W1MX
      Right 2W1LX
    Upper
      Left 2W19X
      Right 2W18X
  Face 2W11X
  Finger
    Left 2W1KX
    Right 2W1JX
  Foot
    Left 2W1TX
    Right 2W1SX
  Hand
    Left 2W1FX
    Right 2W1EX
  Head 2W10X
  Inguinal Region
    Left 2W17X
    Right 2W16X
  Leg
    Lower
      Left 2W1RX
      Right 2W1QX
    Upper
      Left 2W1PX
      Right 2W1NX
  Neck 2W12X
  Thumb
    Left 2W1HX
    Right 2W1GX
  Toe
    Left 2W1VX
    Right 2W1UX
~~Computer-aided assessment, intracranial vascular activity XXE0X07~~
▶**Computer-aided Assessment**
  ▶Cardiac Output XXE2X19
  ▶Intracranial Vascular Activity XXE0X07
Computer-aided guidance, transthoracic echocardiography X2JAX47
Computer-aided mechanical aspiration X2C
Computer-aided triage and notification, pulmonary artery flow XXE3X27
Computer-aided Valve Modeling and Notification, Coronary Artery Flow XXE3X68
Computer-assisted intermittent aspiration see new technology, cardiovascular system X2C
Computer Assisted Procedure
  Extremity
    Lower
      No Qualifier 8E0YXBZ
      With Computerized Tomography 8E0YXBG
      With Fluoroscopy 8E0YXBF
      With Magnetic Resonance Imaging 8E0YXBH
    Upper
      No Qualifier 8E0XXBZ
      With Computerized Tomography 8E0XXBG
      With Fluoroscopy 8E0XXBF
      With Magnetic Resonance Imaging 8E0XXBH
  Head and Neck Region
    No Qualifier 8E09XBZ
    With Computerized Tomography 8E09XBG
    With Fluoroscopy 8E09XBF
    With Magnetic Resonance Imaging 8E09XBH
  Trunk Region
    No Qualifier 8E0WXBZ
    With Computerized Tomography 8E0WXBG
    With Fluoroscopy 8E0WXBF
    With Magnetic Resonance Imaging 8E0WXBH

▶ New ➡ Revised ~~deleted~~ Deleted

C

▶ New ➡ Revised ~~deleted~~ Deleted

Control bleeding in
Abdominal Wall 0W3F
Ankle Region
Left 0Y3L
Right 0Y3K
Arm
Lower
Left 0X3F
Right 0X3D
Upper
Left 0X39
Right 0X38
Axilla
Left 0X35
Right 0X34
Back
Lower 0W3L
Upper 0W3K
Buttock
Left 0Y31
Right 0Y30
Cavity, Cranial 0W31
Chest Wall 0W38
Elbow Region
Left 0X3C
Right 0X3B
Extremity
Lower
Left 0Y3B
Right 0Y39
Upper
Left 0X37
Right 0X36
Face 0W32
Femoral Region
Left 0Y38
Right 0Y37
Foot
Left 0Y3N
Right 0Y3M
Gastrointestinal Tract 0W3P
Genitourinary Tract 0W3R
Hand
Left 0X3K
Right 0X3J
Head 0W30
Inguinal Region
Left 0Y36
Right 0Y35
Jaw
Lower 0W35
Upper 0W34
Knee Region
Left 0Y3G
Right 0Y3F
Leg
Lower
Left 0Y3J
Right 0Y3H
Upper
Left 0Y3D
Right 0Y3C
Mediastinum 0W3C
Nasal Mucosa and Soft Tissue 093K
Neck 0W36
Oral Cavity and Throat 0W33
Pelvic Cavity 0W3J
Pericardial Cavity 0W3D
Perineum
Female 0W3N
Male 0W3M
Peritoneal Cavity 0W3G
Pleural Cavity
Left 0W3B
Right 0W39
Respiratory Tract 0W3Q
Retroperitoneum 0W3H
Shoulder Region
Left 0X33
Right 0X32
Control bleeding in *(Continued)*
Wrist Region
Left 0X3H
Right 0X3G
Control bleeding using tourniquet, external *see* Compression, Anatomical Regions 2W1
Conus arteriosus *use* Ventricle, Right
Conus medullaris *use* Spinal Cord, Lumbar
Convalescent plasma (nonautologous) *see* New Technology, Anatomical Regions XW1
Conversion
Cardiac rhythm 5A2204Z
Gastrostomy to jejunostomy feeding device *see* Insertion of device in, Jejunum 0DHA
Cook Biodesign® Fistula Plug(s) *use* Nonautologous Tissue Substitute
Cook Biodesign® Hernia Graft(s) *use* Nonautologous Tissue Substitute
Cook Biodesign® Layered Graft(s) *use* Nonautologous Tissue Substitute
Cook Zenapro™ Layered Graft(s) *use* Nonautologous Tissue Substitute
Cook Zenith AAA Endovascular Graft
use Intraluminal Device
Cook Zenith® Fenestrated AAA Endovascular Graft
use Intraluminal Device, Branched or Fenestrated, One or Two Arteries in 04V
use Intraluminal Device, Branched or Fenestrated, Three or More Arteries in 04V
Coracoacromial ligament
use Shoulder Bursa and Ligament, Right
use Shoulder Bursa and Ligament, Left
Coracobrachialis muscle
use Upper Arm Muscle, Right
use Upper Arm Muscle, Left
Coracoclavicular ligament
use Shoulder Bursa and Ligament, Right
use Shoulder Bursa and Ligament, Left
Coracohumeral ligament
use Shoulder Bursa and Ligament, Right
use Shoulder Bursa and Ligament, Left
Coracoid process
use Scapula, Right
use Scapula, Left
Cordotomy *see* Division, Central Nervous System and Cranial Nerves 008
Core needle biopsy *see* Biopsy
CoreValve transcatheter aortic valve *use* Zooplastic Tissue in Heart and Great Vessels
Cormet Hip Resurfacing System *use* Resurfacing Device in Lower Joints
Corniculate cartilage *use* Larynx
CoRoent® XL *use* Interbody Fusion Device in Lower Joints
Coronary arteriography
see Plain Radiography, Heart B20
see Fluoroscopy, Heart B21
Corox (OTW) Bipolar Lead
use Cardiac Lead, Pacemaker in 02H
use Cardiac Lead, Defibrillator in 02H
Corpus callosum *use* Brain
Corpus cavernosum *use* Penis
Corpus spongiosum *use* Penis
Corpus striatum *use* Basal Ganglia
Corrugator supercilii muscle *use* Facial Muscle
Cortical strip neurostimulator lead *use* Neurostimulator Lead in Central Nervous System and Cranial Nerves
COSELA™ *use* Trilaciclib
Costatectomy
see Excision, Upper Bones 0PB
see Resection, Upper Bones 0PT
Costectomy
see Excision, Upper Bones 0PB
see Resection, Upper Bones 0PT
Costocervical trunk
use Subclavian Artery, Right
use Subclavian Artery, Left
Costochondrectomy
see Excision, Upper Bones 0PB
see Resection, Upper Bones 0PT
Costoclavicular ligament
use Shoulder Bursa and Ligament, Right
use Shoulder Bursa and Ligament, Left
Costosternoplasty
see Repair, Upper Bones 0PQ
see Replacement, Upper Bones 0PR
see Supplement, Upper Bones 0PU
Costotomy
see Division, Upper Bones 0P8
see Drainage, Upper Bones 0P9
Costotransverse joint *use* Thoracic Vertebral Joint
Costotransverse ligament *use* Rib(s) Bursa and Ligament
Costovertebral joint *use* Thoracic Vertebral Joint
Costoxiphoid ligament *use* Sternum Bursa and Ligament
Counseling
Family, for substance abuse, Other Family Counseling HZ63ZZZ
Group
12-Step HZ43ZZZ
Behavioral HZ41ZZZ
Cognitive HZ40ZZZ
Cognitive-Behavioral HZ42ZZZ
Confrontational HZ48ZZZ
Continuing Care HZ49ZZZ
Infectious Disease
Post-Test HZ4CZZZ
Pre-Test HZ4CZZZ
Interpersonal HZ44ZZZ
Motivational Enhancement HZ47ZZZ
Psychoeducation HZ46ZZZ
Spiritual HZ4BZZZ
Vocational HZ45ZZZ
Individual
12-Step HZ33ZZZ
Behavioral HZ31ZZZ
Cognitive HZ30ZZZ
Cognitive-Behavioral HZ32ZZZ
Confrontational HZ38ZZZ
Continuing Care HZ39ZZZ
Infectious Disease
Post-Test HZ3CZZZ
Pre-Test HZ3CZZZ
Interpersonal HZ34ZZZ
Motivational Enhancement HZ37ZZZ
Psychoeducation HZ36ZZZ
Spiritual HZ3BZZZ
Vocational HZ35ZZZ
Mental Health Services
Educational GZ60ZZZ
Other Counseling GZ63ZZZ
Vocational GZ61ZZZ
Countershock, cardiac 5A2204Z
Corvia IASD® *use* Synthetic Substitute
COVID-19 XW0
COVID-19 Vaccine Dose 1 XW0
COVID-19 Vaccine Dose 2 XW0
Cowper's (bulbourethral) gland *use* Urethra
CPAP (continuous positive airway pressure)
see Assistance, Respiratory 5A09
Craniectomy
see Excision, Head and Facial Bones 0NB
see Resection, Head and Facial Bones 0NT
Cranioplasty
see Repair, Head and Facial Bones 0NQ
see Replacement, Head and Facial Bones 0NR
see Supplement, Head and Facial Bones 0NU
Craniotomy
see Drainage, Central Nervous System and Cranial Nerves 009
see Division, Head and Facial Bones 0N8
see Drainage, Head and Facial Bones 0N9

▶ New ➡ Revised ~~deleted~~ Deleted

C

Creation
  Perineum
    Female 0W4N0
    Male 0W4M0
  Valve
    Aortic 024F0
    Mitral 024G0
    Tricuspid 024J0
Cremaster muscle *use* Perineum Muscle
CRESEMBA® (isavuconazonium sulfate) *use* Other Anti-infective
Cribriform plate
  use Ethmoid Bone, Right
  use Ethmoid Bone, Left
Cricoid cartilage *use* Trachea
Cricoidectomy *see* Excision, Larynx 0CBS
Cricothyroid artery
  use Thyroid Artery, Right
  use Thyroid Artery, Left
Cricothyroid muscle
  use Neck Muscle, Right
  use Neck Muscle, Left
Crisis Intervention GZ2ZZZZ
CRRT (Continuous renal replacement therapy) 5A1D90Z
Crural fascia
  use Subcutaneous Tissue and Fascia, Right Upper Leg
  use Subcutaneous Tissue and Fascia, Left Upper Leg
Crushing, nerve
  Cranial *see* Destruction, Central Nervous System and Cranial Nerves 005
  Peripheral *see* Destruction, Peripheral Nervous System 015
Cryoablation *see* Destruction
Cryotherapy *see* Destruction
Cryptorchidectomy
  see Excision, Male Reproductive System 0VB
  see Resection, Male Reproductive System 0VT
Cryptorchiectomy
  see Excision, Male Reproductive System 0VB
  see Resection, Male Reproductive System 0VT
Cryptotomy
  see Division, Gastrointestinal System 0D8
  see Drainage, Gastrointestinal System 0D9
CT scan *see* Computerized Tomography (CT Scan)
CT sialogram *see* Computerized Tomography (CT Scan), Ear, Nose, Mouth and Throat B92
▶ CTX001™ *use* Exagamglogene Autotemcel
Cubital lymph node
  use Lymphatic, Right Upper Extremity
  use Lymphatic, Left Upper Extremity
Cubital nerve *use* Ulnar Nerve
Cuboid bone
  use Tarsal, Right
  use Tarsal, Left
Cuboideonavicular joint
  use Tarsal Joint, Right
  use Tarsal Joint, Left
Culdocentesis *see* Drainage, Cul-de-sac 0U9F
Culdoplasty
  see Repair, Cul-de-sac 0UQF
  see Supplement, Cul-de-sac 0UUF
Culdoscopy 0UJH8ZZ
Culdotomy *see* Drainage, Cul-de-sac 0U9F
Culmen *use* Cerebellum
Cultured epidermal cell autograft *use* Autologous Tissue Substitute
Cuneiform cartilage *use* Larynx
Cuneonavicular joint
  use Tarsal Joint, Right
  use Tarsal Joint, Left
Cuneonavicular ligament
  use Foot Bursa and Ligament, Right
  use Foot Bursa and Ligament, Left
Curettage
  see Excision
  see Extraction
Cutaneous (transverse) cervical nerve *use* Nerve, Cervical Plexus
CVP (central venous pressure) *see* Measurement, Venous 4A04
Cyclodiathermy *see* Destruction, Eye 085
Cyclophotocoagulation *see* Destruction, Eye 085
CYPHER® Stent *use* Intraluminal Device, Drug-eluting in Heart and Great Vessels
Cystectomy
  see Excision, Bladder 0TBB
  see Resection, Bladder 0TTB
Cystocele repair *see* Repair, Subcutaneous Tissue and Fascia, Pelvic Region 0JQC
Cystography
  see Plain Radiography, Urinary System BT0
  see Fluoroscopy, Urinary System BT1
Cystolithotomy *see* Extirpation, Bladder 0TCB
Cystopexy
  see Repair, Bladder 0TQB
  see Reposition, Bladder 0TSB
Cystoplasty
  see Repair, Bladder 0TQB
  see Replacement, Bladder 0TRB
  see Supplement, Bladder 0TUB
Cystorrhaphy *see* Repair, Bladder 0TQB
Cystoscopy 0TJB8ZZ
Cystostomy *see* Bypass, Bladder 0T1B
Cystostomy tube *use* Drainage Device
Cystotomy *see* Drainage, Bladder 0T9B
Cystourethrography
  see Plain Radiography, Urinary System BT0
  see Fluoroscopy, Urinary System BT1
Cystourethroplasty
  see Repair, Urinary System 0TQ
  see Replacement, Urinary System 0TR
  see Supplement, Urinary System 0TU
▶ CYTALUX® (Pafolacianine), in Fluorescence Guided Procedure *see* Fluorescence Guided Procedure
Cytarabine and Daunorubicin Liposome Antineoplastic XW0

C

D

DBS lead *use* Neurostimulator Lead in Central Nervous System and Cranial Nerves
Daratumumab and Hyaluronidase-fihj XW01318
Darzalex Faspro® *use* Daratumumab and Hyaluronidase-fihj
DeBakey Left Ventricular Assist Device *use* Implantable Heart Assist System in Heart and Great Vessels
Debridement
Excisional *see* Excision
Non-excisional *see* Extraction
Decompression, Circulatory 6A15
Decortication, lung
see Extirpation, Respiratory System 0BC
see Release, Respiratory System 0BN
Deep brain neurostimulator lead *use* Neurostimulator Lead in Central Nervous System and Cranial Nerves
Deep cervical fascia
use Subcutaneous Tissue and Fascia, Right Neck
use Subcutaneous Tissue and Fascia, Left Neck
Deep cervical vein
use Vertebral Vein, Right
use Vertebral Vein, Left
Deep circumflex iliac artery
use External Iliac Artery, Right
use External Iliac Artery, Left
Deep facial vein
use Face Vein, Right
use Face Vein, Left
Deep femoral (profunda femoris) vein
use Femoral Vein, Right
use Femoral Vein, Left
Deep femoral artery
use Femoral Artery, Right
use Femoral Artery, Left
Deep Inferior Epigastric Artery Perforator Flap
Replacement
Bilateral 0HRV077
Left 0HRU077
Right 0HRT077
Transfer
Left 0KXG
Right 0KXF
Deep palmar arch
use Hand Artery, Right
use Hand Artery, Left
Deep transverse perineal muscle *use* Perineum Muscle
DefenCath™ *use* Taurolidine Anti-infective and Heparin Anticoagulant
Deferential artery
use Internal Iliac Artery, Right
use Internal Iliac Artery, Left
Defibrillator Generator
Abdomen 0JH8
Chest 0JH6
▶ **Defibrillator Lead**
▶ Insertion of device in, Mediastinum 0WHC
▶ Removal of device from, Mediastinum 0WPC
▶ Revision of device in, Mediastinum 0WWC
Defibtech Automated Chest Compression (ACC) device 5A1221J
Defitelio *use* Other Substance
Defitelio® infusion *see* Introduction of substance in or on, Physiological Systems and Anatomical Regions 3E0
Delivery
Cesarean *see* Extraction, Products of Conception 10D0
Forceps *see* Extraction, Products of Conception 10D0
Manually assisted 10E0XZZ
Products of Conception 10E0XZZ
Vacuum assisted *see* Extraction, Products of Conception 10D0
Delta frame external fixator
use External Fixation Device, Hybrid in 0PH
use External Fixation Device, Hybrid in 0PS
Delta frame external fixator *(Continued)*
use External Fixation Device, Hybrid in 0QH
use External Fixation Device, Hybrid in 0QS
Delta III Reverse shoulder prosthesis *use* Synthetic Substitute, Reverse Ball and Socket in 0RR
Deltoid fascia
use Subcutaneous Tissue and Fascia, Right Upper Arm
use Subcutaneous Tissue and Fascia, Left Upper Arm
Deltoid ligament
use Ankle Bursa and Ligament, Right
use Ankle Bursa and Ligament, Left
Deltoid muscle
use Shoulder Muscle, Right
use Shoulder Muscle, Left
Deltopectoral (infraclavicular) lymph node
use Lymphatic, Right Upper Extremity
use Lymphatic, Left Upper Extremity
Denervation
Cranial nerve *see* Destruction, Central Nervous System and Cranial Nerves 005
Peripheral nerve *see* Destruction, Peripheral Nervous System 015
Dens *use* Cervical Vertebra
Densitometry
Plain Radiography
Femur
Left BQ04ZZ1
Right BQ03ZZ1
Hip
Left BQ01ZZ1
Right BQ00ZZ1
Spine
Cervical BR00ZZ1
Lumbar BR09ZZ1
Thoracic BR07ZZ1
Whole BR0GZZ1
Ultrasonography
Elbow
Left BP4HZZ1
Right BP4GZZ1
Hand
Left BP4PZZ1
Right BP4NZZ1
Shoulder
Left BP49ZZ1
Right BP48ZZ1
Wrist
Left BP4MZZ1
Right BP4LZZ1
Denticulate (dentate) ligament *use* Spinal Meninges
Depressor anguli oris muscle *use* Facial Muscle
Depressor labii inferioris muscle *use* Facial Muscle
Depressor septi nasi muscle *use* Facial Muscle
Depressor supercilii muscle *use* Facial Muscle
Dermabrasion *see* Extraction, Skin and Breast 0HD
Dermis *see* Skin
Descending genicular artery
use Femoral Artery, Right
use Femoral Artery, Left
Destruction
Acetabulum
Left 0Q55
Right 0Q54
Adenoids 0C5Q
Ampulla of Vater 0F5C
Anal Sphincter 0D5R
Anterior Chamber
Left 08533ZZ
Right 08523ZZ
Anus 0D5Q
Aorta
Abdominal 0450
Thoracic
Ascending/Arch 025X
Descending 025W
Destruction *(Continued)*
Aortic Body 0G5D
Appendix 0D5J
Artery
Anterior Tibial
Left 045Q
Right 045P
Axillary
Left 0356
Right 0355
Brachial
Left 0358
Right 0357
Celiac 0451
Colic
Left 0457
Middle 0458
Right 0456
Common Carotid
Left 035J
Right 035H
Common Iliac
Left 045D
Right 045C
External Carotid
Left 035N
Right 035M
External Iliac
Left 045J
Right 045H
Face 035R
Femoral
Left 045L
Right 045K
Foot
Left 045W
Right 045V
Gastric 0452
Hand
Left 035F
Right 035D
Hepatic 0453
Inferior Mesenteric 045B
Innominate 0352
Internal Carotid
Left 035L
Right 035K
Internal Iliac
Left 045F
Right 045E
Internal Mammary
Left 0351
Right 0350
Intracranial 035G
Lower 045Y
Peroneal
Left 045U
Right 045T
Popliteal
Left 045N
Right 045M
Posterior Tibial
Left 045S
Right 045R
Pulmonary
Left 025R
Right 025Q
Pulmonary Trunk 025P
Radial
Left 035C
Right 035B
Renal
Left 045A
Right 0459
Splenic 0454
Subclavian
Left 0354
Right 0353
Superior Mesenteric 0455

▶ New ➡ Revised ~~deleted~~ Deleted

Destruction *(Continued)*
Artery *(Continued)*
Temporal
Left 035T
Right 035S
Thyroid
Left 035V
Right 035U
Ulnar
Left 035A
Right 0359
Upper 035Y
Vertebral
Left 035Q
Right 035P
Atrium
Left 0257
Right 0256
Auditory Ossicle
Left 095A
Right 0959
Basal Ganglia 0058
Bladder 0T5B
Bladder Neck 0T5C
Bone
Ethmoid
Left 0N5G
Right 0N5F
Frontal 0N51
Hyoid 0N5X
Lacrimal
Left 0N5J
Right 0N5H
Nasal 0N5B
Occipital 0N57
Palatine
Left 0N5L
Right 0N5K
Parietal
Left 0N54
Right 0N53
Pelvic
Left 0Q53
Right 0Q52
Sphenoid 0N5C
Temporal
Left 0N56
Right 0N55
Zygomatic
Left 0N5N
Right 0N5M
Brain 0050
Breast
Bilateral 0H5V
Left 0H5U
Right 0H5T
Bronchus
Lingula 0B59
Lower Lobe
Left 0B5B
Right 0B56
Main
Left 0B57
Right 0B53
Middle Lobe, Right 0B55
Upper Lobe
Left 0B58
Right 0B54
Buccal Mucosa 0C54
Bursa and Ligament
Abdomen
Left 0M5J
Right 0M5H
Ankle
Left 0M5R
Right 0M5Q
Elbow
Left 0M54
Right 0M53

Destruction *(Continued)*
Bursa and Ligament *(Continued)*
Foot
Left 0M5T
Right 0M5S
Hand
Left 0M58
Right 0M57
Head and Neck 0M50
Hip
Left 0M5M
Right 0M5L
Knee
Left 0M5P
Right 0M5N
Lower Extremity
Left 0M5W
Right 0M5V
Perineum 0M5K
Rib(s) 0M5G
Shoulder
Left 0M52
Right 0M51
Spine
Lower 0M5D
Upper 0M5C
Sternum 0M5F
Upper Extremity
Left 0M5B
Right 0M59
Wrist
Left 0M56
Right 0M55
Carina 0B52
Carotid Bodies, Bilateral 0G58
Carotid Body
Left 0G56
Right 0G57
Carpal
Left 0P5N
Right 0P5M
Cecum 0D5H
Cerebellum 005C
Cerebral Hemisphere 0057
Cerebral Meninges 0051
Cerebral Ventricle 0056
Cervix 0U5C
Chordae Tendineae 0259
Choroid
Left 085B
Right 085A
Cisterna Chyli 075L
Clavicle
Left 0P5B
Right 0P59
Clitoris 0U5J
Coccygeal Glomus 0G5B
Coccyx 0Q5S
Colon
Ascending 0D5K
Descending 0D5M
Sigmoid 0D5N
Transverse 0D5L
Conduction Mechanism 0258
Conjunctiva
Left 085TXZZ
Right 085SXZZ
Cord
Bilateral 0V5H
Left 0V5G
Right 0V5F
Cornea
Left 0859XZZ
Right 0858XZZ
Cul-de-sac 0U5F
Diaphragm 0B5T
Disc
Cervical Vertebral 0R53
Cervicothoracic Vertebral 0R55

Destruction *(Continued)*
Duct *(Continued)*
Lumbar Vertebral 0S52
Lumbosacral 0S54
Thoracic Vertebral 0R59
Thoracolumbar Vertebral 0R5B
Duct
Common Bile 0F59
Cystic 0F58
Hepatic
Common 0F57
Left 0F56
Right 0F55
Lacrimal
Left 085Y
Right 085X
Pancreatic 0F5D
Accessory 0F5F
Parotid
Left 0C5C
Right 0C5B
Thoracic 075K
Duodenum 0D59
Dura Mater 0052
Ear
External
Left 0951
Right 0950
External Auditory Canal
Left 0954
Right 0953
Inner
Left 095E
Right 095D
Middle
Left 0956
Right 0955
Endometrium 0U5B
Epididymis
Bilateral 0V5L
Left 0V5K
Right 0V5J
Epiglottis 0C5R
Esophagogastric Junction 0D54
Esophagus 0D55
Lower 0D53
Middle 0D52
Upper 0D51
Eustachian Tube
Left 095G
Right 095F
Eye
Left 0851XZZ
Right 0850XZZ
Eyelid
Lower
Left 085R
Right 085Q
Upper
Left 085P
Right 085N
Fallopian Tube
Left 0U56
Right 0U55
Fallopian Tubes, Bilateral 0U57
Femoral Shaft
Left 0Q59
Right 0Q58
Femur
Lower
Left 0Q5C
Right 0Q5B
Upper
Left 0Q57
Right 0Q56
Fibula
Left 0Q5K
Right 0Q5J
Finger Nail 0H5QXZZ
Gallbladder 0F54

▶ New ➡ Revised ~~deleted~~ Deleted

Destruction *(Continued)*
Thalamus 0059
Thymus 075M
Thyroid Gland
Left Lobe 0G5G
Right Lobe 0G5H
Tibia
Left 0Q5H
Right 0Q5G
Toe Nail 0H5RXZZ
Tongue 0C57
Tonsils 0C5P
Tooth
Lower 0C5X
Upper 0C5W
Trachea 0B51
Tunica Vaginalis
Left 0V57
Right 0V56
Turbinate, Nasal 095L
Tympanic Membrane
Left 0958
Right 0959
Ulna
Left 0P5L
Right 0P5K
Ureter
Left 0T57
Right 0T56
Urethra 0T5D
Uterine Supporting Structure 0U54
Uterus 0U59
Uvula 0C5N
Vagina 0U5G
Valve
Aortic 025F
Mitral 025G
Pulmonary 025H
Tricuspid 025J
Vas Deferens
Bilateral 0V5Q
Left 0V5P
Right 0V5N
Vein
Axillary
Left 0558
Right 0557
Azygos 0550
Basilic
Left 055C
Right 055B
Brachial
Left 055A
Right 0559
Cephalic
Left 055F
Right 055D
Colic 0657
Common Iliac
Left 065D
Right 065C
Coronary 0254
Esophageal 0653
External Iliac
Left 065G
Right 065F
External Jugular
Left 055Q
Right 055P
Face
Left 055V
Right 055T
Femoral
Left 065N
Right 065M
Foot
Left 065V
Right 065T
Gastric 0652
Hand
Left 055H
Right 055G

Destruction *(Continued)*
Vein *(Continued)*
Hemiazygos 0551
Hepatic 0654
Hypogastric
Left 065J
Right 065H
Inferior Mesenteric 0656
Innominate
Left 0554
Right 0553
Internal Jugular
Left 055N
Right 055M
Intracranial 055L
Lower 065Y
Portal 0658
Pulmonary
Left 025T
Right 025S
Renal
Left 065B
Right 0659
Saphenous
Left 065Q
Right 065P
Splenic 0651
Subclavian
Left 0556
Right 0555
Superior Mesenteric 0655
Upper 055Y
Vertebral
Left 055S
Right 055R
Vena Cava
Inferior 0650
Superior 025V
Ventricle
Left 025L
Right 025K
Vertebra
Cervical 0P53
Lumbar 0Q50
Thoracic 0P54
Vesicle
Bilateral 0V53
Left 0V52
Right 0V51
Vitreous
Left 08553ZZ
Right 08543ZZ
Vocal Cord
Left 0C5V
Right 0C5T
Vulva 0U5M
Detachment
Arm
Lower
Left 0X6F0Z
Right 0X6D0Z
Upper
Left 0X690Z
Right 0X680Z
Elbow Region
Left 0X6C0ZZ
Right 0X6B0ZZ
Femoral Region
Left 0Y680ZZ
Right 0Y670ZZ
Finger
Index
Left 0X6P0Z
Right 0X6N0Z
Little
Left 0X6W0Z
Right 0X6V0Z
Middle
Left 0X6R0Z
Right 0X6Q0Z

Detachment *(Continued)*
Ring
Left 0X6T0Z
Right 0X6S0Z
Foot
Left 0Y6N0Z
Right 0Y6M0Z
Forequarter
Left 0X610ZZ
Right 0X600ZZ
Hand
Left 0X6K0Z
Right 0X6J0Z
Hindquarter
Bilateral 0Y640ZZ
Left 0Y630ZZ
Right 0Y620ZZ
Knee Region
Left 0Y6G0ZZ
Right 0Y6F0ZZ
Leg
Lower
Left 0Y6J0Z
Right 0Y6H0Z
Upper
Left 0Y6D0Z
Right 0Y6C0Z
Shoulder Region
Left 0X630ZZ
Right 0X620ZZ
Thumb
Left 0X6M0Z
Right 0X6L0Z
Toe
1st
Left 0Y6Q0Z
Right 0Y6P0Z
2nd
Left 0Y6S0Z
Right 0Y6R0Z
3rd
Left 0Y6U0Z
Right 0Y6T0Z
4th
Left 0Y6W0Z
Right 0Y6V0Z
5th
Left 0Y6Y0Z
Right 0Y6X0Z
Determination, Mental status GZ14ZZZ
Detorsion
see Release
see Reposition
▶**DETOUR® System**
▶*use* Conduit through Femoral Vein to Superficial Femoral Artery in New Technology
▶*use* Conduit through Femoral Vein to Popliteal Artery in New Technology
Detoxification Services, for substance abuse HZ2ZZZZ
Device Fitting F0DZ
Diagnostic Audiology *see* Audiology, Diagnostic
Diagnostic imaging *see* Imaging, Diagnostic
Diagnostic radiology *see* Imaging, Diagnostic
Dialysis
Hemodialysis *see* Performance, Urinary 5A1D
Peritoneal 3E1M39Z
Diaphragma sellae *use* Dura Mater
Diaphragmatic pacemaker generator *use* Stimulator Generator in Subcutaneous Tissue and Fascia
Diaphragmatic Pacemaker Lead
Insertion of device in, Diaphragm 0BHT
Removal of device from, Diaphragm 0BPT
Revision of device in, Diaphragm 0BWT
Digital radiography, plain *see* Plain Radiography

Dilation
Ampulla of Vater 0F7C
Anus 0D7Q
Aorta
Abdominal 0470
Thoracic
Ascending/Arch 027X
Descending 027W
Artery
Anterior Tibial
Left 047Q
Sustained Release Drug-eluting Intraluminal Device X27Q385
Four or More X27Q3C5
Three X27Q3B5
Two X27Q395
Right 047P
Sustained Release Drug-eluting Intraluminal Device X27P385
Four or More X27P3C5
Three X27P3B5
Two X27P395
Axillary
Left 0376
Right 0375
Brachial
Left 0378
Right 0377
Celiac 0471
Colic
Left 0477
Middle 0478
Right 0476
Common Carotid
Left 037J
Right 037H
Common Iliac
Left 047D
Right 047C
Coronary
Four or More Arteries 0273
One Artery 0270
Three Arteries 0272
Two Arteries 0271
External Carotid
Left 037N
Right 037M
External Iliac
Left 047J
Right 047H
Face 037R
Femoral
Left 047L
Sustained Release Drug-eluting Intraluminal Device X27J385
Four or More X27J3C5
Three X27J3B5
Two X27J395
Right 047K
Sustained Release Drug-eluting Intraluminal Device X27H385
Four or More X27H3C5
Three X27H3B5
Two X27H395
Foot
Left 047W
Right 047V
Gastric 0472
Hand
Left 037F
Right 037D
Hepatic 0473
Inferior Mesenteric 047B
Innominate 0372
Internal Carotid
Left 037L
Right 037K
Internal Iliac
Left 047F
Right 047E

Dilation (Continued)
Artery (Continued)
Internal Mammary
Left 0371
Right 0370
Intracranial 037G
Lower 047Y
Peroneal
Left 047U
Sustained Release Drug-eluting Intraluminal Device X27U385
Four or More X27U3C5
Three X27U3B5
Two X27U395
Right 047T
Sustained Release Drug-eluting Intraluminal Device X27T385
Four or More X27T3C5
Three X27T3B5
Two X27T395
Popliteal
Left 047N
Left Distal
Sustained Release Drug-eluting Intraluminal Device X27N385
Four or More X27N3C5
Three X27N3B5
Two X27N395
Left Proximal
Sustained Release Drug-eluting Intraluminal Device X27L385
Four or More X27L3C5
Three X27L3B5
Two X27L395
Right 047M
Right Distal
Sustained Release Drug-eluting Intraluminal Device X27M385
Four or More X27M3C5
Three X27M3B5
Two X27M395
Right Proximal
Sustained Release Drug-eluting Intraluminal Device X27K385
Four or More X27K3C5
Three X27K3B5
Two X27K395
Posterior Tibial
Left 047S
Sustained Release Drug-eluting Intraluminal Device X27S385
Four or More X27S3C5
Three X27S3B5
Two X27S395
Right 047R
Sustained Release Drug-eluting Intraluminal Device X27R385
Four or More X27R3C5
Three X27R3B5
Two X27R395
Pulmonary
Left 027R
Right 027Q
Pulmonary Trunk 027P
Radial
Left 037C
Right 037B
Renal
Left 047A
Right 0479
Splenic 0474
Subclavian
Left 0374
Right 0373
Superior Mesenteric 0475
Temporal
Left 037T
Right 037S
Thyroid
Left 037V
Right 037U

Dilation (Continued)
Artery (Continued)
Ulnar
Left 037A
Right 0379
Upper 037Y
Vertebral
Left 037Q
Right 037P
Bladder 0T7B
Bladder Neck 0T7C
Bronchus
Lingula 0B79
Lower Lobe
Left 0B7B
Right 0B76
Main
Left 0B77
Right 0B73
Middle Lobe, Right 0B75
Upper Lobe
Left 0B78
Right 0B74
Carina 0B72
Cecum 0D7H
Cerebral Ventricle 0076
Cervix 0U7C
Colon
Ascending 0D7K
Descending 0D7M
Sigmoid 0D7N
Transverse 0D7L
Duct
Common Bile 0F79
Cystic 0F78
Hepatic
Common 0F77
Left 0F76
Right 0F75
Lacrimal
Left 087Y
Right 087X
Pancreatic 0F7D
Accessory 0F7F
Parotid
Left 0C7C
Right 0C7B
Duodenum 0D79
Esophagogastric Junction 0D74
Esophagus 0D75
Lower 0D73
Middle 0D72
Upper 0D71
Eustachian Tube
Left 097G
Right 097F
Fallopian Tube
Left 0U76
Right 0U75
Fallopian Tubes, Bilateral 0U77
Hymen 0U7K
Ileocecal Valve 0D7C
Ileum 0D7B
Intestine
Large 0D7E
Left 0D7G
Right 0D7F
Small 0D78
Jejunum 0D7A
Kidney Pelvis
Left 0T74
Right 0T73
Larynx 0C7S
Pharynx 0C7M
Rectum 0D7P
Stomach 0D76 Pylorus 0D77
Trachea 0B71
Ureter
Left 0T77
Right 0T76

Drainage (Continued)
Bursa and Ligament (Continued)
Upper Extremity
Left 0M9B
Right 0M99
Wrist
Left 0M96
Right 0M95
Buttock
Left 0Y91
Right 0Y90
Carina 0B92
Carotid Bodies, Bilateral 0G98
Carotid Body
Left 0G96
Right 0G97
Carpal
Left 0P9N
Right 0P9M
Cavity, Cranial 0W91
Cecum 0D9H
Cerebellum 009C
Cerebral Hemisphere 0097
Cerebral Meninges 0091
Cerebral Ventricle 0096
Cervix 0U9C
Chest Wall 0W98
Choroid
Left 089B
Right 089A
Cisterna Chyli 079L
Clavicle
Left 0P9B
Right 0P99
Clitoris 0U9J
Coccygeal Glomus 0G9B
Coccyx 0Q9S
Colon
Ascending 0D9K
Descending 0D9M
Sigmoid 0D9N
Transverse 0D9L
Conjunctiva
Left 089T
Right 089S
Cord
Bilateral 0V9H
Left 0V9G
Right 0V9F
Cornea
Left 0899
Right 0898
Cul-de-sac 0U9F
Diaphragm 0B9T
Disc
Cervical Vertebral 0R93
Cervicothoracic Vertebral 0R95
Lumbar Vertebral 0S92
Lumbosacral 0S94
Thoracic Vertebral 0R99
Thoracolumbar Vertebral 0R9B
Duct
Common Bile 0F99
Cystic 0F98
Hepatic
Common 0F97
Left 0F96
Right 0F95
Lacrimal
Left 089Y
Right 089X
Pancreatic 0F9D
Accessory 0F9F
Parotid
Left 0C9C
Right 0C9B
Duodenum 0D99
Dura Mater 0092
Ear
External
Left 0991
Right 0990

Drainage (Continued)
Ear (Continued)
External Auditory Canal
Left 0994
Right 0993
Inner
Left 099E
Right 099D
Middle
Left 0996
Right 0995
Elbow Region
Left 0X9C
Right 0X9B
Epididymis
Bilateral 0V9L
Left 0V9K
Right 0V9J
Epidural Space, Intracranial 0093
Epiglottis 0C9R
Esophagogastric Junction 0D94
Esophagus 0D95
Lower 0D93
Middle 0D92
Upper 0D91
Eustachian Tube
Left 099G
Right 099F
Extremity
Lower
Left 0Y9B
Right 0Y99
Upper
Left 0X97
Right 0X96
Eye
Left 0891
Right 0890
Eyelid
Lower
Left 089R
Right 089Q
Upper
Left 089P
Right 089N
Face 0W92
Fallopian Tube
Left 0U96
Right 0U95
Fallopian Tubes, Bilateral 0U97
Femoral Region
Left 0Y98
Right 0Y97
Femoral Shaft
Left 0Q99
Right 0Q98
Femur
Lower
Left 0Q9C
Right 0Q9B
Upper
Left 0Q97
Right 0Q96
Fibula
Left 0Q9K
Right 0Q9J
Finger Nail 0H9Q
Foot
Left 0Y9N
Right 0Y9M
Gallbladder 0F94
Gingiva
Lower 0C96
Upper 0C95
Gland
Adrenal
Bilateral 0G94
Left 0G92
Right 0G93
Lacrimal
Left 089W
Right 089V

Drainage (Continued)
Gland (Continued)
Minor Salivary 0C9J
Parotid
Left 0C99
Right 0C98
Pituitary 0G90
Sublingual
Left 0C9F
Right 0C9D
Submaxillary
Left 0C9H
Right 0C9G
Vestibular 0U9L
Glenoid Cavity
Left 0P98
Right 0P97
Glomus Jugulare 0G9C
Hand
Left 0X9K
Right 0X9J
Head 0W90
Humeral Head
Left 0P9D
Right 0P9C
Humeral Shaft
Left 0P9G
Right 0P9F
Hymen 0U9K
Hypothalamus 009A
Ileocecal Valve 0D9C
Ileum 0D9B
Inguinal Region
Left 0Y96
Right 0Y95
Intestine
Large 0D9E
Left 0D9G
Right 0D9F
Small 0D98
Iris
Left 089D
Right 089C
Jaw
Lower 0W95
Upper 0W94
Jejunum 0D9A
Joint
Acromioclavicular
Left 0R9H
Right 0R9G
Ankle
Left 0S9G
Right 0S9F
Carpal
Left 0R9R
Right 0R9Q
Carpometacarpal
Left 0R9T
Right 0R9S
Cervical Vertebral 0R91
Cervicothoracic Vertebral 0R94
Coccygeal 0S96
Elbow
Left 0R9M
Right 0R9L
Finger Phalangeal
Left 0R9X
Right 0R9W
Hip
Left 0S9B
Right 0S99
Knee
Left 0S9D
Right 0S9C
Lumbar Vertebral 0S90
Lumbosacral 0S93
Metacarpophalangeal
Left 0R9V
Right 0R9U

D

Drainage *(Continued)*
Vein *(Continued)*
Common Iliac
Left 069D
Right 069C
Esophageal 0693
External Iliac
Left 069G
Right 069F
External Jugular
Left 059Q
Right 059P
Face
Left 059V
Right 059T
Femoral
Left 069N
Right 069M
Foot
Left 069V
Right 069T
Gastric 0692
Hand
Left 059H
Right 059G
Hemiazygos 0591
Hepatic 0694
Hypogastric
Left 069J
Right 069H
Inferior Mesenteric 0696
Innominate
Left 0594
Right 0593
Internal Jugular
Left 059N
Right 059M
Intracranial 059L
Lower 069Y
Portal 0698
Renal
Left 069B
Right 0699
Saphenous
Left 069Q
Right 069P
Splenic 0691
Subclavian
Left 0596
Right 0595
Superior Mesenteric 0695
Upper 059Y
Vertebral
Left 059S
Right 059R
Vena Cava, Inferior 0690
Vertebra
Cervical 0P93
Lumbar 0Q90
Thoracic 0P94
Vesicle
Bilateral 0V93
Left 0V92
Right 0V91

Drainage *(Continued)*
Vitreous
Left 0895
Right 0894
Vocal Cord
Left 0C9V
Right 0C9T
Vulva 0U9M
Wrist Region
Left 0X9H
Right 0X9G
Dressing
Abdominal Wall 2W23X4Z
Arm
Lower
Left 2W2DX4Z
Right 2W2CX4Z
Upper
Left 2W2BX4Z
Right 2W2AX4Z
Back 2W25X4Z
Chest Wall 2W24X4Z
Extremity
Lower
Left 2W2MX4Z
Right 2W2LX4Z
Upper
Left 2W29X4Z
Right 2W28X4Z
Face 2W21X4Z
Finger
Left 2W2KX4Z
Right 2W2JX4Z
Foot
Left 2W2TX4Z
Right 2W2SX4Z
Hand
Left 2W2FX4Z
Right 2W2EX4Z
Head 2W20X4Z
Inguinal Region
Left 2W27X4Z
Right 2W26X4Z
Leg
Lower
Left 2W2RX4Z
Right 2W2QX4Z
Upper
Left 2W2PX4Z
Right 2W2NX4Z
Neck 2W22X4Z
Thumb
Left 2W2HX4Z
Right 2W2GX4Z
Toe
Left 2W2VX4Z
Right 2W2UX4Z
Driver stent (RX) (OTW) *use* Intraluminal Device
Drotrecogin alfa, Infusion *see* Introduction of Recombinant Human-activated Protein C

Duct of Santorini *use* Duct, Pancreatic, Accessory
Duct of Wirsung *use* Duct, Pancreatic
Ductogram, mammary *see* Plain Radiography, Skin, Subcutaneous Tissue and Breast BH0
Ductography, mammary *see* Plain Radiography, Skin, Subcutaneous Tissue and Breast BH0
Ductus deferens
use Vas Deferens, Right
use Vas Deferens, Left
use Vas Deferens, Bilateral
use Vas Deferens
Duodenal ampulla *use* Ampulla of Vater
Duodenectomy
see Excision, Duodenum 0DB9
see Resection, Duodenum 0DT9
Duodenocholedochotomy *see* Drainage, Gallbladder 0F94
Duodenocystostomy
see Bypass, Gallbladder 0F14
see Drainage, Gallbladder 0F94
Duodenoenterostomy
see Bypass, Gastrointestinal System 0D1
see Drainage, Gastrointestinal System 0D9
Duodenojejunal flexure *use* Jejunum
Duodenolysis *see* Release, Duodenum 0DN9
Duodenorrhaphy *see* Repair, Duodenum 0DQ9
Duodenoscopy, single-use (aScope™ Duodeno) (EXALT™ Model D) *see* New Technology, Hepatobiliary System and Pancreas XFJ
Duodenostomy
see Bypass, Duodenum 0D19
see Drainage, Duodenum 0D99
Duodenotomy *see* Drainage, Duodenum 0D99
DuraGraft® Endothelial Damage Inhibitor *use* Endothelial Damage Inhibitor
DuraHeart Left Ventricular Assist System *use* Implantable Heart Assist System in Heart and Great Vessels
Dural venous sinus *use* Vein, Intracranial
Dura mater, intracranial *use* Dura Mater
Dura mater, spinal *use* Spinal Meninges
Durata® Defibrillation Lead *use* Cardiac Lead, Defibrillator in 02H
Durvalumab Antineoplastic XW0
DynaClip® (Forte)
use Internal Fixation Device, Sustained Compression in 0RG
use Internal Fixation Device, Sustained Compression in 0SG
DynaNail® (Helix) (Hybrid) (Mini)
use Internal Fixation Device, Sustained Compression in 0RG
use Internal Fixation Device, Sustained Compression in 0SG
Dynesys® Dynamic Stabilization System
use Spinal Stabilization Device, Pedicle-Based in 0RH
use Spinal Stabilization Device, Pedicle-Based in 0SH

D

▶ New ➡ Revised ~~deleted~~ Deleted

E

E-Luminexx™ (Biliary) (Vascular) Stent *use* Intraluminal Device
Earlobe
use External Ear, Right
use External Ear, Left
use External Ear, Bilateral
ECCO2R (Extracorporeal Carbon Dioxide Removal) 5A0920Z
Echocardiogram *see* Ultrasonography, Heart B24
▶ **EchoGo Heart Failure 1.0 software** XXE2X19
Echography *see* Ultrasonography
EchoTip® Insight™ Portosystemic Pressure Gradient Measurement System 4A044B2
ECMO *see* Performance, Circulatory 5A15
ECMO, intraoperative *see* Performance, Circulatory 5A15A
Eculizumab XW0
EDWARDS INTUITY Elite valve system (rapid deployment technique) *see* Replacement, Valve, Aortic 02RF
EEG (electroencephalogram) *see* Measurement, Central Nervous 4A00
EGD (esophagogastroduodenoscopy) 0DJ08ZZ
Eighth cranial nerve *use* Acoustic Nerve
Ejaculatory duct
use Vas Deferens, Right
use Vas Deferens, Left
use Vas Deferens, Bilateral
use Vas Deferens
EKG (electrocardiogram) *see* Measurement, Cardiac 4A02
EKOS™ EkoSonic® Endovascular System *see* Fragmentation, Artery
Eladocagene exuparvovec XW0Q316
Electrical bone growth stimulator (EBGS)
use Bone Growth Stimulator in Head and Facial Bones
use Bone Growth Stimulator in Upper Bones
use Bone Growth Stimulator in Lower Bones
Electrical muscle stimulation (EMS) lead *use* Stimulator Lead in Muscles
Electrocautery
Destruction *see* Destruction
Repair *see* Repair
Electroconvulsive Therapy
Bilateral-Multiple Seizure GZB3ZZZ
Bilateral-Single Seizure GZB2ZZZ
Electroconvulsive Therapy, Other GZB4ZZZ
Unilateral-Multiple Seizure GZB1ZZZ
Unilateral-Single Seizure GZB0ZZZ
Electroencephalogram (EEG) *see* Measurement, Central Nervous 4A00
Electromagnetic Therapy
Central Nervous 6A22
Urinary 6A21
Electronic muscle stimulator lead *use* Stimulator Lead in Muscles
Electrophysiologic stimulation (EPS) *see* Measurement, Cardiac 4A02
Electroshock therapy *see* Electroconvulsive Therapy
Elevation, bone fragments, skull *see* Reposition, Head and Facial Bones 0NS
Eleventh cranial nerve *use* Accessory Nerve
Ellipsys® vascular access system *see* New Technology, Cardiovascular System X2K
▶ **Elranatamab Antineoplastic** XW013L9
Eluvia™ Drug-Eluting Vascular Stent System
use Intraluminal Device, Sustained Release Drug-eluting in New Technology
use Intraluminal Device, Sustained Release Drug-eluting, Two in New Technology
use Intraluminal Device, Sustained Release Drug-eluting, Three in New Technology
use Intraluminal Device, Sustained Release Drug-eluting, Four or More in New Technology
ELZONRIS™
use Tagraxofusp-erzs Antineoplastic
Embolectomy *see* Extirpation
Embolization
see Occlusion
see Restriction
Embolization coil(s) *use* Intraluminal Device
EMG (electromyogram) *see* Measurement, Musculoskeletal 4A0F
Encephalon *use* Brain
Endarterectomy
see Extirpation, Upper Arteries 03C
see Extirpation, Lower Arteries 04C
Endeavor® (III) (IV) (Sprint) Zotarolimus-eluting Coronary Stent System *use* Intraluminal Device, Drug-eluting in Heart and Great Vessels
EndoAVF procedure, using magnetic-guided radiofrequency *see* Bypass, Upper Arteries 031
EndoAVF procedure, using thermal resistance energy *see* New Technology, Cardiovascular System X2K
Endologix AFX® Endovascular AAA System use Intraluminal Device
EndoSure® sensor *use* Monitoring Device, Pressure Sensor in 02H
ENDOTAK RELIANCE® (G) Defibrillation Lead *use* Cardiac Lead, Defibrillator in 02H
Endothelial damage inhibitor, applied to vein graft XY0VX83
Endotracheal tube (cuffed) (double-lumen) *use* Intraluminal Device, Endotracheal Airway in Respiratory System
Endovascular fistula creation, using magnetic-guided radiofrequency *see* Bypass, Upper Arteries 031
Endovascular fistula creation, using thermal resistance energy *see* New Technology, Cardiovascular System X2K
Endurant® Endovascular Stent Graft *use* Intraluminal Device
Endurant® II AAA stent graft system *use* Intraluminal Device
Engineered Allogeneic Thymus Tissue XW020D8
Engineered chimeric antigen receptor T-cell immunotherapy
Allogeneic XW0
Autologous XW0
Enlargement
see Dilation
see Repair
ENROUTE® Transcarotid Neuroprotection System *see* New Technology, Cardiovascular System X2A
EnRhythm *use* Pacemaker, Dual Chamber in 0JH
ENSPRYNG™ *use* Satralizumab-mwge
Enterorrhaphy *see* Repair, Gastrointestinal System 0DQ
Enterra gastric neurostimulator *use* Stimulator Generator, Multiple Array in 0JH
Enucleation
Eyeball *see* Resection, Eye 08T
Eyeball with prosthetic implant *see* Replacement, Eye 08R
▶ **Epcoritamab Monoclonal Antibody** XW013S9
Ependyma *use* Cerebral Ventricle
Epic™ Stented Tissue Valve (aortic) *use* Zooplastic Tissue in Heart and Great Vessels
Epicel® cultured epidermal autograft *use* Autologous Tissue Substitute
Epidermis *use* Skin
Epididymectomy
see Excision, Male Reproductive System 0VB
see Resection, Male Reproductive System 0VT
Epididymoplasty
see Repair, Male Reproductive System 0VQ
see Supplement, Male Reproductive System 0VU
Epididymorrhaphy *see* Repair, Male Reproductive System 0VQ
Epididymotomy *see* Drainage, Male Reproductive System 0V9
Epidural space, spinal use Spinal Canal
Epiphysiodesis
see Insertion of device in, Upper Bones 0PH
see Repair, Upper Bones 0PQ
see Insertion of device in, Lower Bones 0QH
see Repair, Lower Bones 0QQ
Epiploic foramen *use* Peritoneum
Epiretinal Visual Prosthesis
Left 08H105Z
Right 08H005Z
Episiorrhaphy *see* Repair, Perineum, Female 0WQN
Episiotomy *see* Division, Perineum, Female 0W8N
Epithalamus *use* Thalamus
Epitroclear lymph node
use Lymphatic, Right Upper Extremity
use Lymphatic, Left Upper Extremity
EPS (electrophysiologic stimulation) *see* Measurement, Cardiac 4A02
Eptifibatide, infusion *see* Introduction of Platelet Inhibitor
ERCP (endoscopic retrograde cholangiopancreatography) *see* Fluoroscopy, Hepatobiliary System and Pancreas BF1
Erector spinae muscle
use Trunk Muscle, Right
use Trunk Muscle, Left
Erdafitinib Antineoplastic XW0DXL5
ERLEADA™ *use* Apalutamide Antineoplastic
Esketamine Hydrochloride XW097M5
Esophageal artery *use* Upper Artery
Esophageal obturator airway (EOA) *use* Intraluminal Device, Airway in Gastrointestinal System
Esophageal plexus *use* Thoracic Sympathetic Nerve
Esophagectomy
see Excision, Gastrointestinal System 0DB
see Resection, Gastrointestinal System 0DT
Esophagocoloplasty
see Repair, Gastrointestinal System 0DQ
see Supplement, Gastrointestinal System 0DU
Esophagoenterostomy
see Bypass, Gastrointestinal System 0D1
see Drainage, Gastrointestinal System 0D9
Esophagoesophagostomy
see Bypass, Gastrointestinal System 0D1
see Drainage, Gastrointestinal System 0D9
Esophagogastrectomy
see Excision, Gastrointestinal System 0DB
see Resection, Gastrointestinal System 0DT
Esophagogastroduodenoscopy (EGD) 0DJ08ZZ
Esophagogastroplasty
see Repair, Gastrointestinal System 0DQ
see Supplement, Gastrointestinal System 0DU
Esophagogastroscopy 0DJ68ZZ
Esophagogastrostomy
see Bypass, Gastrointestinal System 0D1
see Drainage, Gastrointestinal System 0D9
Esophagojejunoplasty *see* Supplement, Gastrointestinal System 0DU
Esophagojejunostomy
see Bypass, Gastrointestinal System 0D1
see Drainage, Gastrointestinal System 0D9
Esophagomyotomy *see* Division, Esophagogastric Junction 0D84
Esophagoplasty
see Repair, Gastrointestinal System 0DQ
see Replacement, Esophagus 0DR5
see Supplement, Gastrointestinal System 0DU
Esophagoplication *see* Restriction, Gastrointestinal System 0DV
Esophagorrhaphy *see* Repair, Gastrointestinal System 0DQ
Esophagoscopy 0DJ08ZZ

E

Esophagotomy *see* Drainage, Gastrointestinal System 0D9
Esteem® implantable hearing system *use* Hearing Device in Ear, Nose, Sinus
ESWL (extracorporeal shock wave lithotripsy) *see* Fragmentation
Etesevimab monoclonal antibody XW0
Ethmoidal air cell
- *use* Ethmoid Sinus, Right
- *use* Ethmoid Sinus, Left

Ethmoidectomy
- *see* Excision, Ear, Nose, Sinus 09B
- *see* Resection, Ear, Nose, Sinus 09T
- *see* Excision, Head and Facial Bones 0NB
- *see* Resection, Head and Facial Bones 0NT

Ethmoidotomy *see* Drainage, Ear, Nose, Sinus 099
Evacuation
- Hematoma *see* Extirpation
- Other Fluid *see* Drainage

Evera (XT)(S)(DR/VR) *use* Defibrillator Generator in 0JH
Everolimus-eluting coronary stent *use* Intraluminal Device, Drug-eluting in Heart and Great Vessels
▶EV ICD System (Extravascular implantable defibrillator lead) *use* Defibrillator Lead in AnatomicalRegions, General
Evisceration
- Eyeball *see* Resection, Eye 08T
- Eyeball with prosthetic implant *see* Replacement, Eye 08R

Ex-PRESS™ mini glaucoma shunt *use* Synthetic Substitute
▶Exagamglogene Autotemcel XW1
EXALT™ Model D Single-Use Duodenoscope *see* New Technology, Hepatobiliary System and Pancreas XFJ
Examination *see* Inspection
Exchange *see* Change device in
Excision
- Abdominal Wall 0WBF
- Acetabulum
  - Left 0QB5
  - Right 0QB4
- Adenoids 0CBQ
- Ampulla of Vater 0FBC
- Anal Sphincter 0DBR
- Ankle Region
  - Left 0YBL
  - Right 0YBK
- Anus 0DBQ
- Aorta
  - Abdominal 04B0
  - Thoracic
    - Ascending/Arch 02BX
    - Descending 02BW
- Aortic Body 0GBD
- Appendix 0DBJ
- Arm
  - Lower
    - Left 0XBF
    - Right 0XBD
  - Upper
    - Left 0XB9
    - Right 0XB8
- Artery
  - Anterior Tibial
    - Left 04BQ
    - Right 04BP
  - Axillary
    - Left 03B6
    - Right 03B5
  - Brachial
    - Left 03B8
    - Right 03B7
  - Celiac 04B1
  - Colic
    - Left 04B7
    - Middle 04B8
    - Right 04B6

Excision *(Continued)*
- Artery *(Continued)*
  - Common Carotid
    - Left 03BJ
    - Right 03BH
  - Common Iliac
    - Left 04BD
    - Right 04BC
  - External Carotid
    - Left 03BN
    - Right 03BM
  - External Iliac
    - Left 04BJ
    - Right 04BH
  - Face 03BR
  - Femoral
    - Left 04BL
    - Right 04BK
  - Foot
    - Left 04BW
    - Right 04BV
  - Gastric 04B2
  - Hand
    - Left 03BF
    - Right 03BD
  - Hepatic 04B3
  - Inferior Mesenteric 04BB
  - Innominate 03B2
  - Internal Carotid
    - Left 03BL
    - Right 03BK
  - Internal Iliac
    - Left 04BF
    - Right 04BE
  - Internal Mammary
    - Left 03B1
    - Right 03B0
  - Intracranial 03BG
  - Lower 04BY
  - Peroneal
    - Left 04BU
    - Right 04BT
  - Popliteal
    - Left 04BN
    - Right 04BM
  - Posterior Tibial
    - Left 04BS
    - Right 04BR
  - Pulmonary
    - Left 02BR
    - Right 02BQ
  - Pulmonary Trunk 02BP
  - Radial
    - Left 03BC
    - Right 03BB
  - Renal
    - Left 04BA
    - Right 04B9
  - Splenic 04B4
  - Subclavian
    - Left 03B4
    - Right 03B3
  - Superior Mesenteric 04B5
  - Temporal
    - Left 03BT
    - Right 03BS
  - Thyroid
    - Left 03BV
    - Right 03BU
  - Ulnar
    - Left 03BA
    - Right 03B9
  - Upper 03BY
  - Vertebral
    - Left 03BQ
    - Right 03BP
- Atrium
  - Left 02B7
  - Right 02B6
- Auditory Ossicle
  - Left 09BA
  - Right 09B9

Excision *(Continued)*
- Axilla
  - Left 0XB5
  - Right 0XB4
- Back
  - Lower 0WBL
  - Upper 0WBK
- Basal Ganglia 00B8
- Bladder 0TBB
- Bladder Neck 0TBC
- Bone
  - Ethmoid
    - Left 0NBG
    - Right 0NBF
  - Frontal 0NB1
  - Hyoid 0NBX
  - Lacrimal
    - Left 0NBJ
    - Right 0NBH
  - Nasal 0NBB
  - Occipital 0NB7
  - Palatine
    - Left 0NBL
    - Right 0NBK
  - Parietal
    - Left 0NB4
    - Right 0NB3
  - Pelvic
    - Left 0QB3
    - Right 0QB2
  - Sphenoid 0NBC
  - Temporal
    - Left 0NB6
    - Right 0NB5
  - Zygomatic
    - Left 0NBN
    - Right 0NBM
- Brain 00B0
- Breast
  - Bilateral 0HBV
  - Left 0HBU
  - Right 0HBT
  - Supernumerary 0HBY
- Bronchus
  - Lingula 0BB9
  - Lower Lobe
    - Left 0BBB
    - Right 0BB6
  - Main
    - Left 0BB7
    - Right 0BB3
  - Middle Lobe, Right 0BB5
  - Upper Lobe
    - Left 0BB8
    - Right 0BB4
- Buccal Mucosa 0CB4
- Bursa and Ligament
  - Abdomen
    - Left 0MBJ
    - Right 0MBH
  - Ankle
    - Left 0MBR
    - Right 0MBQ
  - Elbow
    - Left 0MB4
    - Right 0MB3
  - Foot
    - Left 0MBT
    - Right 0MBS
  - Hand
    - Left 0MB8
    - Right 0MB7
  - Head and Neck 0MB0
  - Hip
    - Left 0MBM
    - Right 0MBL
  - Knee
    - Left 0MBP
    - Right 0MBN
  - Lower Extremity
    - Left 0MBW
    - Right 0MBV

E

E

E

E

▶ New ➡ Revised ~~deleted~~ Deleted

Extirpation (Continued)
Artery (Continued)
Pulmonary Trunk 02CP
Radial
Left 03CC
Right 03CB
Renal
Left 04CA
Right 04C9
Splenic 04C4
Subclavian
Left 03C4
Right 03C3
Superior Mesenteric 04C5
Temporal
Left 03CT
Right 03CS
Thyroid
Left 03CV
Right 03CU
Ulnar
Left 03CA
Right 03C9
Upper 03CY
Vertebral
Left 03CQ
Right 03CP
Atrium
Left 02C7
Right 02C6
Auditory Ossicle
Left 09CA
Right 09C9
Basal Ganglia 00C8
Bladder 0TCB
Bladder Neck 0TCC
Bone
Ethmoid
Left 0NCG
Right 0NCF
Frontal 0NC1
Hyoid 0NCX
Lacrimal
Left 0NCJ
Right 0NCH
Nasal 0NCB
Occipital 0NC7
Palatine
Left 0NCL
Right 0NCK
Parietal
Left 0NC4
Right 0NC3
Pelvic
Left 0QC3
Right 0QC2
Sphenoid 0NCC
Temporal
Left 0NC6
Right 0NC5
Zygomatic
Left 0NCN
Right 0NCM
Brain 00C0
Breast
Bilateral 0HCV
Left 0HCU
Right 0HCT
Bronchus
Lingula 0BC9
Lower Lobe
Left 0BCB
Right 0BC6
Main
Left 0BC7
Right 0BC3
Middle Lobe, Right 0BC5
Upper Lobe
Left 0BC8
Right 0BC4
Buccal Mucosa 0CC4

Extirpation (Continued)
Bursa and Ligament
Abdomen
Left 0MCJ
Right 0MCH
Ankle
Left 0MCR
Right 0MCQ
Elbow
Left 0MC4
Right 0MC3
Foot
Left 0MCT
Right 0MCS
Hand
Left 0MC8
Right 0MC7
Head and Neck 0MC0
Hip
Left 0MCM
Right 0MCL
Knee
Left 0MCP
Right 0MCN
Lower Extremity
Left 0MCW
Right 0MCV
Perineum 0MCK
Rib(s) 0MCG
Shoulder
Left 0MC2
Right 0MC1
Spine
Lower 0MCD
Upper 0MCC
Sternum 0MCF
Upper Extremity
Left 0MCB
Right 0MC9
Wrist
Left 0MC6
Right 0MC5
Carina 0BC2
Carotid Bodies, Bilateral 0GC8
Carotid Body
Left 0GC6
Right 0GC7
Carpal
Left 0PCN
Right 0PCM
Cavity, Cranial 0WC1
Cecum 0DCH
Cerebellum 00CC
Cerebral Hemisphere 00C7
Cerebral Meninges 00C1
Cerebral Ventricle 00C6
Cervix 0UCC
Chordae Tendineae 02C9
Choroid
Left 08CB
Right 08CA
Cisterna Chyli 07CL
Clavicle
Left 0PCB
Right 0PC9
Clitoris 0UCJ
Coccygeal Glomus 0GCB
Coccyx 0QCS
Colon
Ascending 0DCK
Descending 0DCM
Sigmoid 0DCN
Transverse 0DCL
Computer-aided Mechanical Aspiration X2C
Conduction Mechanism 02C8
Conjunctiva
Left 08CTXZZ
Right 08CSXZZ
Cord
Bilateral 0VCH
Left 0VCG
Right 0VCF

Extirpation (Continued)
Cornea
Left 08C9XZZ
Right 08C8XZZ
Cul-de-sac 0UCF
Diaphragm 0BCT
Disc
Cervical Vertebral 0RC3
Cervicothoracic Vertebral 0RC5
Lumbar Vertebral 0SC2
Lumbosacral 0SC4
Thoracic Vertebral 0RC9
Thoracolumbar Vertebral 0RCB
Duct
Common Bile 0FC9
Cystic 0FC8
Hepatic
Common 0FC7
Left 0FC6
Right 0FC5
Lacrimal
Left 08CY
Right 08CX
Pancreatic 0FCD
Accessory 0FCF
Parotid
Left 0CCC
Right 0CCB
Duodenum 0DC9
Dura Mater 00C2
Ear
External
Left 09C1
Right 09C0
External Auditory Canal
Left 09C4
Right 09C3
Inner
Left 09CE
Right 09CD
Middle
Left 09C6
Right 09C5
Endometrium 0UCB
Epididymis
Bilateral 0VCL
Left 0VCK
Right 0VCJ
Epidural Space, Intracranial 00C3
Epiglottis 0CCR
Esophagogastric Junction 0DC4
Esophagus 0DC5
Lower 0DC3
Middle 0DC2
Upper 0DC1
Eustachian Tube
Left 09CG
Right 09CF
Eye
Left 08C1XZZ
Right 08C0XZZ
Eyelid
Lower
Left 08CR
Right 08CQ
Upper
Left 08CP
Right 08CN
Fallopian Tube
Left 0UC6
Right 0UC5
Fallopian Tubes, Bilateral 0UC7
Femoral Shaft
Left 0QC9
Right 0QC8
Femur
Lower
Left 0QCC
Right 0QCB
Upper
Left 0QC7
Right 0QC6

E

Extirpation (Continued)
Nerve (Continued)
Cervical 01C1
Cervical Plexus 01C0
Facial 00CM
Femoral 01CD
Glossopharyngeal 00CP
Head and Neck Sympathetic 01CK
Hypoglossal 00CS
Lumbar 01CB
Lumbar Plexus 01C9
Lumbar Sympathetic 01CN
Lumbosacral Plexus 01CA
Median 01C5
Oculomotor 00CH
Olfactory 00CF
Optic 00CG
Peroneal 01CH
Phrenic 01C2
Pudendal 01CC
Radial 01C6
Sacral 01CR
Sacral Plexus 01CQ
Sacral Sympathetic 01CP
Sciatic 01CF
Thoracic 01C8
Thoracic Sympathetic 01CL
Tibial 01CG
Trigeminal 00CK
Trochlear 00CJ
Ulnar 01C4
Vagus 00CQ
Nipple
Left 0HCX
Right 0HCW
Omentum 0DCU
Oral Cavity and Throat 0WC3
Orbit
Left 0NCQ
Right 0NCP
Orbital Atherectomy see Extirpation, Heart and Great Vessels 02C
Ovary
Bilateral 0UC2
Left 0UC1
Right 0UC0
Palate
Hard 0CC2
Soft 0CC3
Pancreas 0FCG
Para-aortic Body 0GC9
Paraganglion Extremity 0GCF
Parathyroid Gland 0GCR
Inferior
Left 0GCP
Right 0GCN
Multiple 0GCQ
Superior
Left 0GCM
Right 0GCL
Patella
Left 0QCF
Right 0QCD
Pelvic Cavity 0WCJ
Penis 0VCS
Pericardial Cavity 0WCD
Pericardium 02CN
Peritoneal Cavity 0WCG
Peritoneum 0DCW
Phalanx
Finger
Left 0PCV
Right 0PCT
Thumb
Left 0PCS
Right 0PCR
Toe
Left 0QCR
Right 0QCQ
Pharynx 0CCM
Pineal Body 0GC1

Extirpation (Continued)
Pleura
Left 0BCP
Right 0BCN
Pleural Cavity
Left 0WCB
Right 0WC9
Pons 00CB
Prepuce 0VCT
Prostate 0VC0
Radius
Left 0PCJ
Right 0PCH
Rectum 0DCP
Respiratory Tract 0WCQ
Retina
Left 08CF
Right 08CE
Retinal Vessel
Left 08CH
Right 08CG
Retroperitoneum 0WCH
Ribs
1 to 2 0PC1
3 or More 0PC2
Sacrum 0QC1
Scapula
Left 0PC6
Right 0PC5
Sclera
Left 08C7XZZ
Right 08C6XZZ
Scrotum 0VC5
Septum
Atrial 02C5
Nasal 09CM
Ventricular 02CM
Sinus
Accessory 09CP
Ethmoid
Left 09CV
Right 09CU
Frontal
Left 09CT
Right 09CS
Mastoid
Left 09CC
Right 09CB
Maxillary
Left 09CR
Right 09CQ
Sphenoid
Left 09CX
Right 09CW
Skin
Abdomen 0HC7XZZ
Back 0HC6XZZ
Buttock 0HC8XZZ
Chest 0HC5XZZ
Ear
Left 0HC3XZZ
Right 0HC2XZZ
Face 0HC1XZZ
Foot
Left 0HCNXZZ
Right 0HCMXZZ
Hand
Left 0HCGXZZ
Right 0HCFXZZ
Inguinal 0HCAXZZ
Lower Arm
Left 0HCEXZZ
Right 0HCDXZZ
Lower Leg
Left 0HCLXZZ
Right 0HCKXZZ
Neck 0HC4XZZ
Perineum 0HC9XZZ
Scalp 0HC0XZZ
Upper Arm
Left 0HCCXZZ
Right 0HCBXZZ

Extirpation (Continued)
Skin (Continued)
Upper Leg
Left 0HCJXZZ
Right 0HCHXZZ
Spinal Canal 00CU
Spinal Cord
Cervical 00CW
Lumbar 00CY
Thoracic 00CX
Spinal Meninges 00CT
Spleen 07CP
Sternum 0PC0
Stomach 0DC6
Pylorus 0DC7
Subarachnoid Space, Intracranial 00C5
Subcutaneous Tissue and Fascia
Abdomen 0JC8
Back 0JC7
Buttock 0JC9
Chest 0JC6
Face 0JC1
Foot
Left 0JCR
Right 0JCQ
Hand
Left 0JCK
Right 0JCJ
Lower Arm
Left 0JCH
Right 0JCG
Lower Leg
Left 0JCP
Right 0JCN
Neck
Left 0JC5
Right 0JC4
Pelvic Region 0JCC
Perineum 0JCB
Scalp 0JC0
Upper Arm
Left 0JCF
Right 0JCD
Upper Leg
Left 0JCM
Right 0JCL
Subdural Space, Intracranial 00C4
Tarsal
Left 0QCM
Right 0QCL
Tendon
Abdomen
Left 0LCG
Right 0LCF
Ankle
Left 0LCT
Right 0LCS
Foot
Left 0LCW
Right 0LCV
Hand
Left 0LC8
Right 0LC7
Head and Neck 0LC0
Hip
Left 0LCK
Right 0LCJ
Knee
Left 0LCR
Right 0LCQ
Lower Arm and Wrist
Left 0LC6
Right 0LC5
Lower Leg
Left 0LCP
Right 0LCN
Perineum 0LCH
Shoulder
Left 0LC2
Right 0LC1

E

Extirpation (Continued)
Tendon (Continued)
Thorax
Left 0LCD
Right 0LCC
Trunk
Left 0LCB
Right 0LC9
Upper Arm
Left 0LC4
Right 0LC3
Upper Leg
Left 0LCM
Right 0LCL
Testis
Bilateral 0VCC
Left 0VCB
Right 0VC9
Thalamus 00C9
Thymus 07CM
Thyroid Gland 0GCK
Left Lobe 0GCG
Right Lobe 0GCH
Tibia
Left 0QCH
Right 0QCG
Toe Nail 0HCRXZZ
Tongue 0CC7
Tonsils 0CCP
Tooth
Lower 0CCX
Upper 0CCW
Trachea 0BC1
Tunica Vaginalis
Left 0VC7
Right 0VC6
Turbinate, Nasal 09CL
Tympanic Membrane
Left 09C8
Right 09C7
Ulna
Left 0PCL
Right 0PCK
Ureter
Left 0TC7
Right 0TC6
Urethra 0TCD
Uterine Supporting Structure 0UC4
Uterus 0UC9
Uvula 0CCN
Vagina 0UCG
Valve
Aortic 02CF
Mitral 02CG
Pulmonary 02CH
Tricuspid 02CJ
Vas Deferens
Bilateral 0VCQ
Left 0VCP
Right 0VCN
Vein
Axillary
Left 05C8
Right 05C7
Azygos 05C0
Basilic
Left 05CC
Right 05CB
Brachial
Left 05CA
Right 05C9
Cephalic
Left 05CF
Right 05CD
Colic 06C7
Common Iliac
Left 06CD
Right 06CC
Coronary 02C4
Esophageal 06C3
External Iliac

Extirpation (Continued)
Vein (Continued)
Left 06CG
Right 06CF
External Jugular
Left 05CQ
Right 05CP
Face
Left 05CV
Right 05CT
Femoral
Left 06CN
Right 06CM
Foot
Left 06CV
Right 06CT
Gastric 06C2
Hand
Left 05CH
Right 05CG
Hemiazygos 05C1
Hepatic 06C4
Hypogastric
Left 06CJ
Right 06CH
Inferior Mesenteric 06C6
Innominate
Left 05C4
Right 05C3
Internal Jugular
Left 05CN
Right 05CM
Intracranial 05CL
Lower 06CY
Portal 06C8
Pulmonary
Left 02CT
Right 02CS
Renal
Left 06CB
Right 06C9
Saphenous
Left 06CQ
Right 06CP
Splenic 06C1
Subclavian
Left 05C6
Right 05C5
Superior Mesenteric 06C5
Upper 05CY
Vertebral
Left 05CS
Right 05CR
Vena Cava
Inferior 06C0
Superior 02CV
Ventricle
Left 02CL
Right 02CK
Vertebra
Cervical 0PC3
Lumbar 0QC0
Thoracic 0PC4
Vesicle
Bilateral 0VC3
Left 0VC2
Right 0VC1
Vitreous
Left 08C5
Right 08C4
Vocal Cord
Left 0CCV
Right 0CCT
Vulva 0UCM
Extracorporeal Carbon Dioxide Removal (ECCO2R) 5A0920Z
Extracorporeal shock wave lithotripsy *see* Fragmentation
Extracranial-intracranial bypass (EC-IC) *see* Bypass, Upper Arteries 031

Extraction
Acetabulum
Left 0QD50ZZ
Right 0QD40ZZ
Ampulla of Vater 0FDC
Anus 0DDQ
Appendix 0DDJ
Auditory Ossicle
Left 09DA0ZZ
Right 09D90ZZ
Bone
Ethmoid
Left 0NDG0ZZ
Right 0NDF0ZZ
Frontal 0ND10ZZ
Hyoid 0NDX0ZZ
Lacrimal
Left 0NDJ0ZZ
Right 0NDH0ZZ
Nasal 0NDB0ZZ
Occipital 0ND70ZZ
Palatine
Left 0NDL0ZZ
Right 0NDK0ZZ
Parietal
Left 0ND40ZZ
Right 0ND30ZZ
Pelvic
Left 0QD30ZZ
Right 0QD20ZZ
Sphenoid 0NDC0ZZ
Temporal
Left 0ND60ZZ
Right 0ND50ZZ
Zygomatic
Left 0NDN0ZZ
Right 0NDM0ZZ
Bone Marrow 07DT
Iliac 07DR
Sternum 07DQ
Vertebral 07DS
Brain 00D0
Breast
Bilateral 0HDV0ZZ
Left 0HDU0ZZ
Right 0HDT0ZZ
Supernumerary 0HDY0ZXZ
Bronchus
Lingula 0BD9
Lower Lobe
Left 0BDB
Right 0BD6
Main
Left 0BD7
Right 0BD3
Middle Lobe, Right 0BD5
Upper Lobe
Left 0BD8
Right 0BD4
Bursa and Ligament
Abdomen
Left 0MDJ
Right 0MDH
Ankle
Left 0MDR
Right 0MDQ
Elbow
Left 0MD4
Right 0MD3
Foot
Left 0MDT
Right 0MDS
Hand
Left 0MD8
Right 0MD7
Head and Neck 0MD0
Hip
Left 0MDM
Right 0MDL
Knee
Left 0MDP
Right 0MDN

E

F

Face lift *see* Alteration, Face 0W02
Facet replacement spinal stabilization device
  use Spinal Stabilization Device, Facet Replacement in 0RH
  use Spinal Stabilization Device, Facet Replacement in 0SH
Facial artery *use* Face Artery
Factor Xa Inhibitor Reversal Agent, Andexanet Alfa *use* Coagulation Factor Xa, Inactivated
False vocal cord *use* Larynx
Falx cerebri *use* Dura Mater
Fascia lata
  use Subcutaneous Tissue and Fascia, Right Upper Leg
  use Subcutaneous Tissue and Fascia, Left Upper Leg
Fasciaplasty, fascioplasty
  see Repair, Subcutaneous Tissue and Fascia 0JQ
  see Replacement, Subcutaneous Tissue and Fascia 0JR
Fasciectomy
  see Excision, Subcutaneous Tissue and Fascia 0JB
Fasciorrhaphy *see* Repair, Subcutaneous Tissue and Fascia 0JQ
Fasciotomy
  see Division, Subcutaneous Tissue and Fascia 0J8
  see Drainage, Subcutaneous Tissue and Fascia 0J9
  see Release
Feeding Device
  Change device in
    Lower Intestinal Tract 0D2DXUZ
    Upper Intestinal Tract 0D20XUZ
  Insertion of device in
    Duodenum 0DH9
    Esophagus 0DH5
    Ileum 0DHB
    Intestine, Small 0DH8
    Jejunum 0DHA
    Stomach 0DH6
  Removal of device from
    Esophagus 0DP5
    Intestinal Tract
      Lower Intestinal Tract 0DPD
      Upper Intestinal Tract 0DP0
    Stomach 0DP6
  Revision of device in
    Intestinal Tract
      Lower Intestinal Tract 0DWD
      Upper Intestinal Tract 0DW0
    Stomach 0DW6
Femoral head
  use Upper Femur, Right
  use Upper Femur, Left
Femoral lymph node
  use Lymphatic, Right Lower Extremity
  use Lymphatic, Left Lower Extremity
Femoropatellar joint
  use Knee Joint, Right
  use Knee Joint, Left
  use Knee Joint, Femoral Surface, Right
  use Knee Joint, Femoral Surface, Left
Femorotibial joint
  use Knee Joint, Right
  use Knee Joint, Left
  use Knee Joint, Tibial Surface, Right
  use Knee Joint, Tibial Surface, Left
FETROJA® *use* Cefiderocol Anti-infective
FGS (fluorescence-guided surgery)
  see Fluorescence Guided Procedure
Fibular artery
  use Peroneal Artery, Right
  use Peroneal Artery, Left
Fibular sesamoid
  use Metatarsal, Right
  use Metatarsal, Left
Fibularis brevis muscle
  use Lower Leg Muscle, Right
  use Lower Leg Muscle, Left
Fibularis longus muscle
  use Lower Leg Muscle, Right
  use Lower Leg Muscle, Left
Fifth cranial nerve *use* Trigeminal Nerve
Filum terminale *use* Spinal Meninges
Fimbriectomy
  see Excision, Female Reproductive System 0UB
  see Resection, Female Reproductive System 0UT
Fine needle aspiration
  Fluid or gas *see* Drainage
  Tissue biopsy
    see Extraction
    see Excision
First cranial nerve *use* Olfactory Nerve
First intercostal nerve *use* Brachial Plexus
Fistulization
  see Bypass
  see Drainage
  see Repair
Fitting
  Arch bars, for fracture reduction *see* Reposition, Mouth and Throat 0CS
  Arch bars, for immobilization *see* Immobilization, Face 2W31
  Artificial limb *see* Device Fitting, Rehabilitation F0D
  Hearing aid *see* Device Fitting, Rehabilitation F0D
  Ocular prosthesis F0DZ8UZ
  Prosthesis, limb *see* Device Fitting, Rehabilitation F0D
  Prosthesis, ocular F0DZ8UZ
Fixation, bone
  External, with fracture reduction *see* Reposition
  External, without fracture reduction *see* Insertion
  Internal, with fracture reduction *see* Reposition
  Internal, without fracture reduction *see* Insertion
FLAIR® Endovascular Stent Graft *use* Intraluminal Device
Flexible Composite Mesh *use* Synthetic Substitute
Flexor carpi radialis muscle
  use Lower Arm and Wrist Muscle, Right
  use Lower Arm and Wrist Muscle, Left
Flexor carpi ulnaris muscle
  use Lower Arm and Wrist Muscle, Right
  use Lower Arm and Wrist Muscle, Left
Flexor digitorum brevis muscle
  use Foot Muscle, Right
  use Foot Muscle, Left
Flexor digitorum longus muscle
  use Lower Leg Muscle, Right
  use Lower Leg Muscle, Left
Flexor hallucis brevis muscle
  use Foot Muscle, Right
  use Foot Muscle, Left
Flexor hallucis longus muscle
  use Lower Leg Muscle, Right
  use Lower Leg Muscle, Left
Flexor pollicis longus muscle
  use Lower Arm and Wrist Muscle, Right
  use Lower Arm and Wrist Muscle, Left
▶Flourish® Pediatric Esophageal Atresia Device *use* Magnetic Lengthening Device in Gastrointestinal System
Flow Diverter embolization device
  use Intraluminal Device, Flow Diverter in 03V
FlowSense Noninvasive Thermal Sensor 4B00XW0
Fluorescence Guided Procedure
  Extremity
    Lower 8E0Y
    Upper 8E0X
Fluorescence Guided Procedure *(Continued)*
  Head and Neck Region 8E09
    Aminolevulinic Acid 8E090EM
    No Qualifier 8E090EZ
  ▶Reproductive System, Female, Pafolacianine (CYTALUX®) 8E0U
  ➡Trunk Region
    ▶No Qualifier 8E0W
    ▶Pafolacianine (CYTALUX®) 8E0W
Fluorescent Pyrazine, Kidney XT25XE5
Fluoroscopy
  Abdomen and Pelvis BW11
  Airway, Upper BB1DZZZ
  Ankle
    Left BQ1H
    Right BQ1G
  Aorta
    Abdominal B410
      Laser, Intraoperative B410
    Thoracic B310
      Laser, Intraoperative B310
    Thoraco-Abdominal B31P
      Laser, Intraoperative B31P
  Aorta and Bilateral Lower Extremity Arteries B41D
    Laser, Intraoperative B41D
  Arm
    Left BP1FZZZ
    Right BP1EZZZ
  Artery
    Brachiocephalic-Subclavian
      Right B311
      Laser, Intraoperative B311
    Bronchial B31L
      Laser, Intraoperative B31L
    Bypass Graft, Other B21F
    Cervico-Cerebral Arch B31Q
      Laser, Intraoperative B31Q
    Common Carotid
      Bilateral B315
        Laser, Intraoperative B315
      Left B314
        Laser, Intraoperative B314
      Right B313
        Laser, Intraoperative B313
    Coronary
      Bypass Graft
        Multiple B213
          Laser, Intraoperative B213
        Single B212
          Laser, Intraoperative B212
      Multiple B211
        Laser, Intraoperative B211
      Single B210
        Laser, Intraoperative B210
    External Carotid
      Bilateral B31C
        Laser, Intraoperative B31C
      Left B31B
        Laser, Intraoperative B31B
      Right B319
        Laser, Intraoperative B319
    Hepatic B412
      Laser, Intraoperative B412
    Inferior Mesenteric B415
      Laser, Intraoperative B415
    Intercostal B31L
      Laser, Intraoperative B31L
    Internal Carotid
      Bilateral B318
        Laser, Intraoperative B318
      Left B317
        Laser, Intraoperative B317
      Right B316
        Laser, Intraoperative B316
    Internal Mammary Bypass Graft
      Left B218
      Right B217
    Intra-Abdominal
      Other B41B
      Laser, Intraoperative B41B

F

F

- Fluoroscopy *(Continued)*
  - Vein *(Continued)*
    - Lower Extremity
      - Bilateral B51D
      - Left B51C
      - Right B51B
    - Other B51V
    - Pelvic (Iliac)
      - Left B51G
      - Right B51F
    - Pelvic (Iliac) Bilateral B51H
    - Portal B51T
    - Pulmonary
      - Bilateral B51S
      - Left B51R
      - Right B51Q
    - Renal
      - Bilateral B51L
      - Left B51K
      - Right B51J
    - Spanchnic B51T
    - Subclavian
      - Left B517
      - Right B516
    - Upper Extremity
      - Bilateral B51P
      - Left B51N
      - Right B51M
  - Vena Cava
    - Inferior B519
    - Superior B518
  - Wrist
    - Left BP1M
    - Right BP1L
- **Fluoroscopy, laser intraoperative**
  - *see* Fluoroscopy, Heart B21
  - *see* Fluoroscopy, Upper Arteries B31
  - *see* Fluoroscopy, Lower Arteries B41
- **Flushing** *see* Irrigation
- **Foley catheter** *use* Drainage Device
- **Fontan completion procedure Stage II** *see* Bypass, Vena Cava, Inferior 0610
- **Foramen magnum** *use* Occipital Bone
- **Foramen of Monro (intraventricular)** *use* Cerebral Ventricle
- **Foreskin** *use* Prepuce
- **Formula™ Balloon-Expandable Renal Stent System** *use* Intraluminal Device
- **Fosfomycin Anti-infective** XW0
- **Fosfomycin injection**
  - *use* Fosfomycin Anti-infective
- **Fossa of Rosenmuller** *use* Nasopharynx
- **Fourth cranial nerve** *use* Nerve, Trochlear
- **Fourth ventricle** *use* Cerebral Ventricle
- **Fovea**
  - *use* Retina, Right
  - *use* Retina, Left
- **Fragmentation**
  - Ampulla of Vater 0FFC
  - Anus 0DFQ
  - Appendix 0DFJ
  - Artery
    - Anterior Tibial
      - Left 04FQ3Z
      - Right 04FP3Z
    - Axillary
      - Left 03F63Z
      - Right 03F53Z
    - Brachial
      - Left 03F83Z
      - Right 03F73Z
    - Common Iliac
      - Left 04FD3Z
      - Right 04FC3Z
    - Coronary
      - Four or More Arteries 02F33ZZ
      - One Artery 02F03ZZ
      - Three Arteries 02F23ZZ
      - Two Arteries 02F13ZZ
- Fragmentation *(Continued)*
  - Artery *(Continued)*
    - External Iliac
      - Left 04FD3Z
      - Right 04FH3Z
    - Femoral
      - Left 04FL3Z
      - Right 04FK3Z
    - Innominate 03F23Z
    - Internal Iliac
      - Left 04FF3Z
      - Right 04FE3Z
    - Intracranial 03FG3Z
    - Lower 04FY3Z
    - Peroneal
      - Left 04FU3Z
      - Right 04FT3Z
    - Popliteal
      - Left 04FN3Z
      - Right 04FM3Z
    - Posterior Tibial
      - Left 04FN3Z
      - Right 04FM3Z
    - Pulmonary
      - Left 02FR3Z
      - Right 02FQ3Z
    - Pulmonary Trunk 02FP3Z
    - Radial
      - Left 03FC3Z
      - Right 03FB3Z
    - Subclavian
      - Left 03F43Z
      - Right 03F33Z
    - Ulnar
      - Left 03FA3Z
      - Right 03F93Z
  - Bladder 0TFB
  - Bladder Neck 0TFC
  - Bronchus
    - Lingula 0BF9
    - Lower Lobe
      - Left 0BFB
      - Right 0BF6
    - Main
      - Left 0BF7
      - Right 0BF3
    - Middle Lobe, Right 0BF5
    - Upper Lobe
      - Left 0BF8
      - Right 0BF4
  - Carina 0BF2
  - Cavity, Cranial 0WF1
  - Cecum 0DFH
  - Cerebral Ventricle 00F6
  - Colon
    - Ascending 0DFK
    - Descending 0DFM
    - Sigmoid 0DFN
    - Transverse 0DFL
  - Duct
    - Common Bile 0FF9
    - Cystic 0FF8
    - Hepatic
      - Common 0FF7
      - Left 0FF6
      - Right 0FF5
    - Pancreatic 0FFD
      - Accessory 0FFF
    - Parotid
      - Left 0CFC
      - Right 0CFB
  - Duodenum 0DF9
  - Epidural Space, Intracranial 00F3
  - Esophagus 0DF5
  - Fallopian Tube
    - Left 0UF6
    - Right 0UF5
  - Fallopian Tubes, Bilateral 0UF7
  - Gallbladder 0FF4
  - Gastrointestinal Tract 0WFP
- Fragmentation *(Continued)*
  - Genitourinary Tract 0WFR
  - Ileum 0DFB
  - Intestine
    - Large 0DFE
      - Left 0DFG
      - Right 0DFF
    - Small 0DF8
  - Jejunum 0DFA
  - Kidney Pelvis
    - Left 0TF4
    - Right 0TF3
  - Mediastinum 0WFC
  - Oral Cavity and Throat 0WF3
  - Pelvic Cavity 0WFJ
  - Pericardial Cavity 0WFD
  - Pericardium 02FN
  - Peritoneal Cavity 0WFG
  - Pleural Cavity
    - Left 0WFB
    - Right 0WF9
  - Rectum 0DFP
  - Respiratory Tract 0WFQ
  - Spinal Canal 00FU
  - Stomach 0DF6
  - Subarachnoid Space, Intracranial 00F5
  - Subdural Space, Intracranial 00F4
  - Trachea 0BF1
  - Ureter
    - Left 0TF7
    - Right 0TF6
  - Urethra 0TFD
  - Uterus 0UF9
  - Vein
    - Axillary
      - Left 05F83Z
      - Right 05F73Z
    - Basilic
      - Left 05FC3Z
      - Right 05F73Z
    - Brachial
      - Left 05FC3Z
      - Right 05FB3Z
    - Cephalic
      - Left 05FF3Z
      - Right 05 FD3Z
    - Common Iliac
      - Left 06FD3Z
      - Right 06FC3Z
    - External Iliac
      - Left 06FG3Z
      - Right 06FF3Z
    - Femoral
      - Left 06FN3Z
      - Right 06FM3Z
    - Hypogastric
      - Left 06FJ3Z
      - Right 06FH3Z
    - Innominate
      - Left 05F43Z
      - Right 05F33Z
    - Lower 06FY3Z
    - Pulmonary
      - Left 02FT3Z
      - Right 02FS3Z
    - Saphenous
      - Left 06FQ3Z
      - Right 05F53Z
    - Upper
  - Vitreous
    - Left 08F5
    - Right 08F4
- **Fragmentation, Ultrasonic** *see* Fragmentation, Artery
- **Freestyle (Stentless) Aortic Root Bioprosthesis** *use* Zooplastic Tissue in Heart and Great Vessels
- **Frenectomy**
  - *see* Excision, Mouth and Throat 0CB
  - *see* Resection, Mouth and Throat 0CT

F

Frenoplasty, frenuloplasty
see Repair, Mouth and Throat 0CQ
see Replacement, Mouth and Throat 0CR
see Supplement, Mouth and Throat 0CU
Frenotomy
see Drainage, Mouth and Throat 0C9
see Release, Mouth and Throat 0CN
Frenulotomy
see Drainage, Mouth and Throat 0C9
see Release, Mouth and Throat 0CN
Frenulum labii inferioris *use* Lower Lip
Frenulum labii superioris *use* Upper Lip
Frenulum linguae *use* Tongue
Frenulumectomy
see Excision, Mouth and Throat 0CB
see Resection, Mouth and Throat 0CT
Frontal lobe *use* Cerebral Hemisphere
Frontal vein
use Face Vein, Right
use Face Vein, Left
Frozen elephant trunk (FET) technique, aortic arch replacement
see Replacement, Heart and Great Vessels 02R
see New Technology, Cardiovascular System X2R
Frozen elephant trunk (FET) technique, thoracic aorta restriction
see Restriction, Heart and Great Vessels 02V
see New Technology, Cardiovascular System X2V
FUJIFILM EP-7000X system for oxygen saturation endoscopic imaging (OXEI) *see* New Technology, Gastrointestinal System XD2
Fulguration *see* Destruction
Fundoplication, gastroesophageal *see* Restriction, Esophagogastric Junction 0DV4
Fundus uteri *use* Uterus
Fusion
Acromioclavicular
Left 0RGH
Right 0RGG
Ankle
Left 0SGG
▶Open-truss Design Internal Fixation Device XRGK0B9
Right 0SGF
▶Open-truss Design Internal Fixation Device XRGJ0B9

Fusion *(Continued)*
Carpal
Left 0RGR
Right 0RGQ
Carpometacarpal
Left 0RGT
Right 0RGS
Cervical Vertebral 0RG1
2 or more 0RG2
Cervicothoracic Vertebral 0RG4
Coccygeal 0SG6
Elbow
Left 0RGM
Right 0RGL
Finger Phalangeal
Left 0RGX
Right 0RGW
Hip
Left 0SGB
Right 0SG9
Knee
Left 0SGD
Right 0SGC
Lumbar Vertebral 0SG0
2 or more 0SG1
▶Interbody Fusion Device, Custom-Made Anatomically Designed XRGC
~~Interbody Fusion Device, Customizable XRGC~~
~~Interbody Fusion Device, Customizable XRGD~~
▶Interbody Fusion Device, Custom-Made Anatomically Designed XRGB
Lumbosacral 0SG3
▶Interbody Fusion Device, Custom-Made Anatomically Designed XRGD
Metacarpophalangeal
Left 0RGV
Right 0RGU
Metatarsal-Phalangeal
Left 0SGN
Right 0SGM
Occipital-cervical 0RG0

Fusion *(Continued)*
Sacrococcygeal 0SG5
Sacroiliac
Internal Fixation Device with Tulip Connector XRG
Left 0SG8
Right 0SG7
Shoulder
Left 0RGK
Right 0RGJ
Sternoclavicular
Left 0RGF
Right 0RGE
Tarsal
Left 0SGJ
▶Open-truss Design Internal Fixation Device XRGM0B9
Right 0SGH
▶Open-truss Design Internal Fixation Device XRGL0B9
Tarsometatarsal
Left 0SGL
Right 0SGK
Temporomandibular
Left 0RGD
Right 0RGC
Thoracic Vertebral 0RG6
2 to 7 0RG7
8 or more 0RG8
Thoracolumbar Vertebral 0RGA
~~Interbody Fusion Device, Customizable XRGA~~
▶Interbody Fusion Device, Custom-Made Anatomically Designed XRGA
Toe Phalangeal
Left 0SGQ
Right 0SGP
Wrist
Left 0RGP
Right 0RGN
Fusion screw (compression) (lag) (locking)
use Internal Fixation Device in Upper Joints
use Internal Fixation Device in Lower Joints

F

G

Gait training *see* Motor Treatment, Rehabilitation F07
Galea aponeurotica *use* Subcutaneous Tissue and Fascia, Scalp
Gammaglobulin *use* Globulin
GammaTile™ *use* Radioactive Element, Cesium-131 Collagen Implant in 00H
GAMUNEX-C, for COVID-19 treatment *use* High-Dose Intravenous Immune Globulin
Ganglion impar (ganglion of Walther) *use* Sacral Sympathetic Nerve
Ganglionectomy
Destruction of lesion *see* Destruction
Excision of lesion *see* Excision
Gasserian ganglion *use* Trigeminal Nerve
Gastrectomy
Partial *see* Excision, Stomach 0DB6
Total *see* Resection, Stomach 0DT6
Vertical (sleeve) *see* Excision, Stomach 0DB6
Gastric electrical stimulation (GES) lead *use* Stimulator Lead in Gastrointestinal System
Gastric lymph node *use* Lymphatic, Aortic
Gastric pacemaker lead *use* Stimulator Lead in Gastrointestinal System
Gastric plexus *see* Abdominal Sympathetic Nerve
Gastrocnemius muscle
use Lower Leg Muscle, Right
use Lower Leg Muscle, Left
Gastrocolic ligament *use* Omentum
Gastrocolic omentum *use* Omentum
Gastrocolostomy
see Bypass, Gastrointestinal System 0D1
see Drainage, Gastrointestinal System 0D9
Gastroduodenal artery *use* Hepatic Artery
Gastroduodenectomy
see Excision, Gastrointestinal System 0DB
see Resection, Gastrointestinal System 0DT
Gastroduodenoscopy 0DJ08ZZ
Gastroenteroplasty
see Repair, Gastrointestinal System 0DQ
see Supplement, Gastrointestinal System 0DU
Gastroenterostomy
see Bypass, Gastrointestinal System 0D1
see Drainage, Gastrointestinal System 0D9
Gastroesophageal (GE) junction *use* Esophagogastric Junction
Gastrogastrostomy
see Bypass, Stomach 0D16
see Drainage, Stomach 0D96
Gastrohepatic omentum *use* Omentum
Gastrojejunostomy
see Bypass, Stomach 0D16
see Drainage, Stomach 0D96
Gastrolysis *see* Release, Stomach 0DN6
Gastropexy
see Repair, Stomach 0DQ6
see Reposition, Stomach 0DS6
Gastrophrenic ligament *use* Omentum
Gastroplasty
see Repair, Stomach 0DQ6
see Supplement, Stomach 0DU6
Gastroplication *see* Restriction, Stomach 0DV6
Gastropylorectomy *see* Excision, Gastrointestinal System 0DB
Gastrorrhaphy *see* Repair, Stomach 0DQ6
Gastroscopy 0DJ68ZZ
Gastrosplenic ligament *use* Omentum
Gastrostomy
see Bypass, Stomach 0D16
see Drainage, Stomach 0D96
Gastrotomy *see* Drainage, Stomach 0D96
Gemellus muscle
use Hip Muscle, Right
use Hip Muscle, Left
Geniculate ganglion *use* Facial Nerve
Geniculate nucleus *use* Thalamus
Genioglossus muscle *use* Tongue, Palate, Pharynx Muscle
Genioplasty *see* Alteration, Jaw, Lower 0W05
Genitofemoral nerve *use* Lumbar Plexus
GIAPREZA™ *use* Vasopressor
Gilteritinib Antineoplastic XW0DXV5
Gingivectomy *see* Excision, Mouth and Throat 0CB
Gingivoplasty
see Repair, Mouth and Throat 0CQ
see Replacement, Mouth and Throat 0CR
see Supplement, Mouth and Throat 0CU
Glans penis *use* Prepuce
Glenohumeral joint
use Shoulder Joint, Right
use Shoulder Joint, Left
Glenohumeral ligament
use Shoulder Bursa and Ligament, Right
use Shoulder Bursa and Ligament, Left
Glenoid fossa (of scapula)
use Glenoid Cavity, Right
use Glenoid Cavity, Left
Glenoid ligament (labrum)
use Shoulder Joint, Right
use Shoulder Joint, Left
Globus pallidus *use* Basal Ganglia
Glofitamab Antineoplastic XW0
Glomectomy
see Excision, Endocrine System 0GB
see Resection, Endocrine System 0GT
Glossectomy
see Excision, Tongue 0CB7
see Resection, Tongue 0CT7
Glossoepiglottic fold *use* Epiglottis
Glossopexy
see Repair, Tongue 0CQ7
see Reposition, Tongue 0CS7
Glossoplasty
see Repair, Tongue 0CQ7
see Replacement, Tongue 0CR7
see Supplement, Tongue 0CU7
Glossorrhaphy *see* Repair, Tongue 0CQ7
Glossotomy *see* Drainage, Tongue 0C97
Glottis *use* Larynx
Gluteal Artery Perforator Flap
Replacement
Bilateral 0HRV079
Left 0HRU079
Right 0HRT079
Transfer
Left 0KXG
Right 0KXF
Gluteal lymph node *use* Lymphatic, Pelvis
Gluteal vein
use Hypogastric Vein, Right
use Hypogastric Vein, Left
Gluteus maximus muscle
use Hip Muscle, Right
use Hip Muscle, Left
Gluteus medius muscle
use Hip Muscle, Right
use Hip Muscle, Left
Gluteus minimus muscle
use Hip Muscle, Right
use Hip Muscle, Left
GORE EXCLUDER® AAA Endoprosthesis
use Intraluminal Device, Branched or Fenestrated, One or Two Arteries in 04V
use Intraluminal Device, Branched or Fenestrated, Three or More Arteries in 04V
use Intraluminal Device
GORE EXCLUDER® IBE Endoprosthesis *use* Intraluminal Device, Branched or Fenestrated, One or Two Arteries in 04V
GORE TAG® Thoracic Endoprosthesis *use* Intraluminal Device
GORE® DUALMESH® *use* Synthetic Substitute
Gracilis muscle
use Upper Leg Muscle, Right
use Upper Leg Muscle, Left
Graft
see Replacement
see Supplement
Great auricular nerve *use* Lumbar Plexus
Great cerebral vein *use* Intracranial Vein
Great(er) saphenous vein
use Saphenous Vein, Right
use Saphenous Vein, Left
Greater alar cartilage *use* Nasal Mucosa and Soft Tissue
Greater occipital nerve *use* Cervical Nerve
Greater Omentum *use* Omentum
Greater splanchnic nerve *use* Thoracic Sympathetic Nerve
Greater superficial petrosal nerve *use* Facial Nerve
Greater trochanter
use Upper Femur, Right
use Upper Femur, Left
Greater tuberosity
use Humeral Head, Right
use Humeral Head, Left
Greater vestibular (Bartholin's) gland *use* Vestibular Gland
Greater wing *use* Sphenoid Bone
GS-5734 *use* Remdesivir Anti-infective
Guedel airway *use* Intraluminal Device, Airway in Mouth and Throat
Guidance, catheter placement
EKG *see* Measurement, Physiological Systems 4A0
Fluoroscopy *see* Fluoroscopy, Veins B51
Ultrasound *see* Ultrasonography, Veins B54

H

Hallux
use Toe, 1st, Right
use Toe, 1st, Left
Hamate bone
use Carpal, Right
use Carpal, Left
Hancock Bioprosthesis (aortic) (mitral) valve *use* Zooplastic Tissue in Heart and Great Vessels
Hancock Bioprosthetic Valved Conduit *use* Zooplastic Tissue in Heart and Great Vessels
Harmony™ transcatheter pulmonary valve (TPV) placement 02RH38M
Harvesting, stem cells *see* Pheresis, Circulatory 6A55
hdIVIG (high-dose intravenous immunoglobulin), for COVID-19 treatment *use* High-Dose Intravenous Immune Globulin
Head of fibula
use Fibula, Right
use Fibula, Left
Hearing Aid Assessment F14Z
Hearing Assessment F13Z
Hearing Device
Bone Conduction
Left 09HE
Right 09HD
Insertion of device in
Left 0NH6[034]SZ
Right 0NH5[034]SZ
Multiple Channel Cochlear Prosthesis
Left 09HE
Right 09HD
Removal of device from, Skull 0NP0
Revision of device in, Skull 0NW0
Single Channel Cochlear Prosthesis
Left 09HE
Right 09HD
Hearing Treatment F09Z
Heart Assist System
Implantable
Insertion of device in, Heart 02HA
Removal of device from, Heart 02PA
Revision of device in, Heart 02WA
Short-term External
~~Insertion of device in, Heart 02HA~~
~~Removal of device from, Heart 02PA~~
~~Revision of device in, Heart 02WA~~
▶Insertion of device in
▶Aorta, Thoracic, Descending 02HW3RZ
▶Heart 02HA
▶Removal of device from
▶Aorta, Thoracic, Descending 02PW3RZ
▶Heart 02PA
▶Revision of device in
▶Aorta, Thoracic, Descending 02WW3RZ
▶Heart 02WA
HeartMate 3™ LVAS *use* Implantable Heart Assist System in Heart and Great Vessels
HeartMate II® Left Ventricular Assist Device (LVAD) *use* Implantable Heart Assist System in Heart and Great Vessels
HeartMate XVE® Left Ventricular Assist Device (LVAD) *use* Implantable Heart Assist System in Heart and Great Vessels
HeartMate® implantable heart assist system *see* Insertion of device in, Heart 02HA
Helix
use External Ear, Right
use External Ear, Left
use External Ear, Bilateral
Hematopoietic cell transplant (HCT) *see* Transfusion, Circulatory 302
Hemicolectomy *see* Resection, Gastrointestinal System 0DT
Hemicystectomy *see* Excision, Urinary System 0TB
Hemigastrectomy *see* Excision, Gastrointestinal System 0DB
Hemiglossectomy *see* Excision, Mouth and Throat 0CB
Hemilaminectomy
see Excision, Upper Bones 0PB
see Excision, Lower Bones 0QB
Hemilaminotomy
see Release, Central Nervous System 00N
see Release, Peripheral Nervous System 01N
see Drainage, Upper Bones 0P9
see Excision, Upper Bones 0PB
see Release, Upper Bones 0PN
see Drainage, Lower Bones 0Q9
see Excision, Lower Bones 0QB
see Release, Lower Bones 0QN
Hemilaryngectomy *see* Excision, Larynx 0CBS
Hemimandibulectomy *see* Excision, Head and Facial Bones 0NB
Hemimaxillectomy *see* Excision, Head and Facial Bones 0NB
Hemipylorectomy *see* Excision, Gastrointestinal System 0DB
Hemispherectomy
see Excision, Central Nervous System and Cranial Nerves 00B
see Resection, Central Nervous System and Cranial Nerves 00T
Hemithyroidectomy
see Excision, Endocrine System 0GB
see Resection, Endocrine System 0GT
Hemodialysis *see* Performance, Urinary 5A1D
Hemolung® Respiratory Assist System (RAS) 5A0920Z
Hemospray® Endoscopic Hemostat *use* Mineral-based Topical Hemostatic Agent
Hepatectomy
see Excision, Hepatobiliary System and Pancreas 0FB
see Resection, Hepatobiliary System and Pancreas 0FT
Hepatic artery proper *use* Hepatic Artery
Hepatic flexure *use* Transverse Colon
Hepatic lymph node *use* Aortic Lymphatic
Hepatic plexus *use* Abdominal Sympathetic Nerve
Hepatic portal vein *use* Portal Vein
Hepaticoduodenostomy
see Bypass, Hepatobiliary System and Pancreas 0F1
see Drainage, Hepatobiliary System and Pancreas 0F9
Hepaticotomy *see* Drainage, Hepatobiliary System and Pancreas 0F9
Hepatocholedochostomy *see* Drainage, Duct, Common Bile 0F99
Hepatogastric ligament *use* Omentum
Hepatopancreatic ampulla *use* Ampulla of Vater
Hepatopexy
see Repair, Hepatobiliary System and Pancreas 0FQ
see Reposition, Hepatobiliary System and Pancreas 0FS
Hepatorrhaphy *see* Repair, Hepatobiliary System and Pancreas 0FQ
Hepatotomy *see* Drainage, Hepatobiliary System and Pancreas 0F9
▶**HEPZATO™ KIT (melphalan hydrochloride Hepatic Delivery System)** *use* MelphalanHydrochloride Antineoplastic
Herculink (RX) Elite Renal Stent System *use* Intraluminal Device
Herniorrhaphy
see Repair, Anatomical Regions, General 0WQ
see Repair, Anatomical Regions, Lower Extremities 0YQ
With synthetic substitute
see Supplement, Anatomical Regions, General 0WU
see Supplement, Anatomical Regions, Lower Extremities 0YU
HIG (hyperimmune globulin), for COVID-19 treatment *use* Hyperimmune Globulin
High-dose intravenous immune globulin, for COVID-19 treatment XW1
High-dose intravenous immunoglobulin (hdIVIG), for COVID-19 treatment *use* High-Dose Intravenous Immune Globulin
Hip (joint) liner *use* Liner in Lower Joints
HIPEC (hyperthermic intraperitoneal chemotherapy) 3E0M30Y
HistoSonics® System *see* New Technology, Hepatobiliary System and Pancreas XF5
Histotripsy, liver *see* New Technology, Hepatobiliary System and Pancreas XF5
hIVIG (hyperimmune intravenous immunoglobulin), for COVID-19 treatment *use* Hyperimmune Globulin
Holter monitoring 4A12X45
Holter valve ventricular shunt *use* Synthetic Substitute
➡**Human angiotensin II, synthetic** *use* Vasopressor
Humeroradial joint
use Elbow Joint, Right
use Elbow Joint, Left
Humeroulnar joint
use Elbow Joint, Right
use Elbow Joint, Left
Humerus, distal
use Humeral Shaft, Right
use Humeral Shaft, Left
Hydrocelectomy *see* Excision, Male Reproductive System 0VB
Hydrotherapy
Assisted exercise in pool *see* Motor Treatment, Rehabilitation F07
Whirlpool *see* Activities of Daily Living Treatment, Rehabilitation F08
Hymenectomy
see Excision, Hymen 0UBK
see Resection, Hymen 0UTK
Hymenoplasty
see Repair, Hymen 0UQK
see Supplement, Hymen 0UUK
Hymenorrhaphy *see* Repair, Hymen 0UQK
Hymenotomy
see Division, Hymen 0U8K
see Drainage, Hymen 0U9K
Hyoglossus muscle *use* Tongue, Palate, Pharynx Muscle
Hyoid artery
use Thyroid Artery, Right
use Thyroid Artery, Left
Hyperalimentation *see* Introduction of substance in or on
Hyperbaric oxygenation
Decompression sickness treatment *see* Decompression, Circulatory 6A15
Other treatment see Assistance, Circulatory 5A05
Hyperimmune globulin *use* Globulin
Hyperimmune globulin, for COVID-19 treatment XW1
Hyperimmune intravenous immunoglobulin (hIVIG), for COVID-19 treatment *use* Hyperimmune Globulin
Hyperthermia
Radiation Therapy
Abdomen DWY38ZZ
Adrenal Gland DGY28ZZ
Bile Ducts DFY28ZZ
Bladder DTY28ZZ
Bone, Other DPYC8ZZ
Bone Marrow D7Y08ZZ
Brain D0Y08ZZ
Brain Stem D0Y18ZZ
Breast
Left DMY08ZZ
Right DMY18ZZ
Bronchus DBY18ZZ

Hyperthermia (Continued)
Radiation Therapy (Continued)
Cervix DUY18ZZ
Chest DWY28ZZ
Chest Wall DBY78ZZ
Colon DDY58ZZ
Diaphragm DBY88ZZ
Duodenum DDY28ZZ
Ear D9Y08ZZ
Esophagus DDY08ZZ
Eye D8Y08ZZ
Femur DPY98ZZ
Fibula DPYB8ZZ
Gallbladder DFY18ZZ
Gland
Adrenal DGY28ZZ
Parathyroid DGY48ZZ
Pituitary DGY08ZZ
Thyroid DGY58ZZ
Glands, Salivary D9Y68ZZ
Head and Neck DWY18ZZ
Hemibody DWY48ZZ
Humerus DPY68ZZ
Hypopharynx D9Y38ZZ
Ileum DDY48ZZ
Jejunum DDY38ZZ
Kidney DTY08ZZ
Larynx D9YB8ZZ
Liver DFY08ZZ
Lung DBY28ZZ
Lymphatics
Abdomen D7Y68ZZ
Axillary D7Y48ZZ
Inguinal D7Y88ZZ
Neck D7Y38ZZ
Pelvis D7Y78ZZ
Thorax D7Y58ZZ
Mandible DPY38ZZ
Maxilla DPY28ZZ
Mediastinum DBY68ZZ
Mouth D9Y48ZZ
Nasopharynx D9YD8ZZ
Neck and Head DWY18ZZ

Hyperthermia (Continued)
Radiation Therapy (Continued)
Nerve, Peripheral D0Y78ZZ
Nose D9Y18ZZ
Oropharynx D9YF8ZZ
Ovary DUY08ZZ
Palate
Hard D9Y88ZZ
Soft D9Y98ZZ
Pancreas DFY38ZZ
Parathyroid Gland DGY48ZZ
Pelvic Bones DPY88ZZ
Pelvic Region DWY68ZZ
Pineal Body DGY18ZZ
Pituitary Gland DGY08ZZ
Pleura DBY58ZZ
Prostate DVY08ZZ
Radius DPY78ZZ
Rectum DDY78ZZ
Rib DPY58ZZ
Sinuses D9Y78ZZ
Skin
Abdomen DHY88ZZ
Arm DHY48ZZ
Back DHY78ZZ
Buttock DHY98ZZ
Chest DHY68ZZ
Face DHY28ZZ
Leg DHYB8ZZ
Neck DHY38ZZ
Skull DPY08ZZ
Spinal Cord D0Y68ZZ
Spleen D7Y28ZZ
Sternum DPY48ZZ
Stomach DDY18ZZ
Testis DVY18ZZ
Thymus D7Y18ZZ
Thyroid Gland DGY58ZZ
Tibia DPYB8ZZ
Tongue D9Y58ZZ
Trachea DBY08ZZ
Ulna DPY78ZZ
Ureter DTY18ZZ

Hyperthermia (Continued)
Radiation Therapy (Continued)
Urethra DTY38ZZ
Uterus DUY28ZZ
Whole Body DWY58ZZ
Whole Body 6A3Z
Hyperthermic intraperitoneal chemotherapy (HIPEC) 3E0M30Y
Hypnosis GZFZZZZ
Hypogastric artery
use Internal Iliac Artery, Right
use Internal Iliac Artery, Left
Hypopharynx *use* Pharynx
Hypophysectomy
see Excision, Gland, Pituitary 0GB0
see Resection, Gland, Pituitary 0GT0
Hypophysis *use* Gland, Pituitary
Hypothalamotomy *see* Destruction, Thalamus 0059
Hypothenar muscle
use Hand Muscle, Right
use Hand Muscle, Left
Hypothermia, Whole Body 6A4Z
Hysterectomy
Supracervical *see* Resection, Uterus 0UT9
Total *see* Resection, Uterus 0UT9
Hysterolysis *see* Release, Uterus 0UN9
Hysteropexy
see Repair, Uterus 0UQ9
see Reposition, Uterus 0US9
Hysteroplasty
see Repair, Uterus 0UQ9
Hysterorrhaphy *see* Repair, Uterus 0UQ9
Hysteroscopy 0UJD8ZZ
Hysterotomy
see Drainage, Uterus 0U99
Hysterotrachelectomy
see Resection, Uterus 0UT9
see Resection, Cervix 0UTC
Hysterotracheloplasty
see Repair, Uterus 0UQ9
Hysterotrachelorrhaphy *see* Repair, Uterus 0UQ9

H

I

IABP (Intra-aortic balloon pump) *see* Assistance, Cardiac 5A02
IAEMT (Intraoperative anesthetic effect monitoring and titration) *see* Monitoring, Central Nervous 4A10
IASD® (InterAtrial Shunt Device), Corvia *use* Synthetic Substitute
Idarucizumab, Pradaxa® (dabigatran) reversal agent *use* Other Therapeutic Substance
Ide-cel *use* Idecabtagene Vicleucel Immunotherapy
Idecabtagene vicleucel *use* Idecabtagene Vicleucel Immunotherapy
Idecabtagene vicleucel immunotherapy XW0
iFuse Bedrock™ Granite Implant System *use* Internal Fixation Device with Tulip Connector in New Technology
IGIV-C, for COVID-19 treatment *use* Hyperimmune Globulin
IHD (Intermittent hemodialysis) 5A1D70Z
Ileal artery *use* Superior Mesenteric Artery
Ileectomy
 see Excision, Ileum 0DBB
 see Resection, Ileum 0DTB
Ileocolic artery *use* Superior Mesenteric Artery
Ileocolic vein *use* Colic Vein
Ileopexy
 see Repair, Ileum 0DQB
 see Reposition, Ileum 0DSB
Ileorrhaphy *see* Repair, Ileum 0DQB
Ileoscopy 0DJD8ZZ
Ileostomy
 see Bypass, Ileum 0D1B
 see Drainage, Ileum 0D9B
Ileotomy *see* Drainage, Ileum 0D9B
Ileoureterostomy *see* Bypass, Bladder 0T1B
Iliac crest
 use Pelvic Bone, Right
 use Pelvic Bone, Left
Iliac fascia
 use Subcutaneous Tissue and Fascia, Right Upper Leg
 use Subcutaneous Tissue and Fascia, Left Upper Leg
Iliac lymph node *use* Lymphatic, Pelvis
Iliacus muscle
 use Hip Muscle, Right
 use Hip Muscle, Left
Iliofemoral ligament
 use Hip Bursa and Ligament, Right
 use Hip Bursa and Ligament, Left
Iliohypogastric nerve *use* Lumbar Plexus
Ilioinguinal nerve *use* Lumbar Plexus
Iliolumbar artery
 use Internal Iliac Artery, Right
 use Internal Iliac Artery, Left
Iliolumbar ligament *use* Lower Spine Bursa and Ligament
Iliotibial tract (band)
 use Subcutaneous Tissue and Fascia, Right Upper Leg
 use Subcutaneous Tissue and Fascia, Left Upper Leg
Ilium
 use Pelvic Bone, Right
 use Pelvic Bone, Left
Ilizarov external fixator
 use External Fixation Device, Ring in 0PH
 use External Fixation Device, Ring in 0PS
 use External Fixation Device, Ring in 0QH
 use External Fixation Device, Ring in 0QS
Ilizarov-Vecklich device
 use External Fixation Device, Limb Lengthening in 0PH
 use External Fixation Device, Limb Lengthening in 0QH
Imaging, diagnostic
 see Plain Radiography
 see Fluoroscopy
 see Computerized Tomography (CT Scan)
 see Magnetic Resonance Imaging (MRI)
 see Ultrasonography
Imdevimab (REGN10987) and casirivimab (REGN10933) *use* REGN-COV2 Monoclonal Antibody
IMFINZI® *use* Durvalumab Antineoplastic
IMI/REL
 use Imipenem-cilastatin-relebactam Anti-infective
Imipenem-cilastatin-relebactam Anti-infective XW0
Immobilization
 Abdominal Wall 2W33X
 Arm
  Lower
   Left 2W3DX
   Right 2W3CX
  Upper
   Left 2W3BX
   Right 2W3AX
 Back 2W35X
 Chest Wall 2W34X
 Extremity
  Lower
   Left 2W3MX
   Right 2W3LX
  Upper
   Left 2W39X
   Right 2W38X
 Face 2W31X
 Finger
  Left 2W3KX
  Right 2W3JX
 Foot
  Left 2W3TX
  Right 2W3SX
 Hand
  Left 2W3FX
  Right 2W3EX
 Head 2W30X
 Inguinal Region
  Left 2W37X
  Right 2W36X
 Leg
  Lower
   Left 2W3RX
   Right 2W3QX
  Upper
   Left 2W3PX
   Right 2W3NX
 Neck 2W32X
 Thumb
  Left 2W3HX
  Right 2W3GX
 Toe
  Left 2W3VX
  Right 2W3UX
Immunization *see* Introduction of Serum, Toxoid, and Vaccine
Immunoglobulin *use* Globulin
Immunotherapy *see* Introduction of Immunotherapeutic Substance
Immunotherapy, antineoplastic
 Interferon *see* Introduction of Low-dose Interleukin-2
 Interleukin-2 of high-dose *see* Introduction, High-dose Interleukin-2
 Interleukin-2, low-dose *see* Introduction of Low-dose Interleukin-2
 Monoclonal antibody *see* Introduction of Monoclonal Antibody
 Proleukin, high-dose *see* Introduction of High-dose Interleukin-2
 Proleukin, low-dose *see* Introduction of Low-dose Interleukin-2
▶ **Impella® 5.5 with SmartAssist® System** *use* Conduit to Short-term External Heart Assist System in New Technology
Impella® heart pump *use* Short-term External Heart Assist System in Heart and Great Vessels
Impeller Pump
 Continuous, Output 5A0221D
 Intermittent, Output 5A0211D
Implantable cardioverter-defibrillator (ICD) *use* Defibrillator Generator in 0JH
Implantable drug infusion pump (anti-spasmodic) (chemotherapy) (pain) *use* Infusion Device, Pump in Subcutaneous Tissue and Fascia
Implantable glucose monitoring device *use* Monitoring Device
Implantable hemodynamic monitor (IHM) *use* Monitoring Device, Hemodynamic in 0JH
Implantable hemodynamic monitoring system (IHMS) *use* Monitoring Device, Hemodynamic in 0JH
Implantable Miniature Telescope™ (IMT) use Synthetic Substitute, Intraocular Telescope in 08R
Implantation
 see Replacement
 see Insertion
Implanted (venous) (access) port *use* Vascular Access Device, Totally Implantable in Subcutaneous Tissue and Fascia
IMV (intermittent mandatory ventilation) *see* Assistance, Respiratory 5A09
In Vitro Fertilization 8E0ZXY1
Incision, abscess *see* Drainage
Incudectomy
 see Excision, Ear, Nose, Sinus 09B
 see Resection, Ear, Nose, Sinus 09T
Incudopexy
 see Repair, Ear, Nose, Sinus 09Q
 see Reposition, Ear, Nose, Sinus 09S
Incus
 use Ossicle, Auditory, Right
 use Ossicle, Auditory, Left
Induction of labor
 Artificial rupture of membranes *see* Drainage, Pregnancy 109
 Oxytocin *see* Introduction of Hormone
InDura, intrathecal catheter (1P) (spinal) *use* Infusion Device
Inebilizumab-cdon XW0
Inferior cardiac nerve *use* Thoracic Sympathetic Nerve
Inferior cerebellar vein *use* Intracranial Vein
Inferior cerebral vein *use* Intracranial Vein
Inferior epigastric artery
 use External Iliac Artery, Right
 use External Iliac Artery, Left
Inferior epigastric lymph node *use* Lymphatic, Pelvis
Inferior genicular artery
 use Popliteal Artery, Right
 use Popliteal Artery, Left
Inferior gluteal artery
 use Internal Iliac Artery, Right
 use Internal Iliac Artery, Left
Inferior gluteal nerve *use* Sacral Plexus Nerve
Inferior hypogastric plexus *use* Abdominal Sympathetic Nerve
Inferior labial artery *use* Face Artery
Inferior longitudinal muscle *use* Tongue, Palate, Pharynx Muscle
Inferior mesenteric ganglion *use* Abdominal Sympathetic Nerve
Inferior mesenteric lymph node *use* Mesenteric Lymphatic
Inferior mesenteric plexus *use* Abdominal Sympathetic Nerve
Inferior oblique muscle
 use Extraocular Muscle, Right
 use Extraocular Muscle, Left
Inferior pancreaticoduodenal artery *use* Superior Mesenteric Artery
Inferior phrenic artery *use* Abdominal Aorta

Inferior rectus muscle
use Extraocular Muscle, Right
use Extraocular Muscle, Left
Inferior suprarenal artery
use Renal Artery, Right
use Renal Artery, Left
Inferior tarsal plate
use Lower Eyelid, Right
use Lower Eyelid, Left
Inferior thyroid vein
use Innominate Vein, Right
use Innominate Vein, Left
Inferior tibiofibular joint
use Ankle Joint, Right
use Ankle Joint, Left
Inferior turbinate use Nasal Turbinate
Inferior ulnar collateral artery
use Brachial Artery, Right
use Brachial Artery, Left
Inferior vesical artery
use Internal Iliac Artery, Right
use Internal Iliac Artery, Left
Infraauricular lymph node use Lymphatic, Head
Infraclavicular (deltopectoral) lymph node
use Lymphatic, Right Upper Extremity
use Lymphatic, Left Upper Extremity
Infrahyoid muscle
use Neck Muscle, Right
use Neck Muscle, Left
Infraparotid lymph node use Lymphatic, Head
Infraspinatus fascia
use Subcutaneous Tissue and Fascia, Right Upper Arm
use Subcutaneous Tissue and Fascia, Left Upper Arm
Infraspinatus muscle
use Shoulder Muscle, Right
use Shoulder Muscle, Left
Infundibulopelvic ligament use Uterine Supporting Structure
Infusion see Introduction of substance in or on
Infusion Device, Pump
Insertion of device in
Abdomen 0JH8
Back 0JH7
Chest 0JH6
Lower Arm
Left 0JHH
Right 0JHG
Lower Leg
Left 0JHP
Right 0JHN
Trunk 0JHT
Upper Arm
Left 0JHF
Right 0JHD
Upper Leg
Left 0JHM
Right 0JHL
Removal of device from
Lower Extremity 0JPW
Trunk 0JPT
Upper Extremity 0JPV
Revision of device in
Lower Extremity 0JWW
Trunk 0JWT
Upper Extremity 0JWV
Infusion, glucarpidase
Central vein 3E043GQ
Peripheral vein 3E033GQ
Inguinal canal
use Inguinal Region, Right
use Inguinal Region, Left
use Inguinal Region, Bilateral
Inguinal triangle
see Inguinal Region, Right
see Inguinal Region, Left
see Inguinal Region, Bilateral
Injection see Introduction of substance in or on
Injection reservoir, port use Vascular Access Device, Reservoir in Subcutaneous Tissue and Fascia
Injection reservoir, pump use Infusion Device, Pump in Subcutaneous Tissue and Fascia
Insemination, artificial 3E0P7LZ
Insertion
Antimicrobial envelope see Introduction of Anti-infective
Aqueous drainage shunt
see Bypass, Eye 081
see Drainage, Eye 089
Bone, Pelvic, Internal Fixation Device with Tulip Connector XNH
▶ Conduit to Short-term External Heart Assist System X2H
▶ Intracardiac Pacemaker, Dual-Chamber X2H
▶ Intraluminal Device, Bioprosthetic Valve X2H
Joint
Lumbar Vertebral, Posterior Spinal Motion Preservation Device XRHB018
Lumbosacral, Posterior Spinal Motion Preservation Device XRHD018
Neurostimulator Lead, Sphenopalatine Ganglion X0HK3Q8
Neurostimulator Lead with Paired Stimulation System X0HQ3R8
Products of Conception 10H0
Spinal Stabilization Device
see Insertion of device in, Upper Joints 0RH
see Insertion of device in, Lower Joints 0SH
▶ Tibial Extension with Motion Sensors XNH
Insertion of device in
Abdominal Wall 0WHF
Acetabulum
Left 0QH5
Right 0QH4
Anal Sphincter 0DHR
Ankle Region
Left 0YHL
Right 0YHK
Anus 0DHQ
Aorta
Abdominal 04H0
Thoracic
Ascending/Arch 02HX
Descending 02HW
Arm
Lower
Left 0XHF
Right 0XHD
Upper
Left 0XH9
Right 0XH8
Artery
Anterior Tibial
Left 04HQ
Right 04HP
Axillary
Left 03H6
Right 03H5
Brachial
Left 03H8
Right 03H7
Celiac 04H1
Colic
Left 04H7
Middle 04H8
Right 04H6
Common Carotid
Left 03HJ
Right 03HH
Common Iliac
Left 04HD
Right 04HC
Coronary
Four or More Arteries 02H3
One Artery 02H0
Three Arteries 02H2
Two Arteries 02H1
Insertion of device in *(Continued)*
Artery *(Continued)*
External Carotid
Left 03HN
Right 03HM
External Iliac
Left 04HJ
Right 04HH
Face 03HR
Femoral
Left 04HL
Right 04HK
Foot
Left 04HW
Right 04HV
Gastric 04H2
Hand
Left 03HF
Right 03HD
Hepatic 04H3
Inferior Mesenteric 04HB
Innominate 03H2
Internal Carotid
Left 03HL
Right 03HK
Internal Iliac
Left 04HF
Right 04HE
Internal Mammary
Left 03H1
Right 03H0
Intracranial 03HG
Lower 04HY
Peroneal
Left 04HU
Right 04HT
Popliteal
Left 04HN
Right 04HM
Posterior Tibial
Left 04HS
Right 04HR
Pulmonary
Left 02HR
Right 02HQ
Pulmonary Trunk 02HP
Radial
Left 03HC
Right 03HB
Renal
Left 04HA
Right 04H9
Splenic 04H4
Subclavian
Left 03H4
Right 03H3
Superior Mesenteric 04H5
Temporal
Left 03HT
Right 03HS
Thyroid
Left 03HV
Right 03HU
Ulnar
Left 03HA
Right 03H9
Upper 03HY
Vertebral
Left 03HQ
Right 03HP
Atrium
Left 02H7
Right 02H6
Axilla
Left 0XH5
Right 0XH4
Back
Lower 0WHL
Upper 0WHK
Bladder 0THB
Bladder Neck 0THC

▶ New ➡ Revised ~~deleted~~ Deleted

J

Jakafi® *use* Ruxolitinib
Jejunal artery *use* Superior Mesenteric Artery
Jejunectomy
 see Excision, Jejunum 0DBA
 see Resection, Jejunum 0DTA
Jejunocolostomy
 see Bypass, Gastrointestinal System 0D1
 see Drainage, Gastrointestinal System 0D9
Jejunopexy
 see Repair, Jejunum 0DQA
 see Reposition, Jejunum 0DSA
Jejunostomy
 see Bypass, Jejunum 0D1A
 see Drainage, Jejunum 0D9A
Jejunotomy *see* Drainage, Jejunum 0D9A
Joint fixation plate
 use Internal Fixation Device in Upper Joints
 use Internal Fixation Device in Lower Joints
Joint liner (insert) *use* Liner in Lower Joints
Joint spacer (antibiotic)
 use Spacer in Upper Joints
 use Spacer in Lower Joints
Jugular body *use* Glomus Jugulare
Jugular lymph node
 use Lymphatic, Right Neck
 use Lymphatic, Left Neck

K

Kappa *use* Pacemaker, Dual Chamber in 0JH
Kcentra *use* 4-Factor Prothrombin Complex Concentrate
Keratectomy, kerectomy
 see Excision, Eye 08B
 see Resection, Eye 08T
Keratocentesis *see* Drainage, Eye 089
Keratoplasty
 see Repair, Eye 08Q
 see Replacement, Eye 08R
 see Supplement, Eye 08U
Keratotomy
 see Drainage, Eye 089
 see Repair, Eye 08Q
KEVZARA® *use* Sarilumab
Keystone Heart TriGuard 3™ CEPD (cerebral embolic protection device) X2A6325
Kirschner wire (K-wire)
 use Internal Fixation Device in Head and Facial Bones
 use Internal Fixation Device in Upper Bones
 use Internal Fixation Device in Lower Bones
 use Internal Fixation Device in Upper Joints
 use Internal Fixation Device in Lower Joints
Knee (implant) insert *use* Liner in Lower Joints
KUB x-ray *see* Plain Radiography, Kidney, Ureter and Bladder BT04
Kuntscher nail
 use Internal Fixation Device, Intramedullary in Upper Bones
 use Internal Fixation Device, Intramedullary in Lower Bones
KYMRIAH® *use* Tisagenlecleucel Immunotherapy

L

L

▶ New ➡ Revised ~~deleted~~ Deleted

Left gastric artery *use* Gastric Artery
Left gastroepiploic artery *use* Splenic Artery
Left gastroepiploic vein *use* Splenic Vein
Left inferior phrenic vein *use* Renal Vein, Left
Left inferior pulmonary vein *use* Pulmonary Vein, Left
Left jugular trunk *use* Thoracic Duct
Left lateral ventricle *use* Cerebral Ventricle
Left ovarian vein *use* Renal Vein, Left
Left second lumbar vein *use* Renal Vein, Left
Left subclavian trunk *use* Thoracic Duct
Left subcostal vein *use* Hemiazygos Vein
Left superior pulmonary vein *use* Pulmonary Vein, Left
Left suprarenal vein *use* Renal Vein, Left
Left testicular vein *use* Renal Vein, Left
Lengthening
  Bone, with device *see* Insertion of Limb Lengthening Device
  Muscle, by incision *see* Division, Muscles 0K8
  Tendon, by incision *see* Division, Tendons 0L8
Leptomeninges, intracranial *use* Cerebral Meninges
Leptomeninges, spinal *use* Spinal Meninges
Leronlimab monoclonal antibody XW013K6
Lesser alar cartilage *use* Nasal Mucosa and Soft Tissue
Lesser occipital nerve *use* Cervical Plexus
Lesser Omentum *use* Omentum
Lesser saphenous vein
  use Saphenous Vein, Right
  use Saphenous Vein, Left
Lesser splanchnic nerve *use* Thoracic Sympathetic Nerve
Lesser trochanter
  use Upper Femur, Right
  use Upper Femur, Left
Lesser tuberosity
  use Humeral Head, Right
  use Humeral Head, Left
Lesser wing *use* Sphenoid Bone
Leukopheresis, therapeutic *see* Pheresis, Circulatory 6A55
Levator anguli oris muscle *use* Facial Muscle
Levator ani muscle *use* Perineum Muscle
Levator labii superioris alaeque nasi muscle *use* Facial Muscle
Levator labii superioris muscle *use* Facial Muscle
Levator palpebrae superioris muscle
  use Upper Eyelid, Right
  use Upper Eyelid, Left
Levator scapulae muscle
  use Neck Muscle, Right
  use Neck Muscle, Left
Levator veli palatini muscle *use* Tongue, Palate, Pharynx Muscle
Levatores costarum muscle
  use Thorax Muscle, Right
  use Thorax Muscle, Left
Lifeline ARM Automated Chest Compression (ACC) device 5A1221J
LifeStent® (Flexstar) (XL) Vascular Stent System *use* Intraluminal Device
Lifileucel *use* Lifileucel Immunotherapy
Lifileucel immunotherapy XW0
Ligament of head of fibula
  use Knee Bursa and Ligament, Right
  use Knee Bursa and Ligament, Left
Ligament of the lateral malleolus
  use Ankle Bursa and Ligament, Right
  use Ankle Bursa and Ligament, Left
Ligamentum flavum, cervical *use* Head and Neck Bursa and Ligament
Ligamentum flavum, lumbar *use* Lower Spine Bursa and Ligament
Ligamentum flavum, thoracic *use* Upper Spine Bursa and Ligament
Ligation *see* Occlusion
Ligation, hemorrhoid *see* Occlusion, Lower Veins, Hemorrhoidal Plexus
Light Therapy GZJZZZZ
LigaPASS 2.0™ PJK Prevention System *use* Posterior Vertebral Tether in New Technology
Liner
  Removal of device from
    Hip
      Left 0SPB09Z
      Right 0SP909Z
    Knee
      Left 0SPD09Z
      Right 0SPC09Z
  Revision of device in
    Hip
      Left 0SWB09Z
      Right 0SW909Z
    Knee
      Left 0SWD09Z
      Right 0SWC09Z
  Supplement
    Hip
      Left 0SUB09Z
        Acetabular Surface 0SUE09Z
        Femoral Surface 0SUS09Z
      Right 0SU909Z
        Acetabular Surface 0SUA09Z
        Femoral Surface 0SUR09Z
    Knee
      Left 0SUD09
        Femoral Surface 0SUU09Z
        Tibial Surface 0SUW09Z
      Right 0SUC09
        Femoral Surface 0SUT09Z
        Tibial Surface 0SUV09Z
Lingual artery
  use Artery, External Carotid, Right
  use Artery, External Carotid, Left
Lingual tonsil *use* Pharynx
Lingulectomy, lung
  see Excision, Lung Lingula 0BBH
  see Resection, Lung Lingula 0BTH
Lisocabtagene Maraleucel *use* Lisocabtagene Maraleucel Immunotherapy
Lisocabtagene Maraleucel Immunotherapy XW0
Lithoplasty *see* Fragmentatio
Lithotripsy
  see Fragmentation
  With removal of fragments *see* Extirpation
LITT (laser interstitial thermal therapy)
  see Laser Interstitial Thermal Therapy
  see Destruction
LIVIAN™ CRT-D *use* Cardiac Resynchronization Defibrillator Pulse Generator in 0JH
LIVTENCITY™ *use* Maribavir Anti-infective
Lobectomy
  see Excision, Central Nervous System and Cranial Nerves 00B
  see Excision, Respiratory System 0BB
  see Resection, Respiratory System 0BT
  see Excision, Hepatobiliary System and Pancreas 0FB
  see Resection, Hepatobiliary System and Pancreas 0FT
  see Excision, Endocrine System 0GB
  see Resection, Endocrine System 0GT
Lobotomy *see* Division, Brain 0080
Localization
  see Map
  see Imaging
Locus ceruleus *use* Pons
▶ **Longeviti ClearFit® Cranial Implant** *use* Synthetic Substitute, Ultrasound Penetrable in New Technology
▶ **Longeviti ClearFit® OTS Cranial Implant** *use* Synthetic Substitute, Ultrasound Penetrable in New Technology
Long thoracic nerve *use* Brachial Plexus
Loop ileostomy *see* Bypass, Ileum 0D1B
Loop recorder, implantable *use* Monitoring Device
▶ **Lovotibeglogene Autotemcel** XW1
Lower GI series *see* Fluoroscopy, Colon BD14
Lower Respiratory Fluid Nucleic Acid-base Microbial Detection XXEBXQ6
LTX regional anticoagulant *use* Nafamostat Anticoagulant
LUCAS® chest compression system 5A1221J
Lumbar artery *use* Abdominal Aorta
Lumbar facet joint *use* Lumbar Vertebral Joint
Lumbar ganglion *use* Lumbar Sympathetic Nerve
Lumbar lymph node *use* Lymphatic, Aortic
Lumbar lymphatic trunk *use* Cisterna Chyli
Lumbar splanchnic nerve *use* Lumbar Sympathetic Nerve
Lumbosacral facet joint *use* Lumbosacral Joint
Lumbosacral trunk *use* Lumbar Nerve
Lumpectomy
  see Excision
Lunate bone
  use Carpal, Right
  use Carpal, Left
Lunotriquetral ligament
  use Hand Bursa and Ligament, Right
  use Hand Bursa and Ligament, Left
▶ **LUNSUMIO™** *use* Mosunetuzumab Antineoplastic
Lurbinectedin XW0
Lymphadenectomy
  see Excision, Lymphatic and Hemic Systems 07B
  see Resection, Lymphatic and Hemic Systems 07T
Lymphadenotomy *see* Drainage, Lymphatic and Hemic Systems 079
Lymphangiectomy
  see Excision, Lymphatic and Hemic Systems 07B
  see Resection, Lymphatic and Hemic Systems 07T
Lymphangiogram *see* Plain Radiography, Lymphatic System B70
Lymphangioplasty
  see Repair, Lymphatic and Hemic Systems 07Q
  see Supplement, Lymphatic and Hemic Systems 07U
Lymphangiorrhaphy *see* Repair, Lymphatic and Hemic Systems 07Q
Lymphangiotomy *see* Drainage, Lymphatic and Hemic Systems 079
Lysis *see* Release

L

▶ New ➠ Revised ~~deleted~~ Deleted

M

Macula
use Retina, Right
use Retina, Left
MAGEC® Spinal Bracing and Distraction System *use* Magnetically Controlled Growth Rod(s) in New Technology
Magnet extraction, ocular foreign body *see* Extirpation, Eye 08C
Magnetic-guided radiofrequency endovascular fistula
Radial Artery, Left 031C3ZF
Radial Artery, Right 031B3ZF
Ulnar Artery, Left 031A3ZF
Ulnar Artery, Right 03193ZF
Magnetic Resonance Imaging (MRI)
Abdomen BW30
Ankle
Left BQ3H
Right BQ3G
Aorta
Abdominal B430
Thoracic B330
Arm
Left BP3F
Right BP3E
Artery
Celiac B431
Cervico-Cerebral Arch B33Q
Common Carotid, Bilateral B335
Coronary
Bypass Graft, Multiple B233
Multiple B231
Internal Carotid, Bilateral B338
Intracranial B33R
Lower Extremity
Bilateral B43H
Left B43G
Right B43F
Pelvic B43C
Renal, Bilateral B438
Spinal B33M
Superior Mesenteric B434
Upper Extremity
Bilateral B33K
Left B33J
Right B33H
Vertebral, Bilateral B33G
Bladder BT30
Brachial Plexus BW3P
Brain B030
Breast
Bilateral BH32
Left BH31
Right BH30
Calcaneus
Left BQ3K
Right BQ3J
Chest BW33Y
Coccyx BR3F
Connective Tissue
Lower Extremity BL31
Upper Extremity BL30
Corpora Cavernosa BV30
Disc
Cervical BR31
Lumbar BR33
Thoracic BR32
Ear B930
Elbow
Left BP3H
Right BP3G
Eye
Bilateral B837
Left B836
Right B835
Femur
Left BQ34
Right BQ33
Fetal Abdomen BY33

Magnetic Resonance Imaging (MRI) *(Continued)*
Fetal Extremity BY35
Fetal Head BY30
Fetal Heart BY31
Fetal Spine BY34
Fetal Thorax BY32
Fetus, Whole BY36
Foot
Left BQ3M
Right BQ3L
Forearm
Left BP3K
Right BP3J
Gland
Adrenal, Bilateral BG32
Parathyroid BG33
Parotid, Bilateral B936
Salivary, Bilateral B93D
Submandibular, Bilateral B939
Thyroid BG34
Head BW38
Heart, Right and Left B236
Hip
Left BQ31
Right BQ30
Intracranial Sinus B532
Joint
Finger
Left BP3D
Right BP3C
Hand
Left BP3D
Right BP3C
Temporomandibular, Bilateral BN39
Kidney
Bilateral BT33
Left BT32
Right BT31
Transplant BT39
Knee
Left BQ38
Right BQ37
Larynx B93J
Leg
Left BQ3F
Right BQ3D
Liver BF35
Liver and Spleen BF36
Lung Apices BB3G
Lung, Bilateral, Hyperpolarized Xenon 129 (Xe-129) BB34Z3Z
Nasopharynx B93F
Neck BW3F
Nerve
Acoustic B03C
Brachial Plexus BW3P
Oropharynx B93F
Ovary
Bilateral BU35
Left BU34
Right BU33
Ovary and Uterus BU3C
Pancreas BF37
Patella
Left BQ3W
Right BQ3V
Pelvic Region BW3G
Pelvis BR3C
Pituitary Gland B039
Plexus, Brachial BW3P
Prostate BV33
Retroperitoneum BW3H
Sacrum BR3F
Scrotum BV34
Sella Turcica B039
Shoulder
Left BP39
Right BP38
Sinus
Intracranial B532
Paranasal B932

Magnetic Resonance Imaging (MRI) *(Continued)*
Spinal Cord B03B
Spine
Cervical BR30
Lumbar BR39
Thoracic BR37
Spleen and Liver BF36
Subcutaneous Tissue
Abdomen BH3H
Extremity
Lower BH3J
Upper BH3F
Head BH3D
Neck BH3D
Pelvis BH3H
Thorax BH3G
Tendon
Lower Extremity BL33
Upper Extremity BL32
Testicle
Bilateral BV37
Left BV36
Right BV35
Toe
Left BQ3Q
Right BQ3P
Uterus BU36
Pregnant BU3B
Uterus and Ovary BU3C
Vagina BU39
Vein
Cerebellar B531
Cerebral B531
Jugular, Bilateral B535
Lower Extremity
Bilateral B53D
Left B53C
Right B53B
Other B53V
Pelvic (Iliac) Bilateral B53H
Portal B53T
Pulmonary, Bilateral B53S
Renal, Bilateral B53L
Spanchnic B53T
Upper Extremity
Bilateral B53P
Left B53N
Right B53M
Vena Cava
Inferior B539
Superior B538
Wrist
Left BP3M
Right BP3L
Magnetically Controlled Growth Rod(s)
Cervical XNS3
Lumbar XNS0
Thoracic XNS4
Magnus Neuromodulation System (MNS) X0Z0X18
Malleotomy *see* Drainage, Ear, Nose, Sinus 099
Malleus
use Auditory Ossicle, Right
use Auditory Ossicle, Left
Mammaplasty, mammoplasty
see Alteration, Skin and Breast 0H0
see Repair, Skin and Breast 0HQ
see Replacement, Skin and Breast 0HR
see Supplement, Skin and Breast 0HU
Mammary duct
use Breast, Right
use Breast, Left
use Breast, Bilateral
Mammary gland
use Breast, Right
use Breast, Left
use Breast, Bilateral
Mammectomy
see Excision, Skin and Breast 0HB
see Resection, Skin and Breast 0HT
Mammillary body *use* Hypothalamus

M

Mammography *see* Plain Radiography, Skin, Subcutaneous Tissue and Breast BH0
Mammotomy *see* Drainage, Skin and Breast 0H9
Mandibular nerve *use* Trigeminal Nerve
Mandibular notch
use Mandible, Right
use Mandible, Left
Mandibulectomy
see Excision, Head and Facial Bones 0NB
see Resection, Head and Facial Bones 0NT
Manipulation
Adhesions *see* Release
Chiropractic *see* Chiropractic Manipulation
Manual removal, retained placenta *see* Extraction, Products of Conception, Retained 10D1
Manubrium *use* Sternum
Map
Basal Ganglia 00K8
Brain 00K0
Cerebellum 00KC
Cerebral Hemisphere 00K7
Conduction Mechanism 02K8
Hypothalamus 00KA
Medulla Oblongata 00KD
Pons 00KB
Thalamus 00K9
Mapping
Doppler ultrasound *see* Ultrasonography
Electrocardiogram only *see* Measurement, Cardiac 4A02
Maribavir Anti-infective XW0
Mark IV Breathing Pacemaker System *use* Stimulator Generator in Subcutaneous Tissue and Fascia
MarrowStim™ PAD Kit for CBMA (Concentrated Bone Marrow Aspirate) *use* Other Substance
MarrowStim™ PAD Kit, for injection of concentrated bone marrow aspirate *see* Introduction of substance in or on, Muscle 3E02
Marsupialization
see Drainage
see Excision
Massage, cardiac
External 5A12012
Open 02QA0ZZ
Masseter muscle *use* Head Muscle
Masseteric fascia *use* Subcutaneous Tissue and Fascia, Face
Mastectomy
see Excision, Skin and Breast 0HB
see Resection, Skin and Breast 0HT
Mastoid (postauricular) lymph node
use Lymphatic, Right Neck
use Lymphatic, Left Neck
Mastoid air cells
use Mastoid Sinus, Right
use Mastoid Sinus, Left
Mastoid process
use Temporal Bone, Right
use Temporal Bone, Left
Mastoidectomy
see Excision, Ear, Nose, Sinus 09B
see Resection, Ear, Nose, Sinus 09T
Mastoidotomy *see* Drainage, Ear, Nose, Sinus 099
Mastopexy
see Reposition, Skin and Breast 0HS
see Repair, Skin and Breast 0HQ
Mastorrhaphy *see* Repair, Skin and Breast 0HQ
Mastotomy *see* Drainage, Skin and Breast 0H9
Maxillary artery
use External Carotid Artery, Right
use External Carotid Artery, Left
Maxillary nerve *use* Trigeminal Nerve
Maximo II DR (VR) *use* Defibrillator Generator in 0JH
Maximo II DR CRT-D *use* Cardiac Resynchronization Defibrillator Pulse Generator in 0JH
Measurement
Arterial
Flow
Coronary 4A03
Intracranial 4A03X5D
Peripheral 4A03
Pulmonary 4A03
Pressure
Coronary 4A03
Peripheral 4A03
Pulmonary 4A03
Thoracic, Other 4A03
Pulse
Coronary 4A03
Peripheral 4A03
Pulmonary 4A03
Saturation, Peripheral 4A03
Sound, Peripheral 4A03
Biliary
Flow 4A0C
Pressure 4A0C
Cardiac
Action Currents 4A02
Defibrillator 4B02XTZ
Electrical Activity 4A02
Guidance 4A02X4A
No Qualifier 4A02X4Z
Output 4A02
Pacemaker 4B02XSZ
Rate 4A02
Rhythm 4A02
Sampling and Pressure
Bilateral 4A02
Left Heart 4A02
Right Heart 4A02
Sound 4A02
Total Activity, Stress 4A02XM4
Central Nervous
Cerebrospinal Fluid Shunt, Wireless Sensor 4B00XW0
Conductivity 4A00
Electrical Activity 4A00
Pressure 4A000BZ
Intracranial 4A00
Saturation, Intracranial 4A00
Stimulator 4B00XVZ
Temperature, Intracranial 4A00
Circulatory, Volume 4A05XLZ
Gastrointestinal
Motility 4A0B
Pressure 4A0B
Secretion 4A0B
Lower Respiratory Fluid Nucleic Acid-base Microbial Detection XXEBXQ6
Lymphatic
Flow 4A06
Pressure 4A06
Metabolism 4A0Z
Musculoskeletal
Contractility 4A0F
Pressure 4A0F3BE
Stimulator 4B0FXVZ
Olfactory, Acuity 4A08X0Z
Peripheral Nervous
Conductivity
Motor 4A01
Sensory 4A01
Electrical Activity 4A01
Stimulator 4B01XVZ
Positive Blood Culture Fluorescence Hybridization for Organism Identification, Concentration and Susceptibility XXE5XN6
Products of Conception
Cardiac
Electrical Activity 4A0H
Rate 4A0H
Rhythm 4A0H
Sound 4A0H
Nervous
Conductivity 4A0J
Electrical Activity 4A0J
Pressure 4A0J
Measurement *(Continued)*
Respiratory
Capacity 4A09
Flow 4A09
Pacemaker 4B09XSZ
Rate 4A09
Resistance 4A09
Total Activity 4A09
Volume 4A09
Sleep 4A0ZXQZ
Temperature 4A0Z
Urinary
Contractility 4A0D
Flow 4A0D
Pressure 4A0D
Resistance 4A0D
Volume 4A0D
Venous
Flow
Central 4A04
Peripheral 4A04
Portal 4A04
Pulmonary 4A04
Pressure
Central 4A04
Peripheral 4A04
Portal 4A04
Pulmonary 4A04
Pulse
Central 4A04
Peripheral 4A04
Portal 4A04
Pulmonary 4A04
Saturation, Peripheral 4A04
Visual
Acuity 4A07X0Z
Mobility 4A07X7Z
Pressure 4A07XBZ
Whole Blood Nucleic Acid-base Microbial Detection XXE5XM5
Meatoplasty, urethra *see* Repair, Urethra 0TQD
Meatotomy *see* Drainage, Urinary System 0T9
Mechanical chest compression (mCPR) 5A1221J
Mechanical initial specimen diversion technique using active negative pressure (blood collection) XXE5XR7
Mechanical ventilation *see* Performance, Respiratory 5A19
Medial canthus
use Lower Eyelid, Right
use Lower Eyelid, Left
Medial collateral ligament (MCL)
use Knee Bursa and Ligament, Right
use Knee Bursa and Ligament, Left
Medial condyle of femur
use Lower Femur, Right
use Lower Femur, Left
Medial condyle of tibia
use Tibia, Right
use Tibia, Left
Medial cuneiform bone
use Tarsal, Right
use Tarsal, Left
Medial epicondyle of femur
use Lower Femur, Right
use Lower Femur, Left
Medial epicondyle of humerus
use Humeral Shaft, Right
use Humeral Shaft, Left
Medial malleolus
use Tibia, Right
use Tibia, Left
Medial meniscus
use Knee Joint, Right
use Knee Joint, Left
Medial plantar artery
use Foot Artery, Right
use Foot Artery, Left
Medial plantar nerve *use* Tibial Nerve
Medial popliteal nerve *use* Tibial Nerve

M

Medial rectus muscle
  use Extraocular Muscle, Right
  use Extraocular Muscle, Left
Medial sural cutaneous nerve *use* Tibial Nerve
Median antebrachial vein
  use Basilic Vein, Right
  use Basilic Vein, Left
Median cubital vein
  use Basilic Vein, Right
  use Basilic Vein, Left
Median sacral artery *use* Abdominal Aorta
Mediastinal cavity *use* Mediastinum
Mediastinal lymph node *use* Lymphatic, Thorax
Mediastinal space *use* Mediastinum
Mediastinoscopy 0WJC4ZZ
Medication Management GZ3ZZZZ
  for substance abuse
    Antabuse HZ83ZZZ
    Bupropion HZ87ZZZ
    Clonidine HZ86ZZZ
    Levo-alpha-acetyl-methadol (LAAM) HZ82ZZZ
    Methadone Maintenance HZ81ZZZ
    Naloxone HZ85ZZZ
    Naltrexone HZ84ZZZ
    Nicotine Replacement HZ80ZZZ
    Other Replacement Medication HZ89ZZZ
    Psychiatric Medication HZ88ZZZ
Meditation 8E0ZXY5
Medtronic Endurant® II AAA stent graft system *use* Intraluminal Device
Meissner's (submucous) plexus *use* Abdominal Sympathetic Nerve
Melody® transcatheter pulmonary valve *use* Zooplastic Tissue in Heart and Great Vessels
▶ **Melphalan Hydrochloride Antineoplastic** XW053T9
Membranous urethra *use* Urethra
Meningeorrhaphy
  see Repair, Cerebral Meninges 00Q1
  see Repair, Spinal Meninges 00QT
Meniscectomy, knee
  see Excision, Joint, Knee, Right 0SBC
  see Excision, Joint, Knee, Left 0SBD
Mental foramen
  use Mandible, Right
  use Mandible, Left
Mentalis muscle *use* Facial Muscle
Mentoplasty *see* Alteration, Jaw, Lower 0W05
Meropenem-vaborbactam Anti-infective XW0
Mesenterectomy *see* Excision, Mesentery 0DBV
Mesenteriorrhaphy, mesenterorrhaphy *see* Repair, Mesentery 0DQV
Mesenteriplication *see* Repair, Mesentery 0DQV
Mesoappendix *use* Mesentery
Mesocolon *use* Mesentery
Metacarpal ligament
  use Hand Bursa and Ligament, Right
  use Hand Bursa and Ligament, Left
Metacarpophalangeal ligament
  use Hand Bursa and Ligament, Right
  use Hand Bursa and Ligament, Left
Metal on metal bearing surface *use* Synthetic Substitute, Metal in 0SR
Metatarsal ligament
  use Foot Bursa and Ligament, Right
  use Foot Bursa and Ligament, Left
Metatarsectomy
  see Excision, Lower Bones 0QB
  see Resection, Lower Bones 0QT
Metatarsophalangeal (MTP) joint
  use Metatarsal-Phalangeal Joint, Right
  use Metatarsal-Phalangeal Joint, Left
Metatarsophalangeal ligament
  use Foot Bursa and Ligament, Right
  use Foot Bursa and Ligament, Left
Metathalamus *use* Thalamus
Micro-Driver stent (RX) (OTW) *use* Intraluminal Device
MicroMed HeartAssist *use* Implantable Heart Assist System in Heart and Great Vessels
Micrus CERECYTE microcoil *use* Intraluminal Device, Bioactive in Upper Arteries
Midcarpal joint
  use Carpal Joint, Right
  use Carpal Joint, Left
Middle cardiac nerve *use* Thoracic Sympathetic Nerve
Middle cerebral artery *use* Intracranial Artery
Middle cerebral vein *use* Intracranial Vein
Middle colic vein *use* Colic Vein
Middle genicular artery
  use Popliteal Artery, Right
  use Popliteal Artery, Left
Middle hemorrhoidal vein
  use Hypogastric Vein, Right
  use Hypogastric Vein, Left
▶ **Middle meningeal artery, intracranial portion** *use* Intracranial Artery
Middle rectal artery
  use Internal Iliac Artery, Right
  use Internal Iliac Artery, Left
Middle suprarenal artery *use* Abdominal Aorta
Middle temporal artery
  use Temporal Artery, Right
  use Temporal Artery, Left
Middle turbinate *use* Nasal Turbinate
Mineral-based Topical Hemostatic Agent XW0
MIRODERM™ Biologic Wound Matrix *use* Nonautologous Tissue Substitute
MIRODERM™ skin graft *see* Replacement, Skin and Breast 0HR
MitraClip valve repair system *use* Synthetic Substitute
Mitral annulus *use* Mitral Valve
Mitroflow® Aortic Pericardial Heart Valve *use* Zooplastic Tissue in Heart and Great Vessels
MNS (Magnus Neuromodulation System) X0Z0X18
Mobilization, adhesions *see* Release
Molar gland *use* Buccal Mucosa
MolecuLight i:X® wound imaging *see* Other Imaging, Anatomical Regions BW5
Monitoring
  Arterial
    Flow
      Coronary 4A13
      Peripheral 4A13
      Pulmonary 4A13
    Pressure
      Coronary 4A13
      Peripheral 4A13
      Pulmonary 4A13
    Pulse
      Coronary 4A13
      Peripheral 4A13
      Pulmonary 4A13
    Saturation, Peripheral 4A13
    Sound, Peripheral 4A13
  ▶ Brain Electrical Activity, Computer-aided Detection and Notification XX20X89
  Cardiac
    Electrical Activity 4A12
      Ambulatory 4A12X45
      No Qualifier 4A12X4Z
    Output 4A12
    Rate 4A12
    Rhythm 4A12
    Sound 4A12
    Total Activity, Stress 4A12XM4
    Vascular Perfusion, Indocyanine Green Dye 4A12XSH
  Central Nervous
    Conductivity 4A10
    Electrical Activity
      Intraoperative 4A10
      No Qualifier 4A10
Monitoring *(Continued)*
    Pressure 4A100BZ
      Intracranial 4A10
    Saturation, Intracranial 4A10
    Temperature, Intracranial 4A10
  Gastrointestinal
    Motility 4A1B
    Pressure 4A1B
    Secretion 4A1B
    Vascular Perfusion, Indocyanine Green Dye 4A1BXSH
  Kidney, Fluorescent Pyrazine XT25XE5
  Lymphatic
    Flow
    Indocyanine Green Dye 4A16
    No Qualifier 4A16
    Pressure 4A16
  ▶ Muscle Compartment Pressure, Micro-Electro-Mechanical System XX2F3W9
  Oxygen Saturation Endoscopic Imaging (OXEI) XD2
  Peripheral Nervous
    Conductivity
      Motor 4A11
      Sensory 4A11
    Electrical Activity Intraoperative 4A11
    No Qualifier 4A11
  Products of Conception
    Cardiac
      Electrical Activity 4A1H
      Rate 4A1H
      Rhythm 4A1H
      Sound 4A1H
    Nervous
      Conductivity 4A1J
      Electrical Activity 4A1J
      Pressure 4A1J
  Respiratory
    Capacity 4A19
    Flow 4A19
    Rate 4A19
    Resistance 4A19
    Volume 4A19
  Skin and Breast, Vascular Perfusion, Indocyanine Green Dye 4A1GXSH
  Sleep 4A1ZXQZ
  Temperature 4A1Z
  Urinary
    Contractility 4A1D
    Flow 4A1D
    Pressure 4A1D
    Resistance 4A1D
    Volume 4A1D
  Venous
    Flow
      Central 4A14
      Peripheral 4A14
      Portal 4A14
      Pulmonary 4A14
    Pressure
      Central 4A14
      Peripheral 4A14
      Portal 4A14
      Pulmonary 4A14
    Pulse
      Central 4A14
      Peripheral 4A14
      Portal 4A14
      Pulmonary 4A14
    Saturation
      Central 4A14
      Portal 4A14
      Pulmonary 4A14
Monitoring Device, Hemodynamic
  Abdomen 0JH8
  Chest 0JH6
Mosaic Bioprosthesis (aortic) (mitral) valve *use* Zooplastic Tissue in Heart and Great Vessels
Mosunetuzumab Antineoplastic XW0

M

▶ New ➡ Revised ~~deleted~~ Deleted

Motor Function Assessment F01
Motor Treatment F07
MR Angiography
see Magnetic Resonance Imaging (MRI), Heart B23
see Magnetic Resonance Imaging (MRI), Upper Arteries B33
see Magnetic Resonance Imaging (MRI), Lower Arteries B43
MULTI-LINK (VISION)(MINI-VISION) (ULTRA) Coronary Stent System *use* Intraluminal Device
Multiple sleep latency test 4A0ZXQZ
▶**Muscle Compartment Pressure, Micro-Electro-Mechanical System** XX2F3W9
Musculocutaneous nerve *use* Brachial Plexus Nerve
Musculopexy
see Repair, Muscles 0KQ
see Reposition, Muscles 0KS
Musculophrenic artery
use Internal Mammary Artery, Right
use Internal Mammary Artery, Left
Musculoplasty
see Repair, Muscles 0KQ
see Supplement, Muscles 0KU
Musculorrhaphy *see* Repair, Muscles 0KQ
Musculospiral nerve *use* Radial Nerve
▶**MY01 Continuous Compartmental Pressure Monitor** XX2F3W9
Myectomy
see Excision, Muscles 0KB
see Resection, Muscles 0KT
Myelencephalon *use* Medulla Oblongata
Myelogram
CT *see* Computerized Tomography (CT Scan), Central Nervous System B02
MRI *see* Magnetic Resonance Imaging (MRI), Central Nervous System B03
Myenteric (Auerbach's) plexus *use* Abdominal Sympathetic Nerve
Myocardial Bridge Release *see* Release, Artery, Coronary
Myomectomy *see* Excision, Female Reproductive System 0UB
Myometrium *use* Uterus
Myopexy
see Repair, Muscles 0KQ
see Reposition, Muscles 0KS
Myoplasty
see Repair, Muscles 0KQ
see Supplement, Muscles 0KU
Myorrhaphy *see* Repair, Muscles 0KQ
Myoscopy *see* Inspection, Muscles 0KJ
Myotomy
see Division, Muscles 0K8
see Drainage, Muscles 0K9
Myringectomy
see Excision, Ear, Nose, Sinus 09B
see Resection, Ear, Nose, Sinus 09T
Myringoplasty
see Repair, Ear, Nose, Sinus 09Q
see Replacement, Ear, Nose, Sinus 09R
see Supplement, Ear, Nose, Sinus 09U
Myringostomy *see* Drainage, Ear, Nose, Sinus 099
Myringotomy *see* Drainage, Ear, Nose, Sinus 099

M

N

NA-1 (Nerinitide) *use* Nerinitide
Nafamostat anticoagulant XY0YX37
Nail bed
use Finger Nail
use Toe Nail
Nail plate
use Finger Nail
use Toe Nail
nanoLOCK™ interbody fusion device
use Interbody Fusion Device in Upper Joints
use Interbody Fusion Device in Lower Joints
Narcosynthesis GZGZZZZ
Narsoplimab monoclonal antibody XW0
Nasal cavity *use* Nasal Mucosa and Soft Tissue
Nasal concha *use* Nasal Turbinate
Nasalis muscle *use* Facial Muscle
Nasolacrimal duct
use Lacrimal Duct, Right
use Lacrimal Duct, Left
Nasopharyngeal airway (NPA) *use* Intraluminal Device, Airway in Ear, Nose, Sinus
Navicular bone
use Tarsal, Right
use Tarsal, Left
Near Infrared Spectroscopy, Circulatory System 8E02
Neck of femur
use Upper Femur, Right
use Upper Femur, Left
Neck of humerus (anatomical)(surgical)
use Humeral Head, Right
use Humeral Head, Left
Nelli® Seizure Monitoring System XXE0X48
Neovasc Reducer™ *use* Reduction Device in New Technology
Nephrectomy
see Excision, Urinary System 0TB
see Resection, Urinary System 0TT
Nephrolithotomy *see* Extirpation, Urinary System 0TC
Nephrolysis *see* Release, Urinary System 0TN
Nephropexy
see Repair, Urinary System 0TQ
see Reposition, Urinary System 0TS
Nephroplasty
see Repair, Urinary System 0TQ
see Supplement, Urinary System 0TU
Nephropyeloureterostomy
see Bypass, Urinary System 0T1
see Drainage, Urinary System 0T9
Nephrorrhaphy *see* Repair, Urinary System 0TQ
Nephroscopy, transurethral 0TJ58ZZ
Nephrostomy
see Bypass, Urinary System 0T1
see Drainage, Urinary System 0T9
Nephrotomography
see Plain Radiography, Urinary System BT0
see Fluoroscopy, Urinary System BT1
Nephrotomy
see Division, Urinary System 0T8
see Drainage, Urinary System 0T9
Nerinitide XW0
Nerve conduction study
see Measurement, Central Nervous 4A00
see Measurement, Peripheral Nervous 4A01
Nerve Function Assessment F01
Nerve to the stapedius *use* Facial Nerve
Nesiritide *use* Human B-type Natriuretic Peptide
Neurectomy
see Excision, Central Nervous System and Cranial Nerves 00B
see Excision, Peripheral Nervous System 01B
Neurexeresis
see Extraction, Central Nervous System and Cranial Nerves 00D
see Extraction, Peripheral Nervous System 01D
NeuroBlate™ System *see* Destruction
Neurohypophysis *use* Gland, Pituitary
Neurolysis
see Release, Central Nervous System and Cranial Nerves 00N
see Release, Peripheral Nervous System 01N
Neuromuscular electrical stimulation (NEMS) lead *use* Stimulator Lead in Muscles
Neurophysiologic monitoring *see* Monitoring, Central Nervous 4A10
Neuroplasty
see Repair, Central Nervous System and Cranial Nerves 00Q
see Supplement, Central Nervous System and Cranial Nerves 00U
see Repair, Peripheral Nervous System 01Q
see Supplement, Peripheral Nervous System 01U
Neurorrhaphy
see Repair, Central Nervous System and Cranial Nerves 00Q
see Repair, Peripheral Nervous System 01Q
Neurostimulator Generator
Insertion of device in, Skull 0NH00NZ
Removal of device from, Skull 0NP00NZ
Revision of device in, Skull 0NW00NZ
Neurostimulator generator, multiple channel *use* Stimulator Generator, Multiple Array in 0JH
Neurostimulator generator, multiple channel rechargeable *use* Stimulator Generator, Multiple Array Rechargeable in 0JH
Neurostimulator generator, single channel *use* Stimulator Generator, Single Array in 0JH
Neurostimulator generator, single channel rechargeable *use* Stimulator Generator, Single Array Rechargeable in 0JH
Neurostimulator Lead
Insertion of device in
Brain 00H0
Canal, Spinal 00HU
Cerebral Ventricle 00H6
Nerve
Cranial 00HE
Peripheral 01HY
Spinal Canal 00HU
Spinal Cord 00HV
Vein
Azygos 05H0
Innominate
Left 05H4
Right 05H3
Removal of device from
Brain 00P0
Cerebral Ventricle 00P6
Nerve
Cranial 00PE
Peripheral 01PY
Spinal Canal 00PU
Spinal Cord 00PV
Vein
Azygos 05P0
Innominate
Left 05P4
Right 05P3
Revision of device in
Brain 00W0
Cerebral Ventricle 00W6
Nerve
Cranial 00WE
Peripheral 01WY
Spinal Canal 00WU
Spinal Cord 00WV
Vein
Azygos 05W0
Innominate
Left 05W4
Right 05W3
Sphenopalatine Ganglion, Insertion X0HK3Q8
Neurostimulator Lead with Paired Stimulation System, Insertion X0HQ3R8
Neurostimulator Lead in Oropharynx XWHD7Q7
Neurotomy
see Division, Central Nervous System and Cranial Nerves 008
see Division, Peripheral Nervous System 018
Neurotripsy
see Destruction, Central Nervous System and Cranial Nerves 005
see Destruction, Peripheral Nervous System 015
Neutralization plate
use Internal Fixation Device in Head and Facial Bones
use Internal Fixation Device in Upper Bones
use Internal Fixation Device in Lower Bones
New Technology
Afamitresgene Autoleucel Immunotherapy XW0
Amivantamab Monoclonal Antibody XW0
▶Anacaulase-bcdb XW0
Antibiotic-eluting Bone Void Filler XW0V0P7
Aorta
Thoracic Arch using Branched Synthetic Substitute with Intraluminal Device X2RX0N7
Thoracic Descending using Branched Synthetic Substitute with Intraluminal Device X2VW0N7
Apalutamide Antineoplastic XW0DXJ5
Atezolizumab Antineoplastic XW0
Axicabtagene Ciloleucel Immunotherapy XW0
Bamlanivimab Monoclonal Antibody XW0
Baricitinib XW0
Betibeglogene Autotemcel XW1
Bioengineered Allogeneic Construct, Skin XHRPXF7
~~Brain Electrical Activity, Computer-aided Semiologic Analysis XXE0X48~~
▶Brain Electrical Activity
▶Computer-aided Detection and Notification XX20X89
▶Computer-aided Semiologic Analysis XXE0X48
Brexanolone XW0
Brexucabtagene Autoleucel Immunotherapy XW0
Broad Consortium Microbiota-based Live Biotherapeutic Suspension XW0H7X8
~~Bromelain-enriched Proteolytic Enzyme XW0~~
▶Bypass
▶Conduit through Femoral Vein to Popliteal Artery X2K
▶Conduit through Femoral Vein to Superficial Femoral Artery X2K
Caplacizumab XW0
Cefiderocol Anti-infective XW0
Ceftolozane/Tazobactam Anti-infective XW0
Cerebral Embolic Filtration
Duel Filter X2A5312
Extracorporeal Flow Reversal Circuit X2A
Single Deflection Filter X2A6325
CD24Fc Immunomodulator XW0
Ciltacabtagene Autoleucel XW0
Coagulation Factor Xa, Inactivated XW0
~~Computer-aided Assessment, Intracranial Vascular Activity XXE0X07~~
▶Computer-aided Assessment
▶Cardiac Output XXE2X19
▶Intracranial Vascular Activity XXE0X07
Computer-aided Guidance, Transthoracic Echocardiography X2JAX47
Computer-aided Mechanical Aspiration X2C
Computer-aided Triage and Notification, Pulmonary Artery Flow XXE3X27
Computer-aided Valve Modeling and Notification, Coronary Artery Flow XXE3X68

▶ New ➡ Revised ~~deleted~~ Deleted

N

New Technology *(Continued)*
Reposition
Cervical, Magnetically Controlled Growth Rod(s) XNS3
Lumbar
Magnetically Controlled Growth Rod(s) XNS0
Posterior (Dynamic) Distraction Device XNS0
Thoracic
Magnetically Controlled Growth Rod(s) XNS4
Posterior (Dynamic) Distraction Device XNS4
Ruxolitinib XW0DXT5
▶Rezafungin XW0
▶Sabizabulin XW0
Sarilumab XW0
SARS-CoV-2 Antibody Detection, Serum/Plasma Nanoparticle Fluorescence XXE5XV7
SARS-CoV-2 Polymerase Chain Reaction, Nasopharyngeal Fluid XXE97U7
Satralizumab-mwge XW01397
▶SER-109 XW0DXN9
Single-use Duodenoscope XFJ
Single-use Oversleeve with Intraoperative Colonic Irrigation XDPH8K7
Spesolimab Monoclonal Antibody XW0
▶Sulbactam-Durlobactam XW0
Supplement
▶Arteriovenous Fistula, Extraluminal Support Device X2U
Bursa and Ligament, Spine, Posterior Vertebral Tether XKU
▶Coronary Artery/Arteries, Vein Graft Extraluminal Support Device(s) X2U4079
Vertebra
Lumbar, Mechanically Expandable (Paired) Synthetic Substitute XNU0356
Thoracic, Mechanically Expandable (Paired) Synthetic Substitute XNU4356
~~Synthetic Human Angiotensin II XW0~~
Tabelecleucel Immunotherapy XW0
Tagraxofusp-erzs Antineoplastic XW0
▶Talar Prosthesis Synthetic Substitute XNR
Taurolidine Anti-infective and Heparin Anticoagulant XY0YX28

New Technology *(Continued)*
Teclistamab Antineoplastic XW01348
Terlipressin XW0
Tisagenlecleucel Immunotherapy XW0
Tocilizumab XW0
Treosulfan XW0
Trilaciclib XW0
▶Ultrasound Penetrable Synthetic Substitute, Skull XNR80D9
Uridine Triacetate XW0DX82
Venetoclax Antineoplastic XW0DXR5
Whole Blood Nucleic Acid-base Microbial Detection XXE5XM5
Whole Blood Reverse Transcription and Quantitative Real-time Polymerase Chain Reaction XXE5X38
NexoBrid™ *use* Anacaulase-bcdb
Ninth cranial nerve *use* Glossopharyngeal Nerve
NIRS (Near Infrared Spectroscopy) *see* Physiological Systems and Anatomical Regions
Nitinol framed polymer mesh *use* Synthetic Substitute
Niyad™ *use* Nafamostat Anticoagulant
Non-tunneled central venous catheter *use* Infusion Device
Nonimaging Nuclear Medicine Assay
Bladder, Kidneys and Ureters CT63
Blood C763
Kidneys, Ureters and Bladder CT63
Lymphatics and Hematologic System C76YYZZ
Ureters, Kidneys and Bladder CT63
Urinary System CT6YYZZ
Nonimaging Nuclear Medicine Probe
Abdomen CW50
Abdomen and Chest CW54
Abdomen and Pelvis CW51
Brain C050
Central Nervous System C05YYZZ
Chest CW53
Chest and Abdomen CW54
Chest and Neck CW56
Extremity
Lower CP5PZZZ
Upper CP5NZZZ
Head and Neck CW5B
Heart C25YYZZ
Right and Left C256

Nonimaging Nuclear Medicine Probe *(Continued)*
Lymphatics
Head C75J
Head and Neck C755
Lower Extremity C75P
Neck C75K
Pelvic C75D
Trunk C75M
Upper Chest C75L
Upper Extremity C75N Lymphatics and Hematologic System C75YYZZ
Musculoskeletal System, Other CP5YYZZ
Neck and Chest CW56
Neck and Head CW5B
Pelvic Region CW5J
Pelvis and Abdomen CW51
Spine CP55ZZZ
Nonimaging Nuclear Medicine Uptake
Endocrine System CG4YYZZ
Gland, Thyroid CG42
Nostril *use* Nasal Mucosa and Soft Tissue
Novacor Left Ventricular Assist Device *use* Implantable Heart Assist System in Heart and Great Vessels
Novation® Ceramic AHS® (Articulation Hip System) *use* Synthetic Substitute, Ceramic in 0SR
Nuclear medicine
see Planar Nuclear Medicine Imaging
see Tomographic (Tomo) Nuclear Medicine Imaging
see Positron Emission Tomographic (PET) Imaging
see Nonimaging Nuclear Medicine Uptake
see Nonimaging Nuclear Medicine Probe
see Nonimaging Nuclear Medicine Assay
see Systemic Nuclear Medicine Therapy
Nuclear scintigraphy *see* Nuclear Medicine
NUsurface® Meniscus Implant
use Synthetic Substitute, Lateral Meniscus in New Technology
use Synthetic Substitute, Medial Meniscus in New Technology
Nutrition, concentrated substances
Enteral infusion 3E0G36Z
Parenteral (peripheral) infusion *see* Introduction of Nutritional Substance
NUZYRA™ *use* Omadacycline Anti-infective

▶ New ➠ Revised ~~deleted~~ Deleted

N

O

Obliteration *see* Destruction
Obturator artery
use Internal Iliac Artery, Right
use Internal Iliac Artery, Left
Obturator lymph node *use* Lymphatic, Pelvis
Obturator muscle
use Hip Muscle, Right
use Hip Muscle, Left
Obturator nerve *use* Lumbar Plexus
Obturator vein
use Hypogastric Vein, Right
use Hypogastric Vein, Left
Obtuse margin *use* Heart, Left
Occipital artery
use External Carotid Artery, Right
use External Carotid Artery, Left
Occipital lobe *use* Cerebral Hemisphere
Occipital lymph node
use Lymphatic, Right Neck
use Lymphatic, Left Neck
Occipitofrontalis muscle *use* Facial Muscle
Occlusion
Ampulla of Vater 0FLC
Anus 0DLQ
Aorta
Abdominal 04L0
Thoracic, Descending 02LW
Artery
Anterior Tibial
Left 04LQ
Right 04LP
Axillary
Left 03L6
Right 03L5
Brachial
Left 03L8
Right 03L7
Celiac 04L1
Colic
Left 04L7
Middle 04L8
Right 04L6
Common Carotid
Left 03LJ
Right 03LH
Common Iliac
Left 04LD
Right 04LC
External Carotid
Left 03LN
Right 03LM
External Iliac
Left 04LJ
Right 04LH
Face 03LR
Femoral
Left 04LL
Right 04LK
Foot
Left 04LW
Right 04LV
Gastric 04L2
Hand
Left 03LF
Right 03LD
Hepatic 04L3
Inferior Mesenteric 04LB
Innominate 03L2
Internal Carotid
Left 03LL
Right 03LK
Internal Iliac
Left 04LF
Right 04LE
Internal Mammary
Left 03L1
Right 03L0
Intracranial 03LG

Occlusion *(Continued)*
Artery
Lower 04LY
Peroneal
Left 04LU
Right 04LT
Popliteal
Left 04LN
Right 04LM
Posterior Tibial
Left 04LS
Right 04LR
Pulmonary
Left 02LR
Right 02LQ
Pulmonary Trunk 02LP
Radial
Left 03LC
Right 03LB
Renal
Left 04LA
Right 04L9
Splenic 04L4
Subclavian
Left 03L4
Right 03L3
Superior Mesenteric 04L5
Temporal
Left 03LT
Right 03LS
Thyroid
Left 03LV
Right 03LU
Ulnar
Left 03LA
Right 03L9
Upper 03LY
Vertebral
Left 03LQ
Right 03LP
Atrium, Left 02L7
Bladder 0TLB
Bladder Neck 0TLC
Bronchus
Lingula 0BL9
Lower Lobe
Left 0BLB
Right 0BL6
Main
Left 0BL7
Right 0BL3
Middle Lobe, Right 0BL5
Upper Lobe
Left 0BL8
Right 0BL4
Carina 0BL2
Cecum 0DLH
Cisterna Chyli 07LL
Colon
Ascending 0DLK
Descending 0DLM
Sigmoid 0DLN
Transverse 0DLL
Cord
Bilateral 0VLH
Left 0VLG
Right 0VLF
Cul-de-sac 0ULF
Duct
Common Bile 0FL9
Cystic 0FL8
Hepatic
Common 0FL7
Left 0FL6
Right 0FL5
Lacrimal
Left 08LY
Right 08LX
Pancreatic 0FLD
Accessory 0FLF

Occlusion *(Continued)*
Duct
Parotid
Left 0CLC
Right 0CLB
Duodenum 0DL9
Esophagogastric Junction 0DL4
Esophagus 0DL5
Lower 0DL3
Middle 0DL2
Upper 0DL1
Fallopian Tube
Left 0UL6
Right 0UL5
Fallopian Tubes, Bilateral 0UL7
Ileocecal Valve 0DLC
Ileum 0DLB
Intestine
Large 0DLE
Left 0DLG
Right 0DLF
Small 0DL8
Jejunum 0DLA
Kidney Pelvis
Left 0TL4
Right 0TL3
Left atrial appendage (LAA) *see* Occlusion, Atrium, Left 02L7
Lymphatic
Aortic 07LD
Axillary
Left 07L6
Right 07L5
Head 07L0
Inguinal
Left 07LJ
Right 07LH
Internal Mammary
Left 07L9
Right 07L8
Lower Extremity
Left 07LG
Right 07LF
Mesenteric 07LB
Neck
Left 07L2
Right 07L1
Pelvis 07LC
Thoracic Duct 07LK
Thorax 07L7
Upper Extremity
Left 07L4
Right 07L3
Rectum 0DLP
Stomach 0DL6
Pylorus 0DL7
Trachea 0BL1
Ureter
Left 0TL7
Right 0TL6
Urethra 0TLD
Vagina 0ULG
Valve, Pulmonary 02LH
Vas Deferens
Bilateral 0VLQ
Left 0VLP
Right 0VLN
Vein
Axillary
Left 05L8
Right 05L7
Azygos 05L0
Basilic
Left 05LC
Right 05LB
Brachial
Left 05LA
Right 05L9
Cephalic
Left 05LF
Right 05LD

Occlusion *(Continued)*
Vein
Colic 06L7
Common Iliac
Left 06LD
Right 06LC
Esophageal 06L3
External Iliac
Left 06LG
Right 06LF
External Jugular
Left 05LQ
Right 05LP
Face
Left 05LV
Right 05LT
Femoral
Left 06LN
Right 06LM
Foot
Left 06LV
Right 06LT
Gastric 06L2
Hand
Left 05LH
Right 05LG
Hemiazygos 05L1
Hepatic 06L4
Hypogastric
Left 06LJ
Right 06LH
Inferior Mesenteric 06L6
Innominate
Left 05L4
Right 05L3
Internal Jugular
Left 05LN
Right 05LM
Intracranial 05LL
Lower 06LY
Portal 06L8
Pulmonary
Left 02LT
Right 02LS
Renal
Left 06LB
Right 06L9
Saphenous
Left 06LQ
Right 06LP
Splenic 06L1
Subclavian
Left 05L6
Right 05L5
Superior Mesenteric 06L5
Upper 05LY
Vertebral
Left 05LS
Right 05LR
Vena Cava
Inferior 06L0
Superior 02LV
Occlusion, REBOA (resuscitative endovascular balloon occlusion of the aorta)
02LW3DJ
04L03DJ
Occupational therapy *see* Activities of Daily Living Treatment, Rehabilitation F08
Octagam 10%, for COVID-19 treatment *use* High-Dose Intravenous Immune Globulin
Odentectomy
see Excision, Mouth and Throat 0CB
see Resection, Mouth and Throat 0CT
Odontoid process *use* Cervical Vertebra
Olecranon bursa
use Elbow Bursa and Ligament, Right
use Elbow Bursa and Ligament, Left
Olecranon process
use Ulna, Right
use Ulna, Left
Olfactory bulb *use* Olfactory Nerve
Olumiant® *use* Baricitinib
Omadacycline Anti-infective XW0
Omentectomy, omentumectomy
see Excision, Gastrointestinal System 0DB
see Resection, Gastrointestinal System 0DT
Omentofixation *see* Repair, Gastrointestinal System 0DQ
Omentoplasty
see Repair, Gastrointestinal System 0DQ
see Replacement, Gastrointestinal System 0DR
see Supplement, Gastrointestinal System 0DU
Omentorrhaphy *see* Repair, Gastrointestinal System 0DQ
Omentotomy *see* Drainage, Gastrointestinal System 0D9
Omidubicel XW1
Omnilink Elite Vascular Balloon Expandable Stent System *use* Intraluminal Device
Onychectomy
see Excision, Skin and Breast 0HB
see Resection, Skin and Breast 0HT
Onychoplasty
see Repair, Skin and Breast 0HQ
see Replacement, Skin and Breast 0HR
Onychotomy *see* Drainage, Skin and Breast 0H9
Oophorectomy
see Excision, Female Reproductive System 0UB
see Resection, Female Reproductive System 0UT
Oophoropexy
see Repair, Female Reproductive System 0UQ
see Reposition, Female Reproductive System 0US
Oophoroplasty
see Repair, Female Reproductive System 0UQ
see Supplement, Female Reproductive System 0UU
Oophororrhaphy *see* Repair, Female Reproductive System 0UQ
Oophorostomy *see* Drainage, Female Reproductive System 0U9
Oophorotomy
see Division, Female Reproductive System 0U8
see Drainage, Female Reproductive System 0U9
Oophorrhaphy *see* Repair, Female Reproductive System 0UQ
Open Pivot (mechanical) valve *use* Synthetic Substitute
Open Pivot Aortic Valve Graft (AVG) *use* Synthetic Substitute
▶Open-truss Design Internal Fixation Device
▶Ankle
▶Left XRGK0B9
▶Right XRGJ0B9
▶Tarsal
▶Left XRGM0B9
▶Right XRGL0B9
Ophthalmic artery *use* Intracranial Artery
Ophthalmic nerve *use* Trigeminal Nerve
Ophthalmic vein *use* Intracranial Vein
Opponensplasty
Tendon replacement *see* Replacement, Tendons 0LR
Tendon transfer *see* Transfer, Tendons 0LX
Optic chiasma *use* Optic Nerve
Optic disc
use Retina, Right
use Retina, Left
Optic foramen *use* Sphenoid Bone
Optical coherence tomography, intravascular *see* Computerized Tomography (CT Scan)
Optimizer™ III implantable pulse generator *use* Contractility Modulation Device in 0JH
Orbicularis oculi muscle
use Upper Eyelid, Right
use Upper Eyelid, Left
Orbicularis oris muscle *use* Facial Muscle
Orbital atherectomy *see* Extirpation, Heart and Great Vessels 02C
Orbital fascia *use* Subcutaneous Tissue and Fascia, Face
Orbital portion of ethmoid bone
use Orbit, Right
use Orbit, Left
Orbital portion of frontal bone
use Orbit, Right
use Orbit, Left
Orbital portion of lacrimal bone
use Orbit, Right
use Orbit, Left
Orbital portion of maxilla
use Orbit, Right
use Orbit, Left
Orbital portion of palatine bone
use Orbit, Right
use Orbit, Left
Orbital portion of sphenoid bone
use Orbit, Right
use Orbit, Left
Orbital portion of zygomatic bone
use Orbit, Right
use Orbit, Left
Orchectomy, orchidectomy, orchiectomy
see Excision, Male Reproductive System 0VB
see Resection, Male Reproductive System 0VT
Orchidoplasty, orchioplasty
see Repair, Male Reproductive System 0VQ
see Replacement, Male Reproductive System 0VR
see Supplement, Male Reproductive System 0VU
Orchidorrhaphy, orchiorrhaphy *see* Repair, Male Reproductive System 0VQ
Orchidotomy, orchiotomy, orchotomy *see* Drainage, Male Reproductive System 0V9
Orchiopexy
see Repair, Male Reproductive System 0VQ
see Reposition, Male Reproductive System 0VS
Oropharyngeal airway (OPA) *use* Intraluminal Device, Airway in Mouth and Throat
Oropharynx *use* Pharynx
Ossiculectomy
see Excision, Ear, Nose, Sinus 09B
see Resection, Ear, Nose, Sinus 09T
Ossiculotomy *see* Drainage, Ear, Nose, Sinus 099
Ostectomy
see Excision, Head and Facial Bones 0NB
see Resection, Head and Facial Bones 0NT
see Excision, Upper Bones 0PB
see Resection, Upper Bones 0PT
see Excision, Lower Bones 0QB
see Resection, Lower Bones 0QT
Osteoclasis
see Division, Head and Facial Bones 0N8
see Division, Upper Bones 0P8
see Division, Lower Bones 0Q8
Osteolysis
see Release, Head and Facial Bones 0NN
see Release, Upper Bones 0PN
see Release, Lower Bones 0QN
Osteopathic Treatment
Abdomen 7W09X
Cervical 7W01X
Extremity
Lower 7W06X
Upper 7W07X
Head 7W00X
Lumbar 7W03X
Pelvis 7W05X
Rib Cage 7W08X
Sacrum 7W04X
Thoracic 7W02X

▶ New ➡ Revised ~~deleted~~ Deleted

P

Pacemaker
Dual Chamber
Abdomen 0JH8
Chest 0JH6
Intracardiac
Insertion of device in
Atrium
Left 02H7
Right 02H6
Vein, Coronary 02H4
Ventricle
Left 02HL
Right 02HK
Removal of device from, Heart 02PA
Revision of device in, Heart 02WA
Single Chamber
Abdomen 0JH8
Chest 0JH6
Single Chamber Rate Responsive
Abdomen 0JH8
Chest 0JH6
Packing
Abdominal Wall 2W43X5Z
Anorectal 2Y43X5Z
Arm
Lower
Left 2W4DX5Z
Right 2W4CX5Z
Upper
Left 2W4BX5Z
Right 2W4AX5Z
Back 2W45X5Z
Chest Wall 2W44X5Z
Ear 2Y42X5Z
Extremity
Lower
Left 2W4MX5Z
Right 2W4LX5Z
Upper
Left 2W49X5Z
Right 2W48X5Z
Face 2W41X5Z
Finger
Left 2W4KX5Z
Right 2W4JX5Z
Foot
Left 2W4TX5Z
Right 2W4SX5Z
Genital Tract, Female 2Y44X5Z
Hand
Left 2W4FX5Z
Right 2W4EX5Z
Head 2W40X5Z
Inguinal Region
Left 2W47X5Z
Right 2W46X5Z
Leg
Lower
Left 2W4RX5Z
Right 2W4QX5Z
Upper
Left 2W4PX5Z
Right 2W4NX5Z
Mouth and Pharynx 2Y40X5Z
Nasal 2Y41X5Z
Neck 2W42X5Z
Thumb
Left 2W4HX5Z
Right 2W4GX5Z
Toe
Left 2W4VX5Z
Right 2W4UX5Z
Urethra 2Y45X5Z
Paclitaxel-eluting coronary stent *use* Intraluminal Device, Drug-eluting in Heart and Great Vessels
Paclitaxel-eluting peripheral stent
use Intraluminal Device, Drug-eluting in Upper Arteries
use Intraluminal Device, Drug-eluting in Lower Arteries
Palatine gland *use* Buccal Mucosa
Palatine tonsil *use* Tonsils
Palatine uvula *use* Uvula
Palatoglossal muscle *use* Tongue, Palate, Pharynx Muscle
Palatopharyngeal muscle *use* Tongue, Palate, Pharynx Muscle
Palatoplasty
see Repair, Mouth and Throat 0CQ
see Replacement, Mouth and Throat 0CR
see Supplement, Mouth and Throat 0CU
Palatorrhaphy *see* Repair, Mouth and Throat 0CQ
Palmar (volar) digital vein
use Hand Vein, Right
use Hand Vein, Left
Palmar (volar) metacarpal vein
use Hand Vein, Right
use Hand Vein, Left
Palmar cutaneous nerve
use Radial Nerve
use Median Nerve
Palmar fascia (aponeurosis)
use Subcutaneous Tissue and Fascia, Right Hand
use Subcutaneous Tissue and Fascia, Left Hand
Palmar interosseous muscle
use Hand Muscle, Right
use Hand Muscle, Left
Palmar ulnocarpal ligament
use Wrist Bursa and Ligament, Right
use Wrist Bursa and Ligament, Left
Palmaris longus muscle
use Lower Arm and Wrist Muscle, Right
use Lower Arm and Wrist Muscle, Left
Pancreatectomy
see Excision, Pancreas 0FBG
see Resection, Pancreas 0FTG
Pancreatic artery *use* Splenic Artery
Pancreatic plexus *use* Abdominal Sympathetic Nerve
Pancreatic vein *use* Splenic Vein
Pancreaticoduodenostomy *see* Bypass, Hepatobiliary System and Pancreas 0F1
Pancreaticosplenic lymph node *use* Lymphatic, Aortic
Pancreatogram, endoscopic retrograde *see* Fluoroscopy, Pancreatic Duct BF18
Pancreatolithotomy *see* Extirpation, Pancreas 0FCG
Pancreatotomy
see Division, Pancreas 0F8G
see Drainage, Pancreas 0F9G
Panniculectomy
see Excision, Skin, Abdomen 0HB7
see Excision, Subcutaneous Tissue and Fascia, Abdomen 0JB8
Paraaortic lymph node *use* Lymphatic, Aortic
Paracentesis
Eye *see* Drainage, Eye 089
Peritoneal Cavity *see* Drainage, Peritoneal Cavity 0W9G
Tympanum *see* Drainage, Ear, Nose, Sinus 099
▶ Paradise™ Ultrasound Renal Denervation System X051329
Parapharyngeal space *use* Neck
Pararectal lymph node *use* Lymphatic, Mesenteric
Parasternal lymph node *use* Lymphatic, Thorax
Parathyroidectomy
see Excision, Endocrine System 0GB
see Resection, Endocrine System 0GT
Paratracheal lymph node *use* Lymphatic, Thorax
Paraurethral (Skene's) gland *use* Vestibular Gland
Parenteral nutrition, total *see* Introduction of Nutritional Substance
Parietal lobe *use* Cerebral Hemisphere
Parotid lymph node *use* Lymphatic, Head
Parotid plexus *use* Facial Nerve
Parotidectomy
see Excision, Mouth and Throat 0CB
see Resection, Mouth and Throat 0CT
Pars flaccida
use Tympanic Membrane, Right
use Tympanic Membrane, Left
Partial joint replacement
Hip *see* Replacement, Lower Joints 0SR
Knee *see* Replacement, Lower Joints 0SR
Shoulder *see* Replacement, Upper Joints 0RR
Partially absorbable mesh *use* Synthetic Substitute
Patch, blood, spinal 3E0R3GC
Patellapexy
see Repair, Lower Bones 0QQ
see Reposition, Lower Bones 0QS
Patellaplasty
see Repair, Lower Bones 0QQ
see Replacement, Lower Bones 0QR
see Supplement, Lower Bones 0QU
Patellar ligament
use Knee Bursa and Ligament, Right
use Knee Bursa and Ligament, Left
Patellar tendon
use Knee Tendon, Right
use Knee Tendon, Left
Patellectomy
see Excision, Lower Bones 0QB
see Resection, Lower Bones 0QT
Patellofemoral joint
use Knee Joint, Right
use Knee Joint, Left
use Knee Joint, Femoral Surface, Right
use Knee Joint, Femoral Surface, Left
pAVF (percutaneous arteriovenous fistula), using magnetic-guided radiofrequency *see* Bypass, Upper Arteries 031
pAVF (percutaneous arteriovenous fistula), using thermal resistance energy *see* New Technology, Cardiovascular System X2K
Pectineus muscle
use Upper Leg Muscle, Right
use Upper Leg Muscle, Left
Pectoral (anterior) lymph node
use Lymphatic, Right Axillary
use Lymphatic, Left Axillary
Pectoral fascia *use* Subcutaneous Tissue and Fascia, Chest
Pectoralis major muscle
use Thorax Muscle, Right
use Thorax Muscle, Left
Pectoralis minor muscle
use Thorax Muscle, Right
use Thorax Muscle, Left
Pedicle-based dynamic stabilization device
use Spinal Stabilization Device, Pedicle-Based in 0RH
use Spinal Stabilization Device, Pedicle-Based in 0SH
PEEP (positive end expiratory pressure) *see* Assistance, Respiratory 5A09
PEG (percutaneous endoscopic gastrostomy) 0DH63UZ
PEJ (percutaneous endoscopic jejunostomy) 0DHA3UZ
Pelvic splanchnic nerve
use Abdominal Sympathetic Nerve
use Sacral Sympathetic Nerve
Penectomy
see Excision, Male Reproductive System 0VB
see Resection, Male Reproductive System 0VT
Penumbra Indigo® aspiration system *see* New Technology, Cardiovascular System X2C
Penile urethra *use* Urethra
PERCEPT™ PC neurostimulator *use* Stimulator Generator, Multiple Array in 0JH
Perceval sutureless valve (rapid deployment technique) *see* Replacement, Valve, Aortic 02RF
Perianal skin *use* Skin, Perineum
Percutaneous endoscopic gastrojejunostomy (PEG/J) tube *use* Feeding Device in Gastrointestinal System

▶ New ➡ Revised ~~deleted~~ Deleted

Percutaneous endoscopic gastrostomy (PEG) tube *use* Feeding Device in Gastrointestinal System
Percutaneous nephrostomy catheter *use* Drainage Device
Percutaneous transluminal coronary angioplasty (PTCA) *see* Dilation, Heart and Great Vessels 027
Performance
Biliary
Multiple, Filtration 5A1C60Z
Single, Filtration 5A1C00Z
Cardiac
Continuous
Output 5A1221Z
Pacing 5A1223Z
Intermittent, Pacing 5A1213Z
Single, Output, Manual 5A12012
Circulatory
Continuous
Central Membrane 5A1522F
Peripheral Veno-arterial Membrane 5A1522G
Peripheral Veno-venous Membrane 5A1522H
Intraoperative
Central Membrane 5A15A2F
Peripheral Veno-arterial Membrane 5A15A2G
Peripheral Veno-venous Membrane 5A15A2H
Respiratory
24-96 Consecutive Hours, Ventilation 5A1945Z
Greater than 96 Consecutive Hours, Ventilation 5A1955Z
Less than 24 Consecutive Hours, Ventilation 5A1935Z
Single, Ventilation, Nonmechanical 5A19054
Urinary
Continuous, Greater than 18 hours per day, Filtration 5A1D90Z
Intermittent, Less than 6 Hours Per Day, Filtration 5A1D70Z
Prolonged Intermittent, 6-18 hours per day, Filtration 5A1D80Z
Perfusion *see* Introduction of substance in or on
Perfusion, donor organ
Heart 6AB50BZ
Kidney(s) 6ABT0BZ
Liver 6ABF0BZ
Lung(s) 6ABB0BZ
Pericardiectomy
see Excision, Pericardium 02BN
see Resection, Pericardium 02TN
Pericardiocentesis
see Drainage, Cavity, Pericardial 0W9D
Pericardiolysis *see* Release, Pericardium 02NN
Pericardiophrenic artery
use Internal Mammary Artery, Right
use Internal Mammary Artery, Left
Pericardioplasty
see Repair, Pericardium 02QN
see Replacement, Pericardium 02RN
see Supplement, Pericardium 02UN
Pericardiorrhaphy *see* Repair, Pericardium 02QN
Pericardiostomy *see* Drainage, Cavity, Pericardial 0W9D
Pericardiotomy *see* Drainage, Cavity, Pericardial 0W9D
Perimetrium *use* Uterus
Peripheral Intravascular Lithotripsy (Peripheral IVL) see Fragmentation
Peripheral parenteral nutrition *see* Introduction of Nutritional Substance
Peripherally inserted central catheter (PICC) *use* Infusion Device
Peritoneal dialysis 3E1M39Z
Peritoneocentesis
see Drainage, Peritoneum 0D9W
see Drainage, Cavity, Peritoneal 0W9G
Peritoneoplasty
see Repair, Peritoneum 0DQW
see Replacement, Peritoneum 0DRW
see Supplement, Peritoneum 0DUW
Peritoneoscopy 0DJW4ZZ
Peritoneotomy *see* Drainage, Peritoneum 0D9W
Peritoneumectomy
see Excision, Peritoneum 0DBW
Peroneus brevis muscle
use Lower Leg Muscle, Right
use Lower Leg Muscle, Left
Peroneus longus muscle
use Lower Leg Muscle, Right
use Lower Leg Muscle, Left
Pessary ring *use* Intraluminal Device, Pessary in Female Reproductive System
PET scan *see* Positron Emission Tomographic (PET) Imaging
Petrous part of temoporal bone
use Temporal Bone, Right
use Temporal Bone, Left
Phacoemulsification, lens
With IOL implant *see* Replacement, Eye 08R
Without IOL implant *see* Extraction, Eye 08D
Phagenyx® system XWHD7Q7
Phalangectomy
see Excision, Upper Bones 0PB
see Resection, Upper Bones 0PT
see Excision, Lower Bones 0QB
see Resection, Lower Bones 0QT
Phallectomy
see Excision, Penis 0VBS
see Resection, Penis 0VTS
Phalloplasty
see Repair, Penis 0VQS
see Supplement, Penis 0VUS
Phallotomy *see* Drainage, Penis 0V9S
Pharmacotherapy, for substance abuse
Antabuse HZ93ZZZ
Bupropion HZ97ZZZ
Clonidine HZ96ZZZ
Levo-alpha-acetyl-methadol (LAAM) HZ92ZZZ
Methadone Maintenance HZ91ZZZ
Naloxone HZ95ZZZ
Naltrexone HZ94ZZZ
Nicotine Replacement HZ90ZZZ
Psychiatric Medication HZ98ZZZ
Replacement Medication, Other HZ99ZZZ
Pharyngeal constrictor muscle *use* Tongue, Palate, Pharynx Muscle
Pharyngeal plexus *use* Vagus Nerve
Pharyngeal recess *use* Nasopharynx
Pharyngeal tonsil *use* Adenoids
Pharyngogram *see* Fluoroscopy, Pharynx B91G
Pharyngoplasty
see Repair, Mouth and Throat 0CQ
see Replacement, Mouth and Throat 0CR
see Supplement, Mouth and Throat 0CU
Pharyngorrhaphy *see* Repair, Mouth and Throat 0CQ
Pharyngotomy *see* Drainage, Mouth and Throat 0C9
Pharyngotympanic tube
use Eustachian Tube, Right
use Eustachian Tube, Left
Pheresis
Erythrocytes 6A55
Leukocytes 6A55
Plasma 6A55
Platelets 6A55
Stem Cells
Cord Blood 6A55
Hematopoietic 6A55
Phlebectomy
see Excision, Upper Veins 05B
see Extraction, Upper Veins 05D
see Excision, Lower Veins 06B
see Extraction, Lower Veins 06D
Phlebography
see Plain Radiography, Veins B50
Impedance 4A04X51
Phleborrhaphy
see Repair, Upper Veins 05Q
see Repair, Lower Veins 06Q
Phlebotomy
see Drainage, Upper Veins 059
see Drainage, Lower Veins 069
Photocoagulation
For Destruction *see* Destruction
For Repair *see* Repair
Photopheresis, therapeutic *see* Phototherapy, Circulatory 6A65
Phototherapy
Circulatory 6A65
Skin 6A60
Ultraviolet light see Ultraviolet Light Therapy, Physiological Systems 6A8
Phrenectomy, phrenoneurectomy *see* Excision, Nerve, Phrenic 01B2
Phrenemphraxis *see* Destruction, Nerve, Phrenic 0152
Phrenic nerve stimulator generator *use* Stimulator Generator in Subcutaneous Tissue and Fascia
Phrenic nerve stimulator lead *use* Diaphragmatic Pacemaker Lead in Respiratory System
Phreniclasis *see* Destruction, Nerve, Phrenic 0152
Phrenicoexeresis *see* Extraction, Nerve, Phrenic 01D2
Phrenicotomy *see* Division, Nerve, Phrenic 0182
Phrenicotripsy *see* Destruction, Nerve, Phrenic 0152
Phrenoplasty
see Repair, Respiratory System 0BQ
see Supplement, Respiratory System 0BU
Phrenotomy *see* Drainage, Respiratory System 0B9
Physiatry *see* Motor Treatment, Rehabilitation F07
Physical medicine *see* Motor Treatment, Rehabilitation F07
Physical therapy *see* Motor Treatment, Rehabilitation F07
PHYSIOMESH™ Flexible Composite Mesh *use* Synthetic Substitute
Pia mater, intracranial *use* Cerebral Meninges
Pia mater, spinal *use* Spinal Meninges
PiCSO® Impulse System X2A7358
Pinealectomy
see Excision, Pineal Body 0GB1
see Resection, Pineal Body 0GT1
Pinealoscopy 0GJ14ZZ
Pinealotomy *see* Drainage, Pineal Body 0G91
Pinna
use External Ear, Right
use External Ear, Left
use External Ear, Bilateral
Pipeline™ (flex) embolization device *use* Intraluminal Device, Flow Diverter in 03V
Piriform recess (sinus) *use* Pharynx
Piriformis muscle
use Hip Muscle, Right
use Hip Muscle, Left
PIRRT (Prolonged intermittent renal replacement therapy) 5A1D80Z
Pisiform bone
use Carpal, Right
use Carpal, Left
Pisohamate ligament
use Hand Bursa and Ligament, Right
use Hand Bursa and Ligament, Left
Pisometacarpal ligament
use Hand Bursa and Ligament, Right
use Hand Bursa and Ligament, Left
Pituitectomy
see Excision, Gland, Pituitary 0GB0
see Resection, Gland, Pituitary 0GT0
Plain film radiology *see* Plain Radiography
Plain Radiography
Abdomen BW00ZZZ
Abdomen and Pelvis BW01ZZZ

P

▶ New ➠ Revised ~~deleted~~ Deleted

P

P

▶ New ➠ Revised ~~deleted~~ Deleted

Preputiotomy *see* Drainage, Male Reproductive System 0V9
Pressure support ventilation *see* Performance, Respiratory 5A19
PRESTIGE® Cervical Disc *use* Synthetic Substitute
Pretracheal fascia
use Subcutaneous Tissue and Fascia, Right Neck
use Subcutaneous Tissue and Fascia, Left Neck
Prevertebral fascia
use Subcutaneous Tissue and Fascia, Right Neck
use Subcutaneous Tissue and Fascia, Left Neck
PrimeAdvanced neurostimulator (SureScan) (MRI Safe) *use* Stimulator Generator, Multiple Array in 0JH
Princeps pollicis artery
use Hand Artery, Right
use Hand Artery, Left
Probing, duct
Diagnostic *see* Inspection
Dilation *see* Dilation
PROCEED™ Ventral Patch *use* Synthetic Substitute
Procerus muscle *use* Facial Muscle
Proctectomy
see Excision, Rectum 0DBP
see Resection, Rectum 0DTP
Proctoclysis *see* Introduction of substance in or on, Gastrointestinal Tract, Lower 3E0H
Proctocolectomy
see Excision, Gastrointestinal System 0DB
see Resection, Gastrointestinal System 0DT
Proctocolpoplasty
see Repair, Gastrointestinal System 0DQ
see Supplement, Gastrointestinal System 0DU
Proctoperineoplasty
see Repair, Gastrointestinal System 0DQ
see Supplement, Gastrointestinal System 0DU
Proctoperineorrhaphy *see* Repair, Gastrointestinal System 0DQ
Proctopexy
see Repair, Rectum 0DQP
see Reposition, Rectum 0DSP
Proctoplasty
see Repair, Rectum 0DQP
see Supplement, Rectum 0DUP
Proctorrhaphy *see* Repair, Rectum 0DQP
Proctoscopy 0DJD8ZZ
Proctosigmoidectomy
see Excision, Gastrointestinal System 0DB
see Resection, Gastrointestinal System 0DT
Proctosigmoidoscopy 0DJD8ZZ
Proctostomy *see* Drainage, Rectum 0D9P
Proctotomy *see* Drainage, Rectum 0D9P
Prodisc-C *use* Synthetic Substitute
Prodisc-L *use* Synthetic Substitute
Production, atrial septal defect *see* Excision, Septum, Atrial 02B5
Profunda brachii
use Brachial Artery, Right
use Brachial Artery, Left
Profunda femoris (deep femoral) vein
use Femoral Vein, Right
use Femoral Vein, Left
PROLENE Polypropylene Hernia System (PHS) *use* Synthetic Substitute
Pronator quadratus muscle
use Lower Arm and Wrist Muscle, Right
use Lower Arm and Wrist Muscle, Left
Pronator teres muscle
use Lower Arm and Wrist Muscle, Right
use Lower Arm and Wrist Muscle, Left
▶Prone positioning, intubated *see* Assistance, Respiratory 5A09
Prostatectomy
see Excision, Prostate 0VB0
see Resection, Prostate 0VT0
Prostatic artery
use Internal Iliac Artery, Right
use Internal Iliac Artery, Left
Prostatic urethra *use* Urethra
Prostatomy, prostatotomy *see* Drainage, Prostate 0V90
Protecta XT CRT-D *use* Cardiac Resynchronization Defibrillator Pulse Generator in 0JH
Protecta XT DR (XT VR) *use* Defibrillator Generator in 0JH
Protégé® RX Carotid Stent System *use* Intraluminal Device
Proximal radioulnar joint
use Elbow Joint, Right
use Elbow Joint, Left
Psoas muscle
use Hip Muscle, Right
use Hip Muscle, Left
PSV (pressure support ventilation) *see* Performance, Respiratory 5A19
Psychoanalysis GZ54ZZZ
Psychological Tests
Cognitive Status GZ14ZZZ
Developmental GZ10ZZZ
Intellectual and Psychoeducational GZ12ZZZ
Neurobehavioral Status GZ14ZZZ
Neuropsychological GZ13ZZZ
Personality and Behavioral GZ11ZZZ
Psychotherapy
Family, Mental Health Services GZ72ZZZ
Group
GZHZZZZ
Mental Health Services GZHZZZZ
Individual
see Psychotherapy, Individual, Mental Health Services
for substance abuse
12-Step HZ53ZZZ
Behavioral HZ51ZZZ
Cognitive HZ50ZZZ
Cognitive-Behavioral HZ52ZZZ
Confrontational HZ58ZZZ
Interactive HZ55ZZZ
Interpersonal HZ54ZZZ
Motivational Enhancement HZ57ZZZ
Psychoanalysis HZ5BZZZ
Psychodynamic HZ5CZZZ
Psychoeducation HZ56ZZZ
Psychophysiological HZ5DZZZ
Supportive HZ59ZZZ
Mental Health Services
Behavioral GZ51ZZZ
Cognitive GZ52ZZZ
Cognitive-Behavioral GZ58ZZZ
Interactive GZ50ZZZ
Interpersonal GZ53ZZZ
Psychoanalysis GZ54ZZZ
Psychodynamic GZ55ZZZ
Psychophysiological GZ59ZZZ
Supportive GZ56ZZZ
PTCA (percutaneous transluminal coronary angioplasty) *see* Dilation, Heart and Great Vessels 027
Pterygoid muscle *use* Head Muscle
Pterygoid process *use* Sphenoid Bone
Pterygopalatine (sphenopalatine) ganglion *use* Head and Neck Sympathetic Nerve
Pubis
use Pelvic Bone, Right
use Pelvic Bone, Left
Pubofemoral ligament
use Hip Bursa and Ligament, Right
use Hip Bursa and Ligament, Left
Pudendal nerve *use* Sacral Plexus
Pull-through, laparoscopic-assisted transanal
see Excision, Gastrointestinal System 0DB
see Resection, Gastrointestinal System 0DT
Pull-through, rectal *see* Resection, Rectum 0DTP
Pulmoaortic canal *use* Pulmonary Artery, Left
Pulmonary annulus *use* Pulmonary Valve
Pulmonary artery wedge monitoring *see* Monitoring, Arterial 4A13
Pulmonary plexus
use Vagus Nerve
use Thoracic Sympathetic Nerve
Pulmonic valve *use* Pulmonary Valve
Pulpectomy *see* Excision, Mouth and Throat 0CB
Pulverization *see* Fragmentation
Pulvinar *use* Thalamus
Pump reservoir *use* Infusion Device, Pump in Subcutaneous Tissue and Fascia
Punch biopsy *see* Excision with qualifier Diagnostic
Puncture *see* Drainage
Puncture, lumbar *see* Drainage, Spinal Canal 009U
Pure-Vu® system XDPH8K7
Pyelography
see Plain Radiography, Urinary System BT0
see Fluoroscopy, Urinary System BT1
Pyeloileostomy, urinary diversion *see* Bypass, Urinary System 0T1
Pyeloplasty
see Repair, Urinary System 0TQ
see Replacement, Urinary System 0TR
see Supplement, Urinary System 0TU
Pyeloplasty, dismembered
see Repair, Kidney Pelvis
Pyelorrhaphy *see* Repair, Urinary System 0TQ
Pyeloscopy 0TJ58ZZ
Pyelostomy
see Bypass, Urinary System 0T1
see Drainage, Urinary System 0T9
Pyelotomy *see* Drainage, Urinary System 0T9
Pylorectomy
see Excision, Stomach, Pylorus 0DB7
see Resection, Stomach, Pylorus 0DT7
Pyloric antrum *use* Stomach, Pylorus
Pyloric canal *use* Stomach, Pylorus
Pyloric sphincter *use* Stomach, Pylorus
Pylorodiosis *see* Dilation, Stomach, Pylorus 0D77
Pylorogastrectomy
see Excision, Gastrointestinal System 0DB
see Resection, Gastrointestinal System 0DT
Pyloroplasty
see Repair, Stomach, Pylorus 0DQ7
see Supplement, Stomach, Pylorus 0DU7
Pyloroscopy 0DJ68ZZ
Pylorotomy *see* Drainage, Stomach, Pylorus 0D97
Pyramidalis muscle
use Abdomen Muscle, Right
use Abdomen Muscle, Left

Q

QAngio XA® 3D XXE3X58
QFR® (Quantitative Flow Ratio) analysis of coronary angiography XXE3X58
Quadrangular cartilage *use* Nasal Septum
Quadrant resection of breast *see* Excision, Skin and Breast 0HB
Quadrate lobe *use* Liver
Quadratus femoris muscle
use Hip Muscle, Right
use Hip Muscle, Left
Quadratus lumborum muscle
use Trunk Muscle, Right
use Trunk Muscle, Left
Quadratus plantae muscle
use Foot Muscle, Right
use Foot Muscle, Left
Quadriceps (femoris)
use Upper Leg Muscle, Right
use Upper Leg Muscle, Left
Quantitative Flow Ratio Analysis, Coronary Artery Flow XXE3X58
Quarantine 8E0ZXY6
▶Quizartinib Antineoplastic XW0DXJ9

R

Radial artery arteriovenous fistula, using thermal resistance energy X2K
Radial collateral carpal ligament
  use Wrist Bursa and Ligament, Right
  use Wrist Bursa and Ligament, Left
Radial collateral ligament
  use Elbow Bursa and Ligament, Right
  use Elbow Bursa and Ligament, Left
Radial notch
  use Ulna, Right
  use Ulna, Left
Radial recurrent artery
  use Radial Artery, Right
  use Radial Artery, Left
Radial vein
  use Brachial Vein, Right
  use Brachial Vein, Left
Radialis indicis
  use Hand Artery, Right
  use Hand Artery, Left
Radiation Therapy
  see Beam Radiation
  see Brachytherapy
  see Other Radiation
  see Stereotactic Radiosurgery
Radiation treatment *see* Radiation Therapy
Radiocarpal joint
  use Wrist Joint, Right
  use Wrist Joint, Left
Radiocarpal ligament
  use Wrist Bursa and Ligament, Right
  use Wrist Bursa and Ligament, Left
Radiography *see* Plain Radiography
Radiology, analog *see* Plain Radiography
Radiology, diagnostic *see* Imaging, Diagnostic
Radioulnar ligament
  use Wrist Bursa and Ligament, Right
  use Wrist Bursa and Ligament, Left
Range of motion testing *see* Motor Function Assessment, Rehabilitation F01
Rapid ASPECTS XXE0X07
REALIZE® Adjustable Gastric Band *use* Extraluminal Device
Reattachment
  Abdominal Wall 0WMF0ZZ
  Ampulla of Vater 0FMC
  Ankle Region
    Left 0YML0ZZ
    Right 0YMK0ZZ
  Arm
    Lower
      Left 0XMF0ZZ
      Right 0XMD0ZZ
    Upper
      Left 0XM90ZZ
      Right 0XM80ZZ
  Axilla
    Left 0XM50ZZ
    Right 0XM40ZZ
  Back
    Lower 0WML0ZZ
    Upper 0WMK0ZZ
  Bladder 0TMB
  Bladder Neck 0TMC
  Breast
    Bilateral 0HMVXZZ
    Left 0HMUXZZ
    Right 0HMTXZZ
  Bronchus
    Lingula 0BM90ZZ
    Lower Lobe
      Left 0BMB0ZZ
      Right 0BM60ZZ
    Main
      Left 0BM70ZZ
      Right 0BM30ZZ
    Middle Lobe, Right 0BM50ZZ
    Upper Lobe
      Left 0BM80ZZ
      Right 0BM40ZZ

Reattachment *(Continued)*
  Bursa and Ligament
    Abdomen
      Left 0MMJ
      Right 0MMH
    Ankle
      Left 0MMR
      Right 0MMQ
    Elbow
      Left 0MM4
      Right 0MM3
    Foot
      Left 0MMT
      Right 0MMS
    Hand
      Left 0MM8
      Right 0MM7
    Head and Neck 0MM0
    Hip
      Left 0MMM
      Right 0MML
    Knee
      Left 0MMP
      Right 0MMN
    Lower Extremity
      Left 0MMW
      Right 0MMV
    Perineum 0MMK
    Rib(s) 0MMG
    Shoulder
      Left 0MM2
      Right 0MM1
    Spine
      Lower 0MMD
      Upper 0MMC
    Sternum 0MMF
    Upper Extremity
      Left 0MMB
      Right 0MM9
    Wrist
      Left 0MM6
      Right 0MM5
  Buttock
    Left 0YM10ZZ
    Right 0YM00ZZ
  Carina 0BM20ZZ
  Cecum 0DMH
  Cervix 0UMC
  Chest Wall 0WM80ZZ
  Clitoris 0UMJXZZ
  Colon
    Ascending 0DMK
    Descending 0DMM
    Sigmoid 0DMN
    Transverse 0DML
  Cord
    Bilateral 0VMH
    Left 0VMG
    Right 0VMF
  Cul-de-sac 0UMF
  Diaphragm 0BMT0ZZ
  Duct
    Common Bile 0FM9
    Cystic 0FM8
    Hepatic
      Common 0FM7
      Left 0FM6
      Right 0FM5
    Pancreatic 0FMD
      Accessory 0FMF
  Duodenum 0DM9
  Ear
    Left 09M1XZZ
    Right 09M0XZZ
  Elbow Region
    Left 0XMC0ZZ
    Right 0XMB0ZZ
  Esophagus 0DM5
  Extremity
    Lower
      Left 0YMB0ZZ
      Right 0YM90ZZ

Reattachment *(Continued)*
  Extremity *(Continued)*
    Upper
      Left 0XM70ZZ
      Right 0XM60ZZ
  Eyelid
    Lower
      Left 08MRXZZ
      Right 08MQXZZ
    Upper
      Left 08MPXZZ
      Right 08MNXZZ
  Face 0WM20ZZ
  Fallopian Tube
    Left 0UM6
    Right 0UM5
  Fallopian Tubes, Bilateral 0UM7
  Femoral Region
    Left 0YM80ZZ
    Right 0YM70ZZ
  Finger
    Index
      Left 0XMP0ZZ
      Right 0XMN0ZZ
    Little
      Left 0XMW0ZZ
      Right 0XMV0ZZ
    Middle
      Left 0XMR0ZZ
      Right 0XMQ0ZZ
    Ring
      Left 0XMT0ZZ
      Right 0XMS0ZZ
  Foot
    Left 0YMN0ZZ
    Right 0YMM0ZZ
  Forequarter
    Left 0XM10ZZ
    Right 0XM00ZZ
  Gallbladder 0FM4
  Gland
    Adrenal
      Left 0GM2
      Right 0GM3
  Hand
    Left 0XMK0ZZ
    Right 0XMJ0ZZ
  Hindquarter
    Bilateral 0YM40ZZ
    Left 0YM30ZZ
    Right 0YM20ZZ
  Hymen 0UMK
  Ileum 0DMB
  Inguinal Region
    Left 0YM60ZZ
    Right 0YM50ZZ
  Intestine
    Large 0DME
      Left 0DMG
      Right 0DMF
    Small 0DM8
  Jaw
    Lower 0WM50ZZ
    Upper 0WM40ZZ
  Jejunum 0DMA
  Kidney
    Left 0TM1
    Right 0TM0
  Kidney Pelvis
    Left 0TM4
    Right 0TM3
  Kidneys, Bilateral 0TM2
  Knee Region
    Left 0YMG0ZZ
    Right 0YMF0ZZ
  Leg
    Lower
      Left 0YMJ0ZZ
      Right 0YMH0ZZ
    Upper
      Left 0YMD0ZZ
      Right 0YMC0ZZ

New   Revised   ~~deleted~~ Deleted

Reattachment (Continued)
Lip
Lower 0CM10ZZ
Upper 0CM00ZZ
Liver 0FM0
Left Lobe 0FM2
Right Lobe 0FM1
Lung
Left 0BML0ZZ
Lower Lobe
Left 0BMJ0ZZ
Right 0BMF0ZZ
Middle Lobe, Right 0BMD0ZZ
Right 0BMK0ZZ
Upper Lobe
Left 0BMG0ZZ
Right 0BMC0ZZ
Lung Lingula 0BMH0ZZ
Muscle
Abdomen
Left 0KML
Right 0KMK
Facial 0KM1
Foot
Left 0KMW
Right 0KMV
Hand
Left 0KMD
Right 0KMC
Head 0KM0
Hip
Left 0KMP
Right 0KMN
Lower Arm and Wrist
Left 0KMB
Right 0KM9
Lower Leg
Left 0KMT
Right 0KMS
Neck
Left 0KM3
Right 0KM2
Perineum 0KMM
Shoulder
Left 0KM6
Right 0KM5
Thorax
Left 0KMJ
Right 0KMH
Tongue, Palate, Pharynx 0KM4
Trunk
Left 0KMG
Right 0KMF
Upper Arm
Left 0KM8
Right 0KM7
Upper Leg
Left 0KMR
Right 0KMQ
Nasal Mucosa and Soft Tissue 09MKXZZ
Neck 0WM60ZZ
Nipple
Left 0HMXXZZ
Right 0HMWXZZ
Ovary
Bilateral 0UM2
Left 0UM1
Right 0UM0
Palate, Soft 0CM30ZZ
Pancreas 0FMG
Parathyroid Gland 0GMR
Inferior
Left 0GMP
Right 0GMN
Multiple 0GMQ
Superior
Left 0GMM
Right 0GML
Penis 0VMSXZZ
Perineum
Female 0WMN0ZZ
Male 0WMM0ZZ

Reattachment (Continued)
Rectum 0DMP
Scrotum 0VM5XZZ
Shoulder Region
Left 0XM30ZZ
Right 0XM20ZZ
Skin
Abdomen 0HM7XZZ
Back 0HM6XZZ
Buttock 0HM8XZZ
Chest 0HM5XZZ
Ear
Left 0HM3XZZ
Right 0HM2XZZ
Face 0HM1XZZ
Foot
Left 0HMNXZZ
Right 0HMMXZZ
Hand
Left 0HMGXZZ
Right 0HMFXZZ
Inguinal 0HMAXZZ
Lower Arm
Left 0HMEXZZ
Right 0HMDXZZ
Lower Leg
Left 0HMLXZZ
Right 0HMKXZZ
Neck 0HM4XZZ
Perineum 0HM9XZZ
Scalp 0HM0XZZ
Upper Arm
Left 0HMCXZZ
Right 0HMBXZZ
Upper Leg
Left 0HMJXZZ
Right 0HMHXZZ
Stomach 0DM6
Tendon
Abdomen
Left 0LMG
Right 0LMF
Ankle
Left 0LMT
Right 0LMS
Foot
Left 0LMW
Right 0LMV
Hand
Left 0LM8
Right 0LM7
Head and Neck 0LM0
Hip
Left 0LMK
Right 0LMJ
Knee
Left 0LMR
Right 0LMQ
Lower Arm and Wrist
Left 0LM6
Right 0LM5
Lower Leg
Left 0LMP
Right 0LMN
Perineum 0LMH
Shoulder
Left 0LM2
Right 0LM1
Thorax
Left 0LMD
Right 0LMC
Trunk
Left 0LMB
Right 0LM9
Upper Arm
Left 0LM4
Right 0LM3
Upper Leg
Left 0LMM
Right 0LML

Reattachment (Continued)
Testis
Bilateral 0VMC
Left 0VMB
Right 0VM9
Thumb
Left 0XMM0ZZ
Right 0XML0ZZ
Thyroid Gland
Left Lobe 0GMG
Right Lobe 0GMH
Toe
1st
Left 0YMQ0ZZ
Right 0YMP0ZZ
2nd
Left 0YMS0ZZ
Right 0YMR0ZZ
3rd
Left 0YMU0ZZ
Right 0YMT0ZZ
4th
Left 0YMW0ZZ
Right 0YMV0ZZ
5th
Left 0YMY0ZZ
Right 0YMX0ZZ
Tongue 0CM70ZZ
Tooth
Lower 0CMX
Upper 0CMW
Trachea 0BM10ZZ
Tunica Vaginalis
Left 0VM7
Right 0VM6
Ureter
Left 0TM7
Right 0TM6
Ureters, Bilateral 0TM8
Urethra 0TMD
Uterine Supporting Structure 0UM4
Uterus 0UM9
Uvula 0CMN0ZZ
Vagina 0UMG
Vulva 0UMMXZZ
Wrist Region
Left 0XMH0ZZ
Right 0XMG0ZZ
REBOA (resuscitative endovascular balloon occlusion of the aorta)
02LW3DJ
04L03DJ
Rebound HRD® (Hernia Repair Device) *use* Synthetic Substitute
REBYOTA® *use* Broad Consortium Microbiota-based Live Biotherapeutic Suspension
RECELL® cell suspension autograft *see* Replacement, Skin and Breast 0HR
Recession
see Repair
see Reposition
Reclosure, disrupted abdominal wall 0WQFXZZ
Reconstruction
see Repair
see Replacement
see Supplement
Rectectomy
see Excision, Rectum 0DBP
see Resection, Rectum 0DTP
Rectocele repair
see Repair, Subcutaneous Tissue and Fascia, Pelvic Region 0JQC
Rectopexy
see Repair, Gastrointestinal System 0DQ
see Reposition, Gastrointestinal System 0DS
Rectoplasty
see Repair, Gastrointestinal System 0DQ
see Supplement, Gastrointestinal System 0DU
Rectorrhaphy *see* Repair, Gastrointestinal System 0DQ

R

Rectoscopy 0DJD8ZZ
Rectosigmoid junction *use* Colon, Sigmoid
Rectosigmoidectomy
see Excision, Gastrointestinal System 0DB
see Resection, Gastrointestinal System 0DT
Rectostomy *see* Drainage, Rectum 0D9P
Rectotomy *see* Drainage, Rectum 0D9P
Rectus abdominis muscle
use Abdomen Muscle, Right
use Abdomen Muscle, Left
Rectus femoris muscle
use Upper Leg Muscle, Right
use Upper Leg Muscle, Left
Recurrent laryngeal nerve *use* Vagus Nerve
Reducer™ system *use* Reduction Device in New Technology
Reduction
Dislocation *see* Reposition
Fracture *see* Reposition
Intussusception, intestinal *see* Reposition, Gastrointestinal System 0DS
Mammoplasty *see* Excision, Skin and Breast 0HB
Prolapse *see* Reposition
Torsion *see* Reposition
Volvulus, gastrointestinal *see* Reposition, Gastrointestinal System 0DS
Reduction device, coronary sinus X2V73Q7
Refusion *see* Fusion
REGN-COV2 monoclonal antibody XW0
Rehabilitation
see Speech Assessment, Rehabilitation F00
see Motor Function Assessment, Rehabilitation F01
see Activities of Daily Living Assessment, Rehabilitation F02
see Speech Treatment, Rehabilitation F06
see Motor Treatment, Rehabilitation F07
see Activities of Daily Living Treatment, Rehabilitation F08
see Hearing Treatment, Rehabilitation F09
see Cochlear Implant Treatment, Rehabilitation F0B
see Vestibular Treatment, Rehabilitation F0C
see Device Fitting, Rehabilitation F0D
see Caregiver Training, Rehabilitation F0F
Reimplantation
see Reattachment
see Reposition
see Transfer
Reinforcement
see Repair
see Supplement
Relaxation, scar tissue *see* Release
Release
Acetabulum
Left 0QN5
Right 0QN4
Adenoids 0CNQ
Ampulla of Vater 0FNC
Anal Sphincter 0DNR
Anterior Chamber
Left 08N33ZZ
Right 08N23ZZ
Anus 0DNQ
Aorta
Abdominal 04N0
Thoracic
Ascending/Arch 02NX
Descending 02NW
Aortic Body 0GND
Appendix 0DNJ
Artery
Anterior Tibial
Left 04NQ
Right 04NP
Axillary
Left 03N6
Right 03N5
Brachial
Left 03N8
Right 03N7

Release *(Continued)*
Artery *(Continued)*
Celiac 04N1
Colic
Left 04N7
Middle 04N8
Right 04N6
Common Carotid
Left 03NJ
Right 03NH
Common Iliac
Left 04ND
Right 04NC
Coronary
Four or More Arteries 02N3
One Artery 02N0
Three Arteries 02N2
Two Arteries 02N1
External Carotid
Left 03NN
Right 03NM
External Iliac
Left 04NJ
Right 04NH
Face 03NR
Femoral
Left 04NL
Right 04NK
Foot
Left 04NW
Right 04NV
Gastric 04N2
Hand
Left 03NF
Right 03ND
Hepatic 04N3
Inferior Mesenteric 04NB
Innominate 03N2
Internal Carotid
Left 03NL
Right 03NK
Internal Iliac
Left 04NF
Right 04NE
Internal Mammary
Left 03N1
Right 03N0
Intracranial 03NG
Lower 04NY
Peroneal
Left 04NU
Right 04NT
Popliteal
Left 04NN
Right 04NM
Posterior Tibial
Left 04NS
Right 04NR
Pulmonary
Left 02NR
Right 02NQ
Pulmonary Trunk 02NP
Radial
Left 03NC
Right 03NB
Renal
Left 04NA
Right 04N9
Splenic 04N4
Subclavian
Left 03N4
Right 03N3
Superior Mesenteric 04N5
Temporal
Left 03NT
Right 03NS
Thyroid
Left 03NV
Right 03NU
Ulnar
Left 03NA
Right 03N9

Release *(Continued)*
Artery *(Continued)*
Upper 03NY
Vertebral
Left 03NQ
Right 03NP
Atrium
Left 02N7
Right 02N6
Auditory Ossicle
Left 09NA
Right 09N9
Basal Ganglia 00N8
Bladder 0TNB
Bladder Neck 0TNC
Bone
Ethmoid
Left 0NNG
Right 0NNF
Frontal 0NN1
Hyoid 0NNX
Lacrimal
Left 0NNJ
Right 0NNH
Nasal 0NNB
Occipital 0NN7
Palatine
Left 0NNL
Right 0NNK
Parietal
Left 0NN4
Right 0NN3
Pelvic
Left 0QN3
Right 0QN2
Sphenoid 0NNC
Temporal
Left 0NN6
Right 0NN5
Zygomatic
Left 0NNN
Right 0NNM
Brain 00N0
Breast
Bilateral 0HNV
Left 0HNU
Right 0HNT
Bronchus
Lingula 0BN9
Lower Lobe
Left 0BNB
Right 0BN6
Main
Left 0BN7
Right 0BN3
Middle Lobe, Right 0BN5
Upper Lobe
Left 0BN8
Right 0BN4
Buccal Mucosa 0CN4
Bursa and Ligament
Abdomen
Left 0MNJ
Right 0MNH
Ankle
Left 0MNR
Right 0MNQ
Elbow
Left 0MN4
Right 0MN3
Foot
Left 0MNT
Right 0MNS
Hand
Left 0MN8
Right 0MN7
Head and Neck 0MN0
Hip
Left 0MNM
Right 0MNL

R

Release (Continued)
Joint (Continued)
Sternoclavicular
Left 0RNF
Right 0RNE
Tarsal
Left 0SNJ
Right 0SNH
Tarsometatarsal
Left 0SNL
Right 0SNK
Temporomandibular
Left 0RND
Right 0RNC
Thoracic Vertebral 0RN6
Thoracolumbar Vertebral 0RNA
Toe Phalangeal
Left 0SNQ
Right 0SNP
Wrist
Left 0RNP
Right 0RNN
Kidney
Left 0TN1
Right 0TN0
Kidney Pelvis
Left 0TN4
Right 0TN3
Larynx 0CNS
Lens
Left 08NK3ZZ
Right 08NJ3ZZ
Lip
Lower 0CN1
Upper 0CN0
Liver 0FN0
Left Lobe 0FN2
Right Lobe 0FN1
Lung
Bilateral 0BNM
Left 0BNL
Lower Lobe
Left 0BNJ
Right 0BNF
Middle Lobe, Right 0BND
Right 0BNK
Upper Lobe
Left 0BNG
Right 0BNC
Lung Lingula 0BNH
Lymphatic
Aortic 07ND
Axillary
Left 07N6
Right 07N5
Head 07N0
Inguinal
Left 07NJ
Right 07NH
Internal Mammary
Left 07N9
Right 07N8
Lower Extremity
Left 07NG
Right 07NF
Mesenteric 07NB
Neck
Left 07N2
Right 07N1
Pelvis 07NC
Thoracic Duct 07NK
Thorax 07N7
Upper Extremity
Left 07N4
Right 07N3
Mandible
Left 0NNV
Right 0NNT
Maxilla 0NNR

Release (Continued)
Medulla Oblongata 00ND
Mesentery 0DNV
Metacarpal
Left 0PNQ
Right 0PNP
Metatarsal
Left 0QNP
Right 0QNN
Muscle
Abdomen
Left 0KNL
Right 0KNK
Extraocular
Left 08NM
Right 08NL
Facial 0KN1
Foot
Left 0KNW
Right 0KNV
Hand
Left 0KND
Right 0KNC
Head 0KN0
Hip
Left 0KNP
Right 0KNN
Lower Arm and Wrist
Left 0KNB
Right 0KN9
Lower Leg
Left 0KNT
Right 0KNS
Neck
Left 0KN3
Right 0KN2
Papillary 02ND
Perineum 0KNM
Shoulder
Left 0KN6
Right 0KN5
Thorax
Left 0KNJ
Right 0KNH
Tongue, Palate, Pharynx 0KN4
Trunk
Left 0KNG
Right 0KNF
Upper Arm
Left 0KN8
Right 0KN7
Upper Leg
Left 0KNR
Right 0KNQ
Myocardial Bridge *see* Release, Artery, Coronary
Nasal Mucosa and Soft Tissue 09NK
Nasopharynx 09NN
Nerve
Abdominal Sympathetic 01NM
Abducens 00NL
Accessory 00NR
Acoustic 00NN
Brachial Plexus 01N3
Cervical 01N1
Cervical Plexus 01N0
Facial 00NM
Femoral 01ND
Glossopharyngeal 00NP
Head and Neck Sympathetic 01NK
Hypoglossal 00NS
Lumbar 01NB
Lumbar Plexus 01N9
Lumbar Sympathetic 01NN
Lumbosacral Plexus 01NA
Median 01N5
Oculomotor 00NH
Olfactory 00NF
Optic 00NG
Peroneal 01NH

Release (Continued)
Nerve (Continued)
Phrenic 01N2
Pudendal 01NC
Radial 01N6
Sacral 01NR
Sacral Plexus 01NQ
Sacral Sympathetic 01NP
Sciatic 01NF
Thoracic 01N8
Thoracic Sympathetic 01NL
Tibial 01NG
Trigeminal 00NK
Trochlear 00NJ
Ulnar 01N4
Vagus 00NQ
Nipple
Left 0HNX
Right 0HNW
Omentum 0DNU
Orbit
Left 0NNQ
Right 0NNP
Ovary
Bilateral 0UN2
Left 0UN1
Right 0UN0
Palate
Hard 0CN2
Soft 0CN3
Pancreas 0FNG
Para-aortic Body 0GN9
Paraganglion Extremity 0GNF
Parathyroid Gland 0GNR
Inferior
Left 0GNP
Right 0GNN
Multiple 0GNQ
Superior
Left 0GNM
Right 0GNL
Patella
Left 0QNF
Right 0QND
Penis 0VNS
Pericardium 02NN
Peritoneum 0DNW
Phalanx
Finger
Left 0PNV
Right 0PNT
Thumb
Left 0PNS
Right 0PNR
Toe
Left 0QNR
Right 0QNQ
Pharynx 0CNM
Pineal Body 0GN1
Pleura
Left 0BNP
Right 0BNN
Pons 00NB
Prepuce 0VNT
Prostate 0VN0
Radius
Left 0PNJ
Right 0PNH
Rectum 0DNP
Retina
Left 08NF3ZZ
Right 08NE3ZZ
Retinal Vessel
Left 08NH3ZZ
Right 08NG3ZZ
Ribs
1 to 2 0PN1
3 or More 0PN2
Sacrum 0QN1

R

Release (Continued)
Scapula
Left 0PN6
Right 0PN5
Sclera
Left 08N7XZZ
Right 08N6XZZ
Scrotum 0VN5
Septum
Atrial 02N5
Nasal 09NM
Ventricular 02NM
Sinus
Accessory 09NP
Ethmoid
Left 09NV
Right 09NU
Frontal
Left 09NT
Right 09NS
Mastoid
Left 09NC
Right 09NB
Maxillary
Left 09NR
Right 09NQ
Sphenoid
Left 09NX
Right 09NW
Skin
Abdomen 0HN7XZZ
Back 0HN6XZZ
Buttock 0HN8XZZ
Chest 0HN5XZZ
Ear
Left 0HN3XZZ
Right 0HN2XZZ
Face 0HN1XZZ
Foot
Left 0HNNXZZ
Right 0HNMXZZ
Hand
Left 0HNGXZZ
Right 0HNFXZZ
Inguinal 0HNAXZZ
Lower Arm
Left 0HNEXZZ
Right 0HNDXZZ
Lower Leg
Left 0HNLXZZ
Right 0HNKXZZ
Neck 0HN4XZZ
Perineum 0HN9XZZ
Scalp 0HN0XZZ
Upper Arm
Left 0HNCXZZ
Right 0HNBXZZ
Upper Leg
Left 0HNJXZZ
Right 0HNHXZZ
Spinal Cord
Cervical 00NW
Lumbar 00NY
Thoracic 00NX
Spinal Meninges 00NT
Spleen 07NP
Sternum 0PN0
Stomach 0DN6
Pylorus 0DN7
Subcutaneous Tissue and Fascia
Abdomen 0JN8
Back 0JN7
Buttock 0JN9
Chest 0JN6
Face 0JN1
Foot
Left 0JNR
Right 0JNQ
Hand
Left 0JNK
Right 0JNJ

Release (Continued)
Subcutaneous Tissue and Fascia (Continued)
Lower Arm
Left 0JNH
Right 0JNG
Lower Leg
Left 0JNP
Right 0JNN
Neck
Left 0JN5
Right 0JN4
Pelvic Region 0JNC
Perineum 0JNB
Scalp 0JN0
Upper Arm
Left 0JNF
Right 0JND
Upper Leg
Left 0JNM
Right 0JNL
Tarsal
Left 0QNM
Right 0QNL
Tendon
Abdomen
Left 0LNG
Right 0LNF
Ankle
Left 0LNT
Right 0LNS
Foot
Left 0LNW
Right 0LNV
Hand
Left 0LN8
Right 0LN7
Head and Neck 0LN0
Hip
Left 0LNK
Right 0LNJ
Knee
Left 0LNR
Right 0LNQ
Lower Arm and Wrist
Left 0LN6
Right 0LN5
Lower Leg
Left 0LNP
Right 0LNN
Perineum 0LNH
Shoulder
Left 0LN2
Right 0LN1
Thorax
Left 0LND
Right 0LNC
Trunk
Left 0LNB
Right 0LN9
Upper Arm
Left 0LN4
Right 0LN3
Upper Leg
Left 0LNM
Right 0LNL
Testis
Bilateral 0VNC
Left 0VNB
Right 0VN9
Thalamus 00N9
Thymus 07NM
Thyroid Gland 0GNK
Left Lobe 0GNG
Right Lobe 0GNH
Tibia
Left 0QNH
Right 0QNG
Toe Nail 0HNRXZZ
Tongue 0CN7
Tonsils 0CNP

Release (Continued)
Tooth
Lower 0CNX
Upper 0CNW
Trachea 0BN1
Tunica Vaginalis
Left 0VN7
Right 0VN6
Turbinate, Nasal 09NL
Tympanic Membrane
Left 09N8
Right 09N7
Ulna
Left 0PNL
Right 0PNK
Ureter
Left 0TN7
Right 0TN6
Urethra 0TND
Uterine Supporting Structure 0UN4
Uterus 0UN9
Uvula 0CNN
Vagina 0UNG
Valve
Aortic 02NF
Mitral 02NG
Pulmonary 02NH
Tricuspid 02NJ
Vas Deferens
Bilateral 0VNQ
Left 0VNP
Right 0VNN
Vein
Axillary
Left 05N8
Right 05N7
Azygos 05N0
Basilic
Left 05NC
Right 05NB
Brachial
Left 05NA
Right 05N9
Cephalic
Left 05NF
Right 05ND
Colic 06N7
Common Iliac
Left 06ND
Right 06NC
Coronary 02N4
Esophageal 06N3
External Iliac
Left 06NG
Right 06NF
External Jugular
Left 05NQ
Right 05NP
Face
Left 05NV
Right 05NT
Femoral
Left 06NN
Right 06NM
Foot
Left 06NV
Right 06NT
Gastric 06N2
Hand
Left 05NH
Right 05NG
Hemiazygos 05N1
Hepatic 06N4
Hypogastric
Left 06NJ
Right 06NH
Inferior Mesenteric 06N6
Innominate
Left 05N4
Right 05N3

Release *(Continued)*
Vein *(Continued)*
Internal Jugular
Left 05NN
Right 05NM
Intracranial 05NL
Lesser Saphenous
Left 06NS
Right 06NR
Lower 06NY
Portal 06N8
Pulmonary
Left 02NT
Right 02NS
Renal
Left 06NB
Right 06N9
Saphenous
Left 06NQ
Right 06NP
Splenic 06N1
Subclavian
Left 05N6
Right 05N5
Superior Mesenteric 06N5
Upper 05NY
Vertebral
Left 05NS
Right 05NR
Vena Cava
Inferior 06N0
Superior 02NV
Ventricle
Left 02NL
Right 02NK
Vertebra
Cervical 0PN3
Lumbar 0QN0
Thoracic 0PN4
Vesicle
Bilateral 0VN3
Left 0VN2
Right 0VN1
Vitreous
Left 08N53ZZ
Right 08N43ZZ
Vocal Cord
Left 0CNV
Right 0CNT
Vulva 0UNM
Relocation *see* Reposition
Remdesivir anti-infection XW0
Removal
Abdominal Wall 2W53X
Anorectal 2Y53X5Z
Arm
Lower
Left 2W5DX
Right 2W5CX
Upper
Left 2W5BX
Right 2W5AX
Back 2W55X
Chest Wall 2W54X
Ear 2Y52X5Z
Extremity
Lower
Left 2W5MX
Right 2W5LX
Upper
Left 2W59X
Right 2W58X
Face 2W51X
Finger
Left 2W5KX
Right 2W5JX
Foot
Left 2W5TX
Right 2W5SX
Genital Tract, Female 2Y54X5Z

Removal *(Continued)*
Hand
Left 2W5FX
Right 2W5EX
Head 2W50X
Inguinal Region
Left 2W57X
Right 2W56X
Leg
Lower
Left 2W5RX
Right 2W5QX
Upper
Left 2W5PX
Right 2W5NX
Mouth and Pharynx 2Y50X5Z
Nasal 2Y51X5Z
Neck 2W52X
Thumb
Left 2W5HX
Right 2W5GX
Toe
Left 2W5VX
Right 2W5UX
Urethra 2Y55X5Z
Removal of device from
Abdominal Wall 0WPF
Acetabulum
Left 0QP5
Right 0QP4
Anal Sphincter 0DPR
Anus 0DPQ
▶ Aorta, Thoracic, Descending 02PW3RZ
Artery
Lower 04PY
Upper 03PY
Back
Lower 0WPL
Upper 0WPK
Bladder 0TPB
Bone
Facial 0NPW
Lower 0QPY
Nasal 0NPB
Pelvic
Left 0QP3
Right 0QP2
Upper 0PPY
Bone Marrow 07PT
Brain 00P0
Breast
Left 0HPU
Right 0HPT
Bursa and Ligament
Lower 0MPY
Upper 0MPX
Carpal
Left 0PPN
Right 0PPM
Cavity, Cranial 0WP1
Cerebral Ventricle 00P6
Chest Wall 0WP8
Cisterna Chyli 07PL
Clavicle
Left 0PPB
Right 0PP9
Coccyx 0QPS
Diaphragm 0BPT
Disc
Cervical Vertebral 0RP3
Cervicothoracic Vertebral 0RP5
Lumbar Vertebral 0SP2
Lumbosacral 0SP4
Thoracic Vertebral 0RP9
Thoracolumbar Vertebral 0RPB
Duct
Hepatobiliary 0FPB
Pancreatic 0FPD
Ear
Inner
Left 09PE
Right 09PD

Removal of device from *(Continued)*
Ear *(Continued)*
Left 09PJ
Right 09PH
Epididymis and Spermatic Cord 0VPM
Esophagus 0DP5
Extremity
Lower
Left 0YPB
Right 0YP9
Upper
Left 0XP7
Right 0XP6
Eye
Left 08P1
Right 08P0
Face 0WP2
Fallopian Tube 0UP8
Femoral Shaft
Left 0QP9
Right 0QP8
Femur
Lower
Left 0QPC
Right 0QPB
Upper
Left 0QP7
Right 0QP6
Fibula
Left 0QPK
Right 0QPJ
Finger Nail 0HPQX
Gallbladder 0FP4
Gastrointestinal Tract 0WPP
Genitourinary Tract 0WPR
Gland
Adrenal 0GP5
Endocrine 0GPS
Pituitary 0GP0
Salivary 0CPA
Glenoid Cavity
Left 0PP8
Right 0PP7
Great Vessel 02PY
Hair 0HPSX
Head 0WP0
Heart 02PA
Humeral Head
Left 0PPD
Right 0PPC
Humeral Shaft
Left 0PPG
Right 0PPF
Intestinal Tract
Lower Intestinal Tract 0DPD
Upper Intestinal Tract 0DP0
Jaw
Lower 0WP5
Upper 0WP4
Joint
Acromioclavicular
Left 0RPH
Right 0RPG
Ankle
Left 0SPG
Right 0SPF
Carpal
Left 0RPR
Right 0RPQ
Carpometacarpal
Left 0RPT
Right 0RPS
Cervical Vertebral 0RP1
Cervicothoracic Vertebral 0RP4
Coccygeal 0SP6
Elbow
Left 0RPM
Right 0RPL
Finger Phalangeal
Left 0RPX
Right 0RPW

Removal of device from *(Continued)*
Joint *(Continued)*
Hip
Left 0SPB
Acetabular Surface 0SPE
Femoral Surface 0SPS
Right 0SP9
Acetabular Surface 0SPA
Femoral Surface 0SPR
Knee
Left 0SPD
Femoral Surface 0SPU
Tibial Surface 0SPW
Right 0SPC
Femoral Surface 0SPT
Tibial Surface 0SPV
Lumbar Vertebral 0SP0
Lumbosacral 0SP3
Metacarpophalangeal
Left 0RPV
Right 0RPU
Metatarsal-Phalangeal
Left 0SPN
Right 0SPM
Occipital-cervical 0RP0
Sacrococcygeal 0SP5
Sacroiliac
Left 0SP8
Right 0SP7
Shoulder
Left 0RPK
Right 0RPJ
Sternoclavicular
Left 0RPF
Right 0RPE
Tarsal
Left 0SPJ
Right 0SPH
Tarsometatarsal
Left 0SPL
Right 0SPK
Temporomandibular
Left 0RPD
Right 0RPC
Thoracic Vertebral 0RP6
Thoracolumbar Vertebral 0RPA
Toe Phalangeal
Left 0SPQ
Right 0SPP
Wrist
Left 0RPP
Right 0RPN
Kidney 0TP5
Larynx 0CPS
Lens
Left 08PK3
Right 08PJ3
Liver 0FP0
Lung
Left 0BPL
Right 0BPK
Lymphatic 07PN
Thoracic Duct 07PK
Mediastinum 0WPC
Mesentery 0DPV
Metacarpal
Left 0PPQ
Right 0PPP
Metatarsal
Left 0QPP
Right 0QPN
Mouth and Throat 0CPY
Muscle
Extraocular
Left 08PM
Right 08PL
Lower 0KPY
Upper 0KPX
Nasal Mucosa and Soft Tissue 09PK
Neck 0WP6

Removal of device from *(Continued)*
Nerve
Cranial 00PE
Peripheral 01PY
Omentum 0DPU
Ovary 0UP3
Pancreas 0FPG
Parathyroid Gland 0GPR
Patella
Left 0QPF
Right 0QPD
Pelvic Cavity 0WPJ
Penis 0VPS
Pericardial Cavity 0WPD
Perineum
Female 0WPN
Male 0WPM
Peritoneal Cavity 0WPG
Peritoneum 0DPW
Phalanx
Finger
Left 0PPV
Right 0PPT
Thumb
Left 0PPS
Right 0PPR
Toe
Left 0QPR
Right 0QPQ
Pineal Body 0GP1
Pleura 0BPQ
Pleural Cavity
Left 0WPB
Right 0WP9
Products of Conception 10P0
Prostate and Seminal Vesicles 0VP4
Radius
Left 0PPJ
Right 0PPH
Rectum 0DPP
Respiratory Tract 0WPQ
Retroperitoneum 0WPH
Ribs
1 to 2 0PP1
3 or More 0PP2
Sacrum 0QP1
Scapula
Left 0PP6
Right 0PP5
Scrotum and Tunica Vaginalis 0VP8
Sinus 09PY
Skin 0HPPX
Skull 0NP0
Spinal Canal 00PU
Spinal Cord 00PV
Spleen 07PP
Sternum 0PP0
Stomach 0DP6
Subcutaneous Tissue and Fascia
Head and Neck 0JPS
Lower Extremity 0JPW
Trunk 0JPT
Upper Extremity 0JPV
Tarsal
Left 0QPM
Right 0QPL
Tendon
Lower 0LPY
Upper 0LPX
Testis 0VPD
Thymus 07PM
Thyroid Gland 0GPK
Tibia
Left 0QPH
Right 0QPG
Toe Nail 0HPRX
Trachea 0BP1
Tracheobronchial Tree 0BP0
Tympanic Membrane
Left 09P8
Right 09P7

Removal of device from *(Continued)*
Ulna
Left 0PPL
Right 0PPK
Ureter 0TP9
Urethra 0TPD
Uterus and Cervix 0UPD
Vagina and Cul-de-sac 0UPH
Vas Deferens 0VPR
Vein
Azygos 05P0
Innominate
Left 05P4
Right 05P3
Lower 06PY
Upper 05PY
Vertebra
Cervical 0PP3
Lumbar 0QP0
Thoracic 0PP4
Vulva 0UPM
Renal calyx
use Kidney, Right
use Kidney, Left
use Kidneys, Bilateral
use Kidney
Renal capsule
use Kidney, Right
use Kidney, Left
use Kidneys, Bilateral
use Kidney
Renal cortex
use Kidney, Right
use Kidney, Left
use Kidneys, Bilateral
use Kidney
Renal dialysis *see* Performance, Urinary 5A1D
Renal nerve *use* Abdominal Sympathetic Nerve
Renal plexus *use* Abdominal Sympathetic Nerve
Renal segment
use Kidney, Right
use Kidney, Left
use Kidneys, Bilateral
use Kidney
Renal segmental artery
use Renal Artery, Right
use Renal Artery, Left
Reopening, operative site
Control of bleeding *see* Control bleeding in
Inspection only *see* Inspection
Repair
Abdominal Wall 0WQF
Acetabulum
Left 0QQ5
Right 0QQ4
Adenoids 0CQQ
Ampulla of Vater 0FQC
Anal Sphincter 0DQR
Ankle Region
Left 0YQL
Right 0YQK
Anterior Chamber
Left 08Q33ZZ
Right 08Q23ZZ
Anus 0DQQ
Aorta
Abdominal 04Q0
Thoracic
Ascending/Arch 02QX
Descending 02QW
Aortic Body 0GQD
Appendix 0DQJ
Arm
Lower
Left 0XQF
Right 0XQD
Upper
Left 0XQ9
Right 0XQ8

▶ New ➡ Revised ~~deleted~~ Deleted

R

▶ New ➡ Revised ~~deleted~~ Deleted

Repair (Continued)
Cornea
Left 08Q9XZZ
Right 08Q8XZZ
Cul-de-sac 0UQF
Diaphragm 0BQT
Disc
Cervical Vertebral 0RQ3
Cervicothoracic Vertebral 0RQ5
Lumbar Vertebral 0SQ2
Lumbosacral 0SQ4
Thoracic Vertebral 0RQ9
Thoracolumbar Vertebral 0RQB
Duct
Common Bile 0FQ9
Cystic 0FQ8
Hepatic
Common 0FQ7
Left 0FQ6
Right 0FQ5
Lacrimal
Left 08QY
Right 08QX
Pancreatic 0FQD
Accessory 0FQF
Parotid
Left 0CQC
Right 0CQB
Duodenum 0DQ9
Dura Mater 00Q2
Ear
External
Bilateral 09Q2
Left 09Q1
Right 09Q0
External Auditory Canal
Left 09Q4
Right 09Q3
Inner
Left 09QE
Right 09QD
Middle
Left 09Q6
Right 09Q5
Elbow Region
Left 0XQC
Right 0XQB
Epididymis
Bilateral 0VQL
Left 0VQK
Right 0VQJ
Epiglottis 0CQR
Esophagogastric Junction 0DQ4
Esophagus 0DQ5
Lower 0DQ3
Middle 0DQ2
Upper 0DQ1
Eustachian Tube
Left 09QG
Right 09QF
Extremity
Lower
Left 0YQB
Right 0YQ9
Upper
Left 0XQ7
Right 0XQ6
Eye
Left 08Q1XZZ
Right 08Q0XZZ
Eyelid
Lower
Left 08QR
Right 08QQ
Upper
Left 08QP
Right 08QN
Face 0WQ2
Fallopian Tube
Left 0UQ6
Right 0UQ5

Repair (Continued)
Fallopian Tubes, Bilateral 0UQ7
Femoral Region
Bilateral 0YQE
Left 0YQ8
Right 0YQ7
Femoral Shaft
Left 0QQ9
Right 0QQ8
Femur
Lower
Left 0QQC
Right 0QQB
Upper
Left 0QQ7
Right 0QQ6
Fibula
Left 0QQK
Right 0QQJ
Finger
Index
Left 0XQP
Right 0XQN
Little
Left 0XQW
Right 0XQV
Middle
Left 0XQR
Right 0XQQ
Ring
Left 0XQT
Right 0XQS
Finger Nail 0HQQXZZ
Floor of mouth *see* Repair, Oral Cavity and Throat 0WQ3
Foot
Left 0YQN
Right 0YQM
Gallbladder 0FQ4
Gingiva
Lower 0CQ6
Upper 0CQ5
Gland
Adrenal
Bilateral 0GQ4
Left 0GQ2
Right 0GQ3
Lacrimal
Left 08QW
Right 08QV
Minor Salivary 0CQJ
Parotid
Left 0CQ9
Right 0CQ8
Pituitary 0GQ0
Sublingual
Left 0CQF
Right 0CQD
Submaxillary
Left 0CQH
Right 0CQG
Vestibular 0UQL
Glenoid Cavity
Left 0PQ8
Right 0PQ7
Glomus Jugulare 0GQC
Hand
Left 0XQK
Right 0XQJ
Head 0WQ0
Heart 02QA
Left 02QC
Right 02QB
Humeral Head
Left 0PQD
Right 0PQC
Humeral Shaft
Left 0PQG
Right 0PQF
Hymen 0UQK
Hypothalamus 00QA
Ileocecal Valve 0DQC

Repair (Continued)
Ileum 0DQB
Inguinal Region
Bilateral 0YQA
Left 0YQ6
Right 0YQ5
Intestine
Large 0DQE
Left 0DQG
Right 0DQF
Small 0DQ8
Iris
Left 08QD3ZZ
Right 08QC3ZZ
Jaw
Lower 0WQ5
Upper 0WQ4
Jejunum 0DQA
Joint
Acromioclavicular
Left 0RQH
Right 0RQG
Ankle
Left 0SQG
Right 0SQF
Carpal
Left 0RQR
Right 0RQQ
Carpometacarpal
Left 0RQT
Right 0RQS
Cervical Vertebral 0RQ1
Cervicothoracic Vertebral 0RQ4
Coccygeal 0SQ6
Elbow
Left 0RQM
Right 0RQL
Finger Phalangeal
Left 0RQX
Right 0RQW
Hip
Left 0SQB
Right 0SQ9
Knee
Left 0SQD
Right 0SQC
Lumbar Vertebral 0SQ0
Lumbosacral 0SQ3
Metacarpophalangeal
Left 0RQV
Right 0RQU
Metatarsal-Phalangeal
Left 0SQN
Right 0SQM
Occipital-cervical 0RQ0
Sacrococcygeal 0SQ5
Sacroiliac
Left 0SQ8
Right 0SQ7
Shoulder
Left 0RQK
Right 0RQJ
Sternoclavicular
Left 0RQF
Right 0RQE
Tarsal
Left 0SQJ
Right 0SQH
Tarsometatarsal
Left 0SQL
Right 0SQK
Temporomandibular
Left 0RQD
Right 0RQC
Thoracic Vertebral 0RQ6
Thoracolumbar Vertebral 0RQA
Toe Phalangeal
Left 0SQQ
Right 0SQP
Wrist
Left 0RQP
Right 0RQN

R

R

New Revised ~~deleted~~ Deleted

Repair (Continued)
Sinus
Accessory 09QP
Ethmoid
Left 09QV
Right 09QU
Frontal
Left 09QT
Right 09QS
Mastoid
Left 09QC
Right 09QB
Maxillary
Left 09QR
Right 09QQ
Sphenoid
Left 09QX
Right 09QW
Skin
Abdomen 0HQ7XZZ
Back 0HQ6XZZ
Buttock 0HQ8XZZ
Chest 0HQ5XZZ
Ear
Left 0HQ3XZZ
Right 0HQ2XZZ
Face 0HQ1XZZ
Foot
Left 0HQNXZZ
Right 0HQMXZZ
Hand
Left 0HQGXZZ
Right 0HQFXZZ
Inguinal 0HQAXZZ
Lower Arm
Left 0HQEXZZ
Right 0HQDXZZ
Lower Leg
Left 0HQLXZZ
Right 0HQKXZZ
Neck 0HQ4XZZ
Perineum 0HQ9XZZ
Scalp 0HQ0XZZ
Upper Arm
Left 0HQCXZZ
Right 0HQBXZZ
Upper Leg
Left 0HQJXZZ
Right 0HQHXZZ
Skull 0NQ0
Spinal Cord
Cervical 00QW
Lumbar 00QY
Thoracic 00QX
Spinal Meninges 00QT
Spleen 07QP
Sternum 0PQ0
Stomach 0DQ6
Pylorus 0DQ7
Subcutaneous Tissue and Fascia
Abdomen 0JQ8
Back 0JQ7
Buttock 0JQ9
Chest 0JQ6
Face 0JQ1
Foot
Left 0JQR
Right 0JQQ
Hand
Left 0JQK
Right 0JQJ
Lower Arm
Left 0JQH
Right 0JQG
Lower Leg
Left 0JQP
Right 0JQN
Neck
Left 0JQ5
Right 0JQ4

Repair (Continued)
Subcutaneous Tissue and Fascia (Continued)
Pelvic Region 0JQC
Perineum 0JQB
Scalp 0JQ0
Upper Arm
Left 0JQF
Right 0JQD
Upper Leg
Left 0JQM
Right 0JQL
Tarsal
Left 0QQM
Right 0QQL
Tendon
Abdomen
Left 0LQG
Right 0LQF
Ankle
Left 0LQT
Right 0LQS
Foot
Left 0LQW
Right 0LQV
Hand
Left 0LQ8
Right 0LQ7
Head and Neck 0LQ0
Hip
Left 0LQK
Right 0LQJ
Knee
Left 0LQR
Right 0LQQ
Lower Arm and Wrist
Left 0LQ6
Right 0LQ5
Lower Leg
Left 0LQP
Right 0LQN
Perineum 0LQH
Shoulder
Left 0LQ2
Right 0LQ1
Thorax
Left 0LQD
Right 0LQC
Trunk
Left 0LQB
Right 0LQ9
Upper Arm
Left 0LQ4
Right 0LQ3
Upper Leg
Left 0LQM
Right 0LQL
Testis
Bilateral 0VQC
Left 0VQB
Right 0VQ9
Thalamus 00Q9
Thumb
Left 0XQM
Right 0XQL
Thymus 07QM
Thyroid Gland 0GQK
Left Lobe 0GQG
Right Lobe 0GQH
Thyroid Gland Isthmus 0GQJ
Tibia
Left 0QQH
Right 0QQG
Toe
1st
Left 0YQQ
Right 0YQP
2nd
Left 0YQS
Right 0YQR
3rd
Left 0YQU
Right 0YQT

Repair (Continued)
Toe (Continued)
4th
Left 0YQW
Right 0YQV
5th
Left 0YQY
Right 0YQX
Toe Nail 0HQRXZZ
Tongue 0CQ7
Tonsils 0CQP
Tooth
Lower 0CQX
Upper 0CQW
Trachea 0BQ1
Tunica Vaginalis
Left 0VQ7
Right 0VQ6
Turbinate, Nasal 09QL
Tympanic Membrane
Left 09Q8
Right 09Q7
Ulna
Left 0PQL
Right 0PQK
Ureter
Left 0TQ7
Right 0TQ6
Urethra 0TQD
Uterine Supporting Structure 0UQ4
Uterus 0UQ9
Uvula 0CQN
Vagina 0UQG
Valve
Aortic 02QF
Mitral 02QG
Pulmonary 02QH
Tricuspid 02QJ
Vas Deferens
Bilateral 0VQQ
Left 0VQP
Right 0VQN
Vein
Axillary
Left 05Q8
Right 05Q7
Azygos 05Q0
Basilic
Left 05QC
Right 05QB
Brachial
Left 05QA
Right 05Q9
Cephalic
Left 05QF
Right 05QD
Colic 06Q7
Common Iliac
Left 06QD
Right 06QC
Coronary 02Q4
Esophageal 06Q3
External Iliac
Left 06QG
Right 06QF
External Jugular
Left 05QQ
Right 05QP
Face
Left 05QV
Right 05QT
Femoral
Left 06QN
Right 06QM
Foot
Left 06QV
Right 06QT
Gastric 06Q2
Hand
Left 05QH
Right 05QG

R

▶ New ➡ Revised ~~deleted~~ Deleted

R

Replacement *(Continued)*
  Bursa and Ligament *(Continued)*
    Shoulder
      Left 0MR2
      Right 0MR1
    Spine
      Lower 0MRD
      Upper 0MRC
    Sternum 0MRF
    Upper Extremity
      Left 0MRB
      Right 0MR9
    Wrist
      Left 0MR6
      Right 0MR5
  Carina 0BR2
  Carpal
    Left 0PRN
    Right 0PRM
  Cerebral Meninges 00R1
  Cerebral Ventricle 00R6
  Chordae Tendineae 02R9
  Choroid
    Left 08RB
    Right 08RA
  Clavicle
    Left 0PRB
    Right 0PR9
  Coccyx 0QRS
  Conjunctiva
    Left 08RTX
    Right 08RSX
  Cornea
    Left 08R9
    Right 08R8
  Diaphragm 0BRT
  Disc
    Cervical Vertebral 0RR30
    Cervicothoracic Vertebral 0RR50
    Lumbar Vertebral 0SR20
    Lumbosacral 0SR40
    Thoracic Vertebral 0RR90
    Thoracolumbar Vertebral 0RRB0
  Duct
    Common Bile 0FR9
    Cystic 0FR8
    Hepatic
      Common 0FR7
      Left 0FR6
      Right 0FR5
    Lacrimal
      Left 08RY
      Right 08RX
    Pancreatic 0FRD
      Accessory 0FRF
    Parotid
      Left 0CRC
      Right 0CRB
  Dura Mater 00R2
  Ear
    External
      Bilateral 09R2
      Left 09R1
      Right 09R0
    Inner
      Left 09RE0
      Right 09RD0
    Middle
      Left 09R60
      Right 09R50
  Epiglottis 0CRR
  Esophagus 0DR5
  Eye
    Left 08R1
    Right 08R0
  Eyelid
    Lower
      Left 08RR
      Right 08RQ
    Upper
      Left 08RP
      Right 08RN

Replacement *(Continued)*
  Femoral Shaft
    Left 0QR9
    Right 0QR8
  Femur
    Lower
      Left 0QRC
      Right 0QRB
    Upper
      Left 0QR7
      Right 0QR6
  Fibula
    Left 0QRK
    Right 0QRJ
  Finger Nail 0HRQX
  Gingiva
    Lower 0CR6
    Upper 0CR5
  Glenoid Cavity
    Left 0PR8
    Right 0PR7
  Heart 02RA0
  Hair 0HRSX
  Humeral Head
    Left 0PRD
    Right 0PRC
  Humeral Shaft
    Left 0PRG
    Right 0PRF
  Iris
    Left 08RD3
    Right 08RC3
  Joint
    Acromioclavicular
      Left 0RRH0
      Right 0RRG0
    Ankle
      Left 0SRG
      Right 0SRF
    Carpal
      Left 0RRR0
      Right 0RRQ0
    Carpometacarpal
      Left 0RRT0
      Right 0RRS0
    Cervical Vertebral 0RR10
    Cervicothoracic Vertebral 0RR40
    Coccygeal 0SR60
    Elbow
      Left 0RRM0
      Right 0RRL0
    Finger Phalangeal
      Left 0RRX0
      Right 0RRW0
    Hip
      Left 0SRB
        Acetabular Surface 0SRE
        Femoral Surface 0SRS
      Right 0SR9
        Acetabular Surface 0SRA
        Femoral Surface 0SRR
    Knee
      Left 0SRD
        Femoral Surface 0SRU
        Tibial Surface 0SRW
      Right 0SRC
        Femoral Surface 0SRT
        Tibial Surface 0SRV
    Lumbar Vertebral 0SR00
    Lumbosacral 0SR30
    Metacarpophalangeal
      Left 0RRV0
      Right 0RRU0
    Metatarsal-Phalangeal
      Left 0SRN0
      Right 0SRM0
    Occipital-cervical 0RR00
    Sacrococcygeal 0SR50
    Sacroiliac
      Left 0SR80
      Right 0SR70

Replacement *(Continued)*
  Joint *(Continued)*
    Shoulder
      Left 0RRK
      Right 0RRJ
    Sternoclavicular
      Left 0RRF0
      Right 0RRE0
    Tarsal
      Left 0SRJ0
      Right 0SRH0
    Tarsometatarsal
      Left 0SRL0
      Right 0SRK0
    Temporomandibular
      Left 0RRD0
      Right 0RRC0
    Thoracic Vertebral 0RR60
    Thoracolumbar Vertebral 0RRA0
    Toe Phalangeal
      Left 0SRQ0
      Right 0SRP0
    Wrist
      Left 0RRP0
      Right 0RRN0
  Kidney Pelvis
    Left 0TR4
    Right 0TR3
  Larynx 0CRS
  Lens
    Left 08RK30Z
    Right 08RJ30Z
  Lip
    Lower 0CR1
    Upper 0CR0
  Mandible
    Left 0NRV
    Right 0NRT
  Maxilla 0NRR
  Mesentery 0DRV
  Metacarpal
    Left 0PRQ
    Right 0PRP
  Metatarsal
    Left 0QRP
    Right 0QRN
  Muscle
    Abdomen
      Left 0KRL
      Right 0KRK
    Facial 0KR1
    Foot
      Left 0KRW
      Right 0KRV
    Hand
      Left 0KRD
      Right 0KRC
    Head 0KR0
    Hip
      Left 0KRP
      Right 0KRN
    Lower Arm and Wrist
      Left 0KRB
      Right 0KR9
    Lower Leg
      Left 0KRT
      Right 0KRS
    Neck
      Left 0KR3
      Right 0KR2
    Papillary 02RD
    Perineum 0KRM
    Shoulder
      Left 0KR6
      Right 0KR5
    Thorax
      Left 0KRJ
      Right 0KRH
    Tongue, Palate, Pharynx 0KR4
    Trunk
      Left 0KRG
      Right 0KRF

R

R

Replacement *(Continued)*
Vein *(Continued)*
Colic 06R7
Common Iliac
Left 06RD
Right 06RC
Esophageal 06R3
External Iliac
Left 06RG
Right 06RF
External Jugular
Left 05RQ
Right 05RP
Face
Left 05RV
Right 05RT
Femoral
Left 06RN
Right 06RM
Foot
Left 06RV
Right 06RT
Gastric 06R2
Hand
Left 05RH
Right 05RG
Hemiazygos 05R1
Hepatic 06R4
Hypogastric
Left 06RJ
Right 06RH
Inferior Mesenteric 06R6
Innominate
Left 05R4
Right 05R3
Internal Jugular
Left 05RN
Right 05RM
Intracranial 05RL
Lower 06RY
Portal 06R8
Pulmonary
Left 02RT
Right 02RS
Renal
Left 06RB
Right 06R9
Saphenous
Left 06RQ
Right 06RP
Splenic 06R1
Subclavian
Left 05R6
Right 05R5
Superior Mesenteric 06R5
Upper 05RY
Vertebral
Left 05RS
Right 05RR
Vena Cava
Inferior 06R0
Superior 02RV
Ventricle
Left 02RL
Right 02RK
Vertebra
Cervical 0PR3
Lumbar 0QR0
Thoracic 0PR4
Vitreous
Left 08R53
Right 08R43
Vocal Cord
Left 0CRV
Right 0CRT
Replacement, hip
Partial or total *see* Replacement, Lower Joints 0SR
Resurfacing only *see* Supplement, Lower Joints 0SU
Replacement, knee
Meniscus implant only *see* New Technology, Joints XRR
Partial or total *see* Replacement, Lower Joints 0SR
Replantation *see* Reposition
Replantation, scalp *see* Reattachment, Skin, Scalp 0HM0
Reposition
Acetabulum
Left 0QS5
Right 0QS4
Ampulla of Vater 0FSC
Anus 0DSQ
Aorta
Abdominal 04S0
Thoracic
Ascending/Arch 02SX0ZZ
Descending 02SW0ZZ
Artery
Anterior Tibial
Left 04SQ
Right 04SP
Axillary
Left 03S6
Right 03S5
Brachial
Left 03S8
Right 03S7
Celiac 04S1
Colic
Left 04S7
Middle 04S8
Right 04S6
Common Carotid
Left 03SJ
Right 03SH
Common Iliac
Left 04SD
Right 04SC
Coronary
One Artery 02S00ZZ
Two Arteries 02S10ZZ
External Carotid
Left 03SN
Right 03SM
External Iliac
Left 04SJ
Right 04SH
Face 03SR
Femoral
Left 04SL
Right 04SK
Foot
Left 04SW
Right 04SV
Gastric 04S2
Hand
Left 03SF
Right 03SD
Hepatic 04S3
Inferior Mesenteric 04SB
Innominate 03S2
Internal Carotid
Left 03SL
Right 03SK
Internal Iliac
Left 04SF
Right 04SE
Internal Mammary
Left 03S1
Right 03S0
Intracranial 03SG
Lower 04SY
Peroneal
Left 04SU
Right 04ST
Popliteal
Left 04SN
Right 04SM
Posterior Tibial
Left 04SS
Right 04SR
Reposition *(Continued)*
Artery *(Continued)*
Pulmonary
Left 02SR0ZZ
Right 02SQ0ZZ
Pulmonary Trunk 02SP0ZZ
Radial
Left 03SC
Right 03SB
Renal
Left 04SA
Right 04S9
Splenic 04S4
Subclavian
Left 03S4
Right 03S3
Superior Mesenteric 04S5
Temporal
Left 03ST
Right 03SS
Thyroid
Left 03SV
Right 03SU
Ulnar
Left 03SA
Right 03S9
Upper 03SY
Vertebral
Left 03SQ
Right 03SP
Auditory Ossicle
Left 09SA
Right 09S9
Bladder 0TSB
Bladder Neck 0TSC
Bone
Ethmoid
Left 0NSG
Right 0NSF
Frontal 0NS1
Hyoid 0NSX
Lacrimal
Left 0NSJ
Right 0NSH
Nasal 0NSB
Occipital 0NS7
Palatine
Left 0NSL
Right 0NSK
Parietal
Left 0NS4
Right 0NS3
Pelvic
Left 0QS3
Right 0QS2
Sphenoid 0NSC
Temporal
Left 0NS6
Right 0NS5
Zygomatic
Left 0NSN
Right 0NSM
Breast
Bilateral 0HSV0ZZ
Left 0HSU0ZZ
Right 0HST0ZZ
Bronchus
Lingula 0BS90ZZ
Lower Lobe
Left 0BSB0ZZ
Right 0BS60ZZ
Main
Left 0BS70ZZ
Right 0BS30ZZ
Middle Lobe, Right 0BS50ZZ
Upper Lobe
Left 0BS80ZZ
Right 0BS40ZZ
Bursa and Ligament
Abdomen
Left 0MSJ
Right 0MSH

R

R

▶ New ➡ Revised ~~deleted~~ Deleted

R

R

Resection *(Continued)*
Eustachian Tube
Left 09TG
Right 09TF
Eye
Left 08T1XZZ
Right 08T0XZZ
Eyelid
Lower
Left 08TR
Right 08TQ
Upper
Left 08TP
Right 08TN
Fallopian Tube
Left 0UT6
Right 0UT5
Fallopian Tubes, Bilateral 0UT7
Femoral Shaft
Left 0QT90ZZ
Right 0QT80ZZ
Femur
Lower
Left 0QTC0ZZ
Right 0QTB0ZZ
Upper
Left 0QT70ZZ
Right 0QT60ZZ
Fibula
Left 0QTK0ZZ
Right 0QTJ0ZZ
Finger Nail 0HTQXZZ
Gallbladder 0FT4
Gland
Adrenal
Bilateral 0GT4
Left 0GT2
Right 0GT3
Lacrimal
Left 08TW
Right 08TV
Minor Salivary 0CTJ0ZZ
Parotid
Left 0CT90ZZ
Right 0CT80ZZ
Pituitary 0GT0
Sublingual
Left 0CTF0ZZ
Right 0CTD0ZZ
Submaxillary
Left 0CTH0ZZ
Right 0CTG0ZZ
Vestibular 0UTL
Glenoid Cavity
Left 0PT80ZZ
Right 0PT70ZZ
Glomus Jugulare 0GTC
Humeral Head
Left 0PTD0ZZ
Right 0PTC0ZZ
Humeral Shaft
Left 0PTG0ZZ
Right 0PTF0ZZ
Hymen 0UTK
Ileocecal Valve 0DTC
Ileum 0DTB
Intestine
Large 0DTE
Left 0DTG
Right 0DTF
Small 0DT8
Iris
Left 08TD3ZZ
Right 08TC3ZZ
Jejunum 0DTA
Joint
Acromioclavicular
Left 0RTH0ZZ
Right 0RTG0ZZ
Ankle
Left 0STG0ZZ
Right 0STF0ZZ

Resection *(Continued)*
Joint *(Continued)*
Carpal
Left 0RTR0ZZ
Right 0RTQ0ZZ
Carpometacarpal
Left 0RTT0ZZ
Right 0RTS0ZZ
Cervicothoracic Vertebral 0RT40ZZ
Coccygeal 0ST60ZZ
Elbow
Left 0RTM0ZZ
Right 0RTL0ZZ
Finger Phalangeal
Left 0RTX0ZZ
Right 0RTW0ZZ
Hip
Left 0STB0ZZ
Right 0ST90ZZ
Knee
Left 0STD0ZZ
Right 0STC0ZZ
Metacarpophalangeal
Left 0RTV0ZZ
Right 0RTU0ZZ
Metatarsal-Phalangeal
Left 0STN0ZZ
Right 0STM0ZZ
Sacrococcygeal 0ST50ZZ
Sacroiliac
Left 0ST80ZZ
Right 0ST70ZZ
Shoulder
Left 0RTK0ZZ
Right 0RTJ0ZZ
Sternoclavicular
Left 0RTF0ZZ
Right 0RTE0ZZ
Tarsal
Left 0STJ0ZZ
Right 0STH0ZZ
Tarsometatarsal
Left 0STL0ZZ
Right 0STK0ZZ
Temporomandibular
Left 0RTD0ZZ
Right 0RTC0ZZ
Toe Phalangeal
Left 0STQ0ZZ
Right 0STP0ZZ
Wrist
Left 0RTP0ZZ
Right 0RTN0ZZ
Kidney
Left 0TT1
Right 0TT0
Kidney Pelvis
Left 0TT4
Right 0TT3
Kidneys, Bilateral 0TT2
Larynx 0CTS
Lens
Left 08TK3ZZ
Right 08TJ3ZZ
Lip
Lower 0CT1
Upper 0CT0
Liver 0FT0
Left Lobe 0FT2
Right Lobe 0FT1
Lung
Bilateral 0BTM
Left 0BTL
Lower Lobe
Left 0BTJ
Right 0BTF
Middle Lobe, Right 0BTD
Right 0BTK

Resection *(Continued)*
Lung *(Continued)*
Upper Lobe
Left 0BTG
Right 0BTC
Lung Lingula 0BTH
Lymphatic
Aortic 07TD
Axillary
Left 07T6
Right 07T5
Head 07T0
Inguinal
Left 07TJ
Right 07TH
Internal Mammary
Left 07T9
Right 07T8
Lower Extremity
Left 07TG
Right 07TF
Mesenteric 07TB
Neck
Left 07T2
Right 07T1
Pelvis 07TC
Thoracic Duct 07TK
Thorax 07T7
Upper Extremity
Left 07T4
Right 07T3
Mandible
Left 0NTV0ZZ
Right 0NTT0ZZ
Maxilla 0NTR0ZZ
Metacarpal
Left 0PTQ0ZZ
Right 0PTP0ZZ
Metatarsal
Left 0QTP0ZZ
Right 0QTN0ZZ
Muscle
Abdomen
Left 0KTL
Right 0KTK
Extraocular
Left 08TM
Right 08TL
Facial 0KT1
Foot
Left 0KTW
Right 0KTV
Hand
Left 0KTD
Right 0KTC
Head 0KT0
Hip
Left 0KTP
Right 0KTN
Lower Arm and Wrist
Left 0KTB
Right 0KT9
Lower Leg
Left 0KTT
Right 0KTS
Neck
Left 0KT3
Right 0KT2
Papillary 02TD
Perineum 0KTM
Shoulder
Left 0KT6
Right 0KT5
Thorax
Left 0KTJ
Right 0KTH
Tongue, Palate, Pharynx 0KT4
Trunk
Left 0KTG
Right 0KTF

▶ New ➡ Revised ~~deleted~~ Deleted

R

Restriction (Continued)
Artery (Continued)
Common Carotid
Left 03VJ
Right 03VH
Common Iliac
Left 04VD
Right 04VC
External Carotid
Left 03VN
Right 03VM
External Iliac
Left 04VJ
Right 04VH
Face 03VR
Femoral
Left 04VL
Right 04VK
Foot
Left 04VW
Right 04VV
Gastric 04V2
Hand
Left 03VF
Right 03VD
Hepatic 04V3
Inferior Mesenteric 04VB
Innominate 03V2
Internal Carotid
Left 03VL
Right 03VK
Internal Iliac
Left 04VF
Right 04VE
Internal Mammary
Left 03V1
Right 03V0
Intracranial 03VG
Lower 04VY
Peroneal
Left 04VU
Right 04VT
Popliteal
Left 04VN
Right 04VM
Posterior Tibial
Left 04VS
Right 04VR
Pulmonary
Left 02VR
Right 02VQ
Pulmonary Trunk 02VP
Radial
Left 03VC
Right 03VB
Renal
Left 04VA
Right 04V9
Splenic 04V4
Subclavian
Left 03V4
Right 03V3
Superior Mesenteric 04V5
Temporal
Left 03VT
Right 03VS
Thyroid
Left 03VV
Right 03VU
Ulnar
Left 03VA
Right 03V9
Upper 03VY
Vertebral
Left 03VQ
Right 03VP
Bladder 0TVB
Bladder Neck 0TVC

Restriction (Continued)
Bronchus
Lingula 0BV9
Lower Lobe
Left 0BVB
Right 0BV6
Main
Left 0BV7
Right 0BV3
Middle Lobe, Right 0BV5
Upper Lobe
Left 0BV8
Right 0BV4
Carina 0BV2
Cecum 0DVH
Cervix 0UVC
Cisterna Chyli 07VL
Colon
Ascending 0DVK
Descending 0DVM
Sigmoid 0DVN
Transverse 0DVL
Duct
Common Bile 0FV9
Cystic 0FV8
Hepatic
Common 0FV7
Left 0FV6
Right 0FV5
Lacrimal
Left 08VY
Right 08VX
Pancreatic 0FVD
Accessory 0FVF
Parotid
Left 0CVC
Right 0CVB
Duodenum 0DV9
Esophagogastric Junction 0DV4
Esophagus 0DV5
Lower 0DV3
Middle 0DV2
Upper 0DV1
Heart 02VA
Ileocecal Valve 0DVC
Ileum 0DVB
Intestine
Large 0DVE
Left 0DVG
Right 0DVF
Small 0DV8
Jejunum 0DVA
Kidney Pelvis
Left 0TV4
Right 0TV3
Lymphatic
Aortic 07VD
Axillary
Left 07V6
Right 07V5
Head 07V0
Inguinal
Left 07VJ
Right 07VH
Internal Mammary
Left 07V9
Right 07V8
Lower Extremity
Left 07VG
Right 07VF
Mesenteric 07VB
Neck
Left 07V2
Right 07V1
Pelvis 07VC
Thoracic Duct 07VK
Thorax 07V7

Restriction (Continued)
Lymphatic (Continued)
Upper Extremity
Left 07V4
Right 07V3
Rectum 0DVP
Stomach 0DV6
Pylorus 0DV7
Trachea 0BV1
Ureter
Left 0TV7
Right 0TV6
Urethra 0TVD
Valve, Mitral 02VG
Vein
Axillary
Left 05V8
Right 05V7
Azygos 05V0
Basilic
Left 05VC
Right 05VB
Brachial
Left 05VA
Right 05V9
Cephalic
Left 05VF
Right 05VD
Colic 06V7
Common Iliac
Left 06VD
Right 06VC
Esophageal 06V3
External Iliac
Left 06VG
Right 06VF
External Jugular
Left 05VQ
Right 05VP
Face
Left 05VV
Right 05VT
Femoral
Left 06VN
Right 06VM
Foot
Left 06VV
Right 06VT
Gastric 06V2
Hand
Left 05VH
Right 05VG
Hemiazygos 05V1
Hepatic 06V4
Hypogastric
Left 06VJ
Right 06VH
Inferior Mesenteric 06V6
Innominate
Left 05V4
Right 05V3
Internal Jugular
Left 05VN
Right 05VM
Intracranial 05VL
Lower 06VY
Portal 06V8
Pulmonary
Left 02VT
Right 02VS
Renal
Left 06VB
Right 06V9
Saphenous
Left 06VQ
Right 06VP
Splenic 06V1

R

R

▶ New ➡ Revised ~~deleted~~ Deleted

Revision of device in *(Continued)*
Joint *(Continued)*
Knee
Left 0SWD
Femoral Surface 0SWU
Tibial Surface 0SWW
Right 0SWC
Femoral Surface 0SWT
Tibial Surface 0SWV
Lumbar Vertebral 0SW0
Lumbosacral 0SW3
Metacarpophalangeal
Left 0RWV
Right 0RWU
Metatarsal-Phalangeal
Left 0SWN
Right 0SWM
Occipital-cervical 0RW0
Sacrococcygeal 0SW5
Sacroiliac
Left 0SW8
Right 0SW7
Shoulder
Left 0RWK
Right 0RWJ
Sternoclavicular
Left 0RWF
Right 0RWE
Tarsal
Left 0SWJ
Right 0SWH
Tarsometatarsal
Left 0SWL
Right 0SWK
Temporomandibular
Left 0RWD
Right 0RWC
Thoracic Vertebral 0RW6
Thoracolumbar Vertebral 0RWA
Toe Phalangeal
Left 0SWQ
Right 0SWP
Wrist
Left 0RWP
Right 0RWN
Kidney 0TW5
Larynx 0CWS
Lens
Left 08WK
Right 08WJ
Liver 0FW0
Lung
Left 0BWL
Right 0BWK
Lymphatic 07WN
Thoracic Duct 07WK
Mediastinum 0WWC
Mesentery 0DWV
Metacarpal
Left 0PWQ
Right 0PWP
Metatarsal
Left 0QWP
Right 0QWN
Mouth and Throat 0CWY
Muscle
Extraocular
Left 08WM
Right 08WL
Lower 0KWY
Upper 0KWX
Nasal Mucosa and Soft Tissue 09WK
Neck 0WW6
Nerve
Cranial 00WE
Peripheral 01WY
Omentum 0DWU
Ovary 0UW3
Pancreas 0FWG

Revision of device in *(Continued)*
Parathyroid Gland 0GWR
Patella
Left 0QWF
Right 0QWD
Pelvic Cavity 0WWJ
Penis 0VWS
Pericardial Cavity 0WWD
Perineum
Female 0WWN
Male 0WWM
Peritoneal Cavity 0WWG
Peritoneum 0DWW
Phalanx
Finger
Left 0PWV
Right 0PWT
Thumb
Left 0PWS
Right 0PWR
Toe
Left 0QWR
Right 0QWQ
Pineal Body 0GW1
Pleura 0BWQ
Pleural Cavity
Left 0WWB
Right 0WW9
Prostate and Seminal Vesicles 0VW4
Radius
Left 0PWJ
Right 0PWH
Respiratory Tract 0WWQ
Retroperitoneum 0WWH
Ribs
1 to 2 0PW1
3 or More 0PW2
Sacrum 0QW1
Scapula
Left 0PW6
Right 0PW5
Scrotum and Tunica Vaginalis 0VW8
Septum
Atrial 02W5
Ventricular 02WM
Sinus 09WY
Skin 0HWPX
Skull 0NW0
Spinal Canal 00WU
Spinal Cord 00WV
Spleen 07WP
Sternum 0PW0
Stomach 0DW6
Subcutaneous Tissue and Fascia
Head and Neck 0JWS
Lower Extremity 0JWW
Trunk 0JWT
Upper Extremity 0JWV
Tarsal
Left 0QWM
Right 0QWL
Tendon
Lower 0LWY
Upper 0LWX
Testis 0VWD
Thymus 07WM
Thyroid Gland 0GWK
Tibia
Left 0QWH
Right 0QWG
Toe Nail 0HWRX
Trachea 0BW1
Tracheobronchial Tree 0BW0
Tympanic Membrane
Left 09W8
Right 09W7
Ulna
Left 0PWL
Right 0PWK

Revision of device in *(Continued)*
Ureter 0TW9
Urethra 0TWD
Uterus and Cervix 0UWD
Vagina and Cul-de-sac 0UWH
Valve
Aortic 02WF
Mitral 02WG
Pulmonary 02WH
Tricuspid 02WJ
Vas Deferens 0VWR
Vein
Azygos 05W0
Innominate
Left 05W4
Right 05W3
Lower 06WY
Upper 05WY
Vertebra
Cervical 0PW3
Lumbar 0QW0
Thoracic 0PW4
Vulva 0UWM
Revo MRI™ SureScan® pacemaker *use* Pacemaker, Dual Chamber in 0JH
Rezafungin XW0
rhBMP-2 *use* Recombinant Bone Morphogenetic Protein
Rheos® System device *use* Stimulator Generator in Subcutaneous Tissue and Fascia
Rheos® System lead *use* Stimulator Lead in Upper Arteries
Rhinopharynx *use* Nasopharynx
Rhinoplasty
see Alteration, Nasal Mucosa and Soft Tissue 090K
see Repair, Nasal Mucosa and Soft Tissue 09QK
see Replacement, Nasal Mucosa and Soft Tissue 09RK
see Supplement, Nasal Mucosa and Soft Tissue 09UK
Rhinorrhaphy *see* Repair, Nasal Mucosa and Soft Tissue 09QK
Rhinoscopy 09JKXZZ
Rhizotomy
see Division, Central Nervous System and Cranial Nerves 008
see Division, Peripheral Nervous System 018
Rhomboid major muscle
use Trunk Muscle, Right
use Trunk Muscle, Left
Rhomboid minor muscle
use Trunk Muscle, Right
use Trunk Muscle, Left
Rhythm electrocardiogram *see* Measurement, Cardiac 4A02
Rhytidectomy *see* Alteration, Face 0w02
Right ascending lumbar vein *use* Azygos Vein
Right atrioventricular valve *use* Tricuspid Valve
Right auricular appendix *use* Atrium, Right
Right colic vein *use* Colic Vein
Right coronary sulcus *use* Heart, Right
Right gastric artery *use* Gastric Artery
Right gastroepiploic vein *use* Superior Mesenteric Vein
Right inferior phrenic vein *use* Inferior Vena Cava
Right inferior pulmonary vein *use* Pulmonary Vein, Right
Right jugular trunk *use* Lymphatic, Right Neck
Right lateral ventricle *use* Cerebral Ventricle
Right lymphatic duct *use* Lymphatic, Right Neck
Right ovarian vein *use* Inferior Vena Cava
Right second lumbar vein *use* Inferior Vena Cava
Right subclavian trunk *use* Lymphatic, Right Neck

R

Right subcostal vein *use* Azygos Vein
Right superior pulmonary vein *use* Pulmonary Vein, Right
Right suprarenal vein *use* Inferior Vena Cava
Right testicular vein *use* Inferior Vena Cava
Rima glottidis *use* Larynx
Risorius muscle *use* Facial Muscle
RNS System lead *use* Neurostimulator Lead in Central Nervous System and Cranial Nerves
RNS system neurostimulator generator *use* Neurostimulator Generator in Head and Facial Bones
Robotic Assisted Procedure
  Extremity
    Lower 8E0Y
    Upper 8E0X
  Head and Neck Region 8E09
  Trunk Region 8E0W
~~Robotic Waterjet Ablation, Destruction, Prostate XV508A4~~
Rotation of fetal head
  Forceps 10S07ZZ
  Manual 10S0XZZ
Round ligament of uterus *use* Uterine Supporting Structure
Round window
  use Inner Ear, Right
  use Inner Ear, Left
Roux-en-Y operation
  see Bypass, Gastrointestinal System 0D1
  see Bypass, Hepatobiliary System and Pancreas 0F1
Rupture
  Adhesions *see* Release
  Fluid collection *see* Drainage
Ruxolitinib XW0DWT5

S

S-ICD™ lead *use* Subcutaneous Defibrillator Lead in Subcutaneous Tissue and Fascia
▶Sabizabulin XW0
Sacral ganglion *use* Sacral Sympathetic Nerve
Sacral lymph node *use* Lymphatic, Pelvis
Sacral nerve modulation (SNM) lead *use* Stimulator Lead in Urinary System
Sacral neuromodulation lead *use* Stimulator Lead in Urinary System
Sacral splanchnic nerve *use* Sacral Sympathetic Nerve
Sacrectomy *see* Excision, Lower Bones 0QB
Sacrococcygeal ligament *use* Lower Spine Bursa and Ligament
Sacrococcygeal symphysis *use* Sacrococcygeal Joint
Sacroiliac ligament *use* Lower Spine Bursa and Ligament
Sacrospinous ligament *use* Lower Spine Bursa and Ligament
Sacrotuberous ligament *use* Lower Spine Bursa and Ligament
Salpingectomy
  see Excision, Female Reproductive System 0UB
  see Resection, Female Reproductive System 0UT
Salpingolysis *see* Release, Female Reproductive System 0UN
Salpingopexy
  see Repair, Female Reproductive System 0UQ
  see Reposition, Female Reproductive System 0US
Salpingopharyngeus muscle *use* Tongue, Palate, Pharynx Muscle
Salpingoplasty
  see Repair, Female Reproductive System 0UQ
  see Supplement, Female Reproductive System 0UU
Salpingorrhaphy *see* Repair, Female Reproductive System 0UQ
Salpingoscopy 0UJ88ZZ
Salpingostomy *see* Drainage, Female Reproductive System 0U9
Salpingotomy *see* Drainage, Female Reproductive System 0U9
Salpinx
  use Fallopian Tube, Right
  use Fallopian Tube, Left
Saphenous nerve *use* Femoral Nerve
SAPIEN transcatheter aortic valve *use* Zooplastic Tissue in Heart and Great Vessels
Sarilumab XW0
SARS-CoV-2 antibody detection, serum/plasma nanoparticle fluorescence XXE5XV7
SARS-CoV-2 polymerase chain reaction, nasopharyngeal fluid XXE97U7
Sartorius muscle
  use Upper Leg Muscle, Right
  use Upper Leg Muscle, Left
Satralizumab-mwge XW01397
SAVAL below-the-knee (BTK) drug-eluting stent system
  use Intraluminal Device, Sustained Release Drug-eluting in New Technology
  use Intraluminal Device, Sustained Release Drug-eluting, Two in New Technology
  use Intraluminal Device, Sustained Release Drug-eluting, Three in New Technology
  use Intraluminal Device, Sustained Release Drug-eluting, Four or More in New Technology
Scalene muscle
  use Neck Muscle, Right
  use Neck Muscle, Left
Scan
  Computerized Tomography (CT) *see* Computerized Tomography (CT Scan)
  Radioisotope *see* Planar Nuclear Medicine Imaging
Scaphoid bone
  use Carpal, Right
  use Carpal, Left
Scapholunate ligament
  use Wrist Bursa and Ligament, Right
  use Wrist Bursa and Ligament, Left
Scaphotrapezium ligament
  use Hand Bursa and Ligament, Right
  use Hand Bursa and Ligament, Left
Scapulectomy
  see Excision, Upper Bones 0PB
  see Resection, Upper Bones 0PT
Scapulopexy
  see Repair, Upper Bones 0PQ
  see Reposition, Upper Bones 0PS
Scarpa's (vestibular) ganglion *use* Acoustic Nerve
Sclerectomy *see* Excision, Eye 08B
Sclerotherapy, mechanical *see* Destruction
Sclerotherapy, via injection of sclerosing agent *see* Introduction, Destructive Agent
Sclerotomy *see* Drainage, Eye 089
Scrotectomy
  see Excision, Male Reproductive System 0VB
  see Resection, Male Reproductive System 0VT
Scrotoplasty
  see Repair, Male Reproductive System 0VQ
  see Supplement, Male Reproductive System 0VU
Scrotorrhaphy *see* Repair, Male Reproductive System 0VQ
Scrototomy *see* Drainage, Male Reproductive System 0V9
Sebaceous gland *use* Skin
Second cranial nerve *use* Optic Nerve
Section, cesarean *see* Extraction, Pregnancy 10D
Secura (DR) (VR) *use* Defibrillator Generator in 0JH
Sella turcica *use* Sphenoid Bone
▶Selux Rapid AST Platform XXE5XY9
Semicircular canal
  use Inner Ear, Right
  use Inner Ear, Left
Semimembranosus muscle
  use Upper Leg Muscle, Right
  use Upper Leg Muscle, Left
Semitendinosus muscle
  use Upper Leg Muscle, Right
  use Upper Leg Muscle, Left
Sentinel™ Cerebral Protection System (CPS) X2A5312
Seprafilm *use* Adhesion Barrier
Septal cartilage *use* Nasal Septum
Septectomy
  see Excision, Heart and Great Vessels 02B
  see Resection, Heart and Great Vessels 02T
  see Excision, Ear, Nose, Sinus 09B
  see Resection, Ear, Nose, Sinus 09T
SeptiCyte® RAPID XXE5X38
Septoplasty
  see Repair, Heart and Great Vessels 02Q
  see Replacement, Heart and Great Vessels 02R
  see Supplement, Heart and Great Vessels 02U
  see Repair, Ear, Nose, Sinus 09Q
  see Replacement, Ear, Nose, Sinus 09R
  see Reposition, Ear, Nose, Sinus 09S
  see Supplement, Ear, Nose, Sinus 09U
Septostomy, balloon atrial 02163Z7
Septotomy *see* Drainage, Ear, Nose, Sinus 099
Sequestrectomy, bone *see* Extirpation
▶SER-109 XW0DXN9
Serratus anterior muscle
  use Thorax Muscle, Right
  use Thorax Muscle, Left
Serratus posterior muscle
  use Trunk Muscle, Right
  use Trunk Muscle, Left
Seventh cranial nerve *use* Facial Nerve
Sheffield hybrid external fixator
  use External Fixation Device, Hybrid in 0PH
  use External Fixation Device, Hybrid in 0PS
  use External Fixation Device, Hybrid in 0QH
  use External Fixation Device, Hybrid in 0QS
Sheffield ring external fixator
  use External Fixation Device, Ring in 0PH
  use External Fixation Device, Ring in 0PS
  use External Fixation Device, Ring in 0QH
  use External Fixation Device, Ring in 0QS
Shirodkar cervical cerclage 0UVC7ZZ
Shockwave Intravascular Lithotripsy (Shockwave IVL) *see* Fragmentation
Shock Wave Therapy, Musculoskeletal 6A93
Short gastric artery *use* Splenic Artery
Shortening
  see Excision
  see Repair
  see Reposition
Shunt creation *see* Bypass
Sialoadenectomy
  Complete *see* Resection, Mouth and Throat 0CT
  Partial *see* Excision, Mouth and Throat 0CB
Sialodochoplasty
  see Repair, Mouth and Throat 0CQ
  see Replacement, Mouth and Throat 0CR
  see Supplement, Mouth and Throat 0CU
Sialoectomy
  see Excision, Mouth and Throat 0CB
  see Resection, Mouth and Throat 0CT
Sialography *see* Plain Radiography, Ear, Nose, Mouth and Throat B90
Sialolithotomy *see* Extirpation, Mouth and Throat 0CC
Sigmoid artery *use* Inferior Mesenteric Artery
Sigmoid flexure *use* Sigmoid Colon
Sigmoid vein *use* Inferior Mesenteric Vein
Sigmoidectomy
  see Excision, Gastrointestinal System 0DB
  see Resection, Gastrointestinal System 0DT
Sigmoidorrhaphy *see* Repair, Gastrointestinal System 0DQ
Sigmoidoscopy 0DJD8ZZ
Sigmoidotomy *see* Drainage, Gastrointestinal System 0D9
Single lead pacemaker (atrium) (ventricle) *use* Pacemaker, Single Chamber in 0JH
Single lead rate responsive pacemaker (atrium) (ventricle) *use* Pacemaker, Single Chamber Rate Responsive in 0JH
Single-use duodenoscope XFJ
Single-use oversleeve with intraoperative colonic irrigation XDPH8K7
Sinoatrial node *use* Conduction Mechanism
Sinogram
  Abdominal Wall *see* Fluoroscopy, Abdomen and Pelvis BW11
  Chest Wall *see* Plain Radiography, Chest BW03
  Retroperitoneum *see* Fluoroscopy, Abdomen and Pelvis BW11
Sinus venosus *use* Atrium, Right
Sinusectomy
  see Excision, Ear, Nose, Sinus 09B
  see Resection, Ear, Nose, Sinus 09T
Sinusoscopy 09JY4ZZ
Sinusotomy *see* Drainage, Ear, Nose, Sinus 099
Sirolimus-eluting coronary stent *use* Intraluminal Device, Drug-eluting in Heart and Great Vessels
Sixth cranial nerve *use* Abducens Nerve
Size reduction, breast *see* Excision, Skin and Breast 0HB
SJM Biocor® Stented Valve System *use* Zooplastic Tissue in Heart and Great Vessels
Skene's (paraurethral) gland *use* Vestibular Gland
Sling
  Fascial, orbicularis muscle (mouth) *see* Supplement, Muscle, Facial 0KU1
  Levator muscle, for urethral suspension *see* Reposition, Bladder Neck 0TSC
  Pubococcygeal, for urethral suspension *see* Reposition, Bladder Neck 0TSC
  Rectum *see* Reposition, Rectum 0DSP
Small bowel series *see* Fluoroscopy, Bowel, Small BD13

S

▶SPIKEVAX™
▶*use* COVID-19 Vaccine Dose 1
▶*use* COVID-19 Vaccine Dose 2
▶use COVID-19 Vaccine
▶use COVID-19 Vaccine Dose 3
▶use COVID-19 Vaccine Booster
Spinal cord neurostimulator lead *use* Neurostimulator Lead in Central Nervous System and Cranial Nerves
Spinal growth rods, magnetically controlled *use* Magnetically Controlled Growth Rod(s) in New Technology
Spinal nerve, cervical *use* Cervical Nerve
Spinal nerve, lumbar *use* Lumbar Nerve
Spinal nerve, sacral *use* Sacral Nerve
Spinal nerve, thoracic *use* Thoracic Nerve
Spinal Stabilization Device
Facet Replacement
Cervical Vertebral 0RH1
Cervicothoracic Vertebral 0RH4
Lumbar Vertebral 0SH0
Lumbosacral 0SH3
Occipital-cervical 0RH0
Thoracic Vertebral 0RH6
Thoracolumbar Vertebral 0RHA
Interspinous Process
Cervical Vertebral 0RH1
Cervicothoracic Vertebral 0RH4
Lumbar Vertebral 0SH0
Lumbosacral 0SH3
Occipital-cervical 0RH0
Thoracic Vertebral 0RH6
Thoracolumbar Vertebral 0RHA
Pedicle-Based
Cervical Vertebral 0RH1
Cervicothoracic Vertebral 0RH4
Lumbar Vertebral 0SH0
Lumbosacral 0SH3
Occipital-cervical 0RH0
Thoracic Vertebral 0RH6
Thoracolumbar Vertebral 0RHA
SpineJack® system *use* Synthetic Substitute, Mechanically Expandable (Paired) in New Technology
Spinous process
use Cervical Vertebra
use Thoracic Vertebra
use Lumbar Vertebra
Spiral ganglion *use* Acoustic Nerve
Spiration IBV™ Valve System *use* Intraluminal Device, Endobronchial Valve in Respiratory System
Splenectomy
see Excision, Lymphatic and Hemic Systems 07B
see Resection, Lymphatic and Hemic Systems 07T
Splenic flexure *use* Transverse Colon
Splenic plexus *use* Abdominal Sympathetic Nerve
Splenius capitis muscle *use* Head Muscle
Splenius cervicis muscle
use Neck Muscle, Right
use Neck Muscle, Left
Splenolysis *see* Release, Lymphatic and Hemic Systems 07N
Splenopexy
see Repair, Lymphatic and Hemic Systems 07Q
see Reposition, Lymphatic and Hemic Systems 07S
Splenoplasty *see* Repair, Lymphatic and Hemic Systems 07Q
Splenorrhaphy *see* Repair, Lymphatic and Hemic Systems 07Q
Splenotomy *see* Drainage, Lymphatic and Hemic Systems 079
Splinting, musculoskeletal *see* Immobilization, Anatomical Regions 2W3
SPRAVATO™ *use* Esketamine Hydrochloride
SPY PINPOINT fluorescence imaging system
see Monitoring, Physiological Systems 4A1
see Other Imaging, Hepatobiliary System and Pancreas BF5
SPY system intraoperative fluorescence cholangiography *see* Other Imaging, Hepatobiliary System and Pancreas BF5
SPY system intravascular fluorescence angiography *see* Monitoring, Physiological Systems 4A1
SSO2 (Supersaturated Oxygen) therapy, cardiac intra-arterial 5A0222C
Staged hepatectomy
see Division, Hepatobiliary System and Pancreas 0F8
see Resection, Hepatobiliary System and Pancreas 0FT
Stapedectomy
see Excision, Ear, Nose, Sinus 09B
see Resection, Ear, Nose, Sinus 09T
Stapediolysis *see* Release, Ear, Nose, Sinus 09N
Stapedioplasty
see Repair, Ear, Nose, Sinus 09Q
see Replacement, Ear, Nose, Sinus 09R
see Supplement, Ear, Nose, Sinus 09U
Stapedotomy *see* Drainage, Ear, Nose, Sinus 099
Stapes
use Auditory Ossicle, Right
use Auditory Ossicle, Left
Static Spacer (Antibiotic) *use* Spacer in Lower Joints
STELARA® *use* Other New Technology Therapeutic Substance
Stellate ganglion *use* Head and Neck Sympathetic Nerve
Stem cell transplant *see* Transfusion, Circulatory 302
Stensen's duct
use Parotid Duct, Right
use Parotid Duct, Left
Stent, intraluminal (cardiovascular) (gastrointestinal)(hepatobiliary)(urinary) *use* Intraluminal Device
Stent retriever thrombectomy *see* Extirpation, Upper Arteries 03C
Stented tissue valve *use* Zooplastic Tissue in Heart and Great Vessels
Stereotactic Radiosurgery
Abdomen DW23
Adrenal Gland DG22
Bile Ducts DF22
Bladder DT22
Bone Marrow D720
Brain D020
Brain Stem D021
Breast
Left DM20
Right DM21
Bronchus DB21
Cervix DU21
Chest DW22
Chest Wall DB27
Colon DD25
Diaphragm DB28
Duodenum DD22
Ear D920
Esophagus DD20
Eye D820
Gallbladder DF21
Gamma Beam
Abdomen DW23JZZ
Adrenal Gland DG22JZZ
Bile Ducts DF22JZZ
Bladder DT22JZZ
Bone Marrow D720JZZ
Brain D020JZZ
Brain Stem D021JZZ
Breast
Left DM20JZZ
Right DM21JZZ
Bronchus DB21JZZ
Cervix DU21JZZ
Stereotactic Radiosurgery *(Continued)*
Gamma Beam *(Continued)*
Chest DW22JZZ
Chest Wall DB27JZZ
Colon DD25JZZ
Diaphragm DB28JZZ
Duodenum DD22JZZ
Ear D920JZZ
Esophagus DD20JZZ
Eye D820JZZ
Gallbladder DF21JZZ
Gland
Adrenal DG22JZZ
Parathyroid DG24JZZ
Pituitary DG20JZZ
Thyroid DG25JZZ
Glands, Salivary D926JZZ
Head and Neck DW21JZZ
Ileum DD24JZZ
Jejunum DD23JZZ
Kidney DT20JZZ
Larynx D92BJZZ
Liver DF20JZZ
Lung DB22JZZ
Lymphatics
Abdomen D726JZZ
Axillary D724JZZ
Inguinal D728JZZ
Neck D723JZZ
Pelvis D727JZZ
Thorax D725JZZ
Mediastinum DB26JZZ
Mouth D924JZZ
Nasopharynx D92DJZZ
Neck and Head DW21JZZ
Nerve, Peripheral D027JZZ
Nose D921JZZ
Ovary DU20JZZ
Palate
Hard D928JZZ
Soft D929JZZ
Pancreas DF23JZZ
Parathyroid Gland DG24JZZ
Pelvic Region DW26JZZ
Pharynx D92CJZZ
Pineal Body DG21JZZ
Pituitary Gland DG20JZZ
Pleura DB25JZZ
Prostate DV20JZZ
Rectum DD27JZZ
Sinuses D927JZZ
Spinal Cord D026JZZ
Spleen D722JZZ
Stomach DD21JZZ
Testis DV21JZZ
Thymus D721JZZ
Thyroid Gland DG25JZZ
Tongue D925JZZ
Trachea DB20JZZ
Ureter DT21JZZ
Urethra DT23JZZ
Uterus DU22JZZ
Gland
Adrenal DG22
Parathyroid DG24
Pituitary DG20
Thyroid DG25
Glands, Salivary D926
Head and Neck DW21
Ileum DD24
Jejunum DD23
Kidney DT20
Larynx D92B
Liver DF20
Lung DB22
Lymphatics
Abdomen D726
Axillary D724
Inguinal D728
Neck D723
Pelvis D727
Thorax D725

▶ New ➡ Revised ~~deleted~~ Deleted

S

S

Stimulator Lead (Continued)
Removal of device from (Continued)
Bladder 0TPB
Muscle
Lower 0KPY
Upper 0KPX
Stomach 0DP6
Ureter 0TP9
Revision of device in
Anal Sphincter 0DWR
Artery, Upper 03WY
Bladder 0TWB
Muscle
Lower 0KWY
Upper 0KWX
Stomach 0DW6
Ureter 0TW9
Stoma
Excision
Abdominal Wall 0WBFXZ2
Neck 0WB6XZ2
Repair
Abdominal Wall 0WQFXZ2
Neck 0WQ6XZ2
Stomatoplasty
see Repair, Mouth and Throat 0CQ
see Replacement, Mouth and Throat 0CR
see Supplement, Mouth and Throat 0CU
Stomatorrhaphy see Repair, Mouth and Throat 0CQ
StrataGraft® use Bioengineered Allogeneic Construct
Stratos LV use Cardiac Resynchronization Pacemaker Pulse Generator in 0JH
Stress test
4A02XM4
4A12XM4
Stripping see Extraction
Study
Electrophysiologic stimulation, cardiac see Measurement, Cardiac 4A02
Ocular motility 4A07X7Z
Pulmonary airway flow measurement see Measurement, Respiratory 4A09
Visual acuity 4A07X0Z
Styloglossus muscle use Tongue, Palate, Pharynx Muscle
Stylomandibular ligament use Head and Neck Bursa and Ligament
Stylopharyngeus muscle use Tongue, Palate, Pharynx Muscle
Subacromial bursa
use Shoulder Bursa and Ligament, Right
use Shoulder Bursa and Ligament, Left
Subaortic (common iliac) lymph node use Lymphatic, Pelvis
Subarachnoid space, spinal use Spinal Canal
Subclavicular (apical) lymph node
use Lymphatic, Right Axillary
use Lymphatic, Left Axillary
Subclavius muscle
use Thorax Muscle, Right
use Thorax Muscle, Left
Subclavius nerve use Brachial Plexus Nerve
Subcostal artery use Upper Artery
Subcostal muscle
use Thorax Muscle, Right
use Thorax Muscle, Left
Subcostal nerve use Thoracic Nerve
Subcutaneous Defibrillator Lead
Insertion of device in, Subcutaneous Tissue and Fascia, Chest 0JH6
Removal of device from, Subcutaneous Tissue and Fascia, Trunk 0JPT
Revision of device in, Subcutaneous Tissue and Fascia, Trunk 0JWT
Subcutaneous injection reservoir, port use Vascular Access Device, Totally Implantable in Subcutaneous Tissue and Fascia
Subcutaneous injection reservoir, pump use Infusion Device, Pump in Subcutaneous Tissue and Fascia
Subdermal progesterone implant use Contraceptive Device in Subcutaneous Tissue and Fascia
Subdural space, spinal use Spinal Canal
Submandibular ganglion
use Head and Neck Sympathetic Nerve
use Facial Nerve
Submandibular gland
use Submaxillary Gland, Right
use Submaxillary Gland, Left
Submandibular lymph node use Lymphatic, Head
Submandibular space use Subcutaneous Tissue and Fascia, Face
Submaxillary ganglion use Head and Neck Sympathetic Nerve
Submaxillary lymph node use Lymphatic, Head
Submental artery use Face Artery
Submental lymph node use Lymphatic, Head
Submucous (Meissner's) plexus use Abdominal Sympathetic Nerve
Suboccipital nerve use Cervical Nerve
Suboccipital venous plexus
use Vertebral Vein, Right
use Vertebral Vein, Left
Subparotid lymph node use Lymphatic, Head
Subscapular (posterior) lymph node
use Lymphatic, Right Axillary
use Lymphatic, Left Axillary
Subscapular aponeurosis
use Subcutaneous Tissue and Fascia, Right Upper Arm
use Subcutaneous Tissue and Fascia, Left Upper Arm
Subscapular artery
use Axillary Artery, Right
use Axillary Artery, Left
Subscapularis muscle
use Shoulder Muscle, Right
use Shoulder Muscle, Left
Substance Abuse Treatment
Counseling
Family, for substance abuse, Other Family Counseling HZ63ZZZ
Group
12-Step HZ43ZZZ
Behavioral HZ41ZZZ
Cognitive HZ40ZZZ
Cognitive-Behavioral HZ42ZZZ
Confrontational HZ48ZZZ
Continuing Care HZ49ZZZ
Infectious Disease
Post-Test HZ4CZZZ
Pre-Test HZ4CZZZ
Interpersonal HZ44ZZZ
Motivational Enhancement HZ47ZZZ
Psychoeducation HZ46ZZZ
Spiritual HZ4BZZZ
Vocational HZ45ZZZ
Individual
12-Step HZ33ZZZ
Behavioral HZ31ZZZ
Cognitive HZ30ZZZ
Cognitive-Behavioral HZ32ZZZ
Confrontational HZ38ZZZ
Continuing Care HZ39ZZZ
Infectious Disease
Post-Test HZ3CZZZ
Pre-Test HZ3CZZZ
Interpersonal HZ34ZZZ
Motivational Enhancement HZ37ZZZ
Psychoeducation HZ36ZZZ
Spiritual HZ3BZZZ
Vocational HZ35ZZZ
Detoxification Services, for substance abuse HZ2ZZZZ
Substance Abuse Treatment (Continued)
Medication Management
Antabuse HZ83ZZZ
Bupropion HZ87ZZZ
Clonidine HZ86ZZZ
Levo-alpha-acetyl-methadol (LAAM) HZ82ZZZ
Methadone Maintenance HZ81ZZZ
Naloxone HZ85ZZZ
Naltrexone HZ84ZZZ
Nicotine Replacement HZ80ZZZ
Other Replacement Medication HZ89ZZZ
Psychiatric Medication HZ88ZZZ
Pharmacotherapy
Antabuse HZ93ZZZ
Bupropion HZ97ZZZ
Clonidine HZ96ZZZ
Levo-alpha-acetyl-methadol (LAAM) HZ92ZZZ
Methadone Maintenance HZ91ZZZ
Naloxone HZ95ZZZ
Naltrexone HZ94ZZZ
Nicotine Replacement HZ90ZZZ
Psychiatric Medication HZ98ZZZ
Replacement Medication, Other HZ99ZZZ
Psychotherapy
12-Step HZ53ZZZ
Behavioral HZ51ZZZ
Cognitive HZ50ZZZ
Cognitive-Behavioral HZ52ZZZ
Confrontational HZ58ZZZ
Interactive HZ55ZZZ
Interpersonal HZ54ZZZ
Motivational Enhancement HZ57ZZZ
Psychoanalysis HZ5BZZZ
Psychodynamic HZ5CZZZ
Psychoeducation HZ56ZZZ
Psychophysiological HZ5DZZZ
Supportive HZ59ZZZ
Substantia nigra use Basal Ganglia
Subtalar (talocalcaneal) joint
use Tarsal Joint, Right
use Tarsal Joint, Left
Subtalar ligament
use Foot Bursa and Ligament, Right
use Foot Bursa and Ligament, Left
Subthalamic nucleus use Basal Ganglia
Suction curettage (D&C), nonobstetric see Extraction, Endometrium 0UDB
Suction curettage, obstetric post-delivery see Extraction, Products of Conception, Retained 10D1
▶ SUL-DUR use Sulbactam-Durlobactam
▶ Sulbactam-Durlobactam XW0
Superficial circumflex iliac vein
use Saphenous Vein, Right
use Saphenous Vein, Left
Superficial epigastric artery
use Femoral Artery, Right
use Femoral Artery, Left
Superficial epigastric vein
use Saphenous Vein, Right
use Saphenous Vein, Left
Superficial Inferior Epigastric Artery Flap
Replacement
Bilateral 0HRV078
Left 0HRU078
Right 0HRT078
Transfer
Left 0KXG
Right 0KXF
Superficial palmar arch
use Hand Artery, Right
use Hand Artery, Left
Superficial palmar venous arch
use Hand Vein, Right
use Hand Vein, Left
Superficial temporal artery
use Temporal Artery, Right
use Temporal Artery, Left

S

- **Superficial transverse perineal muscle** *use* Perineum Muscle
- **Superior cardiac nerve** *use* Thoracic Sympathetic Nerve
- **Superior cerebellar vein** *use* Intracranial Vein
- **Superior cerebral vein** *use* Intracranial Vein
- **Superior clunic (cluneal) nerve** *use* Lumbar Nerve
- **Superior epigastric artery**
  - *use* Internal Mammary Artery, Right
  - *use* Internal Mammary Artery, Left
- **Superior genicular artery**
  - *use* Popliteal Artery, Right
  - *use* Popliteal Artery, Left
- **Superior gluteal artery**
  - *use* Internal Iliac Artery, Right
  - *use* Internal Iliac Artery, Left
- **Superior gluteal nerve** *use* Lumbar Plexus Nerve
- **Superior hypogastric plexus** *use* Abdominal Sympathetic Nerve
- **Superior labial artery** *use* Face Artery
- **Superior laryngeal artery**
  - *use* Thyroid Artery, Right
  - *use* Thyroid Artery, Left
- **Superior laryngeal nerve** *use* Vagus Nerve
- **Superior longitudinal muscle** *use* Tongue, Palate, Pharynx Muscle
- **Superior mesenteric ganglion** *use* Abdominal Sympathetic Nerve
- **Superior mesenteric lymph node** *use* Lymphatic, Mesenteric
- **Superior mesenteric plexus** *use* Abdominal Sympathetic Nerve
- **Superior oblique muscle**
  - *use* Extraocular Muscle, Right
  - *use* Extraocular Muscle, Left
- **Superior olivary nucleus** *use* Pons
- **Superior rectal artery** *use* Inferior Mesenteric Artery
- **Superior rectal vein** *use* Inferior Mesenteric Vein
- **Superior rectus muscle**
  - *use* Extraocular Muscle, Right
  - *use* Extraocular Muscle, Left
- **Superior tarsal plate**
  - *use* Upper Eyelid, Right
  - *use* Upper Eyelid, Left
- **Superior thoracic artery**
  - *use* Axillary Artery, Right
  - *use* Axillary Artery, Left
- **Superior thyroid artery**
  - *use* External Carotid Artery, Right
  - *use* External Carotid Artery, Left
  - *use* Thyroid Artery, Right
  - *use* Thyroid Artery, Left
- **Superior turbinate** *use* Nasal Turbinate
- **Superior ulnar collateral artery**
  - *use* Brachial Artery, Right
  - *use* Brachial Artery, Left
- **Superior vesical artery**
  - *use* Internal Iliac Artery, Right
  - *use* Internal Iliac Artery, Left
- ~~Supersaturated Oxygen therapy~~
  - ~~5A0512C~~
  - ~~5A0522C~~
- **Supersaturated Oxygen (SSO2) therapy, cardiac intra-arterial** 5A0222C
- **Supplement**
  - Abdominal Wall 0WUF
  - Acetabulum
    - Left 0QU5
    - Right 0QU4
  - Ampulla of Vater 0FUC
  - Anal Sphincter 0DUR
  - Ankle Region
    - Left 0YUL
    - Right 0YUK
  - Anus 0DUQ

Supplement *(Continued)*
  - Aorta
    - Abdominal 04U0
    - Thoracic
      - Ascending/Arch 02UX
      - Descending 02UW
  - Arm
    - Lower
      - Left 0XUF
      - Right 0XUD
    - Upper
      - Left 0XU9
      - Right 0XU8
  - ▶ Arteriovenous Fistula, Extraluminal Support Device X2U
  - Artery
    - Anterior Tibial
      - Left 04UQ
      - Right 04UP
    - Axillary
      - Left 03U6
      - Right 03U5
    - Brachial
      - Left 03U8
      - Right 03U7
    - Celiac 04U1
    - Colic
      - Left 04U7
      - Middle 04U8
      - Right 04U6
    - Common Carotid
      - Left 03UJ
      - Right 03UH
    - Common Iliac
      - Left 04UD
      - Right 04UC
    - Coronary
      - Four or More Arteries 02U3
      - One Artery 02U0
      - Three Arteries 02U2
      - Two Arteries 02U1
    - External Carotid
      - Left 03UN
      - Right 03UM
    - External Iliac
      - Left 04UJ
      - Right 04UH
    - Face 03UR
    - Femoral
      - Left 04UL
      - Right 04UK
    - Foot
      - Left 04UW
      - Right 04UV
    - Gastric 04U2
    - Hand
      - Left 03UF
      - Right 03UD
    - Hepatic 04U3
    - Inferior Mesenteric 04UB
    - Innominate 03U2
    - Internal Carotid
      - Left 03UL
      - Right 03UK
    - Internal Iliac
      - Left 04UF
      - Right 04UE
    - Internal Mammary
      - Left 03U1
      - Right 03U0
    - Intracranial 03UG
    - Lower 04UY
    - Peroneal
      - Left 04UU
      - Right 04UT
    - Popliteal
      - Left 04UN
      - Right 04UM
    - Posterior Tibial
      - Left 04US
      - Right 04UR

Supplement *(Continued)*
  - Artery *(Continued)*
    - Pulmonary
      - Left 02UR
      - Right 02UQ
    - Pulmonary Trunk 02UP
    - Radial
      - Left 03UC
      - Right 03UB
    - Renal
      - Left 04UA
      - Right 04U9
    - Splenic 04U4
    - Subclavian
      - Left 03U4
      - Right 03U3
    - Superior Mesenteric 04U5
    - Temporal
      - Left 03UT
      - Right 03US
    - Thyroid
      - Left 03UV
      - Right 03UU
    - Ulnar
      - Left 03UA
      - Right 03U9
    - Upper 03UY
    - Vertebral
      - Left 03UQ
      - Right 03UP
  - Atrium
    - Left 02U7
    - Right 02U6
  - Auditory Ossicle
    - Left 09UA
    - Right 09U9
  - Axilla
    - Left 0XU5
    - Right 0XU4
  - Back
    - Lower 0WUL
    - Upper 0WUK
  - Bladder 0TUB
  - Bladder Neck 0TUC
  - Bone
    - Ethmoid
      - Left 0NUG
      - Right 0NUF
    - Frontal 0NU1
    - Hyoid 0NUX
    - Lacrimal
      - Left 0NUJ
      - Right 0NUH
    - Nasal 0NUB
    - Occipital 0NU7
    - Palatine
      - Left 0NUL
      - Right 0NUK
    - Parietal
      - Left 0NU4
      - Right 0NU3
    - Pelvic
      - Left 0QU3
      - Right 0QU2
    - Sphenoid 0NUC
    - Temporal
      - Left 0NU6
      - Right 0NU5
    - Zygomatic
      - Left 0NUN
      - Right 0NUM
  - Breast
    - Bilateral 0HUV
    - Left 0HUU
    - Right 0HUT
  - Bronchus
    - Lingula 0BU9
    - Lower Lobe
      - Left 0BUB
      - Right 0BU6
    - Main
      - Left 0BU7
      - Right 0BU3

S

Supplement *(Continued)*
Vertebra
Cervical 0PU3
Lumbar 0QU0
Mechanically Expandable (Paired)
Synthetic Substitute XNU0356
Thoracic 0PU4
Mechanically Expandable (Paired)
Synthetic Substitute XNU0356
Vesicle
Bilateral 0VU3
Left 0VU2
Right 0VU1
Vocal Cord
Left 0CUV
Right 0CUT
Vulva 0UUM
Wrist Region
Left 0XUH
Right 0XUG
Supraclavicular (Virchow's) lymph node
use Lymphatic, Right Neck
use Lymphatic, Left Neck
Supraclavicular nerve *use* Cervical Plexus
Suprahyoid lymph node *use* Lymphatic, Head
Suprahyoid muscle
use Neck Muscle, Right
use Neck Muscle, Left
Suprainguinal lymph node *use* Lymphatic, Pelvis
Supraorbital vein
use Face Vein, Right
use Face Vein, Left
Suprarenal gland
use Adrenal Gland, Left
use Adrenal Gland, Right
use Adrenal Gland, Bilateral
use Adrenal Gland
Suprarenal plexus *use* Abdominal Sympathetic Nerve
Suprascapular nerve *use* Brachial Plexus Nerve
Supraspinatus fascia
use Subcutaneous Tissue and Fascia, Right Upper Arm
use Subcutaneous Tissue and Fascia, Left Upper Arm
Supraspinatus muscle
use Shoulder Muscle, Right
use Shoulder Muscle, Left
Supraspinous ligament
use Upper Spine Bursa and Ligament
use Lower Spine Bursa and Ligament
Suprasternal notch *use* Sternum
Supratrochlear lymph node
use Lymphatic, Right Upper Extremity
use Lymphatic, Left Upper Extremity
Sural artery
use Popliteal Artery, Right
use Popliteal Artery, Left
Surpass Streamline™ Flow Diverter *use* Intraluminal Device, Flow Diverter in 03V
Suspension
Bladder Neck *see* Reposition, Bladder Neck 0TSC
Kidney *see* Reposition, Urinary System 0TS
Urethra *see* Reposition, Urinary System 0TS
Urethrovesical *see* Reposition, Bladder Neck 0TSC
Uterus *see* Reposition, Uterus 0US9
Vagina *see* Reposition, Vagina 0USG
Sustained Release Drug-eluting Intraluminal Device
Dilation
Anterior Tibial
Left X27Q385
Right X27P385
Femoral
Left X27J385
Right X27H385
Peroneal
Left X27U385
Right X27T385
Popliteal
Left Distal X27N385
Left Proximal X27L385
Right Distal X27M385
Right Proximal X27K385
Posterior Tibial
Left X27S385
Right X27R385
Four or More
Anterior Tibial
Left X27Q3C5
Right X27P3C5
Femoral
Left X27J3C5
Right X27H3C5
Peroneal
Left X27U3C5
Right X27T3C5
Popliteal
Left Distal X27N3C5
Left Proximal X27L3C5
Right Distal X27M3C5
Right Proximal X27K3C5
Posterior Tibial
Left X27S3C5
Right X27R3C5
Three
Anterior Tibial
Left X27Q3B5
Right X27P3B5
Femoral
Left X27J3B5
Right X27H3B5
Peroneal
Left X27U3B5
Right X27T3B5
Popliteal
Left Distal X27N3B5
Left Proximal X27L3B5
Right Distal X27M3B5
Right Proximal X27K3B5
Sustained Release Drug-eluting Intraluminal Device *(Continued)*
Three *(Continued)*
Posterior Tibial
Left X27S3B5
Right X27R3B5
Two
Anterior Tibial
Left X27Q395
Right X27P395
Femoral
Left X27J395
Right X27H395
Peroneal
Left X27U395
Right X27T395
Popliteal
Left Distal X27N395
Left Proximal X27L395
Right Distal X27M395
Right Proximal X27K395
Posterior Tibial
Left X27S395
Right X27R395
Suture
Laceration repair *see* Repair
Ligation *see* Occlusion
Suture Removal
Extremity
Lower 8E0YXY8
Upper 8E0XXY8
Head and Neck Region 8E09XY8
Trunk Region 8E0WXY8
Sutureless valve, Perceval (rapid deployment technique) *see* Replacement, Valve, Aortic 02RF
Sweat gland *use* Skin
Sympathectomy
see Excision, Peripheral Nervous System 01B
SynCardia Total Artificial Heart *use* Synthetic Substitute
SynCardia (temporary) total artificial heart (TAH) *use* Synthetic Substitute, Pneumatic in 02R
Synchra CRT-P *use* Cardiac Resynchronization Pacemaker Pulse Generator in 0JH
SynchroMed pump *use* Infusion Device, Pump in Subcutaneous Tissue and Fascia
Synechiotomy, iris *see* Release, Eye 08N
Synovectomy
Lower joint *see* Excision, Lower Joints 0SB
Upper joint *see* Excision, Upper Joints 0RB
~~Synthetic Human Angiotensin II XW0~~
Systemic Nuclear Medicine Therapy
Abdomen CW70
Anatomical Regions, Multiple CW7YYZZ
Chest CW73
Thyroid CW7G
Whole Body CW7N

S

▶ New ➡ Revised ~~deleted~~ Deleted

T

tab-cel® *use* Tabelecleucel Immunotherapy
Tabelecleucel Immunotherapy XW0
Tagraxofusp-erzs Antineoplastic XW0
Takedown
  Arteriovenous shunt *see* Removal of device from, Upper Arteries 03P
  Arteriovenous shunt, with creation of new shunt *see* Bypass, Upper Arteries 031
  Stoma
    see Excision
    see Reposition
Talent® Converter *use* Intraluminal Device
Talent® Occluder *use* Intraluminal Device
Talent® Stent Graft (abdominal) (thoracic) *use* Intraluminal Device
Talocalcaneal (subtalar) joint
  use Tarsal Joint, Right
  use Tarsal Joint, Left
Talocalcaneal ligament
  use Foot Bursa and Ligament, Right
  use Foot Bursa and Ligament, Left
Talocalcaneonavicular joint
  use Tarsal Joint, Right
  use Tarsal Joint, Left
Talocalcaneonavicular ligament
  use Foot Bursa and Ligament, Right
  use Foot Bursa and Ligament, Left
Talocrural joint
  use Ankle Joint, Right
  use Ankle Joint, Left
Talofibular ligament
  use Ankle Bursa and Ligament, Right
  use Ankle Bursa and Ligament, Left
Talus bone
  use Tarsal, Right
  use Tarsal, Left
TandemHeart® System *use* Short-term External Heart Assist System in Heart and Great Vessels
Tarsectomy
  see Excision, Lower Bones 0QB
  see Resection, Lower Bones 0QT
Tarsometatarsal ligament
  use Foot Bursa and Ligament, Right
  use Foot Bursa and Ligament, Left
Tarsorrhaphy *see* Repair, Eye 08Q
Tattooing
  Cornea 3E0CXMZ
  Skin *see* Introduction of substance in or on Skin 3E00
Taurolidine Anti-infective and Heparin Anticoagulant XY0YX28
TAXUS® Liberté® Paclitaxel-eluting Coronary Stent System *use* Intraluminal Device, Drug-eluting in Heart and Great Vessels
TBNA (transbronchial needle aspiration)
  Fluid or gas *see* Drainage, Respiratory System 0B9
  Tissue biopsy *see* Extraction, Respiratory System 0BD
Tecartus™ *use* Brexucabtagene Autoleucel Immunotherapy
TECENTRIQ® *use* Atezolizumab Antineoplastic
Teclistamab Antineoplastic XW01348
Telemetry
  4A12X4Z
  Ambulatory 4A12X45
Temperature gradient study 4A0ZXKZ
Temporal lobe *use* Cerebral Hemisphere
Temporalis muscle *use* Head Muscle
Temporoparietalis muscle *use* Head Muscle
Tendolysis *see* Release, Tendons 0LN
Tendonectomy
  see Excision, Tendons 0LB
  see Resection, Tendons 0LT
Tendonoplasty, tenoplasty
  see Repair, Tendons 0LQ
  see Replacement, Tendons 0LR
  see Supplement, Tendons 0LU
Tendorrhaphy *see* Repair, Tendons 0LQ
Tendototomy
  see Division, Tendons 0L8
  see Drainage, Tendons 0L9
Tenectomy, tenonectomy
  see Excision, Tendons 0LB
  see Resection, Tendons 0LT
Tenolysis *see* Release, Tendons 0LN
Tenontorrhaphy *see* Repair, Tendons 0LQ
Tenontotomy
  see Division, Tendons 0L8
  see Drainage, Tendons 0L9
Tenorrhaphy *see* Repair, Tendons 0LQ
Tenosynovectomy
  see Excision, Tendons 0LB
  see Resection, Tendons 0LT
Tenotomy
  see Division, Tendons 0L8
  see Drainage, Tendons 0L9
Tensor fasciae latae muscle
  use Hip Muscle, Right
  use Hip Muscle, Left
Tensor veli palatini muscle *use* Tongue, Palate, Pharynx Muscle
Tenth cranial nerve *use* Vagus Nerve
Tentorium cerebelli *use* Dura Mater
Teres major muscle
  use Shoulder Muscle, Right
  use Shoulder Muscle, Left
Teres minor muscle
  use Shoulder Muscle, Right
  use Shoulder Muscle, Left
Terlipressin XW0
TERLIVAZ® *use* Terlipressin
Termination of pregnancy
  Aspiration curettage 10A07ZZ
  Dilation and curettage 10A07ZZ
  Hysterotomy 10A00ZZ
  Intra-amniotic injection 10A03ZZ
  Laminaria 10A07ZW
  Vacuum 10A07Z6
Testectomy
  see Excision, Male Reproductive System 0VB
  see Resection, Male Reproductive System 0VT
Testicular artery *use* Abdominal Aorta
Testing
  Glaucoma 4A07XBZ
  Hearing *see* Hearing Assessment, Diagnostic Audiology F13
  Mental health *see* Psychological Tests
  Muscle function, electromyography (EMG) *see* Measurement, Musculoskeletal 4A0F
  Muscle function, manual *see* Motor Function Assessment, Rehabilitation F01
  Neurophysiologic monitoring, intra-operative *see* Monitoring, Physiological Systems 4A1
  Range of motion *see* Motor Function Assessment, Rehabilitation F01
  Vestibular function *see* Vestibular Assessment, Diagnostic Audiology F15
Thalamectomy *see* Excision, Thalamus 00B9
Thalamotomy
  see Drainage, Thalamus 0099
Thenar muscle
  use Hand Muscle, Right
  use Hand Muscle, Left
Therapeutic Massage
  Musculoskeletal System 8E0KX1Z
  Reproductive System
    Prostate 8E0VX1C
    Rectum 8E0VX1D
Therapeutic occlusion coil(s) *use* Intraluminal Device
Thermography 4A0ZXKZ
Thermotherapy, prostate *see* Destruction, Prostate 0V50
Third cranial nerve *use* Oculomotor Nerve
Third occipital nerve *use* Cervical Nerve
Third ventricle *use* Cerebral Ventricle
Thoracectomy *see* Excision, Anatomical Regions, General 0WB
Thoracentesis *see* Drainage, Anatomical Regions, General 0W9
Thoracic aortic plexus *use* Thoracic Sympathetic Nerve
Thoracic esophagus *use* Esophagus, Middle
Thoracic facet joint *use* Thoracic Vertebral Joint
Thoracic ganglion *use* Thoracic Sympathetic Nerve
Thoracoacromial artery
  use Axillary Artery, Right
  use Axillary Artery, Left
Thoracocentesis *see* Drainage, Anatomical Regions, General 0W9
Thoracolumbar facet joint *use* Thoracolumbar Vertebral Joint
Thoracoplasty
  see Repair, Anatomical Regions, General 0WQ
  see Supplement, Anatomical Regions, General 0WU
Thoracostomy tube *use* Drainage Device
Thoracostomy, for lung collapse *see* Drainage, Respiratory System 0B9
Thoracotomy *see* Drainage, Anatomical Regions, General 0W9
Thoraflex™ hybrid device *use* Branched Synthetic Substitute with Intraluminal Device in New Technology
Thoratec IVAD (Implantable Ventricular Assist Device) *use* Implantable Heart Assist System in Heart and Great Vessels
Thoratec Paracorporeal Ventricular Assist Device *use* Short-term External Heart Assist System in Heart and Great Vessels
Thrombectomy *see* Extirpation
Thrombolysis, Ultrasound assisted *see* Fragmentation, Artery
Thymectomy
  see Excision, Lymphatic and Hemic Systems 07B
  see Resection, Lymphatic and Hemic Systems 07T
Thymopexy
  see Repair, Lymphatic and Hemic Systems 07Q
  see Reposition, Lymphatic and Hemic Systems 07S
Thymus gland *use* Thymus
Thyroarytenoid muscle
  use Neck Muscle, Right
  use Neck Muscle, Left
Thyrocervical trunk
  use Thyroid Artery, Right
  use Thyroid Artery, Left
Thyroid cartilage *use* Larynx
Thyroidectomy
  see Excision, Endocrine System 0GB
  see Resection, Endocrine System 0GT
Thyroidorrhaphy *see* Repair, Endocrine System 0GQ
Thyroidoscopy 0GJK4ZZ
Thyroidotomy *see* Drainage, Endocrine System 0G9
▶ Tibial Extension with Motion Sensors, Insertion XNH
Tibial insert *use* Liner in Lower Joints
Tibial sesamoid
  use Metatarsal, Right
  use Metatarsal, Left
Tibialis anterior muscle
  use Lower Leg Muscle, Right
  use Lower Leg Muscle, Left

T

T

▶**TricValve® Transcatheter Bicaval Valve System** *use* Intraluminal Device, Bioprosthetic Valve in New Technology
Trifacial nerve *use* Trigeminal Nerve
Trifecta™ Valve (aortic) *use* Zooplastic Tissue in Heart and Great Vessels
Trigone of bladder *use* Bladder
TriGuard 3™ CEPD (cerebral embolic protection device) X2A6325
Trilaciclib XW0
Trimming, excisional *see* Excision
Triquetral bone
  use Carpal, Right
  use Carpal, Left
Trochanteric bursa
  use Hip Bursa and Ligament, Right
  use Hip Bursa and Ligament, Left
TUMT (Transurethral microwave thermotherapy of prostate) 0V507ZZ
TUNA (transurethral needle ablation of prostate) 0V507ZZ
Tunneled central venous catheter *use* Vascular Access Device, Tunneled in Subcutaneous Tissue and Fascia
Tunneled spinal (intrathecal) catheter *use* Infusion Device
Turbinectomy
  see Excision, Ear, Nose, Sinus 09B
  see Resection, Ear, Nose, Sinus 09T
Turbinoplasty
  see Repair, Ear, Nose, Sinus 09Q
  see Replacement, Ear, Nose, Sinus 09R
  see Supplement, Ear, Nose, Sinus 09U
Turbinotomy
  see Division, Ear, Nose, Sinus 098
  see Drainage, Ear, Nose, Sinus 099
TURP (transurethral resection of prostate)
  see Excision, Prostate 0VB0
  see Resection, Prostate 0VT0
Twelfth cranial nerve *use* Hypoglossal Nerve
Two lead pacemaker *use* Pacemaker, Dual Chamber in 0JH
Tympanic cavity
  use Middle Ear, Right
  use Middle Ear, Left
Tympanic nerve *use* Glossopharyngeal Nerve
Tympanic part of temoporal bone
  use Temporal Bone, Right
  use Temporal Bone, Left
Tympanogram *see* Hearing Assessment, Diagnostic Audiology F13
Tympanoplasty
  see Repair, Ear, Nose, Sinus 09Q
  see Replacement, Ear, Nose, Sinus 09R
  see Supplement, Ear, Nose, Sinus 09U
Tympanosympathectomy *see* Excision, Nerve, Head and Neck Sympathetic 01BK
Tympanotomy *see* Drainage, Ear, Nose, Sinus 099
TYRX Antibacterial Envelope *use* Anti-Infective Envelope

U

Ultrasonography *(Continued)*
Vena Cava
Inferior, Intravascular B549ZZ3
Superior, Intravascular B548ZZ3
Wrist
Left, Densitometry BP4MZZ1
Right, Densitometry BP4LZZ1
▶Ultrasound Ablation, Destruction, Renal Sympathetic Nerve(s) X051329
Ultrasound bone healing system
use Bone Growth Stimulator in Head and Facial Bones
use Bone Growth Stimulator in Upper Bones
use Bone Growth Stimulator in Lower Bones
▶Ultrasound Penetrable Synthetic Substitute, Skull XNR80D9
Ultrasound Therapy
Heart 6A75
No Qualifier 6A75
Vessels
Head and Neck 6A75
Other 6A75
Peripheral 6A75
Ultraviolet Light Therapy, Skin 6A80
Umbilical artery
use Internal Iliac Artery, Right
use Internal Iliac Artery, Left
use Lower Artery
Uniplanar external fixator
use External Fixation Device, Monoplanar in 0PH
use External Fixation Device, Monoplanar in 0PS
use External Fixation Device, Monoplanar in 0QH
use External Fixation Device, Monoplanar in 0QS
UPLIZNA® *use* Inebilizumab-cdon
Upper GI series *see* Fluoroscopy, Gastrointestinal, Upper BD15
Ureteral orifice
use Ureter, Left
use Ureter
use Ureter, Right
use Ureters, Bilateral
Ureterectomy
see Excision, Urinary System 0TB
see Resection, Urinary System 0TT
Ureterocolostomy *see* Bypass, Urinary System 0T1
Ureterocystostomy *see* Bypass, Urinary System 0T1
Ureteroenterostomy *see* Bypass, Urinary System 0T1
Ureteroileostomy *see* Bypass, Urinary System 0T1
Ureterolithotomy *see* Extirpation, Urinary System 0TC
Ureterolysis *see* Release, Urinary System 0TN
Ureteroneocystostomy
see Bypass, Urinary System 0T1
see Reposition, Urinary System 0TS
Ureteropelvic junction (UPJ)
use Kidney Pelvis, Right
use Kidney Pelvis, Left
Ureteropexy
see Repair, Urinary System 0TQ
see Reposition, Urinary System 0TS
Ureteroplasty
see Repair, Urinary System 0TQ
see Replacement, Urinary System 0TR
see Supplement, Urinary System 0TU
Ureteroplication *see* Restriction, Urinary System 0TV
Ureteropyelography *see* Fluoroscopy, Urinary System BT1
Ureterorrhaphy *see* Repair, Urinary System 0TQ
Ureteroscopy 0TJ98ZZ
Ureterostomy
see Bypass, Urinary System 0T1
see Drainage, Urinary System 0T9
Ureterotomy *see* Drainage, Urinary System 0T9
Ureteroureterostomy *see* Bypass, Urinary System 0T1
Ureterovesical orifice
use Ureter, Right
use Ureter, Left
use Ureters, Bilateral
use Ureter
Urethral catheterization, indwelling 0T9B70Z
Urethrectomy
see Excision, Urethra 0TBD
see Resection, Urethra 0TTD
Urethrolithotomy *see* Extirpation, Urethra 0TCD
Urethrolysis *see* Release, Urethra 0TND
Urethropexy
see Repair, Urethra 0TQD
see Reposition, Urethra 0TSD
Urethroplasty
see Repair, Urethra 0TQD
see Replacement, Urethra 0TRD
see Supplement, Urethra 0TUD
Urethrorrhaphy *see* Repair, Urethra 0TQD
Urethroscopy 0TJD8ZZ
Urethrotomy *see* Drainage, Urethra 0T9D
Uridine Triacetate XW0DX82
Urinary incontinence stimulator lead *use* Stimulator Lead in Urinary System
Urography *see* Fluoroscopy, Urinary System BT1
Ustekinumab *use* Other New Technology Therapeutic Substance
Uterine Artery
use Internal Iliac Artery, Right
use Internal Iliac Artery, Left
Uterine artery embolization (UAE) *see* Occlusion, Lower Arteries 04L
Uterine cornu *use* Uterus
Uterine tube
use Fallopian Tube, Right
use Fallopian Tube, Left
Uterine vein
use Hypogastric Vein, Right
use Hypogastric Vein, Left
Uvulectomy
see Excision, Uvula 0CBN
see Resection, Uvula 0CTN
Uvulorrhaphy *see* Repair, Uvula 0CQN
Uvulotomy *see* Drainage, Uvula 0C9N

U

V

V-Wave Interatrial Shunt System *use* Synthetic Substitute
Vabomere™ *use* Meropenem-vaborbactam Anti-infective
Vaccination *see* Introduction of Serum, Toxoid, and Vaccine
Vacuum extraction, obstetric 10D07Z6
Vaginal artery
use Internal Iliac Artery, Right
use Internal Iliac Artery, Left
Vaginal pessary *use* Intraluminal Device, Pessary in Female Reproductive System
Vaginal vein
use Hypogastric Vein, Right
use Hypogastric Vein, Left
Vaginectomy
see Excision, Vagina 0UBG
see Resection, Vagina 0UTG
Vaginofixation
see Repair, Vagina 0UQG
see Reposition, Vagina 0USG
Vaginoplasty
see Repair, Vagina 0UQG
see Supplement, Vagina 0UUG
Vaginorrhaphy *see* Repair, Vagina 0UQG
Vaginoscopy 0UJH8ZZ
Vaginotomy *see* Drainage, Female Reproductive System 0U9
Vagotomy *see* Division, Nerve, Vagus 008Q
Valiant Thoracic Stent Graft *use* Intraluminal Device
Valvotomy, valvulotomy
see Division, Heart and Great Vessels 028
see Release, Heart and Great Vessels 02N
Valvuloplasty
see Repair, Heart and Great Vessels 02Q
see Replacement, Heart and Great Vessels 02R
see Supplement, Heart and Great Vessels 02U
Valvuloplasty, Alfieri Stitch *see* Restriction, Valve, Mitral 02VG
Vanta™ PC neurostimulator *use* Stimulator Generator, Multiple Array in 0JH
Vascular Access Device
Totally Implantable
Insertion of device in
Abdomen 0JH8
Chest 0JH6
Lower Arm
Left 0JHH
Right 0JHG
Lower Leg
Left 0JHP
Right 0JHN
Upper Arm
Left 0JHF
Right 0JHD
Upper Leg
Left 0JHM
Right 0JHL
Removal of device from
Lower Extremity 0JPW
Trunk 0JPT
Upper Extremity 0JPV
Revision of device in
Lower Extremity 0JWW
Trunk 0JWT
Upper Extremity 0JWV
Tunneled
Insertion of device in
Abdomen 0JH8
Chest 0JH6
Lower Arm
Left 0JHH
Right 0JHG
Lower Leg
Left 0JHP
Right 0JHN
Vascular Access Device *(Continued)*
Tunneled *(Continued)*
Insertion of device in *(Continued)*
Upper Arm
Left 0JHF
Right 0JHD
Upper Leg
Left 0JHM
Right 0JHL
Removal of device from
Lower Extremity 0JPW
Trunk 0JPT
Upper Extremity 0JPV
Revision of device in
Lower Extremity 0JWW
Trunk 0JWT
Upper Extremity 0JWV
Vasectomy *see* Excision, Male Reproductive System 0VB
Vasography
see Plain Radiography, Male Reproductive System BV0
see Fluoroscopy, Male Reproductive System BV1
Vasoligation *see* Occlusion, Male Reproductive System 0VL
Vasorrhaphy *see* Repair, Male Reproductive System 0VQ
Vasostomy *see* Bypass, Male Reproductive System 0V1
Vasotomy
Drainage *see* Drainage, Male Reproductive System 0V9
With ligation *see* Occlusion, Male Reproductive System 0VL
Vasovasostomy *see* Repair, Male Reproductive System 0VQ
VasQ™ External Support device *use* Synthetic Substitute, Extraluminal Support Device in New Technology
Vastus intermedius muscle
use Upper Leg Muscle, Right
use Upper Leg Muscle, Left
Vastus lateralis muscle
use Upper Leg Muscle, Right
use Upper Leg Muscle, Left
Vastus medialis muscle
use Upper Leg Muscle, Right
use Upper Leg Muscle, Left
VCG (vectorcardiogram) *see* Measurement, Cardiac 4A02
Vectra® Vascular Access Graft *use* Vascular Access Device, Tunneled in Subcutaneous Tissue and Fascia
Vein Graft Extraluminal Support Device(s), Supplement, Coronary Artery/Arteries X2U4079
Veklury *use* Remdesivir Anti-infective
Venclexta® *use* Venetoclax Antineoplastic
Venectomy
see Excision, Upper Veins 05B
see Excision, Lower Veins 06B
Venetoclax Antineoplastic XW0DXR5
Venography
see Plain Radiography, Veins B50
see Fluoroscopy, Veins B51
Venorrhaphy
see Repair, Upper Veins 05Q
see Repair, Lower Veins 06Q
Venotripsy
see Occlusion, Upper Veins 05L
see Occlusion, Lower Veins 06L
VenoValve® *use* Intraluminal Device, Bioprosthetic Valve in New Technology
Ventricular fold *use* Larynx
Ventriculoatriostomy *see* Bypass, Central Nervous System and Cranial Nerves 001
Ventriculocisternostomy *see* Bypass, Central Nervous System and Cranial Nerves 001
Ventriculogram, cardiac
Combined left and right heart *see* Fluoroscopy, Heart, Right and Left B216
Left ventricle *see* Fluoroscopy, Heart, Left B215
Right ventricle *see* Fluoroscopy, Heart, Right B214
Ventriculopuncture, through previously implanted catheter 8C01X6J
Ventriculoscopy 00J04ZZ
Ventriculostomy
External drainage *see* Drainage, Cerebral Ventricle 0096
Internal shunt *see* Bypass, Cerebral Ventricle 0016
Ventriculovenostomy *see* Bypass, Cerebral Ventricle 0016
Ventrio™ Hernia Patch *use* Synthetic Substitute
VEP (visual evoked potential) 4A07X0Z
Vermiform appendix *use* Appendix
Vermilion border
use Upper Lip
use Lower Lip
Versa *use* Pacemaker, Dual Chamber in 0JH
Version, obstetric
External 10S0XZZ
Internal 10S07ZZ
Vertebral arch
use Cervical Vertebra
use Thoracic Vertebra
use Lumbar Vertebra
Vertebral artery, intracranial portion *use* Intracranial Artery
Vertebral body
use Cervical Vertebra
use Thoracic Vertebra
use Lumbar Vertebra
Vertebral canal *use* Spinal Canal
Vertebral foramen
use Cervical Vertebra
use Thoracic Vertebra
use Lumbar Vertebra
Vertebral lamina
use Cervical Vertebra
use Thoracic Vertebra
use Lumbar Vertebra
Vertebral pedicle
use Cervical Vertebra
use Thoracic Vertebra
use Lumbar Vertebra
Vesical vein
use Hypogastric Vein, Right
use Hypogastric Vein, Left
Vesicotomy *see* Drainage, Urinary System 0T9
Vesiculectomy
see Excision, Male Reproductive System 0VB
see Resection, Male Reproductive System 0VT
Vesiculogram, seminal *see* Plain Radiography, Male Reproductive System BV0
Vesiculotomy *see* Drainage, Male Reproductive System 0V9
VEST™ Venous External Support device *use* Vein Graft Extraluminal Support Device(s) in New Technology
Vestibular (Scarpa's) ganglion *use* Acoustic Nerve
Vestibular Assessment F15Z
Vestibular nerve *use* Acoustic Nerve
Vestibular Treatment F0C
Vestibulocochlear nerve *use* Acoustic Nerve
VH-IVUS (virtual histology intravascular ultrasound) *see* Ultrasonography, Heart B24

New Revised ~~deleted~~ Deleted

Virchow's (supraclavicular) lymph node
  use Lymphatic, Right Neck
  use Lymphatic, Left Neck
Virtuoso (II) (DR) (VR) *use* Defibrillator Generator in 0JH
Vistogard® *use* Uridine Triacetate
Visualase™ MRI-Guided Laser Ablation System *see* Destruction
Vitrectomy
  see Excision, Eye 08B
  see Resection, Eye 08T
Vitreous body
  use Vitreous, Right
  use Vitreous, Left
Viva (XT)(S) *use* Cardiac Resynchronization Defibrillator Pulse Generator in 0JH
Vivistim® Paired VNS System Lead *use* Neurostimulator Lead with Paired Stimulation System in New Technology
Vocal fold
  use Vocal Cord, Right
  use Vocal Cord, Left
Vocational
  Assessment *see* Activities of Daily Living Assessment, Rehabilitation F02
  Retraining *see* Activities of Daily Living Treatment, Rehabilitation F08
Volar (palmar) digital vein
  use Hand Vein, Right
  use Hand Vein, Left
Volar (palmar) metacarpal vein
  use Hand Vein, Right
  use Hand Vein, Left
Vomer bone *use* Nasal Septum
Vomer of nasal septum *use* Nasal Bone
Voraxaze *use* Glucarpidase
Vulvectomy
  see Excision, Female Reproductive System 0UB
  see Resection, Female Reproductive System 0UT
VYXEOS™ *use* Cytarabine and Daunorubicin Liposome Antineoplastic

W

WALLSTENT® Endoprosthesis *use* Intraluminal Device
Washing *see* Irrigation
WavelinQ EndoAVF system
  Radial Artery, Left 031C3ZF
  Radial Artery, Right 031B3ZF
  Ulnar Artery, Left 031A3ZF
  Ulnar Artery, Right 03193ZF
Wedge resection, pulmonary *see* Excision, Respiratory System 0BB
Whole Blood Nucleic Acid-base Microbial Detection XXE5XM5
Whole Blood Reverse Transcription and Quantitative Real-time Polymerase Chain Reaction XXE5X38
Window *see* Drainage
Wiring, dental 2W31X9Z

X

Xact Carotid Stent System *use* Intraluminal Device
XENLETA™ *use* Lefamulin Anti-infective
X-ray *see* Plain Radiography
X-Spine Axle Cage
  use Spinal Stabilization Device, Interspinous Process in 0RH
  use Spinal Stabilization Device, Interspinous Process in 0SH
X-STOP® Spacer
  use Spinal Stabilization Device, Interspinous Process in 0RH
  use Spinal Stabilization Device, Interspinous Process in 0SH
Xenograft *use* Zooplastic Tissue in Heart and Great Vessels
XENOVIEW™ BB34Z3Z
XIENCE Everolimus Eluting Coronary Stent System *use* Intraluminal Device, Drug-eluting in Heart and Great Vessels
Xiphoid process *use* Sternum
XLIF® System *use* Interbody Fusion Device in Lower Joints
XOSPATA® *use* Gilteritinib Antineoplastic

Y

Yescarta® *use* Axicabtagene Ciloleucel Immunotherapy
Yoga Therapy 8E0ZXY4

Z

Z-plasty, skin for scar contracture *see* Release, Skin and Breast 0HN
Zenith AAA Endovascular Graft
  use Intraluminal Device
Zenith® Fenestrated AAA Endovascular Graft
  use Intraluminal Device, Branched or Fenestrated, One or Two Arteries in 04V
  use Intraluminal Device, Branched or Fenestrated, Three or More Arteries in 04V
Zenith Flex® AAA Endovascular Graft *use* Intraluminal Device
Zenith® Renu™ AAA Ancillary Graft *use* Intraluminal Device
Zenith TX2® TAA Endovascular Graft *use* Intraluminal Device
ZEPZELCA™ *use* Lurbinectedin
ZERBAXA® *use* Ceftolozane/Tazobactam Anti-infective
Zilver® PTX® (paclitaxel) Drug-Eluting Peripheral Stent
  use Intraluminal Device, Drug-eluting in Upper Arteries
  use Intraluminal Device, Drug-eluting in Lower Arteries
Zimmer® NexGen® LPS Mobile Bearing Knee
  use Synthetic Substitute
Zimmer® NexGen® LPS-Flex Mobile Knee *use* Synthetic Substitute
ZINPLAVA™ infusion *see* Introduction with qualifier Other Therapeutic Monoclonal Antibody
Zonule of Zinn
  use Lens, Right
  use Lens, Left
Zotarolimus-eluting coronary stent *use* Intraluminal Device, Drug-eluting in Heart and Great Vessels
ZULRESSO™ *use* Brexanolone
Zygomatic process of frontal bone *use* Frontal Bone
Zygomatic process of temporal bone
  use Temporal Bone, Right
  use Temporal Bone, Left
Zygomaticus muscle *use* Facial Muscle
▶ ZYNTEGLO® *use* Betibeglogene Autotemcel
Zyvox *use* Oxazolidinones

Z

KEYS

Appendices

Appendix A

DEFINITIONS

SECTION-CHARACTER

SECTION Ø - MEDICAL AND SURGICAL
CHARACTER 3 - OPERATION

Alteration	**Definition:** Modifying the anatomic structure of a body part without affecting the function of the body part **Explanation:** Principal purpose is to improve appearance **Includes/Examples:** Face lift, breast augmentation
Bypass	**Definition:** Altering the route of passage of the contents of a tubular body part **Explanation:** Rerouting contents of a body part to a downstream area of the normal route, to a similar route and body part, or to an abnormal route and dissimilar body part. Includes one or more anastomoses, with or without the use of a device **Includes/Examples:** Coronary artery bypass, colostomy formation
Change	**Definition:** Taking out or off a device from a body part and putting back an identical or similar device in or on the same body part without cutting or puncturing the skin or a mucous membrane **Explanation:** All CHANGE procedures are coded using the approach EXTERNAL **Includes/Examples:** Urinary catheter change, gastrostomy tube change
Control	**Definition:** Stopping, or attempting to stop, postprocedural or other acute bleeding **Includes/Examples:** Control of post-prostatectomy hemorrhage, control of intracranial subdural hemorrhage, control of bleeding duodenal ulcer, control of retroperitoneal hemorrhage
Creation	**Definition:** Putting in or on biological or synthetic material to form a new body part that to the extent possible replicates the anatomic structure or function of an absent body part **Explanation:** Used for gender reassignment surgery and corrective procedures in individuals with congenital anomalies **Includes/Examples:** Creation of vagina in a male, creation of right and left atrioventricular valve from common atrioventricular valve
Destruction	**Definition:** Physical eradication of all or a portion of a body part by the direct use of energy, force, or a destructive agent **Explanation:** None of the body part is physically taken out **Includes/Examples:** Fulguration of rectal polyp, cautery of skin lesion

Detachment	**Definition:** Cutting off all or a portion of the upper or lower extremities **Explanation:** The body part value is the site of the detachment, with a qualifier if applicable to further specify the level where the extremity was detached **Includes/Examples:** Below knee amputation, disarticulation of shoulder
Dilation	**Definition:** Expanding an orifice or the lumen of a tubular body part **Explanation:** The orifice can be a natural orifice or an artificially created orifice. Accomplished by stretching a tubular body part using intraluminal pressure or by cutting part of the orifice or wall of the tubular body part **Includes/Examples:** Percutaneous transluminal angioplasty, internal urethrotomy
Division	**Definition:** Cutting into a body part, without draining fluids and/or gases from the body part, in order to separate or transect a body part **Explanation:** All or a portion of the body part is separated into two or more portions **Includes/Examples:** Spinal cordotomy, osteotomy
Drainage	**Definition:** Taking or letting out fluids and/or gases from a body part **Explanation:** The qualifier DIAGNOSTIC is used to identify drainage procedures that are biopsies **Includes/Examples:** Thoracentesis, incision and drainage
Excision	**Definition:** Cutting out or off, without replacement, a portion of a body part **Explanation:** The qualifier DIAGNOSTIC is used to identify excision procedures that are biopsies **Includes/Examples:** Partial nephrectomy, liver biopsy
Extirpation	**Definition:** Taking or cutting out solid matter from a body part **Explanation:** The solid matter may be an abnormal byproduct of a biological function or a foreign body; it may be imbedded in a body part or in the lumen of a tubular body part. The solid matter may or may not have been previously broken into pieces **Includes/Examples:** Thrombectomy, choledocholithotomy
Extraction	**Definition:** Pulling or stripping out or off all or a portion of a body part by the use of force **Explanation:** The qualifier DIAGNOSTIC is used to identify extraction procedures that are biopsies **Includes/Examples:** Dilation and curettage, vein stripping

SECTION Ø - MEDICAL AND SURGICAL
CHARACTER 3 - OPERATION

Fragmentation	**Definition:** Breaking solid matter in a body part into pieces **Explanation:** Physical force (e.g., manual, ultrasonic) applied directly or indirectly is used to break the solid matter into pieces. The solid matter may be an abnormal byproduct of a biological function or a foreign body. The pieces of solid matter are not taken out **Includes/Examples:** Extracorporeal shockwave lithotripsy, transurethral lithotripsy
Fusion	**Definition:** Joining together portions of an articular body part rendering the articular body part immobile **Explanation:** The body part is joined together by fixation device, bone graft, or other means **Includes/Examples:** Spinal fusion, ankle arthrodesis
Insertion	**Definition:** Putting in a nonbiological appliance that monitors, assists, performs, or prevents a physiological function but does not physically take the place of a body part **Includes/Examples:** Insertion of radioactive implant, insertion of central venous catheter
Inspection	**Definition:** Visually and/or manually exploring a body part **Explanation:** Visual exploration may be performed with or without optical instrumentation. Manual exploration may be performed directly or through intervening body layers **Includes/Examples:** Diagnostic arthroscopy, exploratory laparotomy
Map	**Definition:** Locating the route of passage of electrical impulses and/or locating functional areas in a body part **Explanation:** Applicable only to the cardiac conduction mechanism and the central nervous system **Includes/Examples:** Cardiac mapping, cortical mapping
Occlusion	**Definition:** Completely closing an orifice or the lumen of a tubular body part **Explanation:** The orifice can be a natural orifice or an artificially created orifice **Includes/Examples:** Fallopian tube ligation, ligation of inferior vena cava
Reattachment	**Definition:** Putting back in or on all or a portion of a separated body part to its normal location or other suitable location **Explanation:** Vascular circulation and nervous pathways may or may not be reestablished **Includes/Examples:** Reattachment of hand, reattachment of avulsed kidney
Release	**Definition:** Freeing a body part from an abnormal physical constraint by cutting or by the use of force **Explanation:** Some of the restraining tissue may be taken out but none of the body part is taken out **Includes/Examples:** Adhesiolysis, carpal tunnel release
Removal	**Definition:** Taking out or off a device from a body part **Explanation:** If a device is taken out and a similar device put in without cutting or puncturing the skin or mucous membrane, the procedure is coded to the root operation CHANGE. Otherwise, the procedure for taking out a device is coded to the root operation REMOVAL **Includes/Examples:** Drainage tube removal, cardiac pacemaker removal
Repair	**Definition:** Restoring, to the extent possible, a body part to its normal anatomic structure and function **Explanation:** Used only when the method to accomplish the repair is not one of the other root operations **Includes/Examples:** Colostomy takedown, suture of laceration
Replacement	**Definition:** Putting in or on biological or synthetic material that physically takes the place and/or function of all or a portion of a body part **Explanation:** The body part may have been taken out or replaced, or may be taken out, physically eradicated, or rendered nonfunctional during the Replacement procedure. A Removal procedure is coded for taking out the device used in a previous replacement procedure **Includes/Examples:** Total hip replacement, bone graft, free skin graft
Reposition	**Definition:** Moving to its normal location, or other suitable location, all or a portion of a body part **Explanation:** The body part is moved to a new location from an abnormal location, or from a normal location where it is not functioning correctly. The body part may or may not be cut out or off to be moved to the new location **Includes/Examples:** Reposition of undescended testicle, fracture reduction
Resection	**Definition:** Cutting out or off, without replacement, all of a body part **Includes/Examples:** Total nephrectomy, total lobectomy of lung

SECTION Ø - MEDICAL AND SURGICAL
CHARACTER 3 - OPERATION

Restriction	**Definition:** Partially closing an orifice or the lumen of a tubular body part **Explanation:** The orifice can be a natural orifice or an artificially created orifice **Includes/Examples:** Esophagogastric fundoplication, cervical cerclage
Revision	**Definition:** Correcting, to the extent possible, a portion of a malfunctioning device or the position of a displaced device **Explanation:** Revision can include correcting a malfunctioning or displaced device by taking out or putting in components of the device such as a screw or pin **Includes/Examples:** Adjustment of position of pacemaker lead, recementing of hip prosthesis
Supplement	**Definition:** Putting in or on biological or synthetic material that physically reinforces and/or augments the function of a portion of a body part **Explanation:** The biological material is non-living, or is living and from the same individual. The body part may have been previously replaced, and the Supplement procedure is performed to physically reinforce and/or augment the function of the replaced body part **Includes/Examples:** Herniorrhaphy using mesh, mitral valve ring annuloplasty, put a new acetabular liner in a previous hip replacement
Transfer	**Definition:** Moving, without taking out, all or a portion of a body part to another location to take over the function of all or a portion of a body part **Explanation:** The body part transferred remains connected to its vascular and nervous supply **Includes/Examples:** Tendon transfer, skin pedicle flap transfer
Transplantation	**Definition:** Putting in or on all or a portion of a living body part taken from another individual or animal to physically take the place and/or function of all or a portion of a similar body part **Explanation:** The native body part may or may not be taken out, and the transplanted body part may take over all or a portion of its function **Includes/Examples:** Kidney transplant, heart transplant

SECTION Ø - MEDICAL AND SURGICAL
CHARACTER 4 - BODY PART

1st Toe, Left 1st Toe, Right	**Includes:** Hallux
Abdomen Muscle, Left Abdomen Muscle, Right	**Includes:** External oblique muscle Internal oblique muscle Pyramidalis muscle Rectus abdominis muscle Transversus abdominis muscle
Abdominal Aorta	**Includes:** Inferior phrenic artery Lumbar artery Median sacral artery Middle suprarenal artery Ovarian artery Testicular artery
Abdominal Sympathetic Nerve	**Includes:** Abdominal aortic plexus Auerbach's (myenteric) plexus Celiac (solar) plexus Celiac ganglion Gastric plexus Hepatic plexus Inferior hypogastric plexus Inferior mesenteric ganglion Inferior mesenteric plexus Meissner's (submucous) plexus Myenteric (Auerbach's) plexus Pancreatic plexus Pelvic splanchnic nerve Renal nerve Renal plexus Solar (celiac) plexus Splenic plexus Submucous (Meissner's) plexus Superior hypogastric plexus Superior mesenteric ganglion Superior mesenteric plexus Suprarenal plexus

SECTION Ø - MEDICAL AND SURGICAL
CHARACTER 4 - BODY PART

Abducens Nerve	**Includes:** Sixth cranial nerve
Accessory Nerve	**Includes:** Eleventh cranial nerve
Acoustic Nerve	**Includes:** Cochlear nerve Eighth cranial nerve Scarpa's (vestibular) ganglion Spiral ganglion Vestibular (Scarpa's) ganglion Vestibular nerve Vestibulocochlear nerve
Adenoids	**Includes:** Pharyngeal tonsil
Adrenal Gland Adrenal Gland, Left Adrenal Gland, Right Adrenal Glands, Bilateral	**Includes:** Suprarenal gland
Ampulla of Vater	**Includes:** Duodenal ampulla Hepatopancreatic ampulla
Anal Sphincter	**Includes:** External anal sphincter Internal anal sphincter
Ankle Bursa and Ligament, Left Ankle Bursa and Ligament, Right	**Includes:** Calcaneofibular ligament Deltoid ligament Ligament of the lateral malleolus Talofibular ligament
Ankle Joint, Left Ankle Joint, Right	**Includes:** Inferior tibiofibular joint Talocrural joint
Anterior Chamber, Left Anterior Chamber, Right	**Includes:** Aqueous humour
Anterior Tibial Artery, Left Anterior Tibial Artery, Right	**Includes:** Anterior lateral malleolar artery Anterior medial malleolar artery Anterior tibial recurrent artery Dorsalis pedis artery Posterior tibial recurrent artery
Anus	**Includes:** Anal orifice

Aortic Valve	**Includes:** Aortic annulus
Appendix	**Includes:** Vermiform appendix
Atrial Septum	**Includes:** Interatrial septum
Atrium, Left	**Includes:** Atrium pulmonale Left auricular appendix
Atrium, Right	**Includes:** Atrium dextrum cordis Right auricular appendix Sinus venosus
Auditory Ossicle, Left Auditory Ossicle, Right	**Includes:** Incus Malleus Stapes
Axillary Artery, Left Axillary Artery, Right	**Includes:** Anterior circumflex humeral artery Lateral thoracic artery Posterior circumflex humeral artery Subscapular artery Superior thoracic artery Thoracoacromial artery
Azygos Vein	**Includes:** Right ascending lumbar vein Right subcostal vein
Basal Ganglia	**Includes:** Basal nuclei Claustrum Corpus striatum Globus pallidus Substantia nigra Subthalamic nucleus
Basilic Vein, Left Basilic Vein, Right	**Includes:** Median antebrachial vein Median cubital vein
Bladder	**Includes:** Trigone of bladder
Brachial Artery, Left Brachial Artery, Right	**Includes:** Inferior ulnar collateral artery Profunda brachii Superior ulnar collateral artery

SECTION Ø - MEDICAL AND SURGICAL

CHARACTER 4 - BODY PART

Brachial Plexus	**Includes:** Axillary nerve Dorsal scapular nerve First intercostal nerve Long thoracic nerve Musculocutaneous nerve Subclavius nerve Suprascapular nerve
Brachial Vein, Left Brachial Vein, Right	**Includes:** Radial vein Ulnar vein
Brain	**Includes:** Cerebrum Corpus callosum Encephalon
Breast, Bilateral Breast, Left Breast, Right	**Includes:** Mammary duct Mammary gland
Buccal Mucosa	**Includes:** Buccal gland Molar gland Palatine gland
Carotid Bodies, Bilateral Carotid Body, Left Carotid Body, Right	**Includes:** Carotid glomus
Carpal Joint, Left Carpal Joint, Right	**Includes:** Intercarpal joint Midcarpal joint
Carpal, Left Carpal, Right	**Includes:** Capitate bone Hamate bone Lunate bone Pisiform bone Scaphoid bone Trapezium bone Trapezoid bone Triquetral bone
Celiac Artery	**Includes:** Celiac trunk
Cephalic Vein, Left Cephalic Vein, Right	**Includes:** Accessory cephalic vein
Cerebellum	**Includes:** Culmen
Cerebral Hemisphere	**Includes:** Frontal lobe Occipital lobe Parietal lobe Temporal lobe
Cerebral Meninges	**Includes:** Arachnoid mater, intracranial Leptomeninges, intracranial Pia mater, intracranial
Cerebral Ventricle	**Includes:** Aqueduct of Sylvius Cerebral aqueduct (Sylvius) Choroid plexus Ependyma Foramen of Monro (intraventricular) Fourth ventricle Interventricular foramen (Monro) Left lateral ventricle Right lateral ventricle Third ventricle
Cervical Nerve	**Includes:** Greater occipital nerve Spinal nerve, cervical Suboccipital nerve Third occipital nerve
Cervical Plexus	**Includes:** Ansa cervicalis Cutaneous (transverse) cervical nerve Great auricular nerve Lesser occipital nerve Supraclavicular nerve Transverse (cutaneous) cervical nerve
Cervical Spinal Cord	**Includes:** Dorsal root ganglion
Cervical Vertebra	**Includes:** Dens Odontoid process Spinous process Transverse foramen Transverse process Vertebral body Vertebral arch Vertebral foramen Vertebral lamina Vertebral pedicle
Cervical Vertebral Joint	**Includes:** Atlantoaxial joint Cervical facet joint
Cervical Vertebral Joints, 2 or more	**Includes:** Cervical facet joint
Cervicothoracic Vertebral Joint	**Includes:** Cervicothoracic facet joint
Cisterna Chyli	**Includes:** Intestinal lymphatic trunk Lumbar lymphatic trunk

APPENDIX A

SECTION Ø - MEDICAL AND SURGICAL
CHARACTER 4 - BODY PART

Coccygeal Glomus	**Includes:** Coccygeal body
Colic Vein	**Includes:** Ileocolic vein Left colic vein Middle colic vein Right colic vein
Conduction Mechanism	**Includes:** Atrioventricular node Bundle of His Bundle of Kent Sinoatrial node
Conjunctiva, Left Conjunctiva, Right	**Includes:** Plica semilunaris
Dura Mater	**Includes:** Diaphragma sellae Dura mater, intracranial Falx cerebri Tentorium cerebelli
Elbow Bursa and Ligament, Left Elbow Bursa and Ligament, Right	**Includes:** Annular ligament Olecranon bursa Radial collateral ligament Ulnar collateral ligament
Elbow Joint, Left Elbow Joint, Right	**Includes:** Distal humerus, involving joint Humeroradial joint Humeroulnar joint Proximal radioulnar joint
Epidural Space, Intracranial	**Includes:** Extradural space, intracranial
Epiglottis	**Includes:** Glossoepiglottic fold
Esophagogastric Junction	**Includes:** Cardia Cardioesophageal junction Gastroesophageal (GE) junction
Esophagus, Lower	**Includes:** Abdominal esophagus
Esophagus, Middle	**Includes:** Thoracic esophagus
Esophagus, Upper	**Includes:** Cervical esophagus
Ethmoid Bone, Left Ethmoid Bone, Right	**Includes:** Cribriform plate

Ethmoid Sinus, Left Ethmoid Sinus, Right	**Includes:** Ethmoidal air cell
Eustachian Tube, Left Eustachian Tube, Right	**Includes:** Auditory tube Pharyngotympanic tube
External Auditory Canal, Left External Auditory Canal, Right	**Includes:** External auditory meatus
External Carotid Artery, Left External Carotid Artery, Right	**Includes:** Ascending pharyngeal artery Internal maxillary artery Lingual artery Maxillary artery Occipital artery Posterior auricular artery Superior thyroid artery
External Ear, Bilateral External Ear, Left External Ear, Right	**Includes:** Antihelix Antitragus Auricle Earlobe Helix Pinna Tragus
External Iliac Artery, Left External Iliac Artery, Right	**Includes:** Deep circumflex iliac artery Inferior epigastric artery
External Jugular Vein, Left External Jugular Vein, Right	**Includes:** Posterior auricular vein
Extraocular Muscle, Left Extraocular Muscle, Right	**Includes:** Inferior oblique muscle Inferior rectus muscle Lateral rectus muscle Medial rectus muscle Superior oblique muscle Superior rectus muscle
Eye, Left Eye, Right	**Includes:** Ciliary body Posterior chamber
Face Artery	**Includes:** Angular artery Ascending palatine artery External maxillary artery Facial artery Inferior labial artery Submental artery Superior labial artery

SECTION Ø - MEDICAL AND SURGICAL
CHARACTER 4 - BODY PART

Face Vein, Left Face Vein, Right	**Includes:** Angular vein Anterior facial vein Common facial vein Deep facial vein Frontal vein Posterior facial (retromandibular) vein Supraorbital vein
Facial Muscle	**Includes:** Buccinator muscle Corrugator supercilii muscle Depressor anguli oris muscle Depressor labii inferioris muscle Depressor septi nasi muscle Depressor supercilii muscle Levator anguli oris muscle Levator labii superioris alaeque nasi muscle Levator labii superioris muscle Mentalis muscle Nasalis muscle Occipitofrontalis muscle Orbicularis oris muscle Procerus muscle Risorius muscle Zygomaticus muscle
Facial Nerve	**Includes:** Chorda tympani Geniculate ganglion Greater superficial petrosal nerve Nerve to the stapedius Parotid plexus Posterior auricular nerve Seventh cranial nerve Submandibular ganglion
Fallopian Tube, Left Fallopian Tube, Right	**Includes:** Oviduct Salpinx Uterine tube
Femoral Artery, Left Femoral Artery, Right	**Includes:** Circumflex iliac artery Deep femoral artery Descending genicular artery External pudendal artery Superficial epigastric artery
Femoral Nerve	**Includes:** Anterior crural nerve Saphenous nerve
Femoral Shaft, Left Femoral Shaft, Right	**Includes:** Body of femur
Femoral Vein, Left Femoral Vein, Right	**Includes:** Deep femoral (profunda femoris) vein Popliteal vein Profunda femoris (deep femoral) vein
Fibula, Left Fibula, Right	**Includes:** Body of fibula Head of fibula Lateral malleolus
Finger Nail	**Includes:** Nail bed Nail plate
Finger Phalangeal Joint, Left Finger Phalangeal Joint, Right	**Includes:** Interphalangeal (IP) joint
Foot Artery, Left Foot Artery, Right	**Includes:** Arcuate artery Dorsal metatarsal artery Lateral plantar artery Lateral tarsal artery Medial plantar artery
Foot Bursa and Ligament, Left Foot Bursa and Ligament, Right	**Includes:** Calcaneocuboid ligament Cuneonavicular ligament Intercuneiform ligament Interphalangeal ligament Metatarsal ligament Metatarsophalangeal ligament Subtalar ligament Talocalcaneal ligament Talocalcaneonavicular ligament Tarsometatarsal ligament
Foot Muscle, Left Foot Muscle, Right	**Includes:** Abductor hallucis muscle Adductor hallucis muscle Extensor digitorum brevis muscle Extensor hallucis brevis muscle Flexor digitorum brevis muscle Flexor hallucis brevis muscle Quadratus plantae muscle
Foot Vein, Left Foot Vein, Right	**Includes:** Common digital vein Dorsal metatarsal vein Dorsal venous arch Plantar digital vein Plantar metatarsal vein Plantar venous arch
Frontal Bone	**Includes:** Zygomatic process of frontal bone

SECTION Ø - MEDICAL AND SURGICAL
CHARACTER 4 - BODY PART

Gastric Artery	**Includes:** Left gastric artery Right gastric artery
Glenoid Cavity, Left Glenoid Cavity, Right	**Includes:** Glenoid fossa (of scapula)
Glomus Jugulare	**Includes:** Jugular body
Glossopharyngeal Nerve	**Includes:** Carotid sinus nerve Ninth cranial nerve Tympanic nerve
Hand Artery, Left Hand Artery, Right	**Includes:** Deep palmar arch Princeps pollicis artery Radialis indicis Superficial palmar arch
Hand Bursa and Ligament, Left Hand Bursa and Ligament, Right	**Includes:** Carpometacarpal ligament Intercarpal ligament Interphalangeal ligament Lunotriquetral ligament Metacarpal ligament Metacarpophalangeal ligament Pisohamate ligament Pisometacarpal ligament Scaphotrapezium ligament
Hand Muscle, Left Hand Muscle, Right	**Includes:** Hypothenar muscle Palmar interosseous muscle Thenar muscle
Hand Vein, Left Hand Vein, Right	**Includes:** Dorsal metacarpal vein Palmar (volar) digital vein Palmar (volar) metacarpal vein Superficial palmar venous arch Volar (palmar) digital vein Volar (palmar) metacarpal vein
Head and Neck Bursa and Ligament	**Includes:** Alar ligament of axis Cervical interspinous ligament Cervical intertransverse ligament Cervical ligamentum flavum Interspinous ligament, cervical Intertransverse ligament, cervical Lateral temporomandibular ligament Ligamentum flavum, cervical Sphenomandibular ligament Stylomandibular ligament Transverse ligament of atlas
Head and Neck Sympathetic Nerve	**Includes:** Cavernous plexus Cervical ganglion Ciliary ganglion Internal carotid plexus Otic ganglion Pterygopalatine (sphenopalatine) ganglion Sphenopalatine (pterygopalatine) ganglion Stellate ganglion Submandibular ganglion Submaxillary ganglion
Head Muscle	**Includes:** Auricularis muscle Masseter muscle Pterygoid muscle Splenius capitis muscle Temporalis muscle Temporoparietalis muscle
Heart, Left	**Includes:** Left coronary sulcus Obtuse margin
Heart, Right	**Includes:** Right coronary sulcus
Hemiazygos Vein	**Includes** Left ascending lumbar vein Left subcostal vein
Hepatic Artery	**Includes:** Common hepatic artery Gastroduodenal artery Hepatic artery proper
Hip Bursa and Ligament, Left Hip Bursa and Ligament, Right	**Includes:** Iliofemoral ligament Ischiofemoral ligament Pubofemoral ligament Transverse acetabular ligament Trochanteric bursa
Hip Joint, Left Hip Joint, Right	**Includes:** Acetabulofemoral joint
Hip Muscle, Left Hip Muscle, Right	**Includes:** Gemellus muscle Gluteus maximus muscle Gluteus medius muscle Gluteus minimus muscle Iliacus muscle Obturator muscle Piriformis muscle Psoas muscle Quadratus femoris muscle Tensor fasciae latae muscle

SECTION Ø - MEDICAL AND SURGICAL
CHARACTER 4 - BODY PART

Humeral Head, Left Humeral Head, Right	**Includes:** Greater tuberosity Lesser tuberosity Neck of humerus (anatomical) (surgical)
Humeral Shaft, Left Humeral Shaft, Right	**Includes:** Distal humerus Humerus, distal Lateral epicondyle of humerus Medial epicondyle of humerus
Hypogastric Vein, Left Hypogastric Vein, Right	**Includes:** Gluteal vein Internal iliac vein Internal pudendal vein Lateral sacral vein Middle hemorrhoidal vein Obturator vein Uterine vein Vaginal vein Vesical vein
Hypoglossal Nerve	**Includes:** Twelfth cranial nerve
Hypothalamus	**Includes:** Mammillary body
Inferior Mesenteric Artery	**Includes:** Sigmoid artery Superior rectal artery
Inferior Mesenteric Vein	**Includes:** Sigmoid vein Superior rectal vein
Inferior Vena Cava	**Includes:** Postcava Right inferior phrenic vein Right ovarian vein Right second lumbar vein Right suprarenal vein Right testicular vein
Inguinal Region, Bilateral Inguinal Region, Left Inguinal Region, Right	**Includes:** Inguinal canal Inguinal triangle
Inner Ear, Left Inner Ear, Right	**Includes:** Bony labyrinth Bony vestibule Cochlea Round window Semicircular canal
Innominate Artery	**Includes:** Brachiocephalic artery Brachiocephalic trunk
Innominate Vein, Left Innominate Vein, Right	**Includes:** Brachiocephalic vein Inferior thyroid vein
Internal Carotid Artery, Left Internal Carotid Artery, Right	**Includes:** Caroticotympanic artery Carotid sinus
Internal Iliac Artery, Left Internal Iliac Artery, Right	**Includes:** Deferential artery Hypogastric artery Iliolumbar artery Inferior gluteal artery Inferior vesical artery Internal pudendal artery Lateral sacral artery Middle rectal artery Obturator artery Superior gluteal artery Umbilical artery Uterine Artery Vaginal artery
Internal Mammary Artery, Left Internal Mammary Artery, Right	**Includes:** Anterior intercostal artery Internal thoracic artery Musculophrenic artery Pericardiophrenic artery Superior epigastric artery
Intracranial Artery	**Includes:** Anterior cerebral artery Anterior choroidal artery Anterior communicating artery Basilar artery Circle of Willis Internal carotid artery, intracranial portion Middle cerebral artery Middle meningeal artery, intracranial portion Ophthalmic artery Posterior cerebral artery Posterior communicating artery Posterior inferior cerebellar artery (PICA) Vertebral artery, intracranial portion

SECTION Ø - MEDICAL AND SURGICAL
CHARACTER 4 - BODY PART

Intracranial Vein	**Includes:** Anterior cerebral vein Basal (internal) cerebral vein Dural venous sinus Great cerebral vein Inferior cerebellar vein Inferior cerebral vein Internal (basal) cerebral vein Middle cerebral vein Ophthalmic vein Superior cerebellar vein Superior cerebral vein
Jejunum	**Includes:** Duodenojejunal flexure
Kidney	**Includes:** Renal calyx Renal capsule Renal cortex Renal segment
Kidney Pelvis, Left Kidney Pelvis, Right	**Includes:** Ureteropelvic junction (UPJ)
Kidney, Left Kidney, Right Kidneys, Bilateral	**Includes:** Renal calyx Renal capsule Renal cortex Renal segment
Knee Bursa and Ligament, Left Knee Bursa and Ligament, Right	**Includes:** Anterior cruciate ligament (ACL) Lateral collateral ligament (LCL) Ligament of head of fibula Medial collateral ligament (MCL) Patellar ligament Popliteal ligament Posterior cruciate ligament (PCL) Prepatellar bursa
Knee Joint, Femoral Surface, Left Knee Joint, Femoral Surface, Right	**Includes:** Femoropatellar joint Patellofemoral joint
Knee Joint, Left Knee Joint, Right	**Includes:** Femoropatellar joint Femorotibial joint Lateral meniscus Medial meniscus Patellofemoral joint Tibiofemoral joint
Knee Joint, Tibial Surface, Left Knee Joint, Tibial Surface, Right	**Includes:** Femorotibial joint Tibiofemoral joint
Knee Tendon, Left Knee Tendon, Right	**Includes:** Patellar tendon
Lacrimal Duct, Left Lacrimal Duct, Right	**Includes:** Lacrimal canaliculus Lacrimal punctum Lacrimal sac Nasolacrimal duct
Larynx	**Includes:** Aryepiglottic fold Arytenoid cartilage Corniculate cartilage Cuneiform cartilage False vocal cord Glottis Rima glottidis Thyroid cartilage Ventricular fold
Lens, Left Lens, Right	**Includes:** Zonule of Zinn
Liver	**Includes:** Quadrate lobe
Lower Arm and Wrist Muscle, Left Lower Arm and Wrist Muscle, Right	**Includes:** Anatomical snuffbox Brachioradialis muscle Extensor carpi radialis muscle Extensor carpi ulnaris muscle Flexor carpi radialis muscle Flexor carpi ulnaris muscle Flexor pollicis longus muscle Palmaris longus muscle Pronator quadratus muscle Pronator teres muscle
Lower Artery	**Includes:** Umbilical artery
Lower Eyelid, Left Lower Eyelid, Right	**Includes:** Inferior tarsal plate Medial canthus
Lower Femur, Left Lower Femur, Right	**Includes:** Lateral condyle of femur Lateral epicondyle of femur Medial condyle of femur Medial epicondyle of femur

SECTION Ø - MEDICAL AND SURGICAL

CHARACTER 4 - BODY PART

Lower Leg Muscle, Left Lower Leg Muscle, Right	**Includes:** Extensor digitorum longus muscle Extensor hallucis longus muscle Fibularis brevis muscle Fibularis longus muscle Flexor digitorum longus muscle Flexor hallucis longus muscle Gastrocnemius muscle Peroneus brevis muscle Peroneus longus muscle Popliteus muscle Soleus muscle Tibialis anterior muscle Tibialis posterior muscle
Lower Leg Tendon, Left Lower Leg Tendon, Right	**Includes:** Achilles tendon
Lower Lip	**Includes:** Frenulum labii inferioris Labial gland Vermilion border
Lower Spine Bursa and Ligament	**Includes:** Iliolumbar ligament Interspinous ligament, lumbar Intertransverse ligament, lumbar Ligamentum flavum, lumbar Sacrococcygeal ligament Sacroiliac ligament Sacrospinous ligament Sacrotuberous ligament Supraspinous ligament
Lumbar Nerve	**Includes:** Lumbosacral trunk Spinal nerve, lumbar Superior clunic (cluneal) nerve
Lumbar Plexus	**Includes:** Accessory obturator nerve Genitofemoral nerve Iliohypogastric nerve Ilioinguinal nerve Lateral femoral cutaneous nerve Obturator nerve Superior gluteal nerve
Lumbar Spinal Cord	**Includes:** Cauda equina Conus medullaris Dorsal root ganglion
Lumbar Sympathetic Nerve	**Includes:** Lumbar ganglion Lumbar splanchnic nerve
Lumbar Vertebra	**Includes:** Spinous process Transverse process Vertebral arch Vertebral body Vertebral foramen Vertebral lamina Vertebral pedicle
Lumbar Vertebral Joint	**Includes:** Lumbar facet joint
Lumbosacral Joint	**Includes:** Lumbosacral facet joint
Lymphatic, Aortic	**Includes:** Celiac lymph node Gastric lymph node Hepatic lymph node Lumbar lymph node Pancreaticosplenic lymph node Paraaortic lymph node Retroperitoneal lymph node
Lymphatic, Head	**Includes:** Buccinator lymph node Infraauricular lymph node Infraparotid lymph node Parotid lymph node Preauricular lymph node Submandibular lymph node Submaxillary lymph node Submental lymph node Subparotid lymph node Suprahyoid lymph node
Lymphatic, Left Axillary	**Includes:** Anterior (pectoral) lymph node Apical (subclavicular) lymph node Brachial (lateral) lymph node Central axillary lymph node Lateral (brachial) lymph node Pectoral (anterior) lymph node Posterior (subscapular) lymph node Subclavicular (apical) lymph node Subscapular (posterior) lymph node
Lymphatic, Left Lower Extremity	**Includes:** Femoral lymph node Popliteal lymph node
Lymphatic, Left Neck	**Includes:** Cervical lymph node Jugular lymph node Mastoid (postauricular) lymph node Occipital lymph node Postauricular (mastoid) lymph node Retropharyngeal lymph node Supraclavicular (Virchow's) lymph node Virchow's (supraclavicular) lymph node

SECTION Ø - MEDICAL AND SURGICAL
CHARACTER 4 - BODY PART

Lymphatic, Left Upper Extremity	**Includes:** Cubital lymph node Deltopectoral (infraclavicular) lymph node Epitrochlear lymph node Infraclavicular (deltopectoral) lymph node Supratrochlear lymph node
Lymphatic, Mesenteric	**Includes:** Inferior mesenteric lymph node Pararectal lymph node Superior mesenteric lymph node
Lymphatic, Pelvis	**Includes:** Common iliac (subaortic) lymph node Gluteal lymph node Iliac lymph node Inferior epigastric lymph node Obturator lymph node Sacral lymph node Subaortic (common iliac) lymph node Suprainguinal lymph node
Lymphatic, Right Axillary	**Includes:** Anterior (pectoral) lymph node Apical (subclavicular) lymph node Brachial (lateral) lymph node Central axillary lymph node Lateral (brachial) lymph node Pectoral (anterior) lymph node Posterior (subscapular) lymph node Subclavicular (apical) lymph node Subscapular (posterior) lymph node
Lymphatic, Right Lower Extremity	**Includes:** Femoral lymph node Popliteal lymph node
Lymphatic, Right Neck	**Includes:** Cervical lymph node Jugular lymph node Mastoid (postauricular) lymph node Occipital lymph node Postauricular (mastoid) lymph node Retropharyngeal lymph node Right jugular trunk Right lymphatic duct Right subclavian trunk Supraclavicular (Virchow's) lymph node Virchow's (supraclavicular) lymph node
Lymphatic, Right Upper Extremity	**Includes:** Cubital lymph node Deltopectoral (infraclavicular) lymph node Epitrochlear lymph node Infraclavicular (deltopectoral) lymph node Supratrochlear lymph node

Lymphatic, Thorax	**Includes:** Intercostal lymph node Mediastinal lymph node Parasternal lymph node Paratracheal lymph node Tracheobronchial lymph node
Main Bronchus, Right	**Includes:** Bronchus Intermedius Intermediate bronchus
Mandible, Left Mandible, Right	**Includes:** Alveolar process of mandible Condyloid process Mandibular notch Mental foramen
Mastoid Sinus, Left Mastoid Sinus, Right	**Includes:** Mastoid air cells
Maxilla	**Includes:** Alveolar process of maxilla
Maxillary Sinus, Left Maxillary Sinus, Right	**Includes:** Antrum of Highmore
Median Nerve	**Includes:** Anterior interosseous nerve Palmar cutaneous nerve
Mediastinum	**Includes:** Mediastinal cavity Mediastinal space
Medulla Oblongata	**Includes:** Myelencephalon
Mesentery	**Includes:** Mesoappendix Mesocolon
Metatarsal, Left Metatarsal, Right	**Includes:** Fibular sesamoid Tibial sesamoid
Metatarsal-Phalangeal Joint, Left Metatarsal-Phalangeal Joint, Right	**Includes:** Metatarsophalangeal (MTP) joint
Middle Ear, Left Middle Ear, Right	**Includes:** Oval window Tympanic cavity
Minor Salivary Gland	**Includes:** Anterior lingual gland

SECTION Ø - MEDICAL AND SURGICAL

CHARACTER 4 - BODY PART

Mitral Valve	**Includes:** Bicuspid valve Left atrioventricular valve Mitral annulus
Nasal Bone	**Includes:** Vomer of nasal septum
Nasal Mucosa and Soft Tissue	**Includes:** Columella External naris Greater alar cartilage Internal naris Lateral nasal cartilage Lesser alar cartilage Nasal cavity Nostril
Nasal Septum	**Includes:** Quadrangular cartilage Septal cartilage Vomer bone
Nasal Turbinate	**Includes:** Inferior turbinate Middle turbinate Nasal concha Superior turbinate
Nasopharynx	**Includes:** Choana Fossa of Rosenmuller Pharyngeal recess Rhinopharynx
Neck	**Includes:** Parapharyngeal space Retropharyngeal
Neck Muscle, Left Neck Muscle, Right	**Includes:** Anterior vertebral muscle Arytenoid muscle Cricothyroid muscle Infrahyoid muscle Levator scapulae muscle Platysma muscle Scalene muscle Splenius cervicis muscle Sternocleidomastoid muscle Suprahyoid muscle Thyroarytenoid muscle
Nipple, Left Nipple, Right	**Includes:** Areola
Occipital Bone	**Includes:** Foramen magnum
Oculomotor Nerve	**Includes:** Third cranial nerve
Olfactory Nerve	**Includes:** First cranial nerve Olfactory bulb

Omentum	**Includes:** Gastrocolic ligament Gastrocolic omentum Gastrohepatic omentum Gastrophrenic ligament Gastrosplenic ligament Greater omentum Hepatogastric ligament Lesser omentum
Optic Nerve	**Includes:** Optic chiasma Second cranial nerve
Orbit, Left Orbit, Right	**Includes:** Bony orbit Orbital portion of ethmoid bone Orbital portion of frontal bone Orbital portion of lacrimal bone Orbital portion of maxilla Orbital portion of palatine bone Orbital portion of sphenoid bone Orbital portion of zygomatic bone
Pancreatic Duct	**Includes:** Duct of Wirsung
Pancreatic Duct, Accessory	**Includes:** Duct of Santorini
Parotid Duct, Left Parotid Duct, Right	**Includes:** Stensen's duct
Pelvic Bone, Left Pelvic Bone, Right	**Includes:** Iliac crest Ilium Ischium Pubis
Pelvic Cavity	**Includes:** Retropubic space Space of Retzius
Penis	**Includes:** Corpus cavernosum Corpus spongiosum
Perineum Muscle	**Includes:** Bulbospongiosus muscle Cremaster muscle Deep transverse perineal muscle Ischiocavernosus muscle Levator ani muscle Superficial transverse perineal muscle
Peritoneum	**Includes:** Epiploic foramen
Peroneal Artery, Left Peroneal Artery, Right	**Includes:** Fibular artery

APPENDIX A

SECTION Ø - MEDICAL AND SURGICAL
CHARACTER 4 - BODY PART

Peroneal Nerve	**Includes:** Common fibular nerve Common peroneal nerve External popliteal nerve Lateral sural cutaneous nerve
Pharynx	**Includes:** Base of tongue Hypopharynx Laryngopharynx Lingual tonsil Oropharynx Piriform recess (sinus) Tongue, base of
Phrenic Nerve	**Includes:** Accessory phrenic nerve
Pituitary Gland	**Includes:** Adenohypophysis Hypophysis Neurohypophysis
Pons	**Includes:** Apneustic center Basis pontis Locus ceruleus Pneumotaxic center Pontine tegmentum Superior olivary nucleus
Popliteal Artery, Left Popliteal Artery, Right	**Includes:** Inferior genicular artery Middle genicular artery Superior genicular artery Sural artery Tibioperoneal trunk
Portal Vein	**Includes:** Hepatic portal vein
Prepuce	**Includes:** Foreskin Glans penis
Pudendal Nerve	**Includes:** Posterior labial nerve Posterior scrotal nerve
Pulmonary Artery, Left	**Includes:** Arterial canal (duct) Botallo's duct Pulmoaortic canal
Pulmonary Valve	**Includes:** Pulmonary annulus Pulmonic valve
Pulmonary Vein, Left	**Includes:** Left inferior pulmonary vein Left superior pulmonary vein
Pulmonary Vein, Right	**Includes:** Right inferior pulmonary vein Right superior pulmonary vein
Radial Artery, Left Radial Artery, Right	**Includes:** Radial recurrent artery
Radial Nerve	**Includes:** Dorsal digital nerve Musculospiral nerve Palmar cutaneous nerve Posterior interosseous nerve
Radius, Left Radius, Right	**Includes:** Ulnar notch
Rectum	**Includes:** Anorectal junction
Renal Artery, Left Renal Artery, Right	**Includes:** Inferior suprarenal artery Renal segmental artery
Renal Vein, Left	**Includes:** Left inferior phrenic vein Left ovarian vein Left second lumbar vein Left suprarenal vein Left testicular vein
Retina, Left Retina, Right	**Includes:** Fovea Macula Optic disc
Retroperitoneum	**Includes:** Retroperitoneal cavity Retroperitoneal space
Rib(s) Bursa and Ligament	**Includes:** Costoxiphoid ligament
Sacral Nerve	**Includes:** Spinal nerve, sacral
Sacral Plexus	**Includes:** Inferior gluteal nerve Posterior femoral cutaneous nerve Pudendal nerve
Sacral Sympathetic Nerve	**Includes:** Ganglion impar (ganglion of Walther) Pelvic splanchnic nerve Sacral ganglion Sacral splanchnic nerve
Sacrococcygeal Joint	**Includes:** Sacrococcygeal symphysis

SECTION Ø - MEDICAL AND SURGICAL
CHARACTER 4 - BODY PART

Saphenous Vein, Left Saphenous Vein, Right	**Includes:** External pudendal vein Great(er) saphenous vein Lesser saphenous vein Small saphenous vein Superficial circumflex iliac vein Superficial epigastric vein
Scapula, Left Scapula, Right	**Includes:** Acromion (process) Coracoid process
Sciatic Nerve	**Includes:** Ischiatic nerve
Shoulder Bursa and Ligament, Left Shoulder Bursa and Ligament, Right	**Includes:** Acromioclavicular ligament Coracoacromial ligament Coracoclavicular ligament Coracohumeral ligament Costoclavicular ligament Glenohumeral ligament Interclavicular ligament Sternoclavicular ligament Subacromial bursa Transverse humeral ligament Transverse scapular ligament
Shoulder Joint, Left Shoulder Joint, Right	**Includes:** Glenohumeral joint Glenoid ligament (labrum)
Shoulder Muscle, Left Shoulder Muscle, Right	**Includes:** Deltoid muscle Infraspinatus muscle Subscapularis muscle Supraspinatus muscle Teres major muscle Teres minor muscle
Sigmoid Colon	**Includes:** Rectosigmoid junction Sigmoid flexure
Skin	**Includes:** Dermis Epidermis Sebaceous gland Sweat gland
Skin, Chest	**Includes:** Breast procedures, skin only
Sphenoid Bone	**Includes:** Greater wing Lesser wing Optic foramen Pterygoid process Sella turcica

Spinal Canal	**Includes:** Epidural space, spinal Extradural space, spinal Subarachnoid space, spinal Subdural space, spinal Vertebral canal
Spinal Cord	**Includes:** Dorsal root ganglion
Spinal Meninges	**Includes:** Arachnoid mater, spinal Denticulate (dentate) ligament Dura mater, spinal Filum terminale Leptomeninges, spinal Pia mater, spinal
Spleen	**Includes:** Accessory spleen
Splenic Artery	**Includes:** Left gastroepiploic artery Pancreatic artery Short gastric artery
Splenic Vein	**Includes:** Left gastroepiploic vein Pancreatic vein
Sternum	**Includes:** Manubrium Suprasternal notch Xiphoid process
Sternum Bursa and Ligament	**Includes:** Costoxiphoid ligament Sternocostal ligament
Stomach, Pylorus	**Includes:** Pyloric antrum Pyloric canal Pyloric sphincter
Subclavian Artery, Left Subclavian Artery, Right	**Includes:** Costocervical trunk Dorsal scapular artery Internal thoracic artery
Subcutaneous Tissue and Fascia, Chest	**Includes:** Pectoral fascia
Subcutaneous Tissue and Fascia, Face	**Includes:** Chin Masseteric fascia Orbital fascia Submandibular space
Subcutaneous Tissue and Fascia, Left Foot	**Includes:** Plantar fascia (aponeurosis)

APPENDIX A

SECTION Ø - MEDICAL AND SURGICAL
CHARACTER 4 - BODY PART

Subcutaneous Tissue and Fascia, Left Hand	**Includes:** Palmar fascia (aponeurosis)
Subcutaneous Tissue and Fascia, Left Lower Arm	**Includes:** Antebrachial fascia Bicipital aponeurosis
Subcutaneous Tissue and Fascia, Left Neck	**Includes:** Deep cervical fascia Pretracheal fascia Prevertebral fascia
Subcutaneous Tissue and Fascia, Left Upper Arm	**Includes:** Axillary fascia Deltoid fascia Infraspinatus fascia Subscapular aponeurosis Supraspinatus fascia
Subcutaneous Tissue and Fascia, Left Upper Leg	**Includes:** Crural fascia Fascia lata Iliac fascia Iliotibial tract (band)
Subcutaneous Tissue and Fascia, Right Foot	**Includes:** Plantar fascia (aponeurosis)
Subcutaneous Tissue and Fascia, Right Hand	**Includes:** Palmar fascia (aponeurosis)
Subcutaneous Tissue and Fascia, Right Lower Arm	**Includes:** Antebrachial fascia Bicipital aponeurosis
Subcutaneous Tissue and Fascia, Right Neck	**Includes:** Deep cervical fascia Pretracheal fascia Prevertebral fascia
Subcutaneous Tissue and Fascia, Right Upper Arm	**Includes:** Axillary fascia Deltoid fascia Infraspinatus fascia Subscapular aponeurosis Supraspinatus fascia
Subcutaneous Tissue and Fascia, Right Upper Leg	**Includes:** Crural fascia Fascia lata Iliac fascia Iliotibial tract (band)
Subcutaneous Tissue and Fascia, Scalp	**Includes:** Galea aponeurotica
Subcutaneous Tissue and Fascia, Trunk	**Includes:** External oblique aponeurosis Transversalis fascia
Submaxillary Gland, Left Submaxillary Gland, Right	**Includes:** Submandibular gland
Superior Mesenteric Artery	**Includes:** Ileal artery Ileocolic artery Inferior pancreaticoduodenal artery Jejunal artery
Superior Mesenteric Vein	**Includes:** Right gastroepiploic vein
Superior Vena Cava	**Includes:** Precava
Tarsal Joint, Left Tarsal Joint, Right	**Includes:** Calcaneocuboid joint Cuboideonavicular joint Cuneonavicular joint Intercuneiform joint Subtalar (talocalcaneal) joint Talocalcaneal (subtalar) joint Talocalcaneonavicular joint
Tarsal, Left Tarsal, Right	**Includes:** Calcaneus Cuboid bone Intermediate cuneiform bone Lateral cuneiform bone Medial cuneiform bone Navicular bone Talus bone
Temporal Artery, Left Temporal Artery, Right	**Includes:** Middle temporal artery Superficial temporal artery Transverse facial artery
Temporal Bone, Left Temporal Bone, Right	**Includes:** Mastoid process Petrous part of temporal bone Tympanic part of temporal bone Zygomatic process of temporal bone
Thalamus	**Includes:** Epithalamus Geniculate nucleus Metathalamus Pulvinar
Thoracic Aorta, Ascending/Arch	**Includes:** Aortic arch Ascending aorta
Thoracic Duct	**Includes:** Left jugular trunk Left subclavian trunk

SECTION Ø - MEDICAL AND SURGICAL
CHARACTER 4 - BODY PART

Thoracic Nerve	**Includes:** Intercostal nerve Intercostobrachial nerve Spinal nerve, thoracic Subcostal nerve
Thoracic Spinal Cord	**Includes:** Dorsal root ganglion
Thoracic Sympathetic Nerve	**Includes:** Cardiac plexus Esophageal plexus Greater splanchnic nerve Inferior cardiac nerve Least splanchnic nerve Lesser splanchnic nerve Middle cardiac nerve Pulmonary plexus Superior cardiac nerve Thoracic aortic plexus Thoracic ganglion
Thoracic Vertebra	**Includes:** Spinous process Transverse process Vertebral arch Vertebral body Vertebral foramen Vertebral lamina Vertebral pedicle
Thoracic Vertebral Joint	**Includes:** Costotransverse joint Costovertebral joint Thoracic facet joint
Thoracolumbar Vertebral Joint	**Includes:** Thoracolumbar facet joint
Thorax Muscle, Left Thorax Muscle, Right	**Includes:** Intercostal muscle Levatores costarum muscle Pectoralis major muscle Pectoralis minor muscle Serratus anterior muscle Subclavius muscle Subcostal muscle Transverse thoracis muscle
Thymus	**Includes:** Thymus gland
Thyroid Artery, Left Thyroid Artery, Right	**Includes:** Cricothyroid artery Hyoid artery Sternocleidomastoid artery Superior laryngeal artery Superior thyroid artery Thyrocervical trunk
Tibia, Left Tibia, Right	**Includes:** Lateral condyle of tibia Medial condyle of tibia Medial malleolus
Tibial Nerve	**Includes:** Lateral plantar nerve Medial plantar nerve Medial popliteal nerve Medial sural cutaneous nerve
Toe Nail	**Includes:** Nail bed Nail plate
Toe Phalangeal Joint, Left Toe Phalangeal Joint, Right	**Includes:** Interphalangeal (IP) joint
Tongue	**Includes:** Frenulum linguae
Tongue, Palate, Pharynx Muscle	**Includes:** Chrondroglossus muscle Genioglossus muscle Hyoglossus muscle Inferior longitudinal muscle Levator veli palatini muscle Palatoglossal muscle Palatopharyngeal muscle Pharyngeal constrictor muscle Salpingopharyngeus muscle Styloglossus muscle Stylopharyngeus muscle Superior longitudinal muscle Tensor veli palatini muscle
Tonsils	**Includes:** Palatine tonsil
Trachea	**Includes:** Cricoid cartilage
Transverse Colon	**Includes:** Hepatic flexure Splenic flexure
Tricuspid Valve	**Includes:** Right atrioventricular valve Tricuspid annulus
Trigeminal Nerve	**Includes:** Fifth cranial nerve Gasserian ganglion Mandibular nerve Maxillary nerve Ophthalmic nerve Trifacial nerve
Trochlear Nerve	**Includes:** Fourth cranial nerve

SECTION Ø - MEDICAL AND SURGICAL
CHARACTER 4 - BODY PART

Body Part	Includes
Trunk Muscle, Left Trunk Muscle, Right	**Includes:** Coccygeus muscle Erector spinae muscle Interspinalis muscle Intertransversarius muscle Latissimus dorsi muscle Quadratus lumborum muscle Rhomboid major muscle Rhomboid minor muscle Serratus posterior muscle Transversospinalis muscle Trapezius muscle
Tympanic Membrane, Left Tympanic Membrane, Right	**Includes:** Pars flaccida
Ulna, Left Ulna, Right	**Includes:** Olecranon process Radial notch
Ulnar Artery, Left Ulnar Artery, Right	**Includes:** Anterior ulnar recurrent artery Common interosseous artery Posterior ulnar recurrent artery
Ulnar Nerve	**Includes:** Cubital nerve
Upper Arm Muscle, Left Upper Arm Muscle, Right	**Includes:** Biceps brachii muscle Brachialis muscle Coracobrachialis muscle Triceps brachii muscle
Upper Artery	**Includes:** Aortic intercostal artery Bronchial artery Esophageal artery Subcostal artery
Upper Eyelid, Left Upper Eyelid, Right	**Includes:** Lateral canthus Levator palpebrae superioris muscle Orbicularis oculi muscle Superior tarsal plate
Upper Femur, Left Upper Femur, Right	**Includes:** Femoral head Greater trochanter Lesser trochanter Neck of femur
Upper Leg Muscle, Left Upper Leg Muscle, Right	**Includes:** Adductor brevis muscle Adductor longus muscle Adductor magnus muscle Biceps femoris muscle Gracilis muscle Pectineus muscle Quadriceps (femoris) Rectus femoris muscle Sartorius muscle Semimembranosus muscle Semitendinosus muscle Vastus intermedius muscle Vastus lateralis muscle Vastus medialis muscle
Upper Lip	**Includes:** Frenulum labii superioris Labial gland Vermilion border
Upper Spine Bursa and Ligament	**Includes:** Interspinous ligament, thoracic Intertransverse ligament, thoracic Ligamentum flavum, thoracic Supraspinous ligament
Ureter Ureter, Left Ureter, Right Ureters, Bilateral	**Includes:** Ureteral orifice Ureterovesical orifice
Urethra	**Includes:** Bulbourethral (Cowper's) gland Cowper's (bulbourethral) gland External urethral sphincter Internal urethral sphincter Membranous urethra Penile urethra Prostatic urethra
Uterine Supporting Structure	**Includes:** Broad ligament Infundibulopelvic ligament Ovarian ligament Round ligament of uterus
Uterus	**Includes:** Fundus uteri Myometrium Perimetrium Uterine cornu
Uvula	**Includes:** Palatine uvula

SECTION Ø - MEDICAL AND SURGICAL
CHARACTER 4 - BODY PART

Vagus Nerve	**Includes:** Anterior vagal trunk Pharyngeal plexus Pneumogastric nerve Posterior vagal trunk Pulmonary plexus Recurrent laryngeal nerve Superior laryngeal nerve Tenth cranial nerve
Vas Deferens Vas Deferens, Bilateral Vas Deferens, Left Vas Deferens, Right	**Includes:** Ductus deferens Ejaculatory duct
Ventricle, Right	**Includes:** Conus arteriosus
Ventricular Septum	**Includes:** Interventricular septum
Vertebral Artery, Left Vertebral Artery, Right	**Includes:** Anterior spinal artery Posterior spinal artery
Vertebral Vein, Left Vertebral Vein, Right	**Includes:** Deep cervical vein Suboccipital venous plexus
Vestibular Gland	**Includes:** Bartholin's (greater vestibular) gland Greater vestibular (Bartholin's) gland Paraurethral (Skene's) gland Skene's (paraurethral) gland
Vitreous, Left Vitreous, Right	**Includes:** Vitreous body
Vocal Cord, Left Vocal Cord, Right	**Includes:** Vocal fold
Vulva	**Includes:** Labia majora Labia minora
Wrist Bursa and Ligament, Left Wrist Bursa and Ligament, Right	**Includes:** Palmar ulnocarpal ligament Radial collateral carpal ligament Radiocarpal ligament Radioulnar ligament Scapholunate ligament Ulnar collateral carpal ligament
Wrist Joint, Left Wrist Joint, Right	**Includes:** Distal radioulnar joint Radiocarpal joint

SECTION Ø - MEDICAL AND SURGICAL
CHARACTER 5 - APPROACH

External	**Definition:** Procedures performed directly on the skin or mucous membrane and procedures performed indirectly by the application of external force through the skin or mucous membrane
Open	**Definition:** Cutting through the skin or mucous membrane and any other body layers necessary to expose the site of the procedure
Percutaneous	**Definition:** Entry, by puncture or minor incision, of instrumentation through the skin or mucous membrane and any other body layers necessary to reach the site of the procedure
Percutaneous Endoscopic	**Definition:** Entry, by puncture or minor incision, of instrumentation through the skin or mucous membrane and any other body layers necessary to reach and visualize the site of the procedure
Via Natural or Artificial Opening	**Definition:** Entry of instrumentation through a natural or artificial external opening to reach the site of the procedure
Via Natural or Artificial Opening Endoscopic	**Definition:** Entry of instrumentation through a natural or artificial external opening to reach and visualize the site of the procedure
Via Natural or Artificial Opening With Percutaneous Endoscopic Assistance	**Definition:** Entry of instrumentation through a natural or artificial external opening and entry, by puncture or minor incision, of instrumentation through the skin or mucous membrane and any other body layers necessary to aid in the performance of the procedure

SECTION Ø - MEDICAL AND SURGICAL
CHARACTER 6 - DEVICE

Articulating Spacer in Lower Joints	**Includes:** Articulating Spacer (Antibiotic) Spacer, Articulating (Antibiotic)
Artificial Sphincter in Gastrointestinal System	**Includes:** Artificial anal sphincter (AAS) Artificial bowel sphincter (neosphincter)
Artificial Sphincter in Urinary System	**Includes:** AMS 8ØØ® Urinary Control System Artificial urinary sphincter (AUS)
Autologous Arterial Tissue in Heart and Great Vessels	**Includes:** Autologous artery graft
Autologous Arterial Tissue in Lower Arteries	**Includes:** Autologous artery graft
Autologous Arterial Tissue in Lower Veins	**Includes:** Autologous artery graft
Autologous Arterial Tissue in Upper Arteries	**Includes:** Autologous artery graft
Autologous Arterial Tissue in Upper Veins	**Includes:** Autologous artery graft
Autologous Tissue Substitute	**Includes:** Autograft Cultured epidermal cell autograft Epicel® cultured epidermal autograft
Autologous Venous Tissue in Heart and Great Vessels	**Includes:** Autologous vein graft
Autologous Venous Tissue in Lower Arteries	**Includes:** Autologous vein graft
Autologous Venous Tissue in Lower Veins	**Includes:** Autologous vein graft
Autologous Venous Tissue in Upper Arteries	**Includes:** Autologous vein graft
Autologous Venous Tissue in Upper Veins	**Includes:** Autologous vein graft
Biologic with Synthetic Substitute, Autoregulated Electrohydraulic for Replacement in Heart and Great Vessels	**Includes:** Carmat total artificial heart (TAH)
Bone Growth Stimulator in Head and Facial Bones	**Includes:** Electrical bone growth stimulator (EBGS) Ultrasonic osteogenic stimulator Ultrasound bone healing system
Bone Growth Stimulator in Lower Bones	**Includes:** Electrical bone growth stimulator (EBGS) Ultrasonic osteogenic stimulator Ultrasound bone healing system
Bone Growth Stimulator in Upper Bones	**Includes:** Electrical bone growth stimulator (EBGS) Ultrasonic osteogenic stimulator Ultrasound bone healing system
Cardiac Lead in Heart and Great Vessels	**Includes:** Cardiac contractility modulation lead
Cardiac Lead, Defibrillator for Insertion in Heart and Great Vessels	**Includes:** ACUITY™ Steerable Lead Attain Ability® lead Attain StarFix® (OTW) lead Cardiac resynchronization therapy (CRT) lead Corox (OTW) Bipolar Lead Durata® Defibrillation Lead ENDOTAK RELIANCE® (G) Defibrillation Lead
Cardiac Lead, Pacemaker for Insertion in Heart and Great Vessels	**Includes:** ACUITY™ Steerable Lead Attain Ability® Lead Attain StarFix® (OTW) lead Cardiac resynchronization therapy (CRT) lead Corox (OTW) Bipolar Lead
Cardiac Resynchronization Defibrillator Pulse Generator for Insertion in Subcutaneous Tissue and Fascia	**Includes:** COGNIS® CRT-D Concerto II CRT-D Consulta CRT-D CONTAK RENEWAL® 3 RF (HE) CRT-D LIVIAN™ CRT-D Maximo II DR CRT-D Ovatio™ CRT-D Protecta XT CRT-D Viva (XT)(S)
Cardiac Resynchronization Pacemaker Pulse Generator for Insertion in Subcutaneous Tissue and Fascia	**Includes:** Consulta CRT-P Stratos LV Synchra CRT-P
Contraceptive Device in Female Reproductive System	**Includes:** Intrauterine device (IUD)
Contraceptive Device in Subcutaneous Tissue and Fascia	**Includes:** Subdermal progesterone implant
Contractility Modulation Device for Insertion in Subcutaneous Tissue and Fascia	**Includes:** Optimizer™ III implantable pulse generator

SECTION Ø, CHARACTER 6

SECTION Ø - MEDICAL AND SURGICAL
CHARACTER 6 - DEVICE

Defibrillator Generator for Insertion in Subcutaneous Tissue and Fascia	**Includes:** Implantable cardioverter-defibrillator (ICD) Maximo II DR (VR) Protecta XT DR (XT VR) Secura (DR) (VR) Evera (XT)(S)(DR/VR) Virtuoso (II) (DR) (VR)
Defibrillator Lead in Anatomical Regions, General	**Includes:** EV ICD System (Extravascular implantable defibrillator lead)
Diaphragmatic Pacemaker Lead in Respiratory System	**Includes:** Phrenic nerve stimulator lead
Drainage Device	**Includes:** Cystostomy tube Foley catheter Percutaneous nephrostomy catheter Thoracostomy tube
External Fixation Device in Head and Facial Bones	**Includes:** External fixator
External Fixation Device in Lower Bones	**Includes:** External fixator
External Fixation Device in Lower Joints	**Includes:** External fixator
External Fixation Device in Upper Bones	**Includes:** External fixator
External Fixation Device in Upper Joints	**Includes:** External fixator
External Fixation Device, Hybrid for Insertion in Upper Bones	**Includes:** Delta frame external fixator Sheffield hybrid external fixator
External Fixation Device, Hybrid for Insertion in Lower Bones	**Includes:** Delta frame external fixator Sheffield hybrid external fixator
External Fixation Device, Hybrid for Reposition in Upper Bones	**Includes:** Delta frame external fixator Sheffield hybrid external fixator
External Fixation Device, Hybrid for Reposition in Lower Bones	**Includes:** Delta frame external fixator Sheffield hybrid external fixator
External Fixation Device, Limb Lengthening for Insertion in Upper Bones	**Includes:** Ilizarov-Vecklich device
External Fixation Device, Limb Lengthening for Insertion in Lower Bones	**Includes:** Ilizarov-Vecklich device
External Fixation Device, Monoplanar for Insertion in Upper Bones	**Includes:** Uniplanar external fixator
External Fixation Device, Monoplanar for Insertion in Lower Bones	**Includes:** Uniplanar external fixator
External Fixation Device, Monoplanar for Reposition in Upper Bones	**Includes:** Uniplanar external fixator
External Fixation Device, Monoplanar for Reposition in Lower Bones	**Includes:** Uniplanar external fixator
External Fixation Device, Ring for Insertion in Upper Bones	**Includes:** Ilizarov external fixator Sheffield ring external fixator
External Fixation Device, Ring for Insertion in Lower Bones	**Includes:** Ilizarov external fixator Sheffield ring external fixator
External Fixation Device, Ring for Reposition in Upper Bones	**Includes:** Ilizarov external fixator Sheffield ring external fixator
External Fixation Device, Ring for Reposition in Lower Bones	**Includes:** Ilizarov external fixator Sheffield ring external fixator
Extraluminal Device	**Includes:** AtriClip LAA Exclusion System LAP-BAND® adjustable gastric banding system REALIZE® Adjustable Gastric Band
Feeding Device in Gastrointestinal System	**Includes:** Percutaneous endoscopic gastrojejunostomy (PEG/J) tube Percutaneous endoscopic gastrostomy (PEG) tube
Hearing Device in Ear, Nose, Sinus	**Includes:** Esteem® implantable hearing system
Hearing Device in Head and Facial Bones	**Includes:** Bone anchored hearing device

APPENDIX A

SECTION Ø - MEDICAL AND SURGICAL
CHARACTER 6 - DEVICE

Hearing Device, Bone Conduction for Insertion in Ear, Nose, Sinus	**Includes:** Bone anchored hearing device
Hearing Device, Multiple Channel Cochlear Prosthesis for Insertion in Ear, Nose, Sinus	**Includes:** Cochlear implant (CI), multiple channel (electrode)
Hearing Device, Single Channel Cochlear Prosthesis for Insertion in Ear, Nose, Sinus	**Includes:** Cochlear implant (CI), single channel (electrode)
Implantable Heart Assist System in Heart and Great Vessels	**Includes:** Berlin Heart Ventricular Assist Device DeBakey Left Ventricular Assist Device DuraHeart Left Ventricular Assist System HeartMate 3™ LVAS HeartMate II® Left Ventricular Assist Device (LVAD) HeartMate XVE® Left Ventricular Assist Device (LVAD) MicroMed HeartAssist Novacor Left Ventricular Assist Device Thoratec IVAD (Implantable Ventricular Assist Device)
Infusion Device	**Includes:** Ascenda Intrathecal Catheter InDura, intrathecal catheter (1P) (spinal) Non-tunneled central venous catheter Peripherally inserted central catheter (PICC) Tunneled spinal (intrathecal) catheter
Infusion Device, Pump in Subcutaneous Tissue and Fascia	**Includes:** Implantable drug infusion pump (anti-spasmodic) (chemotherapy) (pain) Injection reservoir, pump Pump reservoir Subcutaneous injection reservoir, pump SynchroMed pump
Interbody Fusion Device in Lower Joints	**Includes:** Axial Lumbar Interbody Fusion System AxiaLIF® System CoRoent® XL Direct Lateral Interbody Fusion (DLIF) device EXtreme Lateral Interbody Fusion (XLIF) device Interbody fusion (spine) cage XLIF® System
Interbody Fusion Device in Upper Joints	**Includes:** BAK/C® Interbody Cervical Fusion System Interbody fusion (spine) cage
Internal Fixation Device in Head and Facial Bones	**Includes:** Bone screw (interlocking) (lag) (pedicle) (recessed) Kirschner wire (K-wire) Neutralization plate
Internal Fixation Device in Lower Bones	**Includes:** Bone screw (interlocking) (lag) (pedicle) (recessed) Clamp and rod internal fixation system (CRIF) Kirschner wire (K-wire) Neutralization plate
Internal Fixation Device in Lower Joints	**Includes:** Fusion screw (compression) (lag) (locking) Joint fixation plate Kirschner wire (K-wire)
Internal Fixation Device in Upper Bones	**Includes:** Bone screw (interlocking) (lag) (pedicle) (recessed) Clamp and rod internal fixation system (CRIF) Kirschner wire (K-wire) Neutralization plate
Internal Fixation Device in Upper Joints	**Includes:** Fusion screw (compression) (lag) (locking) Joint fixation plate Kirschner wire (K-wire)
Internal Fixation Device, Intramedullary in Lower Bones	**Includes:** Intramedullary (IM) rod (nail) Intramedullary skeletal kinetic distractor (ISKD) Kuntscher nail
Internal Fixation Device, Intramedullary in Upper Bones	**Includes:** Intramedullary (IM) rod (nail) Intramedullary skeletal kinetic distractor (ISKD) Kuntscher nail
Internal Fixation Device, Intramedullary Limb Lengthening for Insertion in Lower Bones	**Includes:** PRECICE intramedullary limb lengthening system
Internal Fixation Device, Intramedullary Limb Lengthening for Insertion in Upper Bones	**Includes:** PRECICE intramedullary limb lengthening system
Internal Fixation Device, Rigid Plate for Insertion in Upper Bones	**Includes:** Titanium Sternal Fixation System (TSFS)
Internal Fixation Device, Rigid Plate for Reposition in Upper Bones	**Includes:** Titanium Sternal Fixation System (TSFS)

SECTION Ø - MEDICAL AND SURGICAL
CHARACTER 6 - DEVICE

Internal Fixation Device, Sustained Compression for Fusion in Lower Joints	**Includes:** ~~DynaNail Mini®~~ ~~DynaNail®~~ DynaNail® (Helix)(Hybrid)(Mini)
Internal Fixation Device, Sustained Compression for Fusion in Upper Joints	**Includes:** ~~DynaNail Mini®~~ ~~DynaNail®~~ DynaNail® (Helix)(Hybrid)(Mini)
Intracardiac Pacemaker in Heart and Great Vessels	**Includes:** Aveir™ VR, as single chamber
Intraluminal Device	**Includes:** Absolute Pro Vascular (OTW) Self-Expanding Stent System Acculink (RX) Carotid Stent System AFX® Endovascular AAA System AneuRx® AAA Advantage® Assurant (Cobalt) stent Carotid WALLSTENT® Monorail® Endoprosthesis CoAxia NeuroFlo catheter Colonic Z-Stent® Complete (SE) stent Cook Zenith AAA Endovascular Graft Driver stent (RX) (OTW) E-Luminexx™ (Biliary) (Vascular) Stent Embolization coil(s) Endologix AFX® Endovascular AAA System Endurant® Endovascular Stent Graft Endurant® II AAA stent graft system EXCLUDER® AAA Endoprosthesis Express® (LD) Premounted Stent System Express® Biliary SD Monorail® Premounted Stent System Express® SD Renal Monorail® Premounted Stent System FLAIR® Endovascular Stent Graft Formula™ Balloon-Expandable Renal Stent System GORE EXCLUDER® AAA Endoprosthesis GORE TAG® Thoracic Endoprosthesis Herculink (RX) Elite Renal Stent System LifeStent® (Flexstar) (XL) Vascular Stent System Medtronic Endurant® II AAA stent graft system Micro-Driver stent (RX) (OTW) MULTI-LINK (VISION)(MINI-VISION)(ULTRA) Coronary Stent System Omnilink Elite Vascular Balloon Expandable Stent System Protégé® RX Carotid Stent System Stent, intraluminal (cardiovascular) (gastrointestinal)(hepatobiliary)(urinary) Talent® Converter Talent® Occluder Talent® Stent Graft (abdominal) (thoracic) Therapeutic occlusion coil(s) Ultraflex™ Precision Colonic Stent System Valiant Thoracic Stent Graft WALLSTENT® Endoprosthesis Xact Carotid Stent System Zenith AAA Endovascular Graft Zenith Flex® AAA Endovascular Graft Zenith® Renu™ AAA Ancillary Graft Zenith TX2® TAA Endovascular Graft

Intraluminal Device, Airway in Ear, Nose, Sinus	**Includes:** Nasopharyngeal airway (NPA)
Intraluminal Device, Airway in Gastrointestinal System	**Includes:** Esophageal obturator airway (EOA)
Intraluminal Device, Airway in Mouth and Throat	**Includes:** Guedel airway Oropharyngeal airway (OPA)
Intraluminal Device, Bioactive in Upper Arteries	**Includes:** Bioactive embolization coil(s) Micrus CERECYTE microcoil
Intraluminal Device, Branched or Fenestrated, One or Two Arteries for Restriction in Lower Arteries	**Includes:** Cook Zenith® Fenestrated AAA Endovascular Graft EXCLUDER® AAA Endoprosthesis EXCLUDER® IBE Endoprosthesis GORE EXCLUDER® AAA Endoprosthesis GORE EXCLUDER® IBE Endoprosthesis Zenith® Fenestrated AAA Endovascular Graft
Intraluminal Device, Branched or Fenestrated, Three or More Arteries for Restriction in Lower Arteries	**Includes:** Cook Zenith® Fenestrated AAA Endovascular Graft EXCLUDER® AAA Endoprosthesis GORE EXCLUDER® AAA Endoprosthesis Zenith® Fenestrated AAA Endovascular Graft
Intraluminal Device, Drug-eluting in Heart and Great Vessels	**Includes:** CYPHER® Stent Endeavor® (III) (IV) (Sprint) Zotarolimus-eluting Coronary Stent System Everolimus-eluting coronary stent Paclitaxel-eluting coronary stent Sirolimus-eluting coronary stent TAXUS® Liberté® Paclitaxel-eluting Coronary Stent System XIENCE Everolimus Eluting Coronary Stent System Zotarolimus-eluting coronary stent
Intraluminal Device, Drug-eluting in Lower Arteries	**Includes:** Paclitaxel-eluting peripheral stent Zilver® PTX® (paclitaxel) Drug-Eluting Peripheral Stent
Intraluminal Device, Drug-eluting in Upper Arteries	**Includes:** Paclitaxel-eluting peripheral stent Zilver® PTX® (paclitaxel) Drug-Eluting Peripheral Stent
Intraluminal Device, Endobronchial Valve in Respiratory System	**Includes:** Spiration IBV™ Valve System

SECTION Ø - MEDICAL AND SURGICAL
CHARACTER 6 - DEVICE

Intraluminal Device, Endotracheal Airway in Respiratory System	**Includes:** Endotracheal tube (cuffed) (double-lumen)
Intraluminal Device, Flow Diverter for Restriction in Upper Arteries	**Includes:** Flow Diverter embolization device Pipeline™ (Flex) embolization device Surpass Streamline™ Flow Diverter
Intraluminal Device, Pessary in Female Reproductive System	**Includes:** Pessary ring Vaginal pessary
Liner in Lower Joints	**Includes:** Acetabular cup Hip (joint) liner Joint liner (insert) Knee (implant) insert Tibial insert
Magnetic Lengthening Device in Gastrointestinal System	**Includes:** Flourish® Pediatric Esophageal Atresia Device
Monitoring Device	**Includes:** Blood glucose monitoring system Cardiac event recorder Continuous Glucose Monitoring (CGM) device Implantable glucose monitoring device Loop recorder, implantable Reveal (LINQ) (DX) (XT)
Monitoring Device, Hemodynamic for Insertion in Subcutaneous Tissue and Fascia	**Includes:** Implantable hemodynamic monitor (IHM) Implantable hemodynamic monitoring system (IHMS)
Monitoring Device, Pressure Sensor for Insertion in Heart and Great Vessels	**Includes:** CardioMEMS® pressure sensor EndoSure® sensor
Neurostimulator Lead in Central Nervous System and Cranial Nerves	**Includes:** Cortical strip neurostimulator lead DBS lead Deep brain neurostimulator lead RNS System lead Spinal cord neurostimulator lead
Neurostimulator Lead in Peripheral Nervous System	**Includes:** InterStim® Therapy lead
Neurostimulator Generator in Head and Facial Bones	**Includes:** RNS system neurostimulator generator
Nonautologous Tissue Substitute	**Includes:** Acellular Hydrated Dermis Bone bank bone graft Cook Biodesign® Fistula Plug(s) Cook Biodesign® Hernia Graft(s) Cook Biodesign® Layered Graft(s) Cook Zenapro™ Layered Graft(s) Tissue bank graft
Other Device	**Includes:** Alfapump® system
Pacemaker, Dual Chamber for Insertion in Subcutaneous Tissue and Fascia	**Includes:** Advisa (MRI) EnRhythm Kappa Revo MRI™ SureScan® pacemaker Two lead pacemaker Versa
Pacemaker, Single Chamber for Insertion in Subcutaneous Tissue and Fascia	**Includes:** Single lead pacemaker (atrium) (ventricle)
Pacemaker, Single Chamber Rate Responsive for Insertion in Subcutaneous Tissue and Fascia	**Includes:** Single lead rate responsive pacemaker (atrium) (ventricle)
Radioactive Element	**Includes:** Brachytherapy seeds CivaSheet®
Radioactive Element, Cesium-131 Collagen Implant for Insertion in Central Nervous System and Cranial Nerves	Cesium-131 Collagen Implant GammaTile™
Resurfacing Device in Lower Joints	**Includes:** CONSERVE® PLUS Total Resurfacing Hip System Cormet Hip Resurfacing System
Short-term External Heart Assist System in Heart and Great Vessels	Aortix™ System Biventricular external heart assist system BVS 5ØØØ Ventricular Assist Device Centrimag® Blood Pump Impella® heart pump TandemHeart® System Thoratec Paracorporeal Ventricular Assist Device
Spacer in Lower Joints	**Includes:** Joint spacer (antibiotic)
Spacer in Upper Joints	**Includes:** Joint spacer (antibiotic) Spacer, static (antibiotic) Static spacer (antibiotic)
Spinal Stabilization Device, Facet Replacement for Insertion in Upper Joints	**Includes:** Facet replacement spinal stabilization device
Spinal Stabilization Device, Facet Replacement for Insertion in Lower Joints	**Includes:** Facet replacement spinal stabilization device

SECTION Ø - MEDICAL AND SURGICAL
CHARACTER 6 - DEVICE

Spinal Stabilization Device, Interspinous Process for Insertion in Upper Joints	**Includes:** Interspinous process spinal stabilization device X-STOP® Spacer
Spinal Stabilization Device, Interspinous Process for Insertion in Lower Joints	**Includes:** Interspinous process spinal stabilization device X-STOP® Spacer
Spinal Stabilization Device, Pedicle-Based for Insertion in Upper Joints	**Includes:** Dynesys® Dynamic Stabilization System Pedicle-based dynamic stabilization device
Spinal Stabilization Device, Pedicle-Based for Insertion in Lower Joints	**Includes:** Dynesys® Dynamic Stabilization System Pedicle-based dynamic stabilization device
Stimulator Generator in Subcutaneous Tissue and Fascia	**Includes:** Baroreflex Activation Therapy® (BAT®) Diaphragmatic pacemaker generator Mark IV Breathing Pacemaker System Phrenic nerve stimulator generator Rheos® System device
Stimulator Generator, Multiple Array for Insertion in Subcutaneous Tissue and Fascia	**Includes:** Activa PC neurostimulator Enterra gastric neurostimulator Neurostimulator generator, multiple channel PERCEPT™ PC neurostimulator PrimeAdvanced neurostimulator (SureScan) (MRI Safe) Vanta™ PC neurostimulator
Stimulator Generator, Multiple Array Rechargeable for Insertion in Subcutaneous Tissue and Fascia	**Includes:** Activa RC neurostimulator Intellis™ neurostimulator Neurostimulator generator, multiple channel rechargeable RestoreAdvanced neurostimulator (SureScan) (MRI Safe) RestoreSensor neurostimulator (SureScan) (MRI Safe) RestoreUltra neurostimulator (SureScan) (MRI Safe)
Stimulator Generator, Single Array for Insertion in Subcutaneous Tissue and Fascia	**Includes:** Activa SC neurostimulator InterSlim™ II Therapy neurostimulator Itrel (3) (4) neurostimulator Neurostimulator generator, single channel
Stimulator Generator, Single Array Rechargeable for Insertion in Subcutaneous Tissue and Fascia	**Includes:** InterSlim™ II Micro Therapy neurostimulator Neurostimulator generator, single channel rechargeable
Stimulator Lead in Gastrointestinal System	**Includes:** Gastric electrical stimulation (GES) lead Gastric pacemaker lead
Stimulator Lead in Muscles	**Includes:** Electrical muscle stimulation (EMS) lead Electronic muscle stimulator lead Neuromuscular electrical stimulation (NEMS) lead
Stimulator Lead in Upper Arteries	**Includes:** Baroreflex Activation Therapy® (BAT®) Carotid (artery) sinus (baroreceptor) lead Rheos® System lead
Stimulator Lead in Urinary System	**Includes:** Sacral nerve modulation (SNM) lead Sacral neuromodulation lead Urinary incontinence stimulator lead
Subcutaneous Defibrillator Lead in Subcutaneous Tissue and Fascia	**Includes:** S-ICD™ lead
Synthetic Substitute	**Includes:** AbioCor® Total Replacement Heart AMPLATZER® Muscular VSD Occluder Annuloplasty ring Bard® Composix® (E/X) (LP) mesh Bard® Composix® Kugel® patch Bard® Dulex™ mesh Bard® Ventralex™ hernia patch Barricaid® Annular Closure Device (ACD) BRYAN® Cervical Disc System Corvia IASD® Ex-PRESS™ mini glaucoma shunt Flexible Composite Mesh GORE® DUALMESH® Holter valve ventricular shunt IASD® (InterAtrial Shunt Device), Corvia InterAtrial Shunt Device IASD®, Corvia MitraClip valve repair system Nitinol framed polymer mesh Open Pivot (mechanical) valve Open Pivot Aortic Valve Graft (AVG) Partially absorbable mesh PHYSIOMESH™ Flexible Composite Mesh Polymethylmethacrylate (PMMA) Polypropylene mesh PRESTIGE® Cervical Disc PROCEED™ Ventral Patch Prodisc-C Prodisc-L PROLENE Polypropylene Hernia System (PHS) Rebound HRD® (Hernia Repair Device) SynCardia Total Artificial Heart Total artificial (replacement) heart ULTRAPRO Hernia System (UHS) ULTRAPRO Partially Absorbable Lightweight Mesh ULTRAPRO Plug V-Wave Interatrial Shunt System Ventrio™ Hernia Patch Zimmer® NexGen® LPS Mobile Bearing Knee Zimmer® NexGen® LPS-Flex Mobile Knee

SECTION Ø - MEDICAL AND SURGICAL

CHARACTER 6 - DEVICE

Synthetic Substitute, Ceramic for Replacement in Lower Joints	**Includes:** Ceramic on ceramic bearing surface Novation® Ceramic AHS® (Articulation Hip System)
Synthetic Substitute, Intraocular Telescope for Replacement in Eye	**Includes:** Implantable Miniature Telescope™ (IMT)
Synthetic Substitute, Metal for Replacement in Lower Joints	**Includes:** Cobalt/chromium head and socket Metal on metal bearing surface
Synthetic Substitute, Metal on Polyethylene for Replacement in Lower Joints	**Includes:** Cobalt/chromium head and polyethylene socket
Synthetic Substitute, Oxidized Zirconium on Polyethylene for Replacement in Lower Joints	OXINIUM
Synthetic Substitute, Pneumatic for Replacement in Heart and Great Vessels	**Includes:** SynCardia (temporary) total artificial heart (TAH)
Synthetic Substitute, Polyethylene for Replacement in Lower Joints	**Includes:** Polyethylene socket
Synthetic Substitute, Reverse Ball and Socket for Replacement in Upper Joints	**Includes:** Delta III Reverse shoulder prosthesis Reverse® Shoulder Prosthesis
Tissue Expander in Skin and Breast	**Includes:** Tissue expander (inflatable) (injectable)
Tissue Expander in Subcutaneous Tissue and Fascia	**Includes:** Tissue expander (inflatable) (injectable)
Tracheostomy Device in Respiratory System	**Includes:** Tracheostomy tube
Vascular Access Device, Totally Implantable in Subcutaneous Tissue and Fascia	**Includes:** Implanted (venous) (access) port Injection reservoir, port Subcutaneous injection reservoir, port
Vascular Access Device, Tunneled in Subcutaneous Tissue and Fascia	**Includes:** Tunneled central venous catheter Vectra® Vascular Access Graft
Zooplastic Tissue in Heart and Great Vessels	**Includes:** 3f (Aortic) Bioprosthesis valve Bovine pericardial valve Bovine pericardium graft Contegra Pulmonary Valved Conduit CoreValve transcatheter aortic valve Epic™ Stented Tissue Valve (aortic) Freestyle (Stentless) Aortic Root Bioprosthesis Hancock Bioprosthesis (aortic) (mitral) valve Hancock Bioprosthetic Valved Conduit Melody® transcatheter pulmonary valve Mitroflow® Aortic Pericardial Heart Valve Mosaic Bioprosthesis (aortic) (mitral) valve Porcine (bioprosthetic) valve SAPIEN transcatheter aortic valve SJM Biocor® Stented Valve System Stented tissue valve Trifecta™ Valve (aortic) Xenograft

SECTION 1 - OBSTETRICS

CHARACTER 3 - OPERATION

Abortion	**Definition:** Artificially terminating a pregnancy
Change	**Definition:** Taking out or off a device from a body part and putting back an identical or similar device in or on the same body part without cutting or puncturing the skin or a mucous membrane
Delivery	**Definition:** Assisting the passage of the products of conception from the genital canal
Drainage	**Definition:** Taking or letting out fluids and/or gases from a body part by the use of force
Extraction	**Definition:** Pulling or stripping out or off all or a portion of a body part
Insertion	**Definition:** Putting in a nonbiological appliance that monitors, assists, performs, or prevents a physiological function but does not physically take the place of a body part
Inspection	**Definition:** Visually and/or manually exploring a body part **Explanation:** Visual exploration may be performed with or without optical instrumentation. Manual exploration may be performed directly or through intervening body layers

SECTION 1 - OBSTETRICS
CHARACTER 3 - OPERATION

Removal	**Definition:** Taking out or off a device from a body part, region or orifice **Explanation:** If a device is taken out and a similar device put in without cutting or puncturing the skin or mucous membrane, the procedure is coded to the root operation CHANGE. Otherwise, the procedure for taking out a device is coded to the root operation REMOVAL
Repair	**Definition:** Restoring, to the extent possible, a body part to its normal anatomic structure and function **Explanation:** Used only when the method to accomplish the repair is not one of the other root operations
Reposition	**Definition:** Moving to its normal location or other suitable location all or a portion of a body part **Explanation:** The body part is moved to a new location from an abnormal location, or from a normal location where it is not functioning correctly. The body part may or may not be cut out or off to be moved to the new location
Resection	**Definition:** Cutting out or off, without replacement, all of a body part
Transplantation	**Definition:** Putting in or on all or a portion of a living body part taken from another individual or animal to physically take the place and/or function of all or a portion of a similar body part **Explanation:** The native body part may or may not be taken out, and the transplanted body part may take over all or a portion of its function

SECTION 1 - OBSTETRICS
CHARACTER 5 - APPROACH

External	**Definition:** Procedures performed directly on the skin or mucous membrane and procedures performed indirectly by the application of external force through the skin or mucous membrane
Open	**Definition:** Cutting through the skin or mucous membrane and any other body layers necessary to expose the site of the procedure
Percutaneous	**Definition:** Entry, by puncture or minor incision, of instrumentation through the skin or mucous membrane and any other body layers necessary to reach the site of the procedure
Percutaneous Endoscopic	**Definition:** Entry, by puncture or minor incision, of instrumentation through the skin or mucous membrane and any other body layers necessary to reach and visualize the site of the procedure
Via Natural or Artificial Opening	**Definition:** Entry of instrumentation through a natural or artificial external opening to reach the site of the procedure
Via Natural or Artificial Opening Endoscopic	**Definition:** Entry of instrumentation through a natural or artificial external opening to reach and visualize the site of the procedure

SECTION 2 - PLACEMENT
CHARACTER 3 - OPERATION

Change	**Definition:** Taking out or off a device from a body part and putting back an identical or similar device in or on the same body part without cutting or puncturing the skin or a mucous membrane
Compression	**Definition:** Putting pressure on a body region
Dressing	**Definition:** Putting material on a body region for protection
Immobilization	**Definition:** Limiting or preventing motion of a body region
Packing	**Definition:** Putting material in a body region or orifice
Removal	**Definition:** Taking out or off a device from a body part
Traction	**Definition:** Exerting a pulling force on a body region in a distal direction

SECTION 2 - PLACEMENT
CHARACTER 5 - APPROACH

External	**Definition:** Procedures performed directly on the skin or mucous membrane and procedures performed indirectly by the application of external force through the skin or mucous membrane

SECTION 3 - ADMINISTRATION
CHARACTER 3 - OPERATION

Introduction	**Definition:** Putting in or on a therapeutic, diagnostic, nutritional, physiological, or prophylactic substance except blood or blood products
Irrigation	**Definition:** Putting in or on a cleansing substance
Transfusion	**Definition:** Putting in blood or blood products

SECTION 3 - ADMINISTRATION
CHARACTER 5 - APPROACH

External	**Definition:** Procedures performed directly on the skin or mucous membrane and procedures performed indirectly by the application of external force through the skin or mucous membrane
Open	**Definition:** Cutting through the skin or mucous membrane and any other body layers necessary to expose the site of the procedure
Percutaneous	**Definition:** Entry, by puncture or minor incision, of instrumentation through the skin or mucous membrane and any other body layers necessary to reach the site of the procedure
Percutaneous Endoscopic	**Definition:** Entry, by puncture or minor incision, of instrumentation through the skin or mucous membrane and any other body layers necessary to reach and visualize the site of the procedure
Via Natural or Artificial Opening	**Definition:** Entry of instrumentation through a natural or artificial external opening to reach the site of the procedure
Via Natural or Artificial Opening Endoscopic	**Definition:** Entry of instrumentation through a natural or artificial external opening to reach and visualize the site of the procedure

SECTION 3 - ADMINISTRATION
CHARACTER 6 - SUBSTANCE

4-Factor Prothrombin Complex Concentrate	**Includes:** Kcentra
Adhesion Barrier	**Includes:** Seprafilm
Anti-Infective Envelope	**Includes:** AIGISRx Antibacterial Envelope Antibacterial Envelope (TYRX) (AIGISRx) Antimicrobial envelope TYRX Antibacterial Envelope
Clofarabine	**Includes:** Clolar
Globulin	**Includes:** Gammaglobulin Hyperimmune globulin Immunoglobulin Polyclonal hyperimmune globulin
Glucarpidase	**Includes:** Voraxaze
Hematopoietic Stem/ ProgenitorCells, Genetically Modified	**Includes:** OTL-1Ø1 OTL-1Ø3
Human B-type Natriuretic Peptide	**Includes:** Nesiritide
Other Anti-infective	**Includes:** AVYCAZ® (ceftazidime-avibactam) Ceftazidime-avibactam CRESEMBA® (isavuconazonium sulfate) Isavuconazole (isavuconazonium sulfate) Plazomicin
Other Antineoplastic	**Includes:** Blinatumomab BLINCYTO® (blinatumomab)
Other Therapeutic Substance	**Includes:** Idarucizumab, Pradaxa® (dabigatran) reversal agent Praxbind® (idarucizumab), Pradaxa® (dabigatran) reversal agent
Other Thrombolytic	**Includes:** Tissue Plasminogen Activator (tPA)(r-tPA)
Oxazolidinones	**Includes:** Zyvox
Pathogen Reduced Cryoprecipitated Fibrinogen Complex	**Includes:** INTERCEPT Blood System for Plasma Pathogen Reduced Cryoprecipitated Fibrinogen Complex INTERCEPT Fibrinogen Complex
Recombinant Bone Morphogenetic Protein	**Includes:** Bone morphogenetic protein 2 (BMP 2) rhBMP-2
Vasopressor	**Includes:** Angiotensin II GIAPREZA™ Human angiotensin II, synthetic

SECTION 4 - MEASUREMENT AND MONITORING
CHARACTER 3 - OPERATION

Measurement	**Definition:** Determining the level of a physiological or physical function at a point in time
Monitoring	**Definition:** Determining the level of a physiological or physical function repetitively over a period of time

SECTION 4 - MEASUREMENT AND MONITORING
CHARACTER 5 - APPROACH

External	**Definition:** Procedures performed directly on the skin or mucous membrane and procedures performed indirectly by the application of external force through the skin or mucous membrane
Open	**Definition:** Cutting through the skin or mucous membrane and any other body layers necessary to expose the site of the procedure
Percutaneous	**Definition:** Entry, by puncture or minor incision, of instrumentation through the skin or mucous membrane and any other body layers necessary to reach the site of the procedure
Percutaneous Endoscopic	**Definition:** Entry, by puncture or minor incision, of instrumentation through the skin or mucous membrane and any other body layers necessary to reach and visualize the site of the procedure
Via Natural or Artificial Opening	**Definition:** Entry of instrumentation through a natural or artificial external opening to reach the site of the procedure
Via Natural or Artificial Opening Endoscopic	**Definition:** Entry of instrumentation through a natural or artificial external opening to reach and visualize the site of the procedure

APPENDIX A

SECTION 5 - EXTRACORPOREAL OR SYSTEMIC ASSISTANCE AND PERFORMANCE

CHARACTER 3 - OPERATION

Assistance	**Definition:** Taking over a portion of a physiological function by extracorporeal means
Performance	**Definition:** Completely taking over a physiological function by extracorporeal means
Restoration	**Definition:** Returning, or attempting to return, a physiological function to its original state by extracorporeal means.

SECTION 6 - EXTRACORPOREAL OR SYSTEMIC THERAPIES

CHARACTER 3 - OPERATION

Atmospheric Control	**Definition:** Extracorporeal control of atmospheric pressure and composition
Decompression	**Definition:** Extracorporeal elimination of undissolved gas from body fluids
Electromagnetic Therapy	**Definition:** Extracorporeal treatment by electromagnetic rays
Hyperthermia	**Definition:** Extracorporeal raising of body temperature
Hypothermia	**Definition:** Extracorporeal lowering of body temperature
Perfusion	**Definition:** Extracorporeal treatment by diffusion of therapeutic fluid
Pheresis	**Definition:** Extracorporeal separation of blood products
Phototherapy	**Definition:** Extracorporeal treatment by light rays
Shock Wave Therapy	**Definition:** Extracorporeal treatment by shock waves
Ultrasound Therapy	**Definition:** Extracorporeal treatment by ultrasound
Ultraviolet Light Therapy	**Definition:** Extracorporeal treatment by ultraviolet light

SECTION 7 - OSTEOPATHIC

CHARACTER 3 - OPERATION

Treatment	**Definition:** Manual treatment to eliminate or alleviate somatic dysfunction and related disorders

SECTION 7 - OSTEOPATHIC

CHARACTER 5 - APPROACH

External	**Definition:** Procedures performed directly on the skin or mucous membrane and procedures performed indirectly by the application of external force through the skin or mucous membrane

SECTION 8 - OTHER PROCEDURES

CHARACTER 3 - OPERATION

Other Procedures	**Definition:** Methodologies which attempt to remediate or cure a disorder or disease

SECTION 8 - OTHER PROCEDURES
CHARACTER 5 - APPROACH

External	**Definition:** Procedures performed directly on the skin or mucous membrane and procedures performed indirectly by the application of external force through the skin or mucous membrane
Percutaneous	**Definition:** Entry, by puncture or minor incision, of instrumentation through the skin or mucous membrane and any other body layers necessary to reach the site of the procedure
Percutaneous Endoscopic	**Definition:** Entry, by puncture or minor incision, of instrumentation through the skin or mucous membrane and any other body layers necessary to reach and visualize the site of the procedure
Via Natural or Artificial Opening	**Definition:** Entry of instrumentation through a natural or artificial external opening to reach the site of the procedure
Via Natural or Artificial Opening Endoscopic	**Definition:** Entry of instrumentation through a natural or artificial external opening to reach and visualize the site of the procedure

SECTION 9 - CHIROPRACTIC
CHARACTER 3 - OPERATION

Manipulation	**Definition:** Manual procedure that involves a directed thrust to move a joint past the physiological range of motion, without exceeding the anatomical limit

SECTION 9 - CHIROPRACTIC
CHARACTER 5 - APPROACH

External	**Definition:** Procedures performed directly on the skin or mucous membrane and procedures performed indirectly by the application of external force through the skin or mucous membrane

SECTION B - IMAGING
CHARACTER 3 - TYPE

Computerized Tomography (CT Scan)	**Definition:** Computer-reformatted digital display of multiplanar images developed from the capture of multiple exposures of external ionizing radiation
Fluoroscopy	**Definition:** Single plane or bi-plane real-time display of an image developed from the capture of external ionizing radiation on a fluorescent screen. The image may also be stored by either digital or analog means
Magnetic Resonance Imaging (MRI)	**Definition:** Computer reformatted digital display of multiplanar images developed from the capture of radiofrequency signals emitted by nuclei in a body site excited within a magnetic field
Other Imaging	**Definition:** Other specified modality for visualizing a body part
Plain Radiography	**Definition:** Planar display of an image developed from the capture of external ionizing radiation on photographic or photoconductive plate
Ultrasonography	**Definition:** Real-time display of images of anatomy or flow information developed from the capture of reflected and attenuated high-frequency sound waves

APPENDIX A

SECTION C - NUCLEAR MEDICINE
CHARACTER 3 - TYPE

Nonimaging Nuclear Medicine Assay	**Definition:** Introduction of radioactive materials into the body for the study of body fluids and blood elements, by the detection of radioactive emissions
Nonimaging Nuclear Medicine Probe	**Definition:** Introduction of radioactive materials into the body for the study of distribution and fate of certain substances by the detection of radioactive emissions; or, alternatively, measurement of absorption of radioactive emissions from an external source
Nonimaging Nuclear Medicine Uptake	**Definition:** Introduction of radioactive materials into the body for measurements of organ function, from the detection of radioactive emissions
Planar Nuclear Medicine Imaging	**Definition:** Introduction of radioactive materials into the body for single plane display of images developed from the capture of radioactive emissions
Positron Emission Tomographic (PET) Imaging	**Definition:** Introduction of radioactive materials into the body for three-dimensional display of images developed from the simultaneous capture, 180 degrees apart, of radioactive emissions
Systemic Nuclear Medicine Therapy	**Definition:** Introduction of unsealed radioactive materials into the body for treatment
Tomographic (Tomo) Nuclear Medicine Imaging	**Definition:** Introduction of radioactive materials into the body for three-dimensional display of images developed from the capture of radioactive emissions

SECTION F - PHYSICAL REHABILITATION AND DIAGNOSTIC AUDIOLOGY
CHARACTER 3 - TYPE

Activities of Daily Living Assessment	**Definition:** Measurement of functional level for activities of daily living
Activities of Daily Living Treatment	**Definition:** Exercise or activities to facilitate functional competence for activities of daily living
Caregiver Training	**Definition:** Training in activities to support patient's optimal level of function
Cochlear Implant Treatment	**Definition:** Application of techniques to improve the communication abilities of individuals with cochlear implant
Device Fitting	**Definition:** Fitting of a device designed to facilitate or support achievement of a higher level of function
Hearing Aid Assessment	**Definition:** Measurement of the appropriateness and/or effectiveness of a hearing device
Hearing Assessment	**Definition:** Measurement of hearing and related functions
Hearing Treatment	**Definition:** Application of techniques to improve, augment, or compensate for hearing and related functional impairment
Motor and/or Nerve Function Assessment	**Definition:** Measurement of motor, nerve, and related functions
Motor Treatment	**Definition:** Exercise or activities to increase or facilitate motor function
Speech Assessment	**Definition:** Measurement of speech and related functions
Speech Treatment	**Definition:** Application of techniques to improve, augment, or compensate for speech and related functional impairment
Vestibular Assessment	**Definition:** Measurement of the vestibular system and related functions
Vestibular Treatment	**Definition:** Application of techniques to improve, augment, or compensate for vestibular and related functional impairment

SECTION F - PHYSICAL REHABILITATION AND DIAGNOSTIC AUDIOLOGY

CHARACTER 5 - TYPE QUALIFIER

Acoustic Reflex Decay	**Definition:** Measures reduction in size/strength of acoustic reflex over time **Includes/Examples:** Includes site of lesion test
Acoustic Reflex Patterns	**Definition:** Defines site of lesion based upon presence/absence of acoustic reflexes with ipsilateral vs. contralateral stimulation
Acoustic Reflex Threshold	**Definition:** Determines minimal intensity that acoustic reflex occurs with ipsilateral and/or contralateral stimulation
Aerobic Capacity and Endurance	**Definition:** Measures autonomic responses to positional changes; perceived exertion, dyspnea or angina during activity; performance during exercise protocols; standard vital signs; and blood gas analysis or oxygen consumption
Alternate Binaural or Monaural Loudness Balance	**Definition:** Determines auditory stimulus parameter that yields the same objective sensation **Includes/Examples:** Sound intensities that yield same loudness perception
Anthropometric Characteristics	**Definition:** Measures edema, body fat composition, height, weight, length and girth
Aphasia (Assessment)	**Definition:** Measures expressive and receptive speech and language function including reading and writing
Aphasia (Treatment)	**Definition:** Applying techniques to improve, augment, or compensate for receptive/expressive language impairments
Articulation/Phonology (Assessment)	**Definition:** Measures speech production
Articulation/Phonology (Treatment)	**Definition:** Applying techniques to correct, improve, or compensate for speech productive impairment
Assistive Listening Device	**Definition:** Assists in use of effective and appropriate assistive listening device/system
Assistive Listening System/Device Selection	**Definition:** Measures the effectiveness and appropriateness of assistive listening systems/devices
Assistive, Adaptive,Supportive or Protective Devices	**Explanation:** Devices to facilitate or support achievement of a higher level of function in wheelchair mobility; bed mobility; transfer or ambulation ability; bath and showering ability; dressing; grooming; personal hygiene; play or leisure
Auditory Evoked Potentials	**Definition:** Measures electric responses produced by the VIIIth cranial nerve and brainstem following auditory stimulation
Auditory Processing (Assessment)	**Definition:** Evaluates ability to receive and process auditory information and comprehension of spoken language
Auditory Processing (Treatment)	**Definition:** Applying techniques to improve the receiving and processing of auditory information and comprehension of spoken language
Augmentative/Alternative Communication System (Assessment)	**Definition:** Determines the appropriateness of aids, techniques, symbols, and/or strategies to augment or replace speech and enhance communication **Includes/Examples:** Includes the use of telephones, writing equipment, emergency equipment, and TDD
Augmentative/Alternative Communication System (Treatment)	**Includes/Examples:** Includes augmentative communication devices and aids
Aural Rehabilitation	**Definition:** Applying techniques to improve the communication abilities associated with hearing loss
Aural Rehabilitation Status	**Definition:** Measures impact of a hearing loss including evaluation of receptive and expressive communication skills
Bathing/Showering	**Includes/Examples:** Includes obtaining and using supplies; soaping, rinsing, and drying body parts; maintaining bathing position; and transferring to and from bathing positions
Bathing/Showering Techniques	**Definition:** Activities to facilitate obtaining and using supplies, soaping, rinsing and drying body parts, maintaining bathing position, and transferring to and from bathing positions
Bed Mobility (Assessment)	**Definition:** Transitional movement within bed
Bed Mobility (Treatment)	**Definition:** Exercise or activities to facilitate transitional movements within bed
Bedside Swallowing and Oral Function	**Includes/Examples:** Bedside swallowing includes assessment of sucking, masticating, coughing, and swallowing. Oral function includes assessment of musculature for controlled movements, structures and functions to determine coordination and phonation
Bekesy Audiometry	**Definition:** Uses an instrument that provides a choice of discrete or continuously varying pure tones; choice of pulsed or continuous signal

APPENDIX A

SECTION F - PHYSICAL REHABILITATION AND DIAGNOSTIC AUDIOLOGY

CHARACTER 5 - TYPE QUALIFIER

Binaural Electroacoustic Hearing Aid Check	**Definition:** Determines mechanical and electroacoustic function of bilateral hearing aids using hearing aid test box
Binaural Hearing Aid (Assessment)	**Definition:** Measures the candidacy, effectiveness, and appropriateness of hearing aids **Explanation:** Measures bilateral fit
Binaural Hearing Aid (Treatment)	**Explanation:** Assists in achieving maximum understanding and performance
Bithermal, Binaural Caloric Irrigation	**Definition:** Measures the rhythmic eye movements stimulated by changing the temperature of the vestibular system
Bithermal, Monaural Caloric Irrigation	**Definition:** Measures the rhythmic eye movements stimulated by changing the temperature of the vestibular system in one ear
Brief Tone Stimuli	**Definition:** Measures specific central auditory process
Cerumen Management	**Definition:** Includes examination of external auditory canal and tympanic membrane and removal of cerumen from external ear canal
Cochlear Implant	**Definition:** Measures candidacy for cochlear implant
Cochlear Implant Rehabilitation	**Definition:** Applying techniques to improve the communication abilities of individuals with cochlear implant; includes programming the device, providing patients/families with information
Communicative/ Cognitive Integration Skills (Assessment)	**Definition:** Measures ability to use higher cortical functions **Includes/Examples:** Includes orientation, recognition, attention span, initiation and termination of activity, memory, sequencing, categorizing, concept formation, spatial operations, judgment, problem solving, generalization and pragmatic communication
Communicative/ Cognitive Integration Skills (Treatment)	**Definition:** Activities to facilitate the use of higher cortical functions **Includes/Examples:** Includes level of arousal, orientation, recognition, attention span, initiation and termination of activity, memory sequencing, judgment and problem solving, learning and generalization, and pragmatic communication
Computerized Dynamic Posturography	**Definition:** Measures the status of the peripheral and central vestibular system and the sensory/motor component of balance; evaluates the efficacy of vestibular rehabilitation

Conditioned Play Audiometry	**Definition:** Behavioral measures using nonspeech and speech stimuli to obtain frequency-specific and ear-specific information on auditory status from the patient **Explanation:** Obtains speech reception threshold by having patient point to pictures of spondaic words
Coordination/Dexterity (Assessment)	**Definition:** Measures large and small muscle groups for controlled goal-directed movements **Explanation:** Dexterity includes object manipulation
Coordination/Dexterity (Treatment)	**Definition:** Exercise or activities to facilitate gross coordination and fine coordination
Cranial Nerve Integrity	**Definition:** Measures cranial nerve sensory and motor functions, including tastes, smell and facial expression
Dichotic Stimuli	**Definition:** Measures specific central auditory process
Distorted Speech	**Definition:** Measures specific central auditory process
Dix-Hallpike Dynamic	**Definition:** Measures nystagmus following Dix-Hallpike maneuver
Dressing	**Includes/Examples:** Includes selecting clothing and accessories, obtaining clothing from storage, dressing and, fastening and adjusting clothing and shoes, and applying and removing personal devices, prosthesis or orthosis
Dressing Techniques	**Definition:** Activities to facilitate selecting clothing and accessories, dressing and undressing, adjusting clothing and shoes, applying and removing devices, prostheses or orthoses
Dynamic Orthosis	**Includes/Examples:** Includes customized and prefabricated splints, inhibitory casts, spinal and other braces, and protective devices; allows motion through transfer of movement from other body parts or by use of outside forces
Ear Canal Probe Microphone	**Definition:** Real ear measures
Ear Protector Attentuation	**Definition:** Measures ear protector fit and effectiveness
Electrocochleography	**Definition:** Measures the VIIIth cranial nerve action potential
Environmental, Home and Work Barriers	**Definition:** Measures current and potential barriers to optimal function, including safety hazards, access problems and home or office design

SECTION F - PHYSICAL REHABILITATION AND DIAGNOSTIC AUDIOLOGY

CHARACTER 5 - TYPE QUALIFIER

Ergonomics and Body Mechanics	**Definition:** Ergonomic measurement of job tasks, work hardening or work conditioning needs; functional capacity; and body mechanics
Eustachian Tube Function	**Definition:** Measures eustachian tube function and patency of eustachian tube
Evoked Otoacoustic Emissions, Diagnostic	**Definition:** Measures auditory evoked potentials in a diagnostic format
Evoked Otoacoustic Emissions, Screening	**Definition:** Measures auditory evoked potentials in a screening format
Facial Nerve Function	**Definition:** Measures electrical activity of the VIIth cranial nerve (facial nerve)
Feeding/Eating (Assessment)	**Includes/Examples:** Includes setting up food, selecting and using utensils and tableware, bringing food or drink to mouth, cleaning face, hands, and clothing, and management of alternative methods of nourishment
Feeding/Eating (Treatment)	**Definition:** Exercise or activities to facilitate setting up food, selecting and using utensils and tableware, bringing food or drink to mouth, cleaning face, hands, and clothing, and management of alternative methods of nourishment
Filtered Speech	**Definition:** Uses high or low pass filtered speech stimuli to assess central auditory processing disorders, site of lesion testing
Fluency (Assessment)	**Definition:** Measures speech fluency or stuttering
Fluency (Treatment)	**Definition:** Applying techniques to improve and augment fluent speech
Gait and/or Balance	**Definition:** Measures biomechanical, arthrokinematic and other spatial and temporal characteristics of gait and balance
Gait Training/ Functional Ambulation	**Definition:** Exercise or activities to facilitate ambulation on a variety of surfaces and in a variety of environments
Grooming/Personal Hygiene (Assessment)	**Includes/Examples:** Includes ability to obtain and use supplies in a sequential fashion, general grooming, oral hygiene, toilet hygiene, personal care devices, including care for artificial airways
Grooming/Personal Hygiene (Treatment)	**Definition:** Activities to facilitate obtaining and using supplies in a sequential fashion: general grooming, oral hygiene, toilet hygiene, cleaning body, and personal care devices, including artificial airways
Hearing and Related Disorders Counseling	**Definition:** Provides patients/families/ caregivers with information, support, referrals to facilitate recovery from a communication disorder **Includes/Examples:** Includes strategies for psychosocial adjustment to hearing loss for clients and families/caregivers
Hearing and Related Disorders Prevention	**Definition:** Provides patients/families/ caregivers with information and support to prevent communication disorders
Hearing Screening	**Definition:** Pass/refer measures designed to identify need for further audiologic assessment
Home Management (Assessment)	**Definition:** Obtaining and maintaining personal and household possessions and environment **Includes/Examples:** Includes clothing care, cleaning, meal preparation and cleanup, shopping, money management, household maintenance, safety procedures, and childcare/parenting
Home Management (Treatment)	**Definition:** Activities to facilitate obtaining and maintaining personal household possessions and environment **Includes/Examples:** Includes clothing care, cleaning, meal preparation and clean-up, shopping, money management, household maintenance, safety procedures, childcare/ parenting
Instrumental Swallowing and Oral Function	**Definition:** Measures swallowing function using instrumental diagnostic procedures **Explanation:** Methods include videofluoroscopy, ultrasound, manometry, endoscopy
Integumentary Integrity	**Includes/Examples:** Includes burns, skin conditions, ecchymosis, bleeding, blisters, scar tissue, wounds and other traumas, tissue mobility, turgor and texture

APPENDIX A

SECTION F - PHYSICAL REHABILITATION AND DIAGNOSTIC AUDIOLOGY

CHARACTER 5 - TYPE QUALIFIER

Manual Therapy Techniques	**Definition:** Techniques in which the therapist uses his/her hands to administer skilled movements **Includes/Examples:** Includes connective tissue massage, joint mobilization and manipulation, manual lymph drainage, manual traction, soft tissue mobilization and manipulation
Masking Patterns	**Definition:** Measures central auditory processing status
Monaural Electroacoustic Hearing Aid Check	**Definition:** Determines mechanical and electroacoustic function of one hearing aid using hearing aid test box
Monaural Hearing Aid (Assessment)	**Definition:** Measures the candidacy, effectiveness, and appropriateness of a hearing aid **Explanation:** Measures unilateral fit
Monaural Hearing Aid (Treatment)	**Explanation:** Assists in achieving maximum understanding and performance
Motor Function (Assessment)	**Definition:** Measures the body's functional and versatile movement patterns **Includes/Examples:** Includes motor assessment scales, analysis of head, trunk and limb movement, and assessment of motor learning
Motor Function (Treatment)	**Definition:** Exercise or activities to facilitate crossing midline, laterality, bilateral integration, praxis, neuromuscular relaxation, inhibition, facilitation, motor function and motor learning
Motor Speech (Assessment)	**Definition:** Measures neurological motor aspects of speech production
Motor Speech (Treatment)	**Definition:** Applying techniques to improve and augment the impaired neurological motor aspects of speech production
Muscle Performance (Assessment)	**Definition:** Measures muscle strength, power and endurance using manual testing, dynamometry or computer-assisted electromechanical muscle test; functional muscle strength, power and endurance; muscle pain, tone, or soreness; or pelvic-floor musculature **Explanation:** Muscle endurance refers to the ability to contract a muscle repeatedly over time
Muscle Performance (Treatment)	**Definition:** Exercise or activities to increase the capacity of a muscle to do work in terms of strength, power, and/or endurance **Explanation:** Muscle strength is the force exerted to overcome resistance in one maximal effort. Muscle power is work produced per unit of time, or the product of strength and speed. Muscle endurance is the ability to contract a muscle repeatedly over time
Neuromotor Development	**Definition:** Measures motor development, righting and equilibrium reactions, and reflex and equilibrium reactions
Non-invasive Instrumental Status	**Definition:** Instrumental measures of oral, nasal, vocal, and velopharyngeal functions as they pertain to speech production
Nonspoken Language (Assessment)	**Definition:** Measures nonspoken language (print, sign, symbols) for communication
Nonspoken Language (Treatment)	**Definition:** Applying techniques that improve, augment, or compensate spoken communication
Oral Peripheral Mechanism	**Definition:** Structural measures of face, jaw, lips, tongue, teeth, hard and soft palate, pharynx as related to speech production
Orofacial Myofunctional (Assessment)	**Definition:** Measures orofacial myofunctional patterns for speech and related functions
Orofacial Myofunctional (Treatment)	**Definition:** Applying techniques to improve, alter, or augment impaired orofacial myofunctional patterns and related speech production errors
Oscillating Tracking	**Definition:** Measures ability to visually track
Pain	**Definition:** Measures muscle soreness, pain and soreness with joint movement, and pain perception **Includes/Examples:** Includes questionnaires, graphs, symptom magnification scales or visual analog scales
Perceptual Processing (Assessment)	**Definition:** Measures stereognosis, kinesthesia, body schema, right-left discrimination, form constancy, position in space, visual closure, figure-ground, depth perception, spatial relations and topographical orientation

SECTION F - PHYSICAL REHABILITATION AND DIAGNOSTIC AUDIOLOGY

CHARACTER 5 - TYPE QUALIFIER

Perceptual Processing (Treatment)	**Definition:** Exercise and activities to facilitate perceptual processing **Explanation:** Includes stereognosis, kinesthesia, body schema, right-left discrimination, form constancy, position in space, visual closure, figure-ground, depth perception, spatial relations, and topographical orientation **Includes/Examples:** Includes stereognosis, kinesthesia, body schema, right-left discrimination, form constancy, position in space, visual closure, figure-ground, depth perception, spatial relations, and topographical orientation
Performance Intensity Phonetically Balanced Speech Discrimination	**Definition:** Measures word recognition over varying intensity levels
Postural Control	**Definition:** Exercise or activities to increase postural alignment and control
Prosthesis	**Definition:** Artificial substitutes for missing body parts that augment performance or function **Includes/Examples:** Limb prosthesis, ocular prosthesis
Psychosocial Skills (Assessment)	**Definition:** The ability to interact in society and to process emotions **Includes/Examples:** Includes psychological (values, interests, self-concept); social (role performance, social conduct, interpersonal skills, self expression); self-management (coping skills, time management, self-control)
Psychosocial Skills (Treatment)	**Definition:** The ability to interact in society and to process emotions **Includes/Examples:** Includes psychological (values, interests, self-concept); social (role performance, social conduct, interpersonal skills, self expression); self-management (coping skills, time management, self-control)
Pure Tone Audiometry, Air	**Definition:** Air-conduction pure tone threshold measures with appropriate masking
Pure Tone Audiometry, Air and Bone	**Definition:** Air-conduction and bone-conduction pure tone threshold measures with appropriate masking
Pure Tone Stenger	**Definition:** Measures unilateral nonorganic hearing loss based on simultaneous presentation of pure tones of differing volume
Range of Motion and Joint Integrity	**Definition:** Measures quantity, quality, grade, and classification of joint movement and/or mobility **Explanation:** Range of Motion is the space, distance or angle through which movement occurs at a joint or series of joints. Joint integrity is the conformance of joints to expected anatomic, biomechanical and kinematic norms
Range of Motion and Joint Mobility	**Definition:** Exercise or activities to increase muscle length and joint mobility
Receptive/Expressive Language (Assessment)	**Definition:** Measures receptive and expressive language
Receptive/Expressive Language (Treatment)	**Definition:** Applying techniques tot improve and augment receptive/expressive language
Reflex Integrity	**Definition:** Measures the presence, absence, or exaggeration of developmentally appropriate, pathologic or normal reflexes
Select Picture Audiometry	**Definition:** Establishes hearing threshold levels for speech using pictures
Sensorineural Acuity Level	**Definition:** Measures sensorineural acuity masking presented via bone conduction
Sensory Aids	**Definition:** Determines the appropriateness of a sensory prosthetic device, other than a hearing aid or assistive listening system/device
Sensory Awareness/ Processing/Integrity	**Includes/Examples:** Includes light touch, pressure, temperature, pain, sharp/dull, proprioception, vestibular, visual, auditory, gustatory, and olfactory
Short Increment Sensitivity Index	**Definition:** Measures the ear's ability to detect small intensity changes; site of lesion test requiring a behavioral response
Sinusoidal Vertical Axis Rotational	**Definition:** Measures nystagmus following rotation
Somatosensory Evoked Potentials	**Definition:** Measures neural activity from sites throughout the body

SECTION F - PHYSICAL REHABILITATION AND DIAGNOSTIC AUDIOLOGY

CHARACTER 5 - TYPE QUALIFIER

Speech and/or Language Screening	**Definition:** Identifies need for further speech and/or language evaluation
Speech Threshold	**Definition:** Measures minimal intensity needed to repeat spondaic words
Speech-Language Pathology and Related Disorders Counseling	**Definition:** Provides patients/families with information, support, referrals to facilitate recovery from a communication disorder
Speech-Language Pathology and Related Disorders Prevention	**Definition:** Applying techniques to avoid or minimize onset and/or development of a communication disorder
Speech/Word Recognition	**Definition:** Measures ability to repeat/identify single syllable words; scores given as a percentage; includes word recognition/speech discrimination
Staggered Spondaic Word	**Definition:** Measures central auditory processing site of lesion based upon dichotic presentation of spondaic words
Static Orthosis	**Includes/Examples:** Includes customized and prefabricated splints, inhibitory casts, spinal and other braces, and protective devices; has no moving parts, maintains joint(s) in desired position
Stenger	**Definition:** Measures unilateral nonorganic hearing loss based on simultaneous presentation of signals of differing volume
Swallowing Dysfunction	**Definition:** Activities to improve swallowing function in coordination with respiratory function **Includes/Examples:** Includes function and coordination of sucking, mastication, coughing, swallowing
Synthetic Sentence Identification	**Definition:** Measures central auditory dysfunction using identification of third order approximations of sentences and competing messages
Temporal Ordering of Stimuli	**Definition:** Measures specific central auditory process
Therapeutic Exercise	**Definition:** Exercise or activities to facilitate sensory awareness, sensory processing, sensory integration, balance training, conditioning, reconditioning **Includes/Examples:** Includes developmental activities, breathing exercises, aerobic endurance activities, aquatic exercises, stretching and ventilatory muscle training
Tinnitus Masker (Assessment)	**Definition:** Determines candidacy for tinnitus masker
Tinnitus Masker (Treatment)	**Explanation:** Used to verify physical fit, acoustic appropriateness, and benefit; assists in achieving maximum benefit
Tone Decay	**Definition:** Measures decrease in hearing sensitivity to a tone; site of lesion test requiring a behavioral response
Transfer	**Definition:** Transitional movement from one surface to another
Transfer Training	**Definition:** Exercise or activities to facilitate movement from one surface to another
Tympanometry	**Definition:** Measures the integrity of the middle ear; measures ease at which sound flows through the tympanic membrane while air pressure against the membrane is varied
Unithermal Binaural Screen	**Definition:** Measures the rhythmic eye movements stimulated by changing the temperature of the vestibular system in both ears using warm water, screening format
Ventilation, Respiration and Circulation	**Definition:** Measures ventilatory muscle strength, power and endurance, pulmonary function and ventilatory mechanics **Includes/Examples:** Includes ability to clear airway, activities that aggravate or relieve edema, pain, dyspnea or other symptoms, chest wall mobility, cardiopulmonary response to performance of ADL and IAD, cough and sputum, standard vital signs

SECTION F - PHYSICAL REHABILITATION AND DIAGNOSTIC AUDIOLOGY

CHARACTER 5 - TYPE QUALIFIER

Vestibular	**Definition:** Applying techniques to compensate for balance disorders; includes habituation, exercise therapy, and balance retraining
Visual Motor Integration (Assessment)	**Definition:** Coordinating the interaction of information from the eyes with body movement during activity
Visual Motor Integration (Treatment)	**Definition:** Exercise or activities to facilitate coordinating the interaction of information from eyes with body movement during activity
Visual Reinforcement Audiometry	**Definition:** Behavioral measures using nonspeech and speech stimuli to obtain frequency/ear-specific information on auditory status **Includes/Examples:** Includes a conditioned response of looking toward a visual reinforcer (e.g., lights, animated toy) every time auditory stimuli are heard
Vocational Activities and Functional Community or Work Reintegration Skills (Assessment)	**Definition:** Measures environmental, home, work (job/school/play) barriers that keep patients from functioning optimally in their environment **Includes/Examples:** Includes assessment of vocational skill and interests, environment of work (job/school/play), injury potential and injury prevention or reduction, ergonomic stressors, transportation skills, and ability to access and use community resources
Vocational Activities and Functional Community or Work Reintegration Skills (Treatment)	**Definition:** Activities to facilitate vocational exploration, body mechanics training, job acquisition, and environmental or work (job/school/play) task adaptation **Includes/Examples:** Includes injury prevention and reduction, ergonomic stressor reduction, job coaching and simulation, work hardening and conditioning, driving training, transportation skills, and use of community resources
Voice (Assessment)	**Definition:** Measures vocal structure, function and production
Voice (Treatment)	**Definition:** Applying techniques to improve voice and vocal function
Voice Prosthetic (Assessment)	**Definition:** Determines the appropriateness of voice prosthetic/adaptive device to enhance or facilitate communication
Voice Prosthetic (Treatment)	**Includes/Examples:** Includes electrolarynx, and other assistive, adaptive, supportive devices
Wheelchair Mobility (Assessment)	**Definition:** Measures fit and functional abilities within wheelchair in a variety of environments
Wheelchair Mobility (Treatment)	**Definition:** Management, maintenance and controlled operation of a wheelchair, scooter or other device, in and on a variety of surfaces and environments
Wound Management	**Includes/Examples:** Includes non-selective and selective debridement (enzymes, autolysis, sharp debridement), dressings (wound coverings, hydrogel, vacuum-assisted closure), topical agents, etc.

APPENDIX A

SECTION G - MENTAL HEALTH
CHARACTER 3 - TYPE

Biofeedback	**Definition:** Provision of information from the monitoring and regulating of physiological processes in conjunction with cognitive-behavioral techniques to improve patient functioning or well-being **Includes/Examples:** Includes EEG, blood pressure, skin temperature or peripheral blood flow, ECG, electrooculogram, EMG, respirometry or capnometry, GSR/EDR, perineometry to monitor/regulate bowel/bladder activity, electrogastrogram to monitor/regulate gastric motility
Counseling	**Definition:** The application of psychological methods to treat an individual with normal developmental issues and psychological problems in order to increase function, improve well-being, alleviate distress, maladjustment or resolve crises
Crisis Intervention	**Definition:** Treatment of a traumatized, acutely disturbed or distressed individual for the purpose of short-term stabilization **Includes/Examples:** Includes defusing, debriefing, counseling, psychotherapy and/or coordination of care with other providers or agencies
Electroconvulsive Therapy	**Definition:** The application of controlled electrical voltages to treat a mental health disorder **Includes/Examples:** Includes appropriate sedation and other preparation of the individual
Family Psychotherapy	**Definition:** Treatment that includes one or more family members of an individual with a mental health disorder by behavioral, cognitive, psychoanalytic, psychodynamic or psychophysiological means to improve functioning or well-being **Explanation:** Remediation of emotional or behavioral problems presented by one or more family members in cases where psychotherapy with more than one family member is indicated
Group Psychotherapy	**Definition:** Treatment of two or more individuals with a mental health disorder by behavioral, cognitive, psychoanalytic, psychodynamic or psychophysiological means to improve functioning or well-being
Hypnosis	**Definition:** Induction of a state of heightened suggestibility by auditory, visual and tactile techniques to elicit an emotional or behavioral response
Individual Psychotherapy	**Definition:** Treatment of an individual with a mental health disorder by behavioral, cognitive, psychoanalytic, psychodynamic or psychophysiological means to improve functioning or well-being
Light Therapy	**Definition:** Application of specialized light treatments to improve functioning or well-being
Medication Management	**Definition:** Monitoring and adjusting the use of medications for the treatment of a mental health disorder
Narcosynthesis	**Definition:** Administration of intravenous barbiturates in order to release suppressed or repressed thoughts
Psychological Tests	**Definition:** The administration and interpretation of standardized psychological tests and measurement instruments for the assessment of psychological function

SECTION G - MENTAL HEALTH
CHARACTER 4 - QUALIFIER

Behavioral	**Definition:** Primarily to modify behavior **Includes/Examples:** Includes modeling and role playing, positive reinforcement of target behaviors, response cost, and training of self-management skills
Cognitive	**Definition:** Primarily to correct cognitive distortions and errors
Cognitive-Behavioral	**Definition:** Combining cognitive and behavioral treatment strategies to improve functioning **Explanation:** Maladaptive responses are examined to determine how cognitions relate to behavior patterns in response to an event. Uses learning principles and information-processing models
Developmental	**Definition:** Age-normed developmental status of cognitive, social and adaptive behavior skills
Intellectual and Psychoeducational	**Definition:** Intellectual abilities, academic achievement and learning capabilities (including behaviors and emotional factors affecting learning)
Interactive	**Definition:** Uses primarily physical aids and other forms of non-oral interaction with a patient who is physically, psychologically or developmentally unable to use ordinary language for communication **Includes/Examples:** Includes the use of toys in symbolic play
Interpersonal	**Definition:** Helps an individual make changes in interpersonal behaviors to reduce psychological dysfunction **Includes/Examples:** Includes exploratory techniques, encouragement of affective expression, clarification of patient statements, analysis of communication patterns, use of therapy relationship and behavior change techniques
Neurobehavioral and Cognitive Status	**Definition:** Includes neurobehavioral status exam, interview(s), and observation for the clinical assessment of thinking, reasoning and judgment, acquired knowledge, attention, memory, visual spatial abilities, language functions, and planning
Neuropsychological	**Definition:** Thinking, reasoning and judgment, acquired knowledge, attention, memory, visual spatial abilities, language functions, planning
Personality and Behavioral	**Definition:** Mood, emotion, behavior, social functioning, psychopathological conditions, personality traits and characteristics
Psychoanalysis	**Definition:** Methods of obtaining a detailed account of past and present mental and emotional experiences to determine the source and eliminate or diminish the undesirable effects of unconscious conflicts **Explanation:** Accomplished by making the individual aware of their existence, origin, and inappropriate expression in emotions and behavior
Psychodynamic	**Definition:** Exploration of past and present emotional experiences to understand motives and drives using insight-oriented techniques to reduce the undesirable effects of internal conflicts on emotions and behavior **Explanation:** Techniques include empathetic listening, clarifying self-defeating behavior patterns, and exploring adaptive alternatives
Psychophysiological	**Definition:** Monitoring and alteration of physiological processes to help the individual associate physiological reactions combined with cognitive and behavioral strategies to gain improved control of these processes to help the individual cope more effectively
Supportive	**Definition:** Formation of therapeutic relationship primarily for providing emotional support to prevent further deterioration in functioning during periods of particular stress **Explanation:** Often used in conjunction with other therapeutic approaches
Vocational	**Definition:** Exploration of vocational interests, aptitudes and required adaptive behavior skills to develop and carry out a plan for achieving a successful vocational placement **Includes/Examples:** Includes enhancing work related adjustment and/or pursuing viable options in training education or preparation

SECTION H - SUBSTANCE ABUSE TREATMENT
CHARACTER 3 - TYPE

Detoxification Services	**Definition:** Detoxification from alcohol and/or drugs **Explanation:** Not a treatment modality, but helps the patient stabilize physically and psychologically until the body becomes free of drugs and the effects of alcohol
Family Counseling	**Definition:** The application of psychological methods that includes one or more family members to treat an individual with addictive behavior **Explanation:** Provides support and education for family members of addicted individuals. Family member participation is seen as a critical area of substance abuse treatment
Group Counseling	**Definition:** The application of psychological methods to treat two or more individuals with addictive behavior **Explanation:** Provides structured group counseling sessions and healing power through the connection with others
Individual Counseling	**Definition:** The application of psychological methods to treat an individual with addictive behavior **Explanation:** Comprised of several different techniques, which apply various strategies to address drug addiction
Individual Psychotherapy	**Definition:** Treatment of an individual with addictive behavior by behavioral, cognitive, psychoanalytic, psychodynamic or psychophysiological means
Medication Management	**Definition:** Monitoring and adjusting the use of replacement medications for the treatment of addiction
Pharmacotherapy	**Definition:** The use of replacement medications for the treatment of addiction

SECTION X - NEW TECHNOLOGY
CHARACTER 3 - OPERATION

Assistance	**Definition:** Taking over a portion of a physiological function by extracorporeal means
Bypass	**Definition:** Altering the route of passage of the contents of a tubular body part
Destruction	**Definition:** Physical eradication of all or a portion of a body part by the direct use of energy, force, or a destructive agent **Explanation:** None of the body part is physically taken out **Includes/Examples:** Fulguration of rectal polyp, cautery of skin lesion
Dilation	**Definition:** Expanding an orifice or the lumen of a tubular body part **Explanation:** The orifice can be a natural orifice or an artificially created orifice. Accomplished by stretching a tubular body part using intraluminal pressure or by cutting part of the orifice or wall of the tubular body part
Extirpation	**Definition:** Taking or cutting out solid matter from a body part **Explanation:** The solid matter may be an abnormal byproduct of a biological function or foreign body; it may be imbedded in a body part or in the lumen of a tubular body part. The solid matter may or may not have been previously broken into pieces **Includes/Examples:** Thrombectomy, choledocholithotomy
Fusion	**Definition:** Joining together portions of an articular body part rendering the articular body part immobile **Explanation:** The body part is joined together by fixation device, bone graft, or other means **Includes/Examples:** Spinal fusion, ankle arthrodesis
Insertion	**Definition:** Putting in a nonbiological appliance that monitors, assists,performs, or prevents a physiological function but does not physically take the place of a body part
Inspection	**Definition:** Visually and/or manually exploring a body part
Introduction	**Definition:** Putting in or on a therapeutic, diagnostic, nutritional, physiological, or prophylactic substance except blood or blood products
Irrigation	**Definition:** Putting in or on a cleansing substance
Measurement	**Definition:** Determining the level of a physiological or physical function repetitively at a point in time
Monitoring	**Definition:** Determining the level of a physiological or physical function repetitively over a period of time

SECTION X - NEW TECHNOLOGY
CHARACTER 3 - OPERATION

Replacement	**Definition:** Putting in or on biological or synthetic material that physically takes the place and/or function of all or a portion of a body part **Explanation:** The body part may have been taken out or replaced, or may be taken out, physically eradicated, or rendered nonfunctional during the Replacement procedure. A Removal procedure is coded for taking out the device used in a previous replacement procedure **Includes/Examples:** Total hip replacement, bone graft, free skin graft
Reposition	**Definition:** Moving to its normal location, or other suitable location, all or a portion of a body part **Explanation:** The body part is moved to a new location from an abnormal location, or from a normal location where it is not functioning correctly. The body part may or may not be cut out or off to be moved to the new location **Includes/Examples:** Reposition of undescended testicle, fracture reduction
Restriction	Definition: Partially closing an orifice or the lumen of a tubular body part
Supplement	**Definition:** Putting in or on biological or synthetic material that physically reinforces and/or augments the function of a portion of a body part

SECTION X - NEW TECHNOLOGY
CHARACTER 5 - APPROACH

External	**Definition:** Procedures performed directly on the skin or mucous membrane and procedures performed indirectly by the application of external force through the skin or mucous membrane
Open	**Definition:** Cutting through the skin or mucous membrane and any other body layers necessary to expose the site of the procedure
Percutaneous	**Definition:** Entry, by puncture or minor incision, of instrumentation through the skin or mucous membrane and any other body layers necessary to reach the site of the procedure
Percutaneous Endoscopic	**Definition:** Entry, by puncture or minor incision, of instrumentation through the skin or mucous membrane and any other body layers necessary to reach and visualize the site of the procedure
Via Natural or Artificial Opening Endoscopic	**Definition:** Entry of instrumentation through a natural or artificial external opening to reach and visualize the site of the procedure
Via Natural or Artificial Opening	**Definition:** Entry of instrumentation through a natural or artificial external opening to reach the site of the procedure

SECTION X - NEW TECHNOLOGY

CHARACTER 6 - DEVICE / SUBSTANCE / TECHNOLOGY

Anacaulase-bcdb	Bromelain-enriched Proteolytic Enzyme NexoBrid™
Antibiotic-eluting Bone Void Filler	CERAMENT® G
Apalutamide Antineoplastic	ERLEADA™
Atezolizumab Antineoplastic	TECENTRIQ®
Axicabtagene Ciloleucel Immunotherapy	Axicabtagene Ciloleucel Yescarta®
Betibeglogene Autotemcel	ZYNTEGLO®
Bezlotoxumab Monoclonal Antibody	ZINPLAVA™
Bioengineered Allogeneic Construct	StrataGraft®
Branched Synthetic Substitute with Intraluminal Device in Technology	Thoraflex™ Hybrid device
Brexanolone	ZULRESSO™
Brexucabtagene Autoleucel Immunotherapy	Brexucabtagene Autoleucel Tecartus™
~~Bromelain-enriched Proteolytic Enzyme~~	~~NexoBrid™~~
Cefiderocol Anti-infective	FETROJA®
Ceftolozane/Tazobactam Anti-infective	ZEBAXA®
Ciltacabtagene Autoleucel	cilta-cel
Coagulation Factor Xa, Inactivated	Andexanet Alfa, Factor Xa Inhibitor Reversal Agent Andexxa Coagulation Factor Xa, (Recombinant) Factor Xa Inhibitor Reversal Agent, Andexanet Alfa
Concentrated Bone Marrow Aspirate	CBMA (Concentrated Bone Marrow Aspirate)
Conduit through Femoral Vein to Popliteal Artery in New Technology	DETOUR® System
Conduit through Femoral Vein to Superficial Femoral Artery in New Technology	DETOUR® System
Conduit to Short-term External Heart Assist System in New Technology	Impella® 5.5 with SmartAssist(R) System
COVID-19 Vaccine COVID-19 Vaccine Booster COVID-19 Vaccine Dose 1 COVID-19 Vaccine Dose 2 COVID-19 Vaccine Dose 3	COMIRNATY® SPIKEVAX™
Cytarabine and Daunorubicin Liposome Antineoplastic	VYXEOS™
Defibrotide Sodium Anticoagulant	Defitelio
Durvalumab Antineoplastic	IMFINZI®
Eculizumab	Soliris®
Endothelial Damage Inhibitor	DuraGraft® Endothelial Damage Inhibitor
Esketamine Hydrochloride	SPRAVATO™
Fosfomycin Anti-infective	CONTEPO™ Fosfomycin injection
Gilteritinib Antineoplastic	XOSPATA®
High-Dose Intravenous Immune Globulin	GAMUNEX-C, for COVID-19 treatment hdIVIG (high-dose intravenous immunoglobulin), for COVID-19 treatment High-dose intravenous immunoglobulin for COVID-19 treatment Octagam 10%, for COVID-19 treatment
Hyperimmune Globulin	Anti-SARS-CoV-2 hyperimmune globulin HIG (hyperimmune globulin), for COVID-19 treatment hIVIG (hyperimmune intravenous immunoglobulin), for COVID-19 treatment Hyperimmune intravenous immunoglobulin (hIVIG), for COVID-19 treatment IGIV-C, for COVID-19 treatment
Idecabtagene Vicleucel Immunotherapy	ABECMA® Ide-cel Idecabtagene Vicleucel
Imipenem-cilastatin-relebactam Anti-infective	IMI/REL
Interbody Fusion Device,Custom-Made Anatomically Designed in New Technology ~~Interbody Fusion Device, Customizable in New Technology~~	aprevo™
Interbody Fusion Device, Nanotextured Surface in New Technology	nanoLOCK™ interbody fusion device
Interbody Fusion Device, Radiolucent Porous in New Technology	COALESCE® radiolucent interbody fusion device COHERE® radiolucent interbody fusion device
Internal Fixation Device, Open-truss Design in New Technology	Ankle Truss System™ (ATS)

SECTION X - NEW TECHNOLOGY
CHARACTER 6 - DEVICE / SUBSTANCE / TECHNOLOGY

Intracardiac Pacemaker, Dual-Chamber in New Technology	Aveir™ AR, as dual chamber Aveir™ DR, dual chamber
Intraluminal Device, Bioprosthetic Valve in New Technology	TricValve® Transcatheter Bicaval Valve System VenoValve®
Intraluminal Device, Sustained Release Drug-eluting in New Technology	Eluvia™ Drug-Eluting Vascular Stent System SAVAL below-the-knee (BTK) drug-eluting
Intraluminal Device, Sustained Release Drug-eluting, Four or More in New Technology	Eluvia™ Drug-Eluting Vascular Stent System SAVAL below-the-knee (BTK) drug-eluting
Intraluminal Device, Sustained Release Drug-eluting, Three in New Technology	Eluvia™ Drug-Eluting Vascular Stent System SAVAL below-the-knee (BTK) drug-eluting
Intraluminal Device, Sustained Release Drug-eluting, Two in New Technology	Eluvia™ Drug-Eluting Vascular Stent System SAVAL below-the-knee (BTK) drug-eluting
Iobenguane I-131 Antineoplastic	AZEDRA® Iobenguane I-131, High Specific Activity (HSA)
Lefamulin Anti-infective	XENLETA™
Lifileucel Immunotherapy	Lifileucel
Lisocabatagene Maraleucel Immunotherapy	Lisocabtagene Maraleucel
Lurbinectedin	ZEPZELCA™
Magnetically Controlled Growth Rod(s) in New Technology	MAGEC® Spinal Bracing and Distraction System Spinal growth rods, magnetically controlled
Melphalan Hydrochloride Antineoplastic	HEPZATO™ KIT (melphalan hydrochloride Hepatic Delivery System)
Meropenem-vaborbactam Anti-infective	Vabomere™
Mineral-based Topcal Hemostatic Agent	Hemospray® Endoscopic Hemostat
Mosunetuzumab Antineoplastic	LUNSUMIO™
Nafamostat Anticoagulant	LTX Regional Anticoagulant Niyad™
Nerinitide	NA-1 (Nerinitide)
Omadacycline Anti-infective	NUZYRA™
Other New Technology Therapeutic Substance	STELARA® Ustekinumab
Posterior (Dynamic) Distraction Device in New Technology	ApiFix® Minimally Invasive Deformity Correction (MID-C) System
Reduction Device in New Technology	Neovasc Reducer™ Reducer™ System
Ruxolitinib	Jakafi®
Satralizumab-mwge	ENSPRYNG™
Skin Substitute, Porcine Liver Derived in New Technology	MIRODERM™ Biologic Wound Matrix
Sulbactam-Durlobactam	SUL-DUR
~~Synthetic Human Angiotensin II~~	~~Angiotensin II~~ ~~GIAPREZA™~~ ~~Human angiotensin II, synthetic~~
Synthetic Substitute,Extraluminal Support Device in New Technology	VasQ™ External Support device
Synthetic Substitute, Talar Prosthesis in New Technology	Total Ankle Talar Replacement™ (TATR)
Synthetic Substitute,Ultrasound Penetrable in New Technology	Longeviti ClearFit® Cranial Implant Longeviti ClearFit® OTS Cranial Implant
Synthetic Substitute, Mechanically Expandable (Paired) in New Technology	SpineJack® system
Tagraxofusp-erzs Antineoplastic	ELZONRIS™
Terlipressin	TERLIVAZ®
Tibial Extension with Motion Sensors in New Technology	Canturio™ te (Tibial Extension)
Tisagenlecleucel Immunotherapy	KYMRIAH® Tisagenlecleucel
Trilaciclib	COSELA™
Uridine Triacetate	Vistogard®
Vein Graft Extraluminal Support Device(s) in New Technology	VEST™ Venous External Support device
Venetoclax Antineoplastic	Venclexta®
Zooplastic Tissue, Rapid Deployment Technique in New Technology	EDWARDS INTUITY Elite valve system INTUITY Elite valve system, EDWARDS Perceval sutureless valve Sutureless valve, Perceval

BODY PART KEY

Abdominal aortic plexus	**Use:** Abdominal Sympathetic Nerve
Abdominal esophagus	**Use:** Esophagus, Lower
Abductor hallucis muscle	**Use:** Foot Muscle, Right Foot Muscle, Left
Accessory cephalic vein	**Use:** Cephalic Vein, Right Cephalic Vein, Left
Accessory obturator nerve	**Use:** Lumbar Plexus
Accessory phrenic nerve	**Use:** Phrenic Nerve
Accessory spleen	**Use:** Spleen
Acetabulofemoral joint	**Use:** Hip Joint, Right Hip Joint, Left
Achilles tendon	**Use:** Lower Leg Tendon, Right Lower Leg Tendon, Left
Acromioclavicular ligament	**Use:** Shoulder Bursa and Ligament, Right Shoulder Bursa and Ligament, Left
Acromion (process)	**Use:** Scapula, Right Scapula, Left
Adductor brevis muscle	**Use:** Upper Leg Muscle, Right Upper Leg Muscle, Left
Adductor hallucis muscle	**Use:** Foot Muscle, Right Foot Muscle, Left
Adductor longus muscle Adductor magnus muscle	**Use:** Upper Leg Muscle, Right Upper Leg Muscle, Left
Adenohypophysis	**Use:** Pituitary Gland
Alar ligament of axis	**Use:** Head and Neck Bursa and Ligament
Alveolar process of mandible	**Use:** Mandible, Right Mandible, Left
Alveolar process of maxilla	**Use:** Maxilla
Anal orifice	**Use:** Anus
Anatomical snuffbox	**Use:** Lower Arm and Wrist Muscle, Right Lower Arm and Wrist Muscle, Left
Angular artery	**Use:** Face Artery
Angular vein	**Use:** Face Vein, Right Face Vein, Left
Annular ligament	**Use:** Elbow Bursa and Ligament, Right Elbow Bursa and Ligament, Left
Anorectal junction	**Use:** Rectum
Ansa cervicalis	**Use:** Cervical Plexus
Antebrachial fascia	**Use:** Subcutaneous Tissue and Fascia, Right Lower Arm Subcutaneous Tissue and Fascia, Left Lower Arm
Anterior (pectoral) lymph node	**Use:** Lymphatic, Right Axillary Lymphatic, Left Axillary
Anterior cerebral artery	**Use:** Intracranial Artery
Anterior cerebral vein	**Use:** Intracranial Vein
Anterior choroidal artery	**Use:** Intracranial Artery
Anterior circumflex humeral artery	**Use:** Axillary Artery, Right Axillary Artery, Left
Anterior communicating artery	**Use:** Intracranial Artery
Anterior cruciate ligament (ACL)	**Use:** Knee Bursa and Ligament, Right Knee Bursa and Ligament, Left
Anterior crural nerve	**Use:** Femoral Nerve

BODY PART KEY

Anterior facial vein	**Use:** Face Vein, Right Face Vein, Left
Anterior intercostal artery	**Use:** Internal Mammary Artery, Right Internal Mammary Artery, Left
Anterior interosseous nerve	**Use:** Median Nerve
Anterior lateral malleolar artery	**Use:** Anterior Tibial Artery, Right Anterior Tibial Artery, Left
Anterior lingual gland	**Use:** Minor Salivary Gland
Anterior medial malleolar artery	**Use:** Anterior Tibial Artery, Right Anterior Tibial Artery, Left
Anterior spinal artery	**Use:** Vertebral Artery, Right Vertebral Artery, Left
Anterior tibial recurrent artery	**Use:** Anterior Tibial Artery, Right Anterior Tibial Artery, Left
Anterior ulnar recurrent artery	**Use:** Ulnar Artery, Right Ulnar Artery, Left
Anterior vagal trunk	**Use:** Vagus Nerve
Anterior vertebral muscle	**Use:** Neck Muscle, Right Neck Muscle, Left
Antihelix Antitragus	**Use:** External Ear, Right External Ear, Left External Ear, Bilateral
Antrum of Highmore	**Use:** Maxillary Sinus, Right Maxillary Sinus, Left
Aortic annulus	**Use:** Aortic Valve
Aortic arch	**Use:** Thoracic Aorta, Ascending/Arch
Aortic intercostal artery	**Use:** Upper Artery
Apical (subclavicular) lymph node	**Use:** Lymphatic, Right Axillary Lymphatic, Left Axillary

Apneustic center	**Use:** Pons
Aqueduct of Sylvius	**Use:** Cerebral Ventricle
Aqueous humour	**Use:** Anterior Chamber, Right Anterior Chamber, Left
Arachnoid mater	**Use:** Cerebral Meninges Spinal Meninges
Arcuate artery	**Use:** Foot Artery, Right Foot Artery, Left
Areola	**Use:** Nipple, Right Nipple, Left
Arterial canal (duct)	**Use:** Pulmonary Artery, Left
Aryepiglottic fold Arytenoid cartilage	**Use:** Larynx
Arytenoid muscle	**Use:** Neck Muscle, Right Neck Muscle, Left
Ascending aorta	**Use:** Thoracic Aorta, Ascending/Arch
Ascending palatine artery	**Use:** Face Artery
Ascending pharyngeal artery	**Use:** External Carotid Artery, Right External Carotid Artery, Left
Atlantoaxial joint	**Use:** Cervical Vertebral Joint
Atrioventricular node	**Use:** Conduction Mechanism
Atrium dextrum cordis	**Use:** Atrium, Right
Atrium pulmonale	**Use:** Atrium, Left
Auditory tube	**Use:** Eustachian Tube, Right Eustachian Tube, Left
Auerbach's (myenteric) plexus	**Use:** Abdominal Sympathetic Nerve

APPENDIX B

BODY PART KEY

Auricle	**Use:** External Ear, Right External Ear, Left External Ear, Bilateral
Auricularis muscle	**Use:** Head Muscle
Axillary fascia	**Use:** Subcutaneous Tissue and Fascia, Right Upper Arm Subcutaneous Tissue and Fascia, Left Upper Arm
Axillary nerve	**Use:** Brachial Plexus
Bartholin's (greater vestibular) gland	**Use:** Vestibular Gland
Basal (internal) cerebral vein	**Use:** Intracranial Vein
Basal nuclei	**Use:** Basal Ganglia
Base of Tongue	**Use:** Pharynx
Basilar artery	**Use:** Intracranial Artery
Basis pontis	**Use:** Pons
Biceps brachii muscle	**Use:** Upper Arm Muscle, Right Upper Arm Muscle, Left
Biceps femoris muscle	**Use:** Upper Leg Muscle, Right Upper Leg Muscle, Left
Bicipital aponeurosis	**Use:** Subcutaneous Tissue and Fascia, Right Lower Arm Subcutaneous Tissue and Fascia, Left Lower Arm
Bicuspid valve	**Use:** Mitral Valve
Body of femur	**Use:** Femoral Shaft, Right Femoral Shaft, Left
Body of fibula	**Use:** Fibula, Right Fibula, Left
Bony labyrinth	**Use:** Inner Ear, Right Inner Ear, Left
Bony orbit	**Use:** Orbit, Right Orbit, Left
Bony vestibule	**Use:** Inner Ear, Right Inner Ear, Left
Botallo's duct	**Use:** Pulmonary Artery, Left
Brachial (lateral) lymph node	**Use:** Lymphatic, Right Axillary Lymphatic, Left Axillary
Brachialis muscle	**Use:** Upper Arm Muscle, Right Upper Arm Muscle, Left
Brachiocephalic artery Brachiocephalic trunk	**Use:** Innominate Artery
Brachiocephalic vein	**Use:** Innominate Vein, Right Innominate Vein, Left
Brachioradialis muscle	**Use:** Lower Arm and Wrist Muscle, Right Lower Arm and Wrist Muscle, Left
Broad ligament	**Use:** Uterine Supporting Structure
Bronchial artery	**Use:** Upper Artery
Bronchus Intermedius	**Use:** Main Bronchus, Right
Buccal gland	**Use:** Buccal Mucosa
Buccinator lymph node	**Use:** Lymphatic, Head
Buccinator muscle	**Use:** Facial Muscle
Bulbospongiosus muscle	**Use:** Perineum Muscle
Bulbourethral (Cowper's) gland	**Use:** Urethra
Bundle of His Bundle of Kent	**Use:** Conduction Mechanism
Calcaneocuboid joint	**Use:** Tarsal Joint, Right Tarsal Joint, Left
Calcaneocuboid ligament	**Use:** Foot Bursa and Ligament, Right Foot Bursa and Ligament, Left

BODY PART KEY

Calcaneofibular ligament	**Use:** Ankle Bursa and Ligament, Right Ankle Bursa and Ligament, Left
Calcaneus	**Use:** Tarsal, Right Tarsal, Left
Capitate bone	**Use:** Carpal, Right Carpal, Left
Cardia	**Use:** Esophagogastric Junction
Cardiac plexus	**Use:** Thoracic Sympathetic Nerve
Cardioesophageal junction	**Use:** Esophagogastric Junction
Caroticotympanic artery	**Use:** Internal Carotid Artery, Right Internal Carotid Artery, Left
Carotid glomus	**Use:** Carotid Body, Left Carotid Body, Right Carotid Bodies, Bilateral
Carotid sinus	**Use:** Internal Carotid Artery, Right Internal Carotid Artery, Left
Carotid sinus nerve	**Use:** Glossopharyngeal Nerve
Carpometacarpal ligament	**Use:** Hand Bursa and Ligament, Right Hand Bursa and Ligament, Left
Cauda equina	**Use:** Lumbar Spinal Cord
Cavernous plexus	**Use:** Head and Neck Sympathetic Nerve
Celiac (solar) plexus Celiac ganglion	**Use:** Abdominal Sympathetic Nerve
Celiac lymph node	**Use:** Lymphatic, Aortic
Celiac trunk	**Use:** Celiac Artery
Central axillary lymph node	**Use:** Lymphatic, Right Axillary Lymphatic, Left Axillary
Cerebral aqueduct (Sylvius)	**Use:** Cerebral Ventricle
Cerebrum	**Use:** Brain
Cervical esophagus	**Use:** Esophagus, Upper
Cervical facet joint	**Use:** Cervical Vertebral Joint Cervical Vertebral Joints, 2 or more
Cervical ganglion	**Use:** Head and Neck Sympathetic Nerve
Cervical interspinous ligament Cervical intertransverse ligament Cervical ligamentum flavum	**Use:** Head and Neck Bursa and Ligament
Cervical lymph node	**Use:** Lymphatic, Right Neck Lymphatic, Left Neck
Cervicothoracic facet joint	**Use:** Cervicothoracic Vertebral Joint
Choana	**Use:** Nasopharynx
Chondroglossus muscle	**Use:** Tongue, Palate, Pharynx Muscle
Chorda tympani	**Use:** Facial Nerve
Choroid plexus	**Use:** Cerebral Ventricle
Ciliary body	**Use:** Eye, Right Eye, Left
Ciliary ganglion	**Use:** Head and Neck Sympathetic Nerve
Circle of Willis	**Use:** Intracranial Artery
Circumflex iliac artery	**Use:** Femoral Artery, Right Femoral Artery, Left
Claustrum	**Use:** Basal Ganglia
Coccygeal body	**Use:** Coccygeal Glomus
Coccygeus muscle	**Use:** Trunk Muscle, Right Trunk Muscle, Left
Cochlea	**Use:** Inner Ear, Right Inner Ear, Left

BODY PART KEY

Cochlear nerve	**Use:** Acoustic Nerve
Columella	**Use:** Nasal Mucosa and Soft Tissue
Common digital vein	**Use:** Foot Vein, Right Foot Vein, Left
Common facial vein	**Use:** Face Vein, Right Face Vein, Left
Common fibular nerve	**Use:** Peroneal Nerve
Common hepatic artery	**Use:** Hepatic Artery
Common iliac (subaortic) lymph node	**Use:** Lymphatic, Pelvis
Common interosseous artery	**Use:** Ulnar Artery, Right Ulnar Artery, Left
Common peroneal nerve	**Use:** Peroneal Nerve
Condyloid process	**Use:** Mandible, Right Mandible, Left
Conus arteriosus	**Use:** Ventricle, Right
Conus medullaris	**Use:** Lumbar Spinal Cord
Coracoacromial ligament	**Use:** Shoulder Bursa and Ligament, Right Shoulder Bursa and Ligament, Left
Coracobrachialis muscle	**Use:** Upper Arm Muscle, Right Upper Arm Muscle, Left
Coracoclavicular ligament Coracohumeral ligament	**Use:** Shoulder Bursa and Ligament, Right Shoulder Bursa and Ligament, Left
Coracoid process	**Use:** Scapula, Right Scapula, Left
Corniculate cartilage	**Use:** Larynx
Corpus callosum	**Use:** Brain

Corpus cavernosum Corpus spongiosum	**Use:** Penis
Corpus striatum	**Use:** Basal Ganglia
Corrugator supercilii muscle	**Use:** Facial Muscle
Costocervical trunk	**Use:** Subclavian Artery, Right Subclavian Artery, Left
Costoclavicular ligament	**Use:** Shoulder Bursa and Ligament, Right Shoulder Bursa and Ligament, Left
Costotransverse joint	**Use:** Thoracic Vertebral Joint Thoracic Vertebral Joints, 2 to 7 Thoracic Vertebral Joints, 8 or more
Costotransverse ligament	**Use:** Sternum Bursa and Ligament Rib(s) Bursa and Ligament
Costovertebral joint	**Use:** Thoracic Vertebral Joint Thoracic Vertebral Joints, 2 to 7 Thoracic Vertebral Joints, 8 or more
Costoxiphoid ligament	**Use:** Sternum Bursa and Ligament Rib(s) Bursa and Ligament
Cowper's (bulbourethral) gland	**Use:** Urethra
Cremaster muscle	**Use:** Perineum Muscle
Cribriform plate	**Use:** Ethmoid Bone, Right Ethmoid Bone, Left
Cricoid cartilage	**Use:** Trachea
Cricothyroid artery	**Use:** Thyroid Artery, Right Thyroid Artery, Left
Cricothyroid muscle	**Use:** Neck Muscle, Right Neck Muscle, Left

BODY PART KEY

Crural fascia	**Use:** Subcutaneous Tissue and Fascia, Right Upper Leg Subcutaneous Tissue and Fascia, Left Upper Leg
Cubital lymph node	**Use:** Lymphatic, Right Upper Extremity Lymphatic, Left Upper Extremity
Cubital nerve	**Use:** Ulnar Nerve
Cuboid bone	**Use:** Tarsal, Right Tarsal, Left
Cuboideonavicular joint	**Use:** Tarsal Joint, Right Tarsal Joint, Left
Culmen	**Use:** Cerebellum
Cuneiform cartilage	**Use:** Larynx
Cuneonavicular joint	**Use:** Tarsal Joint, Right Tarsal Joint, Left
Cuneonavicular ligament	**Use:** Foot Bursa and Ligament, Right Foot Bursa and Ligament, Left
Cutaneous (transverse) cervical nerve	**Use:** Cervical Plexus
Deep cervical fascia	**Use:** Subcutaneous Tissue and Fascia, Right Neck Subcutaneous Tissue and Fascia, Left Neck
Deep cervical vein	**Use:** Vertebral Vein, Right Vertebral Vein, Left
Deep circumflex iliac artery	**Use:** External Iliac Artery, Right External Iliac Artery, Left
Deep facial vein	**Use:** Face Vein, Right Face Vein, Left
Deep femoral (profunda femoris) vein	**Use:** Femoral Vein, Right Femoral Vein, Left
Deep femoral artery	**Use:** Femoral Artery, Right Femoral Artery, Left
Deep palmar arch	**Use:** Hand Artery, Right Hand Artery, Left
Deep transverse perineal muscle	**Use:** Perineum Muscle
Deferential artery	**Use:** Internal Iliac Artery, Right Internal Iliac Artery, Left
Deltoid fascia	**Use:** Subcutaneous Tissue and Fascia, Right Upper Arm Subcutaneous Tissue and Fascia, Left Upper Arm
Deltoid ligament	**Use:** Ankle Bursa and Ligament, Right Ankle Bursa and Ligament, Left
Deltoid muscle	**Use:** Shoulder Muscle, Right Shoulder Muscle, Left
Deltopectoral (infraclavicular) lymph node	**Use:** Lymphatic, Right Upper Extremity Lymphatic, Left Upper Extremity
Dens	**Use:** Cervical Vertebra
Denticulate (dentate) ligament	**Use:** Spinal Cord
Depressor anguli oris muscle Depressor labii inferioris muscle Depressor septi nasi muscle Depressor supercilii muscle	**Use:** Facial Muscle
Dermis	**Use:** Skin
Descending genicular artery	**Use:** Femoral Artery, Right Femoral Artery, Left
Diaphragma sellae	**Use:** Dura Mater
Distal humerus	**Use:** Humeral Shaft, Right Humeral Shaft, Left
Distal humerus, involving joint	**Use:** Elbow Joint, Right Elbow Joint, Left
Distal radioulnar joint	**Use:** Wrist Joint, Right Wrist Joint, Left
Dorsal digital nerve	**Use:** Radial Nerve

BODY PART KEY

Dorsal metacarpal vein	**Use:** Hand Vein, Right Hand Vein, Left
Dorsal metatarsal artery	**Use:** Foot Artery, Right Foot Artery, Left
Dorsal metatarsal vein	**Use:** Foot Vein, Right Foot Vein, Left
Dorsal scapular artery	**Use:** Subclavian Artery, Right Subclavian Artery, Left
Dorsal scapular nerve	**Use:** Brachial Plexus
Dorsal venous arch	**Use:** Foot Vein, Right Foot Vein, Left
Dorsalis pedis artery	**Use:** Anterior Tibial Artery, Right Anterior Tibial Artery, Left
Duct of Santorini	**Use:** Pancreatic Duct, Accessory
Duct of Wirsung	**Use:** Pancreatic Duct
Ductus deferens	**Use:** Vas Deferens, Right Vas Deferens, Left Vas Deferens, Bilateral Vas Deferens
Duodenal ampulla	**Use:** Ampulla of Vater
Duodenojejunal flexure	**Use:** Jejunum
Dura mater, intracranial	**Use:** Dura Mater
Dura mater, spinal	**Use:** Spinal Meninges
Dural venous sinus	**Use:** Intracranial Vein
Earlobe	**Use:** External Ear, Right External Ear, Left External Ear, Bilateral
Eighth cranial nerve	**Use:** Acoustic Nerve
Ejaculatory duct	**Use:** Vas Deferens, Right Vas Deferens, Left Vas Deferens, Bilateral Vas Deferens
Eleventh cranial nerve	**Use:** Accessory Nerve
Encephalon	**Use:** Brain
Ependyma	**Use:** Cerebral Ventricle
Epidermis	**Use:** Skin
Epidural space, spinal	**Use:** Spinal Canal
Epiploic foramen	**Use:** Peritoneum
Epithalamus	**Use:** Thalamus
Epitrochlear lymph node	**Use:** Lymphatic, Right Upper Extremity Lymphatic, Left Upper Extremity
Erector spinae muscle	**Use:** Trunk Muscle, Right Trunk Muscle, Left
Esophageal artery	**Use:** Upper Artery
Esophageal plexus	**Use:** Thoracic Sympathetic Nerve
Ethmoidal air cell	**Use:** Ethmoid Sinus, Right Ethmoid Sinus, Left
Extensor carpi radialis muscle Extensor carpi ulnaris muscle	**Use:** Lower Arm and Wrist Muscle, Right Lower Arm and Wrist Muscle, Left
Extensor digitorum brevis muscle	**Use:** Foot Muscle, Right Foot Muscle, Left
Extensor digitorum longus muscle	**Use:** Lower Leg Muscle, Right Lower Leg Muscle, Left
Extensor hallucis brevis muscle	**Use:** Foot Muscle, Right Foot Muscle, Left
Extensor hallucis longus muscle	**Use:** Lower Leg Muscle, Right Lower Leg Muscle, Left

BODY PART KEY

External anal sphincter	**Use:** Anal Sphincter
External auditory meatus	**Use:** External Auditory Canal, Right External Auditory Canal, Left
External maxillary artery	**Use:** Face Artery
External naris	**Use:** Nasal Mucosa and Soft Tissue
External oblique aponeurosis	**Use:** Subcutaneous Tissue and Fascia, Trunk
External oblique muscle	**Use:** Abdomen Muscle, Right Abdomen Muscle, Left
External popliteal nerve	**Use:** Peroneal Nerve
External pudendal artery	**Use:** Femoral Artery, Right Femoral Artery, Left
External pudendal vein	**Use:** Saphenous Vein, Right Saphenous Vein, Left
External urethral sphincter	**Use:** Urethra
Extradural space, intracranial	**Use:** Epidural Space, Intracranial
Extradural space, spinal	**Use:** Spinal Canal
Facial artery	**Use:** Face Artery
False vocal cord	**Use:** Larynx
Falx cerebri	**Use:** Dura Mater
Fascia lata	**Use:** Subcutaneous Tissue and Fascia, Right Upper Leg Subcutaneous Tissue and Fascia, Left Upper Leg
Femoral head	**Use:** Upper Femur, Right Upper Femur, Left
Femoral lymph node	**Use:** Lymphatic, Right Lower Extremity Lymphatic, Left Lower Extremity
Femoropatellar joint Femorotibial joint	**Use:** Knee Joint, Right Knee Joint, Left
Fibular artery	**Use:** Peroneal Artery, Right Peroneal Artery, Left
Fibularis brevis muscle Fibularis longus muscle	**Use:** Lower Leg Muscle, Right Lower Leg Muscle, Left
Fifth cranial nerve	**Use:** Trigeminal Nerve
Filum terminale	**Use:** Spinal Meninges
First cranial nerve	**Use:** Olfactory Nerve
First intercostal nerve	**Use:** Brachial Plexus
Flexor carpi radialis muscle Flexor carpi ulnaris muscle	**Use:** Lower Arm and Wrist Muscle, Right Lower Arm and Wrist Muscle, Left
Flexor digitorum brevis muscle	**Use:** Foot Muscle, Right Foot Muscle, Left
Flexor digitorum longus muscle	**Use:** Lower Leg Muscle, Right Lower Leg Muscle, Left
Flexor hallucis brevis muscle	**Use:** Foot Muscle, Right Foot Muscle, Left
Flexor hallucis longus muscle	**Use:** Lower Leg Muscle, Right Lower Leg Muscle, Left
Flexor pollicis longus muscle	**Use:** Lower Arm and Wrist Muscle, Right Lower Arm and Wrist Muscle, Left
Foramen magnum	**Use:** Occipital Bone
Foramen of Monro (intraventricular)	**Use:** Cerebral Ventricle
Foreskin	**Use:** Prepuce
Fossa of Rosenmuller	**Use:** Nasopharynx

BODY PART KEY

Fourth cranial nerve	**Use:** Trochlear Nerve
Fourth ventricle	**Use:** Cerebral Ventricle
Fovea	**Use:** Retina, Right Retina, Left
Frenulum labii inferioris	**Use:** Lower Lip
Frenulum labii superioris	**Use:** Upper Lip
Frenulum linguae	**Use:** Tongue
Frontal lobe	**Use:** Cerebral Hemisphere
Frontal vein	**Use:** Face Vein, Right Face Vein, Left
Fundus uteri	**Use:** Uterus
Galea aponeurotica	**Use:** Subcutaneous Tissue and Fascia, Scalp
Ganglion impar (ganglion of Walther)	**Use:** Sacral Sympathetic Nerve
Gasserian ganglion	**Use:** Trigeminal Nerve
Gastric lymph node	**Use:** Lymphatic, Aortic
Gastric plexus	**Use:** Abdominal Sympathetic Nerve
Gastrocnemius muscle	**Use:** Lower Leg Muscle, Right Lower Leg Muscle, Left
Gastrocolic ligament Gastrocolic omentum	**Use:** Omentum
Gastroduodenal artery	**Use:** Hepatic Artery
Gastroesophageal (GE) junction	**Use:** Esophagogastric Junction
Gastrohepatic omentum Gastrophrenic ligament Gastrosplenic ligament	**Use:** Omentum
Gemellus muscle	**Use:** Hip Muscle, Right Hip Muscle, Left
Geniculate ganglion	**Use:** Facial Nerve
Geniculate nucleus	**Use:** Thalamus
Genioglossus muscle	**Use:** Tongue, Palate, Pharynx Muscle
Genitofemoral nerve	**Use:** Lumbar Plexus
Glans penis	**Use:** Prepuce
Glenohumeral joint	**Use:** Shoulder Joint, Right Shoulder Joint, Left
Glenohumeral ligament	**Use:** Shoulder Bursa and Ligament, Right Shoulder Bursa and Ligament, Left
Glenoid fossa (of scapula)	**Use:** Glenoid Cavity, Right Glenoid Cavity, Left
Glenoid ligament (labrum)	**Use:** Shoulder Bursa and Ligament, Right Shoulder Bursa and Ligament, Left
Globus pallidus	**Use:** Basal Ganglia
Glossoepiglottic fold	**Use:** Epiglottis
Glottis	**Use:** Larynx
Gluteal lymph node	**Use:** Lymphatic, Pelvis
Gluteal vein	**Use:** Hypogastric Vein, Right Hypogastric Vein, Left
Gluteus maximus muscle Gluteus medius muscle Gluteus minimus muscle	**Use:** Hip Muscle, Right Hip Muscle, Left
Gracilis muscle	**Use:** Upper Leg Muscle, Right Upper Leg Muscle, Left

BODY PART KEY

Great auricular nerve	**Use:** Cervical Plexus
Great cerebral vein	**Use:** Intracranial Vein
Greater saphenous vein	**Use:** Saphenous Vein, Right Saphenous Vein, Left
Greater alar cartilage	**Use:** Nasal Mucosa and Soft Tissue
Greater occipital nerve	**Use:** Cervical Nerve
Greater Omentum	**Use:** Omentum
Greater splanchnic nerve	**Use:** Thoracic Sympathetic Nerve
Greater superficial petrosal nerve	**Use:** Facial Nerve
Greater trochanter	**Use:** Upper Femur, Right Upper Femur, Left
Greater tuberosity	**Use:** Humeral Head, Right Humeral Head, Left
Greater vestibular (Bartholin's) gland	**Use:** Vestibular Gland
Greater wing	**Use:** Sphenoid Bone
Hallux	**Use:** 1st Toe, Right 1st Toe, Left
Hamate bone	**Use:** Carpal, Right Carpal, Left
Head of fibula	**Use:** Fibula, Right Fibula, Left
Helix	**Use:** External Ear, Right External Ear, Left External Ear, Bilateral
Hepatic artery proper	**Use:** Hepatic Artery
Hepatic flexure	**Use:** Transverse Colon
Hepatic lymph node	**Use:** Lymphatic, Aortic
Hepatic plexus	**Use:** Abdominal Sympathetic Nerve
Hepatic portal vein	**Use:** Portal Vein
Hepatogastric ligament	**Use:** Omentum
Hepatopancreatic ampulla	**Use:** Ampulla of Vater
Humeroradial joint Humeroulnar joint	**Use:** Elbow Joint, Right Elbow Joint, Left
Humerus, distal	**Use:** Humeral Shaft, Right Humeral Shaft, Left
Hyoglossus muscle	**Use:** Tongue, Palate, Pharynx Muscle
Hyoid artery	**Use:** Thyroid Artery, Right Thyroid Artery, Left
Hypogastric artery	**Use:** Internal Iliac Artery, Right Internal Iliac Artery, Left
Hypopharynx	**Use:** Pharynx
Hypophysis	**Use:** Pituitary Gland
Hypothenar muscle	**Use:** Hand Muscle, Right Hand Muscle, Left
Ileal artery Ileocolic artery	**Use:** Superior Mesenteric Artery
Ileocolic vein	**Use:** Colic Vein
Iliac crest	**Use:** Pelvic Bone, Right Pelvic Bone, Left
Iliac fascia	**Use:** Subcutaneous Tissue and Fascia, Right Upper Leg Subcutaneous Tissue and Fascia, Left Upper Leg

APPENDIX B

BODY PART KEY

Iliac lymph node	**Use:** Lymphatic, Pelvis
Iliacus muscle	**Use:** Hip Muscle, Right Hip Muscle, Left
Iliofemoral ligament	**Use:** Hip Bursa and Ligament, Right Hip Bursa and Ligament, Left
Iliohypogastric nerve Ilioinguinal nerve	**Use:** Lumbar Plexus
Iliolumbar artery	**Use:** Internal Iliac Artery, Right Internal Iliac Artery, Left
Iliolumbar ligament	**Use:** Lower Spine Bursa and Ligament
Iliotibial tract (band)	**Use:** Subcutaneous Tissue and Fascia, Right Upper Leg Subcutaneous Tissue and Fascia, Left Upper Leg
Ilium	**Use:** Pelvic Bone, Right Pelvic Bone, Left
Incus	**Use:** Auditory Ossicle, Right Auditory Ossicle, Left
Inferior cardiac nerve	**Use:** Thoracic Sympathetic Nerve
Inferior cerebellar vein Inferior cerebral vein	**Use:** Intracranial Vein
Inferior epigastric artery	**Use:** External Iliac Artery, Right External Iliac Artery, Left
Inferior epigastric lymph node	**Use:** Lymphatic, Pelvis
Inferior genicular artery	**Use:** Popliteal Artery, Right Popliteal Artery, Left
Inferior gluteal artery	**Use:** Internal Iliac Artery, Right Internal Iliac Artery, Left
Inferior gluteal nerve	**Use:** Sacral Plexus
Inferior hypogastric plexus	**Use:** Abdominal Sympathetic Nerve
Inferior labial artery	**Use:** Face Artery
Inferior longitudinal muscle	**Use:** Tongue, Palate, Pharynx Muscle
Inferior mesenteric ganglion	**Use:** Abdominal Sympathetic Nerve
Inferior mesenteric lymph node	**Use:** Lymphatic, Mesenteric
Inferior mesenteric plexus	**Use:** Abdominal Sympathetic Nerve
Inferior oblique muscle	**Use:** Extraocular Muscle, Right Extraocular Muscle, Left
Inferior pancreaticoduodenal artery	**Use:** Superior Mesenteric Artery
Inferior phrenic artery	**Use:** Abdominal Aorta
Inferior rectus muscle	**Use:** Extraocular Muscle, Right Extraocular Muscle, Left
Inferior suprarenal artery	**Use:** Renal Artery, Right Renal Artery, Left
Inferior tarsal plate	**Use:** Lower Eyelid, Right Lower Eyelid, Left
Inferior thyroid vein	**Use:** Innominate Vein, Right Innominate Vein, Left
Inferior tibiofibular joint	**Use:** Ankle Joint, Right Ankle Joint, Left
Inferior turbinate	**Use:** Nasal Turbinate
Inferior ulnar collateral artery	**Use:** Brachial Artery, Right Brachial Artery, Left
Inferior vesical artery	**Use:** Internal Iliac Artery, Right Internal Iliac Artery, Left

BODY PART KEY

Infraauricular lymph node	**Use:** Lymphatic, Head
Infraclavicular (deltopectoral) lymph node	**Use:** Lymphatic, Right Upper Extremity Lymphatic, Left Upper Extremity
Infrahyoid muscle	**Use:** Neck Muscle, Right Neck Muscle, Left
Infraparotid lymph node	**Use:** Lymphatic, Head
Infraspinatus fascia	**Use:** Subcutaneous Tissue and Fascia, Right Upper Arm Subcutaneous Tissue and Fascia, Left Upper Arm
Infraspinatus muscle	**Use:** Shoulder Muscle, Right Shoulder Muscle, Left
Infundibulopelvic ligament	**Use:** Uterine Supporting Structure
Inguinal canal Inguinal triangle	**Use:** Inguinal Region, Right Inguinal Region, Left Inguinal Region, Bilateral
Interatrial septum	**Use:** Atrial Septum
Intercarpal joint	**Use:** Carpal Joint, Right Carpal Joint, Left
Intercarpal ligament	**Use:** Hand Bursa and Ligament, Right Hand Bursa and Ligament, Left
Interclavicular ligament	**Use:** Shoulder Bursa and Ligament, Right Shoulder Bursa and Ligament, Left
Intercostal lymph node	**Use:** Lymphatic, Thorax
Intercostal muscle	**Use:** Thorax Muscle, Right Thorax Muscle, Left
Intercostal nerve Intercostobrachial nerve	**Use:** Thoracic Nerve
Intercuneiform joint	**Use:** Tarsal Joint, Right Tarsal Joint, Left
Intercuneiform ligament	**Use:** Foot Bursa and Ligament, Right Foot Bursa and Ligament, Left
Intermediate bronchus	**Use:** Main Bronchus, Right
Intermediate cuneiform bone	**Use:** Tarsal, Right Tarsal, Left
Internal (basal) cerebral vein	**Use:** Intracranial Vein
Internal anal sphincter	**Use:** Anal Sphincter
Internal carotid artery, intracranial portion	**Use:** Intracranial Artery
Internal carotid plexus	**Use:** Head and Neck Sympathetic Nerve
Internal iliac vein	**Use:** Hypogastric Vein, Right Hypogastric Vein, Left
Internal maxillary artery	**Use:** External Carotid Artery, Right External Carotid Artery, Left
Internal naris	**Use:** Nasal Mucosa and Soft Tissue
Internal oblique muscle	**Use:** Abdomen Muscle, Right Abdomen Muscle, Left
Internal pudendal artery	**Use:** Internal Iliac Artery, Right Internal Iliac Artery, Left
Internal pudendal vein	**Use:** Hypogastric Vein, Right Hypogastric Vein, Left
Internal thoracic artery	**Use:** Internal Mammary Artery, Right Internal Mammary Artery, Left Subclavian Artery, Right Subclavian Artery, Left
Internal urethral sphincter	**Use:** Urethra
Interphalangeal (IP) joint	**Use:** Finger Phalangeal Joint, Right Finger Phalangeal Joint, Left Toe Phalangeal Joint, Right Toe Phalangeal Joint, Left

BODY PART KEY

Interphalangeal ligament	**Use:** Hand Bursa and Ligament, Right Hand Bursa and Ligament, Left Foot Bursa and Ligament, Right Foot Bursa and Ligament, Left
Interspinalis muscle	**Use:** Trunk Muscle, Right Trunk Muscle, Left
Interspinous ligament	**Use:** Head and Neck Bursa and Ligament Upper Spine Bursa and Ligament Lower Spine Bursa and Ligament
Intertransversarius muscle	**Use:** Trunk Muscle, Right Trunk Muscle, Left
Intertransverse ligament	**Use:** Upper Spine Bursa and Ligament Lower Spine Bursa and Ligament
Interventricular foramen (Monro)	**Use:** Cerebral Ventricle
Interventricular septum	**Use:** Ventricular Septum
Intestinal lymphatic trunk	**Use:** Cisterna Chyli
Ischiatic nerve	**Use:** Sciatic Nerve
Ischiocavernosus muscle	**Use:** Perineum Muscle
Ischiofemoral ligament	**Use:** Hip Bursa and Ligament, Right Hip Bursa and Ligament, Left
Ischium	**Use:** Pelvic Bone, Right Pelvic Bone, Left
Jejunal artery	**Use:** Superior Mesenteric Artery
Jugular body	**Use:** Glomus Jugulare
Jugular lymph node	**Use:** Lymphatic, Right Neck Lymphatic, Left Neck
Labia majora Labia minora	**Use:** Vulva
Labial gland	**Use:** Upper Lip Lower Lip
Lacrimal canaliculus Lacrimal punctum Lacrimal sac	**Use:** Lacrimal Duct, Right Lacrimal Duct, Left
Laryngopharynx	**Use:** Pharynx
Lateral (brachial) lymph node	**Use:** Lymphatic, Right Axillary Lymphatic, Left Axillary
Lateral canthus	**Use:** Upper Eyelid, Right Upper Eyelid, Left
Lateral collateral ligament (LCL)	**Use:** Knee Bursa and Ligament, Right Knee Bursa and Ligament, Left
Lateral condyle of femur	**Use:** Lower Femur, Right Lower Femur, Left
Lateral condyle of tibia	**Use:** Tibia, Right Tibia, Left
Lateral cuneiform bone	**Use:** Tarsal, Right Tarsal, Left
Lateral epicondyle of femur	**Use:** Lower Femur, Right Lower Femur, Left
Lateral epicondyle of humerus	**Use:** Humeral Shaft, Right Humeral Shaft, Left
Lateral femoral cutaneous nerve	**Use:** Lumbar Plexus
Lateral malleolus	**Use:** Fibula, Right Fibula, Left
Lateral meniscus	**Use:** Knee Joint, Right Knee Joint, Left
Lateral nasal cartilage	**Use:** Nasal Mucosa and Soft Tissue
Lateral plantar artery	**Use:** Foot Artery, Right Foot Artery, Left
Lateral plantar nerve	**Use:** Tibial Nerve
Lateral rectus muscle	**Use:** Extraocular Muscle, Right Extraocular Muscle, Left

BODY PART KEY

BODY PART KEY

Lateral sacral artery	**Use:** Internal Iliac Artery, Right Internal Iliac Artery, Left
Lateral sacral vein	**Use:** Hypogastric Vein, Right Hypogastric Vein, Left
Lateral sural cutaneous nerve	**Use:** Peroneal Nerve
Lateral tarsal artery	**Use:** Foot Artery, Right Foot Artery, Left
Lateral temporomandibular ligament	**Use:** Head and Neck Bursa and Ligament
Lateral thoracic artery	**Use:** Axillary Artery, Right Axillary Artery, Left
Latissimus dorsi muscle	**Use:** Trunk Muscle, Right Trunk Muscle, Left
Least splanchnic nerve	**Use:** Thoracic Sympathetic Nerve
Left ascending lumbar vein	**Use:** Hemiazygos Vein
Left atrioventricular valve	**Use:** Mitral Valve
Left auricular appendix	**Use:** Atrium, Left
Left colic vein	**Use:** Colic Vein
Left coronary sulcus	**Use:** Heart, Left
Left gastric artery	**Use:** Gastric Artery
Left gastroepiploic artery	**Use:** Splenic Artery
Left gastroepiploic vein	**Use:** Splenic Vein
Left inferior phrenic vein	**Use:** Renal Vein, Left
Left inferior pulmonary vein	**Use:** Pulmonary Vein, Left
Left jugular trunk	**Use:** Thoracic Duct
Left lateral ventricle	**Use:** Cerebral Ventricle
Left ovarian vein Left second lumbar vein	**Use:** Renal Vein, Left
Left subclavian trunk	**Use:** Thoracic Duct
Left subcostal vein	**Use:** Hemiazygos Vein
Left superior pulmonary vein	**Use:** Pulmonary Vein, Left
Left suprarenal vein Left testicular vein	**Use:** Renal Vein, Left
Leptomeninges, intracranial	**Use:** Cerebral Meninges
Leptomeninges, spinal	**Use:** Spinal Meninges
Lesser alar cartilage	**Use:** Nasal Mucosa and Soft Tissue
Lesser occipital nerve	**Use:** Cervical Plexus
Lesser Omentum	**Use:** Omentum
Lesser saphenous vein	**Use:** Saphenous Vein, Right Saphenous Vein, Left
Lesser splanchnic nerve	**Use:** Thoracic Sympathetic Nerve
Lesser trochanter	**Use:** Upper Femur, Right Upper Femur, Left
Lesser tuberosity	**Use:** Humeral Head, Right Humeral Head, Left
Lesser wing	**Use:** Sphenoid Bone
Levator anguli oris muscle	**Use:** Facial Muscle
Levator ani muscle	**Use:** Perineum Muscle
Levator labii superioris alaeque nasi muscle Levator labii superioris muscle	**Use:** Facial Muscle

APPENDIX B

BODY PART KEY

Levator palpebrae superioris muscle	**Use:** Upper Eyelid, Right Upper Eyelid, Left
Levator scapulae muscle	**Use:** Neck Muscle, Right Neck Muscle, Left
Levator veli palatini muscle	**Use:** Tongue, Palate, Pharynx Muscle
Levatores costarum muscle	**Use:** Thorax Muscle, Right Thorax Muscle, Left
Ligament of head of fibula	**Use:** Knee Bursa and Ligament, Right Knee Bursa and Ligament, Left
Ligament of the lateral malleolus	**Use:** Ankle Bursa and Ligament, Right Ankle Bursa and Ligament, Left
Ligamentum flavum	**Use:** Upper Spine Bursa and Ligament Lower Spine Bursa and Ligament
Lingual artery	**Use:** External Carotid Artery, Right External Carotid Artery, Left
Lingual tonsil	**Use:** Pharynx
Locus ceruleus	**Use:** Pons
Long thoracic nerve	**Use:** Brachial Plexus
Lumbar artery	**Use:** Abdominal Aorta
Lumbar facet joint	**Use:** Lumbar Vertebral Joint Lumbar Vertebral Joints, 2 or more
Lumbar ganglion	**Use:** Lumbar Sympathetic Nerve
Lumbar lymph node	**Use:** Lymphatic, Aortic
Lumbar lymphatic trunk	**Use:** Cisterna Chyli
Lumbar splanchnic nerve	**Use:** Lumbar Sympathetic Nerve
Lumbosacral facet joint	**Use:** Lumbosacral Joint

Lumbosacral trunk	**Use:** Lumbar Nerve
Lunate bone	**Use:** Carpal, Right Carpal, Left
Lunotriquetral ligament	**Use:** Hand Bursa and Ligament, Right Hand Bursa and Ligament, Left
Macula	**Use:** Retina, Right Retina, Left
Malleus	**Use:** Auditory Ossicle, Right Auditory Ossicle, Left
Mammary duct Mammary gland	**Use:** Breast, Right Breast, Left Breast, Bilateral
Mammillary body	**Use:** Hypothalamus
Mandibular nerve	**Use:** Trigeminal Nerve
Mandibular notch	**Use:** Mandible, Right Mandible, Left
Manubrium	**Use:** Sternum
Masseter muscle	**Use:** Head Muscle
Masseteric fascia	**Use:** Subcutaneous Tissue and Fascia, Face
Mastoid (postauricular) lymph node	**Use:** Lymphatic, Right Neck Lymphatic, Left Neck
Mastoid air cells	**Use:** Mastoid Sinus, Right Mastoid Sinus, Left
Mastoid process	**Use:** Temporal Bone, Right Temporal Bone, Left
Maxillary artery	**Use:** External Carotid Artery, Right External Carotid Artery, Left
Maxillary nerve	**Use:** Trigeminal Nerve

BODY PART KEY

Medial canthus	**Use:** Lower Eyelid, Right Lower Eyelid, Left
Medial collateral ligament (MCL)	**Use:** Knee Bursa and Ligament, Right Knee Bursa and Ligament, Left
Medial condyle of femur	**Use:** Lower Femur, Right Lower Femur, Left
Medial condyle of tibia	**Use:** Tibia, Right Tibia, Left
Medial cuneiform bone	**Use:** Tarsal, Right Tarsal, Left
Medial epicondyle of femur	**Use:** Lower Femur, Right Lower Femur, Left
Medial epicondyle of humerus	**Use:** Humeral Shaft, Right Humeral Shaft, Left
Medial malleolus	**Use:** Tibia, Right Tibia, Left
Medial meniscus	**Use:** Knee Joint, Right Knee Joint, Left
Medial plantar artery	**Use:** Foot Artery, Right Foot Artery, Left
Medial plantar nerve Medial popliteal nerve	**Use:** Tibial Nerve
Medial rectus muscle	**Use:** Extraocular Muscle, Right Extraocular Muscle, Left
Medial sural cutaneous nerve	**Use:** Tibial Nerve
Median antebrachial vein Median cubital vein	**Use:** Basilic Vein, Right Basilic Vein, Left
Median sacral artery	**Use:** Abdominal Aorta
Mediastinal lymph node	**Use:** Lymphatic, Thorax
Meissner's (submucous) plexus	**Use:** Abdominal Sympathetic Nerve
Membranous urethra	**Use:** Urethra
Mental foramen	**Use:** Mandible, Right Mandible, Left
Mentalis muscle	**Use:** Facial Muscle
Mesoappendix Mesocolon	**Use:** Mesentery
Metacarpal ligament Metacarpophalangeal ligament	**Use:** Hand Bursa and Ligament, Right Hand Bursa and Ligament, Left
Metatarsal ligament	**Use:** Foot Bursa and Ligament, Right Foot Bursa and Ligament, Left
Metatarsophalangeal (MTP) joint	**Use:** Metatarsal-Phalangeal Joint, Right Metatarsal-Phalangeal Joint, Left
Metatarsophalangeal ligament	**Use:** Foot Bursa and Ligament, Right Foot Bursa and Ligament, Left
Metathalamus	**Use:** Thalamus
Midcarpal joint	**Use:** Carpal Joint, Right Carpal Joint, Left
Middle cardiac nerve	**Use:** Thoracic Sympathetic Nerve
Middle cerebral artery	**Use:** Intracranial Artery
Middle cerebral vein	**Use:** Intracranial Vein
Middle colic vein	**Use:** Colic Vein
Middle genicular artery	**Use:** Popliteal Artery, Right Popliteal Artery, Left
Middle hemorrhoidal vein	**Use:** Hypogastric Vein, Right Hypogastric Vein, Left
Middle rectal artery	**Use:** Internal Iliac Artery, Right Internal Iliac Artery, Left
Middle suprarenal artery	**Use:** Abdominal Aorta

APPENDIX B

BODY PART KEY

Middle temporal artery	**Use:** Temporal Artery, Right Temporal Artery, Left
Middle turbinate	**Use:** Nasal Turbinate
Mitral annulus	**Use:** Mitral Valve
Molar gland	**Use:** Buccal Mucosa
Musculocutaneous nerve	**Use:** Brachial Plexus
Musculophrenic artery	**Use:** Internal Mammary Artery, Right Internal Mammary Artery, Left
Musculospiral nerve	**Use:** Radial Nerve
Myelencephalon	**Use:** Medulla Oblongata
Myenteric (Auerbach's) plexus	**Use:** Abdominal Sympathetic Nerve
Myometrium	**Use:** Uterus
Nail bed Nail plate	**Use:** Finger Nail Toe Nail
Nasal cavity	**Use:** Nasal Mucosa and Soft Tissue
Nasal concha	**Use:** Nasal Turbinate
Nasalis muscle	**Use:** Facial Muscle
Nasolacrimal duct	**Use:** Lacrimal Duct, Right Lacrimal Duct, Left
Navicular bone	**Use:** Tarsal, Right Tarsal, Left
Neck of femur	**Use:** Upper Femur, Right Upper Femur, Left
Neck of humerus (anatomical) (surgical)	**Use:** Humeral Head, Right Humeral Head, Left
Nerve to the stapedius	**Use:** Facial Nerve

Neurohypophysis	**Use:** Pituitary Gland
Ninth cranial nerve	**Use:** Glossopharyngeal Nerve
Nostril	**Use:** Nasal Mucosa and Soft Tissue
Obturator artery	**Use:** Internal Iliac Artery, Right Internal Iliac Artery, Left
Obturator lymph node	**Use:** Lymphatic, Pelvis
Obturator muscle	**Use:** Hip Muscle, Right Hip Muscle, Left
Obturator nerve	**Use:** Lumbar Plexus
Obturator vein	**Use:** Hypogastric Vein, Right Hypogastric Vein, Left
Obtuse margin	**Use:** Heart, Left
Occipital artery	**Use:** External Carotid Artery, Right External Carotid Artery, Left
Occipital lobe	**Use:** Cerebral Hemisphere
Occipital lymph node	**Use:** Lymphatic, Right Neck Lymphatic, Left Neck
Occipitofrontalis muscle	**Use:** Facial Muscle
Odontoid process	**Use:** Cervical Vertebra
Olecranon bursa	**Use:** Elbow Bursa and Ligament, Right Elbow Bursa and Ligament, Left
Olecranon process	**Use:** Ulna, Right Ulna, Left
Olfactory bulb	**Use:** Olfactory Nerve
Ophthalmic artery	**Use:** Intracranial Artery
Ophthalmic nerve	**Use:** Trigeminal Nerve

BODY PART KEY

Ophthalmic vein	**Use:** Intracranial Vein
Optic chiasma	**Use:** Optic Nerve
Optic disc	**Use:** Retina, Right Retina, Left
Optic foramen	**Use:** Sphenoid Bone
Orbicularis oculi muscle	**Use:** Upper Eyelid, Right Upper Eyelid, Left
Orbicularis oris muscle	**Use:** Facial Muscle
Orbital fascia	**Use:** Subcutaneous Tissue and Fascia, Face
Orbital portion of ethmoid bone Orbital portion of frontal bone Orbital portion of lacrimal bone Orbital portion of maxilla Orbital portion of palatine bone Orbital portion of sphenoid bone Orbital portion of zygomatic bone	**Use:** Orbit, Right Orbit, Left
Oropharynx	**Use:** Pharynx
Otic ganglion	**Use:** Head and Neck Sympathetic Nerve
Oval window	**Use:** Middle Ear, Right Middle Ear, Left
Ovarian artery	**Use:** Abdominal Aorta
Ovarian ligament	**Use:** Uterine Supporting Structure
Oviduct	**Use:** Fallopian Tube, Right Fallopian Tube, Left
Palatine gland	**Use:** Buccal Mucosa
Palatine tonsil	**Use:** Tonsils
Palatine uvula	**Use:** Uvula
Palatoglossal muscle Palatopharyngeal muscle	**Use:** Tongue, Palate, Pharynx Muscle
Palmar (volar) digital vein Palmar (volar) metacarpal vein	**Use:** Hand Vein, Right Hand Vein, Left
Palmar cutaneous nerve	**Use:** Median Nerve Radial Nerve
Palmar fascia (aponeurosis)	**Use:** Subcutaneous Tissue and Fascia, Right Hand Subcutaneous Tissue and Fascia, Left Hand
Palmar interosseous muscle	**Use:** Hand Muscle, Right Hand Muscle, Left
Palmar ulnocarpal ligament	**Use:** Wrist Bursa and Ligament, Right Wrist Bursa and Ligament, Left
Palmaris longus muscle	**Use:** Lower Arm and Wrist Muscle, Right Lower Arm and Wrist Muscle, Left
Pancreatic artery	**Use:** Splenic Artery
Pancreatic plexus	**Use:** Abdominal Sympathetic Nerve
Pancreatic vein	**Use:** Splenic Vein
Pancreaticosplenic lymph node Paraaortic lymph node	**Use:** Lymphatic, Aortic
Pararectal lymph node	**Use:** Lymphatic, Mesenteric
Parasternal lymph node Paratracheal lymph node	**Use:** Lymphatic, Thorax
Paraurethral (Skene's) gland	**Use:** Vestibular Gland
Parietal lobe	**Use:** Cerebral Hemisphere
Parotid lymph node	**Use:** Lymphatic, Head
Parotid plexus	**Use:** Facial Nerve
Pars flaccida	**Use:** Tympanic Membrane, Right Tympanic Membrane, Left
Patellar ligament	**Use:** Knee Bursa and Ligament, Right Knee Bursa and Ligament, Left

BODY PART KEY

Patellar tendon	**Use:** Knee Tendon, Right Knee Tendon, Left
Pectineus muscle	**Use:** Upper Leg Muscle, Right Upper Leg Muscle, Left
Pectoral (anterior) lymph node	**Use:** Lymphatic, Right Axillary Lymphatic, Left Axillary
Pectoral fascia	**Use:** Subcutaneous Tissue and Fascia, Chest
Pectoralis major muscle Pectoralis minor muscle	**Use:** Thorax Muscle, Right Thorax Muscle, Left
Pelvic splanchnic nerve	**Use:** Abdominal Sympathetic Nerve Sacral Sympathetic Nerve
Penile urethra	**Use:** Urethra
Pericardiophrenic artery	**Use:** Internal Mammary Artery, Right Internal Mammary Artery, Left
Perimetrium	**Use:** Uterus
Peroneus brevis muscle Peroneus longus muscle	**Use:** Lower Leg Muscle, Right Lower Leg Muscle, Left
Petrous part of temporal bone	**Use:** Temporal Bone, Right Temporal Bone, Left
Pharyngeal constrictor muscle	**Use:** Tongue, Palate, Pharynx Muscle
Pharyngeal plexus	**Use:** Vagus Nerve
Pharyngeal recess	**Use:** Nasopharynx
Pharyngeal tonsil	**Use:** Adenoids
Pharyngotympanic tube	**Use:** Eustachian Tube, Right Eustachian Tube, Left
Pia mater, intracranial	**Use:** Cerebral Meninges
Pia mater, spinal	**Use:** Spinal Meninges
Pinna	**Use:** External Ear, Right External Ear, Left External Ear, Bilateral
Piriform recess (sinus)	**Use:** Pharynx
Piriformis muscle	**Use:** Hip Muscle, Right Hip Muscle, Left
Pisiform bone	**Use:** Carpal, Right Carpal, Left
Pisohamate ligament Pisometacarpal ligament	**Use:** Hand Bursa and Ligament, Right Hand Bursa and Ligament, Left
Plantar digital vein	**Use:** Foot Vein, Right Foot Vein, Left
Plantar fascia (aponeurosis)	**Use:** Subcutaneous Tissue and Fascia, Right Foot Subcutaneous Tissue and Fascia, Left Foot
Plantar metatarsal vein Plantar venous arch	**Use:** Foot Vein, Right Foot Vein, Left
Platysma muscle	**Use:** Neck Muscle, Right Neck Muscle, Left
Plica semilunaris	**Use:** Conjunctiva, Right Conjunctiva, Left
Pneumogastric nerve	**Use:** Vagus Nerve
Pneumotaxic center Pontine tegmentum	**Use:** Pons
Popliteal ligament	**Use:** Knee Bursa and Ligament, Right Knee Bursa and Ligament, Left
Popliteal lymph node	**Use:** Lymphatic, Right Lower Extremity Lymphatic, Left Lower Extremity
Popliteal vein	**Use:** Femoral Vein, Right Femoral Vein, Left
Popliteus muscle	**Use:** Lower Leg Muscle, Right Lower Leg Muscle, Left

BODY PART KEY

Postauricular (mastoid) lymph node	**Use:** Lymphatic, Right Neck Lymphatic, Left Neck
Postcava	**Use:** Inferior Vena Cava
Posterior (subscapular) lymph node	**Use:** Lymphatic, Right Axillary Lymphatic, Left Axillary
Posterior auricular artery	**Use:** External Carotid Artery, Right External Carotid Artery, Left
Posterior auricular nerve	**Use:** Facial Nerve
Posterior auricular vein	**Use:** External Jugular Vein, Right External Jugular Vein, Left
Posterior cerebral artery	**Use:** Intracranial Artery
Posterior chamber	**Use:** Eye, Right Eye, Left
Posterior circumflex humeral artery	**Use:** Axillary Artery, Right Axillary Artery, Left
Posterior communicating artery	**Use:** Intracranial Artery
Posterior cruciate ligament (PCL)	**Use:** Knee Bursa and Ligament, Right Knee Bursa and Ligament, Left
Posterior facial (retromandibular) vein	**Use:** Face Vein, Right Face Vein, Left
Posterior femoral cutaneous nerve	**Use:** Sacral Plexus
Posterior inferior cerebellar artery (PICA)	**Use:** Intracranial Artery
Posterior interosseous nerve	**Use:** Radial Nerve
Posterior labial nerve Posterior scrotal nerve	**Use:** Pudendal Nerve
Posterior spinal artery	**Use:** Vertebral Artery, Right Vertebral Artery, Left
Posterior tibial recurrent artery	**Use:** Anterior Tibial Artery, Right Anterior Tibial Artery, Left

Posterior ulnar recurrent artery	**Use:** Ulnar Artery, Right Ulnar Artery, Left
Posterior vagal trunk	**Use:** Vagus Nerve
Preauricular lymph node	**Use:** Lymphatic, Head
Precava	**Use:** Superior Vena Cava
Prepatellar bursa	**Use:** Knee Bursa and Ligament, Right Knee Bursa and Ligament, Left
Pretracheal fascia Prevertebral fascia	**Use:** Subcutaneous Tissue and Fascia, Right Neck Subcutaneous Tissue and Fascia, Left Neck
Princeps pollicis artery	**Use:** Hand Artery, Right Hand Artery, Left
Procerus muscle	**Use:** Facial Muscle
Profunda brachii	**Use:** Brachial Artery, Right Brachial Artery, Left
Profunda femoris (deep femoral) vein	**Use:** Femoral Vein, Right Femoral Vein, Left
Pronator quadratus muscle Pronator teres muscle	**Use:** Lower Arm and Wrist Muscle, Right Lower Arm and Wrist Muscle, Left
Prostatic urethra	**Use:** Urethra
Proximal radioulnar joint	**Use:** Elbow Joint, Right Elbow Joint, Left
Psoas muscle	**Use:** Hip Muscle, Right Hip Muscle, Left
Pterygoid muscle	**Use:** Head Muscle
Pterygoid process	**Use:** Sphenoid Bone
Pterygopalatine (sphenopalatine) ganglion	**Use:** Head and Neck Sympathetic Nerve

APPENDIX B

BODY PART KEY

Pubis	**Use:** Pelvic Bone, Right Pelvic Bone, Left
Pubofemoral ligament	**Use:** Hip Bursa and Ligament, Right Hip Bursa and Ligament, Left
Pudendal nerve	**Use:** Sacral Plexus
Pulmoaortic canal	**Use:** Pulmonary Artery, Left
Pulmonary annulus	**Use:** Pulmonary Valve
Pulmonary plexus	**Use:** Vagus Nerve Thoracic Sympathetic Nerve
Pulmonic valve	**Use:** Pulmonary Valve
Pulvinar	**Use:** Thalamus
Pyloric antrum Pyloric canal Pyloric sphincter	**Use:** Stomach, Pylorus
Pyramidalis muscle	**Use:** Abdomen Muscle, Right Abdomen Muscle, Left
Quadrangular cartilage	**Use:** Nasal Septum
Quadrate lobe	**Use:** Liver
Quadratus femoris muscle	**Use:** Hip Muscle, Right Hip Muscle, Left
Quadratus lumborum muscle	**Use:** Trunk Muscle, Right Trunk Muscle, Left
Quadratus plantae muscle	**Use:** Foot Muscle, Right Foot Muscle, Left
Quadriceps (femoris)	**Use:** Upper Leg Muscle, Right Upper Leg Muscle, Left
Radial collateral carpal ligament	**Use:** Wrist Bursa and Ligament, Right Wrist Bursa and Ligament, Left
Radial collateral ligament	**Use:** Elbow Bursa and Ligament, Right Elbow Bursa and Ligament, Left

Radial notch	**Use:** Ulna, Right Ulna, Left
Radial recurrent artery	**Use:** Radial Artery, Right Radial Artery, Left
Radial vein	**Use:** Brachial Vein, Right Brachial Vein, Left
Radialis indicis	**Use:** Hand Artery, Right Hand Artery, Left
Radiocarpal joint	**Use:** Wrist Joint, Right Wrist Joint, Left
Radiocarpal ligament Radioulnar ligament	**Use:** Wrist Bursa and Ligament, Right Wrist Bursa and Ligament, Left
Rectosigmoid junction	**Use:** Sigmoid Colon
Rectus abdominis muscle	**Use:** Abdomen Muscle, Right Abdomen Muscle, Left
Rectus femoris muscle	**Use:** Upper Leg Muscle, Right Upper Leg Muscle, Left
Recurrent laryngeal nerve	**Use:** Vagus Nerve
Renal calyx Renal capsule Renal cortex	**Use:** Kidney, Right Kidney, Left Kidneys, Bilateral Kidney
Renal plexus	**Use:** Abdominal Sympathetic Nerve
Renal segment	**Use:** Kidney, Right Kidney, Left Kidneys, Bilateral Kidney
Renal segmental artery	**Use:** Renal Artery, Right Renal Artery, Left
Retroperitoneal lymph node	**Use:** Lymphatic, Aortic
Retroperitoneal space	**Use:** Retroperitoneum

BODY PART KEY

Retropharyngeal lymph node	**Use:** Lymphatic, Right Neck Lymphatic, Left Neck
Retropubic space	**Use:** Pelvic Cavity
Rhinopharynx	**Use:** Nasopharynx
Rhomboid major muscle Rhomboid minor muscle	**Use:** Trunk Muscle, Right Trunk Muscle, Left
Right ascending lumbar vein	**Use:** Azygos Vein
Right atrioventricular valve	**Use:** Tricuspid Valve
Right auricular appendix	**Use:** Atrium, Right
Right colic vein	**Use:** Colic Vein
Right coronary sulcus	**Use:** Heart, Right
Right gastric artery	**Use:** Gastric Artery
Right gastroepiploic vein	**Use:** Superior Mesenteric Vein
Right inferior phrenic vein	**Use:** Inferior Vena Cava
Right inferior pulmonary vein	**Use:** Pulmonary Vein, Right
Right jugular trunk	**Use:** Lymphatic, Right Neck
Right lateral ventricle	**Use:** Cerebral Ventricle
Right lymphatic duct	**Use:** Lymphatic, Right Neck
Right ovarian vein Right second lumbar vein	**Use:** Inferior Vena Cava
Right subclavian trunk	**Use:** Lymphatic, Right Neck
Right subcostal vein	**Use:** Azygos Vein
Right superior pulmonary vein	**Use:** Pulmonary Vein, Right
Right suprarenal vein Right testicular vein	**Use:** Inferior Vena Cava

Rima glottidis	**Use:** Larynx
Risorius muscle	**Use:** Facial Muscle
Round ligament of uterus	**Use:** Uterine Supporting Structure
Round window	**Use:** Inner Ear, Right Inner Ear, Left
Sacral ganglion	**Use:** Sacral Sympathetic Nerve
Sacral lymph node	**Use:** Lymphatic, Pelvis
Sacral splanchnic nerve	**Use:** Sacral Sympathetic Nerve
Sacrococcygeal ligament	**Use:** Lower Spine Bursa and Ligament
Sacrococcygeal symphysis	**Use:** Sacrococcygeal Joint
Sacroiliac ligament Sacrospinous ligament Sacrotuberous ligament	**Use:** Lower Spine Bursa and Ligament
Salpingopharyngeus muscle	**Use:** Tongue, Palate, Pharynx Muscle
Salpinx	**Use:** Fallopian Tube, Right Fallopian Tube, Left
Saphenous nerve	**Use:** Femoral Nerve
Sartorius muscle	**Use:** Upper Leg Muscle, Right Upper Leg Muscle, Left
Scalene muscle	**Use:** Neck Muscle, Right Neck Muscle, Left
Scaphoid bone	**Use:** Carpal, Right Carpal, Left
Scapholunate ligament Scaphotrapezium ligament	**Use:** Hand Bursa and Ligament, Right Hand Bursa and Ligament, Left
Scarpa's (vestibular) ganglion	**Use:** Acoustic Nerve
Sebaceous gland	**Use:** Skin

BODY PART KEY

Second cranial nerve	**Use:** Optic Nerve
Sella turcica	**Use:** Sphenoid Bone
Semicircular canal	**Use:** Inner Ear, Right Inner Ear, Left
Semimembranosus muscle Semitendinosus muscle	**Use:** Upper Leg Muscle, Right Upper Leg Muscle, Left
Septal cartilage	**Use:** Nasal Septum
Serratus anterior muscle	**Use:** Thorax Muscle, Right Thorax Muscle, Left
Serratus posterior muscle	**Use:** Trunk Muscle, Right Trunk Muscle, Left
Seventh cranial nerve	**Use:** Facial Nerve
Short gastric artery	**Use:** Splenic Artery
Sigmoid artery	**Use:** Inferior Mesenteric Artery
Sigmoid flexure	**Use:** Sigmoid Colon
Sigmoid vein	**Use:** Inferior Mesenteric Vein
Sinoatrial node	**Use:** Conduction Mechanism
Sinus venosus	**Use:** Atrium, Right
Sixth cranial nerve	**Use:** Abducens Nerve
Skene's (paraurethral) gland	**Use:** Vestibular Gland
Small saphenous vein	**Use:** Saphenous Vein, Right Saphenous Vein, Left
Solar (celiac) plexus	**Use:** Abdominal Sympathetic Nerve
Soleus muscle	**Use:** Lower Leg Muscle, Right Lower Leg Muscle, Left
Sphenomandibular ligament	**Use:** Head and Neck Bursa and Ligament
Sphenopalatine (pterygopalatine) ganglion	**Use:** Head and Neck Sympathetic Nerve
Spinal nerve, cervical	**Use:** Cervical Nerve
Spinal nerve, lumbar	**Use:** Lumbar Nerve
Spinal nerve, sacral	**Use:** Sacral Nerve
Spinal nerve, thoracic	**Use:** Thoracic Nerve
Spinous process	**Use:** Cervical Vertebra Thoracic Vertebra Lumbar Vertebra
Spiral ganglion	**Use:** Acoustic Nerve
Splenic flexure	**Use:** Transverse Colon
Splenic plexus	**Use:** Abdominal Sympathetic Nerve
Splenius capitis muscle	**Use:** Head Muscle
Splenius cervicis muscle	**Use:** Neck Muscle, Right Neck Muscle, Left
Stapes	**Use:** Auditory Ossicle, Right Auditory Ossicle, Left
Stellate ganglion	**Use:** Head and Neck Sympathetic Nerve
Stensen's duct	**Use:** Parotid Duct, Right Parotid Duct, Left
Sternoclavicular ligament	**Use:** Shoulder Bursa and Ligament, Right Shoulder Bursa and Ligament, Left
Sternocleidomastoid artery	**Use:** Thyroid Artery, Right Thyroid Artery, Left

BODY PART KEY

Sternocleidomastoid muscle	**Use:** Neck Muscle, Right Neck Muscle, Left
Sternocostal ligament	**Use:** Sternum Bursa and Ligament Rib(s) Bursa and Ligament
Styloglossus muscle	**Use:** Tongue, Palate, Pharynx Muscle
Stylomandibular ligament	**Use:** Head and Neck Bursa and Ligament
Stylopharyngeus muscle	**Use:** Tongue, Palate, Pharynx Muscle
Subacromial bursa	**Use:** Shoulder Bursa and Ligament, Right Shoulder Bursa and Ligament, Left
Subaortic (common iliac) lymph node	**Use:** Lymphatic, Pelvis
Subarachnoid space, spinal	**Use:** Spinal Canal
Subclavicular (apical) lymph node	**Use:** Lymphatic, Right Axillary Lymphatic, Left Axillary
Subclavius muscle	**Use:** Thorax Muscle, Right Thorax Muscle, Left
Subclavius nerve	**Use:** Brachial Plexus
Subcostal artery	**Use:** Upper Artery
Subcostal muscle	**Use:** Thorax Muscle, Right Thorax Muscle, Left
Subcostal nerve	**Use:** Thoracic Nerve
Subdural space, spinal	**Use:** Spinal Canal
Submandibular ganglion	**Use:** Facial Nerve Head and Neck Sympathetic Nerve
Submandibular gland	**Use:** Submaxillary Gland, Right Submaxillary Gland, Left
Submandibular lymph node	**Use:** Lymphatic, Head
Submaxillary ganglion	**Use:** Head and Neck Sympathetic Nerve
Submaxillary lymph node	**Use:** Lymphatic, Head
Submental artery	**Use:** Face Artery
Submental lymph node	**Use:** Lymphatic, Head
Submucous (Meissner's) plexus	**Use:** Abdominal Sympathetic Nerve
Suboccipital nerve	**Use:** Cervical Nerve
Suboccipital venous plexus	**Use:** Vertebral Vein, Right Vertebral Vein, Left
Subparotid lymph node	**Use:** Lymphatic, Head
Subscapular (posterior) lymph node	**Use:** Lymphatic, Right Axillary Lymphatic, Left Axillary
Subscapular aponeurosis	**Use:** Subcutaneous Tissue and Fascia, Right Upper Arm Subcutaneous Tissue and Fascia, Left Upper Arm
Subscapular artery	**Use:** Axillary Artery, Right Axillary Artery, Left
Subscapularis muscle	**Use:** Shoulder Muscle, Right Shoulder Muscle, Left
Substantia nigra	**Use:** Basal Ganglia
Subtalar (talocalcaneal) joint	**Use:** Tarsal Joint, Right Tarsal Joint, Left
Subtalar ligament	**Use:** Foot Bursa and Ligament, Right Foot Bursa and Ligament, Left
Subthalamic nucleus	**Use:** Basal Ganglia
Superficial circumflex iliac vein	**Use:** Saphenous Vein, Right Saphenous Vein, Left

BODY PART KEY

Superficial epigastric artery	**Use:** Femoral Artery, Right Femoral Artery, Left
Superficial epigastric vein	**Use:** Saphenous Vein, Right Saphenous Vein, Left
Superficial palmar arch	**Use:** Hand Artery, Right Hand Artery, Left
Superficial palmar venous arch	**Use:** Hand Vein, Right Hand Vein, Left
Superficial temporal artery	**Use:** Temporal Artery, Right Temporal Artery, Left
Superficial transverse perineal muscle	**Use:** Perineum Muscle
Superior cardiac nerve	**Use:** Thoracic Sympathetic Nerve
Superior cerebellar vein Superior cerebral vein	**Use:** Intracranial Vein
Superior clunic (cluneal) nerve	**Use:** Lumbar Nerve
Superior epigastric artery	**Use:** Internal Mammary Artery, Right Internal Mammary Artery, Left
Superior genicular artery	**Use:** Popliteal Artery, Right Popliteal Artery, Left
Superior gluteal artery	**Use:** Internal Iliac Artery, Right Internal Iliac Artery, Left
Superior gluteal nerve	**Use:** Lumbar Plexus
Superior hypogastric plexus	**Use:** Abdominal Sympathetic Nerve
Superior labial artery	**Use:** Face Artery
Superior laryngeal artery	**Use:** Thyroid Artery, Right Thyroid Artery, Left
Superior laryngeal nerve	**Use:** Vagus Nerve
Superior longitudinal muscle	**Use:** Tongue, Palate, Pharynx Muscle
Superior mesenteric ganglion	**Use:** Abdominal Sympathetic Nerve
Superior mesenteric lymph node	**Use:** Lymphatic, Mesenteric
Superior mesenteric plexus	**Use:** Abdominal Sympathetic Nerve
Superior oblique muscle	**Use:** Extraocular Muscle, Right Extraocular Muscle, Left
Superior olivary nucleus	**Use:** Pons
Superior rectal artery	**Use:** Inferior Mesenteric Artery
Superior rectal vein	**Use:** Inferior Mesenteric Vein
Superior rectus muscle	**Use:** Extraocular Muscle, Right Extraocular Muscle, Left
Superior tarsal plate	**Use:** Upper Eyelid, Right Upper Eyelid, Left
Superior thoracic artery	**Use:** Axillary Artery, Right Axillary Artery, Left
Superior thyroid artery	**Use:** External Carotid Artery, Right External Carotid Artery, Left Thyroid Artery, Right Thyroid Artery, Left
Superior turbinate	**Use:** Nasal Turbinate
Superior ulnar collateral artery	**Use:** Brachial Artery, Right Brachial Artery, Left
Supraclavicular (Virchow's) lymph node	**Use:** Lymphatic, Right Neck Lymphatic, Left Neck
Supraclavicular nerve	**Use:** Cervical Plexus
Suprahyoid lymph node	**Use:** Lymphatic, Head
Suprahyoid muscle	**Use:** Neck Muscle, Right Neck Muscle, Left

BODY PART KEY

Suprainguinal lymph node	**Use:** Lymphatic, Pelvis
Supraorbital vein	**Use:** Face Vein, Right Face Vein, Left
Suprarenal gland	**Use:** Adrenal Gland, Left Adrenal Gland, Right Adrenal Glands, Bilateral Adrenal Gland
Suprarenal plexus	**Use:** Abdominal Sympathetic Nerve
Suprascapular nerve	**Use:** Brachial Plexus
Supraspinatus fascia	**Use:** Subcutaneous Tissue and Fascia, Right Upper Arm Subcutaneous Tissue and Fascia, Left Upper Arm
Supraspinatus muscle	**Use:** Shoulder Muscle, Right Shoulder Muscle, Left
Supraspinous ligament	**Use:** Upper Spine Bursa and Ligament Lower Spine Bursa and Ligament
Suprasternal notch	**Use:** Sternum
Supratrochlear lymph node	**Use:** Lymphatic, Right Upper Extremity Lymphatic, Left Upper Extremity
Sural artery	**Use:** Popliteal Artery, Right Popliteal Artery, Left
Sweat gland	**Use:** Skin
Talocalcaneal (subtalar) joint	**Use:** Tarsal Joint, Right Tarsal Joint, Left
Talocalcaneal ligament	**Use:** Foot Bursa and Ligament, Right Foot Bursa and Ligament, Left
Talocalcaneonavicular joint	**Use:** Tarsal Joint, Right Tarsal Joint, Left
Talocalcaneonavicular ligament	**Use:** Foot Bursa and Ligament, Right Foot Bursa and Ligament, Left
Talocrural joint	**Use:** Ankle Joint, Right Ankle Joint, Left
Talofibular ligament	**Use:** Ankle Bursa and Ligament, Right Ankle Bursa and Ligament, Left
Talus bone	**Use:** Tarsal, Right Tarsal, Left
Tarsometatarsal ligament	**Use:** Foot Bursa and Ligament, Right Foot Bursa and Ligament, Left
Temporal lobe	**Use:** Cerebral Hemisphere
Temporalis muscle Temporoparietalis muscle	**Use:** Head Muscle
Tensor fasciae latae muscle	**Use:** Hip Muscle, Right Hip Muscle, Left
Tensor veli palatini muscle	**Use:** Tongue, Palate, Pharynx Muscle
Tenth cranial nerve	**Use:** Vagus Nerve
Tentorium cerebelli	**Use:** Dura Mater
Teres major muscle Teres minor muscle	**Use:** Shoulder Muscle, Right Shoulder Muscle, Left
Testicular artery	**Use:** Abdominal Aorta
Thenar muscle	**Use:** Hand Muscle, Right Hand Muscle, Left
Third cranial nerve	**Use:** Oculomotor Nerve
Third occipital nerve	**Use:** Cervical Nerve
Third ventricle	**Use:** Cerebral Ventricle
Thoracic aortic plexus	**Use:** Thoracic Sympathetic Nerve
Thoracic esophagus	**Use:** Esophagus, Middle

BODY PART KEY

Thoracic facet joint	**Use:** Thoracic Vertebral Joint Thoracic Vertebral Joints, 2 to 7 Thoracic Vertebral Joints, 8 or more
Thoracic ganglion	**Use:** Thoracic Sympathetic Nerve
Thoracoacromial artery	**Use:** Axillary Artery, Right Axillary Artery, Left
Thoracolumbar facet joint	**Use:** Thoracolumbar Vertebral Joint
Thymus gland	**Use:** Thymus
Thyroarytenoid muscle	**Use:** Neck Muscle, Right Neck Muscle, Left
Thyrocervical trunk	**Use:** Thyroid Artery, Right Thyroid Artery, Left
Thyroid cartilage	**Use:** Larynx
Tibialis anterior muscle Tibialis posterior muscle	**Use:** Lower Leg Muscle, Right Lower Leg Muscle, Left
Tibiofemoral joint	**Use:** Knee Joint, Right Knee Joint, Left Knee Joint, Tibial Surface, Right Knee Joint, Tibial Surface, Left
Tongue, base of	**Use:** Pharynx
Tracheobronchial lymph node	**Use:** Lymphatic, Thorax
Tragus	**Use:** External Ear, Right External Ear, Left External Ear, Bilateral
Transversalis fascia	**Use:** Subcutaneous Tissue and Fascia, Trunk
Transverse (cutaneous) cervical nerve	**Use:** Cervical Plexus
Transverse acetabular ligament	**Use:** Hip Bursa and Ligament, Right Hip Bursa and Ligament, Left
Transverse facial artery	**Use:** Temporal Artery, Right Temporal Artery, Left
Transverse foramen	**Use:** Cervical Vertebra
Transverse humeral ligament	**Use:** Shoulder Bursa and Ligament, Right Shoulder Bursa and Ligament, Left
Transverse ligament of atlas	**Use:** Head and Neck Bursa and Ligament
Transverse process	**Use:** Cervical Vertebra Thoracic Vertebra Lumbar Vertebra
Transverse scapular ligament	**Use:** Shoulder Bursa and Ligament, Right Shoulder Bursa and Ligament, Left
Transverse thoracis muscle	**Use:** Thorax Muscle, Right Thorax Muscle, Left
Transversospinalis muscle	**Use:** Trunk Muscle, Right Trunk Muscle, Left
Transversus abdominis muscle	**Use:** Abdomen Muscle, Right Abdomen Muscle, Left
Trapezium bone	**Use:** Carpal, Right Carpal, Left
Trapezius muscle	**Use:** Trunk Muscle, Right Trunk Muscle, Left
Trapezoid bone	**Use:** Carpal, Right Carpal, Left
Triceps brachii muscle	**Use:** Upper Arm Muscle, Right Upper Arm Muscle, Left
Tricuspid annulus	**Use:** Tricuspid Valve
Trifacial nerve	**Use:** Trigeminal Nerve
Trigone of bladder	**Use:** Bladder

BODY PART KEY

Triquetral bone	**Use:** Carpal, Right Carpal, Left
Trochanteric bursa	**Use:** Hip Bursa and Ligament, Right Hip Bursa and Ligament, Left
Twelfth cranial nerve	**Use:** Hypoglossal Nerve
Tympanic cavity	**Use:** Middle Ear, Right Middle Ear, Left
Tympanic nerve	**Use:** Glossopharyngeal Nerve
Tympanic part of temporal bone	**Use:** Temporal Bone, Right Temporal Bone, Left
Ulnar collateral carpal ligament	**Use:** Wrist Bursa and Ligament, Right Wrist Bursa and Ligament, Left
Ulnar collateral ligament	**Use:** Elbow Bursa and Ligament, Right Elbow Bursa and Ligament, Left
Ulnar notch	**Use:** Radius, Right Radius, Left
Ulnar vein	**Use:** Brachial Vein, Right Brachial Vein, Left
Umbilical artery	**Use:** Internal Iliac Artery, Right Internal Iliac Artery, Left Lower Artery
Ureteral orifice	**Use:** Ureter, Right Ureter, Left Ureters, Bilateral Ureter
Ureteropelvic junction (UPJ)	**Use:** Kidney Pelvis, Right Kidney Pelvis, Left
Ureterovesical orifice	**Use:** Ureter, Right Ureter, Left Ureters, Bilateral Ureter
Uterine artery	**Use:** Internal Iliac Artery, Right Internal Iliac Artery, Left
Uterine cornu	**Use:** Uterus
Uterine tube	**Use:** Fallopian Tube, Right Fallopian Tube, Left
Uterine vein	**Use:** Hypogastric Vein, Right Hypogastric Vein, Left
Vaginal artery	**Use:** Internal Iliac Artery, Right Internal Iliac Artery, Left
Vaginal vein	**Use:** Hypogastric Vein, Right Hypogastric Vein, Left
Vastus intermedius muscle Vastus lateralis muscle Vastus medialis muscle	**Use:** Upper Leg Muscle, Right Upper Leg Muscle, Left
Ventricular fold	**Use:** Larynx
Vermiform appendix	**Use:** Appendix
Vermilion border	**Use:** Upper Lip Lower Lip
Vertebral arch Vertebral body	**Use:** Cervical Vertebra Thoracic Vertebra Lumbar Vertebra
Vertebral canal	**Use:** Spinal Canal
Vertebral foramen Vertebral lamina Vertebral pedicle	**Use:** Cervical Vertebra Thoracic Vertebra Lumbar Vertebra
Vesical vein	**Use:** Hypogastric Vein, Right Hypogastric Vein, Left
Vestibular (Scarpa's) ganglion Vestibular nerve Vestibulocochlear nerve	**Use:** Acoustic Nerve
Virchow's (supraclavicular) lymph node	**Use:** Lymphatic, Right Neck Lymphatic, Left Neck

BODY PART KEY

Vitreous body	**Use:** Vitreous, Right Vitreous, Left
Vocal fold	**Use:** Vocal Cord, Right Vocal Cord, Left
Volar (palmar) digital vein Volar (palmar) metacarpal vein	**Use:** Hand Vein, Right Hand Vein, Left
Vomer bone	**Use:** Nasal Septum
Vomer of nasal septum	**Use:** Nasal Bone
Xiphoid process	**Use:** Sternum
Zonule of Zinn	**Use:** Lens, Right Lens, Left
Zygomatic process of frontal bone	**Use:** Frontal Bone
Zygomatic process of temporal bone	**Use:** Temporal Bone, Right Temporal Bone, Left
Zygomaticus muscle	**Use:** Facial Muscle

DEVICE KEY

3f (Aortic) Bioprosthesis valve	**Use:** Zooplastic Tissue in Heart and Great Vessels
AbioCor® Total Replacement Heart	**Use:** Synthetic Substitute
Acellular Hydrated Dermis	**Use:** Nonautologous Tissue Substitute
Acetabular cup	**Use:** Liner in Lower Joints
Activa PC neurostimulator	**Use:** Stimulator Generator, Multiple Array for Insertion in Subcutaneous Tissue and Fascia
Activa RC neurostimulator	**Use:** Stimulator Generator, Multiple Array Rechargeable for Insertion in Subcutaneous Tissue and Fascia
Activa SC neurostimulator	**Use:** Stimulator Generator, Single Array for Insertion in Subcutaneous Tissue and Fascia
ACUITY™ Steerable Lead	**Use:** Cardiac Lead, Pacemaker for Insertion in Heart and Great Vessels Cardiac Lead, Defibrillator for Insertion in Heart and Great Vessels
Advisa (MRI)	**Use:** Pacemaker, Dual Chamber for Insertion in Subcutaneous Tissue and Fascia
AFX® Endovascular AAA System	**Use:** Intraluminal Device
AMPLATZER® Muscular VSD Occluder	**Use:** Synthetic Substitute
AMS 800® Urinary Control System	**Use:** Artificial Sphincter in Urinary System
AneuRx® AAA Advantage®	**Use:** Intraluminal Device
Annuloplasty ring	**Use:** Synthetic Substitute
Artificial anal sphincter (AAS)	**Use:** Artificial Sphincter in Gastrointestinal System
Artificial bowel sphincter (neosphincter)	**Use:** Artificial Sphincter in Gastrointestinal System
Artificial urinary sphincter (AUS)	**Use:** Artificial Sphincter in Urinary System
Assurant (Cobalt) stent	**Use:** Intraluminal Device
AtriClip LAA Exclusion System	**Use:** Extraluminal Device
Attain Ability® lead	**Use:** Cardiac Lead, Pacemaker for Insertion in Heart and Great Vessels Cardiac Lead, Defibrillator for Insertion in Heart and Great Vessels
Attain StarFix® (OTW) lead	**Use:** Cardiac Lead, Pacemaker for Insertion in Heart and Great Vessels Cardiac Lead, Defibrillator for Insertion in Heart and Great Vessels
Autograft	**Use:** Autologous Tissue Substitute
Autologous artery graft	**Use:** Autologous Arterial Tissue in Heart and Great Vessels Autologous Arterial Tissue in Upper Arteries Autologous Arterial Tissue in Lower Arteries Autologous Arterial Tissue in Upper Veins Autologous Arterial Tissue in Lower Veins
Autologous vein graft	**Use:** Autologous Venous Tissue in Heart and Great Vessels Autologous Venous Tissue in Upper Arteries Autologous Venous Tissue in Lower Arteries Autologous Venous Tissue in Upper Veins Autologous Venous Tissue in Lower Veins
Axial Lumbar Interbody Fusion System	**Use:** Interbody Fusion Device in Lower Joints

DEVICE KEY

AxiaLIF® System	**Use:** Interbody Fusion Device in Lower Joints
BAK/C® Interbody Cervical Fusion System	**Use:** Interbody Fusion Device in Upper Joints
Bard® Composix® (E/X) (LP) mesh	**Use:** Synthetic Substitute
Bard® Composix® Kugel® patch	**Use:** Synthetic Substitute
Bard® Dulex™ mesh	**Use:** Synthetic Substitute
Bard® Ventralex™ hernia patch	**Use:** Synthetic Substitute
Baroreflex Activation Therapy® (BAT®)	**Use:** Stimulator Lead in Upper Arteries Cardiac Rhythm Related Device in Subcutaneous Tissue and Fascia
Berlin Heart Ventricular Assist Device	**Use:** Implantable Heart Assist System in Heart and Great Vessels
Bioactive embolization coil(s)	**Use:** Intraluminal Device, Bioactive in Upper Arteries
Biventricular external heart assist system	**Use:** Short-term External Heart Assist System in Heart and Great Vessels
Blood glucose monitoring system	**Use:** Monitoring Device
Bone anchored hearing device	**Use:** Hearing Device, Bone Conduction for Insertion in Ear, Nose, Sinus Hearing Device in Head and Facial Bones
Bone bank bone graft	**Use:** Nonautologous Tissue Substitute
Bone screw (interlocking) (lag) (pedicle) (recessed)	**Use:** Internal Fixation Device in Head and Facial Bones Internal Fixation Device in Upper Bones Internal Fixation Device in Lower Bones
Bovine pericardial valve	**Use:** Zooplastic Tissue in Heart and Great Vessels
Bovine pericardium graft	**Use:** Zooplastic Tissue in Heart and Great Vessels
Brachytherapy seeds	**Use:** Radioactive Element
BRYAN® Cervical Disc System	**Use:** Synthetic Substitute
BVS 5000 Ventricular Assist Device	**Use:** Short-term External Heart Assist System in Heart and Great Vessels
Cardiac contractility modulation lead	**Use:** Cardiac Lead in Heart and Great Vessels
Cardiac event recorder	**Use:** Monitoring Device
Cardiac resynchronization therapy (CRT) lead	**Use:** Cardiac Lead, Pacemaker for Insertion in Heart and Great Vessels Cardiac Lead, Defibrillator for Insertion in Heart and Great Vessels
CardioMEMS® pressure sensor	**Use:** Monitoring Device, Pressure Sensor for Insertion in Heart and Great Vessels
Carotid (artery) sinus (baroreceptor) lead	**Use:** Stimulator Lead in Upper Arteries
Carotid WALLSTENT® Monorail® Endoprosthesis	**Use:** Intraluminal Device
Centrimag® Blood Pump	**Use:** Short-term External Heart Assist System in Heart and Great Vessels
Ceramic on ceramic bearing surface	**Use:** Synthetic Substitute, Ceramic for Replacement in Lower Joints
Cesium-131 Collagen Implant	**Use:** Radioactive Element, Cesium-131 Collagen Implant for Insertion in Central Nervous System and Cranial Nerves
Clamp and rod internal fixation system (CRIF)	**Use:** Internal Fixation Device in Upper Bones Internal Fixation Device in Lower Bones

DEVICE KEY

COALESCE® radiolucent interbody fusion device	**Use:** Interbody Fusion Device, Radiolucent Porous in New Technology
CoAxia NeuroFlo catheter	**Use:** Intraluminal Device
Cobalt/chromium head and polyethylene socket	**Use:** Synthetic Substitute, Metal on Polyethylene for Replacement in Lower Joints
Cobalt/chromium head and socket	**Use:** Synthetic Substitute, Metal for Replacement in Lower Joints
Cochlear implant (CI), multiple channel (electrode)	**Use:** Hearing Device, Multiple Channel Cochlear Prosthesis for Insertion in Ear, Nose, Sinus
Cochlear implant (CI), single channel (electrode)	**Use:** Hearing Device, Single Channel Cochlear Prosthesis for Insertion in Ear, Nose, Sinus
COGNIS® CRT-D	**Use:** Cardiac Resynchronization Defibrillator Pulse Generator for Insertion in Subcutaneous Tissue and Fascia
COHERE® radiolucent interbody fusion device	**Use:** Interbody Fusion Device, Radiolucent Porous in New Technology
Colonic Z-Stent®	**Use:** Intraluminal Device
Complete (SE) stent	**Use:** Intraluminal Device
Concerto II CRT-D	**Use:** Cardiac Resynchronization Defibrillator Pulse Generator for Insertion in Subcutaneous Tissue and Fascia
CONSERVE® PLUS Total Resurfacing Hip System	**Use:** Resurfacing Device in Lower Joints
Consulta CRT-D	**Use:** Cardiac Resynchronization Defibrillator Pulse Generator for Insertion in Subcutaneous Tissue and Fascia
Consulta CRT-P	**Use:** Cardiac Resynchronization Pacemaker Pulse Generator for Insertion in Subcutaneous Tissue and Fascia
CONTAK RENEWAL® 3 RF (HE) CRT-D	**Use:** Cardiac Resynchronization Defibrillator Pulse Generator for Insertion in Subcutaneous Tissue and Fascia
Contegra Pulmonary Valved Conduit	**Use:** Zooplastic Tissue in Heart and Great Vessels
Continuous Glucose Monitoring (CGM) device	**Use:** Monitoring Device
Cook Biodesign® Fistula Plug(s)	**Use:** Nonautologous Tissue Substitute
Cook Biodesign® Hernia Graft(s)	**Use:** Nonautologous Tissue Substitute
Cook Biodesign® Layered Graft(s)	**Use:** Nonautologous Tissue Substitute
Cook Zenapro™ Layered Graft(s)	**Use:** Nonautologous Tissue Substitute
Cook Zenith AAA Endovascular Graft	**Use:** Intraluminal Device, Branched or Fenestrated, One or Two Arteries for Restriction in Lower Arteries Intraluminal Device, Branched or Fenestrated, Three or More Arteries for Restriction in Lower Arteries Intraluminal Device
CoreValve transcatheter aortic valve	**Use:** Zooplastic Tissue in Heart and Great Vessels
Cormet Hip Resurfacing System	**Use:** Resurfacing Device in Lower Joints
CoRoent® XL	**Use:** Interbody Fusion Device in Lower Joints
Corox (OTW) Bipolar Lead	**Use:** Cardiac Lead, Pacemaker for Insertion in Heart and Great Vessels Cardiac Lead, Defibrillator for Insertion in Heart and Great Vessels

APPENDIX C

DEVICE KEY

Cortical strip neurostimulator lead	**Use:** Neurostimulator Lead in Central Nervous System and Cranial Nerves
Cultured epidermal cell autograft	**Use:** Autologous Tissue Substitute
CYPHER® Stent	**Use:** Intraluminal Device, Drug-eluting in Heart and Great Vessels
Cystostomy tube	**Use:** Drainage Device
DBS lead	**Use:** Neurostimulator Lead in Central Nervous System and Cranial Nerves
DeBakey Left Ventricular Assist Device	**Use:** Implantable Heart Assist System in Heart and Great Vessels
Deep brain neurostimulator lead	**Use:** Neurostimulator Lead in Central Nervous System and Cranial Nerves
Delta frame external fixator	**Use:** External Fixation Device, Hybrid for Insertion in Upper Bones External Fixation Device, Hybrid for Reposition in Upper Bones External Fixation Device, Hybrid for Insertion in Lower Bones External Fixation Device, Hybrid for Reposition in Lower Bones
Delta III Reverse shoulder prosthesis	**Use:** Synthetic Substitute, Reverse Ball and Socket for Replacement in Upper Joints
Diaphragmatic pacemaker generator	**Use:** Stimulator Generator in Subcutaneous Tissue and Fascia
Direct Lateral Interbody Fusion (DLIF) device	**Use:** Interbody Fusion Device in Lower Joints
Driver stent (RX) (OTW)	**Use:** Intraluminal Device
DuraHeart Left Ventricular Assist System	**Use:** Implantable Heart Assist System in Heart and Great Vessels
Durata® Defibrillation Lead	**Use:** Cardiac Lead, Defibrillator for Insertion in Heart and Great Vessels
Dynesys® Dynamic Stabilization System	**Use:** Spinal Stabilization Device, Pedicle-Based for Insertion in Upper Joints Spinal Stabilization Device, Pedicle-Based for Insertion in Lower Joints
E-Luminexx™ (Biliary) (Vascular) Stent	**Use:** Intraluminal Device
EDWARDS INTUITY Elite valve system	**Use:** Zooplastic Tissue, Rapid Deployment Technique in New Technology
Electrical bone growth stimulator (EBGS)	**Use:** Bone Growth Stimulator in Head and Facial Bones Bone Growth Stimulator in Upper Bones Bone Growth Stimulator in Lower Bones
Electrical muscle stimulation (EMS) lead	**Use:** Stimulator Lead in Muscles
Electronic muscle stimulator lead	**Use:** Stimulator Lead in Muscles
Embolization coil(s)	**Use:** Intraluminal Device
Endeavor® (III) (IV) (Sprint) Zotarolimus-eluting Coronary Stent System	**Use:** Intraluminal Device, Drug-eluting in Heart and Great Vessels
Endologix AFX® Endovascular AAA System	**Use:** Intraluminal Device
EndoSure® sensor	**Use:** Monitoring Device, Pressure Sensor for Insertion in Heart and Great Vessels
ENDOTAK RELIANCE® (G) Defibrillation Lead	**Use:** Cardiac Lead, Defibrillator for Insertion in Heart and Great Vessels
Endotracheal tube (cuffed) (double-lumen)	**Use:** Intraluminal Device, Endotracheal Airway in Respiratory System
Endurant® Endovascular Stent Graft	**Use:** Intraluminal Device

DEVICE KEY

Endurant® II AAA stent graft system	**Use:** Intraluminal Device
EnRhythm	**Use:** Pacemaker, Dual Chamber for Insertion in Subcutaneous Tissue and Fascia
Enterra gastric neurostimulator	**Use:** Stimulator Generator, Multiple Array for Insertion in Subcutaneous Tissue and Fascia
Epic™ Stented Tissue Valve (aortic)	**Use:** Zooplastic Tissue in Heart and Great Vessels
Epicel® cultured epidermal autograft	**Use:** Autologous Tissue Substitute
Esophageal obturator airway (EOA)	**Use:** Intraluminal Device, Airway in Gastrointestinal System
Esteem® implantable hearing system	**Use:** Hearing Device in Ear, Nose, Sinus
Everolimus-eluting coronary stent	**Use:** Intraluminal Device, Drug-eluting in Heart and Great Vessels
Ex-PRESS™ mini glaucoma shunt	**Use:** Synthetic Substitute
EXCLUDER® AAA Endoprosthesis	**Use:** Intraluminal Device, Branched or Fenestrated, One or Two Arteries for Restriction in Lower Arteries Intraluminal Device, Branched or Fenestrated, Three or More Arteries for Restriction in Lower Arteries
EXCLUDER® IBE Endoprosthesis	**Use:** Intraluminal Device, Branched or Fenestrated, One or Two Arteries for Restriction in Lower Arteries
Express® (LD) Premounted Stent System	**Use:** Intraluminal Device
Express® Biliary SD Monorail® Premounted Stent System	**Use:** Intraluminal Device
Express® SD Renal Monorail® Premounted Stent System	**Use:** Intraluminal Device

External fixator	**Use:** External Fixation Device in Head and Facial Bones External Fixation Device in Upper Bones External Fixation Device in Lower Bones External Fixation Device in Upper Joints External Fixation Device in Lower Joints
EXtreme Lateral Interbody Fusion (XLIF) device	**Use:** Interbody Fusion Device in Lower Joints
Facet replacement spinal stabilization device	**Use:** Spinal Stabilization Device, Facet Replacement for Insertion in Upper Joints Spinal Stabilization Device, Facet Replacement for Insertion in Lower Joints
FLAIR® Endovascular Stent Graft	**Use:** Intraluminal Device
Flexible Composite Mesh	**Use:** Synthetic Substitute
Foley catheter	**Use:** Drainage Device
Formula™ Balloon-Expandable Renal Stent System	**Use:** Intraluminal Device
Freestyle (Stentless) Aortic Root Bioprosthesis	**Use:** Zooplastic Tissue in Heart and Great Vessels
Fusion screw (compression) (lag) (locking)	**Use:** Internal Fixation Device in Upper Joints Internal Fixation Device in Lower Joints
GammaTile™	**Use:** Radioactive Element, Cesium-131 Collagen Implant for Insertion in Central Nervous System and Cranial Nerves
Gastric electrical stimulation (GES) lead	**Use:** Stimulator Lead in Gastrointestinal System
Gastric pacemaker lead	**Use:** Stimulator Lead in Gastrointestinal System

DEVICE KEY

GORE EXCLUDER® AAA Endoprosthesis	**Use:** Intraluminal Device, Branched or Fenestrated, One or Two Arteries for Restriction in Lower Arteries
GORE EXCLUDER® IBE Endoprosthesis	**Use:** Intraluminal Device, Branched or Fenestrated, One or Two Arteries for Restriction in Lower Arteries
GORE TAG® Thoracic Endoprosthesis	**Use:** Intraluminal Device
GORE® DUALMESH®	**Use:** Synthetic Substitute
Guedel airway	**Use:** Intraluminal Device, Airway in Mouth and Throat
Hancock Bioprosthesis (aortic) (mitral) valve	**Use:** Zooplastic Tissue in Heart and Great Vessels
Hancock Bioprosthetic Valved Conduit	**Use:** Zooplastic Tissue in Heart and Great Vessels
HeartMate 3™ LVAS	**Use:** Implantable Heart Assist System in Heart and Great Vessels
HeartMate II® Left Ventricular Assist Device (LVAD)	**Use:** Implantable Heart Assist System in Heart and Great Vessels
HeartMate XVE® Left Ventricular Assist Device (LVAD)	**Use:** Implantable Heart Assist System in Heart and Great Vessels
Hip (joint) liner	**Use:** Liner in Lower Joints
Holter valve ventricular shunt	**Use:** Synthetic Substitute
Ilizarov external fixator	**Use:** External Fixation Device, Ring for Insertion in Upper Bones External Fixation Device, Ring for Reposition in Upper Bones External Fixation Device, Ring for Insertion in Lower Bones External Fixation Device, Ring for Reposition in Lower Bones
Ilizarov-Vecklich device	**Use:** External Fixation Device, Limb Lengthening for Insertion in Upper Bones External Fixation Device, Limb Lengthening for Insertion in Lower Bones
Impella® heart pump	**Use:** Short-term External Heart Assist System in Heart and Great Vessels
Implantable cardioverter-defibrillator (ICD)	**Use:** Defibrillator Generator for Insertion in Subcutaneous Tissue and Fascia
Implantable drug infusion pump (anti-spasmodic) (chemotherapy) (pain)	**Use:** Infusion Device, Pump in Subcutaneous Tissue and Fascia
Implantable glucose monitoring device	**Use:** Monitoring Device
Implantable hemodynamic monitor (IHM)	**Use:** Monitoring Device, Hemodynamic for Insertion in Subcutaneous Tissue and Fascia
Implantable hemodynamic monitoring system (IHMS)	**Use:** Monitoring Device, Hemodynamic for Insertion in Subcutaneous Tissue and Fascia
Implantable Miniature Telescope™ (IMT)	**Use:** Synthetic Substitute, Intraocular Telescope for Replacement in Eye
Implanted (venous) (access) port	**Use:** Vascular Access Device, Totally Implantable in Subcutaneous Tissue and Fascia
InDura, intrathecal catheter (1P) (spinal)	**Use:** Infusion Device
Injection reservoir, port	**Use:** Vascular Access Device, Totally Implantable in Subcutaneous Tissue and Fascia
Injection reservoir, pump	**Use:** Infusion Device, Pump in Subcutaneous Tissue and Fascia

DEVICE KEY

Interbody fusion (spine) cage	**Use:** Interbody Fusion Device in Upper Joints Interbody Fusion Device in Lower Joints
Interspinous process spinal stabilization device	**Use:** Spinal Stabilization Device, Interspinous Process for Insertion in Upper Joints Spinal Stabilization Device, Interspinous Process for Insertion in Lower Joints
InterStim® Therapy lead	**Use:** Neurostimulator Lead in Peripheral Nervous System
InterStim® Therapy neurostimulator	**Use:** Stimulator Generator, Single Array for Insertion in Subcutaneous Tissue and Fascia
Intramedullary (IM) rod (nail)	**Use:** Internal Fixation Device, Intramedullary in Upper Bones Internal Fixation Device, Intramedullary in Lower Bones
Intramedullary skeletal kinetic distractor (ISKD)	**Use:** Internal Fixation Device, Intramedullary in Upper Bones Internal Fixation Device, Intramedullary in Lower Bones
Intrauterine device (IUD)	**Use:** Contraceptive Device in Female Reproductive System
INTUITY Elite valve system, EDWARDS	**Use:** Zooplastic Tissue, Rapid Deployment Technique in New Technology
Itrel (3) (4) neurostimulator	**Use:** Stimulator Generator, Single Array for Insertion in Subcutaneous Tissue and Fascia
Joint fixation plate	**Use:** Internal Fixation Device in Upper Joints Internal Fixation Device in Lower Joints
Joint liner (insert)	**Use:** Liner in Lower Joints
Joint spacer (antibiotic)	**Use:** Spacer in Upper Joints Spacer in Lower Joints
Kappa	**Use:** Pacemaker, Dual Chamber for Insertion in Subcutaneous Tissue and Fascia
Kinetra® neurostimulator	**Use:** Stimulator Generator, Multiple Array for Insertion in Subcutaneous Tissue and Fascia
Kirschner wire (K-wire)	**Use:** Internal Fixation Device in Head and Facial Bones Internal Fixation Device in Upper Bones Internal Fixation Device in Lower Bones Internal Fixation Device in Upper Joints Internal Fixation Device in Lower Joints
Knee (implant) insert	**Use:** Liner in Lower Joints
Kuntscher nail	**Use:** Internal Fixation Device, Intramedullary in Upper Bones Internal Fixation Device, Intramedullary in Lower Bones
LAP-BAND® adjustable gastric banding system	**Use:** Extraluminal Device
LifeStent® (Flexstar) (XL) Vascular Stent System	**Use:** Intraluminal Device
LIVIAN™ CRT-D	**Use:** Cardiac Resynchronization Defibrillator Pulse Generator for Insertion in Subcutaneous Tissue and Fascia
Loop recorder, implantable	**Use:** Monitoring Device
MAGEC® Spinal Bracing and Distraction System	**Use:** Magnetically Controlled Growth Rod(s) in New Technology
Mark IV Breathing Pacemaker System	Stimulator Generator in Subcutaneous Tissue and Fascia
Maximo II DR (VR)	**Use:** Defibrillator Generator for Insertion in Subcutaneous Tissue and Fascia
Maximo II DR CRT-D	**Use:** Cardiac Resynchronization Defibrillator Pulse Generator for Insertion in Subcutaneous Tissue and Fascia

APPENDIX C

DEVICE KEY

Medtronic Endurant® II AAA stent graft system	**Use:** Intraluminal Device
Melody® transcatheter pulmonary valve	**Use:** Zooplastic Tissue in Heart and Great Vessels
Metal on metal bearing surface	**Use:** Synthetic Substitute, Metal for Replacement in Lower Joints
Micro-Driver stent (RX) (OTW)	**Use:** Intraluminal Device
Micrus CERECYTE microcoil	**Use:** Intraluminal Device, Bioactive in Upper Arteries
MIRODERM™ Biologic Wound Matrix	**Use:** Skin Substitute, Porcine Liver Derived in New Technology
MitraClip valve repair system	**Use:** Synthetic Substitute
Mitroflow® Aortic Pericardial Heart Valve	**Use:** Zooplastic Tissue in Heart and Great Vessels
Mosaic Bioprosthesis (aortic) (mitral) valve	**Use:** Zooplastic Tissue in Heart and Great Vessels
MULTI-LINK (VISION)(MINIVISION) (ULTRA) Coronary Stent System	**Use:** Intraluminal Device
nanoLOCK™ interbody fusion device	**Use:** Interbody Fusion Device, Nanotextured Surface in New Technology
Nasopharyngeal airway (NPA)	**Use:** Intraluminal Device, Airway in Ear, Nose, Sinus
Neuromuscular electrical stimulation (NEMS) lead	**Use:** Stimulator Lead in Muscles
Neurostimulator generator, multiple channel	**Use:** Stimulator Generator, Multiple Array for Insertion in Subcutaneous Tissue and Fascia
Neurostimulator generator, multiple channel rechargeable	**Use:** Stimulator Generator, Multiple Array Rechargeable for Insertion in Subcutaneous Tissue and Fascia
Neurostimulator generator, single channel	**Use:** Stimulator Generator, Single Array for Insertion in Subcutaneous Tissue and Fascia
Neurostimulator generator, single channel rechargeable	**Use:** Stimulator Generator, Single Array Rechargeable for Insertion in Subcutaneous Tissue and Fascia
Neutralization plate	**Use:** Internal Fixation Device in Head and Facial Bones Internal Fixation Device in Upper Bones Internal Fixation Device in Lower Bones
Nitinol framed polymer mesh	**Use:** Synthetic Substitute
Non-tunneled central venous catheter	**Use:** Infusion Device
Novacor Left Ventricular Assist Device	**Use:** Implantable Heart Assist System in Heart and Great Vessels
Novation® Ceramic AHS® (Articulation Hip System)	**Use:** Synthetic Substitute, Ceramic for Replacement in Lower Joints
Optimizer™ III implantable pulse generator	**Use:** Contractility Modulation Device for Insertion in Subcutaneous Tissue and Fascia
Oropharyngeal airway (OPA)	**Use:** Intraluminal Device, Airway in Mouth and Throat
Ovatio™ CRT-D	**Use:** Cardiac Resynchronization Defibrillator Pulse Generator for Insertion in Subcutaneous Tissue and Fascia
OXINIUM	**Use:** Synthetic Substitute, Oxidized Zirconium on Polyethylene for Replacement in Lower Joints
Paclitaxel-eluting coronary stent	**Use:** Intraluminal Device, Drug-eluting in Heart and Great Vessels
Paclitaxel-eluting peripheral stent	**Use:** Intraluminal Device, Drug-eluting in Upper Arteries Intraluminal Device, Drug-eluting in Lower Arteries

DEVICE KEY

Device	Use
Partially absorbable mesh	**Use:** Synthetic Substitute
Pedicle-based dynamic stabilization device	**Use:** Spinal Stabilization Device, Pedicle-Based for Insertion in Upper Joints Spinal Stabilization Device, Pedicle-Based for Insertion in Lower Joints
Perceval sutureless valve	**Use:** Zooplastic Tissue, Rapid Deployment Technique in New Technology
Percutaneous endoscopic gastrojejunostomy (PEG/J) tube	**Use:** Feeding Device in Gastrointestinal System
Percutaneous endoscopic gastrostomy (PEG) tube	**Use:** Feeding Device in Gastrointestinal System
Percutaneous nephrostomy catheter	**Use:** Drainage Device
Peripherally inserted central catheter (PICC)	**Use:** Infusion Device
Pessary ring	**Use:** Intraluminal Device, Pessary in Female Reproductive System
Phrenic nerve stimulator generator	**Use:** Stimulator Generator in Subcutaneous Tissue and Fascia
Phrenic nerve stimulator lead	**Use:** Diaphragmatic Pacemaker Lead in Respiratory System
PHYSIOMESH™ Flexible Composite Mesh	**Use:** Synthetic Substitute
Pipeline™ Embolization device (PED)	**Use:** Intraluminal Device
Polyethylene socket	**Use:** Synthetic Substitute, Polyethylene for Replacement in Lower Joints
Polymethylmethacrylate (PMMA)	**Use:** Synthetic Substitute
Polypropylene mesh	**Use:** Synthetic Substitute
Porcine (bioprosthetic) valve	**Use:** Zooplastic Tissue in Heart and Great Vessels
PRESTIGE® Cervical Disc	**Use:** Synthetic Substitute
PrimeAdvanced neurostimulator	**Use:** Stimulator Generator, Multiple Array for Insertion in Subcutaneous Tissue and Fascia
PROCEED™ Ventral Patch	**Use:** Synthetic Substitute
Prodisc-C	**Use:** Synthetic Substitute
Prodisc-L	**Use:** Synthetic Substitute
PROLENE Polypropylene Hernia System (PHS)	**Use:** Synthetic Substitute
Protecta XT CRT-D	**Use:** Cardiac Resynchronization Defibrillator Pulse Generator for Insertion in Subcutaneous Tissue and Fascia
Protecta XT DR (XT VR)	**Use:** Defibrillator Generator for Insertion in Subcutaneous Tissue and Fascia
Protégé® RX Carotid Stent System	**Use:** Intraluminal Device
Pump reservoir	**Use:** Infusion Device, Pump in Subcutaneous Tissue and Fascia
PVAD™ Ventricular Assist Device	**Use:** External Heart Assist System in Heart and Great Vessels
REALIZE® Adjustable Gastric Band	**Use:** Extraluminal Device
Rebound HRD® (Hernia Repair Device)	**Use:** Synthetic Substitute
RestoreAdvanced neurostimulator	**Use:** Stimulator Generator, Multiple Array Rechargeable for Insertion in Subcutaneous Tissue and Fascia
RestoreSensor neurostimulator	**Use:** Stimulator Generator, Multiple Array Rechargeable for Insertion in Subcutaneous Tissue and Fascia

DEVICE KEY

RestoreUltra neurostimulator	**Use:** Stimulator Generator, Multiple Array Rechargeable for Insertion in Subcutaneous Tissue and Fascia
Reveal (DX) (XT)	**Use:** Monitoring Device
Reverse® Shoulder Prosthesis	**Use:** Synthetic Substitute, Reverse Ball and Socket for Replacement in Upper Joints
Revo MRI™ SureScan® pacemaker	**Use:** Pacemaker, Dual Chamber for Insertion in Subcutaneous Tissue and Fascia
Rheos® System device	**Use:** Cardiac Rhythm Related Device in Subcutaneous Tissue and Fascia
Rheos® System lead	**Use:** Stimulator Lead in Upper Arteries
RNS System lead	**Use:** Neurostimulator Lead in Central Nervous System and Cranial Nerves
RNS system neurostimulator generator	**Use:** Neurostimulator Generator in Head and Facial Bones
Sacral nerve modulation (SNM) lead	**Use:** Stimulator Lead in Urinary System
Sacral neuromodulation lead	**Use:** Stimulator Lead in Urinary System
SAPIEN transcatheter aortic valve	**Use:** Zooplastic Tissue in Heart and Great Vessels
Secura (DR) (VR)	**Use:** Defibrillator Generator for Insertion in Subcutaneous Tissue and Fascia
Sheffield hybrid external fixator	**Use:** External Fixation Device, Hybrid for Insertion in Upper Bones External Fixation Device, Hybrid for Reposition in Upper Bones External Fixation Device, Hybrid for Insertion in Lower Bones External Fixation Device, Hybrid for Reposition in Lower Bones
Sheffield ring external fixator	**Use:** External Fixation Device, Ring for Insertion in Upper Bones External Fixation Device, Ring for Reposition in Upper Bones External Fixation Device, Ring for Insertion in Lower Bones External Fixation Device, Ring for Reposition in Lower Bones
Single lead pacemaker (atrium) (ventricle)	**Use:** Pacemaker, Single Chamber for Insertion in Subcutaneous Tissue and Fascia
Single lead rate responsive pacemaker (atrium) (ventricle)	**Use:** Pacemaker, Single Chamber Rate Responsive for Insertion in Subcutaneous Tissue and Fascia
Sirolimus-eluting coronary stent	**Use:** Intraluminal Device, Drug-eluting in Heart and Great Vessels
SJM Biocor® Stented Valve System	**Use:** Zooplastic Tissue in Heart and Great Vessels
Soletra® neurostimulator	**Use:** Stimulator Generator, Single Array for Insertion in Subcutaneous Tissue and Fascia
Spinal cord neurostimulator lead	**Use:** Neurostimulator Lead in Central Nervous System and Cranial Nerves
Spinal growth rods, magnetically controlled	**Use:** Magnetically Controlled Growth Rod(s) in New Technology
Spiration IBV™ Valve System	**Use:** Intraluminal Device, Endobronchial Valve in Respiratory System
Stent (angioplasty) (embolization)	**Use:** Intraluminal Device
Stented tissue valve	**Use:** Zooplastic Tissue in Heart and Great Vessels
Stratos LV	**Use:** Cardiac Resynchronization Pacemaker Pulse Generator for Insertion in Subcutaneous Tissue and Fascia

DEVICE KEY

Subcutaneous injection reservoir, port	**Use:** Vascular Access Device, Totally Implantable in Subcutaneous Tissue and Fascia
Subcutaneous injection reservoir, pump	**Use:** Infusion Device, Pump in Subcutaneous Tissue and Fascia
Subdermal progesterone implant	**Use:** Contraceptive Device in Subcutaneous Tissue and Fascia
Sutureless valve, Perceval	**Use:** Zooplastic Tissue, Rapid Deployment Technique in New Technology
SynCardia Total Artificial Heart	**Use:** Synthetic Substitute
Synchra CRT-P	**Use:** Cardiac Resynchronization Pacemaker Pulse Generator for Insertion in Subcutaneous Tissue and Fascia
Talent® Converter	**Use:** Intraluminal Device
Talent® Occluder	**Use:** Intraluminal Device
Talent® Stent Graft (abdominal) (thoracic)	**Use:** Intraluminal Device
TandemHeart® System	**Use:** Short-term External Heart Assist System in Heart and Great Vessels
TAXUS® Liberté® Paclitaxel-eluting Coronary Stent System	**Use:** Intraluminal Device, Drug-eluting in Heart and Great Vessels
Therapeutic occlusion coil(s)	**Use:** Intraluminal Device
Thoracostomy tube	**Use:** Drainage Device
Thoratec IVAD (Implantable Ventricular Assist Device)	**Use:** Implantable Heart Assist System in Heart and Great Vessels
Thoratec Paracorporeal Ventricular Assist Device	**Use:** Short-term External Heart Assist System in Heart and Great Vessels
Tibial insert	**Use:** Liner in Lower Joints
Tissue bank graft	**Use:** Nonautologous Tissue Substitute
Tissue expander (inflatable) (injectable)	**Use:** Tissue Expander in Skin and Breast Tissue Expander in Subcutaneous Tissue and Fascia
Titanium Sternal Fixation System (TSFS)	**Use:** Internal Fixation Device, Rigid Plate for Insertion in Upper Bones Internal Fixation Device, Rigid Plate for Reposition in Upper Bones
Total artificial (replacement) heart	**Use:** Synthetic Substitute
Tracheostomy tube	**Use:** Tracheostomy Device in Respiratory System
Trifecta™ Valve (aortic)	**Use:** Zooplastic Tissue in Heart and Great Vessels
Tunneled central venous catheter	**Use:** Vascular Access Device, Tunneled in Subcutaneous Tissue and Fascia
Tunneled spinal (intrathecal) catheter	**Use:** Infusion Device
Two lead pacemaker	**Use:** Pacemaker, Dual Chamber for Insertion in Subcutaneous Tissue and Fascia
Ultraflex™ Precision Colonic Stent System	**Use:** Intraluminal Device
ULTRAPRO Hernia System (UHS)	**Use:** Synthetic Substitute
ULTRAPRO Partially Absorbable Lightweight Mesh	**Use:** Synthetic Substitute
ULTRAPRO Plug	**Use:** Synthetic Substitute
Ultrasonic osteogenic stimulator	**Use:** Bone Growth Stimulator in Head and Facial Bones Bone Growth Stimulator in Upper Bones Bone Growth Stimulator in Lower Bones

DEVICE KEY

Ultrasound bone healing system	**Use:** Bone Growth Stimulator in Head and Facial Bones Bone Growth Stimulator in Upper Bones Bone Growth Stimulator in Lower Bones
Uniplanar external fixator	**Use:** External Fixation Device, Monoplanar for Insertion in Upper Bones External Fixation Device, Monoplanar for Reposition in Upper Bones External Fixation Device, Monoplanar for Insertion in Lower Bones External Fixation Device, Monoplanar for Reposition in Lower Bones
Urinary incontinence stimulator lead	**Use:** Stimulator Lead in Urinary System
Vaginal pessary	**Use:** Intraluminal Device, Pessary in Female Reproductive System
Valiant Thoracic Stent Graft	**Use:** Intraluminal Device
Vectra® Vascular Access Graft	**Use:** Vascular Access Device, Tunneled in Subcutaneous Tissue and Fascia
Ventrio™ Hernia Patch	**Use:** Synthetic Substitute
Versa	**Use:** Pacemaker, Dual Chamber for Insertion in Subcutaneous Tissue and Fascia
Virtuoso (II) (DR) (VR)	**Use:** Defibrillator Generator for Insertion in Subcutaneous Tissue and Fascia
WALLSTENT® Endoprosthesis	**Use:** Intraluminal Device
X-STOP® Spacer	**Use:** Spinal Stabilization Device, Interspinous Process for Insertion in Upper Joints Spinal Stabilization Device, Interspinous Process for Insertion in Lower Joints
Xenograft	**Use:** Zooplastic Tissue in Heart and Great Vessels
XIENCE V Everolimus Eluting Coronary Stent System	**Use:** Intraluminal Device, Drug-eluting in Heart and Great Vessels
XLIF® System	**Use:** Interbody Fusion Device in Lower Joints
Zenith Flex® AAA Endovascular Graft	**Use:** Intraluminal Device
Zenith TX2® TAA Endovascular Graft	**Use:** Intraluminal Device
Zenith® Renu™ AAA Ancillary Graft	**Use:** Intraluminal Device
Zilver® PTX® (paclitaxel) Drug-Eluting Peripheral Stent	**Use:** Intraluminal Device, Drug-eluting in Upper Arteries Intraluminal Device, Drug-eluting in Lower Arteries
Zimmer® NexGen® LPS Mobile Bearing Knee	**Use:** Synthetic Substitute
Zimmer® NexGen® LPS-Flex Mobile Knee	**Use:** Synthetic Substitute
Zotarolimus-eluting coronary stent	**Use:** Intraluminal Device, Drug-eluting in Heart and Great Vessels

SUBSTANCE KEY

Term	ICD-10-PCS Value
AIGISRx Antibacterial Envelope Antimicrobial envelope	**Use:** Anti-Infective Envelope
Axicabtagene Ciloeucel	**Use:** Engineered Autologous Chimeric Antigen Receptor T-cell Immunotherapy
Bone morphogenetic protein 2 (BMP 2)	**Use:** Recombinant Bone Morphogenetic Protein
CBMA (Concentrated Bone Marrow Aspirate)	**Use:** Concentrated Bone Marrow Aspirate
Clolar	**Use:** Clofarabine
Defitelio	**Use:** Defibrotide Sodium Anticoagulant
DuraGraft® Endothelial Damage Inhibitor	**Use:** Endothelial Damage Inhibitor
Factor Xa Inhibitor Reversal Agent, Andexanet Alfa	**Use:** Andexanet Alfa, Factor Xa Inhibitor Reversal Agent
Kcentra	**Use:** 4-Factor Prothrombin Complex Concentrate
Nesiritide	**Use:** Human B-type Natriuretic Peptide
rhBMP-2	**Use:** Recombinant Bone Morphogenetic Protein
Seprafilm	**Use:** Adhesion Barrier
STELARA®	**Use:** Other New Technology Therapeutic Substance
Tissue Plasminogen Activator (tPA) (rtPA)	**Use:** Other Thrombolytic
Ustekinumab	**Use:** Other New Technology Therapeutic Substance
Vistogard®	**Use:** Uridine Triacetate
Voraxaze	**Use:** Glucarpidase
VYXEOS™	**Use:** Cytarabine and Daunorubicin Liposome Antineoplastic
ZINPLAVA™	**Use:** Bezlotoxumab Monoclonal Antibody
Zyvox	**Use:** Oxazolidinones

DEVICE AGGREGATION TABLE

Specific Device	for Operation	in Body System	General Device
Autologous Arterial Tissue	All applicable	Heart and Great Vessels Lower Arteries Lower Veins Upper Arteries Upper Veins	**7** Autologous Tissue Substitute
Autologous Venous Tissue	All applicable	Heart and Great Vessels Lower Arteries Lower Veins Upper Arteries Upper Veins	**7** Autologous Tissue Substitute
Cardiac Lead, Defibrillator	Insertion	Heart and Great Vessels	**M** Cardiac Lead
Cardiac Lead, Pacemaker	Insertion	Heart and Great Vessels	**M** Cardiac Lead
Cardiac Resynchronization Defibrillator Pulse Generator	Insertion	Subcutaneous Tissue and Fascia	**P** Cardiac Rhythm Related Device
Cardiac Resynchronization Pacemaker Pulse Generator	Insertion	Subcutaneous Tissue and Fascia	**P** Cardiac Rhythm Related Device
Contractility Modulation Device	Insertion	Subcutaneous Tissue and Fascia	**P** Cardiac Rhythm Related Device
Defibrillator Generator	Insertion	Subcutaneous Tissue and Fascia	**P** Cardiac Rhythm Related Device
Epiretinal Visual Prosthesis	All applicable	Eye	**J** Synthetic Substitute
External Fixation Device, Hybrid	Insertion	Lower Bones Upper Bones	**5** External Fixation Device
External Fixation Device, Hybrid	Reposition	Lower Bones Upper Bones	**5** External Fixation Device
External Fixation Device, Limb Lengthening	Insertion	Lower Bones Upper Bones	**5** External Fixation Device
External Fixation Device, Monoplanar	Insertion	Lower Bones Upper Bones	**5** External Fixation Device
External Fixation Device, Monoplanar	Reposition	Lower Bones Upper Bones	**5** External Fixation Device
External Fixation Device, Ring	Insertion	Lower Bones Upper Bones	**5** External Fixation Device
External Fixation Device, Ring	Reposition	Lower Bones Upper Bones	**5** External Fixation Device
Hearing Device, Bone Conduction	Insertion	Ear, Nose, Sinus	**S** Hearing Device
Hearing Device, Multiple Channel Cochlear Prosthesis	Insertion	Ear, Nose, Sinus	**S** Hearing Device
Hearing Device, Single Channel Cochlear Prosthesis	Insertion	Ear, Nose, Sinus	**S** Hearing Device
Internal Fixation Device, Intramedullary	All applicable	Lower Bones Upper Bones	**4** Internal Fixation Device
Internal Fixation Device, Intramedullary Limb Lengthening	Insertion	Lower Bones Upper Bones	**6** Internal Fixation Device, Intramedullary
Internal Fixation Device, Rigid Plate	Insertion	Upper Bones	**4** Internal Fixation Device
Internal Fixation Device, Rigid Plate	Reposition	Upper Bones	**4** Internal Fixation Device
Intraluminal Device, Flow Diverter	Restriction	Upper Arteries	**D** Intraluminal Device

DEVICE AGGREGATION TABLE

Specific Device	for Operation	in Body System	General Device
Intraluminal Device, Pessary	All applicable	Female Reproductive System	**D** Intraluminal Device
Intraluminal Device, Airway	All applicable	Ear, Nose, Sinus Gastrointestinal System Mouth and Throat	**D** Intraluminal Device
Intraluminal Device, Bioactive	All applicable	Upper Arteries	**D** Intraluminal Device
Intraluminal Device, Branched or Fenestrated, One or Two Arteries	Restriction	Heart and Great Vessels Lower Arteries	**D** Intraluminal Device
Intraluminal Device, Branched or Fenestrated, Three or More Arteries	Restriction	Heart and Great Vessels Lower Arteries	**D** Intraluminal Device
Intraluminal Device, Drug-eluting	All applicable	Heart and Great Vessels Lower Arteries Upper Arteries	**D** Intraluminal Device
Intraluminal Device, Drug-eluting, Four or More	All applicable	Heart and Great Vessels Lower Arteries Upper Arteries	**D** Intraluminal Device
Intraluminal Device, Drug-eluting, Three	All applicable	Heart and Great Vessels Lower Arteries Upper Arteries	**D** Intraluminal Device
Intraluminal Device, Drug-eluting, Two	All applicable	Heart and Great Vessels Lower Arteries Upper Arteries	**D** Intraluminal Device
Intraluminal Device, Endobronchial Valve	All applicable	Respiratory System	**D** Intraluminal Device
Intraluminal Device, Endotracheal Airway	All applicable	Respiratory System	**D** Intraluminal Device
Intraluminal Device, Four or More	All applicable	Heart and Great Vessels Lower Arteries Upper Arteries	**D** Intraluminal Device
Intraluminal Device, Radioactive	All applicable	Heart and Great Vessels	**D** Intraluminal Device
Intraluminal Device, Three	All applicable	Heart and Great Vessels Lower Arteries Upper Arteries	**D** Intraluminal Device
Intraluminal Device, Two	All applicable	Heart and Great Vessels Lower Arteries Upper Arteries	**D** Intraluminal Device
Monitoring Device, Hemodynamic	Insertion	Subcutaneous Tissue and Fascia	**2** Monitoring Device
Monitoring Device, Pressure Sensor	Insertion	Heart and Great Vessels	**2** Monitoring Device
Pacemaker, Dual Chamber	Insertion	Subcutaneous Tissue and Fascia	**P** Cardiac Rhythm Related Device
Pacemaker, Single Chamber	Insertion	Subcutaneous Tissue and Fascia	**P** Cardiac Rhythm Related Device
Pacemaker, Single Chamber Rate Responsive	Insertion	Subcutaneous Tissue and Fascia	**P** Cardiac Rhythm Related Device
Spinal Stabilization Device, Facet Replacement	Insertion	Lower Joints Upper Joints	**4** Internal Fixation Device
Spinal Stabilization Device, Interspinous Process	Insertion	Lower Joints Upper Joints	**4** Internal Fixation Device
Spinal Stabilization Device, Pedicle-Based	Insertion	Lower Joints Upper Joints	**4** Internal Fixation Device

DEVICE AGGREGATION TABLE

Specific Device	for Operation	in Body System	General Device
Spinal Stabilization Device,Vertebral Body Tether	Reposition	Lower Bones Upper Bones	**4** Internal Fixation Device
Stimulator Generator, Multiple Array	Insertion	Subcutaneous Tissue and Fascia	**M** Stimulator Generator
Stimulator Generator, Multiple Array Rechargeable	Insertion	Subcutaneous Tissue and Fascia	**M** Stimulator Generator
Stimulator Generator, Single Array	Insertion	Subcutaneous Tissue and Fascia	**M** Stimulator Generator
Stimulator Generator, Single Array Rechargeable	Insertion	Subcutaneous Tissue and Fascia	**M** Stimulator Generator
Synthetic Substitute, Ceramic	Replacement	Lower Joints	**J** Synthetic Substitute
Synthetic Substitute, Ceramic on Polyethylene	Replacement	Lower Joints	**J** Synthetic Substitute
Synthetic Substitute, Intraocular Telescope	Replacement	Eye	**J** Synthetic Substitute
Synthetic Substitute, Metal	Replacement	Lower Joints	**J** Synthetic Substitute
Synthetic Substitute, Metal on Polyethylene	Replacement	Lower Joints	**J** Synthetic Substitute
Synthetic Substitute, Oxidized Zirconium on Polyethylene	Replacement	Lower Joints	**J** Synthetic Substitute
Synthetic Substitute, Polyethylene	Replacement	Lower Joints	**J** Synthetic Substitute
Synthetic Substitute, Reverse Ball and Socket	Replacement	Upper Joints	**J** Synthetic Substitute

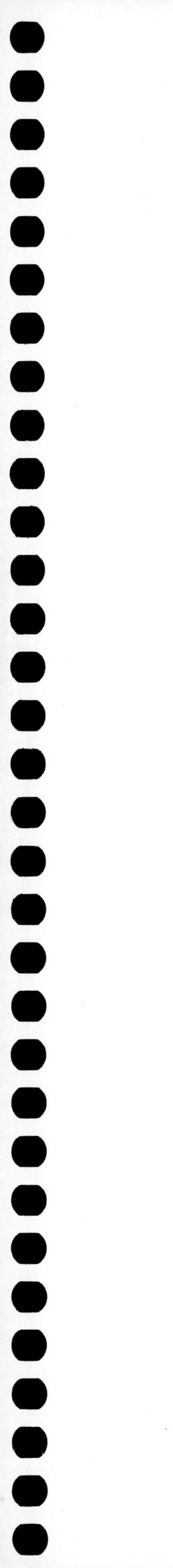